Oncology Nursing Drug Handbook

Oncology Nursing Drug Handbook

Gail M. Wilkes, MSN, APRN-BC, AOCN
Oncology Clinical Instructor
Boston Medical Center
Boston, Massachusetts

Margaret Barton-Burke, PhD, RN
Professor of Oncology Nursing
University of Missouri–St. Louis
St. Louis, Missouri

JONES AND BARTLETT PUBLISHERS
Sudbury, Massachusetts
BOSTON TORONTO LONDON SINGAPORE

World Headquarters
Jones and Bartlett Publishers
40 Tall Pine Drive
Sudbury, MA 01776
978-443-5000
info@jbpub.com
www.jbpub.com

Jones and Bartlett Publishers Canada
6339 Ormindale Way
Mississauga, Ontario L5V 1J2
Canada

Jones and Bartlett Publishers International
Barb House, Barb Mews
London W6 7PA
United Kingdom

Jones and Bartlett's books and products are available through most bookstores and online booksellers. To contact Jones and Bartlett Publishers directly, call 800-832-0034, fax 978-443-8000, or visit our website at www.jbpub.com.

Substantial discounts on bulk quantities of Jones and Bartlett's publications are available to corporations, professional associations, and other qualified organizations. For details and specific discount information, contact the special sales department at Jones and Bartlett via the above contact information or send an email to specialsales@jbpub.com.

ISBN: 978-0-7637-6585-9
ISSN: 1536-0024
6048

Production Credits
Publisher: Kevin Sullivan
Acquisitions Editor: Emily Ekle
Acquisitions Editor: Amy Sibley
Associate Editor: Patricia Donnelly
Editorial Assistant: Rachel Shuster
Supervising Production Editor: Carolyn F. Rogers
Senior Marketing Manager: Barb Bartoszek
Cover Design: Kristin E. Ohlin
V.P., Manufacturing and Inventory Control: Therese Connell
Composition: diacriTech
Printing and Binding: Malloy, Inc.
Cover Printing: Malloy, Inc.

Printed in the United States of America
12 11 10 09 08 10 9 8 7 6 5 4 3 2 1

Contents

Key to Abbreviations *xv*
Preface *xix*
Contributors *xxii*

Section 1 Cancer Treatment 1

Chapter 1 Introduction to Chemotherapy Drugs 2

abarelix for injectable suspension 40
adrenocorticoids 42
altretamine 46
aminoglutethimide 48
amrubicin 51
anastrozole 52
androgens 55
arsenic trioxide 56
asparaginase 63
5-azacytidine 66
bendamustine hydrochloride 69
bicalutamide 73
bleomycin sulfate 75
busulfan 78
busulfan for injection 80
capecitabine 86
carboplatin 89
carmustine 93
chlorambucil 96
cisplatin 98
cladribine 103
clofarabine 107
cyclophosphamide 109
cytarabine, cytosine arabinoside 113

cytarabine, liposome injection 117
dacarbazine 119
dactinomycin 122
daunorubicin citrate liposome injection 125
daunorubicin hydrochloride 128
decitabine 131
docetaxel 135
doxorubicin hydrochloride 144
doxorubicin hydrochloride liposome injection 148
eniluracil 153
epirubicin hydrochloride 155
estramustine 160
estrogens 162
etoposide 165
exemestane 169
floxuridine 171
fludarabine phosphate 174
5-fluorouracil 176
flutamide 179
fulvestrant injection 180
gemcitabine hydrochloride 183
goserelin acetate 187
histrelin implant 190
hydroxyurea 192
idarubicin 195
ifosfamide 198
irinotecan 201
ixabepilone 206
letrozole 213
leuprolide acetate 214
lomustine 217
mechlorethamine hydrochloride 219
melphalan hydrochloride 223
mercaptopurine 226
methotrexate 228
mitomycin 231
mitotane 234
mitoxantrone 236
nelarabine 239
nilutamide 243
oxaliplatin 245

paclitaxel 250
paclitaxel protein-bound particles for injectable suspension 257
patupilone 262
pegasparaginase 263
pemetrexed 266
pentostatin 269
polifeprosan 20 with carmustine (BCNU) implant 272
procarbazine hydrochloride 275
progestational agents 278
raltitrexed 280
rubitecan 282
streptozocin 285
tamoxifen citrate 288
temozolamide 291
teniposide 295
thioguanine 298
thiotepa 300
topotecan hydrochloride for injection 302
toremifene citrate 306
trimetrexate 308
triptorelin pamoate 311
valrubicin 313
vinblastine 315
vincristine 318
vindesine 321
vinorelbine tartrate 324

Chapter 2 Biologic Response Modifier Therapy 329

aldesleukin 334
darbepoetin alfa 339
epoetin alfa 344
filgrastim 348
imiquimod 5% topical cream 349
interferon alfa (α) 351
interferon alfa-2b 355
interferon gamma 359
levamisole hydrochloride 362
megakaryocyte growth and development factor 364
oprelvekin 365
palifermin 368
pegfilgrastim 370

romiplostim 374
sargramostim 375
thyrotropin alfa 377
tumor necrosis factor 380
zoster vaccine live 382

Chapter 3 **Antineoplastic Treatment Agonists: Radiosensitizers, Chemosensitizers, and Chemical Adjuncts 385**

chromic phosphate p32 suspension 387
deferasirox tablets for oral suspension 389
efaproxiral 394
etanidazole 395
fluosol DA (20%) 396
leucovorin calcium 397
levoleucovorin 399
porfirmer 401
tirapazamine 403

Chapter 4 **Cytoprotective Agents 406**

allopurinol sodium 410
amifostine for injection 413
dexrazoxane for injection 416
dexrazoxane for injection 419
glutamine 420
mesna for injection 421
xaliproden 423

Chapter 5 **Molecularly Targeted Therapies 425**

alemtuzumab 471
alitretinoin ge l0.1% 475
axitinib 477
bevacizumab 478
bexarotene 486
bortezomib 491
cediranib 497
cetuximab 498
dasatinib 506
denileukin diftitox 511
elesclomol 516
erlotinib 518

everolimus 521
gefitinib 524
gemtuzumab ozogamicin for injection 528
^{90}Y ibritumomab tiuxetan 533
imatinib mesylate 536
ipilimumab 541
lapatinib ditosylate 544
lenalidomide 548
neovastat 554
nilotinib 555
panitumumab 560
pertuzumab 564
quadrivalent human papillomavirus 566
rituximab 567
sorafenib 572
sunitinib malate 576
temsirolimus 580
thalidomide 584
tipifarnib 588
tositumomab, I^{131} tositumomab 589
trastuzumab 594
trastuzumab-DMI 600
tretinoin 602
liposomal tretinoin 605
vandetanib 610
vatalanib 611
volociximab 613
vorinostat 615

Section 2 Symptom Management 619

Chapter 6 Pain 620

Non-Opioid Analgesics 628
acetaminophen 628
aspirin, acetylsalicylic acid 629
celecoxib 631
choline magnesium trisalicylate 635
clonidine hydrochloride 637
gabapentin 639

ibuprofen 642
indomethacin 645
ketorolac tromethamine 648
pregabalin 652
salsalate 654
ziconotide intrathecal infusion 656
Opioid Analgesics 660
codeine 660
fentanyl buccal tablets 663
fentanyl citrate 667
fentanyl transdermal system 670
hydromorphone 674
levorphanol tartrate opioid 678
meperidine hydrochloride 682
methadone 686
morphine 690
oxycodone 695
oxymorphone hydrochloride 699
oxymorphone hydrochloride extended release 702
Adjuvant Agents 707
modafinil 707

Chapter 7 **Nausea and Vomiting 710**

aprepitant 721
casopitant 723
dexamethasone 724
diphenhydramine hydrochloride 726
dolasetron mesylate 728
dronabinol 731
droperidol 732
fosaprepitant 734
granisetron hydrochloride 736
granisetron hydrochloride transdermal 738
haloperidol 739
metoclopramide hydrochloride 741
nabilone 742
ondansetron hydrochloride 744
palonosetron 746
perphenazine 748
prochlorperazine 749
promethazine hydrochloride 751

scopolamine 753
thiethylperazine 754

Chapter 8 Anorexia and Cachexia 756

dronabinol 759
megestrol acetate 760
thalidomide 762

Chapter 9 Anxiety and Depression 766

alprazolam 773
amitriptyline hydrochloride 775
bupropion hydrochloride 778
buspirone hydrochloride 781
citalopram hydrobromide 783
clonazepam 786
desipramine hydrochloride 789
desvenlafaxine 792
diazepam 797
doxepin hydrochloride 799
duloxetine hydrochloride 802
escitalalopram oxalate 805
fluoxetine hydrochloride 808
imipramine pamoate 812
lorazepam 814
mirtazapine 817
nefazodone HCl 821
nortriptyline hydrochloride 824
oxazepam 827
paroxetine hydrochloride 829
sertraline hydrochloride 832
trazodone hydrochloride 835
venlafaxine hydrochloride 837
zolpidem tartrate 842

Section 3 Complications 845

Chapter 10 Hypercalcemia 846

calcitonin-salmon 851
cinacalcet HCl 853
denosumab 855

etidronate disodium 856
furosemide 858
gallium nitrate 860
pamidronate disodium 861
zoledronic acid 864

Chapter 11 Infection 869

Antibiotics 880
amikacin sulfate 880
amoxicillin 884
ampicillin sodium/sulbactam sodium 887
azithromycin 890
aztreonam 892
carbenicillin indanyl sodium 895
cefaclor 898
cefadroxil 900
cefamandole nafate 902
cefazolin sodium 906
cefdinir 910
cefditoren pivoxil 913
cefepime 914
cefixime 917
cefoperazone sodium 920
cefotaxime sodium 923
cefotetan 926
cefoxitin sodium 928
cefpodoxime proxetil 932
cefprozil 933
ceftazidime 935
ceftibuten 939
ceftriaxone sodium 941
cefuroxime 944
cephalexin 946
cephapirin 948
cephradine 950
ciprofloxacin 953
clarithromycin 956
clindamycin phosphate 959
co-trimoxazole 962
daptomycin 966
demeclocycline hydrochloride 967

dicloxacillin sodium 969
doxycycline hyclate 972
ertapenem sodium 975
erythromycin 977
gatifloxacin 980
gemifloxacin mesylate 983
gentamicin sulfate 986
imipenem/cilastatin sodium 989
kanamycin sulfate 993
levofloxacin 996
linezolid 999
meropenem 1001
metronidazole hydrochloride 1003
mezlocillin sodium 1006
minocycline hydrochloride 1010
moxifloxacin 1013
nafcillin sodium 1016
oxacillin sodium 1019
penicillin G 1022
piperacillin sodium 1025
quinupristin and dalfopristin 1029
rifaximin 1032
streptomycin sulfate 1033
telithromycin 1036
ticarcillin disodium 1038
tigecycline 1042
tobramycin sulfate 1044
vancomycin hydrochloride 1048
Antifungals 1051
amphotericin B, amphotericin B lipid complex 1051
anidulafungin 1055
caspofungin 1057
fluconazole 1059
flucytosine 1061
itraconazole 1064
ketoconazole 1066
micafungin sodium 1068
miconazole nitrate 1070
nystatin 1073
posaconazole 1074
voriconazole 1076

Antivirals 1078
- acyclovir 1078
- cidofovir 1081
- famciclovir 1084
- foscarnet sodium 1086
- ganciclovir 1089
- valacyclovir hydrochloride 1093

Chapter 12 Constipation 1095

- bisacodyl 1096
- docusate calcium, docusate potassium, docusate sodium 1097
- glycerin suppository 1099
- lactulose 1100
- magnesium citrate 1101
- methylcellulose 1102
- methylnaltrexone bromide 1104
- mineral oil 1105
- polyethylene glycol 3350, NF powder 1106
- senna 1108
- sorbitol 1109

Chapter 13 Diarrhea 1111

- deodorized tincture of opium 1113
- diphenoxylate hydrochloride and atropine 1114
- kaolin/pectin 1115
- loperamide hydrochloride 1116
- octreotide acetate 1117

Appendix 1 Controlling Occupational Exposure to Hazardous Drugs 1112

Appendix 2 Common Toxicity Criteria for Adverse Events v 3.0 (CTCAE) 1158

Index 1283

Key to Abbreviations

ABV	doxorubicin (doxorubicin HCl Adriamycin) bleomycin vincristine
ac	“ante cibum”; before meals
ADH	antidiuretic hormone
Afib	atrial fibrillation
AIDS	acquired immunodeficiency syndrome
alkphos	alkaline phosphatase
ALL	acute lymphocytic leukemia
ALT	alanine aminotransferase (formerly SGPT)
AML	acute myelocytic leukemia
ANC	absolute neutrophil count
ANLL	acute nonlymphocytic leukemia
APL	acute promyelocytic leukemia
aPTT	activated partial thromboplastin time
ARDS	adult respiratory distress syndrome
ASA	acetylsalicylic acid
AST	aspartate aminotransferase (formerly SGOT)
AUC	area under curve
bili	bilirubin
BMT	bone marrow transplant
BP	blood pressure
BRM	biologic response modifier
BTP	break through pain
BUN	blood urea nitrogen
Ca	calcium
CAPD	continuous ambulatory periotoneal dialysis
CBC	complete blood count
CFU-GEM	colony forming unit-granulocyte, erythrocyte, megakaryocyte, and macrophage
CHF	congestive heart failure
CLL	chronic lymphocytic leukemia
CPK	creatinine phosphokinase
CR	complete response, e.g., disappearance of all detectable tumor cells

creat	creatinine
CSF	colony-stimulating factor
CTZ	chemoreceptor trigger zone
CVA	cerebrovascular accident
CXR	chest X-ray
D5W	5% dextrose in water
DEHP	diethylhexlphthalate
DHFR	difolate reductase
DLCO	diffusion capacity of the lung for carbon monoxide, which reflects rate of gas transfer across the alveolar-capillary membrane
DMSO	dimethyl sulfoxide
DTIC	dacarbazine
DVT	deep vein thrombosis
EBV	Epstein-Barr virus
EDTA	edetic acid, one of several salts of edetic acid used as a chelating agent
EPS	extra pyramidal side-effects
FAC	fluorouracil-adriamycin-cytoxan combination chemotherapy
FSH	follicle-stimulating hormone
FUDR-MP	5-fluoro-23-deoxyuridine-53-monophosphate
FVC	forced vital capacity
GABA	gamma-aminobutyric acid
GBPS	gated blood pool scan
GFR	glomerular filtration rate
GGT (SGGT)	gamma-glutamine transferase
G6PD	glucose-6-phosphate dehydrogenase
GU	genitourinary
HACA	human anti-chimeric antibody
HAMA	human anti-murine antibody
HCl	hydrochloride
HCT	hematocrit
Hgb	hemoglobin
5-HIAA	5-hydroxyindoleacetic acid
HIV	human immunodeficiency virus
HCC	hepatocellular cancer
Hs	"hora somni;" at bedtime
HSV	herpes simplex virus
5-HT2	5-hydroxytryptamine 2
5-HT3	5-hydroxytryptamine 3
HUS	hemolytic uremic syndrome
ICP	intracranial pressure
ICU	intensive care unit

IFN	interferon
IL	interleukin
I/O	intake/output
IOP	intraocular pressure
IT	intrathecal
IVB	intravenous bolus
IVP	intravenous push; intravenous pyelogram
LAK	lymphocyte activated killer cells
LDH	lactate dehydrogenase
LFTs	liver function tests
LH	luteinizing hormone
LHRH	luteinizing hormone-releasing hormone
LVEF	left ventricular ejection fraction
lytes	electrolytes
MAC	mycobacterium avium complex
MAO	monoamine oxidase
MAOI	monoamine oxidase inhibitor
MCV	mean corpuscular volume
MI	myocardial infarction
MIU	milli international units
MoAbs	monoclonal antibodies
MOPP	mustard-oncovin-prednisone-procarbazine combination chemotherpy for Hodgkin's disease
MTX	methotrexate
MU	milli units
NCI	National Cancer Institute
NHL	non-Hodgkin's lymphoma
NK	natural killer cells
NK1	Neurokinin 1 receptor for Substance P
NMDA	N-methyl-D-aspartate pain receptor
NS	normal saline
NSAIDs	nonsteroidal antiinflammatory drugs
n/v	nausea/vomiting
OS	overall survival
OTC	over-the-counter
PACs	premature atrial contractions
PBPCs	packed red blood cells for transfusion
PCA	patient controlled analgesia
PCP	*pneumocystis carinii* pneumonia
PFS	progression-free survival
PFTs	pulmonary function tests
phos	Phosphorus
plts	Platelets

PML	polymorphonuclear leukocyte
PR	partial response, e.g., reduction in tumor mass by 50% lasting for 3 months or longer
PRN	"pro re nata"; as needed
PSA	prostate-specific antigen
PT	prothrombin time
PTEN	phosphatase and tensin homolog
PTH	parathyroid hormone
PTT	partial thromboplastin time
PVCs	premature ventricular contractions
QID	four times a day
RFTs	renal function tests
RT	radiation therapy
RUQ	right upper quadrant
SBP	systolic blood pressure
sed rate	sedimentation rate
SGPT	serum glutamic-pyruvic transferase
SIADH	syndrome of inappropriate antidiuretic hormone
SPF	skin protection factor
SQ	subcutaneous
SSRI	selective serotonin reuptake inhibitor
Sx	symptom
T	temperature
T4	thyroxine
TCA	tricyclic antidepressants
TFT	thyroid function tests
THC	tetrahydrocannabinol
TIL	tumor infiltrating lymphocytes
TLS	tumor lysis syndrome
TMP-SMX	trimethoprim-sulfamethoxazole
TNF	tumor necrosis factor
TTP/HUS	thrombotic thrombocytopenic purpura/hemolytic anemia syndrome
UA	urinalysis
US	ultrasound
UTI	urinary tract infection
VC	vomiting center
Vfib	ventricular fibrillation
VOD	veno-occlusive disease
VS	vital signs
VSCC	voltage-sensitive calcium channel
VZV	varicella zoster virus
WHO	World Health Organization
XRT	radiation therapy

Preface

Oncology nurses provide expert nursing care to patients with cancer and their families, as the patient moves along the disease trajectory from diagnosis to primary treatment and cure, or to remission, then possible relapse, and death. The nurse uses the nursing process to assess patient and family needs in the 14 high incidence problem areas identified in the Oncology Nursing Society (ONS) standards: prevention and early detection, information, coping, comfort, nutrition, protective mechanisms, mobility, elimination, sexuality, ventilation, oxygenation, complementary and alternative therapies, palliative and end-of-life care, and survivorship.

In 2003, Andrew von Eschenbach, MD, set the elimination of suffering and death due to cancer as the NCI challenge goal. He identified seven major initiatives to accomplish this goal, including development of more effective strategies for prevention and screening; early detection as well as improvement of our understanding of the molecular processes of carcinogenesis; and refinement of molecular targeted therapy (von Eschenbach, 2003). In this view, cancer becomes a chronic disease characterized by periods of exacerbations and remissions. As has been demonstrated in work on angiogenesis, malignant tumors must establish a blood supply when they reach a size of 1–2 mm in order to obtain oxygen and glucose, and to remove cellular waste products. Mortality is caused by metastasis in most people with cancer, and if a malignancy is confined to 1–2 mm with a combination of chemotherapy and anti-angiogenesis drug(s), then indeed, people can "live with cancer." Together, the nurse and patient, along with other members of the healthcare team, develop a plan of care. Since cancer, for many, is a chronic illness with periods of remission and relapse, nursing goals center around promoting self-care and empowering the patient and family to live a high-quality, meaningful life outside the hospital. Nurses are involved in the pharmacologic management of disease (e.g., chemotherapy) and of symptoms that arise during the course of illness (e.g., pain, anxiety, constipation). In addition, as patients receive more aggressive treatment, nurses are deeply involved in the management of complications of disease or treatment, such as infection. As new technologies emerge, such as molecular targeted therapy, nurses need to stay abreast of newly approved agents, their mechanisms of action, and potential side effects. Knowledge of cancer biology and metastases is evolving and offers potential targets. Nurses must keep up with understanding the fundamental molecular flaws to both teach patients and their families, as well as to understand the mechanism of action and potential toxicities. As the paradigm moves to multi-targeted oral agents, the nurse must be creative in developing strategies to promote concordance with treatment regimens and individualize patient care to enhance adherence. For example, nurses are working to establish the evidence base for minimization of toxicity and distress related to EGFR inhibitor rash. Finally, oncology nurses have long said that much of symptom management is in the domain of nursing practice, and they continue to advocate for effective management and symptom resolution. Knowledge of the drugs used in cancer care is critical for today's practicing nurse. In the past, pharmacists wrote drug books for nurses that did not address the application of the nursing process to potential drug toxicities. Today, as the science of cancer treatment is rapidly exploding, it is imperative to keep current with new, emerging therapies.

This book is divided into sections addressing broad areas of nursing practice. There are individual chapters within each section presenting an introductory overview. In 2009 the following new drugs were FDA approved, or were investigational agents being considered by the FDA. These agents include the chemotherapeutic agents bendamustine HCl (Treanda), ixabepilone (Ixempra), and the investiagtional amrubicin. Drugs in the chapter were updated for new indications. In addition, topotecan was updated to include oral administration. Vinorelbine was updated to include the investigational oral drug. Chapter 2 was updated to reflect the ASCO and NCCN Guidelines on growth factor usage and two new drugs, thyrotropin alfa for injection (Thyrogen) and romiplostim, were added. Chapter 3 has been updated, and levoleucovorin (Fusilev) was added. Dexrazoxane for injection (Totect), used to neutralize tissue damage from extravasation of anthracycline chemotherapy, was added to Chapter 4. Chapter 5 has been updated to reflect current thinking about molecular targeted therapy and epigenetics, with the following new drugs included nilotinib (Tasigna) and the following investigational agents: axitinib, elesclomol, everolimus (RAD001), ipilimumab, pertuzumab, patupilone, trastuzumab-DM1, volociximab, were added. Drugs were updated to reflect new indications and changes in safety profiles. Chapter 6 has been updated, as has Chapter 7 with the addition of fosaprepitant (Emend IV), granisetron HCL transdermal, and investigational agent casopitant. Chapter 8 was updated as well. Desvenlafaxine (Pristiq) was added to Chapter 9, and, denosumab was added to Chapter 10. Chapter 11 was updated with the inclusion of the following antimicrobial agents: posaconazole (Noxafil) and anidulafungin (Eraxis). Chapter 12 was updated with the addition of methlynaltrexone bromide. All agents were updated to reflect newly approved indications. Specific drugs are described in terms of their mechanism of action, metabolism, drug interactions, laboratory effects/interference, and special considerations. The most important and common drug side effects are discussed. Chapter 5, Molecularly Targeted Therapies, discusses basic cell biology, carcinogenesis, malignant flaws resulting in abnormal cell division and cell death, invasiveness, and metastases. New additions include a more complete discussion of mTOR inhibitors. This is intended to provide a framework for understanding the new agents that target molecular flaws. Many of these agents inhibit steps in the processes of carcinogenesis and metastases in the areas of signal transduction (growth receptor over expression, ras, tyrosine kinases), cell cycle movement (cyclin-dependent kinases, apoptosis), angiogenesis, invasion, and metastases. In addition, the processes of apoptosis and ubiquitination are further explored. Nursing priorities in the assessment and management of EGFRI skin toxicity are discussed in terms of pathophysiology and consensus management strategies. Standards may change as new scientific knowledge becomes available and as dictated by governmental regulations that affect practice. This book will be updated regularly with new drugs and nursing management strategies to reflect those changes.

The authors, editor, and publisher have made every effort to provide accurate Information. However, they are not responsible for errors, omissions, or for any outcomes related to the use of the contents of this book and take no responsibility for the use of the products and procedures described. Treatment and side effects described in this book may not be applicable to all people; likewise, some people may require a dose or experience a side effect that is not described herein. Drugs and medical devices are discussed that may have limited availability controlled by the Food and Drug Administration (FDA) for use only in a research study or clinical trial. Research, clinical practice, and government regulations often change the accepted standards in this field. When consideration is being given for use of any drug in the clinical setting, the health care provider or reader is responsible for determining FDA status of the drug, reading the package insert, and reviewing prescribing information for the most up-to-date recommendations on dose, precautions, and contraindications, and determining the appropriate usage for the product. This is especially important in the case of drugs that are new or seldom used.

DRUG INFORMATION sections reflect current prescribing practices in the United States, which may differ from clinical practices in Europe and the United Kingdom.

References

American Nurses Association (2004) ANA and ONS: *Standards of Oncology Nursing Practice.* Kansas City; ANA.

von Eschenbach Keynote presentation: Summit series on cancer clinical trials. Executive Summary VIII: Retooling the System: Implementing Solutions. September 29–October 1, 2003.

Contributors

Deborah Berg, BSN, RN
North Londonderry, NH

Catherine K. Bean, BSN, RN, BA
Tampa, FL

Karen Ingwersen, MS, RN
Belmont, MA

Reginald King, PharmD
Philadelphia, PA

Section 1
Cancer Treatment

Chapter 1
Introduction to Chemotherapy Drugs

Chemotherapy drugs interfere with cell division, leading to cell kill, called *cytocidal effects*, or failure to replicate, called *cytostatic effects* (see Figure 1.1, Cell Cycle.) Unfortunately, drugs cannot discriminate between frequently dividing cells that are normal and those that are malignant. Consequently, normal cells as well as malignant cells are injured. Thus, anticipated acute side effects are found also in normal cell populations that divide frequently, i.e., bone marrow, gastrointestinal (GI) mucosa, gonads, and hair follicles. Since normal cells are better able to repair themselves, these side effects are usually reversible. Depending on drug properties, delayed, longer-term toxicities may occur, which may be irreversible. Properties to be aware of include route of administration, dose, excretion, and predilection for uptake by specific organ cells. Examples of toxicities are

- Lung toxicity from bleomycin, busulfan, and the nitrosoureas (BCNU, CCNU)
- Cardiomyopathy from doxorubicin, daunorubicin, mitoxantrone, and paclitaxel
- Renal dysfunction from cisplatin and high-dose methotrexate
- Hemorrhagic cystitis (bladder) from ifosfamide and cyclophosphamide
- Neurotoxicity from the platins, taxanes, and vinca alkaloids
- Development of second malignancies from melphalan, cyclophosphamide, alone, or when certain drugs are combined with radiotherapy

Nurses play a critical role in patient assessment, education, drug administration, and minimization of toxicities. See Table 1.1 for prechemotherapy nursing assessment guidelines. Table 1.2 describes classifications of antineoplastic drugs.

This 12th edition has been updated to include newly approved drugs as well as important investigational agents that should be approved in the near future. This section examines antineoplastic agents and classifies them by their mechanism(s) of action. As knowledge of cancer and its treatment emerges, drugs may be reclassified, such as the anthracycline antitumor antibiotics, which now appear to work by inhibiting topoisomerase II.

As an example, the topoisomerase I inhibitors cause protein-linked DNA single-strand breaks and block DNA and RNA synthesis in dividing cells, thus preventing cells from entering mitosis. To better understand the topoisomerase inhibitors, it is important to go back to the DNA helix. The entire DNA genome consists of two strands wound into a double helix, which measures more 3 feet and is condensed into chromosomes by torsion of the helix. During cell replication, the DNA strands that are coiled in the double helix need to unwind so that they can separate and be copied. This is made possible by the topoisomerase I and II enzymes (Chen and Liu, 1994).

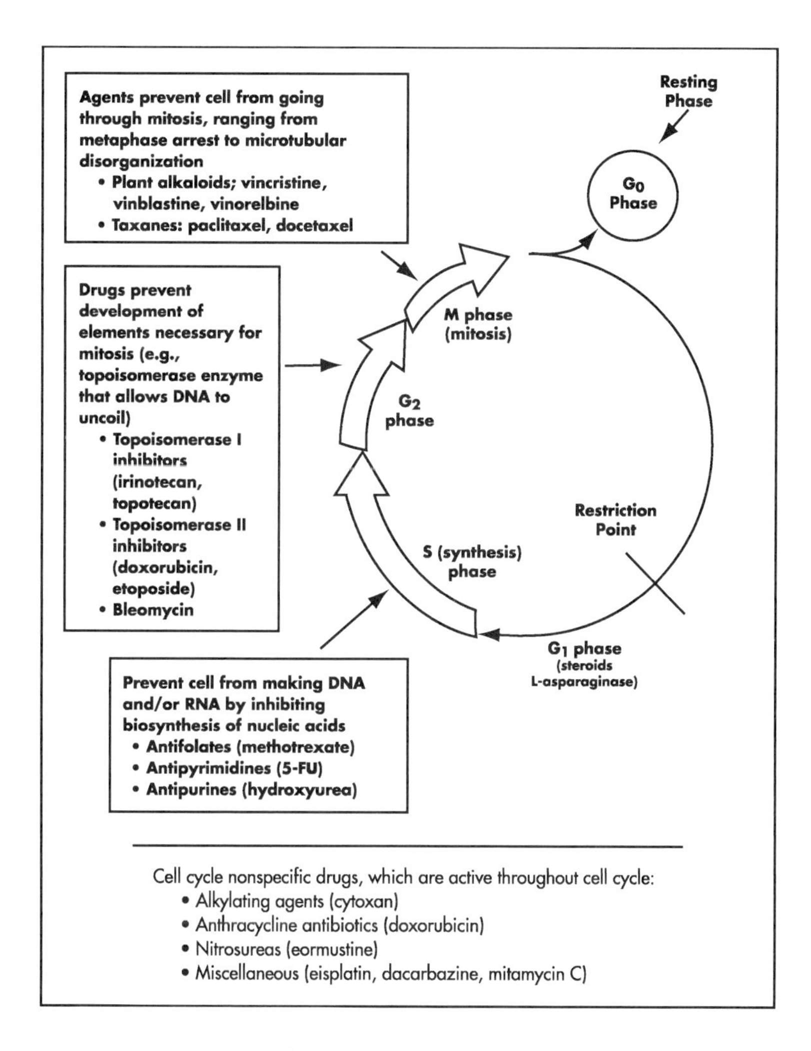

Figure 1.1 Mechanism of Action of Major Chemotherapy Drugs

Topoisomerase I relaxes tension in the DNA helix torsion by causing a transient single-strand break or nick in the DNA when it covalently bonds to the end of one of the DNA strands. The other, intact strand then passes through the break, and relaxation of the DNA helix occurs as the strands swivel at the strand break. The topoisomerase I enzyme then reseals the cleaved strand (religation step), and the enzyme is released from the DNA strand. Transcription (copying of the strands) is then initiated. Interestingly, topoisomerase I is found in greater concentrations in patients with cancers of the colon, non-Hodgkin's lymphoma, and some leukemias (Husain et al, 1994). Drugs

Table 1.1 Prechemotherapy Nursing Assessment Guidelines

Potential Problems/Nursing Diagnoses	Physical Status: Assessment Parameters/ Signs and Symptoms	Drug and Dose-Limiting Factors/Nursing Implications
Hematopoietic System		
1. Impaired tissue perfusion related to chemotherapy-induced anemia, leading to activity intolerance, changes in cardiopulmonary status due to compensatory changes	• Hgb g (norms women, 12–14; men, 14–16) • HCT% (norms women, 38–46; men, 42–54) • Vital signs (↓BP, ↑pulse, ↑respiration) • Pallor (face, palms, conjunctiva) • Fatigue or weakness • Vertigo	Hgb < 8 g HCT < 20% and blood transfusions not initiated • Consider erythropoietin growth factor support when hgb < 10 g/dL when receiving anemia-causing chemotherapy, e.g. cisplatin; do not exceed a target hgb of 12 g/dL (FDA, 2007).
2. Impaired immunocompetence and potential for infection related to chemotherapy-induced neutropenia	• WBC (norm 4500–9000/mm^3); ANC > 2000/mm^3 • Pyrexia/rigor, erythema, swelling, pain any site • Abnormal discharges, draining wounds, skin/mucous membrane lesions • Productive cough, SOB, rectal pain, urinary frequency	WBC ≤ 3,000/mm^3; ANC < 1000/mm^3 Fever > 38.3°C or 101°F • Hold all myelosuppressive agents (exceptions may include leukemia, lymphoma, and/or situations in which there is neoplastic marrow infiltration). • Consider growth factor support to prevent febrile neutropenia if risk > 20% • Febrile neutropenia is a medical emergency • Severe risk of infection ANC < 500 cells/mm^3 • Protective precautions ANC < 500 cells/mm^3

(continued)

Table 1.1 *(Continued)*

Potential Problems/Nursing Diagnoses	Physical Status: Assessment Parameters/Signs and Symptoms	Drug and Dose-Limiting Factors/Nursing Implications
3. Potential for injury (bleeding) related to chemotherapy-induced thrombocytopenia	• Platelet count (150,000–400,000/mm^3) • Spontaneous gingival bleeding or epistaxis • Presence of petechiae or easy bruisability • Hematuria, melena, hematemesis, hemoptysis • Hypermenorrhea • Signs and symptoms of intracranial bleeding (irritability, sensory loss, unequal pupils, headache, ataxia)	Platelet count ≤ 100,000/mm^3 • Hold all myelosuppressive agents (exceptions may include leukemia, lymphoma, and/or situations in which there is neoplastic marrow infiltration) • Platelet transfusion if bleeding • Platelet precaution: platelet count < 50,000 cells/mm^3
Integumentary System		
Alteration in mucous membrane of mouth, nasopharynx, esophagus, rectum, anus, or ostomy stoma related to chemotherapy-induced tissue changes	Mucositis Scale 0 = pink, moist, intact mucosa; absence of pain or burning; can drink and eat +1 = generalized erythema with or without pain or burning +2 = isolated small ulcerations and/or white patches +3 = confluent ulcerations with white patches on ≥25% mucosa; can drink but not eat +4 = hemorrhagic ulcerations; cannot eat or drink	+2 mucositis • Hold antimetabolites (esp. methotrexate, 5-FU) • Hold antitumor antibiotics (esp. doxorubicin, dactinomycin) • Hold Irinotecan • In transplant settings, may require opioid analgesia, aggressive antiemesis • Consider Kepivance™ before transplant chemotherapy
Severe sterile inflammatory rash	• EGFR inhibitor rash • Assess for risk of infection, itching, open areas	• Dose reduce or hold drug • Consider doxycycline 100 mg PO bid, topical clindamycin gel, and steroid taper

(continued)

Table 1.1 *(Continued)*

Potential Problems/Nursing Diagnoses	Physical Status: Assessment Parameters/ Signs and Symptoms	Drug and Dose-Limiting Factors/Nursing Implications
Gastrointestinal System		
Discomfort, nutritional deficiency, and/or fluid and electrolyte disturbances related to chemotherapy-induced:		
1. Anorexia	• Lab values: Albumin and total protein • Normal weight/present weight and % of body weight loss • Normal diet pattern/changes in diet pattern • Alterations in taste sensation • Early satiety	• Manage nutrition impact symptoms • Dietary teaching • Appetite stimulants as needed
2. Nausea and vomiting	• Lab values: Electrolytes • Pattern of n/v (incidence, duration, severity); hydration status • Antiemetic plan: Drug(s), dosage(s), schedule, efficacy: Other (dietary adjustments, relaxation techniques, environmental manipulation)	Intractable n/v × 24 h: IV hydration if unable to take oral fluids • Aggressive combination antiemesis (serotonin antagonist and dexamethasone; or addition of aprepitant to serotonin-antagonist if delayed nausea and vomiting)
3. Bowel disturbances A. Diarrhea	• Normal pattern of bowel elimination • Consistency (loose, watery/bloody stools)	Diarrheal stools × 3/24 h above baseline • Hold antimetabolites (esp. methotrexate, 5-FU); irinotecan

(continued)

Table 1.1 *(Continued)*

Potential Problems/Nursing Diagnoses	Physical Status: Assessment Parameters/ Signs and Symptoms	Drug and Dose-Limiting Factors/Nursing Implications
	• Frequency and duration (no./day and no. of days) • Antidiarrheal drug(s), dosage(s), efficacy	• Teach patient self-administration of antidiarrheal medicine • Antibiotic therapy for unresolved diarrhea per MD
B. Constipation	• Normal pattern of bowel elimination • Consistency (hard, dry, small stools) • Frequency (hours or days beyond normal pattern) • Stool softener(s), laxative(s), efficacy	No BM × 48 h past normal bowel patterns • Hold vinca alkaloids (vinblastine, vincristine) • Teach patient to take stool softener with serotonin-antagonist antiemetic

4. Hepatotoxicity	• Lab values: LDH, ALT, AST, alk phos, bili
	• Pain/tenderness over liver, feeling of fullness
	• Increase in n/v or anorexia
	• Changes in mental status
	• Jaundice
	• High-risk factors:
	  • Hepatic metastasis
	  • Concurrent hepatotoxic drugs
	  • Viral hepatitis
	  • Graft-vs.-host disease
	  • Abdominal XRT
	  • Blood transfusions
		Evidence of chemical hepatitis:
		• Hold hepatotoxic agents (esp. methotrexate, 6-MP), until differential dx established
		• Hold imatinib mesylate if lab thresholds exceeded
		• Hold oxaliplatin if venous occlusive disease suspected
		• Hold or dose reduce drugs metabolized by liver if severe liver dysfunction (e.g., docetaxel, doxorubicin)

(continued)

Table 1.1 *(Continued)*

Potential Problems/Nursing Diagnoses	Physical Status: Assessment Parameters/ Signs and Symptoms	Drug and Dose-Limiting Factors/Nursing Implications
Respiratory System		

Impaired gas exchange or ineffective breathing pattern related to chemotherapy-induced pulmonary fibrosis	• Lab values: PFTs CXR
	• Respirations (rate, rhythm, depth)
	• Chest pain
	• Nonproductive cough
	• Progressive dyspnea
	• Wheezing/stridor
	• High-risk factors:
	  • Total cumulative dose of bleomycin
	  • Age > 60 years
	  • Preexisting lung disease
	  • Concomitant use of other pulmonary toxic drugs
	  • Prior/concomitant XRT
	  • Smoking hx
		• Acute unexplained onset respiratory symptoms
		• Hold all antineoplastic agents until differential dx established (e.g., bleomycin, busulfan, oxaliplatin, gemcitabine)
		• Interstitial Lung Disease (ILD) is a class effect of EGFR antagonists (rare), e.g., gefitinib, cetuximab, erlotinib.
		• Chemotherapy drug may be combined with EGFR antagonists (e.g., gemcitabine and erlotinib). If pulmonary symptoms develop, hold drug until ILD can be ruled out.

Cardiovascular System		
Decreased cardiac output related to chemotherapy-induced: 1. Cardiac arrhythmias 2. Cardiomyopathy 3. Hypertension	• Lab values: cardiac enzymes, electrolytes, ECG, ECHO, MUGA • Vital signs • Presence of arrhythmia (irregular radial/apical pulse)	Acute sx CHF and/or cardiac arrhythmia • Hypertension: risk increased in combination with bevacizumab • Hold all antineoplastic agents until differential dx established • Total dose doxorubicin or daunorubicin > 550 mg/m^2

(continued)

Table 1.1 *(Continued)*

Potential Problems/Nursing Diagnoses	Physical Status: Assessment Parameters/ Signs and Symptoms	Drug and Dose-Limiting Factors/Nursing Implications

	• Signs sx CHF (dyspnea, ankle edema, PND, decrease in LVEF, S_3 gallop, nonproductive cough, rales, cyanosis)
	• High-risk factors:
	  • Total cumulative dose anthracyclines
	  • Preexisting cardiac disease
	  • Prior/concurrent mediastinal XRT
	• Combined anthracycline, cyclophosphamide, trastuzumab, and paclitaxel
		• Risk of CHF increased when chemotherapy given with trastuzumab; hold anthracyclines, trastuzumab, paclitaxel
		• Monitor baseline and serial ejection fractions (LVEF) while receiving treatment with potentially cardiotoxic drugs; evaluate any significant ↓ in LVEF.
		• Severe hypertension: hold bevacizumab until hypertension controlled

Genitourinary System		
1. Alteration in fluid volume (excess) related to chemotherapy-induced: A. Glomerular or renal tubule damage B. Hyperuricemic nephropathy 2. Alteration in comfort related to chemotherapy-induced hemorrhagic cystitis	• Lab values: BUN, creatinine clearance, serum creatinine, uric acid, electrolytes, urinalysis, magnesium, calcium, phosphate • Color, odor, clarity of urine • 24-h fluid intake and output (estimate/actual) • Hematuria; proteinuria • Development of oliguria or anuria • High-risk factors: • Preexisting renal disease Concurrent treatment with nephrotoxic drugs (esp. aminoglycoside antibiotics) • Bevacizumab: rare nephrotic syndrome	• Hold cyclophosphamide, ifosfamide, cisplatin Serum creatinine > 2.0 and/or Creatinine clearance < 70 mL/min Hematuria • Hold cisplatin, streptozotocin Anuria × 24 h • Hold bevacizumab if patient develops nephrotic syndrome or 24-hour urine shows protein more than 2 g • Check BUN/creatinine before treatment • 24 hour urine for protein if spilling protein

(continued)

Table 1.1 *(Continued)*

Potential Problems/Nursing Diagnoses	Physical Status: Assessment Parameters/ Signs and Symptoms	Drug and Dose-Limiting Factors/Nursing Implications
Nervous System		
1. Impaired sensory/motor function related to chemotherapy-induced A. Peripheral neuropathy B. Cranial nerve neuropathy C. Acute oxaliplatin neurotoxicity D. Chemotherapy-induced cognitive changes	• Paresthesias (numbness, tingling in feet, fingertips) • Trigeminal nerve toxicity (severe jaw pain) • Jaw or muscle spasm • Diminished or absent deep tendon reflexes (ankle and knee jerks) • Motor weakness/slapping gait/ataxia • Visual and auditory disturbances • Cold induced paresthesias and dysesthesias lasting < 14 days (oxaliplatin) • Cognitive changes may be influenced by genetics, comorbidities; incidence estimated at 20% of patients receiving standard-dose chemotherapy	Presence of any neurologic signs and symptoms or worsening: • Perform brief nursing neuro exam before each treatment focusing on symptom analysis and functional impairment; consult MD for full neuro exam if signs/symptoms or worsening of existing signs/symptoms • Hold vinca alkaloids, cisplatin, hexamethyl melamine, oxaliplatin, procarbazine until differential dx established • Acute oxaliplatin neurotoxicity: increase length of infusion time to 6 h (decreases peak serum level by 32%); teach patient to avoid cold exposure to hands/feet, oral mucosa for 1–5 days after oxaliplatin drug administration • Assess for motor/sensory changes, impact on function and ability to do ADLs prior to oxaliplatin, taxane or cisplatin administration; hold for grades 3 and 4 toxicity (see Appendix 2)

(continued)

Table 1.1 *(Continued)*

Potential Problems/Nursing Diagnoses	Physical Status: Assessment Parameters/ Signs and Symptoms	Drug and Dose-Limiting Factors/Nursing Implications
		• Teach avoidance of cold for 3–5 days after oxaliplatin administration • Cognitive changes may appear after adjuvant therapy; assess for changes in memory, concentration, effect on work or school performance; reinforce teaching if slower ability to learn new information, following directions

2. Impaired bowel and bladder elimination related to chemotherapy-induced autonomic nerve dysfunction	• Urinary retention
	• Constipation/abdominal cramping and distension
	• High-risk factors:
	  • Changes in diet or mobility
	  • Frequent use of opioid analgesics
	  • Obstructive disease process
		Presence of any neurologic signs and symptoms
		• Hold vinca alkaloids until differential dx established

ALT = alanine aminotransferase; AST = aspartate aminotransferase; bili = bilirubin; BM = bowel movement; CHF = congestive heart failure; CXR = chest X-ray; dx = diagnosis; ECG = electrocardiogram; ECHO = echocardiogram; EGFR = epidermal growth factor receptor; 5-FU = 5-fluorouracil; hx = history; LDH = lactate dehydrogenase; LVEF = left ventricular ejection fraction; MUGA = multigated acquisition (MUGA heart scan); n/v = nausea and vomiting; PFT = pulmonary function test; 6-MP = 6-mercaptopurine; SOB = shortness of breath; sx = symptoms; XRT = radiation therapy *Modified from*: Engleking C 1988 Prechemotherapy Nursing Assessment in Outpatient Settings. *Outpatient Chemotherapy* 3(1):10–11.

TREATMENT

Table 1.2 Classifications of Antineoplastic Drugs

Classification	Mechanism of Action	Examples
	Cell Cycle Specific Agents	
Antimetabolites	Interfere with DNA and RNA synthesis by acting as false metabolites, which are incorporated into the DNA strand, or block essential enzymes, so that DNA synthesis is prevented.	Pemetrexate (Slinta), Cytosine arabinoside (ara-C, Cytosar-U), Eniluracil 5-Fluorouracil (5-FU) Floxuridine (FUDR, 5-FUDR) Hydroxyurea (Hydrea) 6-Mercaptopurine (6-MP, Purinethol) Methotrexate (Amethopterin, Mexate, Folex) 6-Thioguanine (6-TG) Gemcitabine (Gemzar®) Fludarabine (Fludara®) Capecitabine (Xeloda®) Deoxycoformycin (Pentostatin)
Vinca Alkaloids	Crystallize microtubules of mitotic spindle causing metaphase arrest (vincristine, vinblastine, vindesine), role in blocking DNA and preventing cell division in M phase (vinorelbine).	Vincristine (VCR, Oncovin) Vinblastine (VLB, Velban) Vinorelbine (Navelbine®)
Epipodophyllotoxins	Damage the cell prior to mitosis, late S and G_2 phase; inhibit topoisomerase II.	Etoposide (VP-16, Vepesid) Teniposide (VM-26, Vumon)
Taxanes	Promotes early microtubule assembly. Prevents depolymerization, causing cell death (paclitaxel); enhances microtubule assembly and inhibits tubulin depolymerization, thus arresting cell division in metaphase (docetaxel).	Paclitaxel (Taxol®) Docetaxel (Taxotere®) Paclitaxel protein bound

(continued)

Table 1.2 *(Continued)*

Classification	Mechanism of Action	Examples
Epothilones	Naturally occurring microstabilizing agents similar to taxanes; bind tubulin and cause apoptotic cell death.	Ixabepilone (Ixempra) Investigational: Papupilone
Camptothecins Miscellaneous	Act in S phase to inhibit topoisomerase I and cause cell death.	Topotecan (Hycamtin®) Irinotecan (CPT-11, Camptosar®)
Miscellaneous		G_1 phase: L-asparaginase (ELSPAR), Prednisone G_2 phase: Bleomycin (Bleo, Blenoxane)
	Cell Cycle Nonspecific Agents	
Alkylating Agents	Substitute alkyl group for H+ ion causing single- and double-strand breaks in DNA, as well as cross-linkages; thus DNA strands are unable to separate during DNA replication.	Bendamustine (Treanda), Busulfan (Myleran®, oral; Busulfex®, IV), Carboplatin (Paraplatin), *Carmustine (BiCNU, BCNU) Chlorambucil (Leukeran) Cisplatin (*Cis*-Platinum, CDDP, Platinol) Cyclophosphamide (Cytoxan, CTX, Neosar) Dacarbazine (DTIC-Dome, Imidazole) Estramustine phosphate (Estracyte, Emcyt) Ifosfamide (IFEX) *Lomustine (CCNU) Mechlorethamine hydrochloride (nitrogen mustard, mustargen, HN_2) Melphalan (Alkeran, 1-PAM, Phenylalanine Mustard) Oxaliplatin (Eloxatin)

(continued)

Table 1.2 *(Continued)*

Classification	Mechanism of Action	Examples
		*Streptozocin (Streptozotocin, Zanosar), Thiotepa (Triethylene Thiophosphoramide, TSPA)
Antibiotics	Use a variety of mechanisms to prevent cell division and death (DNA strand breakage, intercalation of base pairs, inhibition of RNA and DNA synthesis).	Dactinomycin (Actinomycin D, Cosmegan) Daunorubicin hydrochloride (Daunomycin, Cerubidine) Doxorubicin hydrochloride (Adria, Adriamycin) Epirubicin HCl (Ellenee) Indarubicin (Idamycin) Mithramycin (Mithramycin, Plicamycin) Mitomycin C (Mito, Mutamycin) Mitoxantrone (Novantrone)

*Nitrosoureas (cross blood–brain barrier).

developed within this decade, such as topotecan and irinotecan, work by inhibiting the religation or repair of the single-strand break by binding to topoisomerase I, and cells are arrested in G_2 phase.

Topoisomerase II is also involved in the relaxation of the helix torsion, but it causes a double-strand break to allow crossing of two double-stranded DNA segments. It then causes the closing of the two DNA strand breaks. This permits assembly of chromatin, as well as condensation and decondensation of the chromosomes, and separation of the DNA in the daughter cells during mitosis (Lui et al, 1980). Drugs that are well known to interfere with topoisomerase II are etoposide (non-intercalator, and cell cycle specific for M phase) and doxorubicin (intercalator of base pairs and cell cycle nonspecific) (Eber, 1996).

Descriptions of the drugs in the chapter have been updated to reflect new indications. Agents that have now been approved by the Food and Drug Administration (FDA) for use in cancer treatment have been updated, and investigational agents that are nearing FDA application or appear very promising, are included.

With the promise of increased survival in patients with solid tumors, standard chemotherapy agents are being combined at higher doses for marrow ablation, with subsequent stem cell rescue. However, more severe toxicity is seen (see Table 1.3). In addition, there have been advances in the approval of agents that provide organ protection from drug toxicity (cryoprotectants), which is discussed in Chapter 4.

Emerging Frontiers

As our knowledge of genomics and proteogenomics widens, the possibility of individualized cancer therapy increases. Although the human genome was decoded in 2003, this only opened the door to understanding each of the 35,000 different genes. As each individual has a unique genetic makeup, except for identical twins, so too each individual with cancer has individual genetic features of their tumor. Genetic signatures have emerged showing the different types and responses of colon/rectal, breast, and lung cancers to therapy (Allen and Johnston, 2005; Chen et al, 2007; Marsh and McLeod, 2006; O'Shaughnessy, 2006). Already, microarray technology is used to identify genetic signatures that are likely to respond to given drug therapy and those that are not. For example, a recent review of genomic markers in colorectal cancer revealed that tumors that overexpress thymidylate synthase (TS) and the 3*R/3*R TS gene polymorphism are resistant to 5-FU, whereas those with low TS gene expression have a response with increased survival (Allen and Johnston, 2005). Potti et al (2006) reported that using in vitro drug-sensitivity data together with microarray gene-expression data, they were able to develop gene-expression signatures and predict sensitivity to individual chemotherapy drugs with 80% accuracy. This also allows prediction of effective chemotherapy and targeted therapy combinations. A question that has recently been answered is which women with node-negative, estrogen receptor-positive breast cancer should receive adjuvant chemotherapy. A report by the National Surgical Adjuvant Breast and

Table 1.3 Common Agents Used in Dose-Intensive/High-Dose Chemotherapy and Associated Toxicities

Drug	Toxicity
Doxorubicin	1. Cardiotoxicity leading to degenerative cardiomyopathy over time Standard dose: 60–75 mg/m^2 Current lifetime dose: 450–550 mg/m^2 Current protocol dose ranges: 430–650 mg/m^2 (lifetime) When given over 96 hours in a dilute solution or at low weekly doses, cardiotoxicity appears to decrease. Prior radiation therapy to the chest or prior anthracycline therapy may predispose patient to or enhance cardiotoxicity. 2. Severe mucositis 3. Acute myelosuppression; late onset in children, even at low cumulative doses
Cyclophosphamide	1. Standard dose: 400–1600 mg/m^2 IV; high dose: up to 200 mg/kg 2. High dose: Cardiotoxicity, acute cardiomyopathy Diminished QRS complex on ECG Pulmonary congestion and pleural effusions Cardiomegaly Prior radiation therapy to the chest or prior anthracycline therapy may predispose patient to or enhance cardiotoxicity. Ejection fraction of > 50% not predictive of reduced risk for cardiotoxicity. 3. Hemorrhagic cystitis (occasionally chronic, severe) 4. Acute myelosuppression 5. Acral erythema and sloughing of skin on palms of hands and soles of feet 6. Diffuse hyperpigmentation 7. Gonadal dysfunction Delayed pubertal development Diminished testicular volume in adult males
Cisplatin	1. Standard dose: 15–120 mg/m^2; high dose: 160–200 mg/m^2 2. Renal and hepatic toxicity 3. Eighth cranial nerve damage and ototoxicity 4. Myelosuppression 5. Peripheral neuropathy 6. Intense nausea and vomiting
Carboplatin	1. Standard dose: 400–500 mg/m^2; high dose: 800–1600 mg/m^2 2. Myelosuppression (dose-limiting); pronounced thrombocytopenia

(continued)

Table 1.3 *(Continued)*

Drug	Toxicity
	3. Severe nausea and vomiting 4. Hepatotoxicity 5. Auditory toxicity 6. Mild renal toxicity
Cytosine arabinoside	1. Standard dose: 100–200 mg/m^2; high dose: 2–3 g/m^2 2. Acute neurotoxicity: cerebellar toxicity. Those over 50 at highest risk for minimal recovery from symptoms. Assess prior to each dose for ataxia, nystagmus, and slurred speech; hold dose if any indication of symptomatology (over baseline assessment). 3. Acral erythema and possible sloughing of skin on palms of hands and soles of feet 4. Conjunctivitis: steroid eye drops may prevent or alleviate 5. Intense diarrhea, up to 2–3 liters/24 hours
Busulfan	1. Standard dose: 1–4 mg/m^2; high dose: 16 mg/kg 2. Myelosuppression 3. Severe nausea and vomiting 4. Severe mucositis 5. Pneumonitis, pulmonary fibrosis; "busulfan lung" 6. Hepatic dysfunction leading to veno-occlusive disease 7. Diffuse hyperpigmentation; rare: development of bullae 8. Chronic alopecia
Etoposide	1. Standard dose: 60 mg/m^2; high dose: 60 mg/kg or 80–250 mg/m^2 2. Severe mucositis 3. Acral erythema and sloughing of skin or palms of hands and soles of feet 4. Myelosuppression 5. Severe blood pressure fluctuations 6. Fever and chills during infusion
Methotrexate	1. Standard dose: 10–500 mg/m^2; high dose: 500 mg/m^2 and greater 2. Photosensitivity 3. Diffuse hyperpigmentation 4. Neurotoxicity: seizures, aphasia, cerebellar toxicity (rare; see cytosine arabinoside) 5. Severe diarrhea 6. Renal toxicity 7. Hepatotoxicity and coagulopathies 8. Thrombocytopenia 9. Pulmonary toxicities

(continued)

Table 1.3 *(Continued)*

Drug	Toxicity
Melphalan	1. Standard dose: 6–8 mg/m^2; high dose: 80–140 mg/m^2 2. Severe mucositis 3. Diarrhea 4. Severe nausea, especially in combination with another emetogenic drug 5. Renal toxicity 6. Profound myelosuppression 7. Severe liver toxicity
Carmustine	1. Standard dose: 200–240 mg/m^2; high dose: 600–1200 mg/m^2 2. Hepatic dysfunction leading to veno-occlusive disease 3. Central nervous system changes, including diffuse encephalopathy 4. Mild alopecia
5-Fluorouracil	1. Standard dose: 7–15 mg/kg for five days; high dose: 255–300 mg/m^2 continuous infusion weekly 2. Cardiotoxicity mimicking acute myocardial infarction, angina, cardiogenic shock 3. Photosensitivity and hyperpigmentation 4. Severe diarrhea 5. Cerebellar toxicity

Source: Brown KA, Esper P, Kelleher LO, et al. *Chemotherapy and Biotherapy Guidelines and Recommendations for Practice*. Pittsburgh: Oncology Nursing Society; 2001:60-63. Reproduced with permission from Oncology Nursing Society Publishing.

Bowel Project revealed that a 21-gene recurrence assay is able to quantify and predict the magnitude of benefit from chemotherapy (tamoxifen compared with tamoxifen plus chemotherapy). Women with a low recurrence risk (<18) derived minimal if any benefit from chemotherapy, whereas women with high-risk tumors (>31) derived a large benefit (an absolute decrease in 10-year distant recurrence rate) of 27.6% (mean). Women with intermediate recurrence did not appear to derive a large benefit, but the study could not say there was no benefit to receiving chemotherapy (Paik et al, 2006). As no two people have identical genetic makeups, their ability to metabolize drugs may also differ. Proteogenomics can help predict toxicity based on certain polymorphisms or different variations in a gene that responsible for drug metabolism. For example, for patients receiving irinotecan with a specific polymorphism, they have an increased risk of bone marrow suppression. This is discussed more fully later in the chapter (Lee et al, 2005; McLeod and Watters, 2004).

New technology has permitted a reduction in toxicity and/or increasing dosing from a number of drugs. For instance, the use of nanotechnology to manufacture liposomal delivery vehicles for docetaxel, doxorubicin, daunorubicin, cytarabine, amphotericin, paclitaxel and camptothecins are currently available or being studied. The liposomal "wrapping" of water-soluble or insoluble drugs permits the drug to be preferentially delivered to sites of infection, inflammation, or tumor. Liposomes may pass through gaps in the endothelial lining of blood capillaries within the tumor, where the drug may be unpackaged and released within the tumor. Healthy tissues, on the other hand, have capillary walls that prevent the leakage of liposomes into the tissues, so that toxicity is reduced. The targeting of liposomes for specific tissues or disease sites is accomplished by variation in the number of lipid layers, and the size, charge, and permeability of the layers (Bangham, 1992). The future of nanotechnology has never been brighter, as seven national centers continue their study of different agents in nanotechnology-crafted devices (Jones, 2007). Efforts are being made to try to find agents offering equal efficacy but that can improve quality of life, such as new oral antineoplastic agents, by minimizing trips to the hospital or intrusive administration techniques.

Within the last few years, interest and clinical testing of new approaches to old drugs has occurred. 5-fluorouracil (5-FU) is an old drug that has good efficacy in colorectal cancer and other gastrointestinal cancers. However, it is limited, and increased doses are not necessarily more effective. Also, given by continuous infusion, 5-FU is often more effective because, being cell cycle specific for the S phase, more malignant cells are likely to be exposed to continuous infusion of chemotherapy than if the drug is given by bolus injection.

In an effort to improve the efficacy, new oral fluoropyrimidines have been developed, along with other agents that decrease the breakdown of 5-FU, so that serum drug levels are higher and more sustained, mimicking a continuous infusion. Examples of a prodrug are capecitabine and tegafur, and of an inhibitor of DPD are uracil and eniluracil. In an effort to reduce the toxicity of bolus 5FU/LV deGramont et al (1997) showed that infusional 5FU/LV was equivalent in efficacy but significantly less toxic. This has become the standard way to administer 5FU/LV in the United States at this time.

Capecitabine (Xeloda) is a 5-FU prodrug that is preferentially taken up by tumor cells. The drug has been approved for both the adjuvant treatment of patients with colon cancer as well as patients with advanced metastatic breast and colorectal cancers. Capecitabine has been shown to be equivalent to 5FU/LV and is being studied as a replacement in combination with oxaliplatin, irinotecan, or alone during radiotherapy. It simulates a continuous infusion of 5-FU, and has been shown equivalent to 5FU/LV in both adjuvant and metastatic settings (Cassidy et al, 2004).

As the cancer treatment paradigm shifts toward the administration of oral chemotherapy as well as targeted agents, nurses must focus on patient safety, strategies to enhance adherence to prescribed therapy, and teaching patient/family to provide self-care, including notifying the provider of early toxicity. Meticulous assessment of patient/family learning needs and styles, in addition to close telephone monitoring and triage of telephone calls, is critical to successful treatment. Other strategies such as (1) giving the patient a detailed calendar showing the pill(s) to take each day/time, with small check boxes that the patient can check off as the dose is taken, (2) asking the patient to maintain a diary of dose administration and side effects, or (3) asking the patient to bring their pill bottle with them to each visit for a pill count may be useful in monitoring patient adherence. Studies are underway using electronic methods to monitor patient adherence (Goodin et al, 2007).

Other advances in drug delivery are being used or studied in patients with brain tumors—for example, giving the drug into the tumor through a surgically implanted polymer wafer (interstitial) using implanted microspheres that slowly release chemotherapy, receptor-medicated permeabilizer, which allows administration of drugs that do not cross the blood–brain barrier after the administration of a drug that does such as mannitol, and finally giving chemotherapy through an implanted reservoir in the brain ventricle, which provides chemotherapy distribution into the CSF of the spinal cord (Graham and Cloughesy, 2004).

Planned drug holidays in patients with advanced cancers are another changing paradigm. A number of studies in patients with advanced colorectal cancer (CRC) showed that more aggressive therapy with 5-FU, leucovorin (LV), and oxaliplatin (FOLFOX) for 6 cycles, followed by maintenance using 5-FU/LV only for 12 cycles, and then returning to FOLFOX compared with FOLFOX4 continuously resulted in similar overall survival, but with less neurotoxicity in the group receiving a period of maintenance (OPTIMOX1) (Tournigand et al, 2006); however, completely halting chemotherapy for a period of time resulted in earlier onset of progression. A similar study by Labianca et al (2006) of patients with metastatic CRC looked at intermittent 5-FU, LV, and irinotecan (FOLFIRI) and found similar survival with less toxicity and cost in patients receiving intermittent FOLFIRI compared with those receiving continuous FOLFIRI.

Finally, national evidence-based treatment guidelines based on randomized clinical trials for patients with specific types of cancer have been promulgated, and studies are beginning to document patients who receive therapy based on these guidelines compared with those that do not have lower mortality. Cronin et al (2006) demonstrated that in the year 2000, patients with stage III rectal cancer were less likely to receive guideline-recommended treatment, whereas patients with stage III colon and stage II rectal cancer did with a consequent decrease in their mortality regardless of their comorbidities. Although there did not appear to be any race/ethnicity bias, there were age disparities. There is compelling evidence in the treatment of patients with colon and rectal cancer that older patients derive the same benefit from chemotherapy without greater toxicity (Cronin et al, 2006). Nurses need to advocate for older patients to consider carefully all treatment options to derive the maximal benefit.

Oncology nurses work very hard to prevent or minimize toxicity from chemotherapy agents in their patients. It is now apparent that certain patients have different abilities to metabolize certain drugs, called polymorphisms, or variability in the genes that are responsible for metabolizing the drug. For example, if a patient does not metabolize the drug as well due to a genetic factor, that patient will have more toxicity, such as neutropenia. Pharmacogenetics is an emerging field that will allow the use of knowledge of polymorphisms and drug metabolizing enzymes to maximize the benefit and minimize the risk to patients. For example, 10% of the US population expresses the UGT1A1*28* polymorphism which reduces the metabolism of SN-38, the active metabolite of irinotecan. This results in higher serum levels with more grades 3 and 4 neutropenia in those patients who should receive lower doses of irinotecan. Patients can be tested for this allele, or any patient who has a high bilirubin should be suspected, and a lower dose of the drug should be used initially.

In addition, genetic profiling will assist in predicting responses to certain chemotherapy agents such as 5-FU/cisplatin combinations, 5-FU, oxaliplatin, and other agents (Lenz HJ, 2001).

In the last decade, stimulated by the success of taxanes, epothilones were discovered, and the first, ixabepilone (Ixempra), is now FDA approved for patients with advanced breast cancer who have progressed on paclitaxel. Epothilones are a class of natural substances that cause tubulin polymerization and stabilization similar to paclitaxel. However, these substances have activity in tumor cell lines that are resistant to paclitaxel due to mutations in beta-tubulin (Altmann, 2003). Another agent currently being studied in clinical trials is patupilone (EPO906).

Antineoplastic agents are classified by mechanism of action (see Table 1.2). Cell cycle-specific agents are most active during specific phases of the cell cycle and include antimetabolites (S or synthesis phase), vinca alkaloids (M or mitotic phase), and miscellaneous drugs. Examples of these include L-asparaginase and prednisone (G_1 phase) and bleomycin and etoposide (G_2 phase). In addition, effective drugs such as the taxanes, that have a clear mechanism of action at therapeutic doses, may in fact, have an antiangiogenic effect at lower, more frequent dosing. Endothelial cells appear to be very sensitive to the taxanes. Seidman et al (2004) demonstrated that paclitaxel given weekly at a lower dose (dose density) was superior to an increased dose given every 3 weeks.

Cell cycle nonspecific agents can damage cells in all phases of the cell cycle and include alkylating agents (cyclophosphamide, cisplatin), antitumor/antibiotics (doxorubicin, mitomycin-C), the nitrosoureas (carmustine, lomustine), and others (dacarbazine, procarbazine) (see Table 1.2).

Antineoplastic agents are effective because they interfere with cellular metabolism and replication, resulting in cell death. When malignant cells mutate and develop mechanisms to evade programmed cell death, the tumor cells are no longer sensitive to the drug(s), and resistance emerges. Because of their mechanism of action, it is critical that nurses protect themselves when handling these drugs so that they are not exposed to the potential drug hazards. These drugs can be:

- *Mutagenic*: capable of causing a change in the genetic material within a cell that can be passed on to future cell generations;
- *Teratogenic*: capable of causing damage to a developing fetus exposed to the drug; the greatest risk is during the first trimester of pregnancy when the fetal organ systems are developing;
- *Carcinogenic*: capable of causing malignant change in a cell.

In 1985, the Occupational Safety and Health Administration (OSHA) developed guidelines for the safe handling of antineoplastic agents. These guidelines were revised in 1995 and then in 2004 to include all hazardous drugs (see Appendix I). NIOSH has updated recommendations as of March 2004.

Hormones are used in the management of hormonally sensitive cancers, such as breast and prostate cancers. The hormone changes the hormonal environment, probably affecting growth factors, so that the stimulus for tumor growth is suppressed or removed (see Table 1.4). New Selective Estrogen Receptor Modulators (SERM) and aromatize inhibitors are being developed to improve on the demonstrated success of tamoxifen.

COMPLICATIONS OF DRUG ADMINISTRATION

Hypersensitivity reactions are mediated by an immune mechanism, IgE, and involve the release of vasoactive agents (e.g., histamine, leukotrienes, prostaglandins) by the mast cells in tissue and basophils in the blood *after prior exposure* to the drug, and thus, the immune cells are sensitized. This results in contraction of smooth muscle and dilation of capillaries (Lenz, 2007). The systemic response is characterized by degrees of urticaria, a rash, hypotension, more severe grade 3 bronchospasm (symptomatic, with angioedema), and grade 4 anaphylaxis, with profound vasomotor collapse. In contrast, some patients have a reaction, which may be severe, *on first exposure* to the drug. This reaction is not an immune reaction and is not mediated by IgE, but rather an *anaphylactoid* reaction, in which the drug or vehicle (e.g., Cremaphor with paclitaxel) interacts with the mast cells and basophils, causing a release of the vasoactive agents; however, the end result is the same, and the nursing/medical interventions are the same whether the reaction is immune related or not. Thus, the nurse must be vigilant at all times when administering chemotherapy. Patients who have had hypersensitivity reactions to certain chemotherapy agents may be successfully desensitized and go on to complete their therapy (Feldweg et al, 2005).

All drugs can cause hypersensitivity reactions including anaphylaxis, but only a few drugs cause severe problems. These include the following:

- Paclitaxel (related to carrier vehicle solution CR creme)
- Docetaxel (related to delivery vehicle solution Tween)
- Cisplatin
- Teniposide (VumoM-26)
- Bleomycin (less common; 2% incidence in lymphoma patients)
- Cetuximab (Erbitux, discussed in Chapter 5), 3% incidence with most occurring on the first treatment; may be fatal
- Rituximab (Rituxan, discussed in Chapter 5)

In addition, certain drugs can cause delayed hypersensitivity, such as carboplatin and oxaliplatin, where the patient develops a range of signs and symptoms of hypersensitivity after receiving a number of cycles of the drug, such as 7 cycles of carboplatin (Markman et al, 2003). For nursing management of patients experiencing hypersensitivity or anaphylaxis, as recommended by the Oncology Nursing Society Practice Committee, see Table 1.5.

Table 1.4 Common Hormonal Agents

Classification	Examples
Adrenocorticoids	cortisone hydrocortisone dexamethasone methylprednisone methylprednisolone prednisone prednisolone
Androgens	testosterone propionate (Neo-hombreol, Oreton) fluoxymesterone (Halotestin, Ora-Testryl) testolactone
Estrogens	chlorotrianisene (TACE) diethylstilbestrol (DES) diethylstilbestrol diphosphate (Stilphostrol) ethinyl estradiol (Estinyl) conjugated estrogen (Premarin) Stradiol
Selective Estrogen Receptor Modulators (SERM)	tamoxifen citrate (Nolvadex) toremifene citrate (Fareston) raloxifene (Evista)
Selective aromatase inhibitors • Reversible • Irreversible	anastrozole (Arimidex) letrozole (Femara) exemestane (Aromasin)
Progesterones	medroxyprogesterone acetate (Provera, Depo-Provera) megestrol acetate (Megace, Pallace)
Antitestosterone	leuprolide acetate (Lupron) bicalutamide (Casodex) flutamide (Eulexin) nilutamide (Nilandron)

EXTRAVASATION

Specific chemotherapeutic drugs called *vesicants* may cause severe tissue necrosis if extravasated or inadvertently administered outside the vein. Some of these drugs have antidotes that will minimize or prevent local tissue damage. These are shown in Table 1.6. For a Standardized Nursing Care Plan for management of patients experiencing extravasation, see Table 1.7. It is imperative that the nurse be very careful when

Table 1.5 Management of Hypersensitivity and Anaphylactic Reactions

1. Review the patient's allergy history.
2. Consider prophylactic medications with hydrocortisone or an antihistamine in atopic/allergic individuals. (This requires a physician's order.)
3. *Patient and family education*: Assess the patient's readiness to learn. Inform patient of the potential for an allergic reaction and instruct to report any unusual symptoms such as:
   A. Uneasiness or agitation
   B. Abdominal cramping
   C. Itching
   D. Chest tightness
   E. Light-headedness or dizziness
   F. Chills
4. Ensure that emergency equipment and medications are readily available.
5. Obtain baseline vital signs and note patient's mental status.
6. As appropriate, perform a scratch test, intradermal skin test, or test dose before administering the full dosage (this requires a physician's order). If there is no reaction, the remaining dose can be administered. If an allergic response is suspected, discontinue the test dose (unless it has been completed), maintain the intravenous line, and notify the physician.
7. For a *localized allergic response*:
   A. Evaluate symptoms; observe for urticaria, wheals, localized erythema.
   B. Administer diphenhydramine or hydrocortisone as per physician's order.
   C. Monitor vital signs every 15 minutes for 1 hour.
   D. Continue subsequent dosing or desensitization program according to a physician's order.
   E. If a "flare" reaction appears along the vein with doxorubicin (Adriamycin) or daunorubicin, flush the line with saline.
      a. Ensure that extravasation has not occurred.
      b. Administer hydrocortisone 25–50 mg intravenously with a physician's order, followed by a 0.9% NS flush. This may be adequate to resolve the "flare" reaction.
      c. Once the "flare" reaction has resolved, continue slow infusion of the drug.
      d. Monitor for repeated "flare" episodes. It is preferable to change the intravenous site if possible.
8. For a generalized allergic response, either an *anaphylactoid has never been exposed to the drug before or anaphylaxis (severe hypersensitivity reaction after having received the drug before), assess for following signs or symptoms (these usually occur within the first 15 minutes of the start of the infusion or injection)*:
   A. Subjective signs and symptoms
      a. Generalized itching
      b. Chest tightness
      c. Agitation
      d. Uneasiness
      e. Dizziness
      f. Nausea
      g. Crampy abdominal pain
      h. Anxiety

(continued)

Table 1.5 *(Continued)*

i. Sense of impending doom
j. Desire to urinate or defecate
k. Chills

B. Objective signs
a. Flushed appearance (edema of face, hands, or feet)
b. Localized or generalized urticaria
c. Respiratory distress with or without wheezing
d. Hypotension
e. Cyanosis
f. Difficulty speaking

9. For a *generalized allergic response*:
A. Stop the infusion immediately and notify the physician.
B. Maintain the intravenous line with appropriate solution to expand the vascular space, e.g., NS.
C. If not contraindicated, ensure maximum rate of infusion if the patient is hypotensive.
D. Position the patient to promote perfusion of the vital organs; the supine position is preferred.
E. Monitor vital signs every 2 minutes until stable, then every 5 minutes for 30 minutes, then every 15 minutes as ordered.
F. Reassure the patient and the family.
G. Maintain the airway and anticipate the need for cardiopulmonary resuscitation.
H. All medications must be administered with a physician's order.
I. Anticipate administering the following medications for the following effects:
a. Vasoconstriction to increase cardiac output and blood pressure:
1) epinephrine (1:1000, 0.3–0.5 mL or 0.3–0.5 mg IM or subcutaneous q 10–15 min; or if hypotensive, 1:10,000 concentration giving 0.5–1.0 mL (0.1 mg) IVP in adults; in pediatrics, 1:1000 0.01 mL/kg (up to 0.3 mL)
2) dopamine 2–20 micrograms/kg/min (adults)
b. Antihistamines to stop allergic release of histamines:
1) diphenhydramine: 25–50 mg IVP (adults), 1 mg/kg (max 50 mg, pediatrics)
2) ranitidine 50 mg IV or famotidine 20 mg IV (adults)
c. Bronchodilation: aminophylline 5 mg/kg IV over 30 min (adults)
d. Anti-inflammation/Bronchodilation: steroids. Hydrocortisone 100–500 mg IV (peds 1–2 mg/kg; or Methylprednisolone 30–50 mg IV (peds 0.3–0.5 mg/kg); or dexamethasone 10–20 mg IVP (peds 1–2 mg/kg); or hydrocortisone 100–500 mg IV (peds 1–2 mg/kg)

10. Document the incident in the medical record according to institution policy and procedures.
11. Physician-guided desensitization may be necessary for subsequent dosing.

References: Polovich M, White JM, Kelleher LC, (eds), *Chemotherapy and Biotherapy Guidelines and Recommendations for Practice*. 2nd ed. Pittsburgh, PA: ONS; 2005;86. Barton-Burke, M, Wilkes GM, Ingwersen K. *Cancer Chemotherapy: A Nursing Process Approach*, 3rd ed. Sudbury, MA: Jones and Bartlett Publishers Inc.; 2001. Ellis AK and Day JH. Diagnosis and Management of Anaphylaxis. *Canadian Medical Association Journal* 2003;169(4): 307–312. Sheperd GM. Hypersensitivity Reactions to Chemotherapeutic Drugs. *Allergy and Immunology* 2003;24:253–262.

Table 1.6 Vesicants and Irritants

Vesicants				
Chemotherapeutic Agents	**Antidote**	**Antidote Preparation**	**Local Care**	**Comments**
Alkylating agents				
Mechlorethamine (nitrogen mustard)	Isotonic sodium (NA) thiosulfate	Prepare 1/6 molar solution: 1. If 10% Na thiosulfate solution, mix 4 mL with 6 ml sterile water for injection. 2. If 25% Na thiosulfate solution, mix 1.6 mL with 8.4 ml sterile water.	1. Immediately inject Na thiosulfate through IV cannula, 2 mL for every mg extravasated. 2. Remove needle. 3. Inject antidote into subcutaneous (SC) tissue.	1. Na thiosulfate neutralizes nitrogen mustard, which then is excreted via the kidneys. 2. Time is essential in treating extravasation. 3. Heat and cold not proven effective. 4. Although clinically accepted, reports of the benefits are scant.
Cisplatin (Platinol®[a])	Same as above	Same as above	1. Use 2 ml of the 10% Na thiosulfate for each 100 mg of cisplatin. 2. Remove needle. 3. Inject subcutaneously.	1. Vesicant potential seen with a concentration of more than 20 cc of 0.5 mg/ml extravasates. If less than this, drug is an irritant; no treatment recommended.
Antitumor antibiotics				
Doxorubicin (Adriamycin®[b])	None		1. Apply cold pad with circulating ice water, ice pack, or cryogel pack for 15–20 minutes at least	1. Extravasations of less than 1–2 cc often will heal spontaneously. If greater than 3 cc, ulceration often results.

(continued)

Table 1.6 *(Continued)*

Vesicants				
Chemotherapeutic Agents	**Antidote**	**Antidote Preparation**	**Local Care**	**Comments**
			four times per day for the first 24–48 hours. Elevate site for 48 hrs, then resume normal activity.	2. Protect area from sunlight and heat. 3. Studies suggest benefit of 99% dimethyl sulfoxide (DMSO) 1–2 mL applied to site every 6 hours. Other studies show delayed healing with DMSO.
Daunorubicin (Cerubidine®[c])	None			1. Little information known. 2. In mouse experiments, some benefit from topical DMSO.
Mitomycin-C (mitomycin)	None			1. Protect from sunlight. 2. Delayed skin reactions have occurred in areas far from original IV site. 3. Some research studies show benefit with use of 99% DMSO 1–2 mL applied to site every 6 hours for 14 days. More studies needed.
Dactinomycin (actinomycin-D)	None		1. Apply ice to increase comfort at the site.	1. Heat may enhance tissue damage.

(continued)

Table 1.6 *(Continued)*

Vesicants				
Chemotherapeutic Agents	**Antidote**	**Antidote Preparation**	**Local Care**	**Comments**
			2. Elevate for 48 hours then resume normal activity.	
Mitoxantrone (concentrated dose)	Unknown			1. Antidote and local care measures unknown. 2. Ulceration rare unless concentrated dose infiltrates.
Epirubicin (Ellence®[d])	None			1. Antidote and local care measures unknown. 2. Cold, DMSO, and corticosteroids ineffective in experiments with mice.
Vinca alkaloids/microtubular inhibiting agents				
Vincristine (Oncovin®[e])			1. Apply warm pack for 15–20 minutes at least four times per day for the first 24–48 hours and elevate.	1. These two methods of treatment are very effective for rapid absorption of drug.
Vinblastine (Velban®[e])			Same as above.	Same as above.
Vindesine (Eldisine®)			Same as above.	Same as above.
Vinorebine (Navelbine®[f])			Same as above.	1. Same treatment as vincristine/vinblastine.

(continued)

Table 1.6 *(Continued)*

Vesicants				
Chemotherapeutic Agents	**Antidote**	**Antidote Preparation**	**Local Care**	**Comments**
				2. Moderate vesicant. 3. Manufacturer recommends administering drug over 6–10 minutes into side port of free-flowing IV closest to the IV bag, followed by flush of 75–125 mL of IV solution to reduce incidence of phlebitis and severe back pain.
Taxanes				
Paclitaxel (Taxol®) (concentrated solution)	Ice		Apply ice pack for 15–20 minutes at least four times per day for the first 24 hours.	1. Paclitaxel may have rare vesicant potential (probably due to dilution in 500 cc diluent). 2. Ice and hyaluronidase have been effective in decreasing local tissue damage in a mouse model.

(continued)

Table 1.6 *(Continued)*

Irritants				
Chemotherapeutic Agents	**Antidote**	**Antidote Preparation**	**Local Care**	**Comments**
Alkylating agents Dacarbazine (DTIC)				1. May cause phlebitis. 2. Protect drug from sunlight.
Ifosfamide Carboplatin				1. May cause phlebitis. 2. Antidote or local care measures unknown.
Oxaliplatin (however, has vesicant potential)				1. Oxaliplatin has vesicant potential so is best given via CL. If oxaliplatin given via peripheral line, drug can be diluted in 500 mL D5W (Sanofi Synthelabo, 2004) and infused over 6 hours to decrease discomfort. 2. High dose dexamethasone should be considered as a therapeutic intervention (Kretzschman et al, 2003)
Antitumor Antibiotics				
Daunorubicin citrate (DaunoXome®)				1. May cause pain or burning at IV site. 2. Antidote or local care measures unknown.

(continued)

Table 1.6 *(Continued)*

Irritants				
Chemotherapeutic Agents	**Antidote**	**Antidote Preparation**	**Local Care**	**Comments**
Nitrosoureas				
Carmustine (BCNU)				1. May cause phlebitis. Local care measures are unknown. 2. Antidote or local care measures unknown.
Antitumor Antibiotics				
Doxorubicin liposome (Doxil®)				1. May produce redness and tissue edema. 2. Low ulceration potential. 3. If ulceration begins or pain, redness, or swelling persist, treat like doxorubicin.
Bleomycin (Blenoxane®)				1. May cause irritation to tissue. 2. Little information known.
Epipodophyllotoxin				
Etoposide (VP-16)			1. Apply warm pack.	1. Treatment necessary only if large amount of a concentrated solution extravasates. In this case, treat like vincristine or vinblastine.

(continued)

Table 1.6 *(Continued)*

		Irritants		
Chemotherapeutic Agents	**Antidote**	**Antidote Preparation**	**Local Care**	**Comments**
				2. May cause phlebitis, urticaria, and redness.
Teniposide (VM-26)				Same as above.

[a] *Bristol-Myers-Squibb Oncology, Princeton, NJ*;
[b] *Pharmacia & Upjohn Co, Kalamazoo, MI*;
[c] *Chiron Therapeutics, Emeryville, CA*;
[d] *Andria Laboratories, Dublin, OH*;
[e] *Eli Lilly and Co., Indianapolis, IN*;
[f] *Glaxo Wellcome Oncology/HIV, Research Triangle Park, NC*

Note: Based on information from Bertelli, G., Gozzo, A., Forno, G.B., Vidili, M.G., Silvestro, S., Venturini, M., DelMastro, L., Garrone, O., Rosso, R., and Dini, D., 1995. Topical Dimethylsulfoxide for the Prevention of Soft Tissue Injury after Extravasation of Vesicant Cytotoxic Drugs: A Prospective Clinical Study. *Journal of Clinical Oncology*, 13(11):2851–2855; Lebredo, L., Barrie, R., and Woltering, E.A., 1992. DMSO Protection Against Adriamycin-induced Tissue Necrosis. *Journal of Surgery Research*, 53(1):62–65; Rospond, E.M., and Engel, L.M., 1993. Dimethyl Sulfoxide for Treating Anthracycline Extravasation. *Clinical Pharmatherapeutics* 12(8):560–561. *Source*: Brown KA, Esper P, Kellher LO, et al (2001) *Cancer Chemotherapy Guidelines and Recommendations for Practice*, pp 46–47. Reproduced with permission from Oncology Nursing Society Publishing.

Modified from Polovich M, White Jim, Kellner LO (Eds) (2005) *Chemotherapy and Biotherapy Guidelines and Recommendations for Practice*, 2nd Ed, pp. 79–81. Reproduced with permission from Oncology Nursing Society.

Table 1.7 Standardized Nursing Care Plan for Management of the Patient Experiencing Extravasation (Based on Oncology Nursing Press Cancer Chemotherapy Guidelines)

Nursing Diagnosis	Defining Characteristics	Expected Outcomes	Nursing Interventions
I. Potential alteration in skin integrity related to extravasation.	I. Vesicant drugs may cause erythema, burning, tissue necrosis, tissue sloughing.	I. Extravasation, if it occurs, is detected early with early intervention.	I. Careful technique is used during venipuncture. A. Select venipuncture site away from underlying tendons and blood vessels. B. Secure IV so that catheter/needle site is visible at all times. C. Administer vesicant through freely flowing IV, constantly monitoring IV site and patient response. Nurse should be thoroughly familiar with institutional policy and procedure for administration of a vesicant agent. D. If vesicant drug is administered as a continuous infusion, drug must be given through a patent central line and monitored closely.
II. Potential pain at site of extravasation.	II. Vesicant drugs include: A. Commercial agents 1. dactinomycin 2. daunorubicin 3. doxorubicin 4. mitomycin C 5. estramustine 6. mechlorethamine	II. Skin and underlying tissue damage is minimized.	II. If extravasation is suspected: A. Stop drug administration. B. Aspirate any residual drug and blood from IV tubing, IV catheter/needle IV site if possible. C. Instill antidote, if one exists, through needle if able to remove remaining drug in previous step. If standing orders are not available, notify MD and obtain order.

(continued)

Table 1.7 *(Continued)*

Nursing Diagnosis	Defining Characteristics	Expected Outcomes	Nursing Interventions
	7. vinblastine 8. vincristine 9. vinorelbine 10. idarubicin 11. vindesine 12. epirubicin 13. esorubicin 14. cisplatin (concentrated) 15. mitoxantrone 16. paclitaxel (concentrated) 17. fluorouracil (concentrated) B. Investigational agents 1. amsacrine 2. maytansine 3. bisantrene 4. pyrazofurin 5. adozelesin 6. anti-B4-blocked ricin		D. Remove needle. E. Inject antidote into area of apparent infiltration, if antidote is recommended, using 25-gauge needle into subcutaneous tissue. F. Apply topical cream if recommended. G. Cover lightly with occlusive sterile dressing. H. Apply warm or cold applications as prescribed. I. Elevate arm. J. Assess site regularly for pain, progression of erythema, induration, and for evidence of necrosis: 1. If outpatient, arrange to assess site or teach patient to and to notify provider if condition worsens. Arrange next visit for assessment of site depending on drug, amount infiltrated, extent of potential injury, and patient variables. 2. Discuss with MD the need for plastic-surgical consult if erythema, induration, pain, tissue breakdown occurs.

(continued)

Table 1.7 *(Continued)*

Nursing Diagnosis	Defining Characteristics	Expected Outcomes	Nursing Interventions
			K. When in doubt about whether drug is infiltrating, treat as an infiltration. L. Document precise, concise information in patient's medical record: 1. Date, time 2. Insertion site, needle size and type 3. Drug administration technique, drug sequence, and approximate amount of drug extravasated 4. Appearance of site, patient's subjective response 5. Nursing interventions performed to manage extravasation, and notification of MD 6. Photo documentation if possible 7. Follow-up plan 8. Nurse's signature 9. Institutional policy and procedure for documentation should be adhered to
III. Potential loss of function of extremity related to extravasation			
IV. Potential infection related to skin breakdown			

Source: Barton-Burke M et al (2001) *Cancer Chemotherapy: A Nursing Process Approach*, pp 628–629. Reprinted with permission from Jones and Bartlett Publishers Inc.

administering chemotherapy to minimize the chance of this occurring. The nurse carefully assesses the patient's response, the administration site, and patency of the IV site throughout the administration of the vesicant agent. If ever in doubt whether or not a drug is extravasating, treat it as an extravasation to minimize potential tissue damage to the patient.

When vesicants are administered as a continuous infusion, a central line is required. In addition, it is imperative that the IV insertion site be checked for signs/symptoms of extravasation at least hourly, and that the patient be instructed to tell the nurse immediately if stinging or burning is felt. As many continuous infusions of vesicant chemotherapy occur when the patient is at home, it is again imperative to instruct the patient to pay attention to any changes in sensation at the site, and to call the nurse if any discomfort, stinging, or burning is felt. A number of patients have had extravasation of drug from a needle dislodged from an implanted port onto the surrounding skin, which then caused a necrotic ulcer and necessitated explantation of the subcutaneous port. This year, dexrazoxane for injection (Totect™) was approved for the treatment of doxorubicin extravasations. This agent is the same agent that is used to provide cardioprotection and permit increased doses of doxorubicin in patients with breast cancer who have received maximal doxorubicin. It works as a free radical scavenger and may inhibit topoisomerase II irreversibly (Mouridsen et al, 2007; Schulmeister, 2007); however, the drug in itself is cytotoxic, is expensive, and must be administered within 6 hours of the extravasation. The drug is given as an infusion daily for 3 days. It is unknown whether the drug inactivates the therapeutic dose of the drug that was given before the drug extravasated.

Within the last decade, oncology nurses have been humbled by the reports of significant and lethal errors that have occurred during the chemotherapy prescription, admixing, and administration processes. It is clear that institutional and physician office practices must have systematic review of the entire linked process and steps taken to prevent the occurrence of these errors and tragic consequences through competent checks and balances (Fisher et al, 1996). Fortunately, the series of well-publicized errors have been a "wake-up" call, and oncology nurses, pharmacists, and physicians have worked together to develop safe environments for clinical practice. The Oncology Nursing Society position paper, "Regarding the Preparation of the Professional Registered Nurse Who Administers and Cares for the Individual Receiving Chemotherapy," states that the nurse administering chemotherapy and caring for patients receiving chemotherapy should complete a chemotherapy course and clinical practicum to safely and competently deliver chemotherapy. The course topics should include history of cancer chemotherapy; drug development; principles of cancer chemotherapy; chemotherapy preparation, storage, and transport; nursing assessment; chemotherapy administration; safety precautions during chemotherapy administration; disposal/accidental exposure and spills; and, finally, institutional considerations (ONS Position Paper, revised 6/99: ONS Safe Handling of Hazardous Drugs, 2003; NISOH Safe Handling of Hazardous Drugs, June 2004).

References

Ahles TA, Saykin AJ. Candidate mechanisms for chemotherapy-induced cognitive changes. *Nat Rev Cancer* 2007; 7 192–201

Ajani JA, Dodd LS, Daughtery K, et al. Taxol-Induced Soft-Tissue Injury Secondary to Extravasation: Characterization by Histo-Pathology and Clinical Course. *JNCI* 1994; 86 51–53

Allen WL, Johnston PG. Role of Genomic Markers in Colorectal Cancer Treatment. *J Clin Oncol* 2005; 23(20) 4545–4552

Altmann KH. Epothilone B and its analogs—a new family of anti-cancer agents. *Mini Rev Med Chem* 2003; 3(2) 149–158

Barton-Burke M, Wilkes G, Berg D, et al. *Cancer Chemotherapy: A Nursing Process Approach*, 3rd ed. Sudbury, MA: Jones and Bartlett; 2001

Baylin SB, Herman JG, Graff JR, et al. Alterations in DNA Methylation—A Fundamental Aspect of Neoplasia. *Adv Cancer Res* 1998; 72 141–196

Bower M, Newlands ES, Bleehan NM, et al. Multicenter CRC Phase II Trial of Temozolomide in Recurrent or Progressive High Grade Glioma. *Cancer Chemother Pharmacol* 1997; 40 484–488

Bristol-Myers Squibb Pharmaceutical Research Institute. Investigator Brochure for UFT (Uracil: Ftorafur in a molar ratio of 4:1); 1996

Camp-Sorrell D. Chemotherapy Toxicities and Management. Chapter 17 in Yarbro CH, Frogge MH, Goodman M. *Cancer Nursing: Principles and Practice*, 6th ed. Sudbury, MA: Jones and Bartlett Publishers Inc.; 2005; 412–458

Cassidy J, Scheithauer W, McKendrick J, et al. *Capecitabine (X) vs bolus 5-FU/leucovorin (LV) as adjuvant therapy for colon cancer (the X-ACT study): efficacy results of a phase III trial J Clin Oncol 2004 ASCO Meeting Proceedings*, (Post-Meeting edition) 2004; 22(14S) 3509

Chabner BA, Longo DL. *Cancer Chemotherapy and Biotherapy: Principles and Practice*, 3rd ed. Philadelphia: Lippincott-Raven; 2001

Chang AY, Kuebler JP, Pandya KJ, Pulmonary Toxicity Induced by Mitomycin C Is Highly Responsive to Glucocorticoids. *Cancer* 1986; 57 2285–2290

Chen HY, et al. 5 Gene Pattern Predicts NSCLC Outcome. *New Engl J Med* 2007; 356 11–20

Chen AY, Liu LF. Topoisomerases: Essential Enzymes and Lethal Targets. *Annu Rev Pharmacol Toxicol* 1994; 34 191–218

Cheson BD, Vena DA, Foss FM, Sorenson JM. Neurotoxicity of Purine Analogs: *A Review. J Clin Oncol* 1994; 12(10) 2216–2228

Chiron Therapeutics. *Depocyt Package Insert*. Emeryville, CA, Chiron Therapeutics; 2007

Ciuleanu TE, Brodowicz T, Belani CP, et al. Maintenance Pemetrexed Plus Best Supportive Care (BSC) Versus Placebo Plus BSC: A Phase III Study. *J Clin Oncol* 2008; 26 (May 20 suppl; abstr 8011)

Clinical Trials. *Colorectal Cancer Trials involving Irinotecan and the Saltz Regimen are Temporarily Suspended*. 2001; http://www.cancer.gov/clinicaltrials

Cortes J, Baselga J. Targeting the Microtubules in Breast Cancer Beyond Taxanes: The Epothilones. *The Oncologist* 2007; 12 271–280

Cronin DP, Harlan LC, Potosky AL, et al. Patterns of Care for Adjuvant Therapy in a Random Population-Based Sample of Patients Diagnosed With Colorectal Cancer. *Am J Gastroenterology* 2006; 101(10) 2308–2318

Dang C, Smith K, Fornier M, et al. Updated Cardiac Safety Results with Dose-Dense (DD) Doxorubicin and Cycleophosphamide (AC) Followed by Paclitaxel (T) with Trastuzumab (H) in HER2/neu Overexpressed/Amplified Breast Cancer (BCA). *J Clin Oncol* 2006; 24(18S) 582 (abstract)

de Gramont A, Bossett JF, Milan C, et al. Randomized trial comparing monthly low-dose leucovorin and fluorouracil bolus with bimonthly high-dose leucovorin and fluorouracil bolus plus continuous infusion for advanced colorectal cancer: A French Intergroup study. *J Clin Oncol* 1997; 15 808–815 de Gramont A, Banzi M, Navarro M, et al. Oxaliplatin/5-FU/LV in Adjuvant Colon Cancer: Results of the International Randomized Mosaic Trial. *Proc Am Society Clin Oncol* 2003; abstract 101, 522253

de Gramont A, Boni C, Navarro M, et al. Oxaliplatin/5FU/LV in the adjuvant treatment of stage II and stage III colon cancer: Efficacy results with a median follow-up of 4 years. Oral abstract presented at: ASCO 2005 Gastrointestinal Cancers Symposium; January 27–29, 2005; Hollywood, FL

Dorr RT, Von Hoff DD. *Cancer Chemotherapy Handbook*, 2nd ed. Norwalk, CT: Appleton & Lange; 1994

Ellis AK, Day JH. Diagnosis and Management of Anaphylaxis. *Canadian Medical Association Journal* 2003 169(4) 307–312

Fabian CJ, Molina R, Slavik M, et al. Pyridoxine Therapy for Palmar-Plantar Erythrodysesthesia Associated with Continuous 5-Fluorouracil Infusion. *Invest New Drugs* 1990; 8(1) 57–63

Federal Drug Administration. FDA Advisory Committee Suggests Changes to ESA Use. *NCI Cancer Bulletin* 2007; 4(17)

Feldweg AM, Lee CW, Matulonis UA, Castells M. Rapid Desensitization for Hypersensitivity Reactions to Paclitaxel and Docetaxel: A New Standard Protocol Used in 77 Successful Treatments. *Gynecol Oncol* 2005; 96(3) 824–829

Friedberg JW, Cohen P, Cheson BD, et al. Bendamustine HCL (Treanda) Results in High Rate of Objective Response in Patients with Rituximab-Refractory and Alkylator-Refractory Indolent B-Cell Non-Hodgkins Lymphoma (INHL): Results From a Phase II Multi-Center Single Agent Study (SDX-105-01). *Blood* 2005; 106 70a, abstract 229

George BJ, Ricart AD, Calvo E, et al. Phase I Pharmacokinetic (PK)/Food Effect and Safety Study of Satraplatin in Patients (Pts) With Advanced Solid Tumors. *J Clin Oncol* 2006; 24(18S) 12014 (abstract)

Gianni L, Dombernowsky P, Sledge G, et al. Cardiac Function Following Combination Therapy with Taxol (T) and Doxorubicin (D) for Advanced Breast Cancer (ABC). *Proc Am SocClin Oncol* 1998; 17 115a

Goodin S, Aisner J, Bartel SB, Viele CS. Current Issues Associated With Oral Chemotherapy: A Roundtable Discussion. Am J Health-Syst *Pharm* 2007; 64 (Suppl 5) 533–535

Graham CA, Cloughesy TF. Brain Tumor Treatment: Chemotherapy and Other New Developments. *Semin Oncol Nursing* 2004; 20(4) 260–272

Hainsworth JD, Burris HA, Litchy S, et al. Weekly docetaxel in the treatment of elderly patients with advanced non-small cell lung cancer. *Cancer* 2000; 89(2) 328–333

Harwood KV, Govin K. Short-Term vs Long-Term Local Cooling after Doxorubicin Extravasations: An Eastern Cooperative Oncology Group (ECOG) Study [abstract]. *Proceedings of the American Society of Clinical Oncology* 1994; 13 447

Hong DS, Galsky M, Chiorean E, et al. Phase I Study of the Effects of Renal Impairment on the Pharmacokinetic (PK) and Safety of Satraplatin in Patients (Pts) With Refractory Non-Hematologic Cancer. *J Clin Oncol* 2006; 24(18S) 2044 (abstract)

Hortobagyi GM, et al. Reduction of Skeletal Related Complications in Breast Cancer Patients with Osteolytic Bone Metastases Receiving Chemotherapy by Monthly Pamidronate Sodium Infusion. Proceedings of 32nd Annual ASCO Meeting, Philadelphia, ASCO 1996; abstract 99

Igawa S, Nobuyuki Y, Ueda S, et al. Evaluation of the Recommended Dose and Efficacy of Amrubicin as Second- and Third-Line Chemotherapy for Small Cell Lung Cancer. *J Thoracic Oncol* 2007; 2(8) 741–744

Jones D. Cancer Nanotechnology: Small but Heading for the Big Time. *Nat Rev Drug Disc* 2007; 6(3) 174–175

Labianca R, Floriani I, Cortesi E, et al. Alternating Versus Continuous "FOLFIRI" in Advanced Colorectal Cancer (ACC): A Randomized "GISCAD" Trial. *J Clin Oncol* 2006; 24(18S) 3505

Larson DK. What Is the Appropriate Treatment for Tissue Extravasation by Antitumor Agents? *Plastic and Reconstructive Surgery* 1985; 75 397–405

Laurie SW, Wilson KL, Keinahan DA, et al. Intravenous Extravasation Injuries: The Effectiveness of Hyaluronidase in Their Treatment. *Annals of Plastic Surgery* 1984; 13(3) 191–194

Lee W, Lockhart AC, Kim RB, Rothenberg ML. Cancer Pharmacogenomics: Powerful Tools in Cancer Chemotherapy and Drug Development. *The Oncologist* 2005; 10 104–111

Lenz HL. Resistance to therapy: Molecular markers in GI oncology. State of the Science: GI Oncology, http://www.webtie.org/SOTS/Meetings/Gastrointestinal/March62001/lectures/htm. Accessed May 2006

Lenz HL. Management and Preparedness for Infusion and Hypersensitivity Reactions. *The Oncologist* 2007; 12 601–609

Lui LF, Lui CC, Alberts BM. Type 2 DNA Topoisomerases: Enzymes That Can Unknot a Topologically Knotted DNA Molecule via a Reversible Double-Strand Break. *Cell* 1980; 19 697–707

Mandelli F. Introduction to the Workshop on DNA Methyltransferase Inhibitors. *Leukemia* 1993; 7(Suppl 1) 1–2

Markman M. Prevention of paclitaxel-associated arthralgias and myalgias. *J Support Oncol* 2003; 1 233–234

Markman M, Zanotti L, Peterson G, et al. Expanded experience with an intradermal skin test to predict for the presence or absence of carboplatin sensitivity. *J Clin Oncol* 2003; 21 4611–4614

Marsh S, McLeod HL. Pharmacogenomics: From Bedside to Clinical Practice. *Hum Mol Genet* 2006; 15 R89–R93

McLeod HL, Watters JW. Irinotecan pharmacogenetics: Is it time to intervene? *J Clin Oncol* 2004; 22(8) 9602–963

Minotti G, Saponiero A, Licata S, et al. Paclitaxel and Docetaxel May Enhance the Metabolism of Doxorubicin to Toxic Species in Human Myocardium. *Clin CA Res* 2001; 7 1511–1515

Mouridsen HT, et al. Treatment of Anthracycline Extravasation With Savene (Dexrazoxane). Results From Two Prospective Clinical Multicentre Studies. *Ann Oncol* 2007; 18 546–550

Novotny WF, Holmgren E, Nelson B, et al. Bevacizumab (a monoclonal antibody to vascular endothelial growth factor) does not increase the incidence of venous thromboembolism when added to first-line chemotherapy to treat metastatic colorectal cancer. *Proc Am Soc Clin Oncol* 2004; 2 3252, abstract 3529

Occupational Safety and Health Administration. *Controlling Occupational Exposure to Hazardous Drugs*. 1995; Washington (OSHA Instruction CPL 2-2.20B)

Oncology Nursing Society Board of Directors. *ONS Position Paper: Regarding the Preparation of the Professional Registered Nurse who Administers and Cares for the Individual Receiving Chemotherapy*. Pittsburgh, PA: Oncology Nursing Society; 1999

Onoda S, Masuda N, Seto T, et al. Phase II Trial of Amrubicin for Treatment of Refractory or Relapsed Small-Cell Lung Cancer: Thoracic Oncology Research Group Study 0301. *J Clin Oncol* 2006; 24(34) 5448–5453

O'Shaughnessy JA. Molecular Signatures Predict Outcomes of Breast Cancer. *New Engl J Med* 2006; 355 615–617

Paik S, Tang G, Shak S, et al. Gene Expression and Benefit of Chemotherapy in Women With Node-Negativstrogen Receptor-Positive Breast Cancer. *J Clin Oncol* 2006; 24(23) 3726–3734

Perry MC, (ed). *The Chemotherapy Source Book*, 2nd ed. Baltimore: Williams & Wilkins; 1997

Posner MR, Haddad RI, Wirth LJ. The Evolution of Induction Chemotherapy and Sequential Therapy for Locally Advanced Squamous Cell Cancer of the Head and Neck. *2006 American Society of Clinical Oncology Educational Book,* Alexandria, VA: American Society of Clinical Oncology, 2006, pp 346–352

Potti A, Dressman HK, Bild A, et al. Genomic Signatures to Guide the Use of Chemotherapeutics. *Nat Med* 2006; 12(11) 1294–3000

Polovich M, White JM, Kelleher LO, (eds), *Chemotherapy and Biotherapy Guidelines and Recommendations for Practice*, 2nd ed. Pittsburg, PA: Oncology Nursing Society; 2005

Rittenberg CN, Gralla RJ, Rehmeyer TA. Assessing and Managing Venous Irritation Associated with Vinorelbine Tartare (Navelbine®). *Oncol Nurs Forum* 1995; 22(4) 707–710

Sanofi Synthelabo. Eloxatin Package Insert. New York: Sanofi Synthelabo, Inc.; 2008

Schulmeister L. Totect™: A New Agent for Treating Anthracycline Extravasation. *Clin J Oncol Nurs* 2007; 11(3) 387–395

Seidman AD, Berry D, Cirrincione L, et al. CALGB 9840: Phase III study of weekly (W) paclitaxel (P) via 1-hour (h) infusion versus standard (S) 3 h infusion every third week in the treatment of metastatic breast cancer (MBC), with trastuzumab (T) for HER2 positive MBC and randomized for T in HER2 normal MBC. *Proc Am Soc Clin Oncol* 2004; 236, abstract 512

Sheperd GM. Hypersensitivity Reactions to Chemotherapeutic Drugs. *Allergy and Immunology* 2003; 24 253–262

Tournigand C, Cervantes A, Figer A, et al. OPTIMOX1: A Randomized Study of FOLFOX4 or FOLFOX7 With Oxaliplatin in a Stop-and-Go Fashion in Advanced Colorectal Cancer: A GERCOR Study. *J Clin Oncol* 2006; 24(3) 394–400

Trissel LA, Saenz CA, Ingram DS, Ogundele AB. Compatibility Screening of Oxaliplatin during Simulated Y-site Administration with Other Drugs. *J Oncol Pharm Practice* 2002; 8(1) 33–37

Venook AP, Egorin MJ, Rosner GL, et al. Phase I and Pharmacokinetic Trial of Paclitaxel in Patients with Hepatic Dysfunction: Cancer and Leukemia Group B 9264. *J Clin Oncol* 1998; 16 1811–1819

Vukelja SJ, Lombardo FA, James WD, Weiss RB. Pyridoxine for the Palmar-Plantar Erythrodysesthesia Syndrome [letter]. *Ann Intern Med* 1989; 111 688–689

Wilkes GM. New Therapeutic Options in Colon Cancer: Focus on Oxaliplatin. *Clin J Oncol Nurs* 2002; 3 131–137

Wilkes GM. Therapeutic Options in the Management of Colon Cancer: 2005 Update. *Clin J Oncol Nurs* 2005; 9(1) 31–44

Drug: abarelix for injectable suspension (Plenaxis)

Class: Gonadotropin releasing-hormone (GnRH) antagonist.

Mechanism of Action: Directly and competitively blocks GnRH receptors in the pituitary: suppresses luteinizing hormone (LH) and follicle stimulating hormone (FSH) secretion, and thereby reduces the secretion of testosterone by the testes. There is no initial increase in serum testosterone concentrations.

Metabolism: Following IM administration, drug is slowly absorbed with a mean peak concentration 3 days after injection, and distributes extensively within the body. Drug is highly protein bound (96–99%), and is excreted in the urine, with 13% of drug unchanged.

Dosage/Range:

- 100 mg IM in the buttock days 1, 15, 29 (week 4), and every 4 weeks thereafter
- Assess efficacy by monitoring serum testosterone levels baseline, day 29, and then every 8 weeks thereafter

Drug Preparation:

- Reconstitute drug following manufacturer's recommendations to yield 50 mg/mL
- Administer in the buttock, and rotate sites

Drug Interactions:

- None known.

Lab Effects/Interference:

- LFTs: transaminases may become elevated
- Serum testosterone levels should decrease to < 50 ng/dL. Slight decrease in hemoglobin
- Increase in serum triglycerides by 10%

Special Considerations:

- Drug is indicated for the palliative treatment of men with advanced symptomatic prostate cancer, in whom LHRH agonist therapy is not appropriate and who refuse surgical castration, and have one or more of the following:
  1) risk of neurological compromise due to metastases,
  2) ureteral or bladder outlet obstruction due to local encroachment of metastatic disease, or
  3) severe bone pain from skeletal metastases persisting on opioid analgesia
- Drug achieves castration levels of testosterone 24 hours after IM injection.
- The effectiveness of abarelix in suppressing serum testosterone to castration levels decreases with continued dosing in patients weighing > 225 lbs, and effectiveness beyond 12 months has not been established. Assess total serum testosterone levels just prior to drug administration on day 29, and every 8 weeks thereafter to assure continued response in all patients. Periodic measurement of serum PSA will assist in assessing response.
- Immediate-onset systemic allergic reactions, with hypotension and syncope, may occur; risk increases with increased cumulative dose so patients should be observed for at least 30 minutes following the injection.
- Drug may cause QT interval prolongation in 20% of patients (changes from baseline of > 30 msec, or end-of-treatment QTc values > 450 msec; use cautiously if at all in patients taking class IA (quinidine, procainamide) or class III (amiodarone, sotalol) antiarrhythmic medications.
- Drug is not indicated for women or children; drug may cause fetal harm if administered to a pregnant woman.
- Transaminase levels became clinically significantly elevated in some patients, so levels should be assessed baseline, and periodically during treatment.
- Bone mineral density may decrease with extended treatment with GnRH antagonists and LHRH agonists.

Potential Toxicities/Side Effects and the Nursing Process

I. POTENTIAL FOR INJURY related to HYPERSENSITIVITY REACTION

Defining Characteristics: Allergic reactions can occur immediately after injection, and may result in hypotension and syncope, starting with the initial dose, or occurring later in the course of treatment. Risk increases with the duration of treatment.

Nursing Implications: Assess baseline VS and mental status prior to drug administration, and observe patient for 30 minutes following injection. Recall signs/symptoms of anaphylaxis, and if these occur, notify physician, and assess patient's vital signs. Subjective symptoms are generalized itching, nausea, chest tightness, crampy abdominal pain, difficulty speaking, anxiety, agitation, sense of impending doom, uneasiness, desire to urinate/defecate, dizziness, and chills. Objective signs are flushed appearance; angioedema of face, neck, eyelids, hands, and feet; localized or generalized urticaria; respiratory distress with or without wheezing; hypotension; and cyanosis. Review standing orders or nursing procedures for patient management of anaphylaxis, and be prepared to administer ordered medications, which may include epinephrine 1:1000, hydrocortisone sodium succinate, and diphenhydramine. Teach patient to report any unusual symptoms.

II. ALTERATION IN COMFORT related to HOT FLUSHES, SLEEP DISTURBANCES, PAIN, BREAST ENLARGEMENT/TENDERNESS, HEADACHE, EDEMA, AND DIZZINESS

Defining Characteristics: Signs and symptoms of androgen deprivation are: Hot flushes (79%), sleep deprivation (44%), breast enlargement (30%), breast pain/nipple tenderness (20%). Pain in general occurs in about 31% of patients, as well as back pain (17%).

Nursing Implications: Teach patient that symptoms may occur. Encourage patient to report symptoms early. Develop symptom management plan with patient and physician.

III. ALTERATION IN BOWEL AND BLADDER ELIMINATION related to HORMONAL CHANGES

Defining Characteristics: Diarrhea occurs in about 11% of patients, while constipation occurs in 15%. 10% of patients develop dysuria, micturition frequency, urinary retention, or urinary tract infection.

Nursing Implications: Assess baseline bowel and bladder elimination pattern, and teach patient to report any changes. Teach patient to modify diet to minimize either diarrhea or constipation. Discuss need for referral to urologist if dysuria, urinary retention, or urinary tract infections persist.

Drug: adrenocorticoids (Cortisone, Dexamethasone, Hydrocortisone, Methylprednisolone, Prednisolone, Prednisone)

Class: Hormones.

Mechanism of Action: Cause lysis of lymphoid cells, which leads to their use against lymphatic leukemia, myeloma, malignant lymphoma. May also recruit malignant cells out of G_0 phase, making them vulnerable to damage caused by cell-cycle-phase-specific agents.

Metabolism: Metabolized by the liver, excreted in urine. Prednisone is activated by the liver in its active form, prednisolone.

Dosage/Range:
- Varies according to which preparation is used. Dexamethasone is 25 times the potency of hydrocortisone.
- Cortisone 25 mg.
- Dexamethasone 0.75 mg.
- Hydrocortisone 20 mg.
- Methylprednisolone 4 mg.
- Prednisone, Prednisolone 5 mg.

Drug Preparation:
- None.

Drug Administration:
- Oral.

Drug Interactions:
- May increase K+ loss and hypokalemia when combined with amphotericin B or potassium-depleting diuretics.
- Warfarin (Coumadin) dose may need to be increased.
- Insulin or oral hypoglycemia dose may need to be increased.
- Oral contraceptives may inhibit steroid metabolism.

Lab Effects/Interference:
- Increased Na, decreased K with hypokalemic alkalosis.
- Decreased I^{131} uptake and protein-bound iodine concentration. May cause difficulty monitoring therapeutic response of patients treated for thyroid conditions.
- False-negative results in nitroblue tetrazolium test for systemic bacterial infections.
- May suppress reactions to skin tests.

Special Considerations:
- Chronic steroid use is associated with numerous side effects. Intermittent therapy is safer and in some conditions just as effective as daily therapy.

Potential Toxicities/Side Effects and the Nursing Process

I. ALTERATION IN NUTRITION, LESS THAN BODY REQUIREMENTS, related to GASTRIC IRRITATION, DECREASED CARBOHYDRATE METABOLISM, AND HYPERGLYCEMIA

Defining Characteristics: Steroids can cause increased secretion of hydrochloric acid and decreased secretion of protective gastric mucus, which can exacerbate an existing gastric ulcer. They are insulin antagonists and may cause gluconeogenesis. In addition, steroids may increase appetite and cause weight gain.

Nursing Implications: Administer drugs with meals or an antacid. Instruct patient to report evidence of gastric distress immediately; teach patient to take steroids prior to a meal or with milk or food. Obtain baseline glucose levels and monitor periodic blood sugars throughout therapy. Teach patient to recognize signs/symptoms of hyperglycemia (polyuria, polydipsia, polyphagia), and to report these to the doctor or nurse.

II. POTENTIAL FOR INJURY related to SODIUM AND WATER RETENTION, ALTERATIONS IN FLUID AND ELECTROLYTE BALANCE, AND STEROID-INDUCED IMMUNOSUPPRESSION

Defining Characteristics: Sodium and water retention may occur and lead to CHF, hypertension, and edema in susceptible individuals; hypokalemia and hypocalcemia may occur due to increased excretion of potassium and calcium. Osteoporosis may occur with long-term therapy. Steroids increase susceptibility to infections and tuberculosis, may mask or aggravate infection, and may prolong or delay healing of injuries.

Nursing Implications: Identify patients at risk for complications associated with fluid/sodium retention (i.e., patients with preexisting cardiac, renal, hepatic dysfunction); monitor fluid and electrolyte balance and assess for imbalance. Document baseline cardiac status and monitor through therapy. Instruct patient to report signs/symptoms of hypokalemia (anorexia, muscle twitching, tetany, polyuria, polydipsia) and of hypocalcemia (leg cramps, tingling in fingertips, muscle twitching); monitor electrolytes regularly and discuss abnormal values with physician. Encourage high-potassium, high-calcium diet, and instruct patient in safety measures as needed. Teach patient to report slow healing of wounds, signs/symptoms of infection (erythema, warmth, purulence) of skin areas, as well as sore throat and burning on urination. Reinforce/teach patient hygiene measures for mouth, perineum, and skin.

III. POTENTIAL FOR INJURY related to RAPID WITHDRAWAL OF THERAPY

Defining Characteristics: Long-term therapy leads to suppression of normal adrenal function. Rapid cessation of therapy will lead to adrenal insufficiency, characterized by anorexia, nausea, orthostatic hypotension, dizziness, depression, dyspnea, hypoglycemia, and rebound inflammation (fever, myalgias, arthralgia, malaise). It can be fatal.

Nursing Implications: Discuss with physician the taper of steroids and instruct patient/family carefully. Teach patient to report symptoms of rapid withdrawal to nurse or physician.

IV. POTENTIAL FOR BODY IMAGE DISTURBANCE related to CUSHINGOID CHANGES

Defining Characteristics: Cushingoid state may occur with prolonged use and may be diminished by every-other-day dosing. Changes include moonface, striae, purpura, acne, hirsutism. In addition, increased appetite from steroids may lead to weight gain.

Nursing Implications: Teach patient about potential changes and provide reassurance that they will resolve once therapy ceases; encourage patient to verbalize feelings, and provide emotional support.

V. POTENTIAL FOR SENSORY/PERCEPTUAL ALTERATIONS related to CATARACTS OR GLAUCOMA, AND OCULAR INFECTIONS (increased risk)

Defining Characteristics: Cataracts or glaucoma may develop with prolonged steroid use; risk of ocular infections from virus or fungi is increased.

Nursing Implications: Teach patient to report signs/symptoms of eye infection, such as discharge, erythema, or visual changes; ophthalmologic exams are recommended every two to three months.

VI. INEFFECTIVE COPING related to AFFECTIVE/BEHAVIORAL CHANGES

Defining Characteristics: Emotional lability, insomnia, mood swings, euphoria, and psychosis may occur, causing ineffective coping and role-relationship problems if unprepared.

Nursing Implications: Teach patient and family that affective/behavioral changes may occur and that they will resolve once therapy is discontinued. Encourage patient and family to report these changes, especially if troublesome.

VII. IMPAIRED PHYSICAL MOBILITY related to MUSCULOSKELETAL CHANGES

Defining Characteristics: With chronic, high-dose usage, loss of muscle mass, muscle weakness (steroid myopathy), tendon rupture, osteoporosis, pathologic fractures, and aseptic necrosis of the heads of the humerus and femur can occur.

Nursing Implications: Teach patient that muscle weakness and other effects can occur with therapy and that muscle cramping may occur with discontinuation of therapy. Teach patient to report weakness, cramping, and any musculoskeletal changes. If weakness occurs, therapy may be discontinued.

Drug: altretamine (Hexalen, Hexamethylmelamine)

Class: Alkylating agent.

Mechanism of Action: The exact mechanism of action is unknown. May inhibit incorporation of thymidine and uridine into DNA and RNA, respectively, inhibiting DNA and RNA synthesis. Altretamine is believed not to act as an alkylating agent in vitro, but it may be activated to an alkylating agent in vivo. Also may act as an anti-metabolite with activity in S phase.

Metabolism: Well absorbed orally, although bioavailability is variable. Protein bound with peak plasma concentration in 1 hour. Metabolized extensively in the liver, with majority excreted in the urine. Some of the drug is excreted as respiratory CO_2. Half-life of the parent compound is 4.7–10.2 hours.

Dosage/Range:

- 260 mg/m^2 daily in four equally divided doses × 14 or 21 consecutive days, repeated every 28 days.
- Discontinue for 14 or more days and restart at 200 mg/m^2 daily if any of the following occur: refractory GI intolerance, WBC < 2000 cells/mm^3 or ANC < 1000 cells/mm^3, platelet count < 75,000/mm^3, or progressive neurotoxicity.

Drug Preparation:

- Available in 50-mg capsules.

Drug Administration:

- Oral. Administer dose after meals and at bedtime.

Drug Interactions:

- Concurrent administration of drug with monoamine oxidase inhibitor (MAO) anti-depressants may cause severe orthostatic hypotension.

Lab Effects/Interference:

- Decreased CBC.
- Increased BUN, creatinine.

Special Considerations:

- Nausea and vomiting can be minimized if patient takes dose two hours after meals and at bedtime.
- Nadir three to four weeks after treatment.

Potential Toxicities/Side Effects and the Nursing Process

I. INFECTION AND BLEEDING related to BONE MARROW DEPRESSION

Defining Characteristics: Causes mild to moderate bone marrow suppression, with nadir occurring 21–28 days after beginning treatment, and rapid recovery within one week of cessation of drug. Anemia occurs in 33% of patients and is moderate to severe in 9% of patients.

Nursing Implications: Assess CBC, WBC, differential, and platelet count before each cycle of drug administration, as well as for signs/symptoms of infection or bleeding. Teach patient signs/symptoms of infection and bleeding, and instruct to report them immediately. Teach self-care measures to minimize risk of infection and bleeding, including avoidance of OTC aspirin-containing medications. Assess energy and activity tolerance; discuss blood transfusion with physician as appropriate. Discuss with physician dose interruption and reduction if WBC < 2000/mm^3, ANC < 1000/mm^3, or platelet count < 75,000/mm^3.

II. SENSORY/PERCEPTUAL ALTERATIONS related to PERIPHERAL NEUROPATHY AND CNS EFFECTS

Defining Characteristics: Peripheral sensory neuropathy occurs in 31% of patients and is moderate to severe in 9% of patients. Paresthesia, hyperesthesia, hyperreflexia, and numbness may occur and are reversible. CNS effects of agitation, confusion, hallucinations, depression, mood disorders, and Parkinson-like symptoms may occur, and usually are reversible. Neurologic effects are more common with continuous dosing > 3 months, rather than pulse dosing.

Nursing Implications: Assess baseline neurologic status. Teach patient that possible side effects may occur, and instruct to report them. If neurologic toxicity is severe, drug should be dose reduced, then discontinued if symptoms do not improve.

III. ALTERATION IN NUTRITION, LESS THAN BODY REQUIREMENTS, related to NAUSEA AND VOMITING, DIARRHEA, ABDOMINAL CRAMPS, ANOREXIA

Defining Characteristics: Nausea occurs in 33% of patients and is dose related. Tolerance may develop after three weeks of drug administration. Diarrhea and cramps may be dose-limiting. Anorexia may occur.

Nursing Implications: Premedicate with antiemetics (phenothiazines are usually effective) at least initially, then as needed. Divide dose into four doses, and give

1–2 hours after meals and at bedtime. Instruct patient to report nausea/vomiting, diarrhea, abdominal cramping. Teach self-administration of prescribed antidiarrheals and self-care techniques to manage cramps, e.g., heat pads or position change. If GI side effects are refractory to symptom management, discuss interrupting dose and then dose reduction with physician.

IV. ALTERATION IN SKIN INTEGRITY related to SKIN RASHES

Defining Characteristics: Skin rashes, pruritus, eczematous skin lesions may occur but are rare.

Nursing Implications: Assess for changes in skin color, texture, and integrity. Teach patient to report any changes in skin, and discuss measures to minimize discomfort.

V. ALTERATION IN ELIMINATION related to RENAL DYSFUNCTION

Defining Characteristics: Elevations in BUN (9% of patients) or creatinine (7%) can occur.

Nursing Implications: Assess baseline renal status and monitor renal function studies throughout treatment.

VI. POTENTIAL SEXUAL DYSFUNCTION related to DRUG EFFECTS

Defining Characteristics: Drug is mutagenic, carcinogenic, and teratogenic. Drug causes testicular atrophy and decreased spermatogenesis. It is unknown whether drug is excreted in human milk.

Nursing Implications: Discuss with patient and partner normal sexual patterns and anticipated dysfunction resulting from drug or disease. Provide information, emotional support, and referral for counseling as appropriate.

Drug: aminoglutethimide (Cytadren, Elipten)

Class: Adrenal steroid inhibitor.

Mechanism of Action: Causes "chemical adrenalectomy." Blocks adrenal production of steroids, reducing levels of glucocorticoids, mineralocorticoids, and estrogens. Also inhibits peripheral aromatization of androgens to estrogens.

Metabolism: Well-absorbed orally. Hydroxylated in liver; undergoes enterohepatic circulation. Most of drug is excreted in urine.

Dosage/Range:
- 750–2000 mg PO daily in divided doses.
- 40 mg hydrocortisone daily given to replace glucocorticoid deficiencies.

Drug Preparation:
- None. Available in 250-mg tablets.

Drug Administration:
- Oral.

Drug Interactions:
- Drug enhances dexamethasone metabolism, so hydrocortisone should be used for glucocorticoid replacement.
- Warfarin (Coumadin) dose may need to be increased.
- Alcohol potentiates drug side effects.
- May need to increase doses of theophylline, digitoxin, or medroxyprogesterone.

Lab Effect/Interference:
- Hypothyroidism: monitor TFT.
- Elevated LFTs, especially SGOT, alk phos, bili.

Special Considerations:
- Skin rash may develop within 5–7 days, lasting 8 days, often with malaise and fever (37.7–39°C [100–102°F]). If not resolved in 7–14 days, drug should be discontinued.
- Adjuvant corticosteroids need to be administered.

Potential Toxicities/Side Effects and the Nursing Process

I. ALTERATION IN ENDOCRINE FUNCTION related to ADRENAL INSUFFICIENCY

Defining Characteristics: Drug causes reversible chemical adrenalectomy by blockade of steroid hormone production. Patient will experience signs/symptoms of adrenal insufficiency if enough replacement glucocorticoid steroids are not received. Signs/symptoms of adrenal insufficiency include hyponatremia, hypoglycemia, dizziness, and postural hypotension. In addition, possible ovarian blockade may result in virilization.

Nursing Implications: Teach patient about self-administration of hydrocortisone replacement therapy (i.e., administer in A.M. with breakfast), potential side effects, and tapering schedule; refer to section on adrenocorticoids. Teach patient side effects of hormone replacement and self-assessment techniques, including weekly weights and signs/symptoms of infection. Monitor electrolytes, especially Na+, K+, and Ca++. Assess for signs/symptoms of adrenal insufficiency (fatigue, anorexia, nausea, vomiting, diarrhea, weight loss, weakness, dizziness, and low blood sugar). As appropriate, explore with patient/significant other reproductive and sexuality patterns and impact chemotherapy may have. Recognize that patient may need increased hydrocortisone and mineralocorticoid support if surgery is needed (increased stress requirement).

II. IMPAIRED SKIN INTEGRITY related to DRUG RASH

Defining Characteristics: Area of erythema, pruritus, and unexplained dermatitis may appear within one week of treatment and disappear in 5–8 days. May be accompanied by malaise and low-grade fever.

Nursing Implications: Teach patient to report symptoms and to avoid scratching involved areas if rash develops. Assess skin for any changes and rash development. Consider use of Sarna cream, and use of OTC diphenhydramine.

III. SENSORY/PERCEPTUAL ALTERATIONS related to TRANSIENT SYMPTOMS

Defining Characteristics: Transient symptoms such as drowsiness, lethargy, somnolence, visual blurring, vertigo, and ataxia may occur, as may nystagmus. Lethargy may be severe in elderly patients.

Nursing Implications: Document baseline neurological function and general health assessment. Teach patient possible side effects, self-assessment, and to report symptoms. Discuss with physician possible dose reduction for significant symptoms.

IV. ALTERATION IN NUTRITION related to NAUSEA/VOMITING AND ANOREXIA

Defining Characteristics: Nausea/vomiting and anorexia occur in approximately 10–13% of patients and are mild.

Nursing Implications: Initially, premedicate (and teach patient to) with antiemetics prior to drug administration. Usually symptoms subside within two weeks. Encourage small, frequent feedings.

V. ALTERATION IN OXYGENATION/PERFUSION related to HYPOTENSION

Defining Characteristics: Drug may block aldosterone production leading to orthostatic or persistent hypotension. This is not usually a problem when hydrocortisone replacement is given.

Nursing Implications: Monitor BP regularly. Instruct patient to change position slowly and to report dizziness.

Drug: Amrubicin (investigational)

Class: Topoisomerase II inhibitor.

Mechanism of Action: Drug is a totally synthetic 9-aminoanthracycline. Drug and its active metabolite inhibit the enzyme DNA topoisomerase II, which is involved in relaxing and then rewinding the DNA helix for DNA copying during the synthesis phase. The drug and its metabolite stabilize the topoisomerase II-mediated cleavable complex. They are one-tenth of the strength of doxorubicin as an intercalator of DNA strands; however, the antitumor activity in the lab demonstrated 18 to 220 times more cytotoxicity with rare cardiotoxicity compared with doxorubicin (Onoda et al, 2006).

Metabolism: Drug is metabolized to amrubicinol by reduction of its C-13 ketone group to a hydroxyl group.

Drug Dose/Range: Per protocol, but SCLC studies used 40mg/m^2 IV d 1–3 repeated every three weeks in second-line and 35 mg/m^2 in third-line therapy (Igawa et al, 2007).

Drug Preparation:
- Per protocol.

Drug Administration:
- Per protocol; in one study, IV infusion over 5 min.

Drug Interactions:
- Unknown.

Lab Effects/Interference:
- Neutropenia.
- Thrombocytopenia.
- Anemia.
- Increased AST.
- Hypokalemia, hyponatremia.

Special Considerations:
- Drug is being studied in phase III trials of second-line treatment of SCLC and in first-line treatment for patients with extensive SCLC.
- Major grade 3/4 toxicities were neutropenia, thrombocytopenia, anemia, anorexia, nausea, and vomiting.
- One instance of atrial fibrillation was documented in one patient during trials but no reduction in LVEF (Onoda, 2006).

Potential Toxicities/Side Effects and the Nursing Process

I. POTENTIAL FOR INFECTION AND BLEEDING related to NEUTROPENIA AND THROMBOCYTOPENIA

Defining Characteristics: Incidence of neutropenia was 72% to 78% [grades 3 (28%) and 4 (55%)], thrombocytopenia 14.8% to 20% (grade 3 20%, no grade 4), and anemia

23% in phase II studies; most occurred after cycle 1, and 70% required G-CSF support; 3% of patients had febrile neutropenia in one study.

Nursing Implications: Assess baseline blood counts and platelets. Teach patient to self-assess and report fever, other signs/symptoms of infection, or bleeding right away. Assess medication profile and OTC medications taken. Teach patient to avoid OTC medications containing NSAIDs or aspirin. Teach patient to talk to nurse or physician before beginning any OTC medications. Teach patient to alternate rest and activity to conserve energy.

II. POTENTIAL ALTERATION IN NUTRITION, LESS THAN BODY REQUIREMENTS, related to NAUSEA, ANOREXIA, HYPONATREMIA, ASTHENIA

Defining Characteristics: In clinical studies, nausea affected 26% (gr 3/4: 5%), vomiting 11%, anorexia 39% (gr 3/4: 15%), asthenia 44% (gr 3/4: 15%). Electrolyte abnormalities were hypokalemia (15%) in one study and hyponatremia 8% in another.

Nursing Implications: Assess baseline nutritional status, including appetite, ability to shop or prepare meals, presence of nausea or vomiting, serum electrolytes, and activity tolerance and monitor during treatment. Premedicate with antiemetics. Teach patient self-administration of home anti-emetics as needed and ordered. Encourage small, frequent meals of cool, bland calorie and protein dense foods, and increase fluid intake. Teach dietary changes and medications if ordered for hyponatremia or hypokalemia. Assess oral mucosa prior to drug administration and instruct patient to report changes. Teach patient oral hygiene measures and self-assessment. Notify physician of any abnormalities and discuss implications and management.

Drug: anastrozole (Arimidex)

Class: Nonsteroidal aromatase inhibitor.

Mechanism of Action: Inhibits the enzyme aromatase. Aromatase is one of the P-450 enzymes and is involved in estrogen biosynthesis. Circulating estrogen in postmenopausal women (mainly estradiol) arises from the aromatase-mediated conversion of androstenedione (made by the adrenals) to estrone, then estrone to estradiol, in the peripheral tissues, such as adipose tissue. Anastrozole is highly selective for this enzyme and does not affect steroid synthesis, so that estradiol synthesis is potently suppressed (to undetectable levels) while cortisol and aldosterone levels are unchanged.

Metabolism: Extensively metabolized, with 85% of the drug metabolized by the liver. About 10% of the unchanged drug and 60% of the drug as metabolites are excreted in the urine within 72 hours of drug administration.

Dosage/Range:

- 1 mg PO daily. No dosage adjustment required for mild to moderate hepatic impairment. In an adjuvant study, the treatment duration was 5 years. In patients with metastatic disease, continue until disease progression.

Drug Preparation:

- None. Available as 1-mg tablet.

Drug Administration:

- Take orally with or without food, at approximately the same time daily.

Drug Interactions:

- Tamoxifen: coadministration with anastrozole decreases anastrozole serum levels by 27%.
- Estrogen: coadministration with anastrozole may decrease anastrozole activity; do not use concurrently.
- Herbal estrogen-containing supplements: may decrease drug effect.

Lab Effects/Interference:

- Elevated GGT, especially in patients with liver metastases.
- Decreased total hip and lumbar spine bone mineral density compared with baseline.
- Total cholesterol may be increased.

Special Considerations:

- Indicated for the adjuvant treatment of postmenopausal women with hormone receptor positive early breast cancer; as first-line therapy for postmenopausal women with hormone receptor-positive or hormone receptor-unknown locally advanced or metastatic breast cancer; and for treatment of advanced breast cancer in postmenopausal women with disease progression following tamoxifen therapy.
- In the large Arimidex Tamoxifen Alone or in Combination (ATAC) clinical trial, anastrozole was shown to reduce the relative risk of breast cancer recurrence by 17% over tamoxifen in hormone receptor-positive patients in the adjuvant setting.
- Well-tolerated with low toxicity profile.
- Coadministration of corticosteroids is not necessary.
- Absolutely contraindicated during pregnancy. The drug showed no benefit in ER-negative women.

Potential Toxicities/Side Effects and the Nursing Process

I. SEXUAL DYSFUNCTION related to DECREASED ESTROGEN LEVELS

Defining Characteristics: Hot flashes (12%), asthenia or loss of energy (16%), and vaginal dryness may occur.

Nursing Implications: As appropriate, explore with patient and partner patterns of sexuality and impact therapy may have. Discuss strategies to preserve sexual health.

Teach patient that the vaginal dryness may be from menopause, not the drug, and that the patient SHOULD NOT use estrogen creams. Teach patient to use lubricants.

II. POTENTIAL ALTERATION IN CARDIAC OUTPUT related to THROMBOPHLEBITIS

Defining Characteristics: Thrombophlebitis may occur, but is uncommon.

Nursing Implications: Identify patients at risk. Teach patients to report/come to emergency room for pain, redness, or marked swelling in arms or legs, or if shortness of breath or dizziness occur.

III. ALTERATION IN COMFORT related to HEADACHES, WEAKNESS, JOINT DISORDERS

Defining Characteristics: Headaches are mild and occur in about 13% of patients. Decreased energy and weakness is common. Mild swelling of arms/legs may occur and is mild. Patients receiving anastrozole had more arthrosis, arthralgias, and arthritis.

Nursing Implications: Teach patient that headache and joint disorders are usually relieved by nonprescription analgesics and to report headaches that are unrelieved. Teach patient to elevate extremities when at rest, as needed.

IV. POTENTIAL ALTERATION IN NUTRITION, LESS THAN BODY REQUIREMENTS, related to NAUSEA

Defining Characteristics: Nausea is mild, with a 15% incidence.

Nursing Implications: Determine baseline weight, and monitor at each visit. Teach patient that nausea may occur, and to report this. Discuss strategies to minimize nausea, including diet and dosing time.

V. POTENTIAL ALTERATION IN BOWEL ELIMINATION related to DIARRHEA

Defining Characteristics: Diarrhea is uncommon (9% incidence) and mild.

Nursing Implications: Assess for change in bowel patterns and teach patient to report diarrhea. If diarrhea occurs, teach patient that diarrhea is usually relieved by nonprescription medications, such as loperamide HCl and Kaopectate, and to report unrelieved diarrhea.

Drug: androgens: testosterone propionate (Testex), obfluoxymesterone (Halotestin), obtestolactone (Teslac)

Class: Hormones.

Mechanism of Action: Has stimulatory effect on red blood cells that results in an increased HCT. Other mechanism of action unknown.

Metabolism: Metabolized by the liver; excreted in the urine and feces.

Dosage/Range:
- Fluoxymesterone: 10–30 mg PO daily (3–4 divided doses).
- Testolactone: 100 mg IM 3 × weekly or 250 mg PO 4 × daily.
- Testosterone Propionate: 50–100 mg IM 3 × weekly.

Drug Preparation:
- Drug comes in ready-to-use vials or tablets.

Drug Administration:
- Before IM administration, shake vial vigorously and give injection immediately to avoid solution settling.

Drug Interactions:
- Pharmacological effects of oral anticoagulants may be enhanced; monitor patient and adjust dose.

Lab Effects/Interference:
- LFTs: possible hepatic dysfunction with long-term use.
- Increased serum Ca.
- May cause decreased total serum thyroxine (T_4) concentrations and increased T_3 and T_4.

Special Considerations:
- Fluoxymesterone may increase sensitivity to oral anticoagulants. Should be administered in divided doses because of its short action.

Potential Toxicities/Side Effects and the Nursing Process

I. POTENTIAL FOR INJURY related to SODIUM AND WATER RETENTION, HYPERCALCEMIA, AND OBSTRUCTIVE JAUNDICE

Defining Characteristics: Sodium and water retention may occur, necessitating dose reduction or diuretic use; hypercalcemia may occur initially in patients with bony metastases and needs to be distinguished from disease progression. Obstructive jaundice has occurred with methyltesterone, fluoxymesterone, and oxymetholone.

Nursing Implications: Identify patients most at risk for injury related to sodium and water retention: patients with cardiac, renal, or hepatic dysfunction, as well as patients with low serum albumin. Teach patient about potential side effects and instruct to report any changes to physician or nurse; assess patient at each visit for signs/symptoms of fluid and electrolyte imbalance. Identify patients at risk for hypercalcemia (those with bony metastases) and monitor serum calcium during first few weeks of therapy; hypercalcemia is an indication to discontinue therapy. Teach patient/family signs/symptoms of hypercalcemia (drowsiness, increased thirst, constipation, polyuria) and to notify physician. Monitor LFTs and instruct patient/family to report signs/symptoms of GI distress, diarrhea, jaundice.

II. POTENTIAL FOR SEXUAL DYSFUNCTION related to MASCULINIZATION

Defining Characteristics: Commonly occurs in women receiving drug for > 3 months; with prolonged use masculinization may be irreversible. Symptoms include increased libido, deepening of voice, excessive growth of body (face) hair, acne, and clitoral hypertrophy. In men, priapism (sustained and often painful erections) and reduced ejaculatory volume may occur.

Nursing Implications: Instruct patient to report symptoms of changes in sexual health. Discuss strategies to preserve sexual health; if unacceptable, discuss alternative medications with physician.

III. ALTERATION IN NUTRITION, LESS THAN BODY REQUIREMENTS, related to NAUSEA AND VOMITING

Defining Characteristics: Nausea may occur.

Nursing Implications: Teach patient about possible side effects and administer antiemetics as ordered. Encourage small, frequent feedings and dietary modifications as appropriate.

Drug: arsenic trioxide (Trisenox)

Class: Miscellaneous antineoplastic agent.

Mechanism of Action: Not completely understood, but drug appears to cause changes in DNA with fragmentation typical of apoptosis or programmed cell death. Drug also damages and causes degradation of the fusion protein PMLRAR alpha characteristic of acute promyelocytic leukemia. The gene responsible for the fusion protein is corrected in many cases (cytogenetic complete response), so that immature malignant myelocytic cells mature into normal white blood cells.

Metabolism: Pharmacokinetics continue to be characterized. Drug is metabolized by methylation, primarily in the liver. Arsenic is stored primarily in the liver, kidney, heart, lung, hair, and nails. Drug appears to be excreted in the urine.

Dosage/Range:

Adult:

- Induction dose of 0.15 mg/kg/d IV until bone marrow remission, not to exceed 60 doses.
- Consolidation begins 3–6 weeks after induction therapy is completed, at a dose of 0.15 mg/kg/d IV for 25 doses over a period of up to 5 weeks.

Drug Preparation:

- Drug is available in 10 mL, single-use ampules containing 10 mg of arsenic trioxide, with a concentration of 1 mg/mL, preservative free.
- Further dilute prescribed dose immediately in 100–250 mL 5% dextrose injection, USP or 0.9% sodium chloride injection, USP.
- Administer IV over 1–2 hours, or up to 4 hours if acute vasomotor reactions occur (does not require a central line).
- Drug is chemically and physically stable for 24 hours at room temperature and 48 hours when refrigerated.
- Drug does not contain any preservatives, so unused portions should be discarded.
- Overdosage: If symptoms of serious acute arsenic toxicity appear (seizures, muscle weakness, confusion), discontinue drug immediately and chelation therapy should be considered: dimercaprol 3 mg/kg IM q 4 hours until immediate life-threatening toxicity has subsided, then give penicillamine 250 mg PO up to qid (1 Gm per day).

Drug Interactions:

- Unknown; do not mix with any other medications.
- Drugs that can prolong the QT interval (e.g., certain antiarrhythmics or thioridazine) or lead to electrolyte abnormalities (e.g., diuretics or amphotericin B) should be avoided if possible; otherwise, scrupulous monitoring and correction of abnormalities is critical.

Lab Effects/Interference:

- Hyperkalemia or hypokalemia.
- Hypomagnesemia.
- Hyperglycemia or hypoglycemia.
- Hypocalcemia.
- Increased hepatic transaminases ALT and AST.
- Leukocytosis (50% of patients).
- Anemia (14% of patients).
- Thrombocytopenia (19% of patients).
- Neutropenia (10% of patients).
- Disseminated intravascular coagulation (DIC) (8% of patients).

Special Considerations:

- Drug is indicated for induction of remission and consolidation in patients with acute promyelocytic leukemia (APL) who are refractory to, or have relapsed from, retinoid and anthracycline chemotherapy, and whose APL is characterized by the presence of the t(15;17) translocation or PML/RAR- alpha gene expression.
- Arsenic has been used in medical care for the last 2000 years, and 100 years ago it was used to treat leukemia and infections. However, it was replaced with current chemotherapy and antibiotics. Certain traditional Chinese medicines were found to be anti-leukemic, and the active ingredient was shown to be arsenic trioxide.
- Preliminary studies showed high hematologic complete response rate (55–82%) and cytogenetic conversion to no detection of APL chromosome rearrangement (29–100%) depending on response criteria. This led to a fast track status and early FDA approval. Additional post-approval toxicity reports will help clarify full toxicity profile of this drug.
- Drug may cause APL Differentiation Syndrome similar to the retinoicacidacute Promyelocytic Leukemia (RA-APL), which is characterized by fever, dyspnea, weight gain, pulmonary infiltrates, and pleural or pericardial effusions, with or without leukocytosis. This syndrome can be fatal, and, at the first suggestion, high-dose steroids should be instituted (dexamethasone 10 mg IV bid) for at least 3 days or longer until signs and symptoms abate. The drug manufacturer states that the majority of patients do not require termination of arsenic trioxide therapy during treatment of the syndrome (Cephalon Oncology, Trisenox package insert, July 2006).
- Drug can cause QT interval prolongation and complete atrioventricular block. Prolonged QT interval can progress to a torsade de pointes-type fatal ventricular arrhythmia. Risk factors for development of torsade de pointes are: significant QT prolongation; concomitant administration of drugs that prolong the QT interval; history of torsades de pointes; preexisting QT prolongation; CHF; administration of potassium-wasting diuretics; conditions resulting in hypokalemia or hypomagnesemia, such as concurrent administration of amphotericin B.
- The manufacturer recommends the following: Prior to treatment with arsenic trioxide, the patient should have a baseline 12-lead EKG as well as serum electrolytes and renal function tests. Electrolyte abnormalities should be corrected. Any drugs that prolong the QT interval should be discontinued. If the QT interval prolongation is > 500 msec, this should be corrected prior to drug administration. During arsenic trioxide therapy, serum potassium should be kept > 4.0 mEq/dL and serum magnesium > 1.8 mg/dL. If the QT interval exceeds 500 msec, reassessment and correction of risk factors should occur. The patient should be hospitalized for monitoring if syncope, or rapid or irregular heart rate occurs, and serum electrolytes assessed and any abnormalities corrected. Drug should be stopped until QT interval falls below 460 msec, electrolyte abnormalities corrected, and symptoms resolve.
- Drug is a human carcinogen. Drug should not be used by pregnant or breast-feeding women.
- Standard monitoring: At least 2 times a week, the patient should have electrolyte, hematologic, and coagulation assessed; more frequently if abnormal during the

induction phase, and at least weekly during the consolidation phase. EKGs should be done weekly; more frequently if abnormal.

- Most common side effects are manageable, are reversible, and include: leukocytosis, nausea, vomiting, diarrhea, abdominal pain, fatigue, edema, hyperglycemia, dyspnea, cough, rash, itching, headaches, and dizziness.
- Use with caution in patients with renal insufficiency.

Potential Toxicities/Side Effects and the Nursing Process

I. ALTERATION IN OXYGENATION, POTENTIAL, related to APL DIFFERENTIATION SYNDROME

Defining Characteristics: Drug may cause APL Differentiation Syndrome similar to the retinoic-acid acute Promyelocytic Leukemia (RA-APL), which is characterized by fever, dyspnea, weight gain, pulmonary infiltrates, and pleural or pericardial effusions, with or without leukocytosis. This syndrome develops in response to the differentiation of immature malignant cells into mature normal white blood cells and the increased white blood cell count. The body's response is an inflammatory reaction with fluid retention in the lining of the lungs and heart. This syndrome can be fatal, and at the first suggestion, high-dose steroids should be instituted (dexamethasone 10 mg IV bid) for at least 3 days or longer until signs and symptoms abate. The drug manufacturer states that the majority of patients do not require termination of arsenic trioxide therapy during treatment of the syndrome. The reported incidence is 20%. Leucocytosis, if it occurs, at levels $> 10 \times 10^3/\mu L$ is unrelated to baseline or peak white blood cell counts. Leukocytosis was not treated with chemotherapy, and levels were lower during consolidation than during induction.

Nursing Implications: Assess temperature and VS, oxygen saturation, cardiopulmonary status baseline and at each visit. Assess weight daily, and teach patient to report any SOB, fever, or weight gain immediately. If signs or symptoms develop, notify physician immediately and discuss obtaining CXR, cardiac echo, and focused exam. Discuss CXR, ECHO, and laboratory findings with physician. Be prepared to administer high-dose steroids (e.g., dexamethasone 10 mg IV bid × 3 days or longer depending on symptom resolution). Provide pulmonary and hemodynamic support as necessary. Assess CBC, with focus on white blood cell count and presence of leukocytosis.

II. POTENTIAL ALTERATION IN CARDIAC FUNCTION related to QT PROLONGATION AND ARRHYTHMIA

Defining Characteristics: Drug can cause QT interval prolongation and complete atrioventricular block. Prolonged QT interval can progress to a torsade de pointes-type fatal ventricular arrhythmia. Risk factors for development of torsade de pointes are significant QT prolongation, concomitant administration of drugs that prolong the QT interval, history of torsades de pointes, preexisting QT prolongation, CHF, administration of potassium-wasting diuretics, and conditions resulting in hypokalemia or hypomagnesemia such as concurrent administration of amphotericin B.

Nursing Implications: Assess baseline risk, cardiovascular status, EKG determined QT interval, electrolyte and renal blood studies, and medications the patient is taking that may prolong QT interval, such as serotonin antagonist antiemetics. At least 2 times a week, the patient should have electrolyte, hematologic and coagulation assessed; more frequently if abnormal during the induction phase, and at least weekly during the consolidation phase. EKGs should be done weekly, and more frequently if abnormal. Discuss correction of any electrolyte abnormalities, as well as other risk factors, with physician. Any drugs that prolong the QT interval should be discontinued. If the QT interval prolongation is > 500 msec, this should be corrected prior to drug administration. During arsenic trioxide therapy, serum potassium should be kept > 4.0 mEq/dL and serum magnesium > 1.8 mg/dL. If the QT interval exceeds 500 msec, reassessment and correction of risk factors should occur. The patient should be hospitalized for monitoring if syncope or rapid or irregular heart rate occurs, and serum electrolytes assessed and any abnormalities corrected. Drug should be stopped until QT interval falls below 460 msec, electrolyte abnormalities corrected, and symptoms resolve.

III. ALTERATION IN NUTRITION, LESS THAN BODY REQUIREMENTS, related to GI DYSFUNCTION

Defining Characteristics: Nausea is most common (incidence 75%), followed by vomiting (58%), abdominal pain (58%), diarrhea (53%), constipation (28%), anorexia (23%), dyspepsia (10%), abdominal tenderness or distention (8%), and dry mouth (8%).

Nursing Implications: Assess GI, nutrition status, and presence of GI dysfunction baseline, and with each visit, administer antiemetics, and teach patient self-administration. Discuss risk of serotonin antagonists to prolong QT interval, and contraindication with physician. Teach patient to report signs and symptoms, and evaluate symptom management plan based on effectiveness of symptom control. Assess presence of pain, and discuss pharmacologic and nonpharmacologic analgesic plan with physician.

IV. ALTERATION IN PROTECTIVE MECHANISMS, related to FEVER, ANEMIA, DIC, BLEEDING

Defining Characteristics: Fever affects 63% of patients (13% febrile neutropenia), with 38% of patients having rigors. In clinical studies, 8% of patients had hemorrhage, 14% anemia, 19% thrombocytopenia, 10% neutropenia, and 8% DIC. Patients may develop infections, and in clinical studies, most commonly these were: sinusitis 20%, herpes simplex 13%, upper respiratory tract infection 13%, nonspecific bacterial 8%, herpes zoster 8%, oral candidiasis 5%, and (rarely) sepsis 5%.

Nursing Implications: At least 2 times a week, the patient should have electrolyte, hematologic, and coagulation assessed; more frequently if abnormal during the induction phase, and at least weekly during the consolidation phase. Monitor laboratory results, and discuss abnormalities with physician. Assess patient for fever, signs and symptoms of infection, rigors, and bleeding, and implement management plan to assure patient safety. Transfuse patient as ordered, and monitor closely.

V. ALTERATION IN COMFORT related to HEADACHE, CHEST PAIN, AND INJECTION SITE CHANGES

Defining Characteristics: Headache occurred in approximately 60% of patients while chest pain occurred in 25%. Injection site reactions of pain, erythema, and edema occurred in 20%, 13%, and 10% of patients, respectively.

Nursing Implications: Assess level of comfort, and develop plan for comfort, including pharmacologic, and non-pharmacologic measures. Assess effectiveness, and revise plan as needed. Assess patency of IV site and need for IV catheter change. Assess need for central line. Although not necessary for drug delivery, if patient venous access is limited this may provide enhanced patient comfort.

VI. ALTERATION IN ACTIVITY TOLERANCE related to FATIGUE, MUSCULOSKELETAL PROBLEMS

Defining Characteristics: 63% of patients reported fatigue. In clinical studies, musculoskeletal events were: arthralgias (33%), myalgias (25%), bone pain (23%), back pain (18%), neck pain, and pain in limbs (13%).

Nursing Implications: Assess baseline energy and activity level, and level of comfort. Assess need for assistance with ADLs and home assistance. Assess need for analgesics or local measures to relieve pain and discomfort. Teach patient self-care strategies to minimize exertion and maximize activity, such as clustering activity during shopping, alternating rest and activity periods, diet, gentle exercise. Evaluate success of plan and need for revisions.

VII. ALTERATION IN FLUID AND ELECTROLYTE BALANCE related to HYPOKALEMIA, HYPOMAGNESEMIA, HYPERGLYCEMIA, EDEMA

Defining Characteristics: Hypokalemia occurs in about 50% of patients, hypomagnesemia (45%), hyperglycemia (45%), and edema (40%). Other electrolyte abnormalities are hyperkalemia (18%), hypocalcemia (10%), hypoglycemia (8%), acidosis (5%), and increased transaminases (13–20%).

Nursing Implications: At least 2 times a week, the patient should have electrolyte, hematologic and coagulation assessed; more frequently if abnormal during the induction phase, and at least weekly during the consolidation phase. EKGs should be done weekly, and more frequently if abnormal. Teach patient that edema may occur, and to report it. Assess patient baseline and before each treatment for weight and presence of edema. Discuss abnormalities with physician, correct as ordered, and monitor closely for signs and symptoms of imbalance.

VIII. SENSORY/PERCEPTUAL ALTERATIONS, POTENTIAL, related to PARESTHESIA, DIZZINESS, TREMOR, INSOMNIA

Defining Characteristics: Insomnia occurs in 43% of patients, paresthesia (33%), dizziness (23%), tremor (13%), seizures (8%), somnolence (8%), and (rarely) coma (5%).

Nursing Implications: Assess baseline mental and neurological status, and monitor frequently during therapy. Assess sensory function, and teach patient to report numbness, tingling, dizziness, tremor, seizure, decrease in alertness, and changes in sleep. Assess presence of paresthesias, and motor and sensory function prior to each treatment; discuss presence or worsening with physician. Teach patient self-care strategies, including maintaining safety when walking, getting up, taking a bath, or washing dishes if unable to feel temperature changes. Teach self-care measures to manage sleep problems, and discuss possible need for sleeping medication.

IX. ALTERATION IN GAS EXCHANGE, POTENTIAL, related to COUGH, DYSPNEA, HYPOXIA, PLEURAL EFFUSION

Defining Characteristics: Cough is common, affecting 65% of patients, followed by dyspnea (53%), epistaxis (25%), hypoxia (23%), pleural effusion (20%), postnasal drip (13%), wheezing (13%), decreased breath sounds (10%), crepitations (10%), rales (crackles) (10%), hemoptysis (8%), tachypnea (8%), and rhonchi (8%).

Nursing Implications: Assess baseline pulmonary status, including breath sounds and oxygen saturation, and monitor at least daily during treatment. Teach patient that symptoms may occur and to report them. Discuss management of patients experiencing cough, dyspnea, and other symptoms with physician, and develop individualized management plan.

X. ALTERATION IN SKIN INTEGRITY, POTENTIAL, related to SKIN IRRITATION

Defining Characteristics: Dermatitis affects about 43% of patients, pruritus (33%), ecchymosis (20%), dry skin (13%), erythema (10%), hyperpigmentation (8%), and urticaria (8%).

Nursing Implications: Assess baseline skin integrity and monitor at each visit. Teach patient to report any skin changes or itching. Teach patient symptomatic local measures to manage dermatitis, itch, or other changes. If plan is ineffective, discuss other measures with physician.

Drug: asparaginase (Elspar, L-asparaginase)

Class: Miscellaneous agents (enzyme).

Mechanism of Action: Hydrolyzes serum asparagine, which deprives leukemia cells of the required amino acid. Normal cells are spared because they generally have the ability to synthesize their own asparagine. Cell cycle specific for G_1 postmitotic phase. Some leukemic cells are unable to synthesize asparagine. These cells must obtain asparagine from an exogenous source, the patient's serum. Administration of the enzyme L-asparaginase causes hydrolysis of asparagine to aspartate, resulting in rapid depletion of the asparagine concentration in the patient's serum. The leukemic cells cannot synthesize protein or proliferate.

Metabolism: Metabolism of L-asparaginase is independent of renal and hepatic function. The drug is not recovered in the urine and does not appear to cross the blood–brain barrier.

Dosage/Range:

- IM or IV varies with protocol.
- Typical induction dosing is 200 IU/kg IV daily × 28 days (ALL), or 500–10,000 units/m^2/day × 7 days every 3 weeks, or 10,000–40,000 units every 2–3 weeks.

Drug Preparation:

- IV injection: reconstitute with sterile water for injection or 0.9% sodium chloride injection (without preservative) and use within 8 hours of restoration.
- IV infusion: dilute with 0.9% sodium chloride injection or 5% dextrose injection and use within 8 hours, only if clear; if gelatinous particles develop, filter through a 5.0-μm filter.
- IM: 6000–12,000 units/m^2 dose as a single agent: reconstitute to 10,000 units/mL.
- The lyophilized powder must be stored under refrigeration. The reconstituted solution must also be stored under refrigeration if it is not used immediately. The solution must be discarded 8 hours after preparation.

Drug Administration:

- Test dose: often ordered before first dose or after restarting drug after a break; 0.1–0.2 mL of a 20- to 250-units/mL dose (2–50 units) intradermally and observe patient for 15–30 minutes.
- Use in a hospital setting. Make preparations to treat anaphylaxis at each administration of the drug and have epinephrine, diphenhydramine, and hydrocortisone nearby. Ensure that patent IV is available before giving drugs IM.

Drug Interactions:

- Prednisone: potential additive hyperglycemic effect; monitor blood glucose levels.
- Cyclophosphamide, vincristine, 6-mercaptopurine: may increase or decrease drug's effect (CTX, VCR, 6-MP).
- 6-mercaptopurine: Enhanced hepatotoxicity; monitor LFTs closely.
- Methotrexate: Antagonism if administered immediately prior to methotrexate; when administered some time after methotrexate, may enhance methotrexate activity.
- Synergy with cytosine arabinoside.
- Increased hyperglycemia when given together with prednisone.
- Reduced hypersensitivity when given with 6-mercaptopurine or prednisone.
- Additive neurotoxicity when given with vincristine.
- Asparaginase, when given before vincristine, will decrease vincristine excretion, with resulting increased neurotoxicity; give vincristine 12–24 hours before asparaginase.
- Live vaccines may enhance viral replication and toxicity.

Lab Effects/Interference:

- Increased LFTs.
- Decreased hepatically derived clotting factors.
- Interferes with thyroid function tests after first two days of therapy: effect lasts four weeks.

Special Considerations:

- Potential reduction in antineoplastic effect of methotrexate when given in combination.
- Anaphylaxis is associated with the administration of this drug.
- Intravenous administration of L-asparaginase concurrently with or immediately before prednisone and vincristine administration may be associated with increased toxicity.
- Drug is derived from purified *E. coli* or *Erwinia chrysanthemi*, and if an allergic reaction occurs, the patient may try the other drug. Also, pegylated asparaginase is also available.

Potential Toxicities/Side Effects and the Nursing Process

I. POTENTIAL FOR INJURY related to HYPERSENSITIVITY OR ANAPHYLACTIC REACTIONS

Defining Characteristics: Occurs in 20–30% of patients. Increased incidence after several doses administered, but may occur with first dose. Occurs less often with IM route of administration. May be life-threatening reaction, but is usually mild.

Nursing Implications: Discuss with physician use of test dose prior to drug administration. Assess baseline vital signs and mental status prior to drug administration. Review standing orders or nursing procedure for management of anaphylaxis and be prepared to stop drug immediately if signs/symptoms occur; keep IV line open with 0.9% sodium chloride, notify physician, monitor vital signs, and administer ordered medications, which may include epinephrine 1:1000, hydrocortisone sodium succinate, and diphenhydramine. Teach patient the potential of a hypersensitivity or anaphylactic reaction and to immediately report any unusual symptoms. *Escherichia coli* preparation of L-asparaginase and *Erwinia carotovora* preparation are non-cross-resistant, so if an anaphylactic reaction occurs with one, the other preparation may be used.

II. POTENTIAL FOR INJURY related to HEPATIC DYSFUNCTION OR THROMBOEMBOLISM

Defining Characteristics: Two-thirds of patients have elevated LFTs starting within the first two weeks of treatment: e.g., SGOT, bili, and alk phos. Hepatically derived clotting factors may be depressed, resulting in excessive bleeding or blood clotting. Relatively uncommon.

Nursing Implications: Monitor SGOT, bili, alk phos, albumin, and clotting factors CPT, PTT, fibrinogen. Teach patient of the potential of excessive bleeding or blood clotting, and instruct to report any unusual symptoms. Assess patient for signs/symptoms of bleeding.

III. ALTERED NUTRITION, LESS THAN BODY REQUIREMENTS, related to NAUSEA/VOMITING, ANOREXIA, HYPERGLYCEMIA

Defining Characteristics: 50–60% of patients experience mild to severe nausea and vomiting starting within 4–6 hours after treatment. Anorexia commonly occurs. Hyperglycemia is a transient reaction caused by effects on the pancreas with decreased insulin synthesis. Pancreatitis occurs in 5% of patients.

Nursing Implications: Premedicate with antiemetics and continue prophylactically for 24 hours to prevent nausea and vomiting. Encourage small, frequent meals of cool, bland foods and liquids, as well as favorite foods, especially high-calorie, high-protein foods. Encourage use of spices and do weekly weights. Teach patient about the potential of hyperglycemia and pancreatitis, and instruct to report any unusual symptoms, e.g., increased thirst, urination, and appetite. Monitor serum glucose, amylase, and lipase levels periodically during treatment. Report any laboratory elevations to physician. Treat hyperglycemia issues with diet or insulin as ordered by physician. Treat pancreatitis per physician orders.

IV. SENSORY/PERCEPTUAL ALTERATIONS related to CHANGES IN MENTAL STATUS

Defining Characteristics: 25% of patients experience some changes in mental status—commonly, lethargy, drowsiness, and somnolence; rarely coma. Predominantly seen in adults. Malaise (feeling "blah") occurs in most patients, and generally gets worse with subsequent doses. Drug does not cross BBB.

Nursing Implications: Teach patient about the potential of CNS toxicity, and instruct to report any unusual symptoms. Obtain baseline neurologic and mental function. Assess patient for any neurologic abnormalities and report changes to physician. Discuss with patient the impact of malaise on his/her general sense of well-being and strategies to minimize the distress.

V. POTENTIAL FOR SEXUAL DYSFUNCTION related to REPRODUCTION HAZARD

Defining Characteristics: Drug is teratogenic.

Nursing Implications: As appropriate, explore with patient and partner issues of reproductive and sexual patterns and impact chemotherapy will have. Discuss strategies to preserve sexuality and reproductive health (e.g., sperm banking, contraception).

VI. INFECTION, BLEEDING, AND FATIGUE related to BONE MARROW DEPRESSION

Defining Characteristics: Bone marrow depression is not common. Mild anemia may occur. Serious leukopenia and thrombocytopenia are rare.

Nursing Implications: Monitor CBC, platelet count prior to drug administration, as well as signs/symptoms of infection, bleeding, or anemia. Instruct patient in self-assessment of signs/symptoms of infection, bleeding, or anemia and to report immediately.

Drug: 5-azacytidine (Vidaza)

Class: Antimetabolite.

Mechanism of Action: Azacytidine causes hypomethylation of DNA, which may restore normal gene function to genes responsible for cell division and differentiation of the bone marrow. At higher doses, it also interferes with nucleic acid metabolism by acting as a false metabolite when incorporated into DNA and RNA; cell cycle phase specific for S phase.

Metabolism: Rapidly absorbed following subcutaneous administration, with peak plasma level in 30 minutes. Bioavailability of subcutaneously administered drug is 89% of IV dose. 85% of the total administered dose is excreted in the urine, and < 1% in feces. Mean elimination half-life is about 4 hours in both subcutaneous and IV administered drug.

Dosage/Range:

- 75 mg/m^2 subcutaneous injection daily × 7 days, repeated q 4 weeks for at least 4 cycles.
- Dose may be increased to 100 mg/m^2 after 2 cycles if initial dose ineffective and toxicity manageable (no toxicity except nausea and vomiting).
- Decrease or hold dose if significant bone marrow depression.
- If baseline WBC > 3000/mm^3, ANC > 1500/mm^3, and platelets > 75,000/mm^3, modify dose based on nadir counts.
- ANC < 500/mm^3, platelets < 25,000/mm^3 = 50% dose next course.
- ANC 500–1500/mm^3, platelets 25,000–50,000/mm^3 = 67% of dose next course.
- ANC > 1500/mm^3, platelets > 50,000/mm^3 = 100% dose.
- If baseline WBC < 3000/mm^3, ANC < 1500/mm^3, or platelets < 75,000/mm^3, dose modifications and bone marrow biopsy cellularity at time of nadir used, unless there is clear improvement in differentiation (% mature granulocytes is higher with ANC higher than at onset of treatment)—see package insert.
- Dose modification based on renal function and serum electrolytes.
- If unexplained decreases in serum bicarbonate < 20 mEq/L, dose reduce 50% in next cycle.
- If elevations of BUN or serum creatinine occur, delay next dose until values return to normal or baseline, and reduce dose by 50% in next cycle.

Drug Preparation:

- Drug is a lyophilized powder in 100 mg single-use vials.
- Reconstitute ascetically with 4 mL sterile water for injection, adding diluent slowly into the vial.
- Invert vial 2–3 times and gently rotate, yielding a cloudy suspension containing 25 mg/mL.
- Divide doses greater than 4 mL into 2 syringes and administer within 1 hour of reconstitution at room temperature.
- Reconstituted solution may be kept in the vial or drawn in a syringe(s) and refrigerated immediately for later use for up to 8 hours. After removal from the refrigerator, the suspension may be allowed to equilibrate to room temperature for up to 30 minutes prior to administration.

Drug Administration:

- Invert syringe(s) 2–3 times and gently roll syringe(s) between palms for 30 seconds immediately prior to administration to provide a homogenous suspension.
- Rotate sites for each subcutaneous injection (thigh, abdomen, or upper arm), and give new injection at least 1 inch from old site, and never into areas where site is tender, bruised, red, or hard.

Drug Interactions:

- Bone marrow depressant drugs: increased myelosuppression.

Lab Effects/Interference:

- Decreased ANC, platelets, red blood cell counts.
- Renal tubular acidosis.
- Increased BUN and creatinine.
- Hypokalemia.

Special Considerations:

- Azacytidine is indicated for treatment of patients with all five myelodysplastic subtypes: refractory anemia (RA) or refractory anemia with ringed sideroblasts (RARS) (if accompanied by neutropenia or thrombocytopenia or requiring transfusions), refractory anemia with excess blasts (RAEB), refractory anemia with excess blasts in transformation (RAEB-T), and chronic myelomonocytic leukemia (CMMoL).
- Overall response rate of patients with all patients except those with AML was 15.7% (complete and partial responders).
- Drug is contraindicated in patients with hypersensitivity to mannitol, and in patients with advanced malignant hepatic tumors.
- Drug is fetotoxic and embryotoxic. Women of child-bearing age must use effective contraception methods; men should be advised not to father a child while receiving treatment with azacytidine. Women who are receiving azacytidine should not breast-feed their infant, as drug causes tumors in animals, and has the potential for severe toxicity.
- Monitor renal function closely in elderly patients.
- Use cautiously in patients with preexisting hepatic disease, as patients with extensive liver metastases have rarely been reported to develop coma and death.

Potential Toxicities/Side Effects and the Nursing Process

I. INFECTION AND BLEEDING related to BONE MARROW DEPRESSION

Defining Characteristics: Leukopenia is dose-limiting, with nadir occurring from days 14–17; lasts two weeks, with recovery in 14 days. Thrombocytopenia and anemia also occur. Bone marrow depression lessens once patient has a response to therapy.

Nursing Implications: Monitor CBC, neutrophil, and platelet count prior to drug administration and postchemotherapy; assess for signs/symptoms of infection, bleeding, and anemia. Teach patient/family signs/symptoms of infection, bleeding, and anemia, and instruct to report them to nurse or physician immediately. Teach patient to avoid aspirin-containing OTC medications.

II. ALTERATION IN NUTRITION, LESS THAN BODY REQUIREMENTS, related to NAUSEA AND VOMITING, ANOREXIA, STOMATITIS, CONSTIPATION and DIARRHEA

Defining Characteristics: Nausea/vomiting is dose-related, and occurs in about 70.5%/54.1% of patients, respectively, beginning 1–3 hours postchemotherapy. This tends to be worse in the first 1–2 cycles, and increases in incidence with increasing doses. Diarrhea develops in 36.4% of patients, with incidence increasing as dose increases. Constipation occurs in about 33% of patients and is worse during the first 2 cycles of therapy. Anorexia affects 20% of patients, and stomatitis occurs in 7% of patients.

Nursing Implications: Assess baseline nutritional status, and periodically at visits. Premedicate with antiemetics before injection, and teach patient self-administration of antiemetics at home; encourage small, frequent feedings as tolerated; if severe vomiting occurs, treat with alternative antiemetics and assess for signs/symptoms of fluid and electrolyte imbalance. Monitor serum potassium, as hypokalemia may be a side effect of treatment. Assess baseline bowel elimination status. Instruct patient to report onset of diarrhea and administer antidiarrheals as ordered. If diarrhea is protracted, ensure adequate hydration, monitor total body fluid balance, and teach/reinforce perineal hygiene. Instruct patient to monitor for constipation, and to use measures to prevent constipation if that is a problem. If patient has anorexia, teach patient to identify nutrient-dense foods and to eat small frequent meals, including a bedtime snack. Teach patient strategies to increase appetite, depending upon an individualized assessment. Teach patient to self-assess oral mucosa, and to use a systematic cleansing of teeth/mouth after meals and at bedtime. Monitor LFTs periodically during therapy and discuss abnormalities with physician.

III. ALTERATION IN COMFORT related to FEVER, FATIGUE, ARTHRALGIAS, and INJECTION SITE IRRITATION

Defining Characteristics: Fever occurs in 54% of patients, with rigors affecting about 25%; fatigue in 36% of patients; arthralgias in 22%; and injection site erythema (35%), injection site pain (23%), injection site bruising (14%), injection site reaction (14%). Injection site discomfort was more pronounced during the 1st and 2nd cycles of therapy.

Nursing Implications: Monitor temperature and teach patient to self-assess temperature. Teach patient that pyrexia may occur, and how to self-administer antipyretics. Teach patient to notify nurse/MD if rigors occur and are severe. Teach measures to reduce discomfort related to myalgias if they occur, such as application of heat and NSAIDs. Teach patient strategies to conserve energy, such as alternating activity with reset. Teach patient to rotate sites used for injection, and local measures to increase comfort.

Drug: bendamustine hydrochloride (Treanda)

Class: Alkylating agent; nitrogen mustard derivative.

Mechanism of Action: Bifunctional with both alkylating and purine-like (antimetabolite) action. It causes sustainable double-strand DNA breaks and induces apoptosis, resulting in cell death. It appears to also cause apoptosis-independent cell death. It differs from nitrogen mustard by a benzimidazole ring, which helps to explain why the drug is active in patients who are refractory to other alkylating agents. Drug is active in dividing as well as resting cells.

Metabolism: It undergoes biotransformation in the liver into an active compound; drug's active minor metabolites gamma-hydroxy bendamustine and N-desmethyl-bendamustine are formed via cytochrome P450 CYP1A2. Low plasma protein binding; terminal half-life is 3.5 hours. Excreted via the kidneys as active drug and metabolites. No clinically significant differences in gender, or in geriatric patients, was seen in the adverse reaction profile.

Dosage/Range:
- 100-mg/m^2 IV infusion over 30 minutes on days 1 and 2 of a 28-day cycle, for up to six cycles. Premedicate with antiemetic.
- Delay treatment for grade 4 hematologic toxicity or clinically significant ≥ grade 2 nonhematologic toxicity.
- Dose modifications:
  - Hematologic: grade > 3: reduce dose to 50 mg/m^2 on days 1 and 2; if > grade 3 recurs: dose reduce to 25 mg/m^2 on days 1 and 2 when ANC > 1×10^9/L and platelets > 75×10^9/L.
  - Nonhematologic: clinically significant grade > 3: rereduce dose to 50 mg/m^2 days 1 and 2.
  - May consider dose re-escalation after toxicity resolves and does not recur on lower dose.
  - Discontinue for severe skin reactions, severe infusion, or anaphylactic reactions.
  - Assess patient risk for tumor lysis syndrome and need for prophylaxis (e.g., allopurinol for first few weeks of treatment).

Drug Preparation:
- Aseptically reconstitute each 100 mg of drug with 20 mL of sterile water for injection USP, yielding a concentration of 5 mg/mL. The lyophilized powder should dissolve completely within 5 minutes and be clear without particulate matter.
- Aseptically, withdraw volume of ordered dose, and further dilute in a 500-mL 0.9% sodium chloride for injection infusion bag within 30 minutes of reconstitution. The admixture should be clear and colorless to slightly yellow in color.
- Administer soon after reconstitution if possible, as drug contains no preservatives.
- Once diluted in 0.9% sodium chloride injection USP, the final admixture is stable for 24 hours when refrigerated (2–8°C or 36–47°F) or for 3 hours at room temperature (15–30°C or 59–86°F) and room light.

Drug Administration:
- Assess: ANC > 1×10^9/L and platelets > 75×10^9/L
- Administer as an IV infusion over 30 minutes.
- Assess for rare allergic reactions.

Drug Interactions:
- Synergistic with rituximab.

- Bendamustine drug exposure time may be influenced by CYP1A2 inducers (omeprazole; smoking may decrease plasma concentrations of bendamustine and increase plasma concentrations of the active metabolites) or inhibitors (e.g., ciprofloxacin, fluvoxamine, which may increase plasma concentrations of bendamustine and decrease concentration of active metabolites); consider alternative drugs to avoid CYP1A2 inducers or inhibitors.

Lab Effects/Interference:
- Decreased WBC, platelet counts, hemoglobin.
- Increased LFTs.

Special Considerations:
- FDA indicated for the treatment of patients with chronic lymphocytic leukemia (CLL). Comparative efficacy to first line therapies other than chlorambucil unknown.
- Contraindicated in patients allergic to bendamustine or mannitol and in patients with severe renal (Cr Cl < 40 mL/min) or hepatic impairment.
- Drug is being studied in the treatment of patients with relapsed HD, NHL (low-grade, Mantle cell, high grade), multiple myeloma, and solid tumors such as breast and lung cancers.
- Drug produced a response in 75% of patients with advanced, rituximab-refractory NHL (Friedberg et al, 2005).
- Partial cross-resistance with melphalan and cyclophosphamide; drug may replace cyclophosphamide in the treatment of NHL.
- Drug is carcinogenic and mutagenic. Women should use effective birth control measures to avoid pregnancy while receiving the drug and for 3 months following. Alkylating drugs impair spermatogenesis with azoospermia and total germinal aplasia in men; spermatogenesis may return in several years. Depending on the patient's age, sperm banking may be recommended.
- Rarely, hypertension may occur but is easily managed.
- If overdose is experienced, provide supportive care including monitoring of hematologic parameters and ECGs (QTc prolongation, tachycardia, ST and T wave deviations).

Potential Toxicities/Side Effects and the Nursing Process

I. INFECTION AND BLEEDING related to BONE MARROW DEPRESSION

Defining Characteristics: Myelosuppression is major toxicity, with nadir occurring during the third week after drug administration, and recovery by day 28. Grades 3/4 neutropenia affects 24 with 3% febrile neutropenia. Thrombocytopenia is less common with 3% grades 3/4 and < 1% of patients requiring platelet transfusions. Decreased hemoglobin affects 89% of patients with 13% grades 3/4, and 20% requiring red cell transfusions.

Nursing Implications: Monitor CBC, neutrophil, and platelet count before drug administration and postchemotherapy. Subsequent treatments require ANC $\geq 1 \times 10^9$/L and platelets > 75×10^9/L; assess for signs/symptoms of infection, bleeding, and anemia. Teach patient/family signs/symptoms of infection, bleeding, and anemia, and instruct to report them to nurse or physician immediately. Teach patient to avoid aspirin-containing OTC medications. Teach patient to report increasing fatigue, signs of severe anemia (shortness of breath, chest pain/angina, headaches). Monitor hemoglobin/hematocrit; discuss transfusion or erythrocyte growth factor support with physician if signs/symptoms develop or hematocrit falls < 25 mg/dL. Teach patient about diet high in iron.

II. POTENTIAL FOR INJURY related to INFUSION REACTION AND ANAPHYLAXIS

Defining Characteristics: Infusion reactions occur commonly and are characterized by fever, chills, pruritus, and rash. Fever occurs in 24% of patients and chills in 6%. Rarely, anaphylactoid and anaphylactic reactions may occur, especially on the second and subsequent cycles of therapy. Two percent of patients withdrew from therapy for hypersensitivity reactions.

Nursing Implications: Assess baseline vital signs (VS) and mental status before drug administration. Review standing orders or nursing procedure for patient management of anaphylaxis and be prepared to stop drug immediately if signs/symptoms occur. Keep IV line open with 0.9% sodium chloride; notify physician, monitor VS, and administer ordered medications, which may include epinephrine 1:1000, hydrocortisone sodium succinate, and diphenhydramine. If patients develop a grade 1 or grade 2 reaction, premedicate with antihistamines, antipyretics, and corticosteroids before subsequent cycles. Do not rechallenge, and discontinue therapy for grades 3 or 4 infusion reactions.

III. POTENTIAL FOR INJURY related to TUMOR LYSIS SYNDROME (TLS)

Defining Characteristics: May develop with initial therapy if patient has a large tumor burden; results from rapid lysis of tumor cells. This usually begins 1 to 5 days after initiation of therapy and causes elevations in serum uric acid, potassium, phosphorus, creatinine.

Nursing Implications: For patients with a high tumor burden, expect medical orders to include oral allopurinol and vigorous oral hydration prior to beginning first cycle of therapy, together with IV hydration with the first cycle of therapy. Reinforce teaching about allopurinol and the importance of adhering to therapy as directed for the first few weeks after cycle 1 therapy. Monitor baseline and daily BUN, creatinine, phosphorus, uric acid, and calcium. Monitor for renal, cardiac, neuromuscular signs/symptoms of TLS.

IV. ALTERATION IN NUTRITION, LESS THAN BODY REQUIREMENTS, related to NAUSEA AND VOMITING, DIARRHEA

Defining Characteristics: Nausea and/or vomiting are dose related and occur in 20% and 16% of patients, respectively. Grades 3/4 occur in < 1% of patients. Diarrhea occurs in 9% of patients and is generally mild. Dry mouth, mucositis, stomatitis, and constipation may also occur less commonly.

Nursing Implications: Assess baseline nutritional status and before each treatment. Premedicate with antiemetics before injection, and teach patient self-administration of antiemetics at home; encourage small, frequent feedings as tolerated. If severe vomiting occurs, treat with alternative antiemetics and assess for signs/symptoms of fluid and electrolyte imbalance. Monitor serum potassium, as hypokalemia may be a side effect of treatment. Assess baseline bowel elimination status. Instruct the patient to report the onset of diarrhea and to administer antidiarrheals as ordered. If diarrhea is protracted, ensure adequate hydration, monitor total body fluid balance, and teach/reinforce perineal hygiene. Teach patient dietary modifications, such as the BRAT (bananas, rice, applesauce, toast) diet if diarrhea develops.

V. POTENTIAL FOR IMPAIRED SKIN INTEGRITY related to RASH

Defining Characteristics: Rash occurs in 8% and pruritus in 5% of patients. Rarely, toxic skin reactions and bullous exanthema can occur. Skin reactions may be progressive and increase in severity with further treatment—if this occurs, drug should be withheld or discontinued.

Nursing Implications: Teach patient about possible side effects and self-care measures. Teach patient to report rash, and then monitor patient closely for signs of increase in severity or extent. Discuss with physician symptomatic treatment of skin changes and holding or discontinuing drug if rash is progressive or more severe.

Drug: bicalutamide (Casodex)

Class: Nonsteroidal antiandrogen.

Mechanism of Action: Binds to androgen receptors in the prostate, preventing normal androgen stimulation; affinity is four times greater than that of flutamide.

Metabolism: Extensively metabolized in the liver. Decreased drug excretion in patients with moderate to severe hepatic dysfunction.

Dosage/Range:
- 50 mg PO daily.

Drug Preparation:
- None.

Drug Administration:
- Orally. Usually given with luteinizing hormone-releasing hormone (LHRH) analogue or as a single agent after surgical castration.

Drug Interactions:
- Warfarin: may increase effect; monitor INR closely.

Lab Effects/Interference:
- Increased LFTs.
- Increased BUN, WBC, Hgb.

Special Considerations:
- Use cautiously in patients with moderate to severe hepatic dysfunction. Observe closely for toxicity, as dosage adjustment may be required.
- No dose modification needed for renal dysfunction.

Potential Toxicities/Side Effects and the Nursing Process

I. ALTERATION IN COMFORT, POTENTIAL, related to GYNECOMASTIA AND HOT FLASHES

Defining Characteristics: Gynecomastia occurs in 23% of patients, breast tenderness in 26%, and hot flashes in 9.3%.

Nursing Implications: Teach patient that these side effects may occur, and discuss measures that may offer symptomatic relief.

II. ALTERATION IN NUTRITION, LESS THAN BODY REQUIREMENTS, related to NAUSEA, POTENTIAL

Defining Characteristics: Nausea may occur in 6% of patients.

Nursing Implications: Teach patient that nausea may occur, and instruct to report nausea. Determine baseline weight, and monitor at each visit. Discuss strategies to minimize nausea, including diet modification and time of dosing.

III. ALTERATION IN ELIMINATION, POTENTIAL, related to CONSTIPATION OR DIARRHEA

Defining Characteristics: Incidence of constipation is 6%, while that of diarrhea is 2.5%.

Nursing Implications: Assess baseline elimination pattern. Teach patient that alterations may occur, and instruct to report them if changes do not respond to usual nonprescription management strategies (OTC medications, dietary modifications).

Drug: bleomycin sulfate (Blenoxane)

Class: Antitumor action of bleomycin; isolated from *fungus Streptomyces verticullus.* Possesses both antitumor and antimicrobial actions.

Mechanism of Action: Induces single-strand and double-strand breaks in DNA. DNA synthesis is inhibited.

Metabolism: Excreted via the renal system. About 70% is excreted unchanged in urine; 30–60 minutes after IV infusion, urine levels are 10 times the serum level.

Dosage/Range:
- 5–20 units/m^2 once a week.
- 10–20 units/m^2 twice a week.
- Continuous infusion: 15 units/m^2/day × 4 days.
- Pleural space (for pleurodesis): 50–60 units in 50- to 100-mL diluent, infused into pleural space and followed by change in position every 15 minutes. Give lidocaine 100–200 mg before infusion or mix with bleomycin to maximize comfort.
- Frequency and schedule may vary according to protocol and age.

Drug Preparation:
- Dilute powder in 0.9% sodium chloride or sterile water to prepare 15- or 30-unit vials.

Drug Administration:
- IV, IM, or subcutaneous doses may be administered. Some clinical trial protocols may use 24-hour infusions. There is a risk for anaphylaxis in lymphoma patients and hypotension with higher doses of drug. It may be recommended that a test dose be given before the first dose to detect hypersensitivity in patients with lymphoma.
- Dose reduce if renal insufficiency: creatinine clearance 10–50 mL/min, decrease dose by 25%; creatinine clearance < 10 mL/min, give 50% of dose.
- Maximum lifetime dose is 400 units.

Drug Interactions:
- Cisplatin: may decrease bleomycin excretion with increased toxicity due to renal dysfunction.
- Oxygen: increased risk of pulmonary toxicity; do not use FiO_2 100% oxygen.
- Digoxin dose may need to be increased.
- Phenytoin dose may need to be increased.

Lab Effects/Interference:
- None.

Special Considerations:
- Because of pulmonary toxicities with increasing dose, pulmonary function tests (PFTs) and CXR should be obtained before each course or as outlined by protocol.
- Maximum cumulative lifetime dose: 400 units.

- Oxygen (FiO_2) increases risk of pulmonary toxicity.
- Reduce dose for impaired renal function (urinary creatinine clearance < 40–60 mL/min).
- Risk of pulmonary toxicity increased in elderly (> 70 years old); renal impairment; pulmonary disease or prior chest XRT; exposure to high oxygen concentration (i.e., surgery); cumulative doses > 400 units lifetime.
- May cause chemical fevers up to 39.4–40.5°C (103–105°F) in up to 60% of patients. May need to administer premedications such as acetaminophen, antihistamines, or in some cases steroids.
- Watch for signs/symptoms of hypotension and anaphylaxis with high drug doses; physician may order test dose in patients with lymphoma.
- May cause irritation at site of injection (is considered an irritant, not a vesicant).
- Decreases the oral bioavailability of digoxin when given together.
- Decreases the pharmacologic effects of phenytoin when given in combination.

Potential Toxicities/Side Effects and the Nursing Process

I. POTENTIAL FOR IMPAIRED GAS EXCHANGE related to PULMONARY TOXICITY

Defining Characteristics: Pneumonitis occurs in 10% of patients and is characterized by rales, dyspnea, infiltrate on CXR; in 1% may progress to irreversible pulmonary fibrosis. Risk factors include age > 70, dose > 400 units (but may occur at much lower doses), and concurrent or prior radiotherapy to the chest. Slower, continuous infusion may lower the risk.

Nursing Implications: Discuss with physician the need for PFTs and CXR prior to initiating therapy and monthly during therapy. Assess pulmonary status prior to each treatment (early symptom is dyspnea, and earliest sign is fine crackles). Instruct patient to report cough, dyspnea, shortness of breath. If patient needs surgery, discuss with physician the need to use low FiO_2 during surgery since the lung tissue has been sensitized to bleomycin, and high concentrations of oxygen will cause further lung damage.

II. POTENTIAL FOR INJURY related to ANAPHYLAXIS

Defining Characteristics: Anaphylactoid reaction may occur in 1% of lymphoma patients, characterized by hypotension, confusion, tachycardia, wheezing, and facial edema. Reaction may be immediate or delayed for several hours and may occur after the first or second drug administration.

Nursing Implications: Discuss with physician the use of test dose prior to drug administration in lymphoma patients. Assess baseline vital signs (VS) and mental status prior to drug administration. Review standing orders or nursing procedure for patient management of anaphylaxis, and be prepared to stop drug immediately if signs/symptoms occur. Keep IV line open with 0.9% sodium chloride; notify physician, monitor VS, and administer ordered medications, which may include epinephrine 1:1000, hydrocortisone sodium succinate, and diphenhydramine.

III. POTENTIAL ALTERATION IN COMFORT related to FEVER AND CHILLS, AND PAIN AT TUMOR SITE

Defining Characteristics: Fever (up to 39.4°–40.5°C [103°–105°F]) and chills, occurring in up to 60% of patients, begin 4–10 hours after drug administration and may last 24 hours. There appears to be tolerance with successive doses of bleomycin. Pain may occur at tumor site due to chemotherapy-induced cellular damage.

Nursing Implications: Teach patient that these side effects may occur, and assess patient during and postadministration. If fever occurs, notify physician and administer ordered acetaminophen, antihistamine, or steroid. If tumor pain occurs, reassure patient and discuss with physician the use of acetaminophen as analgesic.

IV. POTENTIAL FOR IMPAIRED SKIN INTEGRITY related to ALOPECIA, SKIN CHANGES, AND NAIL CHANGES

Defining Characteristics: Dose-related alopecia begins 3–4 weeks after first dose and is reversible. Skin changes occur in 50% of patients and include erythema, rash, striae, hyperpigmentation, skin peeling of fingertips, and hyperkeratosis; these are dose-related and begin after 150–200 units have been administered. Skin eruptions include a macular rash over hands and elbows, urticaria, and vesiculations. Pruritus may occur. Nail changes and possible nail loss may occur. Phlebitis at the IV site may occur.

Nursing Implications: Teach patient about possible side effects and self-care measures, including obtaining a wig or cap as appropriate prior to hair loss. Encourage patient to verbalize feelings and provide patient emotional support. Discuss with physician symptomatic treatment of skin changes. Assess IV site for phlebitis and restart IV at alternate site if phlebitis develops.

V. POTENTIAL ALTERATION IN NUTRITION, LESS THAN BODY REQUIREMENTS, related to NAUSEA AND VOMITING, ANOREXIA AND WEIGHT LOSS, AND STOMATITIS

Defining Characteristics: Nausea with or without vomiting may occur; anorexia and weight loss may occur and may continue after treatment is completed; stomatitis may occur and decrease ability and desire to eat.

Nursing Implications: Administer antiemetic prior to initial treatment and revise plan for successive treatments if no nausea/vomiting. Teach patient about possible anorexia and encourage patient to eat high-calorie, high-protein foods. Assess oral mucosa prior to drug administration; teach patient self-assessment and instruct to notify nurse or physician if stomatitis develops. Teach patient oral care prior to drug administration.

VI. POTENTIAL FOR SEXUAL DYSFUNCTION related to REPRODUCTIVE HAZARDS

Defining Characteristics: Drug is mutagenic and probably teratogenic.

Nursing Implications: Discuss with patient and partner both sexuality and reproductive goals, as well as possible impact of chemotherapy. Discuss contraception and sperm banking if appropriate.

Drug: busulfan (Myleran)

Class: Alkylating agent.

Mechanism of Action: Forms carbonium ions through the release of a methane sulfonate group, resulting in the alkylation of DNA. Acts primarily on granulocyte precursors in the bone marrow and is cell cycle phase nonspecific.

Metabolism: Well absorbed orally; almost all metabolites are excreted in the urine. Has a very short half-life.

Dosage/Range:

Chronic myelogenous leukemia:

- 4–8 mg/day PO for 2–3 weeks initially, then maintenance dose of 1–3 mg/m^2 PO daily or 0.05 mg/kg orally daily. Dose titrated based on leukocyte counts. Drug withheld when leukocyte count reaches 15,000/μL; resume when total leukocyte count is 50,000/μL; maintenance dose of 1–3 mg daily used if remission lasts < 3 months.

High doses with bone marrow transplantation:

- See Busulfan for Injection.

Drug Preparation:

- None.

Drug Administration:

- Available in 2-mg scored tablets given orally.

Drug Interactions:

- Combination treatment with thioguanine may cause hepatic dysfunction and the development of esophageal varices in a small number of patients.

Lab Effects/Interference:
- Decreased CBC.
- Increased LFTs.

Special Considerations:
Regular dose:
- If WBC is high, patient is at risk for hyperuricemia. Allopurinol and hydration may be indicated.
- Follow weekly CBC and platelet count initially, then monthly. Dose is decreased to maintenance level when leukocyte count falls below 50,000 mm^3.
- Hyperpigmentation of skin creases may occur due to increased melanin production.
- If given according to accepted guidelines, patients should have minimal side effects.

High dose:
- See Busulfan for Injection.

Potential Toxicities/Side Effects and the Nursing Process

I. POTENTIAL FOR INFECTION, BLEEDING, AND FATIGUE related to BONE MARROW DEPRESSION

Defining Characteristics: The nadir is at 11–30 days following initial drug administration, with recovery in 24–54 days; however, delayed, refractory pancytopenia has occurred.

Nursing Implications: Monitor CBC, WBC differential, and platelets, initially weekly, then at least monthly. Expect drug will be interrupted if counts fall rapidly or steeply. Teach patient to self-assess for signs/symptoms of infection, bleeding, or severe fatigue, and to notify nurse or physician immediately. Teach patient to avoid aspirin-containing OTC medications.

II. POTENTIAL FOR IMPAIRED GAS EXCHANGE related to INTERSTITIAL PULMONARY FIBROSIS

Defining Characteristics: Rarely, bronchopulmonary dysplasia progressing to pulmonary fibrosis can occur, beginning one to many years post-therapy. Symptoms are usually delayed (occurring after four years) and include anorexia, cough, dyspnea, and fever. High-dose corticosteroids may be helpful, but condition may be fatal due to rapid, diffuse fibrosis.

Nursing Implications: Assess pulmonary status routinely in all patients receiving long-term therapy. Discuss plan for regular pulmonary function studies with physician.

III. POTENTIAL FOR SEXUAL AND REPRODUCTIVE DYSFUNCTION related to REPRODUCTIVE HAZARDS

Defining Characteristics: Premenopausal female patients commonly experience ovarian suppression and amenorrhea with menopausal symptoms; men experience sterility, azoospermia, and testicular atrophy. Although successful pregnancies have occurred following busulfan therapy, the drug is potentially teratogenic.

Nursing Implications: Assess patient's/partner's sexual patterns and reproductive goals. Provide information, supportive counseling, and referral as needed. Teach importance of birth control measures as appropriate.

Drug: busulfan for injection (Busulfex)

Class: Alkylating agent.

Mechanism of Action: Forms carbonium ions through the release of a methane sulfonate group, resulting in the alkylation of DNA. Acts primarily on granulocyte precursors in the bone marrow, and is cell cycle, phase non-specific.

Metabolism: After IV administration, drug achieves equal concentrations in the plasma and CSF. Drug is 32% protein-bound. Metabolized in the liver, and excreted in the urine (30%). Appears metabolites may be long-lived.

Dosage/Range:

Conditioning regimen:

- Indicated in combination with cyclophosphamide prior to allogeneic hematopoietic progenitor cell transplantation for chronic myelogenous leukemia.
- 0.8 mg/kg (IBW or actual weight, whichever is lower, or adjusted IBW) IV q 6 h × 4 days (total of 16 doses).
- Cyclophosphamide dose is given on each of 2 days as a 1-hour infusion at a dose of 60 mg/kg beginning on BMT day –3, 6 hours following the 16th dose of IV busulfan.

Drug Preparation:

- Aseptically open ampule, and using the 25-mm, 5-micron nylon membrane syringe filter provided, remove the ordered, calculated drug dose.
- Remove the syringe/filter, replace with a new needle, and dispense the syringe contents into a bag or syringe containing 10 times the volume of the drug, either 0.9% NS injection or 5% dextrose injection. The final concentration of drug should be ≥ 0.5 mg/mL. For example, a 70-kg patient at a dose of 0.8 mg/kg given a concentration of 6 mg/mL would require 9.3 mL (56 mg) busulfan total dose. 9.3 mL of drug × 10 = 93 mL. As the further diluent needed is 0.9% NS inj or D5W inj, the total volume is 9.3 mL + 93 mL = 102.3 mL.

- Mix contents thoroughly.
- Ensure that this meets the recommended drug concentration, e.g., (9.3 mL × 6 mg/mL)/102.3 mL = 0.54 mg/mL.
- Unopened ampules must be refrigerated at 2–8°C (36–46°F).
- Diluted drug is stable at room temperature (25°C) for up to 8 hours, but infusion must be completed within this time. Drug diluted in 0.9% NS Inj, USP, is stable refrigerated (2–8°C) for up to 12 hours, but the infusion must be completed within that time.

Drug Administration:
- Available in a 10-mL, single-use ampule containing 60 mg (6 mg/mL).
- Dilute in 0.9% NS Injection or 5% Dextrose Injection to 10 times volume of drug (see example in Preparation) prior to IV infusion.
- Infuse dose over 2 hours via infusion pump.
- Drug should be administered through a central line.
- All patients should be premedicated with phenytoin, as drug crosses BBB and causes seizures (see Drug Interactions).

Drug Interactions:
- CYP 3A4 inducers: Phenytoin decreases busulfan AUC by 15%, resulting in the target dose. Use carbamazepine, nafcillin, and phenobarbital cautiously.
- Other anticonvulsants may increase busulfan AUC, increasing the risk of veno-occlusive disease or seizures. Monitor busulfan exposure and toxicity closely.
- CYP 3A4 inhibitors: Itraconazole decreases busulfan clearance by up to 25% with potential significant increases in serum busulfan levels. Use ciprofloxacin, clarithromycin, erythromycin, imatinib, and verapamil cautiously.
- Acetaminophen prior to (< 72 hours) or concurrent with busulfan may result in decreased drug clearance and increased serum busulfan levels.
- St. John's Wort: may decrease busulfan serum level; do not use concomitantly.
- Grapefruit juice: may enhance busulfan toxicity as inhibits CYP 3A4 enzymes.

Lab Effects/Interference:
- Profound myelosuppression/aplasia with decreased WBC, neutrophils, Hgb/HCT, and platelet counts.
- If liver veno-occlusive disease develops, increased serum transaminases, alk phos, and bili.
- Creatinine is elevated in 21% of patients.

Special Considerations:
- Drug clearance is best predicted when the busulfan dose is based on adjusted ideal body weight (AIBW).
  - Ideal body weight (IBW in kg): men = 50 + 0.91 × (height in cm – 152); women = 45 + 0.91 × (height in cm – 152).
  - AIBW = IBW + 0.25 × (actual weight – IBW).
- No known antidote if overdose occurs; one report says that drug is dialyzable.

- Drug is metabolized by conjugation with glutathione, so consider administration of same. Drug should only be given in combination with hematopoietic progenitor cell transplantation, as expected toxicity is profound myelosuppression.
- CNS effects including seizures, hepatic veno-occlusive disease (VOD), cardiac tamponade, bronchopulmonary dysplasia with pulmonary fibrosis four months to ten years after therapy.
- Contraindicated in patients with a history of hypersensitivity to drug or its components.
- Women of childbearing age should use effective birth control measures; nursing mothers should interrupt breast-feeding during therapy.
- Drug is for adult use, and has not been studied in patients with hepatic insufficiency.
- Drug may cause cellular dysplasia in many organs (characterized by giant, hyperchromatic nuclei in lymph nodes, pancreas, thyroid, adrenal glands, liver, lungs, and bone marrow), which may cause difficult interpretation of subsequent cytologic examinations in lungs, bladder, and uterine cervix.
- Factors that may increase risk of veno-occlusive disease are history of XRT, more than three cycles of chemotherapy, prior progenitor cell transplantation, or Busulfex dose AUC concentrations of > 1500 μm/min.

Potential Toxicities/Side Effects and the Nursing Process

I. POTENTIAL FOR INFECTION, BLEEDING, AND ANEMIA related to BONE MARROW DEPRESSION

Defining Characteristics: Myelosuppression is profound in 100% of patients. ANC < 500 cells/mm^3 occurred a median of four days posttransplant in 100% of patients. Following progenitor cell infusion, the median recovery of neutrophil count to ≥ 500 cells/mm^3 was day 13 when prophylactic G-CSF was given. 51% of patients experienced 1+ episodes of infection; fever occurred in 80% of patients, with chills in 33%. Thrombocytopenia (< 25,000/mm^3 or requiring platelet transfusion) occurred in 5–6 days in 98% of patients. There was a median of six platelet transfusions per patient in clinical trials. Anemia affected 50% of patients, and the median number of red blood cell transfusions on clinical trials was 4 per patient.

Nursing Implications: Assess WBC, with differential, Hgb/HCT, and platelet count prior to drug administration, and at least daily during treatment. Discuss any abnormalities with physician. Monitor continuously for signs/symptoms of infection or bleeding. Teach patient signs/symptoms of infection and bleeding, self-assessment, and to report signs/symptoms immediately. Teach self-care measures to minimize infection and bleeding, including avoidance of OTC aspirin-containing medications. Discuss with physician use of granulocyte-colony stimulating factor (G-CSF) to prevent febrile neutropenia. Transfuse platelets and red blood cells per physician order.

II. ALTERATION IN CARDIAC OUTPUT, POTENTIAL, related to TACHYCARDIA, THROMBOSIS, HYPERTENSION, VASODILATION

Defining Characteristics: Mild-to-moderate tachycardia has been noted in 44% of patients (11% during drug infusion), and, less commonly, other rhythm disturbances such as arrhythmia (5%), atrial fibrillation (2%), ventricular extrasystoles (2%), and third-degree heart block (2%). Mild-to-moderate thrombosis may occur in 33% of patients, usually associated with a central venous catheter. Hypertension has been seen in 36% of patients and grade 3/4 in 3%. Mild vasodilation (flushing and hot flashes) occurs in 25% of patients. In clinical trials, most commonly in the postcyclophosphamide phase, other less common events were cardiomegaly (5%), mild EKG changes (2%), grades 3 and 4 CHF (2%), and moderate pericardial effusion (2%).

Nursing Implications: Assess baseline cardiac status frequently during shift/care depending upon patient condition, including HR, BP, EKG, and total body fluid balance. Monitor patient for changes in cardiac function throughout treatment course, and report changes immediately. Monitor central venous lines for patency, and use scrupulous care in maintaining catheters; assess for signs/symptoms of venous thrombosis, and discuss management with physician as soon as it is discovered.

III. ALTERATION IN FLUID AND ELECTROLYTE BALANCE, POTENTIAL, related to TREATMENT, CARDIAC RESPONSE

Defining Characteristics: 79% of patients develop edema, hypervolemia, or weight increase, mild or moderate.

Nursing Implications: Assess baseline fluid volume status, weight, orthostatic vital signs, and presence/absence of edema, and assess at least daily, especially after fluid or blood product infusion. Closely monitor I/O and daily total body balance, and discuss abnormalities with physician. Assess renal status, as BUN and creatinine can become elevated in 21% of patients. Assess patient for signs/symptoms of dysuria, oliguria, and hematuria, as hemorrhagic cystis may occur with cyclophosphamide.

IV. POTENTIAL FOR IMPAIRED GAS EXCHANGE related to DYSPNEA AND INTERSTITIAL PULMONARY FIBROSIS

Defining Characteristics: Mild or moderate dyspnea was seen in 25% of study patients, and was severe in 2% (severe hyperventilation). 5% of patients in the study developed alveolar hemorrhage and died. One patient developed nonspecific interstitial fibrosis and died from respiratory failure on BMT day +98. Other reported pulmonary events were mild or moderate, including pharyngitis (18%), hiccup (18%), asthma (8%), atelectasis (2%), pleural effusion (3%), hypoxia (2%), hemoptysis (3%), and sinusitis (3%). As with oral busulfan, pulmonary fibrosis can occur one to many years post-therapy, with the average onset of symptoms four years after therapy (range 4 months to 10 years).

Nursing Implications: Assess pulmonary status, including breath sounds, rate, oxygen saturation, at baseline, and regularly during care. Assess for any underlying problems, such as infection, effusions, and leukemic infiltrates. Teach patient to report any dyspnea, SOB, or other change, and monitor closely. Provide oxygen and support and discuss management plan with physician and implement promptly. After therapy is completed, remind patient that pulmonary fibrosis may develop as a late effect. The patient should have long-term follow-up, and report any dyspnea or SOB, especially in the cold.

V. POTENTIAL FOR ALTERATION IN NUTRITION, LESS THAN BODY REQUIREMENTS, related to NAUSEA/VOMITING, ANOREXIA, STOMATITIS, DIARRHEA, AND ELECTROLYTE ABNORMALITIES

Defining Characteristics: The incidence of GI toxicities is high, but manageable: nausea 98%, vomiting 95%, stomatitis 97%, diarrhea 84%, anorexia 85%, dyspepsia 44%, and mild-to-moderate constipation 38%. Grade 3/4 stomatitis occurred in 26% of patients, severe anorexia in 21%, and grade 3/4 diarrhea in 5%. Additionally, hyperglycemia was seen in 67% of patients, with grade 3/4 in 15%. Hypomagnesemia was mild/moderate in 62%, and severe in 2%; hypokalemia was mild/moderate in 62% and severe in 2%; hypocalcemia was mild/moderate in 46%, and severe in 3%; hypophosphatemia was mild/moderate in 17%, and hyponatremia occurred in 2%.

Nursing Implications: Assess baseline weight, usual weight, and any changes. Assess appetite, and favorite foods. Assess baseline glucose, electrolytes, and minerals, and monitor throughout therapy. Premedicate with aggressive antiemetics (serotonin antagonist) and continue protection throughout treatment. Assess efficacy and modify regimen as needed. Assess oral mucosa and teach patient self-care strategies, including assessment, what to report, oral hygiene regimen. Encourage dietary modifications as needed. Assess bowel elimination pattern baseline and daily during therapy. Teach patient to report diarrhea, and discuss management with physician. Provide comfort measures, and teach patient scrupulous hygiene to prevent infection. Discuss abnormal lab values with physician, correct hyperglycemia, and replete magnesium, potassium, phosphate, calcium, and sodium as ordered.

VI. POTENTIAL FOR SENSORY/PERCEPTUAL ALTERATIONS related to NEUROLOGICAL TOXICITY

Defining Characteristics: Drug crosses BBB, achieving levels equivalent to plasma concentration. Neurologic changes observed in clinical testing were insomnia (84%), anxiety (75%), headaches (65%), dizziness (30%), depression (23%), confusion (11%), lethargy (7%), and hallucinations (5%). Less commonly, delirium occurred in 2%, agitation in 2%, encephalopathy in 2%, and somnolence in 2%. Despite prophylaxis with phenytoin, one patient developed seizures while receiving cyclophosphamide. Especial caution should be used when patients with a history of seizure disorder or head trauma receive the drug.

Nursing Implications: Assess baseline neurologic status and continue to monitor status throughout. Closely monitor patients who have a history of seizure disorder, or head trauma for the development of seizures (seizure precautions). Teach patient to report any changes in usual patterns. Discuss any abnormalities with physician, and develop collaborative symptom-management strategies, including medications. Assess patient interest in relaxation exercises or imagery, or other techniques, and teach self-care strategies. Be prepared to manage seizures as needed.

VII. ALTERATION IN HEPATIC FUNCTION, POTENTIAL, related to VENO-OCCLUSIVE DISEASE (VOD) AND GRAFT-VERSUS-HOST DISEASE (GVHD)

Defining Characteristics: Increased bilirubin occurred in 49% of patients, and grade 3/4 hyperbilirubinemia occurred in 30% within 28 days of transplantation. This was associated with graft-versus-host disease in 6 patients in clinical studies, and with VOD in 8% of patients (5). Severe increases in SGPT occurred in 7%, while mild increases in alkaline phosphatase occurred in 15% of patients. Jaundice occurred in 12%, while hepatomegaly developed in 6%. VOD is a complication of conditioning therapy prior to transplant and occurred in 8% of patients (fatal in 2 of the 5 patients). Factors that may increase risk of veno-occlusive disease are history of XRT, more than three cycles of chemotherapy, prior progenitor cell transplantation, or Busulfex dose AUC concentrations of > 1500 µm/min. Use Jones' criteria to diagnose VOD hyperbilirubinemia, and two of the following: painful hepatomegaly, weight gain > 5%, or ascites. GVHD developed in 18% of patients (severe 3%, mild/moderate 15%, fatal in 3 patients).

Nursing Implications: Assess hepatic function baseline and daily during treatment. Discuss any abnormalities with physician. Teach the patient to report RUQ pain, weight gain, increasing girth, or yellowing of eyes or skin.

VIII. ALTERATION IN COMFORT, POTENTIAL, related to ASTHENIA, PAIN, INJECTION SITE INFLAMMATION, ARTHRALGIAS

Defining Characteristics: Symptoms leading to discomfort include: abdominal pain (mild/moderate 69%, severe 3%), asthenia (mild/moderate 49%, severe 2%), general pain (45%), injection site inflammation or pain (25%), chest or back pain (23–26%), and arthralgia (13%).

Nursing Implications: Assess baseline comfort, and usual strategies to promote comfort. Teach patient to report any pain, weakness, listlessness, injection site discomfort, or any other changes. Discuss strategies to promote comfort, such as use of heat or cold. If discomfort persists, discuss pharmacologic management to reduce symptom distress.

IX. POTENTIAL SEXUAL DYSFUNCTION related to DRUG EFFECTS

Defining Characteristics: Similar to oral busulfan: premenopausal female patients commonly experience ovarian suppression and amenorrhea with menopausal symptoms; men experience sterility, azoospermia, and testicular atrophy. The drug is potentially teratogenic.

Nursing Implications: Assess patient's signs/symptoms and partner's patterns of sexuality and reproductive goals. Teach patient/partner about need for effective contraception and provide other information as appropriate. Provide emotional support, supportive counseling, and referral as needed.

X. ALTERATION IN SKIN INTEGRITY, POTENTIAL, related to SKIN RASH, ALOPECIA

Defining Characteristics: Rash is common (57%) and pruritus less so (28%). Alopecia occurred in 15% of patients. Character of rash ranged from mild vesicular rash (10%), mild/moderate maculopapular rash (8%), vesiculobullous rash (10%), and exfoliative dermatitis (5%). Other skin abnormalities described were erythema nodosum (2%).

Nursing Implications: Assess baseline skin integrity, presence of rashes, itching, and repeat daily. Teach patient skin changes may occur, and to report them. Discuss use of topical agents and antipruritic medications with physician.

Drug: capecitabine (Xeloda, N4-Pentoxycarbonyl-5-deoxy-5-fluorocytidine)

Class: Fluoropyrimidine carbamate.

Mechanism of Action: Metabolites bind to thymidylate synthetase, inhibiting the formation of uracil from thymidylate, and reducing the cell's ability to produce DNA. It also prevents cell division by hindering the formation of RNA, by causing nuclear transcription enzymes to mistakenly incorporate its metabolites in the process of RNA transcription.

Metabolism: Absorbed from the intestinal mucosa as an intact molecule, metabolized in the liver to intermediary metabolite, and then in the liver and tumor tissue to 5-FU precursor. It is then converted through catalytic activation to 5-FU at the tumor site. Metabolites are cleared in the urine.

Dosage/Range:

- 2500 mg/m^2/d PO in two divided doses with food for two weeks, although some patients require starting at 75% of the recommended dose.
- Two-week treatment followed by a 1-week rest period and repeated every three weeks.
- Interrupt for grade 2 nausea, vomiting, diarrhea, stomatitis, or hand-foot syndrome and dose reduce for second and third occurrence; discontinue drug if fourth occurrence.
- Dose reduce for renal dysfunction.
- Adjuvant colon cancer: 1250 mg/m^2 PO bid d 1–14 repeated q 21 days × 8 cycles (24 weeks).
- Breast cancer: In combination with docetaxel: 1250 mg/m^2 PO bid × 14 days, followed by a 7 day rest period, repeated q 3 weeks, with docetaxel 75 mg/m^2 IV over 1 hr day 1, repeated q 3 weeks.
- Combinations with oxaliplatin (CAPOX) and irinotecan (CapIri) are being studied.

Drug Preparation:

- Oral. Available in 150- and 500-mg tablets.
- Administer within 30 min of a meal with a full glass of water.
- Divide daily dose in half; take 12 hours apart.

Drug Interactions:

- Warfarin: ↑ INR, monitor closely and adjust warfarin dose as needed.
- Phenytoin: monitor phenytoin serum level closely and adjust dose as needed.
- Docetaxel: synergy due to up regulation of 5-FU enzyme.
- Leucovorin: synergy and ↑ toxicity; monitor closely.

Lab Effects/Interference:

- Increased bili, alk phos.
- Decreased WBCs.

Special Considerations:

- Indications:

Adjuvant Colon Cancer: In patients who have undergone complete resection of the primary tumor when fluoropyrimidine therapy alone is preferred.

Metastatic Colorectal Cancer: First line treatment when treatment with fluoropyrimidine therapy alone preferred.

Breast Cancer (metastatic): In patients who are resistant to both paclitaxel and an anthracycline-containing regimen, or resistant to paclitaxel in women who cannot receive anthracycline therapy.

Breast Cancer (metastatic): In combination with docetaxel, capecitabine is indicated for the treatment of patients after failure of prior anthracycline-containing chemotherapy.

- Many oncologists begin dosing at 1500 mg/m^2–1875 mg/m^2/d × 14 days.
- Monitor bili baseline and before each cycle, as dose modifications are necessary with hyperbilirubinemia.

- Folic acid should be avoided while taking drug.
- Contraindicated in patients hypersensitive to 5-fluorouracil or patients with creatinine clearance < 30 mL/mm.

Potential Toxicities/Side Effects and the Nursing Process

I. POTENTIAL FOR INFECTION AND BLEEDING related to BONE MARROW DEPRESSION

Defining Characteristics: Commonly causes anemia, neutropenia, and thrombocytopenia.

Nursing Implications: Assess baseline CBC, WBC with differential, and platelet count prior to chemotherapy, as well as for signs/symptoms of infection or bleeding. Teach patient signs/symptoms of infection and bleeding and instruct to report these immediately; teach patient self-care measures to minimize risk of infection and bleeding. This includes avoidance of crowds, proximity to people with infections, and avoidance of OTC aspirin-containing medications.

II. ALTERED NUTRITION, LESS THAN BODY REQUIREMENTS, related to NAUSEA AND VOMITING, STOMATITIS, AND DIARRHEA

Defining Characteristics: Nausea and vomiting occur in 30–50% of patients. Stomatitis and diarrhea also occur in about 50% of patients. Less common with reduced doses. Abdominal pain (35%), constipation (14%), anorexia (26%), dehydration (7%) also occur. Side effects are increased in the old elderly (≥ 80 yrs old).

Nursing Implications: Premedicate patient with antiemetics (phenothiazines usually effective), and continue for 24 hours, at least for first cycle. Encourage small, frequent meals of cool, bland foods. Assess oral mucosa prior to drug administration and teach patient to report changes. Teach patient oral hygiene measures and self-assessment. Instruct patient to report diarrhea, to self-administer prescribed antidiarrheal medications, and to drink adequate fluids. Moderate to severe stomatitis, diarrhea, or nausea and vomiting is an indication to interrupt therapy.

III. ALTERATION IN SKIN INTEGRITY/COMFORT related to HAND/FOOT SYNDROME

Defining Characteristics: Hand and foot syndrome occurs in more than half of patients and is characterized by tingling, numbness, pain, erythema, dryness, rash, swelling, and/or pruritus of hands and feet. Less common with reduced doses.

Nursing Implications: Teach patient about the possibility of this side effect and instruct him or her to stop drug use and inform the physician/nurse immediately should it occur. If patient has pain, expect dose interruption, with dose reduction if this is 2nd or subsequent episode at current dose. Teach patient self-assessment of soles of feet and palms of hands daily for erythema, pain, dry desquamation, and to report pain right away. Teach patients to avoid hot showers, whirlpools, paraffin treatments of nails, vigorous repetitive movements of hands, feet, as well as other body areas; avoid tight fitting shoes and clothes. Teach patients to take cool showers, keep skin surfaces intact and soft with skin emollients. Studies ongoing establishing evidence base for prophylaxis or treatment: vitamin B_6, urea moisturizers, nicotine patch.

IV. ALTERATION IN COMFORT related to FATIGUE, WEAKNESS, DIZZINESS, HEADACHE, FEVER, MYALGIAS, INSOMNIA, AND TASTE PROBLEMS

Defining Characteristics: Fatigue affects approximately 43% of patients, while 42% of patients complained of weakness. Fever was reported in 18% of patients, headache 10%, dizziness 8%, insomnia 7%, and taste problems 6%. Eye irritation was reported by 13% of patients and is related to the drug's excretion via tears.

Nursing Implications: Assess baseline comfort, and teach patient that these symptoms may occur. Teach patient strategies to manage fatigue, such as alternating rest and activity periods, and consolidating tasks. Teach patient to report fever, headache, and eye irritation, and discuss management plan with physician.

Drug: carboplatin (Paraplatin)

Class: Alkylating agent (heavy metal complex).

Mechanism of Action: A second-generation platinum analog. The cytotoxicity is identical to that of the parent, cisplatin, and it is cell cycle phase nonspecific. It reacts with nucleophilic sites on DNA, causing predominantly intrastrand and interstrand crosslinks rather than DNA-protein crosslinks. These crosslinks are similar to those formed with cisplatin but are formed later.

Metabolism: At 24 hours postadministration, approximately 70% of carboplatin is excreted in the urine. The mean half-life is roughly 100 minutes.

Dosage/Range:

- Dose usually given as a function of Area Under the Curve (AUC). Since carboplatin has predictable pharmakinetics based on the drug's excretion by the kidneys, AUC dosing is recommended for this drug. This allows tailoring the drug dose precisely to the individual patient's excretion of the drug (renal function). The Calvert formula is used where:

  The total dose (mg) = target AUC × glomerular filtration rate (GFR) + 25. The GFR is approximated by the urine creatinine clearance, either estimated or actual, and can be calculated by hand. The target AUC is determined by the treatment plan depending on the type of malignancy, such as an AUC of 6 for cancer of unknown primary. Then the dose calculation can be done by hand. Additionally, the manufacturer (Bristol-Myers Squibb Oncology) distributes a calculator to determine the dose.

- As a single agent, 360 mg/m^2 every 4 weeks, or 300 mg/m^2 when combined with cyclophosphamide for advanced ovarian cancer. Delay drug for neutrophil count < 2000/mm^2 or platelets < 100,000/mm^2.
- Drug dose reduction for urine creatinine clearance < 60 mL/minute.
- Autologous bone marrow transplantation: 1600 mg/m^2 IV in divided doses over 4 days (creatinine clearance must be more than 50 mL/min).
- Intraperitoneal: 200–650 mg/m^2 in 2-L IP (ovarian cancer).

Drug Preparation:

- Available as a white powder in amber vial in 50-, 150-, and 450-mg vials.
- Reconstitute with sterile water for injection, 5% dextrose, or 0.9% sodium chloride solution.
- Dilute further in 5% dextrose or 0.9% sodium chloride.
- Injection solution available (10 mg/mL) in 50-, 150-, 450-, and 600-mg vials.
- The solution is chemically stable for 24 hours; discard solution after 8 hours because of the lack of bacteriostatic preservative.

Drug Administration:

- Administered by IV bolus over 15 minutes to 1 hour.
- May also be given as a continuous infusion over 24 hours.
- May be administered intraperitoneally in patients with advanced ovarian cancer.

Drug Interactions:

- Increases renal toxicity when combined with cisplatin.
- Increases bone marrow depression when combined with myelosuppressive drugs.
- Avoid aluminum needles in drug handling.
- Paclitaxel, docetaxel: administer after taxane to maximize cell kill and to minimize the risk of myelosuppression caused by decreased drug excretion.
- Phenytoin: may decrease phenytoin serum levels; monitor levels, and increase drug dose as needed.
- Warfarin: may increase warfarin effect; monitor INR frequently, and dose modify as needed.

Lab Effects/Interference:

- Increased LFTs, RFTs.

Special Considerations:

- Does not have the renal toxicity seen with cisplatin.
- Thrombocytopenia is dose-limiting toxicity, and correlates with GFR.
- Monitor urine creatinine clearance.

Potential Toxicities/Side Effects and the Nursing Process

I. POTENTIAL FOR INFECTION AND BLEEDING related to BONE MARROW DEPRESSION

Defining Characteristics: Myelosuppression is dose-limiting toxicity; platelet nadir is 14–21 days, with usual recovery by day 28; WBC nadir follows 1 week later, but recovery may take 5–6 weeks. The risk of thrombocytopenia is severe, especially when the drug is combined with other myelosuppressive drugs, or if the patient has renal compromise. Anemia may occur with prolonged treatment.

Nursing Implications: Assess CBC, WBC, with differential, and platelet count prior to drug administration. Monitor for signs/symptoms of infection or bleeding. Drug dosage should be reduced if urine creatinine clearance is < 60 mL/min. Drug should be held or dose reduced if absolute neutrophil count (ANC) and/or platelet count is low. Teach the patient signs/symptoms of infection and bleeding, and instruct to report them immediately if they occur. Teach self-care measures to minimize infection and bleeding. Discuss with physician use of granulocyte-colony stimulating factor (G-CSF) to prevent neutropenia in heavily pretreated patients.

II. POTENTIAL FOR ALTERED URINARY ELIMINATION related to NEPHROTOXICITY

Defining Characteristics: The drug does not have the renal toxicity seen with cisplatin (Platinol), so that only minimal hydration is needed. However, the drug is excreted by the kidneys, and concomitant treatment with drugs causing nephrotoxicity (i.e., aminoglycoside antibiotics) can alter renal function studies. Nephrotoxicity does occur at high doses, and patients with renal dysfunction are at risk. In addition, serum electrolyte loss can occur (K^+, Mg^{++}, rarely Ca^{++}). Monitor serum electrolytes prior to treatment and periodically after treatment. Replete electrolytes as ordered.

Nursing Implications: Assess renal function studies, (i.e., urine creatinine clearance, serum blood urea nitrogen [BUN], and creatinine) prior to drug administration. Discuss drug dose modification if creatinine clearance < 60 cc/min, or if other values are abnormal.

III. POTENTIAL FOR ALTERATION IN NUTRITION, LESS THAN BODY REQUIREMENTS, related to NAUSEA/VOMITING, ANOREXIA, STOMATITIS, DIARRHEA, AND HEPATIC DYSFUNCTION

Defining Characteristics: Nausea and vomiting begin 6+ hours after administration and last for < 24 hours, but may be easily prevented by available antiemetics. Anorexia occurs in 10% of patients but is usually mild, lasting 1–2 days. Diarrhea occurs in

10% of patients and is mild. Reversible hepatic dysfunction is mild to moderate, as evidenced by changes in alk phos and SGOT and, rarely, serum glutamic pyruvic transaminase (SGPT) and bili.

Nursing Implications: Premedicate with antiemetics and continue protection for 24 hours, at least for the first cycle. Encourage dietary modifications as needed. Monitor LFTs prior to and periodically during treatment.

IV. POTENTIAL FOR SENSORY/PERCEPTUAL ALTERATIONS related to NEUROLOGICAL CHANGES

Defining Characteristics: Neurologic dysfunction is infrequent, but there is increased risk in patients > 65 years old, or if previously treated with cisplatin and receiving prolonged carboplatin treatment.

Nursing Implications: Assess baseline neurologic status and continue to monitor status throughout treatment, looking for dizziness, confusion, peripheral neuropathy, ototoxicity, visual changes, and changes in taste. Teach patient the potential for side effects, and to report any changes.

V. POTENTIAL SEXUAL DYSFUNCTION related to DRUG EFFECTS

Defining Characteristics: Drug is mutagenic and probably teratogenic. It is unknown whether drug is excreted in breast milk.

Nursing Implications: Assess patient's signs/symptoms and partner's patterns of sexuality and reproductive goals. Teach patient/partner about need for contraception and provide other information as appropriate. Provide emotional support.

VI. POTENTIAL FOR INJURY related to HYPERSENSITIVITY REACTIONS

Defining Characteristics: Drug may cause allergic reactions, ranging from rash, urticaria, erythema, and pruritus to anaphylaxis; they can occur within minutes of drug administration.

Nursing Implications: Assess baseline VS. During drug administration, observe for signs/symptoms of hypersensitivity reaction. If signs/symptoms of anaphylaxis (tachycardia, wheezing, hypotension, facial edema) occur, stop drug immediately. Keep IV patent with 0.9% sodium chloride, notify physician, monitor VS, and be prepared to administer ordered drugs (i.e., steroid, epinephrine, or antihistamines).

Drug: carmustine (BCNU, BiCNU)

Class: Nitrosourea.

Mechanism of Action: Alkylates DNA by causing crosslinks and strand breaks in the same manner as classic mustard agents; it also carbamoylates cellular proteins, thus inhibiting DNA repair. Cell cycle phase nonspecific.

Metabolism: Rapidly distributed and metabolized with a plasma half-life of 1 hour; 70% of IV dose is excreted in urine within 96 hours. Significant concentrations of drug remain in cerebrospinal fluid for 9 hours due to lipid solubility of drug.

Dosage/Range:

Usual:
- 75 100 mg/m^2 IV/day × 2 day OR
- 150–200 mg/m^2 every 6 week OR
- 40 mg/m^2/day on 5 successive days, repeating cycle every 6–8 weeks.
- Polifeprosan 20 with carmustine (BCNU) implant: see "Polifeprosan."

High dose with autologous BMT (*investigational*):
- 450–600 mg/m^2 IV; however, doses of 900 mg/m^2 (in combination with cyclophosphamide) or 1200 mg/m^2 as single agent have been reported.
- These doses are fatal and require AUTOLOGOUS BMT after drug administration.
- Refer to protocol for exact dosages.

Drug Preparation:
- Add sterile alcohol (provided with drug) to vial, then add sterile water for injection.
- May be further diluted with 100–250 mL 5% dextrose or 0.9% sodium chloride.

High dose (*investigational*):
- IV bolus in at least 500 mL of 5% dextrose over 2 hours; can also divide dose into two equal fractions administered 12 hours apart. Refer to protocol for exact information.
- When given for gliomas as a single agent, administer with dexamethasone or mannitol infusion to reduce cerebral edema.
- Usually given in combination with other cytotoxic agents in BMT protocols.

Mycosis fungoides:
- Carmustine topical solution 0.5–3.0 mg/mL may be painted on body after showering, daily × 14 days (investigational).

Drug Interactions:
- Cimetidine may increase myelosuppression when given concurrently. AVOID IF POSSIBLE.
- Possible increased cellular uptake of drug when administered in combination with amphotericin B.
- Carmustine may decrease the pharmacologic effects of phenytoin.
- Avoid concomitant administration of renally or hepatically toxic drugs, as these may increase carmustine-induced renal or hepatic dysfunction.

Lab Effects/Interference:
- Pulmonary, hepatic, and renal function tests.

Special Considerations:
- Drug is an irritant; avoid extravasation.
- Pain at the injection site or along the vein is common. Treat by applying ice pack above the injection site and decreasing the infusion flow rate.
- Patient may act inebriated related to the alcohol diluent and may experience flushing.

High dose:
- Pulmonary toxicity related to higher systemic levels (higher AUC).

Potential Toxicities/Side Effects and the Nursing Process

I. POTENTIAL FOR INFECTION AND BLEEDING related to BONE MARROW DEPRESSION

Defining Characteristics: Delayed myelosuppression is dose-limiting toxicity and is cumulative. WBC nadir 3–5 weeks after dose and persists 1–2 weeks; platelet nadir at 4 weeks, persisting 1–2 weeks. Drug should not be dosed more frequently than once every 6 weeks.

Nursing Implications: Assess baseline CBC, WBC with differential, and platelet count prior to chemotherapy and at least weekly postchemotherapy for the first cycle. Discuss dose reductions with physician for subsequent cycles if counts are lower than normal since bone marrow depression is cumulative. Teach patient and family self-assessment for signs/symptoms of infection and bleeding, and instruct to report them immediately. Teach self-care measures to minimize risk of infection and bleeding, including avoidance of aspirin-containing medicines.

II. POTENTIAL FOR IMPAIRED GAS EXCHANGE related to PULMONARY FIBROSIS

Defining Characteristics: Pulmonary toxicity appears to be dose-related, with risk greatest in patients receiving total doses > 1400 mg (although it can occur at lower doses). Other risk factors include patients with abnormal PFTs prior to drug administration; i.e., baseline forced vital capacity (FVC) < 70% of predicted; carbon monoxide diffusion capacity (DLCO) < 70% of predicted; or if patient is receiving concurrent cyclophosphamide or thoracic radiation. Presents as insidious cough and dyspnea, or may be the sudden onset of respiratory failure. CXR shows interstitial infiltrates. Incidence is 20–30% of patients, with a mortality of 24–80%.

Nursing Implications: Assess patient's risk and baseline pulmonary function prior to chemotherapy, as well as the results of pulmonary function testing periodically during treatment, for evidence of pulmonary dysfunction. Teach patient to report any changes in respiratory pattern.

III. ALTERATION IN NUTRITION, LESS THAN BODY REQUIREMENTS, related to NAUSEA/VOMITING AND LIVER DYSFUNCTION

Defining Characteristics: Severe nausea and vomiting may occur 2 hours after administration and last 4–6 hours. Reversible liver dysfunction, although rare, is related to subacute hepatitis and is characterized by abnormal LFTs, painless jaundice, and (rarely) coma.

Nursing Implications: Premedicate with antiemetics and continue antiemetic protection for 24 hours, at least for the first treatment. Encourage small, frequent feedings of cool, bland foods, and liquids. Infuse drug over 60–120 minutes. Monitor LFTs (SGOT, SGPT, lactic dehydrogenase [LDH], alk phos, bili) during treatment and discuss any abnormalities with physician.

IV. ALTERATION IN COMFORT related to DRUG ADMINISTRATION

Defining Characteristics: Drug diluent is absolute alcohol, so irritation may result in pain along the vein path. Thrombosis is rare, but venospasms and flushing of skin or burning of the eyes can occur with rapid drug infusion.

Nursing Implications: Administer drug only through patent IV and dilute drug in 250 mL of 5% dextrose or 0.9% sodium chloride and infuse over 1–2 hours. If pain along vein occurs, use ice packs above injection site, decrease infusion rate, or further dilute drug. If patient will receive ongoing therapy, consider venous access device.

V. ALTERED URINARY ELIMINATION related to NEPHROTOXICITY

Defining Characteristics: Increase in BUN occurs in 10% of patients and is usually reversible. However, decreased kidney size, progressive azotemia, and renal failure have occurred in patients receiving large cumulative doses over long periods.

Nursing Implications: Assess baseline renal function and monitor BUN and creatinine prior to each successive cycle. Since drug is excreted by the kidneys, drug dosage should be reduced if renal dysfunction exists. If abnormalities occur and persist, discuss discontinuing drug with physician.

VI. POTENTIAL SEXUAL DYSFUNCTION related to DRUG EFFECTS

Defining Characteristics: Drug is mutagenic and teratogenic.

Nursing Implications: Assess patient's and partner's pattern of sexuality and reproductive goals. Teach patient and partner the need for contraception as appropriate. Provide emotional support and counseling, or referral as appropriate.

VII. SENSORY/PERCEPTUAL ALTERATIONS related to OCULAR TOXICITY

Defining Characteristics: Infarcts of optic nerve fiber, retinal hemorrhage, and neuroretinitis have been associated with high-dose therapy.

Nursing Implications: Assess baseline vision and appearance of eyes. Instruct patient to report any visual changes to physician or nurse.

Drug: chlorambucil (Leukeran)

Class: Alkylating agent.

Mechanism of Action: Alkylates DNA by causing strand breaks and crosslinks in the DNA. The drug is a derivative of a nitrogen mustard.

Metabolism: Pharmacokinetics are poorly understood. It is well absorbed orally, with a plasma half-life of 1.5 hours. Degradation is slow; it appears to be eliminated by metabolic transformation, with 60% excreted in urine in 24 hours.

Dosage/Range:
- 0.1–0.2 mg/kg/day (equals 4–8 mg/m^2/day) to initiate treatment for 3–6 week OR
- 14 mg/m^2/day × 5 days with a repeat every 21–28 days, depending on platelet count and WBC.

Drug Preparation:
- 2-mg tablets.

Drug Administration:
- Oral.

Drug Interactions:
- None significant.
- Simultaneous administration of barbiturates may increase toxicity of chlorambucil due to hepatic drug activation.

Lab Effects/Interference:
- BUN, uric acid.
- LFTs, especially alk phos and AST (SGOT).
- CBC, especially WBC with differential.

Special Considerations:

- None.

Potential Toxicities/Side Effects and the Nursing Process

I. POTENTIAL FOR INFECTION related to BONE MARROW DEPRESSION

Defining Characteristics: Neutropenia after third week of treatment lasting for 10 days after the last dose. Neutropenia and thrombocytopenia occur with prolonged use and may be irreversible occasionally (especially if high total doses are given; i.e., > 6.5 mg/kg). Increased toxicity may occur with prior barbiturate use.

Nursing Implications: Assess baseline CBC, including WBC with differential, and platelet count prior to dosing, as well as weekly for the first cycle of therapy. Discuss dose reduction with physician if blood values are abnormal. Teach patient self-assessment of signs/symptoms of infection and bleeding and instruct to report them immediately. Teach self-care measures to minimize risk of infection and bleeding, including avoidance of OTC aspirin-containing medications.

II. POTENTIAL FOR SEXUAL DYSFUNCTION related to REPRODUCTIVE HAZARD

Defining Characteristics: Drug is mutagenic, teratogenic, and suppresses gonadal function with consequent temporary or permanent sterility. Amenorrhea occurs in females, and oligospermia/azoospermia occurs in males.

Nursing Implications: Assess patient's and partner's sexual patterns and reproductive goals. Provide teaching and emotional support; encourage birth control measures as appropriate.

III. POTENTIAL FOR ALTERATION IN NUTRITION, LESS THAN BODY REQUIREMENTS, related to NAUSEA/VOMITING, ANOREXIA/WEIGHT LOSS, AND HEPATIC DYSFUNCTION

Defining Characteristics: Nausea and vomiting are rare. Anorexia and weight loss may occur and be prolonged. Hepatotoxicity with jaundice is rare, but abnormal LFTs may occur.

Nursing Implications: Administer antiemetics as needed and instruct patient in self-administration. Suggest weekly weights and dietary instruction if patient develops anorexia and weight loss. Monitor LFTs baseline and periodically during treatment. Discuss any abnormalities with physician and consider dose modification.

IV. POTENTIAL FOR IMPAIRED GAS EXCHANGE related to PULMONARY FIBROSIS

Defining Characteristics: Bronchopulmonary dysplasia and pulmonary fibrosis may occur rarely with long-term use.

Nursing Implications: Assess patients at risk: increased risk with cumulative dose > 1 g/m^2, preexisting lung disease, concurrent treatment with cyclophosphamide or thoracic radiation. Assess pulmonary status prior to chemotherapy and at each visit, notifying physician of dyspnea. Monitor PFTs periodically for evidence of pulmonary dysfunction. Teach patient to report any changes in pulmonary pattern, such as dyspnea.

V. POTENTIAL FOR SENSORY/PERCEPTUAL ALTERATIONS related to OCULAR DISTURBANCES, CNS ABNORMALITIES

Defining Characteristics: Ocular disturbances may occur, e.g., diplopia, papilledema, retinal hemorrhage. Tremors, muscular twitching, confusion, agitation, ataxia, flaccid paresis, and hallucinations have been described. Seizures, although uncommon, have occurred in adults and children during normal dosing, as well as with overdosing.

Nursing Implications: Assess baseline neurologic status prior to treatment and at each visit. Instruct patient to report any abnormalities.

Drug: cisplatin (Platinol)

Class: Heavy metal that acts like alkylating agent.

Mechanism of Action: Inhibits DNA synthesis by forming inter- and intrastrand crosslinks and by denaturing the double helix, preventing cell replication. Cell cycle phase nonspecific; the chemical properties are similar to those of bifunctional alkylating agents.

Metabolism: Rapidly distributed to tissues (predominately the liver and kidneys) with less than 10% in the plasma 1 hour after infusion. Clearance from plasma proceeds slowly after the first 2 hours due to platinum's covalent bonding with serum proteins; 20–74% of administered drug is excreted in the urine within 24 hours.

Dosage/Range:
- 50–100 mg/m^2 every 3–4 weeks, OR
- 15–30 mg/m^2 × 5 repeated every 3–4 weeks.
- Radiosensitizing effect: Administer 1–3 times per week at doses of 15–50 mg/m^2 (total weekly dose 50 mg/m^2) with concomitant radiotherapy.
- Intraperitoneal: 100 mg/m^2 every 3 weeks for ovarian cancer.

Drug Preparation:

- 10-mg and 50-mg vials. Add sterile water to develop a concentration of 1 mg/mL.
- Further dilute solution with 250 mL or more of 0.9% sodium chloride (recommended) or 5% dextrose (D_5 ½ NS) sodium chloride.
- Never mix with 5% dextrose, as a precipitate will form. Drug stability increased in 0.9% sodium chloride.
- Available as an aqueous solution.
- Do not refrigerate.

Drug Administration:

- Avoid aluminum needles when administering, as precipitate will form.

Drug Interactions:

- Decreases pharmacologic effect of phenytoin, so dose may need to be increased.
- Possible increase in ototoxicity when combined with loop diuretics.
- Increased renal toxicity with concurrent use of aminoglycosides, amphotericin B.
- Cisplatin reduces drug clearance of high-dose methotrexate (MTX) and standard-dose bleomycin by increasing the drugs' half-life; enhances toxicity of ifosfamide (myelosuppression) and etoposide.
- Synergy when cisplatin is combined with etoposide.
- Radiosensitizing effect.
- Sodium thiosulfate and mesna: Each directly inactivates cisplatin.
- Taxanes: Administer cisplatin *after* taxanes (paclitaxel, docetaxel) to prevent delayed taxane excretion with subsequent increased bone marrow depression.

Lab Effects/Interference:

- Decreased M, Ca, phos.
- Increased creatinine, uric acid.

Special Considerations:

- Administer cautiously, if at all, to patients with renal dysfunction, hearing impairment, peripheral neuropathy, or prior allergic reaction to cisplatin.
- Hydrate vigorously before and after administering drug. Urine output should be at least 100–150 mL/hour. Mannitol or furosemide diuresis may be needed to ensure this output.
- Hypersensitivity reactions have occurred, manifested by wheezing, flushing, hypotension, tachycardia. Usually occurs within minutes of starting infusion. Treat with epinephrine, corticosteroids, antihistamines.
- Drug causes potassium and magnesium wasting. Some ideas to help increase magnesium follow.

  To help increase absorption, it is recommended that excessive milk, cheese, or other high-calcium products be limited when eating foods high in magnesium. Calcium and magnesium compete to gain entrance to the body in the intestines, so a high-calcium

diet increases requirements for dietary magnesium. Foods high in magnesium are those with 100 mg or greater per 100 grams, including:
Nuts:
Almonds
Brazil nuts
Cashews
Peanut butter
Peanuts
Pecans
Walnuts
Peas and beans:
Red beans
Split peas
White beans
Other good sources:
Blackstrap molasses
Brewer's yeast
Chocolate (bitter)
Cocoa (dry breakfast)
Cornmeal
Instant coffee and tea
Oatmeal
Shredded wheat
Wheat germ
Whole wheat breads and cereals

- Phase I studies are ongoing, evaluating an oral platinum (JM-216) agent in small-cell lung cancer.
- Amifostine has been shown to be renally protective in patients at risk for renal toxicity from cisplatin; in addition, drug offers protection from neurotoxicity. Other agents being studied, e.g., BNP7787.

Potential Toxicities/Side Effects and the Nursing Process

I. POTENTIAL ALTERATION IN URINARY ELIMINATION related to DRUG-INDUCED RENAL DAMAGE

Defining Characteristics: Dose-limiting toxicity, which may be cumulative. The drug accumulates in the kidneys, causing necrosis of proximal and distal renal tubules. Damage to renal tubules prevents reabsorption of Mg^{++}, Ca^{++}, and K^{+}, with resultant decreased serum levels. Renal damage becomes most obvious 10–20 days after treatment, is reversible, and can be prevented by adequate hydration and diuresis, as well as slower infusion time. Hyperuricemia may occur due to impaired tubular transport of uric acid, but it is responsive to allopurinol. Concurrent administration of nephrotoxic agents is not recommended.

Nursing Implications: Assess renal function studies prior to administration (BUN, creatinine, 24-hour creatinine clearance) and discuss any abnormalities with physician. Assess cardiac and pulmonary status in terms of tolerance of aggressive hydration. Anticipate vigorous hydration regimen with or without forced diuresis (i.e., mannitol, lasix). The typical hydration schedule is 0.9% sodium chloride or D_5 ½ NS at 250 mL/hr × 3–5 hours prechemotherapy and 3–5 hours postchemotherapy (total hydration 3 L). Outpatient hydration of 1–2 L over 1–2 hours prechemotherapy and 1 L postchemotherapy, is typical. Strictly monitor I/O and total body fluid balance. Assess for signs/symptoms of fluid overload and notify physician for supplemental furosemide or other diuretic as needed. Monitor serum electrolytes (Na+, K+, Mg++, Ca++, PO_4) and replete as ordered by physician. Teach patient and family the need for increased oral fluids on discharge—up to 3 L or more for 5 days posttherapy.

II. ALTERATION IN NUTRITION, LESS THAN BODY REQUIREMENTS, related to SEVERE NAUSEA AND VOMITING, TASTE ALTERATIONS

Defining Characteristics: Nausea and vomiting may be severe and will occur in 100% of patients if antiemetics are not given. They begin 1 or more hours postchemotherapy and last 8–24 hours. Since the drug is slowly excreted over five days, delayed nausea and vomiting may occur 24–72 hours after dose. Taste alterations and anorexia occur with long-term use.

Nursing Implications: Premedicate with combination antiemetics (i.e., serotonin antagonist plus dexamethasone), especially for high-dose cisplatin, and continue antiemetics for up to five days with dopamine antagonist. Encourage small, frequent intake of cool, bland foods as tolerated. Infuse cisplatin over at least 1 hour to minimize emesis, since slower infusion rates decrease emesis. Taste alterations may be improved with the use of spices and zinc dietary supplementation. Refer the patient for dietary consultation as needed.

III. POTENTIAL FOR INJURY related to ANAPHYLAXIS

Defining Characteristics: Anaphylaxis has occurred, characterized by wheezing, bronchoconstriction, tachycardia, hypotension, and facial edema, in patients who have previously received the drug.

Nursing Implications: Assess baseline VS and continue to assess patient during infusion. Prior to drug administration, review standing orders or protocols for nursing management of anaphylaxis: stop infusion; keep line open with 0.9% sodium chloride; notify physician; monitor VS; be prepared to administer epinephrine, antihistamines, corticosteroids.

IV. POTENTIAL FOR SENSORY/PERCEPTUAL ALTERATIONS related to NEUROLOGIC TOXICITY

Defining Characteristics: Severe neuropathy may occur in patients receiving high doses or prolonged treatment and may be irreversible, and is seen in stocking-and-glove distribution, with numbness, tingling, and sensory loss in arms and legs. Areflexia, loss of proprioception and vibratory sense, and loss of motor function can occur. Ototoxicity, beginning with loss of high-frequency hearing, affects > 30% of patients. It may be preceded by tinnitus, is dose related, and can be unilateral or bilateral. The damage results from destruction of hair cells lining the organ of Corti and is cumulative and may be permanent. Rarely, ocular toxicity has occurred, but it is reversible (optic neuritis, papilledema, cerebral blindness).

Nursing Implications: Assess baseline neurologic, motor, and sensory functions prior to drug administration. Discuss use of neuroprotector in high-risk patients. Discuss baseline audiogram with physician as appropriate. Instruct patient to report changes in function or sensation, as well as diminished hearing. Discuss with physician risks vs benefits of continuing therapy if/when symptoms develop. If severe neuropathies develop, provide teaching related to activity, emotional support, and referral to physical/occupational therapy as appropriate. Discuss use of neuroprotector in high-risk patients.

V. POTENTIAL FOR ACTIVITY INTOLERANCE related to ANEMIA

Defining Characteristics: Drug may interfere with renal erythropoietin production, resulting in late development of anemia.

Nursing Implications: Teach patient to report increasing fatigue, signs of severe anemia (shortness of breath, chest pain/angina, headaches). Monitor hemoglobin/hematocrit; discuss transfusion with physician if signs/symptoms develop or hematocrit falls < 25 mg/dL. Teach patient about diet high in iron. Exogenous erythropoietin (epoetin alpha) may be helpful.

VI. INFECTION AND BLEEDING related to BONE MARROW DEPRESSION

Defining Characteristics: Bone marrow depression is mild with low to moderate doses, but may be significant when high doses are used, or when drug is given in combination with radiation as a radiation-sensitizer. Nadir is in 2–3 weeks, with recovery in 4–5 weeks.

Nursing Implications: Assess CBC, WBC, differential, and platelet count, as well as any signs/symptoms of infection or bleeding, prior to drug administration. Teach patient to self-assess for signs/symptoms of infection and bleeding. Teach self-care measures to minimize infection and bleeding, including avoidance of aspirin-containing medications.

VII. POTENTIAL SEXUAL DYSFUNCTION related to DRUG EFFECTS

Defining Characteristics: Drug is mutagenic and probably teratogenic.

Nursing Implications: Assess patient's and partner's sexual patterns and reproductive goals. Provide emotional support and discuss strategies to preserve sexual and reproductive health (i.e., contraception and sperm banking).

VIII. POTENTIAL FOR ALTERATIONS IN CARDIOVASCULAR FUNCTION related to CISPLATIN-CONTAINING COMBINATION CHEMOTHERAPY

Defining Characteristics: Angina, myocardial infarction, cerebrovascular accident, thrombotic microangiopathy, cerebral arteritis, and Raynaud's phenomenon have occurred, although they are uncommon. Combination drugs include bleomycin, vinblastine, vincristine, and etoposide.

Nursing Implications: Assess cardiopulmonary status, especially if patient has pre-existing cardiac disease, both prior to and throughout treatment.

Drug: cladribine (Leustatin, 2-CdA)

Class: Antimetabolite.

Mechanism of Action: Selectively damages normal and malignant lymphocytes and monocytes that have large amounts of deoxycytidine kinase but small amounts of deoxynucleotidase. The drug, a chlorinated purine nucleoside, enters passively through the cell membrane, is phosphorylated into the active metabolite 2-CdATP, and accumulates in the cell. 2-CdATP interferes with DNA synthesis and prevents repair of DNA strand breaks in both actively dividing and normal cells. The process may also involve programmed cell death (apoptosis).

Metabolism: Drug is 20% protein-bound and is cleared from the plasma within 1–3 days after cessation of treatment.

Dosage/Range:

- 0.09 mg/kg/day IV as a continuous infusion for 7 days for one course of therapy of hairy-cell leukemia.

Drug Preparation:

- Available in 10 mg/10 mL preservative-free, single-use vials (1 mg/mL), which must be further diluted in 0.9% sodium chloride injection. Diluted drug stable at room

temperature for at least 24 hours in normal light. Once prepared, the solution may be refrigerated up to 8 hours prior to use.
- Single daily dose: add calculated drug dose to 500 mL of 0.9% sodium chloride injection, and administer over 24 hours; repeat daily for a total of 7 days.
- 7-day continuous infusion by ambulatory infusion pump: add calculated drug dose for 7 days to infusion reservoir using a sterile 0.22-μm hydrophilic syringe filter. Then add, again using 0.22-μm filter, sufficient sterile bacteriostatic 0.9% sodium chloride injection containing 0.9% benzyl alcohol to produce 100 mL in the infusion reservoir.
- Do not use 5% dextrose, as it accelerates degradation of drug.

Drug Administration:
- Dilute in minimum of 100 mL.
- Administer as continuous infusion over 24 hours for 7 days.

Drug Interactions:
- Bone marrow-suppressing drugs: increased bone marrow suppression.

Lab Effects/Interference:
- Decreased CBC, platelets.
- Increased LFTs, RFTs.

Special Considerations:
- Indicated for the treatment of active hairy-cell leukemia.
- Unstable in 5% dextrose; should not be used as diluent or infusion fluid.
- Store unopened vials in refrigerator and protect from light.
- Drug may precipitate when exposed to low temperatures. Allow solution to warm to room temperature and shake vigorously. DO NOT HEAT OR MICROWAVE.
- Drug is structurally similar to pentostatin and fludarabine.
- Contraindicated in patients who are hypersensitive to the drug.
- Administer with caution in patients with renal or hepatic insufficiency.
- Embryotoxic; women of childbearing age should use contraception.

Potential Toxicities/Side Effects and the Nursing Process

I. INFECTION AND BLEEDING related to BONE MARROW DEPRESSION

Defining Characteristics: Neutropenia occurs in 70% of patients with nadir 1–2 weeks after infusion, recovery by weeks 4–5. Incidence of infection 28%, with 40% caused by bacterial infection of lungs and venous access sites. Prolonged hypocellularity of bone marrow occurs in 34% of patients, and may last for at least four months. Infections most common in patients with pancytopenia and lymphopenia due to hairy-cell leukemia. Lymphopenia is common with decreased CD4 (helper T-cells) and CD8 (suppressor T-cells), with recovery by weeks 26–34. Common infectious agents are viral (20%)

and fungal (20%). Thrombocytopenia occurs commonly, along with purpura (10%), petechiae (8%), and epistaxis (5%). Platelet recovery occurs by day 12, but 14% of patients require platelet support.

Nursing Implications: Monitor CBC, platelet count prior to therapy, and periodically posttherapy at expected time of nadir. Monitor for, and teach patient self-assessment of signs/symptoms of infection, bleeding. Instruct patient to call physician or nurse or go to emergency room if temperature (T) is greater than 101°F (38.3°C) or bleeding. Transfuse platelets per physician order.

II. ALTERATION IN COMFORT related to FEVER, HEADACHES

Defining Characteristics: Fever (> 100°F [37.5°C]) occurs in 66% of patients during the month following treatment due either to infection (47%) or the release of endogenous pyrogen from lysed lymphocytes. Other symptoms include chills (9%), diaphoresis (9%), malaise (7%), dizziness (9%), insomnia (7%), myalgia (7%), arthralgias (5%). Headaches occur in 22% of patients.

Nursing Implications: Assess patient for fever, chills, diaphoresis during visits; assess signs/symptoms of infection. Teach patient self-assessment, how to report this, and measures to reduce fever. Anticipate laboratory and X-ray tests to rule out infection and perform according to physician order.

III. POTENTIAL IMPAIRMENT OF SKIN INTEGRITY related to RASH

Defining Characteristics: Rash occurs in 27–50% of patients. Other symptoms include pruritus (6%), erythema (6%), injection site reactions (erythema, swelling, pain, phlebitis).

Nursing Implications: Assess skin for any cutaneous changes, such as rash or changes at injection site, and any associated symptoms such as pruritus; discuss with physician. Instruct patient in self-care measures, including avoiding abrasive skin products and clothing; avoiding tight-fitting clothing; use of skin emollients appropriate to specific skin alteration; measures to avoid scratching involved areas. Consider venous access device if skin is at risk for reaction.

IV. FATIGUE related to ANEMIA

Defining Characteristics: Fatigue occurs in 45% of patients. Red cell recovery is by week 8, but 40% of patients require red cell transfusion.

Nursing Implications: Monitor Hgb and HCT and transfuse per physician order. Administer erythropoietin per physician order and teach patient self-administration.

Teach patient about diet and instruct to alternate rest and activity; stress reduction/relaxation techniques may improve energy level.

V. ALTERATION IN ELIMINATION related to DIARRHEA, CONSTIPATION

Defining Characteristics: Diarrhea occurs in 10% of patients while constipation occurs in 9%. Abdominal pain affects 6% of patients.

Nursing Implications: Encourage patient to report onset of change in bowel habits (diarrhea or constipation) and assess factors contributing to changes. Administer or teach patient self-administration of antidiarrheal medication or cathartic as ordered. Teach patient diet modification regarding foods that minimize diarrhea or constipation.

VI. POTENTIAL FOR IMPAIRED GAS EXCHANGE related to COUGH

Defining Characteristics: Cough affects 10%, while abnormal breath sounds occur in 11% and shortness of breath in 7%.

Nursing Implications: Assess baseline pulmonary status, including breath sounds, presence of cough, shortness of breath. Instruct patient to report symptoms of cough, shortness of breath, other abnormalities.

VII. ALTERATION IN NUTRITION, LESS THAN BODY REQUIREMENTS, related to NAUSEA, VOMITING

Defining Characteristics: Nausea is mild and occurs in 28% of patients, while vomiting may occur in 13%. If antiemetics are required, nausea/vomiting is easily controlled by phenothiazines. Renal and hepatic function studies are rarely affected.

Nursing Implications: Premedicate with antiemetics. If nausea and/or vomiting occur, teach patient to self-administer antiemetics per physician order. Encourage small, frequent feedings of cool, bland foods and liquids. Teach patient to record diet history for 2–3 days and weekly weights. If patient has decreased appetite, assess food preferences (encourage or discourage) and suggest use of spices.

VIII. POTENTIAL ALTERATION IN CARDIAC OUTPUT related to TACHYCARDIA

Defining Characteristics: Occurs rarely, with edema and tachycardia each affecting 6% of patients.

Nursing Implications: Assess baseline cardiac status, including apical heart rate, presence of peripheral edema. Instruct patient to report rapid heartbeat or swelling of ankles.

Drug: clofarabine (Clolar)

Class: Purine nucleoside anti-metabolite.

Mechanism of Action: Drug inhibits DNA and DNA repair, causing cell death of both cycling and quiescent cancer cells. In addition, it breaks down the mitochondrial membranes, releasing cytochrome C and apoptosis-inducing factor, leading to programmed cell death.

Metabolism: Drug is 47% protein bound (mostly to albumin), with a terminal half-life of 5.2 hours. 49–60% of the dose is excreted unchanged in the urine. Other non-renal excretion is unknown.

Dosage/Range: 52 mg/m^2 IV over 2 hr daily × 5, to be repeated after recovery of all baseline organ function, about q 2–6 weeks. IV hydration should be continued during the 5 days of treatment.

Drug Preparation: Drug is supplied as a 20 mg in 20 mL vial. Withdraw drug using a sterile 0.2 μm syringe filter and then further dilute with 5% dextrose injection USP or 0.9% sodium chloride injection USP prior to IV infusion. This admixture may be stored at room temperature but must be used within 24 hr of preparation.

Drug Administration: Administer IV over 2 hours; if hyperuricemia (tumor lysis syndrome), patient should receive allopurinol, and may need urine alkalinization and aggressive hydration as well.

Drug Interactions: Concurrent administration with other renally cleared drugs may alter drug levels so should be avoided during the 5 days of treatment; avoid other hepatotoxic drugs, as well as those affecting blood pressure or cardiac function if possible during drug administration.

Lab Effects/Interference: Severe bone marrow depression with decreased white blood cells, neutrophils, red blood cells, and platelets. Drug may cause tumor lysis syndrome with increased levels of potassium, phosphate, uric acid, creatinine, and changes in other electrolyte values. Renal and hepatic function studies should be monitored during the 5 days of drug treatment.

Special Considerations:

- Drug is indicated for the treatment of pediatric patients aged 1–21 years old with relapsed or refractory acute lymphoblastic leukemia after at least 2 prior regimens.
- Treatment results in the rapid lysis of peripheral leukemia cells.

- Drug is fetotoxic so all patients should be taught to use effective contraceptive measures to prevent pregnancy; female patients should be taught not to breast-feed during treatment.
- Drug may cause dehydration, hypotension, capillary leak syndrome.

Potential Toxicities/Side Effects and the Nursing Process

I. INFECTION AND BLEEDING related to BONE MARROW DEPRESSION

Defining Characteristics: Bone marrow depression is dose limiting. Febrile neutropenia occurs in 57% of patients. Pyrexia affects 41% of patients, while 38% experience rigors. Infections include bacteremia, cellulites, herpes simplex, oral candidiasis, pneumonia, sepsis, and staphylococcal infections.

Nursing Implications: Assess WBC, neutrophil, and platelet count, and discuss any abnormalities with physician prior to drug administration; assess for signs/symptoms of skin infections (all mucosal surfaces, body orifices) and bleeding; instruct patient in signs/symptoms of infection and bleeding, as well as to report them or come to emergency room. Teach patient self-care measures to minimize risk of infection and bleeding, including avoidance of OTC aspirin-containing medications. Assess patient's Hgb/HCT and signs/symptoms of fatigue; teach patient self-assessment and to alternate rest and activity as needed.

II. ALTERED NUTRITION, LESS THAN BODY REQUIREMENTS, related to NAUSEA AND VOMITING, ANOREXIA, DIARRHEA, and HEPATOTOXICITY

Defining Characteristics: Nausea and vomiting occur in 75% and 83% of patients, respectively, and can be successfully prevented with combination antiemetics. Anorexia occurs in about 1/3 of patients. Diarrhea is frequent, affecting about 50% of patients. Constipation affects 21% of patients. Hepatotoxicity and jaundice occur in 15% of patients.

Nursing Implications: Premedicate with antiemetics depending on dose, using aggressive, combination antiemetics, and continue throughout chemotherapy. If patient develops nausea/vomiting, assess fluid and electrolyte balance and the need for replacements. Assess oral mucosa prior to chemotherapy and teach patient oral hygiene regimen and self-assessment; encourage patient to report diarrhea, discuss use of antidiarrheals with physician, and teach self-care PRN. Because patients become neutropenic, all mucosal surfaces need to be assessed for infection, and patients must be taught scrupulous perineal hygiene. Monitor LFTs prior to, during, and posttherapy.

III. IMPAIRED SKIN/MUCOSAL INTEGRITY related to RASH, ANAL INFLAMMATION/ULCERATION, ALOPECIA

Defining Characteristics: Maculopapular rash, with or without fever, myalgia, bone pain, occasional chest pain, conjunctivitis, and malaise (cytarabine syndrome) may occur. Syndrome is not common, but occurs 6–12 hours after drug administration; corticosteroids have been helpful in treating/preventing syndrome. Mucosal inflammation and ulceration of anus/rectum may occur, especially in patients with prior hemorrhoids or history of abscesses. Alopecia occurs less frequently.

Nursing Implications: Assess baseline skin and mucous membranes prior to chemotherapy and identify patients at risk for problems. Consider including corticosteroid in antiemetic regimen, especially for high-dose therapy, and discuss with physician prophylactic use of dexamethasone eye drops to prevent conjunctivitis. Teach patient scrupulous perineal hygiene, instruct to report any rectal discomfort, and assess rectal mucosa daily with high-dose therapy. Discuss with patient potential coping strategies if alopecia occurs (i.e., wig, scarves).

IV. ALTERATION IN COMFORT, POTENTIAL, related to EDEMA, FATIGUE, LETHARGY, PAIN

Defining Characteristics: In clinical studies, the frequency of occurrence of these symptoms was: edema 20%, fatigue 36%, injection site pain 14%, pain 19%, arthralgia 11%, back pain 13%, myalgia 14%, pain in limb 29%, dermatitis 41%, erythema 18%, pruritus 47%, palmar plantar erythrodysesthesia syndrome (PPE) 13%, and flushing 18%.

Nursing Implications: Teach patient that these symptoms may occur and to report them. Teach patient self-care measures to reduce discomfort, such as application of heat or cold for pain, arthralgias and myalgias. Teach patient to report redness and pain on palms of hands or soles of feet as this may be PPE, and would require close monitoring and follow-up to prevent moist desquamation. Instruct patient to report any symptoms that do not resolve or improve with self-care measures.

Drug: cyclophosphamide (Cytoxan)

Class: Alkylating agent.

Mechanism of Action: Causes cross-linkage in DNA strands, thus preventing DNA synthesis and cell division. Cell cycle phase nonspecific.

Metabolism: Inactive until converted by microsomes in liver and serum enzymes (phosphamidases). Both cyclophosphamide and its metabolites are excreted by the kidneys.

Plasma half-life: 6–12 hours, with 25% of drug excreted after 8 hours. Prolonged plasma half-life in patients with renal failure results in increased myelosuppression.

Dosage/Range:

- 400 mg/m^2 IV × 5 days.
- 100 mg/m^2 PO × 14 days every 4 weeks.
- 500–1500 mg/m^2 IV every 3–4 weeks.

High dose with BMT (*investigational*):

- 1.8–7 gm/m^2 in combination with other cytotoxic agents.

Drug Preparation:

- Available in 25- and 50-mg tablets; powder for injection: 100-mg, 200-mg, 500-mg, 1-g, and 2-g vials.
- Dilute vials with sterile water. Shake well. Allow solution to clear if lyophilized preparation is not used. Do not use solution unless crystals are fully dissolved.

Drug Administration:

- Oral use: Administer in morning or early afternoon to allow adequate excretion time. Should be taken with meals.
- IV use: For doses > 500 mg, pre- and posthydration to total 500–3000 mL is needed to ensure adequate urine output and to avoid hemorrhagic cystitis. Administer drug over at least 20 minutes for doses > 500 mg.
- Mesna given with high-dose cyclophosphamide to prevent hemorrhagic cystitis.
- Solution is stable for 24 hours at room temperature, 6 days if refrigerated.
- Rapid infusion may result in dizziness, nasal stuffiness, rhinorrhea, sinus congestion during or soon after infusion.

Drug Interactions:

- Increases chloramphenicol half-life.
- Increases duration of leukopenia when given in combination with thiazide diuretics.
- Increases effect of anticoagulant drugs.
- Decreases digoxin level, so dose may need to be increased.
- Potentiation of doxorubicin-induced cardiomyopathy.
- Increased succinylcholine action with prolonged neuromuscular blockage.
- Increased drug action of barbiturates; induction of hepatic microsomes.

Lab Effects/Interference:

- Increased K, uric acid secondary to tumor lysis.
- Monitor electrolytes for symptoms of SIADH.
- Decreased CBC, platelets.

Special Considerations:

- Metabolic and leukopenic toxicity is increased by simultaneous administration of barbiturates, corticosteroids, phenytoin, and sulfonamides.
- Activity and toxicity of both cyclophosphamide and the specific drug may be altered by allopurinol, chloroquine, phenothiazides, potassium iodide, chloramphenicol, imipramine, vitamin A, warfarin, succinylcholine, digoxin, thiazide diuretics.

- Test urine for occult blood.
- High-dose cyclophosphamide therapy may require catheterization and constant bladder irrigation. Mesna should be given, either as a continuous infusion or in bolus doses, around drug administration. Consult protocol. See Chapter 4.
- Monitor patients with hepatic dysfunction closely for toxicity.

Potential Toxicities/Side Effects and the Nursing Process

I. INFECTION AND BLEEDING related to BONE MARROW DEPRESSION

Defining Characteristics: Leukopenia nadir occurs days 7–14, with recovery in 1–2 weeks; thrombocytopenia is less frequent and anemia is mild. Drug is a potent immunosuppressant.

Nursing Implications: Assess CBC, WBC with differential, platelet count, and signs/symptoms of infection and bleeding prior to treatment. Teach patient signs/symptoms of infection and instruct to report them if they occur. Teach patient self-care measures to minimize infection and bleeding. Increased risk of bone marrow depression in patients with prior radiation or chemotherapy.

II. ALTERED URINARY ELIMINATION related to HEMORRHAGIC CYSTITIS

Defining Characteristics: Metabolites of drug, if allowed to accumulate in the bladder, irritate bladder wall capillaries, causing hemorrhagic cystitis. This occurs in 7–40% of patients, is evidenced by microscopic or gross hematuria, is common with high doses, and is preventable. Long-term drug exposure may lead to bladder fibrosis.

Nursing Implications: Monitor BUN and creatinine prior to drug dose and as drug is excreted by the kidneys. Assess for signs/symptoms of hematuria, urinary frequency, or dysuria; instruct patient to report these if they occur. Instruct patient to take in at least 3 L of fluid per day and to empty bladder every 2–3 hours, as well as at bedtime. If patient is receiving a high dose, ensure vigorous hydration prior to drug administration. Bladder irrigation per protocol. Instruct patient to take oral cyclophosphamide early in the day to prevent drug accumulation in bladder during the night.

III. ALTERATION IN NUTRITION, LESS THAN BODY REQUIREMENTS, related to NAUSEA AND VOMITING, ANOREXIA, STOMATITIS, DIARRHEA, AND HEPATOTOXICITY

Defining Characteristics: Nausea and vomiting are dose-related and begin 2–4 hours after dose, peak in 12 hours, and may last 24 hours. Anorexia is common; stomatitis, if it occurs, is mild; and diarrhea is mild and infrequent. Hepatotoxicity is rare.

Nursing Implications: Premedicate with antiemetics prior to drug administration and continue prophylactically for 24 hours, at least for the first cycle. Encourage small feedings of bland foods and liquids. Encourage favorite foods and consult dietitian regarding anorexia if needed. Assess oral mucosa prior to drug administration; teach patient self-assessment techniques and oral care. Monitor LFTs before, during, and after therapy.

IV. ALTERED BODY IMAGE related to ALOPECIA, CHANGES IN NAILS AND SKIN

Defining Characteristics: Alopecia occurs in 30–50% of patients, especially with IV dosing, but some degree of hair loss occurs in all patients. Hair loss begins after 3+ weeks; hair may grow back while on therapy, but will grow back after therapy is discontinued (may be softer in texture). Hyperpigmentation of nails and skin, as well as transverse ridging of nails (banding), may occur.

Nursing Implications: Teach patient about potential hair loss and other changes. Discuss impact of hair loss on patient and strategies to minimize it (i.e., wig, scarf, cap) prior to drug administration. Assess ongoing coping during treatment. If nail changes are distressing, discuss the use of nail polish or other measures.

V. POTENTIAL SEXUAL DYSFUNCTION related to DRUG EFFECTS

Defining Characteristics: Drug is mutagenic and teratogenic. Amenorrhea often occurs in females, and testicular atrophy, possibly with reversible oligospermia/azoospermia, occurs in males. Drug is excreted in breast milk.

Nursing Implications: Assess patient's/partner's sexual patterns and reproductive goals. Discuss strategies to preserve sexual and reproductive health, including contraception and sperm banking, as appropriate. Mothers receiving cyclophosphamide should not breast-feed.

VI. POTENTIAL FOR INJURY related to ACUTE WATER INTOXICATION (SIADH) AND SECOND MALIGNANCY

Defining Characteristics: SIADH may occur with high-dose administration (> 50 mg/kg). Prolonged therapy may cause bladder cancer and acute leukemia.

Nursing Implications: Assess patients receiving high-dose cyclophosphamide: monitor serum Na+, osmolality, and urine osmolality and electrolytes; strictly monitor I/O, total body fluid balance, and daily weight. Screen patients who are receiving prolonged cyclophosphamide therapy for secondary malignancies.

VII. ALTERATION IN CARDIAC OUTPUT related to HIGH-DOSE CYCLOPHOSPHAMIDE

Defining Characteristics: Cardiomyopathy may occur with high doses as well as hemorrhagic cardiac necrosis, transmural hemorrhage, and coronary artery vasculitis at doses of 120–240 mg/kg. The mechanism is endothelial injury with subsequent hemorrhagic necrosis. The incidence is 22%, with 11% mortality, which may be decreased by dividing the dose into two split daily infusions. The risk at standard doses is increased by coadministration of doxorubicin (Adriamycin).

Nursing Implications: Assess cardiac status, especially if patient is receiving a high dose. Discuss baseline cardiac function test (GBPS) and assess for signs/symptoms of cardiomyopathy as treatment continues. Instruct patient to report dyspnea, shortness of breath, or other changes.

VIII. POTENTIAL FOR IMPAIRED GAS EXCHANGE related to PULMONARY TOXICITY

Defining Characteristics: Rare, but may occur with prolonged, high-dose therapy or continuous, low-dose therapy. Onset is insidious and appears as interstitial pneumonitis, which may progress to fibrosis. May respond to steroids.

Nursing Implications: Assess patients receiving high-dose or continuous low-dose cyclophosphamide for signs/symptoms of pulmonary dysfunction. Discuss pulmonary function studies with physician. Assess lung sounds prior to drug administration and periodically during treatment. Teach patient to report dyspnea, cough, or any abnormalities.

Drug: cytarabine, cytosine arabinoside (Ara-C, Cytosar-U)

Class: Antimetabolite.

Mechanism of Action: Incorporated into DNA, slowing its synthesis and causing defects in the linkages to new DNA fragments. Also, cells exposed to cytarabine in the S phase reinitiate DNA synthesis when the drug, a pyrimidine analogue, is removed, resulting in erroneous duplication of the early portions of the DNA strands. Most effective when cells are undergoing rapid DNA synthesis.

Metabolism: Inactivated by liver enzymes in biphasic manner: half-lives 10–15 minutes and 2–3 hours. Crosses the BBB with cerebrospinal fluid concentration of 50% that of plasma; 70% of dose excreted in urine as Ara-U; 4–10% excreted 12–24 hours after administration.

Dosage/Range:

- Varies depending on disease.
- Leukemia: 100 mg/m^2/day IV continuous infusion × 5–10 days; 100 mg/m^2 every 12 h × 1–3 weeks IV or subcutaneous.
- Head and neck: 1 mg/kg every 12 h × 5–7 days IV or subcutaneous.
- High dose: 1–3 g/m^2 IV every 12 h × 4–12 doses to treat refractory acute leukemia.
- Differentiation: 10 mg/m^2 subcutaneous every 12 h × 15–21 days.
- Intrathecal: 5–75 mg/m^2 every 2–7 days until CSF is clear.
- Bone marrow transplant conditioning regimen: 1.5 mg/m^2 IV as continuous infusion over 48 hours.

Drug Preparation:

- 100-mg vials: add water with benzyl alcohol then dilute with 0.9% sodium chloride or 5% dextrose.
- 500-mg vials: add water with benzyl alcohol then dilute with 0.9% sodium chloride or 5% dextrose.
- For intrathecal use and high dose: use preservative-free diluent.
- Reconstituted drug is stable 48 hours at room temperature and 7 days refrigerated.

Drug Administration:

- Doses of 100–200 mg can be given subcutaneous.
- Doses less than 1 g: Administer via pump over 10–20 minutes.
- Doses over 1 g: Administer over 2 hours or longer.

Drug Interactions:

- May be a decreased bioavailability of digoxin when given in combination.

Lab Effects/Interference:

- Decreased CBC.
- Increased LFTs, RFTs.
- Increased uric acid due to tumor lysis.

Special Considerations:

- Thrombophlebitis, pain at the injection site, should be treated with warm compresses.
- Dizziness has occurred with too rapid IV infusions.
- Use with caution if hepatic dysfunction exists.
- Drug is excreted in tears requiring protection of eye conjunctiva (corticosteroid eye drops such as dexamethasone 0.1% ophthalmic drops) with high-dose therapy.

Potential Toxicities/Side Effects and the Nursing Process

I. INFECTION AND BLEEDING related to BONE MARROW DEPRESSION

Defining Characteristics: Bone marrow depression is related to dose and duration of therapy. WBC depression is biphasic. After a 5-day continuous infusion at doses of 50–600 mg/m^2, WBC begins to fall within 24 hours, reaching nadir in 7–9 days, briefly rises around day 12, and begins to fall again, reaching nadir at days 15–24, with recovery within 10 days. Platelet drop begins day 5, reaching nadir at days 12–15, with recovery within 10 days. Anemia is seen frequently, with megaloblastic changes common in the bone marrow. Potent but transient suppression of primary and secondary antibody responses occur.

Nursing Implications: Assess WBC, neutrophil, and platelet count, and discuss any abnormalities with physician prior to drug administration; assess for signs/symptoms of skin infections (all mucosal surfaces, body orifices) and bleeding; instruct patient in signs/symptoms of infection and bleeding, as well as to report them or come to emergency room. Teach patient self-care measures to minimize risk of infection and bleeding, including avoidance of OTC aspirin-containing medications. Assess patient's Hgb/HCT and signs/symptoms of fatigue; teach patient self-assessment and to alternate rest and activity as needed.

II. ALTERED NUTRITION, LESS THAN BODY REQUIREMENTS, related to NAUSEA AND VOMITING, ANOREXIA, STOMATITIS, DIARRHEA, HEPATOTOXICITY

Defining Characteristics: Nausea and vomiting occurs in 50% of patients, is dose related, and lasts for several hours. Can be successfully prevented with combination antiemetics. Anorexia commonly occurs. Stomatitis occurs 7–10 days after therapy is initiated, occurs in 15% of patients, and is dose related. May be preceded by angular stomatitis (reddened area at juncture of lips). Diarrhea is infrequent and mild. Hepatotoxicity is usually mild and reversible, but drug should be used cautiously in patients with impaired hepatic function.

Nursing Implications: Premedicate with antiemetics depending on dose, using aggressive, combination antiemetics for high-dose therapy, and continue throughout chemotherapy. If patient develops nausea/vomiting, assess fluid and electrolyte balance and the need for replacements. Assess oral mucosa prior to chemotherapy and teach patient oral hygiene regimen and self-assessment; encourage patient to report diarrhea, discuss use of antidiarrheals with physician, and teach self-care PRN. Since patients become neutropenic, all mucosal surfaces need to be assessed for infection, and patients must be taught scrupulous perineal hygiene. Monitor LFTs prior to, during, and posttherapy.

III. IMPAIRED SKIN/MUCOSAL INTEGRITY related to RASH, ANAL INFLAMMATION/ULCERATION, ALOPECIA

Defining Characteristics: Maculopapular rash, with or without fever, myalgia, bone pain, occasional chest pain, conjunctivitis, and malaise (cytarabine syndrome) may occur. Syndrome is not common, but occurs 6–12 hours after drug administration; corticosteroids have been helpful in treating/preventing syndrome. Mucosal inflammation and ulceration of anus/rectum may occur, especially in patients with prior hemorrhoids or history of abscesses. Alopecia occurs less frequently.

Nursing Implications: Assess baseline skin and mucous membranes prior to chemotherapy and identify patients at risk for problems. Consider including corticosteroid in antiemetic regimen, especially for high-dose therapy, and discuss with physician prophylactic use of dexamethasone eye drops to prevent conjunctivitis. Teach patient scrupulous perineal hygiene, instruct to report any rectal discomfort, and assess rectal mucosa daily with high-dose therapy. Discuss with patient potential coping strategies if alopecia occurs (i.e., wig, scarves).

IV. POTENTIAL FOR INJURY related to NEUROTOXICITY

Defining Characteristics: Neurotoxicity can occur at high doses. If cerebellar toxicity (characterized by nystagmus, dysarthria, ataxia, slurred speech, and/or dysdiadochokinesia or inability to make fine, coordinated movements) develops, it is an indication to terminate therapy. Onset usually 6–8 days after first dose, lasts 3–7 days. Lethargy and somnolence have resulted from rapid infusion of the drug. Incidence of CNS toxicity is 10% and may be related to total cumulative drug dose, impaired renal function, and/or age > 50 years old. Ocular toxicity may occur, characterized by injection of conjunctive, corneal opacities, decreased visual acuity. This may be a result of inhibition of DNA synthesis of corneal epithelium. Conjunctivitis occurs due to excretion of drug in lacrimal tearing and can be prevented by corticosteroid eye drops. Other visual symptoms that may occur are increased lacrimation, blurred vision, photophobia, eye pain.

Nursing Implications: Assess baseline neurologic status and cerebellar function (coordinated movements such as handwriting and gait) prior to and during therapy. Teach patient to self-assess and report changes in coordination, control of eye movement, handwriting. Monitor patient for somnolence and lethargy during infusion, and infuse drug according to established guidelines. With high-dose therapy, discuss with physician use of prophylactic corticosteroid eye drops. Assess and teach patient self-assessment of eyes and instruct to report increased lacrimation, blurred vision, photophobia, eye pain.

V. POTENTIAL FOR INJURY related to TUMOR LYSIS SYNDROME (TLS)

Defining Characteristics: May develop with initial therapy if patient has a large tumor burden; results from rapid lysis of tumor cells. This usually begins 1–5 days after initiation of therapy and causes elevations in serum uric acid, potassium, phosphorus, BUN, creatinine.

Nursing Implications: If this is induction therapy for a patient with acute leukemia or high tumor burden, expect medical orders to include IV hydration at 150 mL/hour with or without alkalinization, oral allopurinol, strict monitoring of I/O, daily weight, and total body fluid balance determination. Monitor baseline and daily BUN, creatinine, K+, phosphorus, uric acid, and calcium. Monitor for renal, cardiac, neuromuscular signs/symptoms of TLS.

VI. POTENTIAL SEXUAL DYSFUNCTION related to DRUG EFFECTS

Defining Characteristics: Drug is mutagenic and probably teratogenic. Although normal babies have been delivered by mothers receiving drug in first trimester, other babies have had congenital defects. It is unknown whether the drug is excreted in breast milk.

Nursing Implications: Discuss with patient and partner sexuality and reproductive goals and possible impact of chemotherapy. Discuss contraception and sperm banking if appropriate. Discourage breast-feeding if the mother is receiving chemotherapy.

Drug: cytarabine, liposome injection (DepoCyt)

Class: Antimetabolite.

Mechanism of Action: Drug is converted to the metabolite ara-CTP intracellularly. Ara-CTP is thought to inhibit DNA polymerase, thereby affecting DNA synthesis. Incorporation into DNA and RNA may also contribute to cytarabine cellular toxicity.

Metabolism: With systemically administered cytarabine, the drug is metabolized to an inactive compound, ara-U, and is then renally excreted. In the CSF, however, conversion to the ara-U is negligible, because CNS tissue and CSF lack the enzyme necessary for the conversion to occur. Liposomal formulation gives sustained effect over 2 weeks, with a half-life in the CSF of 100–263 hours.

Dosage/Range: Indicated for the intrathecal treatment of lymphomatous meningitis only. To be given as follows:

- Induction therapy: DepoCyt, 50 mg, administered intrathecally (intraventricular or lumbar puncture) every 14 days for 2 doses (weeks 1 and 3).
- Consolidation therapy: DepoCyt, 50 mg, administered intrathecally (intraventricular or lumbar puncture) every 14 days for 3 doses (weeks 5, 7, and 9) followed by 1 additional dose at week 13.
- Maintenance therapy: DepoCyt, 50 mg, administered intrathecally (intraventricular or lumbar puncture) every 28 days for 4 doses (weeks 17, 21, 25, and 29).

- If drug-related neurotoxicity develops, the dose should be reduced to 25 mg. If toxicity persists, treatment with DepoCyt should be terminated.
- Dexamethasone 4 mg PO twice daily × 5 days should begin on day of liposomal cytarabine injection.

Drug Preparation:

- Drug is supplied in single-use vials containing 10 mg/mL and comes as a white to off-white suspension in 5 mL of fluid, preservative free.
- Drug is to be withdrawn immediately before use and should not be used later than 4 hours from the time of withdrawal from vial.
- DepoCyt should be administered directly into the CSF over 1–5 minutes. Patients should lie flat for 1 hour after administration.
- Patients should be started on dexamethasone 4 mg bid either PO or IV for 5 days beginning on the day of DepoCyt injection.

Drug Interactions:

- No formal drug interaction studies of DepoCyt and other drugs have been done.
- Expect increased neurotoxicity if drug is administered at same time as other intrathecal, cytotoxic agents.

Lab Effects/Interference:

- DepoCyt particles are similar in size and appearance to white blood cells, so care must be taken when interpreting CSF samples.

Special Considerations:

- Do not use inline filters with DepoCyt; administer directly into CSF.
- Must be administered with concurrent dexamethasone as described above.
- Granted full FDA approval in 2007 based on two RCTs showing significantly more patients treated with DepoCyt had absence of neurologic progression of disease and significantly higher complete cytologic response (clearing of malignant cells from CSF) compared with standard intrathecal cytarabine.

Potential Toxicities/Side Effects and the Nursing Process

I. ALTERATION IN NUTRITION, LESS THAN BODY REQUIREMENTS, related to NAUSEA AND VOMITING

Defining Characteristics: Nausea, vomiting, and headache are common, and are physical manifestations of chemical arachnoiditis.

Nursing Implications: Administer dexamethasone throughout treatment course as described above. Observe patient for at least 1 hour after administration for toxicity. Administer antiemetics as ordered. Encourage small, frequent feedings of cool, bland foods. Instruct patient to report nausea and vomiting and to self-administer antiemetics as ordered.

II. ALTERATION IN COMFORT related to HEADACHE, NECK AND/OR BACK PAIN, FEVER, NAUSEA, AND VOMITING

Defining Characteristics: Some degree of chemical arachnoiditis is expected in about one-third of patients: incidence approaches 100% of patients when dexamethasone is NOT given with DepoCyt. Causes headache, neck pain, and/or rigidity, back pain, fever, nausea, and vomiting, which are reversible.

Nursing Implications: Instruct patient in dexamethasone self-administration and to report to physician if oral doses are not tolerated. Patients should lie flat for one hour after lumbar puncture and should be observed for immediate toxic reactions. Administer medications to treat pain.

Drug: dacarbazine (DTIC-Dome, Dimethyl-triazeno-imidazolecarboxamide)

Class: Alkylating agent.

Mechanism of Action: Appears to methylate nucleic acids (particularly DNA) causing cross-linkage and breaks in DNA strands, which inhibits RNA and DNA synthesis. Also interacts with sulfhydryl groups to inhibit protein synthesis. Generally, cell cycle phase nonspecific.

Metabolism: Thought to be activated by liver microsomes; 15% of the drug crosses the blood–brain barrier. Undergoes metabolism in liver and biliary excretion, with 18–63% of drug excreted unchanged in the urine. Plasma half-life of 0.65 hour, and terminal half-life of 5 hours.

Dosage/Range:
- 375 mg/m^2 every 2 weeks OR
- 150–250 mg/m^2/day × 5 days, repeat every 3–4 weeks

Drug Preparation:
- Available in 100-, 200-, or 500-mg vials.
- Add sterile water or 0.9% sodium chloride to vial.

Drug Administration:
- Administer via pump over 20 minutes or give via IV push over 2–3 minutes.
- Stable for 8 hours at room temperature, for 72 hours if refrigerated. Store lyophilized drug in refrigerator and protect from light. Drug decomposition is denoted by a change in color from yellow to pink.

Drug Interactions:
- Increased drug metabolism with concurrent administration of Dilantin, phenobarbital; potential increased toxicity with Imuran and 6-MP.

Lab Effects/Interference:
- Decreased CBC.
- Increased LFTs.

Special Considerations:
- Irritant—avoid extravasation.
- Pain may occur above site: Usually unrelieved by slowing IV, but may be relieved by applying ice to painful area. May cause venospasm; slow rate if this occurs.
- Anaphylaxis has occurred with infusion of dacarbazine.

Potential Toxicities/Side Effects and the Nursing Process

I. INFECTION AND BLEEDING related to BONE MARROW DEPRESSION

Defining Characteristics: Nadir occurs days 14–28 following drug administration; anemia may occur with long-term treatment.

Nursing Implications: Evaluate WBC, neutrophil, and platelet count and discuss any abnormalities with physician prior to drug administration; assess for signs/symptoms of infection or bleeding; instruct patient in identifying signs/symptoms of infection and bleeding, and to report them. Teach patient self-care measures to minimize risk of infection and bleeding, including avoidance of OTC aspirin-containing medications. Assess patient's Hgb/HCT and signs/symptoms of fatigue; teach patient self-assessment and instruct to alternate rest and activity as needed.

II. ALTERATION IN NUTRITION, LESS THAN BODY REQUIREMENTS, related to NAUSEA AND VOMITING, DIARRHEA, ANOREXIA, HEPATOTOXICITY

Defining Characteristics: Nausea/vomiting occurs in 90% of patients and is moderate to severe, beginning 1–3 hours after dose. Nausea and vomiting decrease with each consecutive day the drug is given. Preventable by aggressive combination antiemetics. Diarrhea is uncommon. Anorexia is common, occurring in 90% of patients; drug may also cause a metallic taste. Hepatotoxicity is rare, but hepatic veno-occlusive disease has been described (hepatic vein thrombosis and hepatocellular necrosis).

Nursing Implications: Premedicate with combination antiemetics and continue protection during infusions. Administer drug over at least one hour. Use relaxation exercises, imagery, or other techniques; teach patient exercises prior to drug treatment. Teach patient to report diarrhea and administer antidiarrheal medication as ordered, or teach patient self-administration as appropriate. Encourage small, frequent feedings of favorite foods; teach patient/caregiver to make foods ahead of time so patient will have them ready for snacks when hungry; encourage use of spices if food tastes bland; encourage patient to weigh self weekly. Monitor LFTs and discuss abnormalities with physician.

III. ALTERATION IN COMFORT related to FLU-LIKE SYNDROME, PAIN AT INJECTION SITE

Defining Characteristics: Flu-like syndrome may occur, characterized by malaise, headache, myalgia, hypotension; may occur up to 7 days after first dose, lasting 7–21 days, and may recur with subsequent doses of drug. Drug is an irritant and may cause phlebitis of vein.

Nursing Implications: Teach patient flu-like symptoms may occur; suggest symptom management using acetaminophen as needed; encourage fluid intake of > 3 L/day and rest, as determined by healthcare team. Assess patient vein selection prior to drug administration and suggest venous access device early on if patient is to receive ongoing treatment with dacarbazine (DTIC). Administer drug in 100–250-mL IV fluid and infuse slowly over 1 hour. Consider premedications when drug is given peripherally and discuss with physician: hydrocortisone IVP (DTIC forms precipitate with hydrocortisone sodium succinate [Solu-Cortef] but not with hydrocortisone), lidocaine 1–2% IVP, or heparin IVP to minimize vein trauma prior to DTIC infusion. Apply heat or ice above injection site to reduce venous burning.

IV. IMPAIRED SKIN INTEGRITY related to ALOPECIA, FACIAL FLUSHING, ERYTHEMA, URTICARIA

Defining Characteristics: Alopecia occurs in 90% of patients. Facial flushing occurs rarely and is self-limiting; erythema and urticaria may occur around injection site. High dose-related photosensitization may occur, with resulting severe reaction to sunlight, e.g., burning, pain.

Nursing Implications: Teach patient about expected hair loss; encourage patient to verbalize feelings regarding anticipated/actual hair loss and discuss strategies to minimize impact of alopecia. Encourage female patients to obtain wig prior to hair loss; ask male patients to identify how they will manage hair loss. Provide emotional support. In cold climates, encourage patient to wear cap at night to prevent loss of body heat. Teach patient receiving high-dose therapy to cover body, head, and hands when exposed to sunlight, or to avoid direct sunlight. Patient should also use sunblock.

V. POTENTIAL FOR SENSORY/PERCEPTUAL ALTERATIONS related to FACIAL PARESTHESIA, PHOTOSENSITIVITY

Defining Characteristics: Photosensitivity may occur in bright sunlight or ultraviolet light. Facial paresthesias may occur.

Nursing Implications: Instruct patient to report facial paresthesias and in self-care measures if sensory changes occur; wear sunglasses in strong sunlight; wear sunscreens when out in the sun, as well as protective clothing, including a hat; avoid UV or strong sunlight exposure if possible.

VI. POTENTIAL SEXUAL DYSFUNCTION related to DRUG EFFECTS

Defining Characteristics: Drug is teratogenic. It is unknown whether drug is excreted in breast milk. Drug is probably carcinogenic.

Nursing Implications: Assess patient's and partner's patterns of sexuality and reproductive goals. Teach need for contraception and provide information and referral as appropriate. Encourage verbalization of feelings and provide emotional support. Discourage breast-feeding if patient is a lactating mother.

Drug: dactinomycin (Actinomycin D, Cosmegen)

Class: Antitumor antibiotic isolated from *Streptomyces* fungus.

Mechanism of Action: Binds to guanine portion of DNA and blocks the ability of DNA to act as a template for both DNA and RNA. At lower drug doses, the predominant action inhibits RNA, whereas at higher doses both RNA and DNA are inhibited. Cell cycle specific for G_1 and S phases.

Metabolism: Most of drug is excreted unchanged in bile and urine. There is a rapid clearance of drug from plasma (approximately 36 hours). Dose reduction in the presence of liver or renal failure may be needed.

Dosage/Range:
- 10–15 μg/kg/day × 5 days q 3–4 weeks.
- 15–30 μg/kg/week, OR 15 μg/kg/day for 5 days IV.
- Frequency and schedule may vary according to protocol and age.

Drug Preparation:
- Add sterile water for a concentration of 500 μg/mL. Use preservative-free water, as precipitate may develop otherwise.

Drug Administration:
- IV: Drug is a vesicant and should be given through a running IV to avoid extravasation, which can lead to ulceration, pain, and necrosis. Be sure to check the nursing policy and procedure for administration of vesicants.

Drug Interactions:
- None significant.

Lab Effects/Interference:
- Decreased CBC.
- Increased LFTs.
- Decreased calcium.

Special Considerations:

- Drug is a vesicant. Give through a running IV to avoid extravasation, which may develop into ulceration, necrosis, and pain.
- Nausea and vomiting are moderate to severe. Usually occurs 2–5 hours after administration; may persist up to 24 hours.
- Potent myelosuppressive agent: Severity of nadir is dose-limiting toxicity.
- GI toxicity: Mucositis, diarrhea, and abdominal pain.
- Skin changes: Radiation recall phenomenon. Skin discoloration along vein used for injection.
- Alopecia.
- Malaise, fatigue, mental depression.
- Contraindicated in patients with chickenpox or herpes zoster, as life-threatening systemic disease may develop.

Potential Toxicities/Side Effects and the Nursing Process

I. POTENTIAL FOR INFECTION AND BLEEDING related to BONE MARROW DEPRESSION

Defining Characteristics: Myelosuppression often dose-limiting toxicity. Onset of decreasing WBC and platelets in 7–10 days, with nadir 14–21 days after dose and recovery in 21–28 days. Delayed anemia.

Nursing Implications: Assess CBC, WBC, differential, and platelet count prior to drug administration, as well as for signs/symptoms of infection and bleeding, and discuss any abnormalities with physician prior to drug administration. Instruct patient in signs/symptoms of infection and bleeding, and instruct to report this; teach patient self-care measures to minimize risk of infection and bleeding, including avoidance of OTC aspirin-containing medications. Assess patient's Hgb/HCT and signs/symptoms of fatigue; teach patient self-assessment and instruct to alternate rest and activity as needed.

II. ALTERATION IN NUTRITION, LESS THAN BODY REQUIREMENTS, related to NAUSEA/VOMITING, DIARRHEA, ANOREXIA

Defining Characteristics: Nausea/vomiting may be severe and begins 2–5 hours after dose, lasting 24 hours. Diarrhea with/without cramps occurs in 30% of patients. Anorexia occurs frequently.

Nursing Implications: Use combination antiemetics to prevent nausea and vomiting. Nausea/vomiting may be prevented by aggressive, combination antiemetics, such as serotonin antagonist plus dexamethasone. Encourage small, frequent feedings of bland foods. Encourage patient to eat favorite foods and use seasonings on foods if anorexia persists; refer to dietitian as needed.

III. ALTERATION IN MUCOUS MEMBRANES related to STOMATITIS, ESOPHAGITIS, AND PROCTITIS

Defining Characteristics: Irritation and ulceration may occur along the entire GI mucosa.

Nursing Implications: Assess baseline oral mucosa and presence of irritation along GI tract. Instruct patient in self-assessment and teach patient to report irritation; instruct regarding oral hygiene regimen.

IV. POTENTIAL IMPAIRED SKIN INTEGRITY related to RADIATION RECALL, RASH, ALOPECIA, AND DRUG EXTRAVASATION

Defining Characteristics: Recalls damage to skin from previous radiation, resulting in erythema or increased pigmentation at the radiation site. Acne-like rash and alopecia can occur in 47% of patients. Drug is a potent vesicant.

Nursing Implications: Conduct baseline skin, hair assessment. Discuss with patient impact of potential changes on body image, as well as possible coping/adaptive strategies (e.g., obtain wig prior to hair loss). When administering the drug, ensure use of a patent vein to avoid extravasation; consider the use of venous access device early. Be familiar with institution's policy and procedure for administration of a vesicant and management of extravasation.

V. ALTERATION IN COMFORT related to FLU-LIKE SYMPTOMS

Defining Characteristics: Flu-like symptoms can occur, including symptoms of malaise, myalgia, fever, depression.

Nursing Implications: Inform patient this may occur. Assess for occurrence during and after treatment. Discuss with physician symptomatic management.

VI. POTENTIAL FOR ALTERATION IN METABOLISM related to HEPATOTOXICITY AND RENAL TOXICITY

Defining Characteristics: Hepatotoxicity is related to drug metabolism in liver; renal toxicity is related to drug excretion by kidneys.

Nursing Implications: Monitor LFTUN, and creatinine. Discuss abnormalities with physician, as drug doses may need to be reduced.

VII. POTENTIAL FOR SEXUAL DYSFUNCTION

Defining Characteristics: Drug is carcinogenic, mutagenic, and teratogenic. It is unknown if drug is excreted in breast milk.

Nursing Implications: Assess patient's/partner's sexual patterns and reproductive goals. Provide information, supportive counseling, and referral as needed. Teach importance of birth control measures as appropriate. Discourage breast-feeding if patient is a lactating mother.

Drug: daunorubicin citrate liposome injection (DaunoXome)

Class: Anthracycline antibiotic that is isolated from streptomycin products, in particular the rhodomycin products, and encapsulated in a liposome.

Mechanism of Action: No clearly defined mechanism. Intercalates DNA, therefore blocking DNA, RNA, and protein synthesis. Binds to DNA and inhibits DNA replication and DNA-dependent RNA synthesis. Drug is encapsulated within liposomes (lipid vesicles) and is preferentially delivered to solid tumor sites. The liposomal encapsulated drug is protected from chemical and enzymatic degradation, protein binding, and uptake by normal tissues while circulating in the blood. The exact mechanism for selective targeting of tumor sites is unknown but is believed to be related to increased permeability of the tumor neovasculature. Once delivered to the tumor, the drug is slowly released and exerts its antineoplastic action.

Metabolism: Cleared from the plasma at 17 mL/min with a small steady-state volume of distribution. As compared to standard IV daunorubicin, the liposomal encapsulated daunorubicin has higher daunorubicin exposure (plasma area under the curve, ARC). The elimination half-life (4.4 hours) is shorter than standard daunorubicin.

Dosage/Range:
- 20–40 mg/m^2/day IV bolus over 60 minutes every 2 weeks.
- Dosage adjustment if hepatic dysfunction or renal dysfunction.

Drug Preparation:
- Drug is available as 50 mg of daunorubicin base in a total volume of 25 mL (2 mg/mL).
- Visually inspect for particulate matter and discoloration (drug appears as a translucent dispersion of liposomes that scatters light, but should not be opaque or have precipitate or foreign matter present).
- Withdraw the calculated volume of drug and add to an equal volume of 5% dextrose to deliver a 1:1, or 1 mg/mL solution.
- Administer immediately, or may be stored in the refrigerator at 2–8°C (36–46°F) for 6 hours.

- Use ONLY 5% dextrose, NOT 0.9% sodium chloride or any other solution.
- Drug contains no preservatives.
- Unopened drug vials should be stored in the refrigerator at 2–8°C (36–46°F), but should not be frozen. Protect from light.

Drug Administration:
- IV bolus over 60 minutes, repeated every 2 weeks.
- Do not use an inline filter.
- Drug is an irritant, not a vesicant.
- Dose should be reduced in patients with renal or hepatic dysfunction.
- Hold dose if absolute granulocyte count is < 750 cells/mm^3.

Drug Interactions:
- Colchicine, allopurinol, other antigout medications: may have increased effects.
- Bone marrow suppressant agents: increased bone marrow depression.

Lab Effects/Interference:
- Increased LFTs, RFTs (especially if elevated prior to administration).
- Increased uric acid secondary to tumor lysis.

Special Considerations:
- Drug is embryotoxic, so female patients should use contraceptive measures as appropriate.
- Back pain, flushing, and chest tightness may occur during the first 5 minutes of drug administration and resolve with cessation of the infusion. Most patients do not experience recurrence when the infusion is restarted at a slower rate.
- Drug indicated in the treatment of Kaposi's sarcoma. Activity reported to be equivalent to treatment with ABV (doxorubicin, vincristine, bleomycin) but with less alopecia, cardiotoxicity, and neurotoxicity.

Potential Toxicities/Side Effects and the Nursing Process

I. POTENTIAL FOR INFECTION AND BLEEDING related to BONE MARROW DEPRESSION

Defining Characteristics: Myelosuppression can be severe and affects the granulocytes primarily. Incidence of neutropenia of 36% is similar to that of patients receiving ABV (doxorubicin, vincristine, bleomycin), which is 35%. Neutropenia with < 500 cells/mm^3 occurs in 15% of patients (vs 5% in patients receiving ABV). Fever incidence is 47%. Concurrent antiretroviral and antiviral agents received for HIV infection may enhance this. Patients are immunocompromised; therefore, monitoring for opportunistic infection is essential. Platelets and RBCs are less affected.

Nursing Implications: Monitor CBC, WBC, differential, and platelet count prior to drug administration, and discuss any abnormalities with physician. Drug should not be given if ANC is < 750 cells/mm^3. Assess for signs/symptoms of infection or bleeding, and instruct patient in self-assessment and to report signs/symptoms immediately.

Teach patient self-care measures to minimize risk of infection and bleeding, including avoidance of OTC aspirin-containing medications. Drug dosage must be reduced if patient has hepatic dysfunction: 75% of drug dose if serum bili 1.2–3.0 mg/dL, 50% reduction if bili is > 3.0 mg/dL. Drug dosage must be reduced if patient has renal impairment: creatinine > 3 mg/dL, give 50% of normal dose.

II. ALTERATION IN COMFORT related to TRIAD OF BACK PAIN, FLUSHING, CHEST TIGHTNESS

Defining Characteristics: This occurs in 13.8% of patients and is mild to moderate. The syndrome resolves with cessation of the infusion, and does not usually recur when the infusion is resumed at a slower infusion rate.

Nursing Implications: Infuse drug at prescribed rate over 60 minutes. Assess for, and teach patient to report, back pain, flushing, and chest tightness. Stop infusion if this occurs, and once symptoms subside, resume infusion at a slower rate.

III. POTENTIAL FOR ALTERATION IN SKIN INTEGRITY related to ALOPECIA, CHANGES IN SKIN

Defining Characteristics: Mild alopecia occurs in 6% of patients and moderate alopecia in 2% of patients, as compared to 36% of patients receiving ABV chemotherapy. The drug is considered an irritant, NOT a vesicant. Folliculitis, seborrhea, and dry skin occur in < 5% of patients.

Nursing Implications: Teach patient that hair loss is unlikely, and to report this or any skin changes.

IV. POTENTIAL FOR ALTERATION IN NUTRITION, LESS THAN BODY REQUIREMENTS, related to NAUSEA AND VOMITING, ANOREXIA, DIARRHEA

Defining Characteristics: Mild nausea occurs in 35% of patients, moderate nausea in 16% of patients, and severe nausea in 3% of patients. Vomiting is less common, with 10% experiencing mild, 10% experiencing moderate, and 3% experiencing severe vomiting. Anorexia may occur (21%) or increased appetite may occur in < 5% of patients. Diarrhea may occur in 38% of patients. Other GI problems, occurring < 5% of the time, are dysphagia, gastritis, hemorrhoids, hepatomegaly, dry mouth, and tooth caries.

Nursing Implications: Premedicate with antiemetics. Encourage small, frequent feedings of bland foods. If patient has anorexia, teach patient or caregiver to make foods ahead of time, use spices, and encourage weekly weights. Instruct patient to report diarrhea, and to use self-management strategies (medications as ordered, diet modification). Instruct patient to report other GI problems.

V. POTENTIAL FOR ALTERATION IN CARDIAC OUTPUT related to CARDIAC CHANGES

Defining Characteristics: Daunorubicin may cause cardiotoxicity and CHF, but studies with liposomal daunorubicin show rare clinical cardiotoxicity at cumulative doses > 600 mg/m^2. However, especially in patients with preexisting cardiac disease or prior anthracycline treatment, assessment of cardiac function (history and physical) should be performed prior to each dose. In addition, testing of cardiac ejection fraction and echocardiogram should be performed at cumulative doses of 320 mg/m^2, 480 mg/m^2, and every 160 mg/m^2 thereafter.

Nursing Implications: Assess cardiac status prior to chemotherapy administration: signs/symptoms of CHF, quality/regularity and rate of heartbeat, results of prior tests of left ventricular ejection fraction (LVEF) or echocardiogram, if performed. Instruct patient to report dyspnea, palpitations, swelling in extremities. Maintain accurate records of total dose, and expect GBPS to be repeated periodically during treatment and the drug to be discontinued if there is a significant drop in heart function.

VI. POTENTIAL FOR ACTIVITY INTOLERANCE related to FATIGUE

Defining Characteristics: Fatigue occurs in 49% of patients.

Nursing Implications: Assess baseline activity level. Instruct patient to report fatigue and activity intolerance. Teach self-management strategies, including alternating rest and activity periods, and stress reduction.

Drug: daunorubicin hydrochloride (Cerubidine, Daunomycin HCl, Rubidomycin)

Class: Anthracycline antibiotic isolated from streptomycin products, in particular the rhodomycin products.

Mechanism of Action: No clearly defined mechanism. Intercalates DNA, therefore blocking DNA, RNA, and protein synthesis. Binds to DNA and inhibits DNA replication and DNA-dependent RNA synthesis.

Metabolism: Site of significant metabolism is in the liver. Doses need to be modified in presence of abnormal liver function. Excreted in urine and bile.

Dosage/Range:

- 30–60 mg/m^2/day IV for 3 consecutive days.
- AML induction: 45 mg/m^2/day IV × 3 days with cytosine arabinoside 100 mg/m^2/day IV continuous infusion × 7 days.
- Adjust dose for hepatic dysfunction (25% dose reduction [DR]), BR 1.2–3 mg/dL; 50% DR BR > 3.0 mg/dL.

Drug Preparation:

- Available in 20- and 50-mg vials for injection or 20- and 50-mg vials containing lyophilized powder.
- Add sterile water to produce liquid. Drug will form a precipitate when mixed with heparin and is incompatible with dexamethasone.

Drug Administration:

- IV: This drug is a potent vesicant. Give through a running IV to avoid extravasation, which can lead to ulceration, pain, and necrosis. Check individual hospital policy and procedure on administration of a vesicant.

Drug Interactions:

- Incompatible with heparin (forms a precipitate).
- Other bone marrow suppressive drugs: increased bone marrow depression.
- Trastuzumab: may increase cardiotoxicity.

Lab Effects/Interference:

- Increased bili, AST, alk phos.
- Increased uric acid secondary to tumor lysis.

Special Considerations:

- Drug is a potent vesicant. Give through running IV to avoid/minimize risk of extravasation.
- Moderate to severe nausea and vomiting occur in 50% of patients within first 24 hours.
- Causes discoloration of urine (pink to red for up to 48 hours after administration).
- Potent myelosuppressive agent. Nadir occurs within 10–14 days.
- Alopecia.
- Cardiac toxicity: Dose limit at 550 mg/m^2. Patients may exhibit irreversible CHF. Acute toxicity may be seen within hours after administration. This is unrelated to cumulative dose and may manifest symptoms of pump or conduction dysfunction. Rarely, transient EKG abnormalities, CHF; pericardial effusion (whole syndrome referred to as myocarditis-pericarditis syndrome) may occur, which may lead to death.
- Dose reduction necessary in patients with impaired liver function.
- Available in liposomal encapsulated vehicle (Daunoxome) that has less myelosuppression and cardiotoxicity. Drug is currently approved for therapy of Kaposi's sarcoma.

Potential Toxicities/Side Effects and the Nursing Process

I. POTENTIAL FOR INFECTION AND BLEEDING related to BONE MARROW DEPRESSION

Defining Characteristics: WBC and platelet counts begin to decrease in 7 days, with nadir 10–14 days after drug dose; recovery in 21–28 days. Dose reduction indicated with renal or hepatic dysfunction as drug is excreted by these routes.

Nursing Implications: Evaluate WBC, neutrophil, and platelet count and discuss any abnormalities with physician prior to drug administration; assess for signs/symptoms of infection and bleeding; instruct patient in signs/symptoms of infection and bleeding and to report these immediately. Teach patient self-care measures to minimize risk of infection and bleeding, including avoidance of OTC aspirin-containing medications.

II. POTENTIAL FOR ALTERATION IN CARDIAC OUTPUT related to ACUTE AND CHRONIC CARDIAC CHANGES

Defining Characteristics: Acute effects (i.e., EKG changes, atrial arrhythmias) occur in 6–30% of patients 1–3 days after dose and are not life-threatening. Chronic myofibril damage resulting in irreversible cardiomyopathy is life-threatening and dose-related. Cumulative dose should not exceed 550 mg/m^2 or 450 mg/m^2 if patient is receiving/has received radiation to chest or with concurrent administration of cyclophosphamide or other cardiotoxic agent. CHF may develop 1–16 months after therapy ceases if cumulative dose is exceeded.

Nursing Implications: Assess baseline cardiac status, quality and regularity of heartbeat, and baseline EKG. Patient should have baseline GBPS or other measure of left ventricular ejection fraction at baseline, and periodically during treatment. If there is a significant drop in ejection fraction, then drug should be stopped. Maintain accurate documentation of doses administered so that cumulative dose is known. Instruct patient to report dyspnea, shortness of breath, edema, orthopnea.

III. ALTERATION IN NUTRITION, LESS THAN BODY REQUIREMENTS, related to NAUSEA AND VOMITING, STOMATITIS

Defining Characteristics: Mild nausea and vomiting on the day of therapy occur in 50% of patients and can be prevented with antiemetics. Stomatitis is infrequent but may occur 3–7 days after dose.

Nursing Implications: Premedicate with antiemetics, and continue for 24 hours for protection. Assess oral mucosa prior to chemotherapy, teach patient oral hygiene regimen and self-assessment; encourage patient to report burning or oral irritation. Assess pain in mouth, and administer analgesics as needed and ordered.

IV. POTENTIAL FOR IMPAIRED SKIN INTEGRITY related to ALOPECIA, HYPERPIGMENTATION OF FINGERNAILS AND TOENAILS, RADIATION RECALL, AND DRUG EXTRAVASATION

Defining Characteristics: Reversible total alopecia occurs 3–4 weeks after treatment begins; nail beds become hyperpigmented. Drug is a potent vesicant and will result in severe soft tissue damage if extravasated. Damage to skin from prior irradiation may be reactivated (radiation recall). Rash may occur, as may onycholysis (nail loosening from nail bed).

Nursing Implications: Teach patient that alopecia will occur and discuss impact hair loss will have on body image. Discuss coping strategies, including obtaining wig or cap prior to hair loss. Encourage patient to verbalize feelings and provide patient with emotional support. Drug dose may be decreased with prior irradiation; assess for skin changes from radiation recall. Hyperpigmentation of nail beds may cause body image problem; discuss with patient and identify measures to minimize distress. Ensure that drug is administered only through a patent IV and that nurse is familiar with institution's policy for vesicant administration and management of extravasation. Manufacturer recommends aspiration of any remaining drug from IV tubing, discontinuing IV, and applying ice. Assess need for venous access device early.

V. POTENTIAL SEXUAL DYSFUNCTION related to DRUG EFFECTS

Defining Characteristics: Drug is mutagenic and teratogenic. Drug may cause testicular atrophy and azoospermia. It is unknown whether drug is excreted in breast milk.

Nursing Implications: Assess patient's and partner's sexual patterns and reproductive goals. Provide information, supportive counseling, and referral as needed. Male patients may wish to try sperm banking. Teach importance of birth control measures as appropriate. Women receiving the drug should not breast-feed.

VI. POTENTIAL FOR ALTERATION IN COMFORT related to ABDOMINAL PAIN, FEVER, CHILLS

Defining Characteristics: Abdominal pain may occur but is uncommon. Fever and chills, with or without rash, occur rarely.

Nursing Implications: Assess patient for occurrence and provide symptomatic management.

Drug: decitabine (Dacogen, 5-Aza-2-deoxycytidine)

Class: Antimetabolite, molecular/genetic modulator.

Mechanism of Action: Drug is a pyrimidine analogue, and prevents DNA synthesis in the S phase, leading to cell death. Drug is incorporated into DNA and inhibits DNA methyltransferase, causing hypomethylation and cellular differentiation or apoptosis (programmed cell death). Methyltransferase is an enzyme necessary for the expression of cellular genes. The cells in tumors that have progressed or that are resistant to therapy, characteristically have DNA *hyper*-methylation. Decitabine "traps" DNA methyltransferase, thus greatly reducing its activity, which results in the synthesis of DNA that is *hypo*methylated. DNA hypomethylation results in activating genes that have been silent, causing the cell to differentiate, and then to die (cell death through disorganized gene expression or extinction of clones of cells that were terminally differentiated). Research has shown that the drug modulates Tumor Suppressor Genes, the expression of tumor antigens, other genes, and overall cell differentiation.

Metabolism: Biphasic distribution, with mean terminal phase elimination half-life of .5 ± .31 hr. Drug is not plasma bound to serum proteins. Metabolism not fully characterized, but appears to involve deamination in the liver, granulocytes, intestinal epithelium, and whole blood.

Dosage/Range:

- MDS first treatment cycle: 15 mg/m^2 IV continuous infusion over 3 hours, repeated every 8 hours for 3 days.
- Subsequent treatment cycles: Repeat initial cycle every 6 weeks for a minimum of 4 cycles (a CR or PR may take more than 4 cycles).

Dose modifications:

- Delay next cycle until ANC ≥ 1000/μL and platelets ≥ 50,000 μL and dose reduce as follows:
- Recovery requiring more than 6 but less than 8 weeks, delay drug up to 2 weeks and then temporarily reduce dose to 11 mg/m^2 every 8 hours (33/m^2 per day, 99 mg/m^2 per cycle) upon restarting therapy.
- Recovery requiring more than 8 but less than 10 weeks: assess BM for disease progression; if no progression, delay dose up to 2 more weeks and reduce dose to 11 mg/m^2 every 8 hours (33 mg/m^2 per day, 99 mg/m^2 per cycle) upon restarting therapy; maintain or dose increase in subsequent cycles as clinically indicated.
- If any of the non-hematologic toxicities are present, do not restart until toxicity has resolved: serum creatinine ≥ 2 mg/dL, SGPT ≥ 2 times ULN; total bilirubin > 2 times ULN; active or uncontrolled infection.

Drug Preparation:

- Drug supplied for injection as a sterile lyophilized white to almost white powder in a single dose vial containing 50 mg of decitabine. Store vials at 25°C (77°F) with excursions up to 15–30°C (59–86°F) permitted.
- Aseptically add 10 mL sterile water for injection (USP); upon reconstitution, each mL contains approximately 5.0 mg of decitabine at pH 6.7–7.3. Immediately after reconstitution, further dilute with 0.9% sodium chloride injection, 5% dextrose injection, or Lactated Ringer's injection to a final drug concentration of 0.1–1.0 mg/mL. Use within 15 min of reconstitution, or must use cold infusion fluids (2–8°C)

to further dilute the drug, then store at 2–8°C (36–46°F) for up to a maximum of 7 hours until administration.

Drug Administration:
- IV continuous infusion over 3 hours repeated every 8 hours for 3 days.

Drug Interactions:
- Appears to be synergistic with biological agents such as interferons and retinoids (retinoic acid).
- Synergistic cytotoxic effects when given together with each of the following: cisplatin, 4-hydroperoxycyclophosphamide, 3-deazauridine, cyclopentenyl cytosine, cytosine arabinoside, topotecan, and thymidine.
- Does not appear to affect P450 hepatic microenzymes.

Lab Effects/Interference:
- Neutropenia, thrombocytopenia, anemia.
- Hyperglycemia, hyperbilirubinemia.
- Increased creatinine, AST.

Special Considerations:
- Contraindicated in patients with a history of hypersensitivity reactions to the drug or any of its components.
- Indicated for the treatment of patients with myelodysplastic syndrome (MDS), including untreated and previously treated, as well as patients with secondary MDS (refractory anemia, chronic myelomonocytic leukemia), and Intermediate 1, 2, and high-risk International Prognostic Scoring System patients.
- May cause fetal harm; women of childbearing potential should be advised to avoid pregnancy, and if pregnancy occurs, the patient should be apprised of the potential hazard to the fetus.
- Serious adverse events that occurred in patients receiving decitabine, regardless of causality, included cardiac events (MI, CHF, cardiopulmonary arrest, cardiomyopathy, atrial fibrillarin, supraventricular tachycardia); fungal infection, bronchopulmonary aspergillosiycobacterium avium complex infection; intracranial hemorrhage.
- Men should be advised not to father children during treatment and for 2 months afterward.

Potential Toxicities/Side Effects and the Nursing Process

I. POTENTIAL FOR INFECTION AND BLEEDING related to BONE MARROW DEPRESSION

Defining Characteristics: Dose-limiting factor is bone marrow suppression. In MDS studies, the incidence of neutropenia was 90% with 29% of patients developing febrile neutropenia. Thrombocytopenia occurred in 89% of patients. Drug is extensively metabolized in the liver, and partially excreted by the kidneys. Anemia occurs in 82% of patients.

Nursing Implications: Assess baseline CBC and differential, and platelet count, renal and hepatic function tests, prior to initial and subsequent cycles of chemotherapy. Drug should be held if ANC < 1000/μL platelets, 50,000/μL, BR > 2.0 times ULN, AST >, 2 times ULN, creatinine > 2.0 mg/dL (see Dosage). Assess for signs/symptoms of infection, bleeding, and fatigue. Teach patient signs/symptoms of infection or bleeding, to report these immediately, and to come to the emergency room or clinic if febrile or bleeding. Teach patient self-care measures to minimize risk of infection and bleeding. This includes avoidance of crowds and proximity to people with infections, and avoidance of OTC aspirin-containing medications.

II. ALTERED NUTRITION, LESS THAN BODY REQUIREMENTS, related to NAUSEA AND VOMITING, STOMATITIS

Defining Characteristics: Nausea and vomiting may occur, are mild to moderate, and are preventable by antiemetic medicines. Nausea occurs in 42% of patients and vomiting in 25% of patients. Stomatitis occurs in 12% of patients.

Nursing Implications: Premedicate patient with antiemetic. If patient develops nausea and/or vomiting, encourage small, frequent intake of cool, bland foods. Instruct patient to report nausea, and teach self-administration of antiemetic medications. If nausea/vomiting occur and are severe, assess for signs/symptoms of fluid/electrolyte imbalance. Teach patient to self-administer antidiarrheal medications if needed. Assess baseline oral mucous membranes. Teach patient oral assessment, hygiene measures, and to report any alterations.

III. ALTERATION IN COMFORT related to LETHARGY, FEVER, EDEMA, PAIN, RIGORS, ARTHRALGIAS

Defining Characteristics: Pyrexia affects 53% of patients, with rigors in 22% of patients. Peripheral edema affects 25%, arthralgias 20%, and pain 13%. Catheter site pain, erythema, and injection site swelling occurred in 5% of patients.

Nursing Implications: Assess comfort level, symptoms experience at baseline and prior to each dose, then prior to each cycle. Teach patient to alternate rest and activity periods. Teach patient to report fevers > 100.5°F, rigors right away, and to come to the clinic or ED. Teach patient symptomatic management of pain. Assess catheter and injection sites to rule out infection, and to manage comfort.

Drug: docetaxel (Taxotere)

Class: Taxoid, mitotic spindle poison.

Mechanism of Action: Enhances microtubule assembly and inhibits disassembly. Disrupts microtubule network that is essential for mitotic and interphase cellular function. Drug binds to free tubulin and promotes the assembly of tubulin into stable microtubules and also prevents their disassembly. Stabilization of microtubules inhibits mitosis. At low weekly doses, drug may have antiangiogenic properties.

Metabolism: Drug is extensively protein-bound (94–97%). Triphasic elimination. Metabolism involves P-450 3A (CYP3A4) isoenzyme system (in vitro testing). Fecal elimination is main route, accounting for excretion of 75% of the drug and its metabolites within seven days; 80% of the fecal excretion occurs during the first 48 hours. Mild to moderate liver impairment (SGOT and/or SGPT > 1.5 times normal and alk phos > 2.5 times normal) results in decreased clearance of drug by an average of 27%, resulting in a 38% increase in systemic exposure (AUC).

Dosage/Range:

- Adjuvant breast cancer: docetaxel 75 mg/m^2 IV 1 hour after doxorubicin 50 mg/m^2 IVP and cyclophamide 500 mg/m^2 IV q 3 weeks × 6 courses, with G-CSF support PRN.
- Locally advanced or metastatic breast cancer: 60–100 mg/m^2 IV as a 1-hour infusion every 3 weeks.
- Non-small-cell lung cancer, locally advanced or metastatic: (1) 75 mg/m^2 as a 1-hour infusion as a single agent, (2) 75 mg/m^2 as a 1-hour infusion, immediately followed by cisplatin over 30–60 minutes every 3 weeks; or (3) weekly docetaxel 36 mg/m^2 IV × 6 weeks, followed by 2 week rest, repeated q 8 weeks (Hainsworth et al, 2000).
- Hormone refractory prostate cancer: docetaxel 75 mg/m^2 day 1 repeated q 21 days, in combination with prednisone 5 mg PO bid continuously, to be repeated for 10 cycles.
- Advanced gastric cancer: 75 mg/m^2 as a 1-hour infusion followed by cisplatin 75mg/m^2 over 1–3 hr (both on day 1 only), followed by fluorouracil 750 mg/m^2 per day as a 24-hr IV infusion (days 1–5), starting at the end of cisplatin infusion.
- Squamous cell cancer of head and neck (SCCHN) induction therapy followed by RT: 75 mg/m^2 IV (day 1) followed by cisplatin 75 mg/m^2 followed by fluorouracil 750 mg/m^2 per day as a 24-hr IV infusion (days 1–5), starting at end of cisplatin infusion, for four cycles.
- SCCHN induction therapy followed by chemoradiation: 75 mg/m^2 IV (day 1), followed by cisplatin 100 mg/m^2 followed by fluorouracil 1000 mg/m^2 per day as a 24-hr IV infusion (days 1–5), starting at end of cisplatin infusion, for three cycles.
- Dose reductions for nadir ANC < 500 cells/mm^3 for > 1 week, or severe and cumulative cutaneous reactions, or moderate neurosensory signs and/or symptoms, should have a dose reduction when symptoms resolve (see package insert).

- Premedication regimen with corticosteroids: e.g., dexamethasone 8 mg PO bid × 3 days, starting 1 day prior to docetaxel to reduce the incidence and severity of fluid retention and hypersensitivity reactions. For patients with prostate cancer receiving prednisone, the doses of oral dexamethasone are: 8 mg at 12 hours, 3 hours, and 1 hour prior to docetaxel dose.

Drug Preparation (requires 2 dilutions prior to administration):

- Vials available as 80-mg and 20-mg concentrate as single-dose blister packs with diluent. Do not reuse single-dose vials. Drug contains polysorbate 80.
- Unopened vials require protection from bright light. May be stored at room temperature or in refrigerator (36–77°F). Allow to stand at room temperature for at least 5 minutes prior to reconstitution.
- Reconstitute 20-mg and 80-mg vials with the entire contents of accompanying diluent vial (13% ethanol in water for injection). Reconstituted vials contain 10 mg/mL docetaxel (initial diluted solution).
- Gently invert repeatedly, but do not shake the initial diluted solution for approximately 45 seconds.
- Reconstituted vials (10 mg/mL initial diluted solution) are stable for 8 hours at either room temperature or under refrigeration.
- Use only glass or polypropylene or polyolefin plastic (bag) IV containers.
- Withdraw ordered dose, and further dilute in 250 mL volume of 5% dextrose or 0.9% sodium chloride to a final concentration of 0.3–0.74 mg/mL. Thoroughly mix by manual rotation.
- Inspect for any particulate matter or discoloration, and if found, discard.
- Use infusion solution immediately or within 4 hours (including the 1-hour IV administration time).

Drug Administration:

- ANC ≥ 1500 cells/m^2; BR must be < ULN; SGOT and/or SGPT < 1.5 × ULN concomitant with alkaline phosphatase < 2.5 × ULN. Assess patient's ANC and liver function studies, and if abnormal, discuss with physician. See Special Considerations.
- Use only glass or polypropylene bottles, or polypropylene or polyolefin plastic bags for drug infusion, and administer infusion ONLY through polyethylene-lined administration sets.
- Patient should receive corticosteroid premedication (e.g., dexamethasone 8 mg bid) for 3 days beginning 1 day before drug administration to reduce the incidence and severity of fluid retention and hypersensitivity reactions.
- Infuse drug over 1 hour.

Drug Interactions:

- Radiosensitizing effect.
- Theoretically, CYP3A4 inhibitors, such as ketoconazole, erythromycin, troleandomycin, cyclosporine, terfenadine, and nifedipine, can inhibit docetaxel metabolism and result in elevated serum levels of docetaxel; use together with caution or not at all.

- Theoretically, CYP3A4 inducers, such as anticonvulsants and St. John's Wort, may increase metabolism, and decrease serum levels of docetaxel.
- Capecitabine: synergistic effect.
- Calcitriol (high dosN-101): suggested increase in patient survival without added toxicity in patients with prostate cancer (Beer et al, 2007).

Lab Effects/Interference:

- Decreased CBC.

Special Considerations:

- Indicated for the treatment of (1) adjuvant treatment of operable node-positive breast cancer; (2) in combination with trastuzumab in the treatment of HER2 over-expressing node positive or high-risk node negative (ER/PR negative with one high risk feature) (a) as part of a treatment regimen containing doxorubicin, cyclophosphamide, and either paclitaxel or docetaxel OR (b) with docetaxel and carboplatin; (3) locally advanced or metastatic breast cancer after failure of prior chemotherapy; (4) as a single agent in locally advanced or metastatic non-small-cell lung cancer (NSCLC) after failure of prior platinum-based chemotherapy; (5) in combination with cisplatin, in patients with unresectable locally advanced or metastatic NSCLC who have not received prior chemotherapy; (6) in combination with prednisone for the treatment of androgen-independent (hormone-refractory) metastatic prostate; (7) in combination with cisplatin and 5-FU in patients with advanced gastric adenocarcinoma (including gastroesophageal junction) who have not received prior chemotherapy, and (8) as an induction treatment in combination with cisplatin and 5-FU in patients with inoperable locally advanced squamous cell cancer of the head and neck.
- Contraindicated in patients with history of severe hypersensitivity reactions to docetaxel or to other drugs formulated with polysorbate 80; drug should not be used in patients with neutrophil counts of < 1500 cells/mm^3. Drug should not be used in pregnant or breast-feeding women; women of childbearing age should use effective birth control measures.
- Docetaxel generally should not be administered to patients with bilirubin > upper limit of normal (ULN) or to patients with SGOT and/or SGPT > 1.5 × ULN concomitant with alkaline phosphatase > 2.5 × ULN. Patients treated with elevated bilirubin or abnormal transaminases plus alkaline phosphatase have an increased risk of grade 4 neutropenia, febrile neutropenia, severe stomatitis, infections, severe thrombocytopenia, severe skin toxicity, and toxic death. Serum bilirubin, SGOT or SGPT, and alkaline phosphatase should be obtained and reviewed by the treating physician before each cycle of docetaxel treatment.
- Dose modifications during treatment: (1) Patients with breast cancer dosed initially at 100 mg/m^2 who experience either febrile neutropenia, ANC < 500/mm^3 for > 1 week, or severe or cumulative cutaneous reactions, or other grade 3/4 nonhematologic toxicity, should have dose reduced to 75 mg/m^2. If reactions continue at the reduced dose, further reduce to 55 mg/m^2 or discontinue drug. Patients dosed

initially at 60 mg/m^2 who do not experience febrile neutropenia, ANC < 500/mm^3 for > 1 week, nadir platelets < 25,000 cells/mm^3, or severe cutaneous reactions, or severe peripheral neuropathy during drug therapy may tolerate higher drug doses and may be dose-escalated. Patients who develop ≥ grade 3 peripheral neuropathy should have drug discontinued. (2) Patients receiving adjuvant treatment of breast cancer who experience febrile neutropenia should receive G-CSF in all subsequent cycles; if febrile neutropenia recurs, continue G-CSF and dose reduce docetaxel to 60 mg/m^2. Patients who develop grade 3/4 or who develop severe or cumulative cutaneous reactions or moderate neurosensory signs and/or symptoms should have docetaxel dose reduced to 60 mg/m^2. If patient continues to experience these reactions on the reduced dose, treatment should be discontinued. (3) Patients with NSCLC receiving monotherapy, dosed initially at 75 mg/m^2 who experience febrile neutropenia, ANC < 500 mg/m^2 for > 1 week, nadir platelets < 25,000 cells/mm^3, or severe or cumulative cutaneous reactions, or other nonhematologic toxicity grades 3 or 4 should have treatment withheld until toxicity resolves and then have dose reduced to 55 mg/m^2; patients who develop grade ≥ 3 peripheral neuropathy should discontinue docetaxel chemotherapy. (4) Patients with NSCLC receiving combination therapy who are initially dosed at 75 mg/m^2 in combination with cisplatin and whose platelet nadir count during the previous course of therapy is < 25,000 cells/mm^3 or who develop febrile neutropenia or who develop serious non-hematologic toxicities should have a docetaxel dose reduction to 65 mg/m^2 in subsequent cycles. If a further dose reduction is necessary, reduce dose to 50 mg/m^2. (5) Patients with prostate cancer who experience febrile neutropenia, ANC < 500/mm^3 for > 1 week, or severe or cumulative cutaneous reactions, or moderate neuro-sensory signs and/or symptoms during docetaxel therapy should have dose reduced from 75 mg/m^2 to 60 mg/m^2. If the same symptoms arise at the reduced dosage, the drug should be discontinued. (6) Patients with gastric or SCCHN receiving docetaxel in combination with cisplatin and fluorouracil must receive antiemetics and appropriate hydration. G-CSF is recommended for second and subsequent cycles if the patient develops febrile neutropenia, neutropenic infection, or neutropenia lasting more than 7 days. If neutropenic fever, infection, or prolonged neutropenia occur despite G-CSF, reduce docetaxel dose from 75 mg/m^2 to 60 mg/m^2; if neutropenic complications continue to occur despite dose reduction and G-CSF, reduce dose to 45 mg/m^2. In the case of grade 4 thrombocytopenia, dose reduce docetaxel from 75 mg/m^2 to 60 mg/m^2. Retreatment with docetaxel requires that neutrophils recover to > 1500 cells/mm^3 and platelets recover to > 100,000 cells/mm^3. Drug should be discontinued if toxicities persist. Dose modifications of fluorouracil (5-FU): Grade 3 diarrhea, reduce 5-FU dose by 20%; if it occurs a second time, reduce docetaxel dose by 20% as well. If grade 4 diarrhea occurs, reduce 5-FU and docetaxel doses by 20%. If it occurs again, discontinue treatment; grade 3 stomatitis/mucositis: first episode, reduce 5-FU dose by 20%; second episode, stop 5-FU only in this and all subsequent cycles; third episode, dose reduce docetaxel by 20%; grade 4 stomatitis/mucositis: first episode, stop 5-FU only in this and all subsequent cycles; second episode, dose reduce docetaxel by 20%. See package insert for docetaxel dose modifications for abnormal LFTs, as well as those for cisplatin and HFS from 5-FU.

- Patients should receive dexamethasone premedication (such as 8 mg bid × 3 days starting 1 day prior to Taxotere).
- Severe hypersensitivity, including very rare fatal anaphylaxis, has been reported despite dexamethasone premedication.
- Acute myeloid leukemia or MDS may rarely occur after treatment with the drug.
- Administration of docetaxel in Europe is not subject to United States Federal Drug Administration recommendations—non-PVC containers and tubing are not required.
- Incomplete cross-resistance between paclitaxel and docetaxel in many tumor types.
- Studies are ongoing to determine the effectiveness of docetaxel 25–40 mg/m^2 weekly in breast cancer, lung cancer, prostate cancer, and other cancers as drug given in this "dose-dense" fashion. Weekly dose schedules being studied include 3 weeks of treatment followed by 1 week of rest every 4 weeks, and 6 weekly treatments followed by 2 weeks off every 8 weeks. Docetaxel is administered as a 15–30-minute infusion. Hematologic side effects are uncommon with these schedules, and there may be less neuropathy, fatigue, and peripheral edema. Nonhematologic side effects of weekly therapy include asthenia, fluid retention, nail changes, and increased lacrimation. Corticosteroid premedication is often dexamethasone 4 or 8 mg PO q 12 h × 3 doses beginning the day before treatment.
- Incidence of treatment related death increased in patients (1) with elevated LFTs, (2) receiving higher doses (100 mg/m^2), and (3) with NSCLC who have received prior cisplatin and are receiving docetaxel at 100 mg/m^2.

Potential Toxicities/Side Effects and the Nursing Process

I. POTENTIAL FOR INJURY related to HYPERSENSITIVITY OR ANAPHYLAXIS REACTIONS

Defining Characteristics: Severe hypersensitivity reactions characterized by hypotension, dyspnea and/or bronchospasm, or generalized rash/erythema occurred in 2.2% (2 of 92) patients who received 3-day dexamethasone premedication. If patient experiences a severe hypersensitivity reaction, patient should not be rechallenged with docetaxel (e.g., patients with bronchospasm, angioedema, systolic BP < 80 mmHg, generalized urticaria). Minor allergic reactions are characterized by flushing, chest tightness, or low back pain.

Nursing Implications: Ensure that patient has taken premedication (e.g., dexamethasone 8 mg bid starting 1 day prior to chemotherapy). Assess baseline VS and mental status prior to drug administration, especially first and second doses of the drug. Monitor VS every 15 minutes, and remain with patient during first 15 minutes of drug infusion, as most reactions occur during the first 10 minutes.

Stop drug if cardiac arrhythmia (irregular apical pulse) or hypo- or hypertension occur and discuss continuance of infusion with physician. Recall signs/symptoms of anaphylaxis, and if these occur, stop drug immediately and notify physician. Subjective symptoms are generalized itching, nausea, chest tightness, crampy abdominal pain, difficulty speaking, anxiety, agitation, sense of impending doom, uneasiness, desire to urinate/defecate, dizziness, chills. Objective signs are flushed appearance; angioedema of face, neck, eyelids, hands, feet; localized or generalized urticaria; respiratory distress with or without wheezing, hypotension, cyanosis. Review standing orders or nursing procedure for patient management of anaphylaxis, and be prepared to stop drug immediately if signs/symptoms occur, keep IV line open with 0.9% sodium chloride, notify physician, monitor VS, and administer ordered medications, which may include epinephrine 1:1000, hydrocortisone sodium succinate, and diphenhydramine. Teach patient the potential of a hypersensitivity or anaphylactic reaction and to immediately report any unusual symptoms. Depending upon severity of reaction, when planning subsequent treatment discuss with physician administration of antihistamine prior to docetaxel and also gradual increase in infusion rate, e.g., starting at 8-hour rate × 5 minutes, then increasing to 4-hour rate × 5 minutes, then 2-hour rate × 5 minutes, and finally 1-hour infusion rate.

II. POTENTIAL FOR INFECTION AND BLEEDING related to BONE MARROW DEPRESSION

Defining Characteristics: Neutropenia may be severe, is dose-related, is the dose-limiting toxicity, and is noncumulative. Nadir is day 7, with recovery by day 15. Incidence of grade 4 neutropenia (ANC < 500 mm^3) in 2045 patients (any tumor type) with normal hepatic function was 75% at a dose of 100 mg/m^2. Incidence of febrile neutropenia requiring IV antibiotics and/or hospitalization in these patients was 11% and the incidence of septic deaths was 1.6%. Severe thrombocytopenia was less common (8%). However, fatal GI bleeding has been reported in patients with severe hepatic impairment who received docetaxel.

Nursing Implications: Assess LFTs, as dose generally should not be given if SGOT, SGPT, alk phos, or bili suggest moderate to severe hepatic dysfunction (see Special Considerations section). Assess baseline CBC and differential to ensure that ANC is > $1500/mm^3$, and platelet count is > $100{,}000/mm^3$ prior to chemotherapy, as well as for signs/symptoms of infection or bleeding. Teach patient signs/symptoms of infection or bleeding and to report these immediately, and teach patient self-care measures to minimize risk of infection and bleeding. This includes avoidance of crowds and proximity to people with infections, and avoidance of OTC aspirin-containing medications. Teach patient self-administration of G-CSF as ordered to prevent severe neutropenia, and EPO as ordered to prevent severe anemia/transfusion requirements.

Instruct patient to alternate rest and activity periods, and to report increased fatigue, shortness of breath, or chest pain that might herald severe anemia.

III. POTENTIAL ALTERATION IN ACTIVITY TOLERANCE related to ASTHENIA, FATIGUE, MYALGIA, ANEMIA

Defining Characteristics: Fatigue, weakness, and malaise may last from a few days to several weeks, but is rarely severe enough to be dose-limiting. Incidence of asthenia (all grades) is 50–66%. Incidence of anemia is 90%, with grades of 3 and 4 occurring in 8% at doses of 100 mg/m^2 and in 9% at doses of 75 mg/m^2.

Nursing Implications: Assess Hgb/HCT prior to each treatment and at nadir counts. Assess patient activity tolerance and ability to do ADLs. Teach patient self-care strategies to minimize exertion, and maximize activity, such as clustering activity during shopping, alternating rest and activity periods, diet, gentle exercise. Teach self-administration of EPO, if ordered, to prevent severe anemia/transfusion requirements. Instruct patient to alternate rest and activity periods, and to report increased fatigue, shortness of breath, or chest pain that might herald severe anemia.

IV. POTENTIAL ALTERATION IN FLUID BALANCE related to FLUID RETENTION

Defining Characteristics: Fluid retention is a cumulative toxicity that may occur in docetaxel treated patients. Peripheral edema usually begins in the lower extremities and may become generalized with weight gain (2 kg average). Fluid retention is not associated with cardiac, renal, or hepatic impairment and may be minimized by use of dexamethasone 8 mg bid for 3 days beginning the day prior to therapy. Severe fluid retention may occur in up to 6.5% of patients despite premedication, and is characterized by generalized edema, poorly tolerated peripheral edema, pleural effusion requiring drainage, dyspnea at rest, cardiac tamponade, or abdominal distention (due to ascites). Fluid retention usually resolves completely within 16 weeks of last docetaxel dose (range, 0–42+ weeks).

Nursing Implications: Ensure that patient takes corticosteroids as ordered to minimize risk of developing fluid retention. Assess baseline weight and skin turgor, especially in the extremities. Assess respiratory status, including breath sounds. Instruct patient to report any alterations in breathing patterns, swelling in the extremities, and weight gain. If patient has preexisting effusion, monitor effusion closely during treatment. If fluid retention occurs, instruct patient to elevate extremities while at rest. Teach patient not to use added salt when eating or cooking. Discuss with physician use of diuretics for new-onset edema, progression of edema, and weight gain, e.g., > 2 lb.

V. POTENTIAL IMPAIRMENT OF SKIN INTEGRITY related to RASH, ALOPECIA, NAIL CHANGES

Defining Characteristics: Maculopapular, violaceous/erythematous, and pruritic rash may occur, usually on the feet and/or hands, but may also occur on arms, face, or thorax. These localized eruptions usually occur within one week of last docetaxel treatment, and are reversible and usually resolve prior to next treatment. Overall, about 50% of patients experience skin problems. Palmarplantar erythrodysesthia (hand-foot syndrome) may occur but can be minimized by adherence to three-day corticosteroid premedication. Drug extravasation may cause skin discoloration, but no necrosis. Most patients on every-3-week schedules experience alopecia (75% at dose of 100 mg/m^2 and 56% at dose of 75%). Changes in nails may occur in 11–40% of patients, and be severe in 1–2% of patients (hypo- or hyperpigmentation, onycholysis [loss of nail]).

Nursing Implications: Assess skin for any cutaneous changes, such as rash, and any associated symptoms, such as pruritus, and discuss management with physician. If patient develops severe or cumulative skin toxicity, docetaxel dose should be reduced (see Special Considerations). Instruct patient in self-care measures such as avoidance of abrasive skin products and clothing, avoidance of tight-fitting clothes, use of skin emollients appropriate for skin problem, and measures to prevent itching. Discuss potential impact of hair loss prior to drug administration, coping strategies, and plan to minimize body image distortion (e.g., wig, scarf, cap). Assess patient for signs/symptoms of hair loss. Assess patient's response and use of coping strategies; help patient to build on effective strategies. Teach patient self-care measures to preserve hair, such as washing hair with warm water, use of a gentle shampoo and conditioner, use of a soft-bristle brush, cutting hair short to reduce pressure on hair shaft, and use of a satin pillowcase to minimize friction on hair shaft. Teach patient to wear a wide-brimmed hat and sunglasses when outside, and to use sunscreen (at least SPF 15) on scalp when outdoors without a hat. Assess nails baseline, and teach patient to report changes. Teach patient to keep nails clean and trimmed, not to wear nail polish or imitation nails, and to wear protective gloves when doing house cleaning, and gardening. Teach patient to use a nail hardener if nails appear soft, and to use Lotrimin cream if ordered. Severe skin problems require a dose reduction.

VI. SENSORY/PERCEPTUAL ALTERATIONS related to SENSORY NEUROPATHY

Defining Characteristics: Grade 1–4 peripheral neuropathy may affect up to 49% of patients (severe 5.5%). Sensory alterations are paresthesias in a glove and stocking distribution, and numbness. There may be loss of sensation symmetrically, of vibration, and of proprioception. Risk is increased in patients receiving both docetaxel and cisplatin, or in patients with prior neuropathy from diabetes mellitus or alcohol. Extremity weakness or transient myalgia may also occur. Patients described spontaneous reversal of symptoms in a median of 9 weeks from onset (range 0–106).

Nursing Implications: Assess baseline neurologic status. Instruct patient to report signs/symptoms of pins and needle sensation, numbness, pain, increased discomfort with certain sensations, especially in the extremities, or motor weakness. Identify patients at risk: prior cisplatin, or having preexisting neuropathies (ethanol- and diabetes mellitus-related). Assess sensory and motor function prior to each treatment, and if abnormality found, assess impact on patient's function, safety, independence, and quality of life. Test patient's ability to button a shirt, or pick up a dime from a flat surface. If severely impacting safety or quality of life, discuss with patient and physician drug discontinuance or use of cytoprotective agent. Teach self-care strategies, including maintaining safety when walking, getting up, taking bath, or washing dishes and unable to sense temperature, and the need to keep extremities warm in cold weather. Docetaxel should be discontinued if patient develops grades 3 or 4 peripheral neuropathy (see NCI Common Toxicity Criteria, Appendix II). Grade 3 motor = objective weakness, interfering with ADLs; grade 3 sensory = sensory loss or paresthesia interfering with ADLs; grade 4 motor = paralysis; grade 4 sensory = permanent sensory loss that interferes with function.

VII. ALTERED NUTRITION, LESS THAN BODY REQUIREMENTS, related to NAUSEA AND VOMITING, DIARRHEA, CONSTIPATION, DYSGEUSIA, ANOREXIA, STOMATITIS

Defining Characteristics: Nausea and vomiting may occur, but are mild and preventable with antiemetics. Diarrhea occurs and is mild; incidence of any grade of nausea is 33–42%, vomiting 22%, and diarrhea 22–42%. Incidence of stomatitis is 26–51% (severe 5.5%). Only 1.1% of breast cancer patients who received three-day corticosteroid treatment developed severe mucositis.

Nursing Implications: Premedicate patient with antiemetic. If patient develops nausea and/or vomiting, encourage small, frequent intake of cool, bland foods. Instruct patient to report nausea, and teach self-administration of antiemetic medications. If nausea/vomiting occur and are severe, assess for signs/symptoms of fluid/electrolyte imbalance. Encourage patient to report onset of diarrhea. Teach patient to self-administer antidiarrheal medications if needed. Assess baseline oral mucous membranes. Ensure that patient takes three-day corticosteroid regimen. Teach patient oral assessment, hygiene measures, and to report any alterations.

VIII. ALTERATION IN VISION, POTENTIAL, related to HYPERLACRIMATION

Defining Characteristics: Epiphora or hyperlacrimation occurs as a result of lacrimal duct stenosis. There is inflammation of the conjunctiva and ductal epithelium, which occurs chronically, especially with weekly docetaxel therapy. This appears related to cumulative dose, usually about 300 mg/m^2 and resolves after treatment is stopped. Stenosis of tear ducts is reversible.

Nursing Implications: Assess baseline vision and function of tear ducts. Teach patient that this may occur, and to report it. If this occurs, teach patient to use "artificial tears" frequently throughout day, or saline eyewash. Discuss with physician use of prophylactic steroid ophthalmic solution, such as prednisolone acetate 2 gtt bid × 3 days, beginning the day before docetaxel treatment, if patient does not have a history of herpetic eye infection. If the patient is on weekly therapy, discuss with physician treatment break × 2 weeks for symptoms to resolve, and resumption of therapy on a three-week-on, one-week-off schedule.

Drug: doxorubicin hydrochloride (Adriamycin)

Class: Anthracycline antibiotic isolated from streptomycin products, in particular from the rhodomycin products.

Mechanism of Action: Topoisomerase-II inhibitor; antitumor antibiotic binds directly to DNA base pairs (intercalates) and inhibits DNA and DNA-dependent RNA synthesis, as well as protein synthesis; also binds to lipid cellular membrane and disrupts cellular functions, as well as creating hydroxyl free radicals (causes cardiotoxicity in heart cells). Both actions result in programmed cell death (apoptosis). Cell cycle specific for S phase.

Metabolism: Excretion of drug predominates in the liver; renal clearance is minor. Alteration in liver function requires modification of doses, whereas with renal failure there is no need to alter doses. Terminal half-life is 20–48 hours. Drug does not cross the blood–brain barrier. Drug is excreted through urine and may discolor urine from 1–48 hours after administration.

Dosage/Range:
- 60–75 mg/m^2 IV every 2 weeks (dose dense) or 20 mg/m^2 IV weekly.
- 30–75 mg/m^2 IV every 3–4 weeks.
- 20–30 mg/m^2/IV for 3 consecutive days.
- For bladder instillation: 3–60 mg/m^2.
- For interperitoneal instillation: 40 mg in 2 L dialysate (no heparin).
- Continuous infusion: Varies with individual protocol.
- Dose reduce for hepatic dysfunction (50% DR BR 1.2–3 mg/dL; 75 % DR BR > 3.0 mg/dL).

Drug Preparation:
- Available powder for injection (RDF, 10-, 20-, 50-, or 150-mg vials), lyophilized powder (Rubex, 50- or 100-mg vials), solution for injection (PFS, 2 mg/mL), and preservative-free solution (PFS, 2 mg/mL).
- Drug will form a precipitate if mixed with heparin or 5-FU. Dilute with 0.9% sodium chloride (preservative-free) to produce 2-mg/mL concentration.

Drug Administration:

- This drug is a potent vesicant. Give through a patent, running IV to avoid extravasation, which may lead to ulceration, pain, and necrosis. Be sure to check nursing procedure for administration of a vesicant. ANC must be ≥ 1500 cells/m^3.

Drug Interactions:

- Barbiturates: increased plasma clearance of doxorubicin.
- Phenytoin: reduced phenytoin levels.
- Cyclophosphamide: risk of hemorrhage and increased cardiotoxicity.
- Mitomycin: increased risk of cardiotoxicity.
- Trastuzumab: increased risk of cardiotoxicity, avoid concomitant administration.
- Paclitaxel: increased risk of cardiotoxicity; give sequentially.
- Digoxin: decreased serum levels of digoxin; avoid concomitant administration.
- Mercaptopurine: increased risk of hepatotoxicity.
- Incompatible with heparin, forming a precipitate.
- Progesterone (high doses): increased neutropenia and thrombocytopenia.
- Verapamil: in mice, increased cardiotoxicity.
- Cyclosporine: increased toxicity, coma; do not use concurrently.

Lab Effects/Interference:

- Decreased CBC.
- Increased LFTs.
- Increased uric acid secondary to tumor lysis.

Special Considerations:

- Drug is a potent vesicant. Give through patent, running IV to avoid extravasation and tissue necrosis.
- Indicated for the treatment of (1) adjuvant treatment of lymph node positive breast cancer in combination with other agents after surgical resection of primary tumor, and (2) drug has been used in the treatment of acute lymphoblastic leukemia, acute myeloblastic leukemia, Wilms' tumor, neuroblastoma, soft tissue and bone sarcomas, Hodgkin's disease, malignant lymphoma, and cancers of the breast, ovary, bladder (transitional cell), and lung (bronchiogenic).
- Contraindications: ANC < 1500 cells/m^3, severe hepatic impairment, recent myocardial infarction, severe arrhythmias, prior lifetime cumulative doses of anthracyclines, hypersensitivity to doxorubicin.
- Give through central line if drug is to be given by continuous infusion.
- Nausea and vomiting are dose-related. Occur in 50% of patients and begin 1–3 hours after administration.
- Causes discoloration of urine (from pink to red for up to 48 hours).
- Skin changes: May cause radiation recall phenomenon—recalls reaction in previously irradiated tissue.
- Potent myelosuppressive agent causes GI toxicities: mucositis, esophagitis, and diarrhea.

- Cardiac toxicity: Dose limit at 550 mg/m^2. Patients may exhibit irreversible CHF. Acute toxicity may be seen within hours after administration. This is unrelated to cumulative dose and may manifest symptoms of pump or conduction dysfunction. Rarely, transient EKG abnormalities, CHF, pericardial effusion (whole syndrome referred to as *myocarditis-pericarditis syndrome*) may occur, which may lead to death of patient.
- Vein discoloration.
- Increased pigmentation in black patients.
- Drug dosage reductions necessary for hepatic dysfunction: 50% dose given for serum bili 1.2–2.9 mg/dL, 25% dose given for serum bili 3 mg/dL.
- Prior chest radiation therapy (XRT): reduce total lifetime dose to 300–350 mg/m^2.
- Concomitant cyclophosphamide administration: may limit to 450 mg/m^2.
- Obesity: use ideal body weight table found in nutrition books to calculate dose.
- Dexrazoxane available for patients at risk for cardiotoxicity but for whom doxorubicin continues to be effective. See Chapter 4.
- Secondary acute myelocytic leukemia (AML) or myelodysplastic syndrome (MDS); often refractory when results from combination chemotherapy or radiation therapy.
- Delayed cardiotoxicity when used in children.

Potential Toxicities/Side Effects and the Nursing Process

I. POTENTIAL FOR INFECTION AND BLEEDING related to BONE MARROW DEPRESSION

Defining Characteristics: WBC and platelet nadir 10–14 days after drug dose, with recovery from days 15–21. Myelosuppression may be severe but is less severe with weekly dosing.

Nursing Implications: Monitor CBC, WBC, differential, and platelet count prior to drug administration; discuss any abnormalities with physician. Assess for signs/symptoms of infection or bleeding; instruct patient in self-assessment and to report signs/symptoms immediately. Teach patient self-care measures to minimize risk of infection and bleeding, including avoidance of OTC aspirin-containing medications. Drug dosage must be reduced if patient has hepatic dysfunction: 50% reduction of drug dose if bili is 1.2–3.0 mg/dL; 75% reduction if bili is > 3.0 mg/dL.

II. POTENTIAL FOR ALTERATION IN CARDIAC OUTPUT related to ACUTE AND CHRONIC CARDIAC CHANGES

Defining Characteristics: Acutely, pericarditis-myocarditis syndrome may occur during infusion or immediately after (non–life-threatening EKG changes of flat T waves, ST segment changes, PVCs). With high cumulative doses > 550 mg/m^2

(450 mg/m^2 if concurrent treatment with cardiotoxic drugs or radiation to the chest), cardiomyopathy may occur. Risk is decreased if drug given as continuous infusion.

Nursing Implications: Assess cardiac status prior to chemotherapy administration: signs/symptoms of CHF, quality/regularity and rate of heartbeat, results of prior GBPS or other test of LVEF (stop drug if 10% decrease below LLN, LVEF of 45%, or decrease in LVEF of 20% at any level). Instruct patient to report dyspnea, palpitations, swelling in extremities. Maintain accurate records of total dose; expect GBPS to be repeated periodically during treatment and the drug to be discontinued if there is a significant drop in heart function.

III. POTENTIAL FOR ALTERATION IN NUTRITION, LESS THAN BODY REQUIREMENTS, related to NAUSEA AND VOMITING, ANOREXIA, STOMATITIS

Defining Characteristics: Nausea/vomiting occurs in 50% of patients, is moderate to severe, and is preventable with combination antiemetics. Onset 1–3 hours after drug dose and lasts 24 hours. Anorexia occurs frequently, and stomatitis occurs in 10% of patients.

Nursing Implications: Premedicate with combination antiemetics and continue protection for 24 hours. If patient has a central line, slower infusion of drug over 1 hour decreases nausea/vomiting. Encourage small, frequent feedings of bland foods. Anorexia occurs frequently: teach patient or caregiver to make foods ahead of time and use spices; encourage taking weekly weight. Stomatitis occurs in 10% of patients, and esophagitis may occur in patients who have received prior radiation to the chest. Perform oral assessment prior to drug administration and during posttreatment visits. Teach patient oral hygiene and self-assessment techniques.

IV. POTENTIAL ALTERATION IN SKIN INTEGRITY related to ALOPECIA, RADIATION RECALL, NAIL AND SKIN CHANGES, AND DRUG EXTRAVASATION

Defining Characteristics: Complete alopecia occurs with doses > 50 mg/m^2, occurring after therapy begins. Regrowth usually begins a few months after drug is stopped. Hyperpigmentation of nail beds and dermal creases of hands is greatest in dark-skinned individuals. Skin damage from prior radiation may be reactivated. Adriamycin "flare" may occur during peripheral drug administration, often with urticaria and pruritus, and is due to local allergic reaction. Drug is a potent vesicant and causes SEVERE tissue destruction if drug extravasates.

Nursing Implications: Discuss with patient hair loss, anticipated impact, and strategies to decrease distress, e.g., obtaining wig prior to hair loss. Assess body disturbance from hyperpigmentation and discuss strategies to minimize this, e.g., nail polish for dark nail beds. Drug must be administered via patent IV. If flare occurs, this must be distinguished from extravasation, where there is leakage of drug into the perivascular tissue. Stop or slow drug injection and flush with plain IV solution. Wait to see whether reaction will resolve. If confirmed flare, consider diphenhydramine 25 mg IVP to resolve pruritus and/or urticaria, and then resume administration of drug slowly into freely flowing IV. Assess need for venous access device early. If drug administered as a continuous infusion, IT MUST BE GIVEN VIA A CENTRAL LINE.

V. POTENTIAL SEXUAL DYSFUNCTION related to DRUG EFFECT

Defining Characteristics: Drug is teratogenic, mutagenic, and carcinogenic.

Nursing Implications: Assess patient's/partner's sexual patterns and reproductive goals. Provide information, supportive counseling, and referral as needed. Teach importance of birth control measures as appropriate. Male patients may wish to use a sperm bank prior to therapy.

Drug: doxorubicin hydrochloride liposome injection (Doxil)

Class: Anthracycline antibiotic isolated from streptomycin products.

Mechanism of Action: Topoisomerase-inhibitor; antitumor antibiotic binds directly to DNA base pairs (intercalates) and inhibits DNA and DNA-dependent RNA synthesis, as well as protein synthesis. Cytotoxic in all phases of cell cycle but maximally in S phase. Cell cycle nonspecific. Drug is encapsulated in STEALTH liposomes, which have surface-bound methoxypolyethylene glycol to protect the liposome from detection by blood phagocytes, and thus prolong circulation time. It is believed that the liposomal-encapsulated drug is able to penetrate the tumor through abnormal capillaries (tumor neovasculature) and then, once inside the tumor, accumulates and the drug is released.

Metabolism: Slower clearance from the body than doxorubicin (0.041 L/h/m^2 vs 24–35 L/h/m^2) with resulting larger AUC than a similar dose of doxorubicin. Half-life is approximately 55 hours. Has preferential uptake in Kaposi's sarcoma tumors.

Dosage/Range:

- Treatment of metastatic carcinoma of the ovary: 50 mg/m^2 IV every 4 weeks for a minimum of 4 cycles, or until disease progression or toxicity.
- Treatment of multiple myeloma in combination with bortezomib: 30 mg/m^2 IV over 1 hour on day 4 (after bortezomib dose) of a 21-day treatment cycle. Bortezomib 1.3 mg/m^2 IV on days 1, 4, 8, and 11 of a 21-day cycle.
- AIDS/Kaposi's sarcoma: 20 mg/m^2 IV over 30 minutes once every 3 weeks.
- Dose-reduce for palmar-plantar erythrodysesthesia, hematologic toxicity, or stomatitis.

Drug Preparation:

- Drug is available as vials containing 20-mg and 50-mg doxorubicin HCl in a 2-mg/mL concentration.
- Inspect drug for any particulate matter or discoloration; drug is translucent, with red liposomal dispersion.
- Further dilute drug (dose up to 90 mg) in 250 mL 5% dextrose USP ONLY; use 500 mL 5% dextrose USP for doses > 90 mg.
- Administer at once or store diluted drug for 24 hours refrigerated at 2–8°C (36–46°F).

Drug Administration:

- Administer IV at an initial rate of 1 mg/min to minimize risk of infusion reaction; if no reaction, increase rate to complete administration over 1 hour.
- Treat if ANC > 1500 cells/mm^3 and platelets > 75,000/mm^3.
- Dose-reduce for hepatic dysfunction: 50% dose reduction for bilirubin 1.2–3.0 mg/dL; 75% dose reduction if bilirubin > 3.0 mg/dL.
- Delay next dose and dose reduce for grade 3/4 hand-foot syndrome, hematologic toxicity.
- Do not use inline filter.
- Monitor for infusion reactions if drug is infused too rapidly.
- DO NOT ADMINISTER IM OR SUBCUTANEOUS. DO NOT SUBSTITUTE for doxorubicin (nonliposomal).

Drug Interactions:

- Doxorubicin may potentiate the toxicity of (1) cyclophosphamide-induced hemorrhagic cystitis; (2) hepatotoxicity of 6-mercaptopurine; (3) radiation toxicity to heart, mucous membranes, skin, liver.

Lab Effects/Interference:

- Decreased CBC.

Special Considerations:

- Drug is an irritant, not a vesicant.
- Acute, infusion-associated reactions may occur (7% incidence) during drug infusion, characterized by flushing, shortness of breath, facial swelling, headache, chills, back pain, chest or throat tightness, and/or hypotension. Infusion should be stopped. If symptoms are minor, infusion may be resumed at a slower rate, but discontinue if symptoms resume.
- Assessment for cardiac toxicity similar to that for doxorubicin should be done since limited information is available as to cardiotoxicity of liposomal doxorubicin at high cumulative doses.
- FDA-approved for treatment of: (1) patients with ovarian cancer whose disease has progressed or recurred after platinum-based chemotherapy, (2) progressive AIDS-related Kaposi's sarcoma in patients whose disease has progressed on prior combination chemotherapy or in patients unable to tolerate combination chemotherapy,

(3) in combination with bortezomib for the treatment of patients with multiple myeloma who have received one prior treatment, not including bortezomib.
- Drug has been used for the treatment of breast cancer.

Potential Toxicities/Side Effects and the Nursing Process

I. POTENTIAL FOR INFECTION AND BLEEDING related to BONE MARROW DEPRESSION

Defining Characteristics: Leukopenia occurs in 91% of patients, with anemia and thrombocytopenia (< 150,000/mm^3) less common (55% and 60%, respectively). Neutropenia (< 2000/mm^3) occurred in 85% and ANC (< 500/mm^3) occurred in 13% of patients. In ovarian cancer patients, incidence of neutropenia (< 2000 cells/mm^3) was 51%, but ANC < 500 cells/mm^3 was only 8.3%. Thrombocytopenia (< 150,000/mm^3) occurred in 24%, while severe (< 25,000/mm^3) occurred in 1.1% of patients with ovarian cancer. Dose-limiting toxicity in the treatment of HIV-infected patients, possibly because of HIV disease and/or concomitant medications. Anemia may also occur.

Nursing Implications: Monitor CBC, WBC, differential, and platelet count prior to drug administration, and discuss any abnormalities with physician. Assess for signs/symptoms of infection or bleeding, and instruct patient in self-assessment and to report signs/symptoms immediately. Teach patient self-care measures to minimize risk of infection and bleeding, including avoidance of OTC aspirin-containing medications. See drug dosage reductions in Special Considerations section.

II. POTENTIAL FOR ALTERATION IN CARDIAC OUTPUT related to ACUTE AND CHRONIC CARDIAC CHANGES

Defining Characteristics: Experience and data is limited in the cardiotoxicity of liposomal doxorubicin at high cumulative doses. Therefore, the manufacturer recommends the adoption of cardiotoxicity warnings made for doxorubicin HCl. With high cumulative doses > 550 mg/m^2 (400 mg/m^2 if concurrent treatment with cardiotoxic drugs such as cyclophosphamide, or radiation to the chest), cardiomyopathy may occur. In clinical trials, the incidence of "possibly or probably related" cardiac-related adverse events, including cardiomyopathy, arrhythmia, heart failure, pericardial effusion, and tachycardia, was 1–5% in patients with AIDS/Kaposi's sarcoma and < 1% in ovarian cancer patients. In patients with multiple myeloma, the incidence of heart failure events similar in treatment arms (3%), with decreases in LVEF 13% in combination arm compared with 8% in the bortezomib arm alone.

Nursing Implications: Assess patient risk (history of prior anthracycline chemotherapy, history of cardiovascular disease). Assess cardiac status prior to chemotherapy administration: signs/symptoms of CHF, quality/regularity and rate of heartbeat, results of prior GBPS or other test of LVEF. Instruct patient to report dyspnea, palpitations, swelling in extremities. Maintain accurate records of total dose. Expect GBPS to be repeated periodically during treatment and the drug to be discontinued if there is a significant drop in heart function.

III. POTENTIAL FOR INJURY related to ALLERGIC INFUSION REACTION TO LIPOSOMAL COMPONENT(S)

Defining Characteristics: During the initial infusion, patients may experience an acute reaction characterized by flushing, shortness of breath, facial swelling, headache, chills, back pain, chest or throat tightness, and/or hypotension. Incidence is 5–6%. Reactions generally resolve after the immediate termination of the infusion in several hours to a day, or in some patients, after slowing of the infusion rate. Of those patients who experienced reactions, many were able to tolerate subsequent treatment without problem; however, some patients terminated therapy with liposomal doxorubicin because of the reaction.

Nursing Implications: Assess baseline comfort, vital signs, general condition. Infuse liposomal doxorubicin at 1 mg/min to minimize risk of acute reaction. Teach patient to report signs/symptoms of reaction immediately during infusion, and assess patient frequently during initial infusion. If signs/symptoms occur, stop infusion immediately. Discuss with the physician, but anticipate that if signs/symptoms are mild, infusion will resume at slower rate, and if signs/symptoms are severe, patient may not receive additional liposomal doxorubicin.

IV. POTENTIAL ALTERATIONS IN COMFORT AND ACTIVITY related to PALMAR-PLANTAR ERYTHRODYSESTHESIA (HAND-FOOT SYNDROME)

Defining Characteristics: Incidence is approximately 3.4% in patients receiving a dose of 20 mg/m^2 and 37% in patients with ovarian cancer (16% grades 3 and 4). Toxicity becomes dose-limiting in clinical studies at doses of 60 mg/m^2, or when treatment is administered more frequently than every three weeks. Signs/symptoms are swelling, pain, erythema, possibly progressing to desquamation of the skin on hands and feet, and usually occur after six weeks of treatment. Reaction is generally mild, not requiring treatment delays. However, in some patients, reaction can be severe and debilitating, necessitating discontinuance of treatment.

Nursing Implications: Assess baseline skin of patients' hands and feet, and in women with ovarian cancer, skin under areas of pressure, such as under the breasts of women with large breasts or skin folds, before each treatment. Teach patient to report signs/symptoms of reaction (e.g., tingling or burning, redness, flaking of skin in areas of pressure such as soles of feet, under breasts in large-breasted women, small blisters, or small sores on the palms of hands or soles of feet). If signs/symptoms occur, discuss treatment, treatment delays, or discontinuance. Do not use hydrocortisone cream as this will cause greater desquamation of skin.

V. POTENTIAL FOR ALTERATION IN NUTRITION, LESS THAN BODY REQUIREMENTS, related to NAUSEA AND VOMITING, STOMATITIS, DIARRHEA, ANOREXIA

Defining Characteristics: Nausea and/or vomiting occur in 17% and 8% of patients, respectively, are mild to moderate, and are preventable with antiemetics. Stomatitis occurs in 7% of patients. Incidence of diarrhea is 8%. Anorexia may affect 1–5% of patients.

Nursing Implications: Premedicate with antiemetic (dopamine antagonist or serotonin antagonist). Encourage small, frequent feeding of bland foods. Stomatitis occurs in 7% of patients. Perform oral assessment prior to drug administration, and during posttreatment visits. Dose reductions or delay necessary for grades 2–4 stomatitis. Teach patient oral hygiene, and self-assessment techniques. Instruct patient to report diarrhea, and teach self-management strategies for diarrhea.

VI. POTENTIAL FOR ALTERATION IN SKIN INTEGRITY related to ALOPECIA, RASH, PRURITUS, AND RADIATION RECALL

Defining Characteristics: Incidence of alopecia significantly less with liposomal delivery of doxorubicin, and is about 9% in AIDS/Kaposi's sarcoma patients and 15% in women with ovarian cancer. Skin damage from prior radiation may be reactivated. Rash and itching occur in 1–5% of the patients. Rarely, significant skin reactions may occur, such as exfoliative dermatitis. Drug is an irritant, but extravasation should be avoided.

Nursing Implications: Discuss with patient low incidence of hair loss, and to report hair thinning if it occurs. At that time, discuss impact and strategies to decrease distress. Instruct patient to report skin rash or itching, and discuss significance and management with physician. Teach patient to assess for skin changes in prior radiated sites, including mucous membranes, and to report this immediately. Assess and develop management strategies depending on site and extent. Use caution to avoid drug extravasation; if infiltration occurs, stop infusion, apply ice for 30 minutes, and restart a new IV elsewhere.

VII. POTENTIAL ALTERATION IN NUTRITION related to NAUSEA AND/OR VOMITING, STOMATITIS

Defining Characteristics: Nausea occurs in 37% (severe, grade 3/4 in 8%) of ovarian cancer patients and 17% of AIDS/Kaposi's sarcoma patients. Vomiting occurs in

22% of ovarian cancer patients and 7.8% of patients with AIDS/Kaposi's sarcoma. Stomatitis occurs in 37% of women with ovarian cancer and is severe in 7.7%; overall incidence in AIDS/Kaposi's sarcoma patients is 6.8%.

Nursing Implications: Assess baseline nutritional status. Teach patient that these side effects may occur and teach self-care measures, including self-assessment, oral hygiene regimen, and to report occurrence of symptoms. Administer antiemetic prior to chemotherapy, especially in ovarian cancer patients, and assess efficacy after treatment. Revise antiemetic regimen as needed to provide complete protection from nausea and/or vomiting. Assess oral mucosa prior to each treatment. If stomatitis develops, dose reduction should be considered.

VIII. POTENTIAL SEXUAL DYSFUNCTION related to DRUG EFFECTS

Defining Characteristics: Drug is embryotoxic. Doxorubicin has been shown to be carcinogenic and mutagenic.

Nursing Implications: Assess patient's/partner's sexual pattern and reproductive goals. Provide information, supportive counseling, and referral as needed. Teach importance of birth control measures for female patients of childbearing age. Mothers who are nursing should discontinue nursing during treatment.

IX. ACTIVITY INTOLERANCE related to ASTHENIA AND FATIGUE

Defining Characteristics: Anemia is the most common hematologic event, affecting 52.6% of women with ovarian cancer, but only 25% experienced severe anemia (Hgb < 8 gm/dL). Incidence for patients with AIDS/Kaposi's syndrome overall is 55%, with 4% experiencing severe anemia. Asthenia is more common in women with ovarian cancer, affecting 33%, while patients with AIDS/Kaposi's syndrome had an incidence of 9.9%.

Nursing Implications: Assess activity tolerance, and HCT/Hgb baseline, and prior to each treatment. Teach patients to report any changes in energy and activity level. Teach patients self-care strategies to maximize energy use and conservation. Evaluate efficacy of strategies at each visit, and if ineffective, assist patient to problem solve other alternative solutions, such as friends, volunteers, to help with activities such as shopping, food preparation.

Drug: eniluracil (776C85)

Class: Dihydropyrimidine dehydrogenase inhibitor. When used with 5-fluorouracil (5-FU), together they become dihydropyrimidine dehydrogenase inhibitory fluoropyrimidines.

Mechanism of Action: Dihydropyrimidine dehydrogenase (DPD) is the rate limiting enzyme in the degradation of 5-FU. By inhibiting DPD, eniluracil permits higher and longer sustained serum levels of 5-FU. In early studies, a single dose of eniluracil increased plasma half-life of oral 5-FU 6 times, and produced 100% bioavailability (Smith et al, 2000).

Metabolism: Unclear.

Dosage/Range:
- Per protocol.
- Advanced breast cancer: 10 mg/m^2 bid daily × 28 days, with oral 5-FU 1.0 mg/m^2 bid daily × 28 days, then rest × 7 days, cycle repeated q 35 days.
- Dose reduce for hematologic or gastrointestinal toxicity.

Drug Preparation:
- None, oral, available as 2.5-mg and 10-mg tablets.

Drug Administration:
- Take with large amount of water (e.g., 180 mL) at least 1 hour before or after eating.

Drug Interactions:
- Significantly increases 5-FU serum level and half-life, mimicking continuous 5-FU infusions.

Lab Effects/Interference:
- Unknown.

Special Considerations:
- Eniluracil dose is in 10:1 ratio with 5-FU.
- In study of patients with advanced breast cancer, using oral 5-FU concurrently with eniluracil, incidence of grade 1 hand-foot syndrome was 15% and neuropathy 9%, grade 1 only.
- Concurrent oral eniluracil and oral 5-FU well tolerated with low toxicity profile.

Potential Toxicities/Side Effects and the Nursing Process (when used together with oral 5-FU in study on advanced breast cancer)

I. POTENTIAL FOR INFECTION AND BLEEDING related to BONE MARROW DEPRESSION

Defining Characteristics: Neutropenia and thrombocytopenia are dose-related and occur rarely. In the advanced breast cancer trial of oral eniluracil and 5-FU, 30% of patients had granulocytopenia (6% grade 3, 1 patient had neutropenic sepsis), and 42% had thrombocytopenia (3% grade 3). 36% of patients had anemia. Toxicity is enhanced when combined with leucovorin calcium.

Nursing Implications: Assess baseline CBC, WBC, differential, and platelet count prior to chemotherapy, as well as for signs/symptoms of infection or bleeding. Teach patient signs/symptoms of infection or bleeding, and instruct to report these immediately. Teach patient self-care measures to minimize risk of infection and bleeding, including avoidance of crowds, proximity to people with infections, and OTC aspirin-containing medications.

II. ACTIVITY INTOLERANCE, POTENTIAL, related to ASTHENIA, FATIGUE, MALAISE

Defining Characteristics: Malaise and fatigue were reported in 45% of patients, grades 1–2. Anemia occurred in 36% of patients, all grades 1–2.

Nursing Implications: Assess baseline activity level, tolerance, and self-care ability. Teach patients that these side effects are common, but manageable. Assess need for home care assistance and arrange if possible. If not, and needed, involve social worker to assist in coordinating care. Teach patient to alternate rest and activity periods, and strategies to conserve energy.

III. ALTERED NUTRITION, LESS THAN BODY REQUIREMENTS, related to NAUSEA AND VOMITING, STOMATITIS, AND DIARRHEA

Defining Characteristics: Nausea occurred in 27% and vomiting in 12% of patients but was mild. Mucositis was uncommon, affecting 6% of patients, all grades 1–2. Diarrhea can be severe, and in prolonged courses is the dose-limiting toxicity.

Nursing Implications: Premedicate patient with antiemetics (phenothiazines are usually effective), and continue for 24 hours, at least for the first cycle. Encourage small, frequent meals of cool, bland foods. Assess oral mucosa prior to drug administration and instruct patient to report changes. Teach patient oral hygiene measures and self-assessment. Instruct patient to report diarrhea, to self-administer prescribed antidiarrheal medications, and to drink adequate fluids.

Drug: epirubicin hydrochloride (Ellence, Farmorubicin(e), Farmorubicina, Pharmorubicin)

Class: Anthracycline antitumor antibiotic analogue.

Mechanism of Action: Drug complexes with DNA by intercalation of planar rings between DNA base pairs; this inhibits nucleic acid (DNA and RNA) and protein synthesis. This also causes cleavage of DNA by topoisomerase II, causing cell death. Drug also prevents enzymatic separation of DNA, interfering with replication and transcription. Drug also causes the production of cytotoxic free radicals.

Metabolism: Following IV administration, drug rapidly disperses into body tissues and into red blood cells; drug is 77% bound to plasma proteins. Drug is rapidly and extensively metabolized in the liver, excreted primarily through the biliary system, and to a lesser extent in the urine. Drug clearance is reduced in elderly women (35% lower in women aged ≥ 70 years old). Drug clearance is reduced 30% in mild hepatic dysfunction, and 50% in moderate hepatic dysfunction. Drug clearance is reduced (50%) in patients with severe renal impairment (serum creatinine ≥ 5 mg/dL). Dose reductions should be made for patients with hepatic dysfunction and patients with severe renal dysfunction.

Dosage/Range:

FDA indication:

Starting dose as part of adjuvant therapy in patients with axillary node positive breast cancer: 100 mg/m^2 to 120 mg/m^2 IV every 3–4 weeks.

- Drug dose may be given in one day (100 mg/m^2), or divided equally (60 mg/m^2) and given on day 1 and day 8.
- Other dosing schedules that have been studied: 20 mg IV q week; intravesicular dose of 50 mg weekly as a 0.1% solution × 8 weeks, with dose reduction for chemical cystitis.

Dose modifications:

- Bone marrow dysfunction: Consider dose of 75–90 mg/m^2 if patient heavily pre-treated (e.g., with existing BMD or bone marrow infiltration by tumor).
- Hepatic dysfunction: Bilirubin 1.2–3 mg/dL or AST 2–4 × Upper Limit of Normal (ULN) = 50% of recommended starting dose; bilirubin > 3 mg/dL or AST > 4 × ULN = 25% of recommended starting dose.
- Renal dysfunction: Consider lower doses if serum creatinine > 5 mg/dL.
- Dosage adjustment after first treatment cycle: Platelet count < 50,000/mm^3, ANC < 250/mm^3, neutropenic fever, or grades 3/4 nonhematologic toxicity: day 1 dose should be 75% of prior day 1 dose. Delay day 1 chemo until platelet count ≥ 100,000/mm^3, ANC ≥ 1500/mm^3, and nonhematologic toxicities have recovered to ≤ grade 1. If patient is receiving dose divided into day 1 and 8, day 8 dose should be 75% of day 1 dose if platelet counts are 75,000/mm^3–100,000/mm^3 and ANC is 1000–1499/mm^3. If day 8 platelet counts are < 75,000/mm^3, ANC < 1000, or grade 3/4 nonhematologic toxicity has occurred, omit the day 8 dose.
- Patients receiving dose of 120 mg/m^2 regimen should also receive prophylactic antibiotic therapy with trimethoprim-sulfamethoxazole or a fluoroquinolone.

Drug Preparation:

- Drug is provided as a preservative-free, ready-to-use solution (50-mg/25-mL and 200-mg/100-mL single-use vials).
- Use within 24 hours of penetration of rubber stopper; discard any unused drug.
- Store unopened vials in refrigerator between 36–46°F (2–8°C).

Drug Administration:

- Drug is a vesicant, so vesicant precautions should be used (check nursing procedure for administration of a vesicant).
- ANC must be > 1500 cells/mm^3, platelets > 100,000/mm^3.

- Administer via slow IVP into the tubing of a freely flowing IV infusion of 0.9% NS or 5% dextrose solution over 3–5 minutes, checking blood return every few milliliters of drug.

Drug Interactions:
- Cytotoxic drugs: Additive toxicity (hematologic and gastrointestinal).
- Cardioactive drugs (e.g., calcium channel blockers): May increase risk of congestive heart failure; use together cautiously, and monitor cardiac function closely during treatment.
- Radiation therapy: Tissue sensitization to cytotoxic effects of radiation therapy; when drug is given after prior radiation therapy, a radiation recall inflammatory reaction may occur at site of prior radiation.
- Cimetidine: Increases drug AUC by 50%, DO NOT use together. Hold cimetidine during treatment with epirubicin.
- Other drugs extensively metabolized by the liver: Changes in hepatic function caused by concomitant therapies may affect clearance of epirubicin; use together with caution, if at all, and monitor for hematologic and gastrointestinal toxicity closely during treatment.
- Bone marrow-suppressing drugs: increased bone marrow depression.
- Taxanes: separate administration by at least 24 hours to minimize risk of toxicity.

Lab Effects/Interference:
- Decreased white blood and neutrophil cell counts, platelet counts.

Special Considerations:
- Drug is a vesicant, and severe local tissue necrosis will occur if drug infiltrates; avoid IV sites over joints, into small veins, or in veins on arms that have compromised venous or lymphatic drainage.
- Drug should never be given intramuscularly.
- Myocardial toxicity (e.g., CHF) may occur during therapy or months to years after cessation of therapy, and risk increases according to dose. Cumulative doses > 900 mg/m^2 should generally not be exceeded. Risk increases with prior anthracycline or anthracenedione therapy, past or concurrent radiation therapy to mediastinal/pericardial area, active or history of cardiovascular disease, or concomitant use of other cardiotoxic drugs.
- Rarely, secondary cancers (e.g., acute myelogenous leukemia) have been reported, and risk is increased when given in combination with other cytotoxic drugs or when doses of anthracycline chemotherapy have been escalated. The estimated risk is 0.2% at three years, and 0.8% at five years.
- Myelosuppression is the dose-limiting toxicity, and severe myelosuppression may occur.
- Doses must be reduced in patients with hepatic dysfunction.
- Drug is mutagenic, carcinogenic, and genotoxic. Men and women of childbearing age should use effective birth control measures.

- Nursing mothers should not breast-feed during chemotherapy treatment.
- Teach patients that urine will be pink-red for the first 1–2 days following drug administration.

Potential Toxicities/Side Effects and the Nursing Process

I. POTENTIAL FOR INFECTION, BLEEDING, FATIGUE related to BONE MARROW DEPRESSION

Defining Characteristics: WBC and platelet nadir 10–14 days after drug dose, with recovery by day 21. Leukopenia and neutropenia may be severe, especially when given with other myelosuppressive chemotherapy. Thrombocytopenia may be severe, and anemia may occur.

Nursing Implications: Monitor CBC, WBC, differential, and platelet count prior to drug administration; discuss any abnormalities with physician. Assess for signs/symptoms of infection or bleeding; instruct patient in self-assessment and to report signs/symptoms immediately. Teach patient self-care measures to minimize risk of infection and bleeding, including avoidance of company of people with colds and OTC aspirin-containing medications. Dose reduction necessary in patients with hepatic dysfunction, as decreased metabolism of drug results in increased serum levels of drug and hematologic toxicity. Patients receiving 120 mg/m^2 dose should also receive prophylactic antibiotic therapy with trimethoprim-sulfamethoxazole or a fluoroquinolone antibiotic.

II. POTENTIAL FOR ALTERATION IN CARDIAC OUTPUT related to ACUTE AND CHRONIC CARDIAC CHANGES

Defining Characteristics: Cardiotoxicity is dose-related, cumulative, and may occur during or months to years after cessation of therapy. The estimated probability of developing clinically evident CHF is 0.9% at a cumulative dose of 500 mg/m^2, 1.6% at 700 mg/m^2, and 3.3% at a cumulative dose of 900 mg/m^2. The risk of CHF increases rapidly with cumulative doses in excess of 900 mg/m^2. Risk of developing cardiotoxicity is increased by history of cardiovascular disease, prior anthracycline or anthrocenedione therapy, prior or concomitant radiation therapy to mediastinum and/or pericardial area, and concomitant use of other cardiotoxic drugs. Cardiotoxicity may be acute (early) or delayed (late). Signs/symptoms of early toxicity are not usually of clinical significance, do not predict late cardiotoxicity, and usually do not require change in epirubicin therapy. These include: sinus tachycardia and EKG abnormalities (nonspecific ST–T wave changes, and, rarely, PVCs, VT, bradycardia, atrioventricular and bundle branch block). Delayed cardiotoxicity is related to cardiomyopathy, characterized by decreased left ventricular ejection fraction (LVEF) and classic signs/symptoms of CHF (tachycardia, dyspnea, pulmonary edema, dependent edema, hepatomegaly, ascites, pleural effusion, gallop rhythm). If late cardiotoxicity occurs, it is in the late stages of treatment or within months following treatment, and is cumulative dose-related.

Nursing Implications: Assess cardiac status prior to chemotherapy administration: risk factors and signs/symptoms of CHF, quality/regularity and rate of heartbeat, results of baseline and periodic prior gated blood pool scan (GBPS), multigated radionuclide angiography (MUGA), echocardiogram (ECHO), or other test of LVEF. Instruct patient to report dyspnea, palpitations, and swelling in extremities. Maintain accurate records of total dose; expect GBPS or measure of LVEF to be repeated periodically during treatment and the drug to be discontinued if there is a significant drop in heart function as evidenced by LVEF falling below normal range.

III. POTENTIAL FOR ALTERATION IN NUTRITION, LESS THAN BODY REQUIREMENTS, related to NAUSEA AND VOMITING, DIARRHEA, STOMATITIS

Defining Characteristics: Nausea/vomiting occurs in > 90% of patients, can be moderate to severe especially when drug is given together with other emetogenic chemotherapy, and is preventable with combination antiemetics. Onset 1–3 hours after drug dose and lasts 24 hours. Mucositis may occur; stomatitis is most common. Esophagitis is less common but may occur, especially if patient has had prior radiotherapy to the chest. Drug dose must be reduced in patients with hepatic dysfunction; otherwise, increased gastrointestinal toxicity will occur.

Nursing Implications: Assess baseline LFTs, and discuss with physician dose reduction if abnormal. Premedicate with combination antiemetics and continue protection for 24 hours. If patient has a central line, slower infusion of drug over 1 hour decreases nausea/vomiting. Encourage small, frequent feedings of bland foods. Perform oral assessment prior to drug administration and during posttreatment visits. Teach patient oral hygiene and self-assessment techniques. Teach patient to report pain, burning sensation, erythema, erosions, ulcerations, bleeding, or oral infections.

IV. POTENTIAL ALTERATION IN SKIN INTEGRITY related to ALOPECIA, RADIATION RECALL, FACIAL FLUSHING, FLARE REACTION, NAIL/SKIN/ORAL MUCOUS MEMBRANE HYPERPIGMENTATION, AND DRUG EXTRAVASATION

Defining Characteristics: Alopecia is universal, but is reversible, with hair regrowth in two to three months following cessation of therapy. Skin damage and inflammation from prior radiation may be reactivated when drug is given. Drug may cause "flare" reaction or streaking along vein during peripheral drug administration, often with facial flushing, and may be related to excessively rapid drug administration. If it occurs, slow drug administration time, flush line with plain IV solution, and slowly complete therapy. This must be distinguished from extravasation, where there is leakage of drug into the perivascular tissue. Skin and nail hyperpigmentation may occur.

Nursing Implications: Discuss with patient hair loss, anticipated impact, and strategies to decrease distress, e.g., obtaining wig prior to hair loss. Assess body disturbance from hyperpigmentation and discuss strategies to minimize this, e.g., nail polish for dark nail beds. Drug must be administered via patent IV. Local phlebitis or thrombophlebitis may follow a flare reaction, so assess vein path closely, and teach patient to report any pain, erythema, or swelling following drug administration. Drug is a potent vesicant and causes SEVERE tissue destruction if drug extravasates. Teach patient to report any stinging or burning during drug administration, and stop administration if there is any question at all. Assess need for venous access device early.

V. POTENTIAL FOR SEXUAL DYSFUNCTION related to REPRODUCTIVE HAZARD

Defining Characteristics: Drug is genotoxic, mutagenic, and carcinogenic. In laboratory animals receiving very high doses of the drug, testicular atrophy occurred. Drug may cause irreversible amenorrhea in premenopausal women (premature menopause).

Nursing Implications: Assess patient's/partner's sexual patterns and reproductive goals. Provide information, supportive counseling, and referral as needed. Teach importance of birth control measures as appropriate. Male patients may wish to use a sperm bank, and women may wish to investigate cryopreservation of oocytes prior to therapy.

Drug: estramustine (Estracyte, Emcyt)

Class: Alkylating agent.

Mechanism of Action: Acts as a weak alkylator at usual therapeutic concentrations. A chemical combination of mechlorethamine and estradiol phosphate, estramustine is believed to selectively enter cells with estrogen receptors, where the drug acts as an alkylating agent due to bischloroethyl side-chain and liberated estrogens. Believed to have antimicrotubule activity. Cell cycle nonspecific.

Metabolism: Well-absorbed orally, metabolized in liver, partly excreted in urine. Induces a marked decline in serum calcium and phosphate levels.

Dosage/Range:
- 600 mg/m^2 (15 mg/kg) orally daily in three divided doses (range, 10–16 mg/kg/day in most studies with evaluation after 30–90 days).
- IV: Available for investigational use; 150 mg IV initially, then may increase to 300 mg/day per protocol.

Drug Preparation:
- Available in 140-mg capsules.

- Store in refrigerator (2–8°C [36–46°F]); may be stored at room temperature for 24–48 hours.
- IV: Dissolve in at least 10 mL sterile water.

Drug Administration:
- Oral with water, at least 1 hour before or 2 hours after meals.
- IV (investigational): Slow IVP via IV containing 5% dextrose.

Drug Interactions:
- Drug/food: milk, milk products, and Ca^{2+}-rich foods may decrease drug absorption.
- Calcium-containing antacids: may impair drug absorption, take 1 hour before, or 2 hours after drug dose.
- Synergy with vinblastine.

Lab Effects/Interference:
- Changes in Ca.
- Increased serum glucose, LDH, triglyceride levels.
- Increased LFTs, RFTs.
- May affect certain endocrine (e.g., thyroid function tests, prolactin, cortisol) and LFTs because it contains estrogen.

Special Considerations:
- Avoid taking drug with milk, milk products, and calcium-rich foods (e.g., antacids), as this will delay or impair drug absorption.
- Contraindicated or to be used with great caution in patients who are children or who have thrombophlebitis or thromboembolic disorders, peptic ulcers, severe hepatic dysfunction, cardiac disease, hypertension, or diabetes. Drug may increase the risk of embolic events; physician may recommend prophylactic warfarin or aspirin.
- IV preparation is a vesicant; avoid extravasation.
- Transient perineal itching and pain after IV administration.

Potential Toxicities/Side Effects and the Nursing Process

I. POTENTIAL ALTERATION IN TISSUE PERFUSION related to THROMBOPHLEBITIS, THROMBOSIS

Defining Characteristics: Increased risk of clot formation, with risk for development of thrombophlebitis, pulmonary emboli, myocardial infarction, and cerebrovascular accident.

Nursing Implications: Assess patient risk; drug is contraindicated in patients with thrombophlebitis or thromboembolic disorders, unless caused by the malignancy. Should be used cautiously in these patients, and in those patients with coronary artery disease. Drug may worsen CHF. Assess baseline cardiac and peripheral vascular status, including signs/symptoms of CHF. Monitor blood pressure and glucose tolerance during therapy. Instruct patient to report immediately any signs/symptoms, e.g., dyspnea, edema, pain, and erythema in legs.

II. BODY IMAGE DISTURBANCE related to GYNECOMASTIA

Defining Characteristics: Mild to moderate breast enlargement may occur, with nipple tenderness initially.

Nursing Implications: Teach patient about potential side effects; discuss potential impact on body image and comfort. Encourage patient to verbalize feelings; provide information and emotional support.

III. POTENTIAL ALTERATION IN COMFORT related to PERINEAL SYMPTOMS, HEADACHE, RASH, URTICARIA, TRANSIENT PARESTHESIAS (IV)

Defining Characteristics: Perineal itching and pain, as well as transient paresthesias of the mouth, may occur after IV administration (investigational). Other symptoms that may accompany oral dosing are rash, pruritus, dry skin, peeling skin of fingertips, thinning hair, night sweats, lethargy, pain in eyes, and breast tenderness.

Nursing Implications: Assess patient for occurrence of symptoms and discuss measures for symptomatic relief.

IV. POTENTIAL FOR ALTERATION IN NUTRITION, LESS THAN BODY REQUIREMENTS, related to NAUSEA AND VOMITING, DIARRHEA, HEPATIC DYSFUNCTION

Defining Characteristics: Nausea and vomiting occur at higher dosing; tolerance may develop, but dose may need to be reduced. Nausea and vomiting may be delayed but become intractable and necessitate discontinuance of the drug. Diarrhea occurs occasionally. Mild elevations in liver function tests may occur (LDH, SGOT, bili) with or without jaundice, but are usually self-limiting. Abnormal Ca++ and P levels may occur.

Nursing Implications: Assess baseline nutritional fluid and electrolyte status. Premedicate with antiemetics prior to drug administration and continue through treatment. Assess baseline LFTs and Ca++ and P levels; monitor during therapy and discuss any abnormalities with physician. Monitor daily or weekly weights.

Drug: estrogens: diethylstilbestrol (DES), ethinyl estradiol (Estinyl), conjugated estrogen (Premarin), chlorotrianisene (Tace)

Class: Hormones.

Mechanism of Action: Unknown; estrogens change the hormonal milieu of the body.

Metabolism: Metabolized mainly in the liver. Undergoes enterohepatic recirculation. DES is metabolized more slowly than natural estrogens.

Dosage/Range:
- DES: Prostate cancer: 1–3 mg PO daily; breast cancer: 5 mg PO tid.
- Diethylstilbestrol diphosphate: Prostate cancer: 50–200 mg PO tid, 0.5–1.0 g IV daily × 5 days, then 250–1000 mg each week.
- Chlorotrianisene: 1–10 mg PO tid.
- Ethinyl estradiol: 0.5–1.0 mg PO tid.

Drug Preparation:
- None.

Drug Administration:
- Oral.

Drug Interactions:
- None significant.

Lab Effects/Interference:
- Increased Ca.
- Increased T_4 levels.
- Increased clotting factors.
- Decreased serum folate.

Special Considerations:
- Long-term dosage of DES in men has been associated with cardiovascular deaths. Maximum dose should be 1 mg tid for prostate cancer.
- Can cause inaccurate laboratory results (liver, adrenal, thyroid).
- Causes rapid rise in serum calcium in patients with bony metastases; watch for symptoms of hypercalcemia.

Potential Toxicities/Side Effects and the Nursing Process

I. POTENTIAL FOR INJURY related to THROMBOEMBOLIC COMPLICATIONS, HYPERCALCEMIA, SODIUM AND WATER RETENTION, AND CARDIOTOXICITY

Defining Characteristics: Thromboembolic complications are infrequent but serious, and increased risk occurs with long-term use and higher doses. Hypercalcemia occurs in 5–10% of women with breast cancer metastatic to bone, appears in first two weeks of therapy, and is aggravated by preexisting renal disease. There is an increased risk of cardiovascular-related deaths, especially in men on high-dose estrogens for prostate cancer. Drug should be used cautiously, if at all, in patients with underlying cardiac, renal, or hepatic disease.

Nursing Implications: Assess risk (preexisting cardiac, hepatic, and renal disease), baseline cardiac, and vascular status; discuss abnormalities with physician. Monitor status during therapy. Teach patient to report signs/symptoms of edema, dyspnea, localized swelling, pain, tenderness, erythema, and CNS changes. Teach female patient signs/symptoms of hypercalcemia (drowsiness, increased thirst, constipation, increased urine output) and to report this. Monitor Ca++ level in women with metastatic breast cancer closely during first few weeks of therapy.

II. ALTERATION IN NUTRITION, LESS THAN BODY REQUIREMENTS, related to NAUSEA AND VOMITING

Defining Characteristics: Occurs in 25% of patients; intensity is related to specific drug and dose. Tolerance occurs after a few weeks of therapy.

Nursing Implications: Inform patient that this may occur; teach self-administration of antiemetics prior to drug administration per physician order, and to take drug at bedtime to decrease nausea. Discuss with physician starting patient at low dose, with increase as tolerated.

III. ALTERATION IN MALE SEXUAL FUNCTION related to GYNECOMASTIA, LOSS OF LIBIDO, IMPOTENCE, AND VOICE CHANGE

Defining Characteristics: Gynecomastia may be prevented by pretreatment of breast with low dose of radiotherapy. Feminine characteristics disappear when therapy is stopped.

Nursing Implications: Explore with patient and partner reproductive and sexual patterns and impact that chemotherapy may have. Provide information, supportive counseling, and referral as indicated. Since alternative, superior hormonal manipulative drugs are available, discuss these with physician.

IV. POTENTIAL FOR FEMALE SEXUAL DYSFUNCTION related to BREAST TENDERNESS/ENGORGEMENT, UTERINE PROLAPSE, AND URINARY INCONTINENCE

Defining Characteristics: Breast engorgement may occur in postmenopausal women; uterine prolapse and exacerbation of preexisting uterine fibroids with possible uterine bleeding may occur, as may urinary incontinence.

Nursing Implications: Explore with patient sexual and reproductive patterns, and any impact the drug may have. Provide information, supportive counseling, and referral as needed. Discuss with physician alternative hormonal manipulative drugs as needed.

Drug: etoposide (VP-16, VePesid, Etopophos)

Class: Plant alkaloid, a derivative of the mandrake plant (mayapple plant).

Mechanism of Action: Inhibits DNA synthesis in S and G_2 so that cells do not enter mitosis. Causes single-strand breaks in DNA. Cell cycle specific for S and G_2 phases.

Metabolism: Etoposide is rapidly excreted in the urine and, to a lesser extent, in the bile. About 30% of drug is excreted unchanged. Binds to serum albumin (94%) and then becomes extensively tissue-bound.

Dosage/Range:

- 50–100 mg/m^2 IV daily × 5 days (testicular cancer) every 3–4 weeks.
- 75–200 mg/m^2 IV daily × 3 days (small-cell lung cancer) every 3–4 weeks.
- Many other doses based on tumor type being treated (e.g., lymphomas, ANLL, bladder, prostate, uterus, Kaposi's sarcoma).
- Oral dose is twice the intravenous dose, rounded to the nearest 50 mg; can take with or without food.
- High dose (bone marrow transplantation): 750–2400 mg/m^2 IV, or 10–60 mg/kg over 1–4 hours to 24 hours, usually combined with other cytotoxic agents or total body irradiation.
- Dose modification if renal or hepatic dysfunction (see Special Considerations section).

Drug Preparation:

- Available in 5-cc (100-mg) vial as VePesid; the 100-mg Etopophos vial is reconstituted with 5 mL or 10 mL normal saline, D5W, sterile water, bacteriostatic sterile water, or bacteriostatic normal saline with benzyl alcohol to 20 mg/mL or 10 mg/mL, respectively. May be further diluted with NS or D5W to 0.1 mg/mL final concentration.
- Oral capsules are available in 50-mg and 100-mg capsules, and should be stored in the refrigerator.

Drug Administration:

- IV infusion: VePesid over 30–60 minutes to minimize risk of hypotension and bronchospasm (wheezing). In some instances, a test dose may be infused slowly (0.5 mL in 50 0.9% sodium chloride) and the remaining drug infused if no untoward reaction after 5 minutes. Etopophos: IVB over 5 minutes as drug is significantly less likely to cause hypotension.
- Stability: Drug must be diluted with either 5% dextrose injection USP or 0.9% sodium chloride solution and is stable 96 hours in glass and 48 hours in plastic containers at room temperature (25°C [77°F]) under normal fluorescent light at a concentration of 0.2 mg/mL.
- Inspect for clarity of solution prior to administration.
- Oral administration: may give as a single dose up to 400 mg; otherwise, divide dose into 2–4 doses.

Drug Interactions:
- Enhances warfarin action by increasing prothrombin time (PT); need to monitor closely.
- Increased toxicity of methotrexate when given concurrently.
- Cyclosporin: additive cytotoxicity when given concurrently.
- CYP3A4 inducers (e.g., phenytoin) may decrease etoposide level, while CYP3A4 inhibitors (e.g., ketoconazole) may increase etoposide level.
- St. John's Wort: may decrease etoposide level, do not use concurrently.

Lab Effects/Interference:
- Increased PT with patients on warfarin.
- Increased LFTs, metabolic acidosis with higher doses.

Special Considerations:
- Nadir 7–14 days after treatment.
- Dose modifications: reduce drug dose by 50% if bili > 1.5 mg/dL, by 75% if bili > 3.0 mg/dL. Reduce drug 25% if creatinine clearance 10–50 mL/min; reduce by 50% if creatinine clearance < 10 mL/min.
- Synergistic drug effect in combination with cisplatin.
- Radiation recall may occur when combined therapies are used.
- Patients receiving high-dose therapy are at risk for the development of second malignancy or ethanol intoxication (injection contains polyethylene glycol with absolute alcohol).
- VePesid: drug stability is concentration-dependent, while Etopophos is prepared as a phosphate ester, which negates the need for concentration-dependent stability (equally stable for 24 hours at concentrations of 20 mg/mL to 0.1 mg/mL).

Etoposide concentration (mg/mL)	5% Dextrose	0.9% Sodium Chloride
2	0.5 hour*	0.5 hour*
1	2 hours	2 hours
0.6	8 hours	8 hours
0.4	48 hours	48 hours
0.2	96 hours	96 hours

*Check for fine precipitate.
Source: Data from Dorr RT, Von Hoff DD (1994) *Cancer Chemotherapy Handbook* (2nd ed.). Norwalk, CT: Appleton & Lange, p. 462.

Potential Toxicities/Side Effects and the Nursing Process

I. POTENTIAL FOR INJURY related to ALLERGIC REACTION, HYPOTENSION, ANAPHYLAXIS DURING DRUG INFUSION

Defining Characteristics: Bronchospasm (wheezing) may occur, with or without fever, chills; hypotension may occur during rapid infusion. Anaphylaxis may occur, but is rare.

Nursing Implications: Infuse drug over at least 30–60 minutes in correct amount of IV solution (stability related to volume). Monitor temperature, vital signs prior to drug administration, and periodically during treatment. Remain with patient during first 15 minutes of infusion and assess for signs/symptoms of bronchospasm. Discontinue drug and notify physician if bronchospasm or signs/symptoms of anaphylactic-like reaction occur. Maintain patent IV, monitor VS, and have ready epinephrine, diphenhydramine, and hydrocortisone, as well as emergency equipment. Be familiar with institution's practice guidelines for management of anaphylaxis.

II. POTENTIAL FOR INFECTION AND BLEEDING related to BONE MARROW DEPRESSION

Defining Characteristics: Nadir 10–14 days after drug dose, with recovery on days 21–22. Neutropenia may be severe. Profound bone marrow suppression when given in high doses for bone marrow/stem cell rescue.

Nursing Implications: Monitor CBC, WBC, differential, and platelet count prior to chemotherapy and at expected nadir. Assess for signs/symptoms of infection or bleeding prior to drug administration; instruct patient in self-assessment and to report signs/symptoms immediately. Teach patient self-care measures to minimize risk of infection and bleeding, including avoidance of OTC aspirin-containing medications.

III. ALTERED NUTRITION, LESS THAN BODY REQUIREMENTS, related to NAUSEA AND VOMITING, ANOREXIA

Defining Characteristics: Nausea and vomiting are usually mild, occurring soon after infusion. Oral dosing has higher incidence of nausea/vomiting. Anorexia is mild but may be severe with oral dosing. Severe nausea and vomiting when given in high doses, requiring aggressive, maximal antiemesis. In addition, hepatitis, stomatitis, and metabolic acidosis may occur with high-dose therapy.

Nursing Implications: Premedicate with antiemetics and continue prophylactically for at least 4–6 hours after drug administration. Encourage small feedings of bland, cool foods and liquids; encourage spices as desired. Consult dietitian if anorexia is severe. Patients receiving high-dose therapy should have baseline and periodic assessment of laboratory parameters (e.g., LFTs and chemistries), as well as assessment of oral mucosa. Teach patients self-care, including oral assessment, use of oral hygiene regimen, and to report pain, burning, oral lesions.

IV. BODY IMAGE DISTURBANCE related to ALOPECIA

Defining Characteristics: Incidence is 20–90% and is dose-dependent; regrowth may occur between drug cycles.

Nursing Implications: Discuss with patient possible hair loss and potential coping strategies, including obtaining wig or cap. If hair loss is complete, instruct patient to wear cap or scarf at night to prevent loss of body heat in cold climates.

V. POTENTIAL SEXUAL DYSFUNCTION related to DRUG EFFECTS

Defining Characteristics: Drug is mutagenic and teratogenic.

Nursing Implications: Explore with patient and partner sexual patterns and reproductive goals. Teach about need for contraception as appropriate. Provide information, emotional support, and referral as needed.

VI. ALTERED SKIN INTEGRITY related to RADIATION RECALL, PERIVASCULAR IRRITATION IF DRUG INFILTRATES, AND SKIN LESIONS WITH HIGH-DOSE THERAPY

Defining Characteristics: Drug is a radiosensitizer and an irritant. Patients receiving high-dose therapy may develop bullae on the skin (similar to Stevens-Johnson syndrome).

Nursing Implications: Assess skin in area of prior radiation when combined therapies are given as well as mucous membranes. Drug may need to be withheld until skin healing occurs if radiation recall results in skin breakdown. Teach patient wound-management techniques. Use careful venipuncture and infuse drug through patent IV over 30–60 minutes, diluted according to manufacturer's specifications. Teach patients receiving high-dose therapy to report any skin changes.

VII. ALTERATION IN CARDIAC OUTPUT related to RARE MYOCARDIAL INFARCTION, ARRHYTHMIAS

Defining Characteristics: Rare myocardial infarction has been reported after prior mediastinal XRT in patients receiving etoposide-containing regimens. Arrhythmias are uncommon but may occur, especially in patients with preexisting coronary artery disease.

Nursing Implications: Monitor patient during infusion and instruct patient to report any unusual sensations. Discuss any abnormalities with physician.

VIII. SENSORY/PERCEPTUAL ALTERATION related to NEUROTOXICITY

Defining Characteristics: Peripheral neuropathies may occur but are uncommon and mild.

Nursing Implications: Assess motor and sensory function prior to drug administration. Instruct patient to report any changes in sensation or function. Discuss any abnormalities with physician. Encourage patient to verbalize feelings about discomfort and sensory loss, and discuss alternative coping strategies.

Drug: exemestane (Aromasin)

Class: Steroidal aromatase inactivator.

Mechanism of Action: Aromatase converts adrenal and ovarian androgens into estrogen, peripherally, in postmenopausal women. Exemestane acts as a false substrate (looks like androstenedione) and binds irreversibly to the aromatase enzyme, making it inactive ("suicide inhibition"). This results in a significant decrease (up to 95%) in circulating estrogen levels in postmenopausal women without affecting other adrenal enzymes. In the absence of estrogen, the stimulus for breast cancer growth is removed.

Metabolism: Oral drug is rapidly absorbed from the GI tract, with plasma levels increased by about 40% if taken after a high-fat breakfast. Drug is extensively distributed into the tissues, and is highly protein-bound (90%). Drug is extensively metabolized in the liver by the P450 3A4 (CYP 3A4) isoenzyme system, and excreted equally in urine and feces. After a single dose of 25 mg, maximal suppression of circulating estrogen occurs 2–3 days after the dose, and lasts for 4–5 days. In patients with either hepatic or renal insufficiency, the dose of exemestane was three times higher than in patients with normal liver or renal function. This does not require dosage adjustment, but studies looking at the safety of chronic dosing in these groups of patients have not been done.

Dosage/Range:
- 25 mg tab PO daily.

Drug Preparation:
- None. Store tablets at 77°F (25°C).

Drug Administration:
- Oral, once daily, after a meal.

Drug Interactions:
- Although metabolized by the P450 3A4 (CYP 3A4) isoenzyme system, it is unlikely that inhibitors of this system will significantly increase exemestane serum levels; however, manufacturer cautions that known inducers of the enzyme system (e.g., carbamazepine, nafcillin, phenobarbital, phenytoin) may decrease serum levels, and should be used together cautiously.
- St. John's wort: may decrease serum drug level; do not use concurrently.

Lab Effects/Interference:
- Lymphopenia (20% incidence).
- Elevated LFTs (AST, ALT, alk phos, GGT) rarely.

Special Considerations:

- Drug is indicated for the (1) adjuvant treatment of postmenopausal women with ER positive early breast cancer who received 2–3 years of tamoxifen and who are switched to exemestane for completion of a total of five consecutive years of adjuvant hormonal therapy and (2) treatment of advanced breast cancer in postmenopausal women ONLY, whose disease has progressed following tamoxifen therapy. Drug should not be used for premenopausal women as the presence of estrogen may interfere with exemestane action.
- Drug should not be given to pregnant women.
- Drug is well tolerated, with mild to moderate side effects.
- Differs from other selective aromatase inhibitors in that drug irreversibly binds to aromatase, and androgens cannot displace drug from this enzyme. Body must synthesize new aromatase to start estrogen production again.
- Drug similar to or superior to megestrol acetate after tamoxifen failure in metastatic breast cancer (Kaufmann et al, 2000).

Potential Toxicities/Side Effects and the Nursing Process

I. ALTERATION IN ACTIVITY related to FATIGUE

Defining Characteristics: Overall incidence in studies is 22%, while incidence considered drug-related or of indeterminate cause is 8%.

Nursing Implications: Assess baseline activity tolerance, and self-care ability. Teach patient that fatigue may occur, but is usually mild to moderate. Teach patient to alternate rest and activity. Teach patient to manage activities of daily living using energy-saving strategies, e.g., shopping, cooking. Teach patient to accept assistance from friends and family as needed.

II. ALTERATION IN COMFORT related to HOT FLASHES, INCREASED SWEATING, PAIN

Defining Characteristics: Incidence of events attributable to exemestane were hot flashes, 13%, and increased sweating, 4%. In total evaluation of all adverse events, all patients, pain was reported in 13%.

Nursing Implications: Assess patient baseline comfort, and incidence and tolerance of hot flashes and increased sweating. Assess whether patient has any pain, and effectiveness of current pain-management regimen. Teach patient self-care strategies to maximize comfort, to keep cool (e.g., light, loose clothing, fans, cool drinks) and dry (e.g., use of corn starch after bathing, fan), and to minimize any painful discomfort (e.g., depending upon type and location of pain, OTC analgesics, application of heat, cold, Tiger Balm).

III. ALTERATION IN NUTRITION, POTENTIAL, related to NAUSEA, INCREASED APPETITE

Defining Characteristics: Nausea appeared drug-related or of indeterminate cause in 9% of patients, and 3% of patients noted an increased appetite. 8% of patients receiving drug complained of weight gain (greater than 10% of baseline). These side effects are mild to moderate if they occur.

Nursing Implications: Assess baseline nutritional status, optimal and desired weight, and any changes. Teach patient to report nausea or weight gain. Teach patient strategies to minimize nausea (e.g., dietary modification, taking drug after meals) if it occurs, and discuss with physician antiemetic medication if dietary modification not effective. If patient experiences weight gain, discuss patient interest in gentle exercising, such as progressive muscle resistance, which would encourage weight gain as lean body mass rather than fat.

IV. SENSORY/PERCEPTION ALTERATIONS, POTENTIAL, related to DEPRESSION, INSOMNIA

Defining Characteristics: While not reported as side effects considered drug-related or of indeterminate cause, depression and insomnia occurred in 13% and 11%, respectively, of patients participating in the clinical trials.

Nursing Implications: Assess baseline effect, use of effective coping strategies in dealing with disease and treatment, and usual sleep patterns. Teach patient to report changes in mood, such as depression, and difficulty falling asleep, or early awakening. If this occurs, further assess symptom, and suggest self-care strategies to minimize symptom. If nonpharmacologic measures are ineffective, discuss use of antidepressant or sleeping medication with physician, depending upon assessment.

Drug: floxuridine (FUDR, 2′-Deoxy-5-fluorouridine)

Class: Antimetabolite.

Mechanism of Action: Antimetabolite (fluorinated pyrimidine) that is metabolized to 5-FU when given by IV bolus, or metabolized to 5-FUDR-MP 5-fluoro-2′-deoxyuridine-5′-monophosphate when smaller doses are given, by continuous infusion intra-arterially. FUDR-MP is four times more effective in inhibiting the enzyme thymidine synthetase than 5-FU. The inhibition prevents the synthesis of thymidine, an essential component of DNA, resulting in interruption of DNA synthesis and cell death. Other FUDR metabolites inhibit RNA synthesis. Drug is cell cycle specific, with activity during the S phase.

Metabolism: When given IV, drug is transformed to 5-FU; 70–90% of drug is extracted by liver on first pass. Metabolites are excreted by kidneys and lungs. Continuous infusion decreases metabolism of drug with more of the drug being converted to the active metabolite FUDR-MP.

Dosage/Range:
- Intra-arterially (hepatic) by slow infusion pump: 0.1–0.6 mg/kg/day × 7–14 days.

Drug Preparation:
- Reconstitute 500-mg vial of lyophilized powder with 5-mL sterile water (100 mg/mL), then dilute with 0.9% sodium chloride or D5W to volume appropriate for intra-arterial pump.

Drug Administration:
- Usually administered by slow intra-arterial infusion using a surgically placed catheter or percutaneous catheter in a major artery.
- H_2 antagonist antihistamine (i.e., ranitidine 150 mg PO bid) administered concurrently during intra-arterial infusion to prevent development of peptic ulcer disease.

Drug Interactions:
- None significant.

Lab Effects/Interference:
- Decreased WBC, platelets.
- PT, total protein, sedimentation rate (abnormal values).
- Increased LFTs.

Special Considerations:
- Higher doses of the drug increase the risk of biliary sclerosis and fibrosis.
- Drug usually given for 14 days, then heparinized saline for 14 days to maintain line patency.
- Dose reductions or infusion breaks may be necessary depending on toxicity.
- FDA-approved for intrahepatic arterial infusion only.

Potential Toxicities/Side Effects and the Nursing Process

I. ALTERED NUTRITION, LESS THAN BODY REQUIREMENTS, related to NAUSEA/VOMITING, ANOREXIA, STOMATITIS/ESOPHOPHARYNGITIS, DIARRHEA, GASTRITIS, HEPATIC DYSFUNCTION

Defining Characteristics: Nausea and vomiting occur infrequently and are mild; anorexia is common. Mucositis is milder than 5-FU when administered intrahepatically, but more severe when given via carotid artery. Diarrhea is mild to moderately severe. Gastritis may occur, with abdominal cramping and pain. Incidence is greater in patients receiving hepatic artery infusion. Duodenal ulcers may occur in 10% of patients, be painless, and lead to gastric outlet obstruction and vomiting. Chemical hepatitis may be severe, with increased alk phos in patients receiving drug via hepatic artery infusions.

Nursing Implications: Premedicate with antiemetics as ordered and teach patient in self-administration of prescribed antiemetics. Encourage small, frequent feedings of cool, bland foods. If intractable nausea and vomiting, severe diarrhea, or severe cramping occur, notify physician, stop drug, and infuse heparinized saline. Teach patient oral assessment and oral hygiene regimen, and instruct to report any signs/symptoms of stomatitis, esophopharyngitis. Instruct patient to report diarrhea. Teach self-care measures, including diet modification and self-administration of prescribed antidiarrheal medication. Assess for signs/symptoms of abdominal stress, cramping prior to and during infusion. Discuss with physician use of antacids and antisecretory medications. Catheter placement should be verified prior to each infusion cycle, and inadvertent drug infusion into gastric/duodenal-supplying arteries should be investigated. Monitor LFTs prior to drug initiation, during treatment, and at end of 14-day cycle. Discuss abnormalities and dose reductions with physician. Assess patient for signs/symptoms of liver dysfunction: lethargy, weakness, malaise, anorexia, fever, jaundice, icterus.

II. POTENTIAL FOR INJURY related to INTRA-ARTERIAL CATHETER PROBLEMS

Defining Characteristics: Catheter problems that may occur include leakage, arterial ischemia or aneurysm, bleeding at catheter site, catheter occlusion, thrombosis or embolism of artery, vessel perforation or dislodged catheter, infection, and biliary sclerosis.

Nursing Implications: Assess catheter carefully prior to each cycle of therapy for patency, signs/symptoms of infection. Ensure that catheter position and patency are determined prior to each cycle of therapy; do not force flushing solution—reassess and try again. If still unsuccessful, notify physician.

III. SENSORY/PERCEPTUAL ALTERATIONS related to HAND-AND-FOOT SYNDROME AND OTHER CNS SYMPTOMS

Defining Characteristics: Hand-and-foot syndrome occurs in 30–40% of patients (numbness, sensory changes in hands and feet). Uncommonly, cerebellar ataxia, vertigo, nystagmus, seizures, depression, hemiplegia, hiccups, lethargy, and blurred vision may occur.

Nursing Implications: Assess baseline neurologic status prior to and during therapy. Teach patient that hand-foot syndrome may occur and instruct to report signs/symptoms. Discuss with physician use of pyridoxine 50 mg tid to prevent hand-foot syndrome. Assess ability to do activities of daily living and level of comfort.

IV. ALTERATION IN SKIN INTEGRITY related to LOCALIZED ERYTHEMA, DERMATITIS, NONSPECIFIC SKIN TOXICITY, OR RASH

Defining Characteristics: Erythema, dermatitis, pruritus, or rash may occur.

Nursing Implications: Assess for skin changes. Assess impact on comfort and body image. Teach patient self-care.

V. POTENTIAL FOR INFECTION AND BLEEDING related to BONE MARROW DEPRESSION

Defining Characteristics: Occurs rarely when FUDR is given as a single agent via continuous intra-arterial infusion.

Nursing Implications: Assess baseline WBC, neutrophil count, and platelets, during treatment and at completion of 14-day infusion. Discontinue drug infusion if WBC $< 3500/mm^3$ or if platelet count $< 100,000/mm^3$, or per established physician orders; refill pump with heparinized saline.

Drug: fludarabine phosphate (Fludara)

Class: Antimetabolite.

Mechanism of Action: Inhibits DNA synthesis, probably by inhibiting DNA-polymerase-alpha, ribonucleotide reductase, and DNA primase.

Metabolism: Drug is rapidly converted to the active metabolite 2-fluoroara-A when given intravenously. The drug's half-life is about 10 hours. The major route of elimination is via the kidneys, and approximately 23% of the active drug is excreted unchanged in the urine.

Dosage/Range:
- 25 mg/m^2 IV over 30 minutes daily × 5 days, repeated every 28 days.
- Dose reduce 20% for creatinine clearance 30–70 mL/min and hold drug if creatinine clearance < 30 mL/min.

Drug Preparation:
- Aseptically add 2 mL sterile water for injection USP to the 50-mg vial, resulting in a final concentration of 25 mg/mL. The drug may then be diluted further in 100 mL of 5% dextrose or 0.9% sodium chloride. Once reconstituted, the drug should be used within 8 hours.

Drug Administration:
- IV infusion over 30 minutes.

Drug Interactions:
- Pentostatin: increased risk for severe, potentially fatal, pulmonary toxicity; do not administer concomitantly.

Lab Effects/Interference:

- Decreased CBC.
- Tumor lysis syndrome.

Special Considerations:

- Indicated for the treatment of patients with B-cell chronic lymphocytic leukemia (CLL) who have not responded to treatment with at least one standard alkylating agent-containing regimen, or who have progressed on treatment.
- Dose-dependent toxicity: overdosage (four times recommended dose) has been associated with delayed blindness, coma, and death.
- Do not administer in combination with pentostatin, as fatal pulmonary toxicity can occur.
- Administer cautiously in patients with renal insufficiency.
- Drug is teratogenic.
- Drug may cause severe bone marrow depression.

Potential Toxicities/Side Effects and the Nursing Process

I. INFECTION AND BLEEDING related to BONE MARROW DEPRESSION

Defining Characteristics: Severe and cumulative bone marrow depression may occur; nadir, 13 days (range, 3–25 days).

Nursing Implications: Monitor CBC, platelet count prior to drug administration, as well as signs/symptoms of infection and bleeding. Instruct patient in self-assessment of signs/symptoms of infection and bleeding as well as self-care measures, including avoidance of OTC aspirin-containing medication.

II. POTENTIAL FOR ACTIVITY INTOLERANCE related to ANEMIA-INDUCED FATIGUE

Defining Characteristics: Bone marrow depression often includes red cell line.

Nursing Implications: Monitor HgCT; discuss transfusion with physician if HCT does not recover postchemotherapy. Teach patient high-iron diet as appropriate.

III. SENSORY/PERCEPTUAL ALTERATIONS related to CNS EFFECTS, PERIPHERAL NEUROPATHIES

Defining Characteristics: Agitation, confusion, visual disturbances, and coma have occurred. Objective weakness has been reported (9–65%), as have paresthesias (4–12%).

Nursing Implications: Assess baseline neurologic status; monitor neurologic vital signs. Teach patient signs/symptoms and instruct to report them if they occur. Evaluate these changes with physician and discuss continuation of therapy.

IV. POTENTIAL FOR IMPAIRED GAS EXCHANGE related to PULMONARY TOXICITY

Defining Characteristics: Pneumonia occurs in 16–22% of patients. Pulmonary hypersensitivity reaction characterized by dyspnea, cough, interstitial pulmonary infiltrate has been observed. Fatal pulmonary toxicity has occurred when drug is given in combination with pentostatin (Deoxycoformycin).

Nursing Implications: Instruct patient in possible side effects and to report dyspnea, cough, signs of breathlessness following exertion. Assess lung sounds prior to chemotherapy administration. DO NOT administer drug in combination with pentostatin.

V. POTENTIAL FOR SEXUAL DYSFUNCTION, related to TERATOGENICITY

Defining Characteristics: Drug is teratogenic; may cause testicular atrophy. It is unknown whether drug is excreted in breast milk.

Nursing Implications: As appropriate, explore with patient and partner issues of reproduction and sexuality patterns, and impact chemotherapy may have. Discuss strategies to preserve sexual and reproductive health (sperm banking, contraception). Mothers receiving drug should not breast-feed.

VI. ALTERED NUTRITION, LESS THAN BODY REQUIREMENTS, related to NAUSEA/VOMITING, DIARRHEA

Defining Characteristics: Nausea/vomiting occurs in about 30% of patients and can be prevented with standard antiemetics; diarrhea occurs in 15% of patients.

Nursing Implications: Premedicate with antiemetics; evaluate response to emetic protection. Encourage small, frequent meals of cool, bland foods and liquids. If vomiting occurs, assess for signs/symptoms of fluid/electrolyte imbalance; monitor I/O and daily weights, lab results. Encourage patient to report onset of diarrhea; teach patient to administer antidiarrheal medication as ordered.

Drug: 5-fluorouracil (Fluorouracil, Adrucil, 5-FU, Efudex [topical])

Class: Pyrimidine antimetabolite.

Mechanism of Action: Acts as a "false" pyrimidine, inhibiting the formation of an enzyme (thymidine synthetase) necessary for the synthesis of DNA. Also incorporates into RNA, causing abnormal synthesis. Methotrexate given prior to 5-FU results in synergism and enhanced efficacy.

Metabolism: Metabolized by the liver; most is excreted as respiratory CO_2, remainder is excreted by the kidneys. Plasma half-life is 20 minutes.

Dosage/Range:
- 12–15 mg/kg IV once per week, OR
- 12 mg/kg IV every day × 5 days every 4 week, OR
- 500 mg/m^2 every week or every week × 5 weeks.
- Hepatic infusion: 22 mg/kg in 100 mL 5% dextrose infused into hepatic artery over 8 hours for 5–21 consecutive days.
- Head and neck: 1000 mg/m^2 day × 4–5 days as continuous infusion.
- Colon cancer: Adjuvant:
  - Roswell Park: 5-FU 500 mg/m^2 IVB 1 hour into 2 hour infusion of leucovorin 500 mg/m^2, weekly for 6 weeks, repeated q 8 weeks for a total of 3 cycles (6 months).
  - De Gramont (LV5-FU2): *Day 1*: Leucovorin 200 mg/m^2 IV over 2 hours d 1, 2; 5-FU 400 mg/m^2 IVB followed by 600 mg/m^2 IV infusion × 22 hours d 1, 2.
  - FLOX and FOLFOX regimens: See oxaliplatin.
- Metastatic CRC: A variety of regimens, together with leucovorin, in combination with oxaliplatin, irinotecan, bevacizumab.
- Topical: multiple actinic or solar keratoses: apply twice daily.

Drug Preparation:
- No dilution required. Can be added to 0.9% sodium chloride or 5% dextrose.
- Store at room temperature; protect from light. Solution should be clear: if crystals do not disappear after holding vial under hot water, discard vial.

Drug Administration:
- Given via IV push or bolus (slow drip), or as continuous infusion.
- Topical: As cream.

Drug Interactions:
- Warfarin: may increase anticoagulant effect; monitor INR closely and dose warfarin based on result.
- When given with cimetidine, there are increased pharmacologic effects of fluorouracil.
- When given with thiazide diuretics, there is increased risk of myelosuppression.
- Leucovorin causes increased 5-fluorouracil cytotoxicity.

Lab Effects/Interference:
- Decreased CBC.

Special Considerations:
- Cutaneous side effects occur, e.g., skin sensitivity to sun, splitting of fingernails, dry flaky skin, and hyperpigmentation on face, palms of hands.
- Patients who have had adrenalectomy may need higher doses of prednisone while receiving 5-FU, or dose of 5-FU may be reduced in postadrenalectomy patients.

- Reduce dose in patients with compromised hepatic, renal, or bone marrow function and malnutrition.
- Inspect solution for precipitate prior to continuous infusion.

Potential Toxicities/Side Effects and the Nursing Process

I. POTENTIAL FOR INFECTION AND BLEEDING related to BONE MARROW DEPRESSION

Defining Characteristics: Nadir 10–14 days after drug dose; neutropenia, thrombocytopenia are dose-related. Toxicity is enhanced when combined with leucovorin calcium.

Nursing Implications: Assess baseline CBC, WBC, differential, and platelet count prior to chemotherapy, as well as for signs/symptoms of infection or bleeding. Teach patient signs/symptoms of infection or bleeding, and instruct to report these immediately; teach patient self-care measures to minimize risk of infection and bleeding. This includes avoidance of crowds, proximity to people with infections, and avoidance of OTC aspirin-containing medications.

II. ALTERED NUTRITION, LESS THAN BODY REQUIREMENTS, related to NAUSEA AND VOMITING, STOMATITIS, AND DIARRHEA

Defining Characteristics: Nausea and vomiting occur in 30–50% of patients and severity is dose-dependent. Stomatitis can be severe, with onset in 5–8 days; and may herald severe bone marrow depression. Diarrhea can be severe, and in combination with leucovorin calcium is the dose-limiting toxicity.

Nursing Implications: Premedicate patient with antiemetics (phenothiazines are usually effective), and continue for 24 hours, at least for the first cycle. Encourage small, frequent meals of cool, bland foods. Assess oral mucosa prior to drug administration and instruct patient to report changes. Teach patient oral hygiene measures and self-assessment. Instruct patient to report diarrhea, to self-administer prescribed antidiarrheal medications, and to drink adequate fluids. Moderate to severe stomatitis or diarrhea is an indication to interrupt therapy.

III. ALTERATION IN SKIN INTEGRITY related to ALOPECIA, CHANGES IN NAILS AND SKIN

Defining Characteristics: Alopecia is more common with five-day course and involves diffuse thinning of scalp hair, eyelashes, and eyebrows. Brittle nail cracking and loss may occur. Photosensitivity occurs. Chemical phlebitis may occur during continuous infusion with higher doses (pH > 8.0).

Nursing Implications: Teach patient about possible hair loss and skin changes; discuss possible impact on body image. Assess patient's risk for hair loss and skin changes during the therapy and discuss with patient strategies to minimize distress (wig, scarf, nail polish). Instruct patient to use sunblock when outdoors. Suggest implanted venous access device for continuous infusion of 5-FU, especially if patient will receive ongoing therapy.

IV. SENSORY/PERCEPTUAL ALTERATIONS related to PHOTOPHOBIA, CEREBELLAR ATAXIA, OCULAR CHANGES

Defining Characteristics: Photophobia may occur. Occasional cerebellar ataxia may occur and will disappear once drug is stopped. Drug is excreted in tears. Ocular changes that may occur are conjunctivitis, increased lacrimation, photophobia, oculomotor dysfunction, and blurred vision.

Nursing Implications: Assess baseline neurologic status, including vision. Instruct patient to report any changes. Teach patient safety precautions as needed.

Drug: flutamide (Eulexin)

Class: Antiandrogen.

Mechanism of Action: Inhibits androgen uptake or inhibits nuclear binding of androgen in target tissues or both.

Metabolism: Rapidly and completely absorbed. Excreted mainly via urine. Biologically active metabolite reaches maximum plasma levels in approximately 2 hours. Plasma half-life is 6 hours. Largely plasma-bound.

Dosage/Range:
- 250 mg every 8 hours.

Drug Preparation:
- None (available in 125-mg tablets).

Drug Administration:
- Oral.

Drug Interactions:
- Alcohol: increased facial flushing.
- Warfarin: may increase risk of bleeding; monitor INR closely.

Lab Effects/Interference:
- Increased LFTs.
- Increased BUN, creatinine.
- Monitor PSA for changes.

Special Considerations:

- Indicated for the treatment of men with prostate cancer in combination with an LHRH agonist.
- Contraindicated in patients with severe hepatic dysfunction.
- Drug may cause acute hepatic failure within the first 3 months of treatment and is reversible after discontinuation. Teach patient to report jaundice, nausea, vomiting, abdominal (RUQ) tenderness, fatigue, and anorexia and to have liver function evaluated.

Potential Toxicities/Side Effects and the Nursing Process

I. POTENTIAL SEXUAL DYSFUNCTION related to DRUG EFFECTS

Defining Characteristics: Decreased libido and impotence can occur in 33% of patients; gynecomastia occurs in 10% of patients.

Nursing Implications: Assess patient's sexual pattern, any alterations, and patient response. Encourage patient to verbalize feelings; provide information, emotional support, and referral for counseling as available and appropriate.

II. ALTERATION IN COMFORT related to HOT FLASHES

Defining Characteristics: Hot flashes occur commonly.

Nursing Implications: Teach patient that this may occur, and encourage patient to report symptoms. Provide symptomatic support.

III. ALTERED NUTRITION, LESS THAN BODY REQUIREMENTS, related to DIARRHEA, NAUSEA AND VOMITING

Defining Characteristics: Diarrhea and nausea/vomiting occur in 10% of patients.

Nursing Implications: Teach patient that these may occur, and instruct to report them. Assess for occurrence; teach patient self-administration of prescribed antidiarrheal or antiemetic medications.

Drug: fulvestrant injection (Faslodex)

Class: Estrogen Downregulator.

Mechanism of Action: Fulvestrant is an estrogen receptor antagonist that binds to the estrogen receptor of cells that are dependent upon estrogen for growth, including breast cancer cells that are hormone positive. There is no agonist effect as with other antiestrogens, such as tamoxifen. In addition, the estrogen receptor is also degraded so that it is lost from the cell. Because of this, there is no chance that the hormone receptor can be stimulated by low concentrations of estrogen, as with other antiestrogens, and this theoretically reduces the development of resistance.

Metabolism: When given IM, it takes 7 days for the drug to reach maximal plasma levels, which are maintained for at least one month. Half-life is about 40 days, and after 3–6 monthly doses, steady-state plasma area under the curve levels are reached at 2.5 times that of a single-dose injection. Drug undergoes biotransformation similar to endogenous steroids (oxidation, aromatic hydroxylation, conjugation), and oxidative pathway is via cytochrome P-450 (CYP 3A4). Drug is metabolized by the liver and rapidly cleared from the plasma via the hepatobiliary route. 90% is excreted via the feces; renal excretion is < 1%. There were no pharmacokinetic differences found in the elderly and younger adults, men and women, different races, patients with renal impairment, and patients with mild hepatic impairment. However, patients with moderate to severe liver dysfunction have not been studied.

Dosage/Range:
- 250 mg given IM into the buttock monthly as either one 5 mL slow injection or 2 separate 2.5-mL slow injections into each buttock.

Drug Preparation:
- Drug available in refrigerated 5 ml/250 mg, and 2.5 ml/125 mg prefilled syringes; concentration is 50 mg/mL.
- Unopened vials should be stored in the refrigerator at 2–8°C (36–46°F), but do not freeze. Drug can be left at room temperature for a short period of time prior to injection to increase patient comfort.
- Remove glass syringe barrel from tray and ensure it is undamaged.
- Open Safety Glide needle and attach to luer lock end of the syringe.
- Expel any air.

Drug Administration:
- Administer slow IM in one buttock 5 mL (250 mg) or 2.5 mL (125 mg) into each buttock as solution is viscous.
- Z-track administration is recommended to prevent drug leakage into subcutaneous tissue.
- Following drug injection, activate needle protection device when withdrawing needle from patient by pushing lever arm completely forward until needle tip is fully covered.
- If unable to activate, drop into sharps disposal container.

Drug Interactions:
- None significant, as drug does not significantly inhibit the major CYP isoenzymes, including rifampin.
- Herbals that contain estrogen may decrease the drug effect.

Lab Effects/Interference: None.

Special Considerations:
- Indicated for the treatment of hormone receptor positive metastatic breast cancer in postmenopausal women with disease progression following antiestrogen therapy.
- Contraindicated in pregnancy or in patients hypersensitive to the drug or its components.
- Drug should not be used by breast-feeding mothers.
- Injection site reactions more common when drug is given in two divided doses.

Potential Toxicities/Side Effects and the Nursing Process

I. ALTERATION IN COMFORT related to INJECTION SITE REACTION, ABDOMINAL PAIN, BACK PAIN

Defining Characteristics: Injection site reactions (pain and inflammation) occurred in 7% of patients receiving a single 5-mL injection (European Trial) as compared to 27% of patients (North American Trial) receiving two 2.5-mL injections, one in each buttock. Back and bone pain occurred in 15.8% of patients, while abdominal pain occurred in 11.8% of patients and often was associated with other gastrointestinal symptoms.

Nursing Implications: Teach patient this may occur and to report it. Consider using Z-track method, and if using 2 separate injections of 2.5 mL, try a single-dose injection to see if discomfort is reduced. Teach patient to report bone and/or back pain. Teach patient to use over-the-counter analgesics such as acetaminophen or nonsteroidal anti-inflammatory drugs as appropriate to bleeding history or risk factors. Discuss alternatives with physician if ineffective in symptom management.

II. ALTERATION IN NUTRITION, POTENTIAL, related to NAUSEA, VOMITING, CONSTIPATION, DIARRHEA

Defining Characteristics: Nausea occurs in 26%, vomiting 13%, constipation 12.5%, diarrhea 12.3%, and anorexia 9%.

Nursing Implications: Assess baseline appetite, presence of nausea and/or vomiting, and bowel elimination pattern. Teach patient that these side effects may occur, self-care measures to minimize nausea and vomiting such as dietary modification, and to report these side effects. Discuss antiemetics with physician if dietary modification is ineffective. Teach patient to use dietary modification to relieve constipation or diarrhea and, if ineffective, to use over-the-counter laxatives or anti-diarrheal medicine. If ineffective, discuss pharmacologic management with physician.

III. ALTERATION IN SKIN INTEGRITY, POTENTIAL, related to HOT FLASHES AND PERIPHERAL EDEMA

Defining Characteristics: Vasodilation or hot flashes occurred in 17.7% of patients, and peripheral edema in 9% of patients.

Nursing Implications: Assess baseline skin integrity, history of hot flashes in postmenopausal patients, and presence of peripheral edema. Teach patient these side effects may occur and to report them. If hot flashes are severe, review common hot flash management including wearing loose, layered clothing that can be removed when the woman becomes hot, sipping cold beverages throughout the day, sleeping with light nightgown and window open, avoiding triggers such as caffeine or alcohol, and if ineffective, discuss use of venlafaxine (Effexor) or fluoxetine (Paxil) to reduce intensity and frequency of hot flashes (Loprinski et al, 2000). Teach patient self-assessment of peripheral edema, to wear loose stockings and shoes, to keep skin moisturized to prevent cracking, and comfort measures. Teach patient to report increasing edema or related problems.

Drug: gemcitabine hydrochloride (Gemzar, Difluorodeoxycitidine)

Class: Antimetabolite.

Mechanism of Action: Inhibits DNA synthesis by inhibiting DNA polymerase activity through a process called *masked chain termination*. It is a prodrug, structurally similar to ara-C, needing intracellular phosphorylation. It then inhibits DNA synthesis. Cell cycle specific for S phase, causing cells to accumulate at the G_1-S boundary.

Metabolism: Pharmacokinetics vary by age, gender, and infusion time. Half-life for short infusions ranges from 32–94 minutes, while that of long infusions ranges from 245–638 minutes. Following short infusions (< 70 minutes), the drug is not extensively tissue-bound; following long infusions (70–285 minutes), the drug slowly equilibrates within tissues. The terminal half-life of the parent drug, gemcitabine, is 17 minutes. There is negligible binding to serum proteins. Drug and metabolites are excreted in the urine, with 92–98% of the drug dose recovered in the urine within one week. Mean systemic clearance is 90 L/h/m^2. Clearance is about 30% lower in women than in men, and also reduced in the elderly, but this does not necessarily require a dose reduction.

Dosage/Range:

Adults:

- Breast cancer: 1250 mg/m^2 IV over 30 minutes d 1, 8 q 21 days, in combination with paclitaxel 175 mg/m^2 IV over 3 hr administered prior to gemcitabine, day 1 repeated q 21 days. Dose reduce 25% day 8 dose for ANC 1000–1199/mm^3 or platelets 50,000–75,000 × 10^6/L; dose reduce 50% for ANC 700–999/mm^3 and platelets ≥ 50,000 × 10^6/L but hold drug if ANC 700–999/mm^3 and platelets < 50,000 × 10^6/L. Hold drug if ANC < 500/mm^3 or platelets < 50,000 × 10^6/L.
- Pancreatic cancer: 1000 mg/m^2 IV infusion over 30 min every week for up to 7 weeks (or until toxicity necessitates dose reduction or delay), then followed by 1-week break. Treatment then continues weekly for 3 weeks, followed by 1 week off (i.e., treatment 3 weeks out of 4). For patients who complete the initial 7 weeks, or a subsequent 3-week cycle at a dose of 1000 mg/m^2, the dose may be increased by 25% to 1250 mg/m^2 if the following conditions are met: the ANC NADIR is > 1500 × 10/L, platelet count NADIR is > 100,000 × 10/L, and nonhematologic toxicity has not been greater than WHO grade 1. If patient tolerates this course well, the dose for the next cycle can be increased an additional 20% if the above three criteria are met. Dose reduce 25% if ANC 500–999/mm^3 or platelets 50–99,000 × 10^6/L, and hold if ANC < 500/mm^3 of platelets < 50,000 × 10^6/L.
- Non–small-cell lung cancer (inoperable, locally advanced Stage IIIA and IIIB or metastatic) in combination with cisplatin: 4-week cycle: 1000 mg/m^2 IV over 30 minutes on day 1, 8, 15, repeat q 28 days, with cisplatin 100 mg/m^2 IV on day 1 after the gemcitabine infusion; or as a 3-week cycle, with gemcitabine 1250 mg/m^2 IV over 30 minutes on day 1, 8; cisplatin 100 mg/m^2 IV is given following gemcitabine infusion on day 1, repeated q 3 weeks. Dose reduce 25% if ANC 500–999/mm^3 or platelets 50–99,000 × 10^6/L, and hold if ANC < 500/mm^3 of platelets < 50,000 × 10^6/L. Dose reduce 50% for grade 3/4 nonhematologic toxicities when gemcitabine given with cisplatin.
- Ovarian cancer: 1000 mg/m^2 IV over 30 minutes on days 1, 8 of each 21-day cycle, together with carboplatin AUC 4 IV on day 1 **after** gemcitabine administration; ANC must be ≥ 1500 × 10^6/L and a platelet count of ≥ 100,000 × 10^6/L prior to each cycle. Grade 3/4 non-hematologic toxicity = 50% dose reduction. Dose modify day 8 if ANC 1000–1499/mm^3 and/or platelet 75–99,999 × 10^6/L 187 = 50% of dose; hold dose if values are lower than this. Modify dose in subsequent cycles to 800 mg/m^2 on days 1,8 if ANC < 500/mm^3 for > 5 day, ANC < 100/mm^3 > 3 days, febrile neutropenia, platelets < 25,000 × 10^6/L, or cycle delay of > 1 week due to toxicity.

Drug Preparation:

- Drug available in single-use vials of 200 mg/10 mL and 1 g/50 mL. Use 0.9% sodium chloride USP and reconstitute the 200-mg vial with 5 mL, and the 1-g vial with 25 mL. Shake to dissolve the powder. This results in a concentration of 38 mg/mL. Withdraw recommended dose and further dilute in 0.9% sodium chloride injection. Discard unused portion. Inspect solution for particulate matter or discoloration and do not use if these occur. Stable 24 hours at room temperature (20–25°C [68–77°F]). DO NOT refrigerate, as drug crystallization may occur.

Drug Administration:

- ANC ≥ $1500/mm^3$ and platelets > $100{,}000 \times 10^6$/L for day 1 treatment.
- Administer IV over 30 minutes. Infusion time > 60 minutes or dosing more frequently than weekly is associated with greater toxicity.
- Administer gemcitabine before cisplatin.
- Administer gemcitabine after paclitaxel.

Drug Interactions:

- Administer cisplatin after gemcitabine to enhance renal drug clearance; paclitaxel should be administered before gemcitabine.

Lab Effects/Interference:

- Decreased CBC.
- Increased LFTs.

Special Considerations:

- FDA-approved for (1) first-line treatment of patients with locally advanced (nonresectable stage II or III), or metastatic (stage IV) adenocarcinoma of the pancreas or in patients previously treated with 5-FU; (2) in combination with paclitaxel, as first-line therapy for treatment of women with metastatic breast cancer who have failed prior anthracycline adjuvant chemotherapy, unless anthracyclines are contraindicated; (3) first-line treatment of patients with unresectable, locally advance stage IIIA and IIIB non-small-cell lung cancer (NSCLC), in combination with cisplatin, or metastatic NSCLC; and (4) in combination with carboplatin for the treatment of women with advanced ovarian cancer who have relapsed at least 6 months after completion of platinum-based therapy.
- Monitor liver and renal function at baseline and throughout therapy; use cautiously in patients with renal or hepatic dysfunction and monitor closely; drug may aggravate hepatic dysfunction.
- Dose reduction or delay required for hematologic toxicity.
- Assess for onset of rare pulmonary toxicity, especially in combination with erlotinib. Hold dose and evaluate pulmonary symptoms before resuming therapy.
- Hemolytic uremic syndrome (HUS) and/or renal failure have been reported rarely.
- Drug is a radiosensitizer, and radiation recall may occur.
- Monitoring labs: hepatic and renal function baseline and periodically during treatment; CBC/differential before each dose; serum creatinine, potassium, calcium, magnesium during combination with cisplatin.
- Use with caution in patients with impaired renal function or hepatic dysfunction. (Studies have not been done to identify risks in this population.)
- Rarely, HUS (hemolytic uremic syndrome) has occurred. Discontinue drug if signs/symptoms occur (rapid decrease in hemoglobin and thrombocytopenia, together with elevated BUN/creatinine). Observe for elevation of serum bili or LDH.

- Drug can rarely cause severe pulmonary toxicity (interstitial pneumonitis, pulmonary fibrosis, pulmonary edema, adult respiratory distress syndrome), occurring up to 2 weeks following the last gemcitabine infusion. If patients develop dyspnea, with or without bronchospasm, stop gemcitabine until further pulmonary evaluation can proceed; discontinue drug if related to gemcitabine.
- Drug may cause sedation in 10% of patients; caution patient not to drive or operate heavy machinery until it is determined whether patient develops this side effect.
- Drug is embryotoxic; women of childbearing age should avoid pregnancy while receiving the drug.
- Drug may be irritating to the vein, requiring local heat; may require a central line for (long-term) administration.

Potential Toxicities/Side Effects and the Nursing Process

I. POTENTIAL FOR INFECTION AND BLEEDING related to BONE MARROW DEPRESSION

Defining Characteristics: Myelosuppression is dose-limiting toxicity. Incidence of leukopenia is 63%, thrombocytopenia 36%, and anemia 73%. Dose reductions required are shown in the Special Considerations section. Grades 3–4 thrombocytopenia are more common in the elderly, and grades 3–4 neutropenia and thrombocytopenia are more common in women (especially older women). Older women were less able to complete subsequent courses of therapy. Myelosuppression is usually short-lived with recovery within one week. Approximately 19% of patients require RBC transfusions.

Nursing Implications: Assess baseline CBC, WBC, differential, and platelet count prior to chemotherapy, as well as for signs/symptoms of infection or bleeding. Discuss dose reductions or delay based on neutrophil and platelet counts. Teach patient signs/symptoms of infection or bleeding, and instruct to report these immediately. Teach patient self-care measures to minimize risk of infection and bleeding. This includes avoidance of crowds, proximity to people with infections, and OTC aspirin-containing medications. Transfuse red blood cells and platelets as needed per physician order.

II. POTENTIAL ALTERATION IN NUTRITION, LESS THAN BODY REQUIREMENTS, related to NAUSEA AND VOMITING, DIARRHEA, STOMATITIS, AND ALTERATIONS IN LFTS

Defining Characteristics: Nausea and vomiting occur in 69% of patients, and of these, < 15% are severe. Nausea and vomiting are usually mild to moderate and are easily prevented or controlled by antiemetics. Diarrhea may occur (19% incidence), as may stomatitis (11% incidence). Abnormalities in liver transaminases occur in two-thirds of patients; rarely does this require drug discontinuance.

Nursing Implications: Premedicate patient with antiemetics (phenothiazides are usually effective). Encourage small, frequent meals of cool, bland foods. Teach patient self-administration of prescribed antiemetic medications, and to drink adequate fluids. Assess oral mucosa prior to drug administration, and instruct patient to report changes. Teach patient oral hygiene measures and self-assessment. Instruct patient to report diarrhea, to self-administer prescribed antidiarrheal medications, and to drink adequate fluids. Monitor LFTs baseline and periodically during therapy. Notify physician of any abnormalities and discuss implications. Drug should be used cautiously in any patient with hepatic dysfunction.

III. POTENTIAL ALTERATION IN COMFORT related to FLU-LIKE SYMPTOMS

Defining Characteristics: Flu-like symptoms occur in 20% of patients with first treatment dose. Transient febrile episodes occur in 41% of patients.

Nursing Implications: Encourage patient to report flu-like symptoms. Treat fevers with acetaminophen per physician. Assess for alterations in comfort, and discuss symptomatic measures. If severe, discuss drug discontinuance with physician.

IV. IMPAIRED SKIN INTEGRITY related to ALOPECIA, RASH, PRURITUS, EDEMA

Defining Characteristics: Skin rash occurs in about 30% of patients, often within 2–3 days of starting drug. The rash is erythematous, pruritic, and/or maculopapular, and may occur on the neck and extremities. Edema occurs in about 30% of patients, and is primarily peripheral but can rarely be facial or pulmonary. Edema is reversible after drug is discontinued, and appears unrelated to cardiac, renal, or hepatic impairment. Edema is usually mild to moderate. Minimal hair loss occurs in 15% of patients, and is reversible.

Nursing Implications: Assess skin integrity and presence of rash, pruritus, alopecia, and edema prior to dosing. Assess impact of these alterations on patient, and develop plan to manage symptom distress and promote skin integrity. Instruct patient to report rash, itching; discuss treatment of rash with topical corticosteroids. Teach patient self-assessment of signs/symptoms of edema, and instruct to notify healthcare provider if swelling occurs. If severe, discuss drug discontinuance with physician.

Drug: goserelin acetate (Zoladex)

Class: Synthetic analogue of luteinizing hormone-releasing hormone (LHRH).

Mechanism of Action: Inhibits pituitary gonadotropin, achieving a chemical orchiectomy in 2–4 weeks. Sustained-release medication provides continuous drug diffusion from the depot into subcutaneous tissue. This permits monthly injection instead of daily.

Metabolism: Absorbed slowly for first 8 days, then more rapid and constant absorption for remaining 28 days. Time to peak concentration 12–15 days for males and 8–22 days for females.

Dosage/Range:

Adults:

- Subcutaneous: 3.6-mg dose into the anterior upper abdominal wall below the navel line every 28 days or the 10.8-mg depot every 3 months.

Drug Preparation:

- Inspect package for damage. Open package and inspect drug in translucent chamber.
- Select site on upper abdomen.
- Prepare site with alcohol swab, cleansing from center outward.
- Administer local anesthetic as ordered.
- Aseptically, stretch skin at site with nondominant hand, and insert needle into subcutaneous tissue with dominant hand at 45-degree angle.
- Redirect needle so it is parallel to the abdominal wall. Advance needle forward until hub touches skin. Withdraw needle 1 cm (approximately ½ inch).
- Depress plunger fully, expelling depot into prepared site.
- Withdraw needle carefully. Apply gentle pressure bandage to site. Confirm that tip of plunger is visible within needle tip.
- Document in chart.

Drug Interactions:

- None.

Lab Effects/Interference:

- Hypercalcemia in patients with bone metastases.
- Tests of pituitary/gonadal function may be inaccurate while on therapy due to suppression of pituitary/gonadal system.

Special Considerations:

- Compliance to 28-day injection schedule is important.
- Indicated for (1) palliative treatment of advanced prostate cancer; (2) treatment of stage B2 (locally advanced) prostate cancer in combination with flutamide; (3) palliative treatment of advanced breast cancer in premenopausal or perimenopausal women; (4) for the treatment of endometriosis; and (5) endometrial thinning before endometrial ablation for dysfunctional uterine bleeding.
- Initially, there is transient increase in serum testosterone levels, with flare of symptoms.
- Premenopausal women must use effective contraception during and for 12 weeks after treatment with the drug. The drug is contraindicated in mothers who are nursing.
- Well-tolerated treatment.

Potential Toxicities/Side Effects and the Nursing Process

I. SEXUAL DYSFUNCTION related to DECREASED TESTOSTERONE LEVELS

Defining Characteristics: Hot flashes, sexual dysfunction, and decreased erections can occur.

Nursing Implications: Assess normal sexual pattern. Refer as needed for sexual counseling.

II. POTENTIAL ALTERATION IN CARDIAC OUTPUT related to ARRYTHMIA, CARDIOVASCULAR DYSFUNCTION

Defining Characteristics: Arrhythmia, cerebrovascular accident (CVA), hypertension, myocardial infarction, peripheral vascular disease, chest pain may occur in 1–5% of patients.

Nursing Implications: Assess heart rate, blood pressure, peripheral pulses. Teach patient to report palpitations, shortness of breath, chest pain, or leg pain immediately. Evaluate abnormalities with physician.

III. SENSORY/PERCEPTUAL ALTERATION related to ANXIETY, DEPRESSION, HEADACHE

Defining Characteristics: Anxiety, depression, headache may occur (< 5%).

Nursing Implications: Assess baseline effect, comfort. Instruct patient to report mood disorder. Encourage patient to verbalize feelings, provide patient with emotional support. Assess efficacy of supportive care, and if needed, discuss pharmacologic management of symptoms with physician.

IV. ALTERATION IN NUTRITION, LESS THAN BODY REQUIREMENTS, related to VOMITING, HYPERGLYCEMIA

Defining Characteristics: Vomiting may occur (< 5%); also increased weight, ulcer, hyperglycemia.

Nursing Implications: Teach patient to report GI disturbances. Assess severity and discuss management with physician. Assess serum glucose, and if abnormal, discuss dietary or pharmacologic management, depending upon severity, with physician.

V. ALTERATION IN BOWEL ELIMINATION related to CONSTIPATION OR DIARRHEA

Defining Characteristics: Constipation or diarrhea may occur (< 5%).

Nursing Implications: Instruct patient to report problems in elimination. Teach symptomatic management.

VI. ALTERATION IN URINARY ELIMINATION related to OBSTRUCTION OR INFECTION

Defining Characteristics: Urinary obstruction, urinary tract infection, renal insufficiency may occur.

Nursing Implications: Monitor baseline urinary elimination pattern, baseline kidney function tests, and continue to monitor through therapy. Instruct patient to report signs/symptoms of urinary tract infection (UTI).

VII. ALTERATION IN COMFORT related to FEVER, CHILLS, TENDERNESS

Defining Characteristics: Chills, fever, breast swelling, and tenderness. Also, discomfort may result from injection, as a 16-gauge needle is used to inject depot.

Nursing Implications: Instruct patient to report discomfort. Discuss strategies to increase comfort. Administer local anesthetic prior to injection of medication (per physician's order).

Drug: histrelin implant (Vantas)

Class: Synthetic analogue of gonadotropin releasing factor (GnRH) or luteinizing hormone-releasing hormone (LHRH).

Mechanism of Action: Histrelin inhibits pituitary gonadotropin, achieving a chemical orchiectomy.

Metabolism: Implant delivers histrelin continuously for 12 months at 50–60 micrograms per day. Drug serum concentration 50% higher in patients with severe renal dysfunction, but this is not considered clinically significant.

Dosage/Range:
Adults:
- Histrelin implant (50 mg) is aseptically inserted subcutaneously under skin on upper, inner arm using implant tool; at 12 months, implant must be removed before new one is implanted.

Drug Preparation:
- Keep implant refrigerated until implant.
- Select site on upper inner arm, and follow guidelines in package insert using aseptic technique and implant tool.
- Implant is NOT radio-opaque so care must be given to carefully secure the implant as directed.

Drug Interactions:
- Unknown.

Lab Effects/Interference:
- Hypercalcemia in patients with bone metastases.
- Tests of pituitary/gonadal function may be inaccurate while on therapy due to suppression of pituitary/gonadal system.
- Decreased serum testosterone to below castrate levels (< ng/dL)

Special Considerations:
- Indicated for palliative treatment of advanced prostate cancer.
- Initially (1st week of treatment), there is transient increase in serum testosterone levels, with flare of symptoms or onset of new symptoms such as bone pain, neuropathy, hematuria, or ureteral/bladder outlet obstruction. If severe (rarely spinal cord compression, ureteral obstruction), these should be managed immediately.
- Patients with metastatic vertebral and/or urinary tract obstruction should be monitored very closely during the first few weeks of treatment.
- Generally well-tolerated treatment.
- Contraindicated in children and women.

Potential Toxicities/Side Effects and the Nursing Process

I. SEXUAL DYSFUNCTION related to DECREASED TESTOSTERONE LEVELS

Defining Characteristics: Hot flashes (66% with 2.3% severe), testicular atrophy (5.3%), gynecomastica (4.1%), decreased libido (2.3%), and erectile dysfunction (3.5%) can occur.

Nursing Implications: Assess normal sexual pattern. Encourage patient to verbalize feelings to assess impact of symptoms on sexual function; refer as needed for sexual counseling. Teach patient self-care strategies to reduce distress of hot flashes.

II. ALTERATION IN BOWEL ELIMINATION related to CONSTIPATION

Defining Characteristics: Constipation may occur (< 5%).

Nursing Implications: Instruct patient to report problems in elimination. Teach symptomatic management.

III. ALTERATION IN URINARY ELIMINATION related to OBSTRUCTION OR INFECTION

Defining Characteristics: Urinary obstruction, urinary tract infection, renal insufficiency may occur. Renal impairment occurs in 4.7% of patients.

Nursing Implications: Monitor baseline urinary elimination pattern, baseline kidney function tests, and continue to monitor through therapy. Instruct patient to report signs/symptoms of urinary tract infection (UTI).

IV. ALTERATION IN COMFORT related to IMPLANT SITE IRRITATION, ASTHENIA, AND INSOMNIA

Defining Characteristics: Implantation site reactions occur in at least 5.8% of patients: these include bruising, pain/soreness/tenderness after insertion or removal; rarely, erythema, and swelling may occur. Asthenia occurs in about 10% of patients, and insomnia 2.9% of patients.

Nursing Implications: Instruct patient to report discomfort. Discuss strategies to increase comfort. Teach patient to self-assess and reassure local effects will resolve. Teach patient to report any signs/symptoms of infection.

Drug: hydroxyurea (Hydrea, Droxia)

Class: Miscellaneous/antimetabolite.

Mechanism of Action: Prevents conversion of ribonucleotides to deoxyribonucleotides by inhibiting the converting enzyme ribonucleoside diphosphate reductase. DNA synthesis is thus inhibited. Cell cycle phase specific for S phase. May also sensitize cells to the effects of radiation therapy, although the process is not clearly understood.

Metabolism: Rapidly absorbed from GI tract. Peak plasma level reached in 2 hours, with plasma half-life of 3–4 hours. About half the drug is metabolized in the liver and half is excreted in urine as urea and unchanged drug. Some of the drug is eliminated as respiratory CO_2. Crosses BBB.

Dosage/Range:
- 500–3000 mg PO daily (dose reduced in renal dysfunction).
- 20–30 mg/kg/day PO as a continuous dose.
- 100 mg/kg IV daily × 3 days.
- Radiation sensitization: 80 mg/kg as a single dose every 3rd day starting at least 7 days before initiation of radiation.
- Sickle cell disease: To prevent painful crises, initial 15 mg/kg/day, increased by 5 mg/kg every 12 weeks to a maximum dose of 35 mg/kg/day as tolerated.

Drug Preparation:
- None. Hydrea available in 500-mg capsules or Droxia in 200-mg, 300-mg, and 400-mg tablets.

Drug Administration:
- Oral.
- High-dose IV continuous infusions are being studied with doses of 0.5–1 g/m^2/day × 5–12 weeks (investigational).

Drug Interactions:
- None significant.

Lab Effects/Interference:
- Decreased CBC.
- Increased BUN, creatinine, uric acid.
- Increased hepatic enzymes

Special Considerations:
- Hydroxyurea has a side effect of dramatically lowering the WBC in a relatively short period of time (24–48 hours). In leukemia patients endangered by the potential complication of leukostasis, this is the desired effect.
- May need to pretreat with allopurinol to protect patient from tumor lysis syndrome.
- Dermatologic radiation recall phenomena may occur.
- In combination with radiation therapy, mucosal reactions in the radiation field may be severe and require dose interruption.
- Drug used in the treatment of chronic myelogenous leukemia (CML) in chronic phase, as a radiosensitizer (primary brain tumors, head and neck cancer, cancer of the cervix or uterus, non–small-cell lung cancer), and in sickle cell anemia.
- Drug should not be used during pregnancy, or by breast-feeding mothers as drug is excreted in breast milk.
- Dose modification in renal dysfunction: Reduce dose by 50% if creatinine clearance 10–50 mL/min; reduce dose 80% (give only 20% of dose) if creatinine clearance < 10 mL/min.

Potential Toxicities/Side Effects and the Nursing Process

I. INFECTION AND BLEEDING related to BONE MARROW DEPRESSION

Defining Characteristics: WBC begins to decrease 24–48 hours after beginning therapy, with nadir in 10 days and recovery within 10–30 days. Leukopenia more common than thrombocytopenia and anemia, and is dose-related.

Nursing Implications: Assess CBC, WBC with differential, and platelet count prior to drug administration, as well as for signs/symptoms of infection or bleeding. Doses may need to be reduced if patient has undergone prior radiotherapy or chemotherapy.

Dose must be reduced if patient has renal dysfunction. Discuss any abnormalities with physician prior to drug administration. Teach patient signs/symptoms of infection and bleeding, and instruct to report them immediately. Teach self-care measures to minimize risk of infection and bleeding, including avoidance of OTC aspirin-containing medications.

II. ALTERED NUTRITION, LESS THAN BODY REQUIREMENTS, related to NAUSEA AND VOMITING, DIARRHEA, STOMATITIS, ANOREXIA, HEPATIC DYSFUNCTION

Defining Characteristics: Nausea and vomiting are uncommon, anorexia is mild to moderate, stomatitis is uncommon, diarrhea is uncommon, and hepatic dysfunction is rare, although abnormal LFTs may occur.

Nursing Implications: Premedicate with antiemetics as needed. Teach self-administration of prescribed medications. Instruct patient to report nausea/vomiting, diarrhea, anorexia, and stomatitis. Teach patient oral hygiene regimen and assess baseline oral mucosa. Monitor baseline LFTs, and monitor them periodically during therapy.

III. POTENTIAL ALTERATION IN FLUID/ELECTROLYTES/RENAL ELIMINATION STATUS related to TUMOR LYSIS SYNDROME

Defining Characteristics: When drug is first started in patients with high tumor burden, e.g., CML with high WBC, this often results in rapid death of a large number of malignant cells. The lysis or breakdown of these cells results in the release of intracellular contents into the systemic circulation. The resulting metabolic abnormalities are hyperkalemia, hyperphosphatemia, hypocalcemia, and hyperuricemia. If these persist, renal failure with oliguria can result.

Nursing Implications: Assess baseline chemistries, including metabolic panel, renal function. Expect that if the patient is at risk for the development of tumor lysis syndrome, the patient will begin allopurinol 200–300 mg/m^2/day prior to therapy, and receive hydration with alkalization (e.g., 50–100 mEq bicarbonate added per liter) to deliver 3 liters/m^2/day. Assess serum potassium, phosphate, calcium, uric acid, and BUN and creatinine at least daily, and discuss any abnormalities with physician to revise current regimen. Monitor I/O, weights, and total body balance carefully, and at least daily.

IV. SENSORY/PERCEPTUAL ALTERATIONS related to DROWSINESS, HALLUCINATIONS, OTHER CNS EFFECTS

Defining Characteristics: Drug crosses the BBB, so CNS effects may occur, such as drowsiness, confusion, disorientation, headache, vertigo; symptoms last < 24 hours.

Nursing Implications: Assess baseline mental status and neurologic functioning. Instruct patient to report signs/symptoms, and reassure that they will resolve. If symptoms persist, discuss interrupting drug with physician.

V. POTENTIAL SEXUAL/REPRODUCTIVE DYSFUNCTION related to DRUG EFFECTS

Defining Characteristics: Drug is mutagenic and teratogenic. Drug is excreted in breast milk.

Nursing Implications: Assess patient's sexual patterns and reproductive goals. Discuss with patient and partner potential toxicity and impact on sexuality. Provide information, emotional support, and referral as needed. Patient should use contraceptive measures; a mother receiving the drug should not breast-feed.

Drug: idarubicin (Idamycin, 4-Demethoxydaunorubicin)

Class: Antitumor antibiotic.

Mechanism of Action: Cell cycle phase specific for S phase. Analogue of daunorubicin. Has a marked inhibitory effect on RNA synthesis.

Metabolism: Excreted primarily in the bile and urine, with approximately 25% of the intravenous dose accounted for over 5 days. The half-life is 6–9.4 hours.

Dosage/Range:
- Induction: 12 mg/m^2 daily slow IVP × 3 days in combination with ara-C 100 mg/m^2 continuous infusion × 7 days, with consolidation using 10–12 mg/m^2/day × 2 days.

Drug Preparation:
- Available as a red powder.
- The drug is reconstituted with 0.9% sodium chloride injection to give a final concentration of 1 mg/1 mL.

Drug Administration:
- Drug is a vesicant. Administer IV over 10 to 15 minutes into the sidearm of a patent, freely running IV.
- Dose reduction (25%) recommended if renal dysfunction (serum creatinine > 2 mg/dL) or for severe mucositis.

Drug Interactions:
- Other myelosuppressive drugs: additive bone marrow suppression; monitor patient closely.
- Incompatible with heparin—causes precipitant.

Lab Effects/Interference:

- Decreased CBC.
- Increased LFTs, RFTs.

Special Considerations:

- Vesicant.
- Discolored urine (pink to red) may occur up to 48 hours after administration.
- Cardiomyopathy is less common and less severe than with doxorubicin and daunorubicin.
- Drug is light-sensitive.
- Dose-reduce for renal dysfunction.
- Dose-reduce for hepatic dysfunction: give 50% of dose if serum bili is 2.5 mg/dL; do not give dose if serum bili is > 5 mg/dL.

Potential Toxicities/Side Effects and the Nursing Process

I. INFECTION AND BLEEDING related to BONE MARROW DEPRESSION

Defining Characteristics: Hematologic toxicity is dose limiting. Leukopenia nadir 10–20 days with recovery in 1–2 weeks. Thrombocytopenia usually follows leukopenia and is mild. Bone marrow toxicity is not cumulative.

Nursing Implications: Evaluate WBC, neutrophil, and platelet count and discuss any abnormalities with physician prior to drug administration. Assess for signs/symptoms of infection or bleeding and instruct patient in signs/symptoms of infection and bleeding and to report them immediately. Suggest strategies to minimize risk of infection and bleeding, including avoidance of OTC aspirin-containing medications.

II. ALTERATION IN CARDIAC OUTPUT related to CUMULATIVE DOSES OF IDARUBICIN

Defining Characteristics: Cardiac toxicity is similar characteristically but less severe than that seen with daunorubicin and doxorubicin; CHF due to cardiomyopathy seen after large cumulative doses.

Nursing Implications: Assess cardiac status prior to chemotherapy administration: signs/symptoms of CHF, quality/regularity and rate of heartbeat, results of prior GBPS or other test of LVEF. Teach patient to report dyspnea, palpitations, swelling in extremities. Maintain accurate records of total dose; expect GBPS to be repeated periodically during treatment and the drug to be discontinued if there is a significant drop in heart function.

III. ALTERED NUTRITION, LESS THAN BODY REQUIREMENTS, related to NAUSEA/VOMITING, ANOREXIA, STOMATITIS, DIARRHEA, AND HEPATIC DYSFUNCTION

Defining Characteristics: Nausea/vomiting is usually mild to moderate, although it is seen to some degree in most patients; anorexia commonly occurs; stomatitis is mild; diarrhea is infrequent and mild; hepatitis is rare but may occur, and there are also disturbances in LFTs.

Nursing Implications: Premedicate with combination antiemetics and continue protection for 24 hours. If patient has a central line, slower infusion of drug over 1 hour decreases nausea/vomiting. Encourage small, frequent meals of bland foods. Anorexia occurs frequently: teach patient or caregiver to make foods ahead of time and use spices; encourage weekly weights. Stomatitis and esophagitis may occur in patients who have received prior radiation and during posttreatment visits. Teach patient oral hygiene regimen and self-assessment techniques. Encourage patient to report onset of diarrhea; administer or teach patient to self-administer antidiarrheal medications. Monitor SGOT, SGPT, LDH, alk phos, and bili periodically during treatment. Notify physician of any elevations.

IV. ALTERATION IN SKIN INTEGRITY related to ALOPECIA, SKIN CHANGES

Defining Characteristics: Alopecia occurs in about 30% of patients after oral drug and can be partial after IV drug; begins after 3+ weeks and hair may grow back while on therapy; may be slight to diffuse thinning. Skin changes include darkening of nail beds, skin ulcer/necrosis, sensitivity to sunlight, skin itching at irradiated areas, radiation recall, and potential necrosis with extravasation.

Nursing Implications: Discuss with patient hair loss, anticipated impact, and strategies to decrease distress, e.g., obtaining wig prior to hair loss. Assess disturbance of body image from hyperpigmentation and discuss strategies to minimize this, e.g., nail polish. Drug must be administered via patent IV. Assess need for venous access device early. If drug administered as continuous infusion, IT MUST BE GIVEN VIA A CENTRAL LINE.

V. POTENTIAL SEXUAL/REPRODUCTIVE DYSFUNCTION related to DRUG EFFECTS

Defining Characteristics: Gonadal function and fertility may be affected (may be permanent or transient). Reported to be excreted in breast milk.

Nursing Implications: As appropriate, explore with patient and partner issues of reproductive and sexuality patterns and impact chemotherapy will have; discuss strategies to preserve sexuality and reproductive health (e.g., contraception, sperm banking).

Drug: ifosfamide (Ifex)

Class: Alkylating agent.

Mechanism of Action: Destroys DNA throughout the cell cycle by binding to protein and by DNA crosslinking and causing chain scission as well as inhibition of DNA synthesis. Analogue of cyclophosphamide and is cell cycle phase nonspecific. Ifosfamide has been shown to be effective in tumors previously resistant to cyclophosphamide. Activated by microsomes in the liver.

Metabolism: Only about 50% of the drug is metabolized, with much of the drug excreted in the urine almost completely unchanged. Up to 70–86% of the drug dose is recoverable in the urine. Half-life is 13.8 hours for high dose vs 3–10 hours for lower doses.

Dosage/Range:

- All doses given with 2-L hydration/day and Mesna.
- 700 mg–2 grams/m^2/day × 5 days, every 3 weeks.
- Continuous infusion: 1200 mg/m^2/day × 5 days.
- Dose-reduce by 25–50% if serum creatinine is 2.1–3.0 mg/dL and hold if creatinine > 3.0 mg/dL.
- High dose (bone marrow transplant/stem cell rescue): 7.5–16 grams/m^2 IV in divided doses over several days.

Drug Preparation:

- Available as a powder in 1- and 3-g vials and should be reconstituted with sterile water for injection.
- Solution is chemically stable for 7 days, but discard after 8 hours due to lack of bacteriostatic preservative in the solution.
- May be diluted further in either 5% dextrose or 0.9% sodium chloride.

Drug Administration:

- IV bolus: Administer over 30 minutes. Mesna (20% of ifosfamide dose) should be administered with ifosfamide: mesna is begun 15 minutes prior to ifosfamide and repeated at 4 and 8 hours after the ifosfamide (see drug sheet on mesna). Mesna, ascorbic acid, and mucomycin have been used to protect the bladder. Pre- and posthydration (1500–2000 mL/day) or continuous bladder irrigations are recommended to prevent hemorrhagic cystitis.
- Continuous infusion: Administer intravenously for 5 days. Mesna is mixed with ifosfamide in equal amounts (1:1 mix). Prior to initiating continuous infusion, mesna is given IVB (10% of total ifosfamide dose). Following completion of the infusion, mesna alone should be infused for 12–24 hours to protect from delayed drug excretion activity against the bladder.

Drug Interactions:

- Activity/toxicity affected by allopurinol, chloroquine, phenothiazides, potassium iodide, chloramphenicol, imipramine, vitamin A, corticosteroids, succinylcholine.
- Bone marrow-depressant drugs: additive bone marrow depression.
- Mesna binds to and inactivates ifosfamide metabolite, thus preventing bladder toxicity.

Lab Effects/Interference:

- Decreased CBC.
- Increased RFTs, LFTs (AST and ALT).

Special Considerations:

- Metabolic toxicity is increased by simultaneous administration of barbiturates.
- Renal function: BUN, serum creatinine, and creatinine clearance must be determined prior to treatment.
- Therapy requires the concomitant administration of a uroprotector such as mesna and pre- and posthydration; may also require catheterization and constant bladder irrigation, and/or ascorbic acid.
- Test urine for occult blood.
- Dose-limiting toxicity has been renal and bladder dysfunction.
- Increased risk for toxicity in patients who have received prior or concurrent radiotherapy or other antineoplastic agents.
- Drug active in cancers of lung, breast, ovary, pancreas, and stomach; Hodgkin's and NHL, acute and chronic lymphocytic leukemias.

Potential Toxicities/Side Effects and the Nursing Process

I. ALTERED URINARY ELIMINATION related to HEMORRHAGIC CYSTITIS AND RENAL TOXICITY

Defining Characteristics: Symptoms of bladder irritation; hemorrhagic cystitis with hematuria, dysuria, urinary frequency; preventable with uroprotection and hydration. Symptoms of renal toxicity; increased BUN and serum creatinine, decreased urine creatinine clearance (usually reversible); acute tubular necrosis, pyelonephritis, glomerular dysfunction; metabolic acidosis.

Nursing Implications: Assess presence of RBC in urine prior to successive doses, especially if symptoms are present, as well as BUN and creatinine. Administer drug with concomitant uroprotector (e.g., mesna). Encourage prehydration: oral intake of 2–3 L/day prior to chemotherapy; posthydration: increase oral fluids to 2–3 L for 2 days after chemotherapy. If possible, administer drug in morning to minimize drug accumulation in bladder during sleep. Instruct patient to empty bladder every 2–3 hours, before bedtime, and during night when awake. Monitor urinary output and total body balance. Assess urinary elimination pattern prior to each drug dose. If rigorous regimen is adhered to, minimal renal toxicity will result. Monitor BUN and creatinine.

II. ALTERED NUTRITION, LESS THAN BODY REQUIREMENTS, related to NAUSEA AND VOMITING, HEPATOTOXICITY

Defining Characteristics: Nausea and vomiting occur in 58% of patients; dose and schedule-dependent, with increased severity with higher dose and rapid injection. Occurs within a few hours of drug administration and may last 3 days. Elevations of serum transaminase and alk phos may occur; usually transient and resolve spontaneously without apparent sequelae.

Nursing Implications: Premedicate with antiemetics and continue prophylactically to prevent nausea and vomiting for 24 hours at least for the first treatment. Encourage small, frequent feedings of cool, bland foods and liquids. Refer to section on nausea and vomiting. Monitor LFTs during treatment.

III. INFECTION AND BLEEDING related to BONE MARROW DEPRESSION

Defining Characteristics: Leukopenia is mild to moderate. Thrombocytopenia and anemia are rare. Dosage adjustment may be necessary when ifosfamide is combined with other chemotherapy agents. Patients at risk for bone marrow depression include patients with impaired renal function and decreased bone marrow reserve (bone marrow metastases, prior XRT).

Nursing Implications: Evaluate WBC, with neutrophil, and platelet count and discuss any abnormalities with physician prior to drug administration. Assess for signs/symptoms of infection or bleeding and instruct patient in signs/symptoms of infection and bleeding, and to report them immediately; discuss strategies to minimize risk of infection and bleeding, including avoidance of OTC aspirin-containing medications. Assess patient's Hgb/HCT and signs/symptoms of fatigue; teach patient self-assessment and to alternate rest and activity as needed.

IV. ALTERATION IN SKIN INTEGRITY related to ALOPECIA, STERILE PHLEBITIS, SKIN CHANGES

Defining Characteristics: The incidence of alopecia is 83%, with 50% experiencing severe hair loss in 2–4 weeks. Sterile phlebitis may occur at injection site; irritation occurs with extravasation. Hyperpigmentation, dermatitis, and nail ridging may occur.

Nursing Implications: Discuss with patient anticipated impact of hair loss; suggest wig, as appropriate, prior to actual hair loss. Explore with patient response to hair loss and alternative strategies to minimize distress. Carefully monitor injection site during drug administration for signs/symptoms of phlebitis, irritation, vein patency. Assess skin integrity. Assess impact of skin changes on body image. Discuss strategies to minimize distress.

V. POTENTIAL SEXUAL/REPRODUCTIVE DYSFUNCTION related to DRUG EFFECTS

Defining Characteristics: Drug is carcinogenic, mutagenic, and teratogenic. Drug is excreted in breast milk.

Nursing Implications: As appropriate, explore with patient and partner issues of reproductive and sexual patterns, and impact chemotherapy will have. Discuss strategies to preserve sexuality and reproductive health (e.g., sperm banking, contraception).

VI. SENSORY/PERCEPTUAL ALTERATIONS related to CONFUSION, ACTIVITY INTOLERANCE, FATIGUE

Defining Characteristics: Intact drug passes easily into CNS; however, active metabolites do not. Lethargy and confusion may be seen with high doses, lasting 1–8 hours, usually spontaneously reversible. CNS side effects occur in about 12% of patients treated, including somnolence, confusion, depressive psychosis, hallucinations. Less frequent side effects: dizziness, disorientation, cranial nerve dysfunction, seizures, and coma. Incidence of CNS side effects may be higher in patients with compromised renal function, as well as in patients receiving high doses. In most instances, CNS changes are reversible.

Nursing Implications: Identify patients at risk (decreased renal function) and observe closely. Assess neurologic and mental status prior to and during drug administration and on follow-up. Instruct patient to report any alterations in behavior, sensation, perception. Develop a plan of care with patient and family if side effects develop to manage distress and promote safety. Drug should be stopped if confusion, hallucinations, and coma occur.

Drug: irinotecan (Camptosar, Camptothecan-11, CPT-11)

Class: Topoisomerase I inhibitor.

Mechanism of Action: Induces protein-linked DNA single-strand breaks and blocks DNA and RNA synthesis in dividing cells, thus preventing cells from entering mitosis. The active metabolite, SN-38, prevents repair (relegation) of previous, reversible single-strand breaks in DNA by binding to topoisomerase I. Topoisomerase I is an enzyme that relaxes tension in the DNA helix torsion by initially causing this single-strand break in DNA so that DNA replication can occur. Topoisomerases I and II then work together to bring about replication, transcription, and recombination of DNA material. Topoisomerase I is found in higher-than-normal concentrations in certain malignant cells, such as colon adenocarcinoma cells and non-Hodgkin's lymphoma cells.

Metabolism: Metabolized to its active metabolite SN-38 in the liver; 11–20% of the drug is excreted in the urine, and 5–39% in the bile over a 48-hour period. Mean terminal half-life is 6 hours, while that of SN-38 is 10 hours. Drug is moderately protein-bound (30–68%), while SN-38 is highly protein-bound (95%).

Dosage/Range:

Metastatic colorectal cancers

- FOLFIRI Day 1: Irinotecan 180 mg/m^2 IV over 90 minutes, at the same time as Leucovorin 200 mg/m^2 IV over 2 hours through separate arms of a Y-tubing, followed by 5-FU 400 mg/m^2 IVB and then 23-hour 5-FU 1200 mg/m^2 IV continuous infusion (CI), d 1, 2. Total 5-FU CI dose is 2400 mg/m^2 over 46–48 hours. Repeat q 2 weeks.
- *Douillard* Day 1: Irinotecan 180 mg/m^2 IV over 90 minutes, at the same time as Leucovorin 200 mg/m^2 IV over 2 hours through separate arms of a Y-tubing, followed by 5-FU 400 mg/m^2 IVB and then 22-hour 5-FU 600 mg/m^2 IV continuous infusion (CI). Day 2: leucovorin 200 mg/m^2 IV over 2 hours and then 5-FU 400 mg/m^2 IVB and then 22-hour 5-FU 600 mg/m^2 IV continuous infusion (CI). Repeat q 2 weeks.
- *IFL regimen*: Metastatic colorectal cancer (in combination with 5-FU and leucovorin): Irinotecan 125 mg/m^2 IV over 90 minutes (days 1, 8, 15, and 22); leucovorin 20 mg/m^2 IVB immediately after irinotecan (days 1, 8, 15, and 22); 5-FU 500 mg/m^2 IVB immediately after leucovorin (days 1, 8, 15, and 22), followed by 2-week rest period (total, 6-week cycle). Requires *very* close monitoring and supportive care, and thus, bolus 5-FU/LV (IFL) is rarely used in favor of infusional 5-FU/LV; see FOLFIRI or Douillard regimen.
- 350-mg/m^2 IV day 1 repeated every 21 days (300 mg/m^2 for patients > 70 years old, those who have received prior pelvic/abdominal radiotherapy, or those with an ECOG performance status of 2).
- CapIri: Capecitabine 1000 mg/m^2 po bid d 1–14; Irinotecan 80 mg/m^2 IV d 1, 8. Repeat q 22 days.

Drug Preparation:

- Store unopened vials at room temperature and protect from light.
- Dilute and mix drug in 5% dextrose (preferred) or 0.9% sodium chloride to a final concentration of 0.12–1.1 mg/mL. Commonly, the drug is diluted in 500 mL 5% dextrose.
- Diluted drug is stable 24 hours at room temperature. If diluted in 5% dextrose, the drug is stable for 48 hours if refrigerated (2–8°C [36–46°F]) and protected from light.

Drug Administration:

- Administer IV bolus over 90 minutes.

Drug Interactions:

- Vinorelbine, St. John's Wort: inhibits SN38 catabolism by CYP 3A4 with increased serum levels and subsequent toxicity of irinotecan.
- 5-FU: additive or synergistic effect.

Lab Effects/Interference:

- Decreased CBC.
- UGT1A1*28* allele polymorphism occurs in 10% of population; results in decreased metabolism of SN38 and subsequent increased risk of neutropenia, other toxicities.

Special Considerations:

- IFL (Saltz) regimen may result in increased deaths. Use cautiously and monitor patients closely, especially patients with ↓ Performance Status (2), elderly, or patients with prior pelvic/abdominal radiation, or with hepatic dysfunction. Assess for s/s dehydration, febrile neutropenia, diarrhea. Modify dose per manufacturer's guidelines.
  - Independent expert panel reviewed clinical trial data and did not recommend changes in starting doses; potential life-threatening toxicity was highlighted, especially severe myelosuppression, and both *early* and late diarrhea.
  - Patient must have weekly assessment for toxicity.
  - Patient must have dose reduction as recommended; drug should not be administered if the patient is neutropenic or has diarrhea.
  - Patient must be taught to notify provider if toxicity develops, and how to manage diarrhea, nausea, vomiting, potential infection (www.asco.org/people/nr/html/jco-early.htm).
- Drug is indicated for first-line treatment of metastatic colon or rectal cancer in combination with 5-FU and leucovorin, and as a single agent for colorectal cancer recurring or progressing after treatment with 5-FU.
- Dose-limiting toxicities are diarrhea and severe myelosuppression.
- Drug is teratogenic and thus contraindicated in pregnant women; women of childbearing age should be taught and encouraged to use birth control.
- Drug is an irritant. If extravasation occurs, the manufacturer recommends flushing the IV site with sterile water, and then applying ice.
- All patients should receive self-care instructions on management of diarrhea, self-administration of loperamide for delayed diarrhea, and assessment of the patient's ability to purchase loperamide, and ability to comply with instructions.
- Patient response to treatment is usually apparent within two courses of therapy (12 weeks).
- Flushing (vasodilation) may occur during drug infusion, and usually does not require intervention.
- Patient educational material is available from Pharmacia/Upjohn Co.
- Rarely, patients may lack an enzyme necessary for drug metabolism, resulting in increased toxicity (Gilbert's syndrome, abnormal glucuronidation of bilirubin).

- Dose reductions must be made for neutropenia and severe diarrhea, and are different for combination therapy (irinotecan/5-FU/leukovorin) and irinotecan as a single agent.
- Contraindications: serum BR > 2.0 mg/dL although no studies done, grades 3/4 neutropenia occurred in patients with BR 1–2 mg/dL.

Potential Toxicities/Side Effects and the Nursing Process

I. ALTERATION IN ELIMINATION related to DIARRHEA

Defining Characteristics: Diarrhea may be early or late. Early diarrhea is characterized by onset within 24 hours of drug dose and is mediated by cholinergic pathway(s), as the metabolite SN-38 inhibits acetylcholinesterase; diaphoresis and abdominal cramping may precede diarrhea, and may be prevented by atropine. Other cholinergic effects that may appear are salivation, lacrimation, visual disturbances, piloerection, and bradycardia. This can be managed effectively with atropine 0.25–1.0 mg IV or scopolamine. Late diarrhea occurs > 24 hours after the drug dose, can be severe, prolonged, and lead to dehydration and electrolyte imbalance; the etiology appears related to changes in intestinal mucosal epithelium that prevent the reabsorption of water and electrolytes, which are then lost during diarrhea. 88% of patients may experience late diarrhea, and 31% have severe, or grade 3/4 diarrhea. Loperamide is effective in halting late diarrhea. Irinotecan should be held for grade 3 diarrhea (7–9 stools/day, incontinence, or severe cramping) and grade 4 (> 10 stools/day, grossly bloody stool, or need for parenteral support). Once recovered, decrease drug dose at next treatment per manufacturer's guidelines and per physician order.

Nursing Implications: Acute diarrhea: teach patient to report diarrhea, sweating, and abdominal cramping during or after drug administration. Administer atropine 0.25–1 mg IVP per physician order, unless contraindicated, to prevent diarrhea. Delayed diarrhea: teach patient self-management of diarrhea (diet, fluids, avoidance of laxatives), and to notify nurse or physician of vomiting, fever, or if signs/symptoms of dehydration occur (fainting, light-headedness, dizziness). Teaching about diet should include drinking 8–10 large glasses of fluid/day, including soup/broth, soda, Gatorade; avoiding dairy products; eating small meals often; using BRAT diet (bananas, rice, applesauce, toast); and adding other foods as tolerated, such as bland, low-fiber foods, white chicken meat without skin, scrambled eggs, crackers, or pasta without sauce. Also teach patient to avoid foods that worsen diarrhea (fatty, fried, or greasy foods, high-fiber foods with bran, raw fruits and vegetables, popcorn, beans, nuts, chocolate). Review patient's medication profile, including over-the-counter medicines, and teach patient to stop taking any laxatives. Teach patient to avoid cigarette smoking to promote comfort. Instruct patient to record stools, and to take loperamide, not as indicated on the medication package, but as instructed: At the first episode of late-onset diarrhea, take 4 mg (2 [2-mg] capsules) of loperamide, then 2 mg (1 capsule) every 2 hours until free of diarrhea for at least 12 hours. Take a 4-mg dose (2 [2-mg] capsules) at bedtime (Camptosar recommendations). Patient should notify doctor or nurse if diarrhea is unrelieved by loperamide taken as instructed. Assess patient's ability to purchase loperamide if impoverished, and identify other sources that can provide the medication prior to patient's discharge from clinic after drug therapy. Review patient's medication profile to ensure that the patient is not taking any cathartics. Diarrhea must be monitored closely and managed aggressively to prevent morbidity and mortality.

II. POTENTIAL FOR INFECTION, ANEMIA related to BONE MARROW DEPRESSION

Defining Characteristics: Leukopenia has been noted in 63% of patients on single-dose schedules, with an overall neutropenia incidence of 54%, and grade 3/4 neutropenia occurring in 26% of patients. Thrombocytopenia is uncommon, occurring in about 3% of patients. Anemia is common (61%). Nadir is commonly on day 6–9.

Nursing Implications: Evaluate WBC, with neutrophil, and platelet count, and discuss any abnormalities with physician prior to drug administration. Refer to Special Considerations section for dosage modifications based on hematologic toxicity. Assess patient tolerance of chemotherapy and nadir blood counts, especially Cycle 1. Assess for signs/symptoms of infection or bleeding; instruct patient in signs/symptoms of infection and bleeding, and to report them immediately. If febrile neutropenia develops, assess and begin antibiotic therapy ASAP. Instruct in measures to minimize risk of infection and bleeding, including avoidance of OTC aspirin-containing medications. Assess patient's Hgb/HCT and signs/symptoms of fatigue; teach patient self-assessment and to alternate rest and activity as needed.

III. POTENTIAL ALTERATION IN NUTRITION, LESS THAN BODY REQUIREMENTS, related to NAUSEA AND VOMITING, DEHYDRATION

Defining Characteristics: Moderate to severe nausea and vomiting occur in 35–60% of patients, with 17% experiencing NCI grade 3/4 nausea and 13% experiencing NCI grade 3/4 vomiting. Aggressive combination antiemetics are effective in preventing nausea/vomiting.

Nursing Implications: Premedicate with aggressive combination antiemetics such as serotonin antagonist (dolasetron, granisetron, or ondansetron) plus dexamethasone 10 mg IV 30 minutes prior to chemotherapy to prevent nausea and vomiting. Encourage small, frequent meals of cool, bland foods and liquids. Teach patients to monitor their fluid intake, and take daily weights if nausea/vomiting occurs. Assess for signs/symptoms of fluid and electrolyte imbalance. Teach patients self-assessment, and instruct to notify doctor or nurse if these occur. Late-onset nausea and vomiting may occur, and dopamine antagonists such as prochlorperazine are then recommended. If dehydration develops, replace fluid and electrolytes to prevent worsening dehydration and cardiovascular complications.

IV. POTENTIAL FOR IMPAIRED GAS EXCHANGE, POTENTIAL related to DYSPNEA, PULMONARY INFILTRATES, FEVER

Defining Characteristics: Pulmonary effects may occur in up to 22% of patients, ranging from transient dyspnea to pulmonary infiltrates, fever, increased cough, and decreased DLCO in a small number of patients.

Nursing Implications: Assess baseline pulmonary status, and teach patient to report any changes. Assess pulmonary status prior to each treatment and at visits between treatment. If patient develops dyspnea, discuss patient having PFTs with physician, and evaluating whether related to drug. Teach patient to manage dyspnea if it occurs, including alternating activity and rest periods.

Drug: ixabepilone (Ixempra)

Class: Epothilone B analogue.

Mechanism of Action: Normally, cells need to have flexibility in making the structures for mitosis, such as tubulin and the microtubules; the tubulin needs to be able to polymerize and then depolymerize. Ixabepilone binds to the beta-tubulin subunits on microtubules, and strongly promotes tubulin polymerization and stabilization, similar to paclitaxel but at a different binding site; the drug causes the cell to stop cycling (mitotic arrest) at the G_2/M phase of the cell cycle and to die (cytotoxicity). The drug avoids multiple tumor-resistance mechanisms, including efflux transporters and P-glycoprotein; thus, it has effectiveness against tumors that possess these mechanisms resulting in refractoriness to taxanes, anthracyclines, and vinca alkaloids. Ixabepilone also has antiangiogenic activity.

Metabolism: Drug is a semisynthetic analogue of epothilone B. It is a macrolide fermentation product of the myxobacterium *Sorangium cellulosum.* Drug has linear pharmacokinetics, with 67–77% binding to serum proteins. Drug is extensively metabolized in the liver, primarily via oxidative metabolism by CYP 3A4/5 microenzyme system (hepatic microsomes). This produces > 30 inactive metabolites, which are then excreted in the urine (65%) and feces (21%). Eighty-six percent of the dose is eliminated in 7 days. The terminal half-life of the drug is 52 hours, with no accumulation in the plasma when given every 3 weeks. It is unlikely that ixabepilone affects serum levels of drugs that are substrates of CYP enzymes.

Dosage/Range:

- 40 mg/m^2 IV over 3 hours every 21 days.
- In breast cancer, given with capecitabine 1000 mg/m^2 PO twice daily × 14 days, repeated every 3 weeks.
- Do not exceed maximum dose calculated at BSA 2.2 m^2.
- Dose reduce for mild hepatic dysfunction, severe neutropenia, or severe thrombocytopenia; contraindicated in severe hepatic dysfunction (see Special Considerations).
- *Hematologic (ixabepilone)*: When recovered (ANC ≥ 1500 cells/mm^3 and platelets ≥ 100,000 cells/mm^3), decrease dose by 20% for neutrophils < 500 cells/mm^3 for > 7 days, febrile neutropenia, or platelets < 25,000 cells/mm^3 or platelets < 50,000 cells/mm^3 with bleeding.
- *Hematologic (capecitabine)*: For platelets < 25,000 cells/mm^3 or < 50,000 cells/mm^3 with bleeding, hold capecitabine for concurrent diarrhea or stomatitis until platelet count > 50,000 cells/mm^3 then continue at same dose; for neutrophils < 500 cells/mm^3 for > 7 days or febrile neutropenia, hold capecitabine for concurrent diarrhea or stomatitis until ANC > 1000 cells/mm^3 then continue at same dose.
- *Nonhematologic (ixabepilone)*: When toxicity improved to grade 1, decrease by 20% for moderate grade 2 neuropathy (moderate) lasting ≥ 7 days; grade 3 neuropathy (severe) lasting < 7 days; any grade 3 toxicity (severe) other than neuropathy. Discontinue drug for grade 3 neuropathy (severe) lasting ≥ 7 days or any grade 4 toxicity (disabling).
- *Nonhematologic (capecitabine)*: Follow capecitabine label.
- *Hepatic impairment (ixabepilone monotherapy)*: Mild (AST and ALT ≤ 2.5 × ULN and bilirubin ≤ 1 × ULN), give full dose; AST or ALT ≤ 10 × ULN and ≤ 1.5 × ULN give 32 mg/m^2; moderate (AST and ALT ≤ 10 × ULN and bilirubin > 1.5 × ULN ≤ 3 × ULN), give 20–30 mg/m^2.

Drug Preparation:

- Available as Ixempra 15 mg for injection supplied with 8-mL diluent and Ixempra 45 mg with 23.5-mL diluent. Reconstituted solution delivers ixabepilone concentration of 2 mg/mL. This must be further diluted with Lactated Ringer's Injection USP to a final concentration of 0.2–0.6 mg/mL. Drug is stable only in solution with a pH in the range of 6–7.5.
- Reconstituted solution is stable for 1 hour in a syringe at room temperature and light but should be further diluted as soon as possible following reconstitution. After further diluted in Lactated Ringer's, the infusion must be completed within 6 hours of preparation.
- IXEMPRA kit contains 2 vials (vial containing 16 mg drug powder [labeled 15 mg] or 47 mg [labeled 45 mg] and vial of diluent containing dehydrated alcohol). Kit must be stored in a refrigerator (2–8°C [36–46°F]) in original packaging to protect

from light. Remove from refrigerator 30 minutes before mixing; this will also give time for any white precipitate in the diluent to dissolve.

  - Reconstitute by aseptically withdrawing diluent and slowly injecting into vial containing IXEMPRA drug; gently swirl and invert vial until completely dissolved. Aspirate ordered dose (2 mg/mL).
  - Further dilute in 250-mL Lactated Ringers (or larger if needed to deliver a final concentration of 0.2–0.6 mg/mL)—bag must be DEHP free (e.g., non-PVC). Gently invert bag to mix (manual rotation).
- Administer via DEHP-free tubing with DEHP-free final filter 0.2–1.2 microns.
- The drug infusion must be completed within 6 hours of preparation.

Drug Administration:

- ANC must be ≥ 1500 cells/mm^3 and platelets ≥ cells/mm^3.
- Administer as IV infusion over 3 hours. Premedicate with an H_1 antagonist (e.g., diphenhydramine 50 mg PO) and H_2 antagonist (e.g., ranitidine 150–300 mg PO) 1 hour before chemotherapy to minimize hypersensitivity reaction.
- If patient has had a hypersensitivity reaction to ixabepilone in the prior cycle, add a corticosteroid (e.g., dexamethasone 20 mg IV 30 minutes or PO 60 minutes before chemotherapy) to premedications.
- Drug contains dehydrated alcohol; thus, assess patient's neurologic status during and after infusion.

Drug Interactions:

- Capecitabine: synergy, so used together to increase tumor cell kill.
- Strong CYP3A4 inhibitors decrease the metabolism, thus increasing plasma level of ixabepilone and thus should be avoided (Ketoconazole, Itraconazole, clarithromycin, atazanavir, nefazodone, saquinavir, telithromycin, ritonavir, amprenavir, indinavir, nelfinavir, delavirdine, voriconazole, grapefruit juice); if a strong CYP3A4 inhibitor must be given concurrently, reduce ixabepilone dose to 20 mg/m^2; after the strong inhibitor is discontinued, wait 1 week (washout period) before increasing the ixabepilone dose to indicated dose.

Lab Effects/Interference:

- Neutropenia, thrombocytopenia, anemia.

Special Considerations:

- Drug is 3–20 times more potent than paclitaxel.
- Drug is able to overcome p-glycoprotein–related drug resistance.
- Drug is indicated in the treatment of patients with metastatic or locally advanced breast cancer.
- As monotherapy in patients whose tumors are resistant or refractory to anthracyclines, taxanes, and capecitabine.
- In combination with capecitabine in patients whose tumors are resistant to treatment with an anthracycline and a taxane or whose cancer is taxane resistant and for whom further anthracycline therapy is contraindicated (anthracycline resistance

is defined as progression on therapy or within 6 months of adjuvant therapy or 3 months in the metastatic setting; taxane resistance is defined as progression on therapy or within 12 months in the adjuvant setting, or 4 months in the metastatic setting).

- Drug is contraindicated in patients who are hypersensitive to Cremaphor® EL or its derivatives (polyoxyethylated castor oil), patients with a baseline ANC < 1500 cells/mm^3 or platelet count < 100,000 cells/mm^3, or when given in combination with capecitabine, in patients with hepatic dysfunction (AST or ALT > 2.5 × ULN or bilirubin > 1 × ULN due to increased risk of neutropenia related death and other toxicity).
- As a single agent, use cautiously in patients with hepatic dysfunction (AST or ALT > 5 × ULN); do not use in patients with AST or ALT > 10 × ULN or bilirubin > 3 × ULN.
- Use cautiously and assess frequently in patients with preexisting moderate to severe peripheral neuropathy or diabetes mellitus.
- Drug is fetotoxic: Teach women of childbearing age to use effective contraception.
- Toxicity profile similar to paclitaxel.
- A randomized phase III trial in patients with refractory breast cancer showed that patients who received ixabepilone and capecitabine had significantly longer progression-free survival (5.8 months) compared with patients receiving capecitabine alone (4.2 months, $p < 0.0003$). The objective response rate was 35% in the combination group compared with 14% in the single-agent group (Vahdat et al, 2007).

Potential Toxicities/Side Effects and the Nursing Process

I. POTENTIAL FOR INFECTION AND BLEEDING related to BONE MARROW DEPRESSION

Defining Characteristics: Myelosuppression is dose dependent, expressed primarily as neutropenia. Incidence of neutropenia is 68% with grade 3/4 54% (incidence of febrile neutropenia 3% as monotherapy and 5% when given with capecitabine, with infection occurring in 5–6% of patients, respectively). Neutropenic deaths occurred in 1.9% of patients receiving ixabepilone in combination with capecitabine, with normal hepatic function or mild hepatic dysfunction, and in 0.4% in patients receiving monotherapy. Drug is contraindicated in patients with severe hepatic dysfunction (see Special Considerations), and in patients with ANC < 1500 cells/mm^3 or platelets < 100,000 cells/mm^3. Grades 3/4 thrombocytopenia occur in 7% (monotherapy) and 8% (combination therapy) of patients, and anemia in 8% (mono) and 10% (combination). Fatigue is common, affecting 56% (mono) and 60% (combination).

Nursing Implications: Assess baseline CBC, WBC, differential, and platelet count prior to chemotherapy, as well as signs/symptoms of infection or bleeding, and assure

ANC ≥ 1500 cells/mm^3 and platelet count ≥ 100,000 cells/mm^3. If patient experienced severe neutropenia or thrombocytopenia, discuss dose reduction with physician. Teach patient the signs/symptoms of infection or bleeding, and to report these immediately, such as temperature ≥ 100.5°F. Teach patient self-care measures to minimize risk of infection and bleeding. This includes avoidance of crowds, proximity to people with infections, and OTC aspirin-containing medications. Assess baseline activity and energy level. Teach patient that fatigue may occur, and ways to minimize exertion and energy expenditure by alternating rest and activity, and organizing chores so that they are done as efficiently as possible.

II. POTENTIAL FOR INJURY related to HYPERSENSITIVITY REACTIONS

Defining Characteristics: In studies, 1% of patients had severe hypersensitivity reactions (HSRs), including anaphylaxis. The risk of HSRs is reduced by premedication with H_1 and H_2 antagonists.

Nursing Implications: Assess baseline VS and mental status before drug administration. Administer H_1 antagonist (e.g., diphenhydramine 50 mg PO) and H_2 antagonist 30–60 minutes before starting drug. If patient has had a prior reaction, administer ordered corticosteroid (e.g., dexamethasone 20-mg IV or PO) in addition. Remain with patient during first 15 minutes of infusion, and monitor frequently during infusion. Teach patient to report any itching, rash, any new sensations or symptoms. Recall signs/symptoms of HSR. If these occur, stop drug immediately, and notify physician. Subjective symptoms are generalized itching, nausea, chest tightness, crampy abdominal pain, difficulty speaking, anxiety, agitation, sense of impending doom, uneasiness, desire to urinate/defecate, dizziness, chills. Objective signs are flushed appearance; fever, chills, bronchospasm, angioedema of face, neck, eyelids, hands, feet; localized or generalized urticaria; respiratory distress with or without wheezing, hypotension, cyanosis. Review standing orders or nursing procedure for patient management of anaphylaxis and be prepared to stop drug immediately. Notify physician. Monitor VS, and administer ordered medications, which may include epinephrine 1:1000, hydrocortisone sodium succinate, and diphenhydramine.

III. SENSORY/PERCEPTUAL ALTERATIONS related to SENSORY NEUROPATHY

Defining Characteristics: Peripheral neuropathy is common, with sensory neuropathy affecting 62–65% of patients, and motor neuropathy affecting 10–16% of patients. It occurs early with 75% of new onset and worsening neuropathy occurring during first three cycles. Dose reduction results in improvement or no worsening in neuropathy in most patients. About 10% of patients receiving monotherapy and 23% of patients receiving combination with capecitabine developed grade 3/4 peripheral neuropathy. Median number of cycles to onset of grade 3/4 neuropathy was four cycles in both groups, with a median time to improvement of grade 3/4 to baseline or grade 1 of 4–6 weeks for patients receiving monotherapy and 6 weeks for patients receiving combination. Neuropathy is cumulative and reversible (Vahdat et al, 2007).

Nursing Implications: Assess baseline neurologic status. Instruct patient to report signs/symptoms of pins and needles sensation, numbness, burning sensation, pain, increased discomfort with certain sensations, especially in the extremities, or motor weakness. Identify patients at risk: prior cisplatin, or having preexisting neuropathies (ethanol- and diabetes mellitus-related). Assess sensory and motor function prior to each treatment, and if abnormality found, assess impact on patient function, safety, independence, ability to do activities of daily living (ADLs), and quality of life. Test patient's ability to button a shirt, or pick up a dime from a flat surface. If impacting ability to do ADLs, safety, or quality of life, discuss with patient and physician drug reduction (20% for grade 2 lasting ≥ 7 days or grade 3 lasting < 7 days). If grade 3 neuropathy lasts ≥ 7 days, the drug should be discontinued. Teach self-care strategies, including maintaining safety when walking, getting up, taking a bath, or washing dishes; discuss inability to sense temperature, and the need to keep extremities warm in cold weather. See NCI Common Toxicity Criteria in Appendix II: grade 2 motor = symptomatic weakness interfering with function but not ADLs; grade 2 sensory = sensory alteration or paresthesia interfering with function but not ADLs; grade 3 motor = objective weakness, interfering with ADLs; grade 3 sensory = sensory loss or paresthesia interfering with ADLs; grade 4 motor = paralysis; grade 4 sensory = permanent sensory loss that interferes with function.

IV. ALTERATION IN SKIN INTEGRITY related to ALOPECIA, NAIL CHANGES

Defining Characteristics: Alopecia affects 31–48% of patients in clinical trials and is reversible; 9–24% of patients developed nail changes during clinical trials. Palmar plantar erythrodysesthesia (hand-foot syndrome) occurred in 64% of patients receiving capecitabine with ixabepilone.

Nursing Implications: Discuss potential impact of hair loss prior to drug administration. Discuss coping strategies and a plan to minimize body image distortion (e.g., wig, scarf, cap). Assess patient for signs/symptoms of hair loss. Assess patient's response and use of coping strategies, and help patient to build on effective strategies.

Assess patient's fingernails and toenails, and teach patients changes may occur and to report them. Develop plan of care with patient if changes are severe. Refer to capecitabine drug sheet for the assessment, prevention, and management of palmar plantar erythrodysesthesia.

V. ALTERATION IN COMFORT related to ARTHRALGIAS AND MYALGIAS

Defining Characteristics: Arthralgias and myalgias affect about 39–49% of patients, and musculoskeletal pain affected 20–23% of patients.

Nursing Implications: Arthralgias and myalgias may be troublesome, and can be managed with NSAIDs, application of warmth, and other comfort measures. Some patients report that swimming is helpful in minimizing discomfort. Studies of gabapentin, glutamine, and steroids have been disappointing. Opioids may be needed if severe.

VI. ALTERATION IN NUTRITION, LESS THAN BODY REQUIREMENTS, related to NAUSEA, VOMITING, DIARRHEA

Defining Characteristics: Nausea and vomiting occur in approximately 42–53% and 29–39% of patients, respectively. It is mild and preventable with antiemetics. Diarrhea occurs in 22–44% of patients and is mild. Drug appears to cause diarrhea by direct injury to the intestinal mucosa (necrosis of cells) causing inflammation of the bowel wall and decreased absorption. Stomatitis and mucositis occur in 29–31% of patients. Constipation occurs in 16–22% of patients.

Nursing Implications: Assess patient's nutritional status, as well as elimination status. Premedicate patient with antiemetic prior to chemotherapy and give antiemetic to take at home if needed. Encourage small, frequent meals of cool, bland foods. Instruct patient to report nausea unrelieved with antiemetics, and teach self-administration of antiemetics as most patients will receive the drug as an outpatient. If nausea/vomiting occur and are severe, assess for signs/symptoms of fluid/electrolyte imbalance and bring to clinic for aggressive antiemesis. Encourage patient to report onset of diarrhea and to self-administer antidiarrheal medications; review dietary changes to reduce bowel irritation (e.g., avoid spicy, high-fat, high-insoluble fiber foods and increase fluids to 3 L/day). If patient develops constipation, review measures and dietary changes to relieve constipation. Assess baseline oral mucous membranes. Teach patient oral assessment and to report any alterations. Assess LFTs prior to drug administration and periodically during treatment.

Drug: letrozole (Femara)

Class: Nonsteroidal aromatase inhibitor.

Mechanism of Action: Highly selective, potent agent that significantly suppresses (90%) serum estradiol levels within 14 days, without interfering with other steroid hormone synthesis. Binds to the heme group of aromatase, a cytochrome P-450 enzyme necessary for the conversion of androgens to estrogens. Aromatase is thus inhibited, leading to a significant reduction in plasma estradiol, estrone, and estrone sulfate. After six weeks of therapy, there is 97% suppression of estradiol.

Metabolism: Rapidly and completely absorbed after oral administration, with a terminal half-life of 2 days. Metabolized in the liver and excreted in the urine.

Dosage/Range:
- 2.5 mg PO daily.
- Dose reduction recommended in patients with cirrhosis and severe hepatic dysfunction.

Drug Preparation:
- Oral.

Drug Interactions:
- Tamoxifen: coadministration with tamoxifen decreased letrozole plasma levels by 38% but not significant when letrozole was administered immediately after tamoxifen.
- Estrogen: may decrease drug effect.

Lab Effects/Interference:
- Liver transaminases may be transiently elevated.
- Increase in total cholesterol (non-fasting, adjuvant studies).

Special Considerations:
- Indicated for (1) adjuvant treatment of postmenopausal women with hormone receptor positive early breast cancer, (2) the extended adjuvant treatment of early breast cancer in postmenopausal women who have received 5 years of adjuvant tamoxifen therapy; (3) the first-line treatment of post-menopausal women with hormone receptor positive or unknown, locally advanced or metastatic breast cancer; (4) treatment of advanced breast cancer in postmenopausal women with disease progression following antiestrogen therapy.
- Letrozole was compared to tamoxifen in postmenopausal women and found to be superior in terms of response (30% vs 20%), time to disease progression (41 weeks vs 25 weeks), and rate of clinical benefit (49% vs 38%) (Mouridsen et al, 2001).
- Potent aromatase inhibitor with response rate of 20%.
- Drug is contraindicated in premenopausal women, as it has not been evaluated in this population.
- About 200 times more potent than aminoglutethimide.
- Letrozole may cause fetal harm when administered to pregnant women, as drug is embryotoxic and fetotoxic in lab animals. If there is exposure to letrozole during

pregnancy, the patient should be apprised of the potential hazard to the fetus and potential risk for loss of the pregnancy.

Potential Toxicities/Side Effects and the Nursing Process

I. ALTERATION IN COMFORT related to PAIN, FATIGUE, AND HOT FLASHES

Defining Characteristics: Most common side effects were musculoskeletal pain (21%: muscle, skeletal, back, arm, leg), arthralgia (8%), headache (9%), fatigue (8%), and chest pain (6%). Hot flashes occur in approximately 6% of patients.

Nursing Considerations: Assess baseline comfort levels, and teach patient that this discomfort may occur. Teach patient symptomatic measures, and instruct to report if symptoms are unrelieved.

II. ALTERATION IN NUTRITION, LESS THAN BODY REQUIREMENTS, related to NAUSEA/VOMITING, ANOREXIA

Defining Characteristics: Nausea occurs in 13% of patients, with less frequent vomiting and anorexia.

Nursing Implications: Determine baseline weight, and monitor at each visit. Teach patient that these side effects may occur, and instruct to report this. Discuss strategies to minimize nausea, including diet and dosing time.

III. ALTERATION IN BOWEL ELIMINATION related to DIARRHEA AND CONSTIPATION

Defining Characteristics: Diarrhea or constipation occurs in about 6% of patients.

Nursing Implications: Assess for change in bowel patterns, and instruct patient to report diarrhea or constipation. Teach patient that diarrhea or constipation is usually relieved by nonprescription medications such as Kaolin pectate combinations (Kaopectate) for diarrhea, and stool softeners or Psyllium for constipation. Instruct patient to report unrelieved diarrhea or constipation.

Drug: leuprolide acetate (Lupron, Viadur)

Class: Antihormone.

Mechanism of Action: It is a luteinizing hormone-releasing hormone (LHRH) analogue that suppresses the secretion of gonadotropins, including follicle-stimulating hormone (FSH) and luteinizing hormone (LH) from the pituitary gland. There is an initial rise in gonadal steroids and then a significant decrease. The decrease in LH causes the Leydig cells to reduce testosterone production to castrate levels.

Metabolism: Ninety-five percent of the drug is absorbed after subcutaneous injection, with 85–100% of the drug being absorbed after IM or subcutaneous injection. Drug is slightly protein bound (43–49%).

Dosage/Range:

- For palliative treatment of prostate cancer: Depot suspension 7.5 mg IM every month, OR 22.5 mg IM every 3 months, OR 30 mg IM every 4 months, OR Viadur implant 65 mg every 12 months, OR 1 mg/day subcutaneous injection.

Drug Preparation:

- Use syringes, diluent, kit provided by manufacturer.
- Injection: 5 mg/mL; kit 5 mg/mL for 7.5-mg, 22.5-mg doses.
- Powder for injection: 7.5 mg.
- Viadur implant kit contains implant, implanter, and sterile field/supplies. Sterile gloves must be added. Procedure is sterile, and uses a special implant technology.

Drug Administration:

- Depot is administered IM or subcutaneous.
- Daily solution is given subcutaneous.
- Viadur: Kit contains specific directions for insertion of implant, removal, and reinsertion of subsequent dose after 1 year.

Drug Interactions:

- None reported.

Lab Effects/Interference:

- Decreased PSA, testosterone levels; increased calcium, decreased WBC, decreased serum total protein.
- Injection: Increased BUN and creatinine.
- Depot: Increased LDH, alk phos, AST, uric acid, cholesterol, LDL, triglycerides, glucose, WBC, phosphate; decreased potassium, platelets.

Special Considerations:

- Patient should be instructed in proper administration techniques, and in signs/symptoms of infection at site. Sites should be rotated. For Viadur, patient has implant inserted by MD/RN once yearly.
- Initially, drug causes increased LH secretion, resulting in increased testosterone secretion and tumor flare. Usually disappears after 2 weeks.
- Drug has been studied in the treatment of breast and islet cell cancers.
- Studies on Viadur show that implant delivers 120 micrograms of leuprolide acetate per day over 12 months, reducing testosterone levels to castration levels within 2–4 weeks after insertion.

Potential Toxicities/Side Effects and the Nursing Process

I. ALTERATION IN COMFORT related to HOT FLASHES, TUMOR FLARE, EDEMA

Defining Characteristics: Headache, dizziness, and hot flashes may occur. Vasodilation most common, with 67.9% incidence. Sweating may affect 5% of patients. Tumor flare may also occur initially (bone and tumor pain, transient increase in tumor size due to transient increase in testosterone levels). Breast tenderness has been reported. Peripheral edema may occur in 8% of patients.

Nursing Implications: Inform patient that symptoms may occur, that flare reaction will subside after the initial two weeks of therapy. Encourage patient to report symptoms early. Develop symptom management plan with patient and physician.

II. POTENTIAL SEXUAL DYSFUNCTION related to LIBIDO, IMPOTENCE

Defining Characteristics: Frequently causes decreased libido and erectile impotence in men. Gynecomastia occurs in 3–6.9% of patients. In women, amenorrhea occurs after ten weeks of therapy.

Nursing Implications: As appropriate, explore with patient and significant other issues of reproductive and sexual patterns and the impact chemotherapy may have on them. Discuss strategies to preserve sexuality and reproductive health.

III. DEPRESSION, POTENTIAL, related to DRUG EFFECT

Defining Characteristics: Depression may affect up to 5.3% of patients, and less commonly, patients may develop emotional lability, insomnia, nervousness, anxiety.

Nursing Implications: Assess baseline affect and usual coping strategies. Teach patient to report change in affect. Assess effectiveness of coping strategies, encourage patient to verbalize feelings, and provide emotional support. Assess need for referral to psychiatric nurse specialist or social worker if supportive efforts ineffective.

IV. ALTERED NUTRITION, LESS THAN BODY REQUIREMENTS, related to GI SIDE EFFECTS

Defining Characteristics: Anorexia, nausea, and vomiting may occur rarely, with an incidence of < 5%.

Nursing Implications: If patients experience symptoms, encourage small, frequent feedings of favorite foods, especially high-calorie, high-protein foods. Monitor weight weekly. Assess incidence and pattern of nausea, vomiting, or anorexia if they occur. Discuss need for antiemetic with physician and patient.

V. ALTERATION IN SKIN INTEGRITY, POTENTIAL, related to INSERTION, REMOVAL OF 12-MONTH IMPLANT

Defining Characteristics: Insertion and removal of implant caused local site bruising (34.8%) and burning (5.6%). In general, the reactions lasted two weeks, and then resolved completely. In about 10% of patients, reactions lasted longer than two weeks, or reactions didn't develop until after two weeks.

Nursing Implications: Assess baseline skin integrity after implant insertion, or removal. Teach patient that these reactions may occur, and will resolve, usually within two weeks. Teach patients to use local measures to minimize feeling of burning.

Drug: lomustine (CCNU, CeeNU)

Class: Alkylating agent (nitrosourea).

Mechanism of Action: Nitrosourea alkylates DNA with a reactive chloroethyl carbonium ion, producing strand breaks and crosslinks that inhibit RNA and DNA synthesis. Interferes with enzymes and histidine utilization. Is cell cycle phase nonspecific.

Metabolism: Completely absorbed from GI tract. Metabolized rapidly, partly protein-bound. Undergoes hepatic recirculation. Lipid soluble: crosses BBB; 75% excreted in urine within 4 days.

Dosage/Range:
- 130 mg/m^2 PO every 6 weeks.
- 100 mg/m^2 if given with other myelosuppressive drugs.

Drug Preparation:
- Oral: Available in 10-mg, 30-mg, and 100-mg capsules.

Drug Administration:
- Administer on an empty stomach at bedtime.

Drug Interactions:
- Myelosuppressive drugs increase hematologic toxicity; reduce dose.

Lab Effects/Interference:
- Decreased CBC.
- Increased LFTs, RFTs.

Special Considerations:

- Give orally on an empty stomach.
- Consumption of alcohol should be avoided for a short period after taking CCNU.
- Absorbed 30–60 minutes after administration; consequently, vomiting does not usually affect efficacy.

Potential Toxicities/Side Effects and the Nursing Process

I. INFECTION AND BLEEDING related to MYELOSUPPRESSION

Defining Characteristics: Nadir of platelets: 26–34 days, lasting 6–10 days; nadir of WBC: 41–46 days, lasting 9–14 days. Delayed and cumulative bone marrow depression with successive dosing: recovery takes 6–8 weeks. Bone marrow depression is dose-limiting toxicity.

Nursing Implications: Drug should be administered every 6–8 weeks due to delayed nadir and recovery. Monitor CBC, platelets prior to drug administration (WBC > $4000/mm^3$ and platelets > $100,000/mm^3$). Dispense only one dose at a time.

II. ALTERATION IN NUTRITION, LESS THAN BODY REQUIREMENTS, related to NAUSEA/VOMITING, ANOREXIA, DIARRHEA

Defining Characteristics: Onset of nausea/vomiting occurs 2–6 hours after taking dose; may be severe. Anorexia may last for several days. Diarrhea is uncommon.

Nursing Implications: Administer drug on an empty stomach at bedtime. Premedicate with antiemetic and sedative or hypnotic to promote sleep. Discourage food or fluid intake for two hours after drug administration. Encourage small, frequent feedings of favorite foods. Encourage high-calorie, high-protein foods; monitor weekly weights. Encourage patient to report onset of diarrhea. Administer or teach patient to self-administer antidiarrheal medication.

III. ALTERATION IN URINARY ELIMINATION related to RENAL COMPROMISE

Defining Characteristics: After prolonged therapy with high cumulative doses, tubular atrophy, glomerular sclerosis, and interstitial nephritis have occurred, leading to renal failure.

Nursing Implications: Monitor BUN, creatinine prior to dosing, especially in patients receiving prolonged or high cumulative dose therapy. If abnormalities are noted, a creatinine clearance should be determined.

IV. POTENTIAL FOR SEXUAL DYSFUNCTION related to MUTAGENIC AND TERATOGENIC QUALITIES OF CCNU

Defining Characteristics: Drug is teratogenic, mutagenic, and carcinogenic.

Nursing Implications: As appropriate, discuss birth control measures.

V. ACTIVITY INTOLERANCE related to LETHARGY, CONFUSION

Defining Characteristics: Neurologic dysfunction may occur rarely: confusion, lethargy, disorientation, ataxia.

Nursing Implications: Perform neurologic assessment as part of prechemotherapy assessment. Assess orientation and level of consciousness, gait, activity tolerance.

VI. POTENTIAL SENSORY/PERCEPTUAL ALTERATIONS (VISUAL) related to OCULAR DAMAGE

Defining Characteristics: Ocular damage may occur rarely: optic neuritis, retinopathy, blurred vision.

Nursing Implications: Assess vision during prechemotherapy assessment. Encourage patient to report any visual changes.

Drug: mechlorethamine hydrochloride (Mustargen, Nitrogen Mustard, HN_2)

Class: Alkylating agent.

Mechanism of Action: Produces interstrand and intrastrand cross-linkages in DNA, causing miscoding, breakage, and failures of replication. Cell cycle phase nonspecific.

Metabolism: Undergoes chemical transformation after injection with less than 0.01% excreted unchanged in urine. Drug is rapidly inactivated by body fluids. 50% of the inactive metabolites are excreted in the urine within 24 hours.

Dosage/Range:
- IV: 0.4 mg/kg, or 12–16 mg/m^2 IV as single agent; 6 mg/m^2 IV days 1 and 8 of 28-day cycle with MOPP regimen.
- Topical: Dilute 10 mg in 60 mL sterile water; apply with rubber gloves.
- Intracavitary: Pleural, peritoneal, pericardial: 0.2–0.4 mg/kg.

Drug Preparation:
- Add sterile water or 0.9% sodium chloride to each vial. Wear eye and hand protection when mixing.
- Administer via sidearm or rapidly running IV.
- Drug must be used within 15 minutes of reconstitution.

Drug Administration:
- Intravenous: This drug is a potent vesicant. Give through a freely running IV to avoid extravasation, which can lead to ulceration, pain, and necrosis. Check hospital's policy and procedure for administration of a vesicant.

Drug Interactions:
- Myelosuppressive drugs: Additive hematologic toxicity; dose reduce or monitor patient closely.
- Sodium thiosulfate: inactivates drug.

Lab Effects/Interference:
- Decreased CBC.
- Increased uric acid, RFTs.

Special Considerations:
- Drug is a vesicant. Give through a running IV to avoid extravasation. Antidote is sodium thiosulfate: dilute 4 mL sodium thiosulfate injection USP (10%) with 6 mL sterile water for injection, USP and inject subcutaneous in area of infiltration.
- Nadir is 6–8 days after treatment.
- Side effects occur in the reproductive system, such as amenorrhea and azoospermia.
- Severe nausea and vomiting.
- Systemic toxic effects may occur with intracavitary drug administration.

Potential Toxicities/Side Effects and the Nursing Process

I. ALTERATION IN NUTRITION, LESS THAN BODY REQUIREMENTS, related to NAUSEA AND VOMITING, ANOREXIA, DIARRHEA

Defining Characteristics: Nausea and vomiting occur in ~100% of patients, within 30 minutes to 2 hours of drug administration, and up to 8 hours afterward. Nausea and vomiting can be severe, but can be prevented by the use of combination antiemetics such as serotonin antagonist (granisetron or ondansetron) and dexamethasone. Anorexia and taste distortion (metallic taste) occur commonly. Diarrhea may occur up to several days after drug administration.

Nursing Implications: Premedicate with combination antiemetics such as serotonin antagonist (granisetron or ondansetron) and dexamethasone. Continue prophylactically. Antiemetic and sedative may need to be started the evening before if patient develops anticipatory nausea and vomiting. Encourage small, frequent feedings of cool, bland foods, dry toast, crackers. Monitor I/O to detect fluid volume deficit. Notify physician of the need for more aggressive antiemetic if vomitus > 750 mL. Encourage small, frequent feedings of high-calorie, high-protein foods. Encourage use of spices for anorexia; weekly weights. Encourage patient to report onset of diarrhea. Administer or teach patient to self-administer antidiarrheal medication and teach diet modifications (low residue) as appropriate.

II. INFECTION AND BLEEDING related to BONE MARROW DEPRESSION

Defining Characteristics: Potent myelosuppressant with nadir 6–8 days, recovery in 4 weeks. Patients at risk for profound bone marrow depression are those with previous extensive XRT, previous chemotherapy, or compromised bone marrow function. Lymphocyte depression occurs within 24 hours of drug dose.

Nursing Implications: Evaluate WBC, with neutrophil, and platelet count, and discuss any abnormalities with physician prior to drug administration. Assess for signs/symptoms of infection or bleeding; instruct patient in signs/symptoms of infection and bleeding, and to notify nurse or physician if they arise. Teach patient self-care measures to minimize risk of infection and bleeding, including avoidance of OTC aspirin-containing medications. Assess patient's Hgb/HCT and signs/symptoms of fatigue; teach patient self-assessment and to alternate rest and activity as needed. Transfuse red blood cells and platelets per physician order.

III. IMPAIRED SKIN INTEGRITY related to ALOPECIA, DRUG EXTRAVASATION

Defining Characteristics: Alopecia usually occurs as diffuse thinning. Drug is a potent vesicant, causing tissue necrosis and sloughing if extravasation occurs. Thrombosis or thrombophlebitis may occur despite all precautions, and venous access device may be required. Delayed cutaneous hypersensitivity is seen with topical application.

Nursing Implications: Discuss with patient hair loss, anticipated impact, and strategies to decrease distress, e.g., obtaining wig prior to hair loss. Assess body disturbance from hyperpigmentation and discuss strategies to minimize this, e.g., nail polish. Drug must be administered via patent IV. Assess need for venous access device early. Delayed cutaneous hypersensitivity (topical application) is not an indication to stop the drug. Discuss symptomatic management with physician. If extravasation is suspected, stop drug; aspirate any residual drug and blood from IV tubing, IV catheter/needle, and IV site if possible; instill antidote, sodium thio-sulfate (1/6 molar), into area of apparent infiltration as per physician orders and institutional policy and procedure; apply cold or topical medication as per physician orders and institutional policy and procedure. Assess site regularly for pain, progression of erythema, induration, and for evidence of necrosis. When in doubt about whether drug is infiltrating, TREAT AS AN INFILTRATION. Teach patient to assess site, and instruct to notify physician if condition worsens. Arrange next clinic visit for assessment of site depending on drug, amount infiltrated, extent of potential injury, and patient variables. Document in patient's record as per institutional policy. Warm packs may decrease discomfort of phlebitis. Have standing orders and sodium thiosulfate injection USP (10%) close by in the event of actual infiltration of drug; dilute sodium thiosulfate with sterile water for injection and inject subcutaneous in area of infiltration.

IV. ALTERATION IN COMFORT related to CHILLS, FEVER, DIARRHEA

Defining Characteristics: Chills, fever, diarrhea may occur after drug administration. Also weakness, drowsiness, headache may occur.

Nursing Implications: Assess patient for these symptoms during hour following treatment. Instruct patient to report these symptoms and teach self-management at home if outpatient. Provide symptomatic management per physician with acetaminophen, antidiarrheal medication.

V. POTENTIAL SEXUAL DYSFUNCTION related to DRUG EFFECTS

Defining Characteristics: Drug is teratogenic, carcinogenic. Amenorrhea occurs in females. Impaired spermatogenesis occurs in males. If administered to pregnant patients, spontaneous abortion or fetal abnormalities may occur.

Nursing Implications: As appropriate, explore with patient and partner issues of reproductive and sexual patterns, and anticipated impact chemotherapy will have. Discuss strategies to preserve sexuality and reproductive health (sperm banking, contraception).

VI. POTENTIAL FOR SENSORY/PERCEPTUAL ALTERATIONS related to CRANIAL NERVE INJURY

Defining Characteristics: Tinnitus, deafness, and other signs of eighth cranial nerve damage occur rarely, with high drug doses or regional perfusion techniques. Temporary aphasia and paresis occurs very rarely.

Nursing Implications: Assess hearing ability, presence of tinnitus prior to drug doses. If high doses of drug are given, or regional perfusion used, schedule patient for periodic audiometry. Instruct patient to report signs/symptoms of hearing loss.

Drug: melphalan hydrochloride (Alkeran, L-Phenylalanine Mustard, L-PAM, L-Sarcolysin)

Class: Alkylating agent.

Mechanism of Action: Prevents cell replication by causing breaks and cross-linkages in DNA strands with subsequent miscoding and breakage. Cell cycle phase nonspecific. Drug is derivative of nitrogen mustard.

Metabolism: Variable bioavailability after oral administration, especially if taken with food. Therefore, dose is titrated to WBC count; 20–50% of drug is excreted in feces over 6 days, 50% excreted in urine within 24 hours. After IV administration, parent compound disappears from plasma, with a half-life of about 2 hours.

Dosage/Range:

- Multiple myeloma: Several regimens, including 0.25 mg/kg/day × 4 days, in combination with prednisone 2 mg/kg/day, repeated every 6 weeks; OR 6 mg/m^2 orally daily × 5 days every 6 weeks for myeloma; OR 0.1 mg/kg PO × 2–3 weeks, then maintenance of 2–4 mg daily when bone marrow has recovered.
- Bone marrow transplantation: 50–60 mg/m^2 IV, but may be as high as 140–200 mg/m^2 (investigational).

Drug Preparation:

- Oral: Available in 2-mg tablets. Take on empty stomach.
- IV: Reconstitute 50-mg vial with 10 mL of provided diluent resulting in concentration of 5 mg/mL. Further dilute in 100–150 mL to produce a final concentration ≤ 2 mg/mL in 0.9% sodium chloride. Use provided 0.45-3m filter. Administer over 30–45 minutes. Stable for 1 hour at room temperature.

Drug Administration:

- Serious hypersensitivity reactions reported with IV administration.
- IV drug can cause anaphylaxis.
- IV drug is an irritant—avoid extravasation.

Drug Interactions:

- Myelosuppressive chemotherapy: Increases hematologic toxicity; dose-reduce or monitor patient very carefully.
- Cyclosporine: Increases nephrotoxicity.
- H_2 blockers: may decrease oral melphalan bioavailability.

Lab Effects/Interference:

- Decreased CBC.

Special Considerations:

- Nadir is 14–21 days after treatment.
- Increased risk of nephrotoxicity when given with cyclosporine.
- Drug dose reductions are recommended in patients with renal compromise.
- Drug is used in regional perfusion.

Potential Toxicities/Side Effects and the Nursing Process

I. INFECTION AND BLEEDING related to BONE MARROW DEPRESSION

Defining Characteristics: Bone marrow depression may be pronounced; leukopenia and thrombocytopenia occur 14–21 days after intermittent dosing schedules. May be delayed in onset, and cumulative with nadir extended to 5–6 weeks. Combined immunosuppression from disease (e.g., multiple myeloma) and drug may prolong vulnerability to infection. Thrombocytopenia may be persistent.

Nursing Implications: Evaluate WBC, with neutrophil, and platelet count and discuss any abnormalities with physician prior to drug administration. Assess for signs/symptoms of infection or bleeding; instruct patient in signs/symptoms of infection and bleeding, and to notify nurse or physician if they arise. Teach patient self-care measures to minimize risk of infection and bleeding, including avoidance of OTC aspirin-containing medications. Assess patient for Hgb/HCT and signs/symptoms of fatigue; teach patient self-assessment and to alternate rest and activity as needed. Transfuse packed red blood cells and platelets per physician order.

II. ALTERATION IN NUTRITION, LESS THAN BODY REQUIREMENTS, related to NAUSEA AND VOMITING, ANOREXIA

Defining Characteristics: Nausea and vomiting are mild at low, continuous dosing; severe following high doses. Anorexia occurs rarely.

Nursing Implications: Administer drug (oral) on empty stomach. Premedicate with antiemetic (oral) one hour before oral dose. Use aggressive antiemetic regimen for IV Alkeran. Encourage small, frequent feedings of favorite foods, especially high-calorie, high-protein foods. Encourage use of spices; weekly weights.

III. ALTERATION IN CARDIAC OUTPUT, PERFUSION related to ANAPHYLAXIS

Defining Characteristics: Severe hypersensitivity reactions can occur with IV administration, including diaphoresis, hypotension, and cardiac arrest.

Nursing Implications: Review standing orders for management of patient in anaphylaxis and identify location of anaphylaxis kit containing epinephrine 1:1000, hydrocortisone sodium succinate (Solu-Cortef), diphenhydramine HCl (Benadryl), aminophylline, and others. Prior to drug administration, obtain baseline vital signs and record mental status. Administer drug slowly, diluted as per physician's order. Observe for following signs/symptoms, usually occurring within first 15 minutes of infusion. Subjective signs are generalized itching, nausea, chest tightness, crampy abdominal pain, difficulty speaking, anxiety, agitation, sense of impending doom, uneasiness, desire to urinate/defecate, dizziness, chills. Objective signs are flushed appearance (angioedema of face, neck, eyelids, hands, feet), localized or generalized urticaria, respiratory distress ± wheezing, hypotension, cyanosis. For generalized allergic reaction, stop infusion and notify physician. Place patient in supine position to promote perfusion of visceral organs. Monitor VS. Provide emotional reassurance to patient and family. Maintain patent airway and have CPR equipment ready if needed. Document incident. Discuss with physician desensitization for further dosing vs drug discontinuance.

IV. POTENTIAL SEXUAL DYSFUNCTION related to DRUG EFFECTS

Defining Characteristics: Potentially mutagenic and teratogenic.

Nursing Implications: Encourage patient to verbalize goals about family; discuss options, such as sperm banking. As appropriate, discuss or refer for counseling about birth control measures during therapy.

V. POTENTIAL FOR INJURY related to SECOND MALIGNANCY

Defining Characteristics: Acute myelogenous and myelomonocytic leukemias may occur after continuous long-term dosing, especially in patients with ovarian cancer and multiple myeloma. Heralded by preleukemic pancytopenia of several weeks' duration. Chromosomal abnormalities characteristic of acute leukemia.

Nursing Implications: Patients receiving prolonged continuous therapy should be closely followed during and after treatment.

VI. POTENTIAL FOR IMPAIRED GAS EXCHANGE related to PULMONARY TOXICITY

Defining Characteristics: Rare, but may occur, especially with continued chronic dosing. Bronchopulmonary dysplasia and pulmonary fibrosis.

Nursing Implications: Assess pulmonary status for signs/symptoms of pulmonary dysfunction. Assess lung sounds prior to dosing. Instruct patient to report cough or dyspnea. Discuss PFTs to be performed periodically with physician. Long-term follow-up is important.

VII. IMPAIRED SKIN INTEGRITY related to ALOPECIA, MACULOPAPULAR RASH, URTICARIA

Defining Characteristics: Alopecia is minimal if it occurs at all. Maculopapular rash and urticaria are infrequent.

Nursing Implications: Assess skin integrity and presence of rash, urticaria, alopecia prior to dosing. Assess impact of these alterations on patient and develop plan to manage symptom distress.

Drug: mercaptopurine (Purinethol, 6-MP)

Class: Antimetabolite.

Mechanism of Action: One of two thiopurine antimetabolites (with 6-TG) that are converted to monophosphate nucleotides and inhibit de novo purine synthesis. The nucleotides are also incorporated into DNA. Cell cycle phase specific for S phase.

Metabolism: Metabolized by the enzyme xanthine oxidase in the kidney and liver; 50% of the drug is excreted in the urine. Plasma half-life is 20–40 minutes.

Dosage/Range:
- Induction: 2.5 mg/kg PO daily.
- Maintenance: 1.5–2.5 mg/kg PO daily.

Drug Preparation:
- Oral: none; available in 50-mg tablets.

Drug Administration:
- Oral.

Drug Interactions:
- Allopurinol: increased mercaptopurine levels; reduce dose to 25–35% of normal.
- Hepatotoxic drugs: additive hepatotoxicity; monitor LFTs closely.
- Warfarin: decreases or increases INR; monitor INR closely.
- Nonpolarizing muscle relaxants: decreased neuromuscular blockage; use together cautiously.

Lab Effects/Interference:
- Decreased CBC.
- Increased LFTs.
- Increased RFTs: tumor lysis.

Special Considerations:
- Elevated serum glucose levels and elevated serum uric acid levels could be related to the effects of medication.

- Reduce dose in cases of hepatic or renal dysfunction.
- Because xanthine oxidase is inhibited by allopurinol, concurrent use of the latter necessitates a dose reduction of 6-MP to ¼ the normal dose.

Potential Toxicities/Side Effects and the Nursing Process

I. POTENTIAL FOR INFECTION AND BLEEDING related to BONE MARROW DEPRESSION

Defining Characteristics: Nadir varies from 5 days to 6 weeks after treatment. Leukopenia more prominent than thrombocytopenia. Blood counts may continue to fall after therapy is stopped.

Nursing Implications: Evaluate WBC, with neutrophil, and platelet count, and discuss any abnormalities with physician prior to drug administration. Assess for signs/symptoms of infection or bleeding; instruct patient to notify nurse or physician if they arise. Teach patient self-care measures to minimize risk of infection and bleeding, including avoidance of OTC aspirin-containing medications. Assess patient's Hgb/HCT and signs/symptoms of fatigue; teach patient self-assessment and to alternate rest and activity as needed.

II. ALTERATION IN NUTRITION, LESS THAN BODY REQUIREMENTS, related to HEPATOTOXICITY, GI SYMPTOMS

Defining Characteristics: Reversible cholestatic jaundice may develop after 2–5 months of treatment. Hepatic necrosis may develop. Nausea, vomiting, anorexia, diarrhea are infrequent. Stomatitis uncommon, but appears as white patchy areas similar to thrush.

Nursing Implications: Monitor SGOT, SGPT, LDH, alk phos, and bili periodically during treatment. Notify physician of any elevations. Hepatic toxicity may be an indication for discontinuing treatment. Instruct patient to report GI side effects and to perform self-care measures as appropriate.

III. POTENTIAL FOR IMPAIRED SKIN INTEGRITY related to RASH

Defining Characteristics: Skin eruptions; rash may occur.

Nursing Implications: Advise patient these changes may occur. Instruct patient in symptomatic care if distress related to skin reactions occurs.

Drug: methotrexate (Amethopterin, Mexate, Folex)

Class: Antimetabolite, folic acid antagonist.

Mechanism of Action: Blocks the enzyme dihydrofolate reductase (DHFR), which inhibits the conversion of folic acid to tetrahydrofolic acid, resulting in an inhibition of the key precursors of DNA, RNA, and cellular proteins. May synchronize malignant cells in the S phase: at high plasma levels, passive entry of the drug into tumor cells can potentially overcome drug resistance.

Metabolism: Bound to serum albumin; concurrent use of drugs that displace methotrexate from serum albumin should be avoided. Salicylates, sulfonamideilantin, some antibacterials—including tetracycline, chloramphenicol, paraaminobenzoic acid—and alcohol should be avoided, as they will delay excretion. Drug is absorbed from GI tract and peaks in 1 hour. Plasma half-life is 2 hours; 50–100% of dose is excreted into the systemic circulation, with peak concentration 3–12 hours after administration.

Dosage/Range:
- IV: Low: 10–50 mg/m^2; med: 100–500 mg/m^2; high: 500 mg/m^2 and above with leucovorin rescue.
- IT: 10–15 mg/m^2.
- IM: 25 mg/m^2.

Drug Preparation:
- 5-, 50-, 100-, and 200-mg vials are available already reconstituted.
- Powder is available in vials without preservative for IT and high-dose administration (reconstitute with preservative-free 0.9% sodium chloride).

Drug Administration:
- 5–149 mg: slow IVP.
- 150–499 mg: IV drip over 20 minutes.
- 500–1500 mg: infusion, per protocol, with leucovorin rescue.

Drug Interactions:
- Protein-bound drugs (aspirin, sulfonamides, sulfonylureas, phenytoin, tetracycline, chloramphenicol) increase toxicity; give together cautiously and monitor patient closely.
- NSAIDs (nonsteroidal anti-inflammatory drugs, e.g., indomethacin, ketoprofen) increased and prolonged methotrexate levels; DO NOT administer concurrently with high doses of methotrexate; monitor patients closely who are receiving moderate or low-dose methotrexate.
- Cotrimoxazole increased methotrexate serum level; DO NOT use concurrently.
- Omeprazole increased the methotrexate serum level; DO NOT use concurrently.
- Warfarin: anticoagulant effect may increase; monitor INR closely.
- 5-FU: enhanced antitumor effect of 5-FU when methotrexate is given 24 hours before 5-FU.
- Folic acid: may reduce antitumor effect of methotrexate; do not co-administer.

- Thymidine, leucovorin: rescues normal cells from methotrexate effect; may nullify antitumor effect if given close to the time of methotrexate; usually given 24 hours after methotrexate.
- L-asparaginase: reduces methotrexate antitumor effects.

Lab Effects/Interference:
- Decreased CBC.
- Increased LFTs, RFTs.

Special Considerations:
- High doses cross the BBB; reconstitute with preservative-free 0.9% sodium chloride.
- With high doses (1–7.5 gm/m^2), urine should be alkalinized both before and after administration, as the drug is a weak acid and can crystallize in the kidneys at an acid pH. Alkalinize with bicarbonate; add to pre- and posthydration. High doses should only be given under the direction of a qualified oncologist at an institution that can provide rapid serum methotrexate level readings.
- Leucovorin rescue must be given on time per orders to prevent excessive toxicity and to achieve maximum therapeutic response (see Leucovorin Calcium).
- Avoid folic acid and its derivatives during methotrexate therapy. Kidney function must be adequate to excrete drug and avoid excessive toxicity. Check BUN and creatinine before each dose.

Potential Toxicities/Side Effects and the Nursing Process

I. ALTERATION IN NUTRITION, LESS THAN BODY REQUIREMENTS, related to GI SIDE EFFECTS

Defining Characteristics: Nausea and vomiting are uncommon with low dose; more common (39%) with high dose; may occur during drug administration and last 24–72 hours. Anorexia is mild. Stomatitis is a common indication for interruption of therapy: occurs in 3–5 days with high dose, 3–4 weeks with low dose; appears initially at corners of mouth. Stomatitis precedes bone marrow depression. Diarrhea is common and is an indication for interruption of therapy, as enteritis and intestinal perforation may occur; melena, hematemesis may occur. Hepatotoxicity is usually subclinical and reversible, but can lead to cirrhosis; increased risk of hepatotoxicity when given with other agents, like alcohol; transient increase in LFTs with high dose 1–10 days after treatment—may cause jaundice.

Nursing Implications: Premedicate with antiemetics if giving high-dose methotrexate; continue prophylactically for 24 hours (at least) to prevent nausea and vomiting. Encourage small, frequent feedings of cool, bland foods and liquids. Assess for symptoms of fluid and electrolyte imbalance: monitor I/O, daily weights if administered to inpatient. Assess oral cavity every day. Teach patient oral assessment and mouth care regimens. Encourage patient to report early stomatitis. Provide pain relief measures, if indicated. Explore patient compliance to rescue; discuss increase in rescue dose if moderate GI toxicity. Assess patient for diarrhea: guaiac all stools; encourage patient to report onset of diarrhea. Administer or teach patient to self-administer antidiarrheal medications. Monitor LFTs prior to drug dose, especially with high-dose methotrexate. Assess patient prior to and during treatment for signs/symptoms of hepatotoxicity.

II. POTENTIAL FOR INFECTION AND BLEEDING related to BONE MARROW DEPRESSION

Defining Characteristics: Nadir is seen 4–7 days after drug administration, with recovery by day 14. Bone marrow depression occurs in about 10% of patients.

Nursing Implications: Monitor CBC and platelet count prior to drug administration, as well as signs/symptoms of infection or bleeding. Instruct patient in self-assessment of signs/symptoms of infection or bleeding measures to decrease risk. Administer leucovorin calcium as ordered.

III. POTENTIAL FOR ALTERATION IN URINARY ELIMINATION related to RENAL TOXICITY

Defining Characteristics: As an organic acid, methotrexate is insoluble in acid urine. At doses greater than 1 gm/m^2 (i.e., high dose), drug may precipitate in renal tubules, causing acute renal tubular necrosis (ATN).

Nursing Implications: Prehydrate patient with alkaline solution for several hours prior to drug administration. Maintain high urine output with a urine pH greater than 7.0 (hydration fluid may need further alkalinization); dipstick each void. Record I/O. Monitor BUN and serum creatinine before, during, and after drug administration. Increases in these values may require methotrexate dose reductions or leucovorin dose increases.

IV. POTENTIAL FOR IMPAIRED GAS EXCHANGE related to PULMONARY TOXICITY

Defining Characteristics: Pneumothorax (high dose): rare, occurs within first 48 hours after drug administration in patients with pulmonary metastasis. Allergic pneumonitis (high dose): rare but accompanied by eosinophilia, patchy pulmonary infiltrates, fever, cough, shortness of breath. Occurs 1–5 months after initiation of treatment. Pneumonitis (low dose) symptoms usually disappear within a week, with or without use of steroids; interstitial pneumonitis may be a fatal complication.

Nursing Implications: Assess for signs/symptoms of pulmonary dysfunction before each dose and between doses (see Defining Characteristics section). Discuss PFTs to be performed periodically with physician. Assess lung sounds prior to drug administration. Instruct patient to report cough or dyspnea.

V. POTENTIAL FOR ALTERATION IN SKIN INTEGRITY related to ALOPECIA, DERMATITIS

Defining Characteristics: Alopecia and dermatitis are uncommon. Pruritus, urticaria may occur. Photosensitivity, sunburnlike rash 1–5 days after treatment; also, patient can develop radiation recall reaction.

Nursing Implications: Assess patient for signs/symptoms of hair loss. Discuss with patient impact of hair loss and strategies to minimize distress. Instruct patient to avoid sun if possible and to stay covered or wear sunblock if sun exposure is unavoidable.

VI. POTENTIAL FOR SENSORY AND PERCEPTUAL ALTERATIONS related to CNS CHANGES

Defining Characteristics: CNS effects: dizziness, malaise, blurred vision. IT administration may increase CSF pressure. Brain XRT followed by IV methotrexate may also cause neurologic changes.

Nursing Implications: Monitor for CNS effects of drug: dizziness, blurred vision, malaise. Monitor for symptoms of increased CSF pressure: seizures, paresis, headache, nausea and vomiting, brain atrophy, fever. If IV methotrexate follows brain XRT, monitor for symptoms of increased CSF pressure.

VII. POTENTIAL FOR ALTERATIONS IN COMFORT related to PAIN

Defining Characteristics: Sometimes causes back pain during administration.

Nursing Implications: Monitor patient for back and flank pain. Slow down infusion rate if it occurs. Administer analgesics if pain occurs (must avoid aspirin-containing products, as they displace methotrexate from serum albumin).

Drug: mitomycin (Mitomycin C, Mutamycin, 3 Mitozytrex)

Class: Antitumor antibiotic.

Mechanism of Action: Drug acts as alkylating agent and inhibits DNA synthesis by crosslinking of DNA. Alkylating and crosslinking mitomycin metabolites interfere with structure and function of DNA.

Metabolism: Drug is rapidly cleared by the liver. May need to modify dose in presence of liver abnormalities; 10% of drug is excreted unchanged.

Dosage/Range:
- Ten mg/m^2 IV every 8 weeks, with 5-FU and doxorubicin (FAM regimen).
- Bladder instillations 20–40 mg in 20–40 mL of water.
- May be used at different dosages for autologous bone marrow transplant.

Drug Preparation:
- Depending on vial size, dilute with sterile water to obtain concentration of 0.5 mg/mL.

Drug Administration:
- IV: Drug is potent vesicant.
- Give through the sidearm of a patent, running IV to avoid extravasation, which can lead to ulceration, pain, and necrosis. Check individual hospital policy for administration of a vesicant.

Drug Interactions:
- Myelosuppressive agents: Additive toxicity if overlapping nadirs; use cautiously.

Lab Effects/Interference:
- Decreased CBC, especially WBC and platelets.
- Hemolytic uremic syndrome (rare): Decreased hemoglobin, platelets, and increased creatinine.

Special Considerations:
- Indicated for treatment of disseminated adenocarcinoma of the stomach or pancreas in proven combinations with other approved chemotherapeutic agents and as palliative treatment when other modalities have failed.
- May cause interstitial pneumonitis; monitor patient for acute dyspnea and bronchospasm. Risk increases after a cumulative dose of > 60 mg.
- If patient requires surgery and has received mitomycin C together with other antineoplastics, the patient is at risk for ARDS. FiO_2 should be < 50%, and fluidstatus should be monitored closely.
- Rarely, hemolytic uremic syndrome can occur (characterized by rapid fall in hemoglobin, renal failure, severe thrombocytopenia) and progress to pulmonary edema and hypotension. The risk increases as the cumulative dose exceeds 60 mg.
- Drug may be given intra-arterially.
- Manufacturer's recommendations on dosage modification based on hematologic toxicity (NADIR AFTER PRIOR DOSE).

Potential Toxicities/Side Effects and the Nursing Process

I. POTENTIAL FOR INFECTION related to MYELOSUPPRESSION

Defining Characteristics: Myelosuppression is the dose-limiting toxicity. Toxicity is delayed and cumulative. Initial nadir occurs at approximately 4–6 weeks. Usually by the third course, 50% drug modifications are necessary.

Nursing Implications: Monitor WBC, HCT, platelets prior to drug administration. Monitor patients for signs/symptoms of infection. Teach patient self-assessment. Drug dosage should be reduced or held for lower-than-normal blood values.

II. ALTERATION IN NUTRITION, LESS THAN BODY REQUIREMENTS, related to NAUSEA, VOMITING, ANOREXIA, STOMATITIS

Defining Characteristics: Mild-to-moderate nausea and vomiting occur within 1–2 hours, lasting up to 3 days, but may be prevented by adequate premedication. Anorexia occurs commonly, and stomatitis may occur.

Nursing Implications: Premedicate with aggressive antiemetics, i.e., serotonin antagonist to prevent nausea and vomiting at least for the first treatment. Encourage small, frequent feedings of cool, bland foods and liquids. Teach patient and family member preparation of meals in advance, and encourage the use of spices when patient has little appetite. Teach patient oral assessment and oral hygiene regimen, and encourage patient to report early stomatitis.

III. POTENTIAL FOR ACTIVITY INTOLERANCE related to FATIGUE

Defining Characteristics: Fatigue is common.

Nursing Implications: Assess baseline activity level. Teach patient to report fatigue and activity intolerance. Teach self-management strategies, including alternating rest and activity periods, as well as stress reduction.

IV. POTENTIAL FOR IMPAIRED SKIN INTEGRITY related to DRUG EXTRAVASATION, ALOPECIA

Defining Characteristics: Extravasation of drug can cause severe tissue necrosis, erythema, burning, tissue sloughing. Delayed erythema or ulceration has been reported weeks to months after drug dose, at the injection site or distant from it, and despite the fact that there was no evidence of extravasation. Alopecia occurs frequently.

Nursing Implications: Use scrupulous IV technique to prevent extravasation of the drug. If there is doubt as to whether drug has infiltrated, treat as an infiltration, aspirate any drug in the tubing, and discontinue IV. IV line must be patent. Assess for need of venous access device early. Refer to hospital policy for management of extravasation. (If unclear what best strategy is, application of 1–2 mL 99% DMSO to the site every 6 hours × 14 days may offer some benefit [Alberts and Dorr, 1991].) Assess site regularly for pain, progression of erythema, induration, and evidence of necrosis. Discuss with patient hair loss, anticipated impact, and strategies to decrease distress, e.g., obtaining wig prior to hair loss.

V. POTENTIAL FOR INJURY related to HEMOLYTIC UREMIC SYNDROME

Defining Characteristics: 2% of patients may experience significant increase in creatinine unrelated to total dose or duration of therapy. Hold drug if creatinine is > 1.7 mg/dL. Thrombotic microangiopathy may occur with anemia, thrombocytopenia. Blood transfusions may exacerbate condition. Can often be fatal.

Nursing Implications: Monitor renal function, HCT, and platelets prior to each drug dose; hold dose if serum creatinine is > 1.7 mg/dL. If renal failure occurs, hemofiltration or dialysis may be necessary. Discuss risks and benefits with physician and patient if renal insufficiency is present and blood transfusion(s) is required.

VI. POTENTIAL ALTERATION IN OXYGENATION related to INTERSTITIAL PNEUMONITIS

Defining Characteristics: Rarely, interstitial pneumonitis occurs and can be quite severe (ARDS). Signs/symptoms include nonproductive cough, dyspnea, hemoptysis, pneumonia, pulmonary infiltrates on X-ray. Incidence may be reduced by dexamethasone 20 mg IV prior to dose (Chang et al, 1986).

Nursing Implications: Assess baseline pulmonary status, and monitor prior to each drug dose. Teach patient to report dyspnea, new onset cough, or any respiratory symptoms. Discuss abnormalities with physician, and plan for further diagnostic workup.

VII. POTENTIAL FOR INJURY related to VENO-OCCLUSIVE DISEASE OF THE LIVER AFTER BONE MARROW TRANSPLANT

Defining Characteristics: Hepatic veno-occlusive disease has been reported in patients who have received mitomycin C and autologous bone marrow transplant. Signs/symptoms are abdominal pain, hepatomegaly, and liver failure.

Nursing Implications: Assess baseline LFTs, and monitor periodically during therapy. Notify physician of any abnormalities, and discuss further diagnostic workup and management. Refer to autologous bone marrow transplant protocol.

Drug: mitotane (o, p′-DDD, Lysodren)

Class: Antihormone.

Mechanism of Action: Adrenocortical suppressant with direct cytotoxic effect on mitochondria of adrenal cortical cells. Forces a drop in steroid secretion and alters the peripheral metabolism of steroids.

Metabolism: 34–45% of oral dose is absorbed from the GI tract. Metabolized partly in the liver and kidneys to a water-soluble metabolite that is then excreted in the bile and urine. Small amount of drug passes into the CSF.

Dosage/Range:
- Dose ranges from 2–16 g/day PO.
- Usual doses 2–10 g/day.
- Treatment usually begins with low doses (2 g/day) and gradually increases.
- Daily dose is divided into 3–4 doses.
- Reduce dose in patients with hepatic dysfunction.

Drug Preparation:
- None.

Drug Administration:
- Oral. Available as a 500 mg tablet.

Drug Interactions:
- Neurotoxic drugs may have additive toxicity; use cautiously.
- Warfarin: may decrease anticoagulant effect; monitor INR and increase dose as needed.
- Spirolactone: may decrease mitotane effectiveness; do not use together.
- Steroids: decreased steroid effect requiring increased steroid dose.
- Phenytoin, cyclophosphamide, barbiturates: assess effect and need for dose adjustment.

Lab Effects/Interference:
- None.

Special Considerations:
- Hypersensitivity reactions are rare but have occurred.
- Use cautiously in patients with hepatic dysfunction.
- If patient undergoes stress (infection, trauma, shock), requires IV steroids.
- Drug may cause lethargy and somnolence; teach patient not to operate heavy equipment or drive until the effect of the drug is known.

Potential Toxicities/Side Effects and the Nursing Process

I. ALTERATION IN NUTRITION, LESS THAN BODY REQUIREMENTS, related to GI SIDE EFFECTS

Defining Characteristics: Nausea and vomiting occur in 75% of patients and may be dose-limiting toxicity. Anorexia may also occur. Diarrhea occurs in 20% of patients.

Nursing Implications: Nausea and vomiting may be reduced by beginning therapy with a low dose and increasing it as tolerated. Premedicate with antiemetics to prevent nausea and vomiting; continue as needed. Encourage small, frequent meals of cool, bland foods and liquids. Inform patient that nausea and vomiting can occur; encourage patient to report onset. Encourage patient to report onset of diarrhea. Administer or teach administration of antidiarrheal medication. If diarrhea is protracted, ensure adequate hydration, monitor I/O and electrolytes, teach perineal hygiene.

II. POTENTIAL FOR INJURY related to NEUROLOGIC TOXICITY

Defining Characteristics: Lethargy and somnolence are most common; resolve with discontinuation of therapy. Dizziness, vertigo occur in about 15% of patients. Other CNS manifestations are depression, muscle tremors, confusion, headache.

Nursing Implications: Teach the patient and family about possible neurologic toxicity; assess safety of planned activities (e.g., patient should avoid activities that require alertness). Encourage patient and family to report onset of symptoms, as they may necessitate discontinuing therapy.

III. POTENTIAL FOR IMPAIRED SKIN INTEGRITY related to RASH

Defining Characteristics: Skin irritation or rash occurs in about 15% of patients. Sometimes resolves during treatment.

Nursing Implications: Inform patient that rash is expected and will resolve when treatment is finished. Assess skin for integrity; recommend measures to decrease irritation, if indicated.

Drug: mitoxantrone (Novantrone)

Class: New class of antineoplastics—anthracenediones. Antitumor antibiotic.

Mechanism of Action: Inhibits both DNA and RNA synthesis regardless of the phase of cell division. Intercalates between base pairs, thus distorting DNA structure. DNA-dependent RNA synthesis and protein synthesis are also inhibited.

Metabolism: Excreted in both the bile and urine for 24–36 hours as virtually unchanged drug. Mean half-life is 5.8 hours. Peak levels achieved immediately. FDA-approved for acute nonlymphocytic leukemia in adults.

Dosage/Range:
- 12 mg/m^2 IV daily for 3 days, in combination with cytosine arabinoside 100 mg/m^2/day × 7 days continuous infusion for induction therapy of ANLL.
- 12 mg/m^2 IV day 1 every 21 days for prostate cancer, in combination with prednisone 5 mg PO twice a day.
- Multiple sclerosis: 12 mg/m^2 IV every 3 months, maximum lifetime dose 140 mg/m^2.

Drug Preparation:

- Available as dark-blue solution in 2-mg/mL vials: 10-mL (20-mg), 12.5-mL (25-mg), and 15-mL (30-mg) multi-dose vials.
- May be diluted in 5% dextrose, 0.9% sodium chloride, or 5% dextrose in 0.9% sodium chloride.
- Solution is chemically stable at room temperature for at least 48 hours.
- Intact vials should be stored at room temperature. If refrigerated, a precipitate may form. This precipitate can be redissolved when vial is warmed to room temperature.

Drug Administration:

- IV push over 3 minutes through the sidearm of a patent, freely running infusion.
- IV bolus over 5–30 minutes.

Drug Interactions:

- Myelosuppressive agents: Increased hematologic toxicity if nadir overlaps; use together cautiously.

Lab Effects/Interference:

- Decreased CBC.
- Decreased electrolytes.
- Increased LFTs, uric acid.

Special Considerations:

- Nonvesicant. There have been rare reports of tissue necrosis after drug infiltration.
- Incompatible with admixtures containing heparin.
- Patient may experience blue-green urine for 24 hours after drug administration.
- Cardiotoxicity is less than that of doxorubicin or daunorubicin, but risk increases with a cumulative dose of 140 mg/m^2 in patients without a history of prior anthracycline use, and 120 mg/m^2 if prior anthracycline treatment. Monitor LVEF, and discontinue drug if there is a 15–20% decrease in LVEF.

Potential Toxicities/Side Effects and the Nursing Process

I. POTENTIAL FOR INJURY related to BONE MARROW DEPRESSION

Defining Characteristics: Potent bone marrow depression; nadir 9–10 days. Granulocytopenia is usually the dose-limiting toxicity, and toxicity may be cumulative. Thrombocytopenia uncommon, but can be severe when it occurs. Hypersensitivity has been reported occasionally with hypotension, urticaria, dyspnea, rashes.

Nursing Implications: Monitor WBC, HCT, platelets prior to drug administration. Instruct patient in self-assessment for signs/symptoms of infection. Drug dosage should be reduced or held for lower-than-normal blood values. Instruct patient in self-assessment of signs/symptoms of bleeding. Prior to drug administration, obtain baseline vital signs. Observe for signs/symptoms of allergic reaction. Subjective signs/symptoms: generalized itching, dizziness. Objective signs/symptoms: flushed appearance (angioedema of face, neck, eyelids, hands, feet), localized or generalized urticaria. Document incident. Discuss with physician desensitization for future dose vs drug discontinuance.

II. POTENTIAL FOR ALTERATION IN CARDIAC OUTPUT related to CARDIOTOXICITY

Defining Characteristics: CHF with decreased LVEF occurs in about 3% of patients. Increased cardiotoxicity with cumulative dose greater than 180 mg/m^2; cumulative lifetime dose must be reduced if patient has had previous anthracycline therapy.

Nursing Implications: Assess for signs/symptoms of cardiomyopathy. Assess quality and regularity of heartbeat. Baseline EKG. Instruct patient to report dyspnea, shortness of breath, swelling of extremities, orthopnea. Discuss frequency of GBPS with physician.

III. ALTERATION IN NUTRITION, LESS THAN BODY REQUIREMENTS, related to NAUSEA/VOMITING AND MUCOSITIS

Defining Characteristics: Nausea and vomiting are typically not severe and occur in 30% of patients. Mucositis is more common with prolonged dosing; occurs in 5% of patients, usually within one week of therapy.

Nursing Implications: Premedicate with antiemetic and continue prophylactically for 24 hours to prevent nausea and vomiting, at least for the first treatment. Encourage small, frequent feedings of cool, bland foods and liquids. Teach patient oral assessment and oral hygiene regimen. Encourage patient to report early stomatitis.

IV. POTENTIAL FOR IMPAIRED SKIN INTEGRITY related to ALOPECIA AND EXTRAVASATION

Defining Characteristics: Alopecia is mild to moderate; occurs in 20% of patients. Drug is not a vesicant. Stains skin blue without ulcers. There have been rare reports of tissue necrosis following extravasation.

Nursing Implications: Discuss with patient impact of hair loss. Suggest wig as appropriate prior to actual hair loss. Explore with patient response to actual hair loss and plan strategies to minimize distress, e.g., wig, scarf, cap. Use careful technique during venipuncture and IV administration. Administer drug through freely flowing IV, constantly monitoring IV site and patient response.

V. POTENTIAL FOR ANXIETY related to ABNORMAL COLOR OF URINE SCLERA

Defining Characteristics: Urine will be green-blue for 24 hours. Sclera may become discolored blue.

Nursing Implications: Explain to patient changes that may occur with therapy and that they are only temporary.

VI. POTENTIAL SEXUAL DYSFUNCTION related to DRUG EFFECT

Defining Characteristics: Drug is mutagenic and teratogenic.

Nursing Implications: As appropriate, explore with patient and partner issues of reproductive and sexuality patterns and impact chemotherapy may have. Discuss strategies to preserve sexual and reproductive health (e.g., sperm banking, contraception).

Drug: nelarabine (Arranon)

Class: Anti-metabolite.

Mechanism of Action: Drug is a pro-drug of deoxyguanosine analogue of ara-G (9-ß-arabinofuranosylguanine), a cytotoxic agent. It is demethylated and converted into the active 5′-triphosphate ara-GTP. Ara-GTP accumulates in leukemic blasts and enters DNA where it causes inhibition of DNA synthesis and cell death. It may have other mechanisms as well.

Metabolism: Nelarabine and ara-G are rapidly eliminated from the plasma with a half-life of about 30 minutes and 3 hours, respectively. Both are extensively distributed throughout the body, and are not substantially bound to plasma proteins. Nelarabine and ara-G are partially excreted via the kidneys, 5–10% and 20–30%, respectively.

Dosage/Range:

- *Adult*: 1,500 mg/m^2 IV over 2 hours on days 1, 3, 5, repeated every 3 weeks.
- *Pediatric*: 650 mg/m^2 IV over 1 hour on days 1, 2, 3, 4, 5, repeated every 3 weeks.
- Duration of treatment has not been determined; in clinical trials, treatment continued until disease progression, unacceptable toxicity, or patient became a candidate for a bone marrow transplant.

Drug Preparation:

- Drug available in 250-mg vials, 5 mg/mL.
- Appropriate (undiluted) dose of nelarabine should be transferred into polyvinyl chloride (PVC) infusion bags or glass containers, and administered as a 2-hour infusion in adults and a 1-hour infusion in pediatric patients. Drug is stable for 8 hours at up to 30°C in PVC infusion bags. Drug should not be used in patients with creatinine clearance of < 50 mL/minute. Drug should be discontinued for grade 2 or higher neurotoxicity (CTCAE), and dosage should be delayed for other toxicity, including hematologic toxicity.

Drug Interactions: None known.

Lab Effects/Interference:

- *Pediatric patients*: ↑ serum transaminases, bilirubin, creatinine; ↓ serum potassium, albumin, calcium, glucose, magnesium.
- *Adults*: ↑ glucose, AST.
- *Both*: anemia, neutropenia, thrombocytopenia.

Special Considerations:

- Nelarabine is indicated for the treatment of patients with T-cell acute lymphoblastic leukemia and T-cell lymphoblastic lymphoma whose disease has not responded to or has relapsed following treatment with at least two chemotherapy regimens.
- Drug is a potent antineoplastic with potentially significant neurotoxicity, which is dose-limiting, characterized by somnolence, confusion, convulsions, ataxia, paresthesias, and hypoesthesia. Severe neurotoxicity includes coma, status epilepticus, craniospinal demyelination, or ascending neuropathy (like Guillain-Barré syndrome).
- Drug is a potent teratogen. Women of childbearing potential should avoid pregnancy. If drug is used during pregnancy or if patient becomes pregnant while taking the drug, the patient should be warned of potential hazard to the fetus. Nursing mothers should not breast-feed while receiving the drug.
- The risk of adverse events may be increased in patients with severe hepatic impairment (bilirubin > 3.0 mg/dL); closely monitor these patients for toxicities.
- The most common side effects in pediatric patients were bone marrow depression, headache, and vomiting; most common in adult patients were fatigue, nausea, vomiting, constipation, bone marrow depression, cough and dyspnea, somnolence and dizziness, and fever.

Potential Toxicities/Side Effects and the Nursing Process

I. POTENTIAL FOR INJURY related to TUMOR LYSIS SYNDROME (TLS)

Defining Characteristics: May develop with initial therapy if patient has a large tumor burden; results from rapid lysis of tumor cells. This usually begins 1–5 days after initiation of therapy, and causes elevations in serum uric acid, potassium, phosphorus, BUN, creatinine.

Nursing Implications: If this is induction therapy for a patient with acute leukemia or high tumor burden, expect medical orders to include IV hydration at 150 mL/hour with urine alkalinization, allopurinol prophylaxis, strict monitoring of I/O, daily weight, and total body fluid balance determination. Monitor baseline and daily BUN, creatinine, K+, phosphorus, uric acid, and calcium. Monitor for renal, cardiac, neuromuscular signs/symptoms of TLS.

II. INFECTION AND BLEEDING related to BONE MARROW DEPRESSION

Defining Characteristics: In pediatric patients, bone marrow depression is very common anemia 95% (45% grade 3), neutropenia 94% (17% grade 3), and thrombocytopenia 88% (27% grade 3). In adults, anemia affects 99% of patients (20% grade 3), thrombocytopenia 86% (37% grade 3), and neutropenia 81% (14% grade 3), and 12% had febrile neutropenia.

Nursing Implications: Assess WBC, neutrophil, and platelet count, and discuss any abnormalities with physician prior to drug administration; assess for signs/symptoms of skin infections (all mucosal surfaces, body orifices) and bleeding; instruct patient in signs/symptoms of infection and bleeding, as well as to report them or come to the emergency room. Teach patient self-care measures to minimize risk of infection and bleeding, including avoidance of OTC aspirin-containing medications. Assess patient's Hgb/HCT and signs/symptoms of fatigue; teach patient self-assessment and to alternate rest and activity as needed.

III. POTENTIAL FOR INJURY related to NEUROTOXICITY

Defining Characteristics: Neurologic events occurred in 64% of patients. In pediatric studies, most common events were headache (17%), peripheral neuropathy (12%, sensory and/or motor), somnolence (7%), hypoesthesia (6%), seizures (6%, including grand mal and status epilepticus), paresthesia (4%), tremor (4%). Rare grade 3/4 events were status epilepticus (1 fatal), hypertonia, and 3rd nerve paralysis. In adults, somnolence was most common (23%), followed by dizziness (21%), peripheral neuropathy (21%, including motor and/or sensory), hypoesthesia (17%), headache (15%), paresthesia (15%), ataxia (9%), depressed level of consciousness (6%), tremor (5%), blurred vision (4%), amnesia (3%). Grade 3 events in adults were rare and included aphasia, convulsion, hemiparesis, loss of consciousness, while grade 4 events included cerebral hemorrhage, coma, intracranial hemorrhage, leukoencephalopathy.

Nursing Implications: Assess baseline neurologic status, including sedation level, blurred vision, presence of numbness or tingling, difficulty with fine motor movement, such as buttoning clothes, unsteadiness when walking, or tripping. Teach patient that serious neurological side effects may occur: Pediatric: extreme sleepiness, seizures, coma, peripheral neuropathy, weakness and paralysis; adult: sleepiness, dizziness, peripheral neuropathy, rarely seizure, aphasia, hemiparesis, loss of consciousness. Teach patient to notify the provider/go to ED immediately if they occur. Teach adult patient not to drive or operate heavy machinery if sleepiness occurs.

IV. ALTERED NUTRITION, LESS THAN BODY REQUIREMENTS, related to NAUSEA AND VOMITING, STOMATITIS, DIARRHEA, CONSTIPATION, HEPATOTOXICITY

Defining Characteristics: Nausea and vomiting are common in adults, but less common in children (10%). In adults, nausea affects 41%, vomiting 22%, diarrhea 22%, and constipation 21%. In adults, 8% of patients developed stomatitis. Nausea and vomiting can be successfully prevented with combination antiemetics. Rarely dysgeusia can occur. Drug should be used cautiously in patients with impaired hepatic function, and the patient monitored closely for toxicity.

Nursing Implications: Premedicate with antiemetics and revise regimen based on prior response to treatment. If patient develops nausea/vomiting, assess fluid and electrolyte balance and the need for replacements. Assess oral mucosa prior to chemotherapy, and teach patient oral hygiene regimen and self-assessment; encourage patient to report diarrhea, discuss use of antidiarrheals with physician, and teach self-care PRN. Since patients become neutropenic, all mucosal surfaces need to be assessed for infection, and patients must be taught scrupulous perineal hygiene. Monitor LFTs prior to, during, and posttherapy.

V. ALTERATION IN COMFORT related to FATIGUE, FEVER, ASTHENIA, EDEMA, PAIN, RIGORS, MYALGIAS

Defining Characteristics: Fatigue affects 50% of adults, and can be severe in 10%. Pyrexia affects 23% and asthenia 17%. Peripheral edema affects 15%, pain 11%, rigors 8%, myalgias 13%, arthralgias 9%, muscular weakness 8%.

Nursing Implications: Assess comfort level/symptoms experienced at baseline and prior to each dose, then prior to each cycle. Teach patient to alternate rest and activity periods to manage or prevent fatigue. Teach patient to report fevers (> 100.5°F) and rigors right away, and to come to the clinic or ED. Teach patient symptomatic management of myalgias, arthralgias (e.g., local application of heat, acetaminophen if permitted).

Drug: nilutamide (Nilandron)

Class: Antiandrogen.

Mechanism of Action: Irreversibly binds to androgen receptors and inhibits androgen binding. Unlike steroidal antiandrogens, nilutamide binds specifically to adrenal androgen receptor in the nucleus of androgen-sensitive prostate cancer cells. It does not interact with progestin or glucocorticoid receptors.

Metabolism: Following oral administration, nilutamide is rapidly and completely absorbed, with 80% plasma protein binding. Steady-state levels are achieved after about two weeks. Though the drug is extensively metabolized in the liver, it appears that the parent drug is the active compound. The drug is excreted in the urine as metabolites. Renal impairment does not alter the properties of the drug.

Dosage/Range:
- 300 mg/day orally for 30 days and then 150 mg/day.

Drug Preparation/Administration:
- Oral. Start the day of or day after surgical castration.

Drug Interactions:
- Has been shown to inhibit the liver cytochrome P-450 isoenzymes and may decrease the metabolism of compounds requiring these systems. Monitor patients closely for toxicity if the patient is also taking phenytoin or theophylline.
- Warfarin: nilutamide may decrease warfarin metabolism, resulting in increased anticoagulation; monitor INR closely and the dose accordingly.
- Alcohol: rare disulfiram reaction (flushing, throbbing in head and neck, headache, dyspnea, nausea/vomiting, sweating, chest pain, palpitation, hypotension, vertigo, uneasiness, and confusion).

Contraindications:
- In patients with severe hepatic impairment (baseline hepatic enzymes should be evaluated prior to treatment).
- In patients with severe respiratory insufficiency.
- In patients with hypersensitivity to nilutamide or any component of this preparation.

Lab Effects/Interference:
- Causes increased liver enzymes (see below); may cause increased serum glucose.

Special Considerations:
- Monitor LFTs baseline and during therapy. If transaminases rise to greater than 2–3 times the upper limit of normal, therapy should be discontinued.

- Monitor PFTs and CXR baseline and during therapy. If interstitial pneumonitis suspected (CXR or 20–25% decrease in DLCO and FVC), nilutamide should be discontinued.
- Rarely, aplastic anemia may occur.

Potential Toxicities/Side Effects and the Nursing Process

I. ALTERATION IN NUTRITION, LESS THAN BODY REQUIREMENTS, related to NAUSEA, ANOREXIA, CONSTIPATION, CHANGES IN LFTs

Defining Characteristics: Nausea, anorexia occur infrequently. Constipation and increased LFTs are common, affecting 10–50% of patients.

Nursing Implications: Teach patient to report occurrence of loss of appetite or nausea. Encourage small, frequent feedings and consider antiemetic if necessary. Teach the patient to monitor bowel status and to eat foods high in roughage and prunes, to hydrate well, and to take stool softeners as needed to prevent constipation. Monitor baseline and during treatment. Discuss change in treatment if AST, ALT increase by 2–3 times ULN.

II. ALTERATION IN CARDIAC OUTPUT related to HYPERTENSION, ANGINA

Defining Characteristics: Angina occurs in 2% of patients; unclear whether increased incidence of hypertension (9%) due to drug alone.

Nursing Implications: Instruct patient in signs and symptoms of angina, and to report to physician if they occur. Monitor BP on follow-up visits.

III. ALTERATION IN COMFORT related to DIZZINESS, HOT FLASHES, DYSPNEA, VISUAL CHANGES

Defining Characteristics: Hot flashes occur in 28% of patients and are the most common side effect. Dyspnea is rare but is related to interstitial pneumonitis, a serious side effect of the drug; if it occurs, it is usually during the first 3 months of treatment. Patients of Asian heritage are at risk. Many patients experience impaired adaptation to light and, less commonly, changes in color vision.

Nursing Implications: Inform patient that side effects may occur and to report dyspnea immediately to physician, as therapy must be discontinued if it occurs. Baseline chest X-ray and PFTs should be done prior to treatment; if interstitial pneumonitis is suspected, the drug should be discontinued. Patients should be discouraged from driving at night because of visual changes and may find it helpful to wear tinted glasses during the day.

Drug: oxaliplatin (Eloxatin)

Class: Alkylating agent (3rd-generation platinum analogue).

Mechanism of Action: Blocks DNA replication and transcription into RNA by causing intrastrand and interstrand crosslinks in DNA strands. It is cell cycle non-specific. DNA mismatch repair enzymes are unable to repair these errors, and the cell dies. Drug may also bind to proteins in the cell nucleus and cytoplasm to further injure the cell.

Metabolism: Heavily bound (98%) to plasma proteins; following 2-hour drug infusion, 15% of drug is found in plasma and 85% in tissue or excreted in the urine; 40% of the drug binds irreversibly in red blood cells within 2–5 hours of administration. The drug concentrates in the kidney and spleen, and is excreted as platinum-containing metabolites.

Dosage/Range:

- FOLFOX4: *Day 1*: Oxaliplatin 85 mg/m^2 IV infusion in 250–500 ml 5% dextrose in water and leucovorin 200 mg IV infusion in 5% dextrose in water, each over 2 hours simultaneously in different bags connected by a Y-line, followed by 5-FU 400 mg/m^2 IVB over 2–4 minutes, followed by 5-FU 600 mg/m^2 in 250–500 mL D5W as a 22-hour continuous infusion. *Day 2*: Leucovorin 200 mg/m^2 IVB over 2 hours, followed by 5-FU 400 mg/m^2 IVB over 2–4 minutes, followed by 5-FU 600 mg/m^2 in 250–500 mL D5W as a 22-hour continuous infusion.
- FOLFOX6: *Day 1*: Oxaliplatin 85 mg/m^2 IV infusion in 250–500 mL 5% dextrose in water and leucovorin 400 mg IV infusion in 5% dextrose in water, each over 2 hours simultaneously in different bags connected by a Y-line, followed by 5-FU 600 mg/m^2 IVB over 2–4 minutes, followed by 5-FU 2400 mg/m^2 in 250–500 mL D5W as a 46-hour continuous infusion; repeat q 2 weeks.
- FOLFOX7: *Day 1*: Oxaliplatin 130 mg/m^2 IV infusion in 250–500 mL 5% dextrose in water and leucovorin 400 mg IV infusion in 5% dextrose in water, each over 2 hours simultaneously in different bags connected by a Y-line, followed by 5-FU 2400 mg/m^2 in 250–500 mL D5W as a 46-hour continuous infusion; repeat q 2 weeks.
- OPTIMOX1: 6 cycles of FOLFOX7, then 12 cycles of infusional 5-FU/LV, then resume FOLFOX7, if not previously resumed due to progression.
- FLOX: Oxaliplatin 85 mg/m^2 IV over 2 hours d 1, 15, 29; Leucovorin 500 mg/m^2 IV d 1, 8, 15, 22, 29, 36; 5-FU 500 mg/m^2 IVB d 1, 8, 15, 22, 29, 36; repeat q 8 weeks × 3 cycles (adjuvant colon cancer).
- CAPOX: Oxaliplatin 130 mg/m^2 IV over 2–6 hours, d 1; capecitabine 850 mg/m^2 PO bid d 1–14; repeat cycle q 22 days.

Dose Reduction:

- Persistent grade 2 neurotoxicity: Reduce oxaliplatin to 65 mg/m^2 in patients with metastatic CRC, and 75 mg/m^2 in patients receiving adjuvant therapy.
- Grade 3 neurotoxicity: Discontinue oxaliplatin.

- Grades 3–4 gastrointestinal toxicity: Decrease oxaliplatin dose to 65 mg/m^2 and 5-FU by 20% (300 mg/m^2 IVB and 500 mg/m^2 CI).
- Grades 3–4 hematological toxicity (ANC < 1500/mm^3, platelets < 100,000/mm^3): Decrease oxaliplatin dose to 65 mg/m^2 and 5-FU by 20% (300 mg/m^2 IVB and 500 mg/m^2 CI).
- Nausea, vomiting, or other acute symptoms: Infuse oxaliplatin over a period of up to 6 hours, as this lowers peak serum levels by 32%; revise antiemetic regimen.

Drug Preparation:
- Add 10 mL bacteriostatic water for injection or 5% dextrose injection to the 50-mg vial of lyophilized powder and 20 mL to the 100-mg vial. Further dilute in 250–500 mL of 5% dextrose injection.
- DO NOT use chloride-containing solutions.
- DO NOT use aluminum needles or infusion sets containing aluminum.

Drug Administration:
- Administer IV infusion over 2 or more hours through central line, preferably.
- Drug classified as an irritant, but extravasations have resulted in induration and formation of nodule lasting 9 months or more.
- If given peripherally, it may cause infusion site pain; relieve this by further diluting the drug in 500 mL 5% dextrose in water.

Drug Interactions:
- Incompatible with 5-FU and other highly alkaline solutions.
- Incompatible with chloride-containing solutions (forms precipitate).
- Physically incompatible with diazepam (forms precipitate).
- Incompatible with cefepime, cefoperazone, dantrolene.
- Nephrotoxic drugs: renal excretion of oxaliplatin could be reduced with increased serum levels of oxaliplatin.
- 5-FU: At high doses (130 mg/m^2), increases plasma levels of 5-FU by 20%.
- Bevacizumab: increased response rate and survival in metastatic CRC when combined with FOLFOX.

Lab Effects/Interference:
- Decreased CBC, especially WBC and platelets.
- Elevated LFTs.

Special Considerations:
- Indicated for the (1) adjuvant treatment of patients with Stage III colon cancer (FOLFOX4), and (2) first- and second-line treatment of metastatic colon and rectal cancers in combination with infusional 5-fluorouracil (5-FU) and leucovorin (LV) for the treatment of patients with metastatic carcinoma of the colon or rectum.
  - In the MOSAIC study of 2246 patients receiving adjuvant chemotherapy for colon cancer, stage III patients receiving FOLFOX4 had a superior survival compared with patients receiving 5-FU/LV alone (24% risk reduction for recurrence)

4 years out (de Gramont, 2007). In addition, 99% of patients with grade 3 neurotoxicity had resolved or decreased by 1-year posttreatment (de Gramont et al, 2003).

- Peripheral neuropathy (sensory) is dose-limiting toxicity (DLT). Two distinct neurotoxicity syndromes: acute, lasting less than 14 days, and chronic persistent peripheral neuropathy (PN) similar to cisplatin, which is the DLT.
- Rare pulmonary fibrosis and veno-occlusive disease of the liver occur.

Potential Toxicities/Side Effects and the Nursing Process

I. SENSORY/PERCEPTUAL ALTERATIONS related to ACUTE SENSORY NEUROPATHY

Defining Characteristics: Acute neurotoxicity appears related to ion channelopathy. It is common, affecting up to 85% of patients. It is temporary, and occurs during, within hours of, or up to 14 days following oxaliplatin administration. Often precipitated by exposure to cold and characterized by dysesthesias, transient paresthesias, or hypesthesias of the hands, feet, perioral area, and throat. Acute events can be minimized by slower infusion of oxaliplatin, increasing the infusion time from 2 to 6 hours, as this lowers peak serum levels. Studies are ongoing to determine whether glutamine can prevent these, and also studies exploring 1 gm calcium/1 gm magnesium IVB prior to and after the oxaliplatin infusion. Most frightening for patients is pharyngolaryngeal dysesthesia characterized by a sensation of discomfort or tightness in the back of the throat and inability to breathe. It may be accompanied by jaw pain, and is often precipitated by exposure to cold. Cramping of muscles, such as fisted hand, occurs due to prolonged action potential. Rarely, dysarthria (difficulty articulating words), eye pain, and a feeling of chest pressure can occur.

Nursing Implications: Teach patient that acute neurotoxicity can occur but is not dangerous. Teach patient to minimize occurrence by avoiding exposure to cold during and for 3–5 days after drug administration, such as wearing scarves over the face in the winter, warm gloves if going outside or reaching into the refrigerator or freezer. Teach patient to avoid exposure to cold and cold liquids, if lip paresthesias present. Teach patient to use straw if drinking cool liquids. Teach patient to avoid cold air conditioning in the car or home during the summer. Teach patient how to reassure themselves they are breathing if pharyngolaryngeal dysesthesia occurs (cup hands in front of mouth or hold mirror so that breath can be felt or seen on the mirror). Teach patient to warm area, such as fingers or toes, if they become cold, such as running warm water over affected area, as this may help resolve the feeling. Do not use ice chips before and during 5-FU infusions to prevent stomatitis.

II. SENSORY/PERCEPTUAL ALTERATIONS related to PERSISTENT, CHRONIC SENSORY NEUROPATHY

Defining Characteristics: Peripheral neurotoxicity affects about 48% of patients, and risk increases as cumulative doses > 800 mg/m^2. Symptoms include paresthesias, dysesthesias, hypoesthesias, in a stocking and glove distribution, and altered proprioception (knowing where body parts are in relation to the whole). This can become manifested as difficulty writing, walking, swallowing, and buttoning buttons. IF allowed to progress, motor pathways will become involved. When drug is stopped, symptoms may get worse, but in general, symptoms resolve in 4–6 months in many patients. Ongoing studies in patients with advanced CRC are looking at temporarily stopping the drug when grade 2 or 3 neurotoxicity occurs, continuing the 5-FU/LV as maintenance or stopping chemotherapy drugs and resuming after 12 cycles of maintenance or when disease progression occurs. This has shown to reduce the incidence and intensity of PN (OPTIMOX trial). In the MOSAIC trial, an adjuvant trial, although 23% of patients developed grade 3 neurotoxicity after 6 months, all patients except 1% had complete resolution of grade 3 toxicity (de Gramont, 2003).

Nursing Implications: Assess baseline neurologic status (sensory and motor); instruct patient to report signs/symptoms. Identify patients at risk: those with preexisting neuropathies (e.g., ethanol- and diabetes mellitus-related). Assess sensory and motor function, and monitor over time prior to each treatment, such as picking up a dime from a smooth/flat surface, buttoning shirt, and writing name. Specifically, assess whether function impaired, as this necessitates a dose reduction. If the patient is unable to perform activities of daily living, this necessitates drug cessation. In either case, discuss with physician as complete neurological exam should be performed before treatment decision as to drug holiday or discontinuance based on grade of neurotoxicity. Assess impact on patient and quality of life.

III. POTENTIAL FOR INFECTION, BLEEDING, and FATIGUE related to BONE MARROW DEPRESSION

Defining Characteristics: Mild leukopenia, and mild to moderate thrombocytopenia occur. Febrile neutropenia is very uncommon. Anemia is common.

Nursing Implications: Assess baseline CBC, WBC, differential, and platelet count prior to chemotherapy as well as signs/symptoms of infection, bleeding, or fatigue. Teach patient signs/symptoms of infection or bleeding, and to report these immediately. Teach patient self-care measures to minimize risk of infection and bleeding. This includes avoidance of crowds, proximity to people with infections, and OTC aspirin-containing medications. Teach energy-conserving techniques and ways to minimize fatigue, such as gentle exercise as tolerated.

IV. ALTERATION IN NUTRITION, LESS THAN BODY REQUIREMENTS, related to NAUSEA AND VOMITING, DIARRHEA, HEPATOTOXICITY

Defining Characteristics: Nausea and vomiting occur commonly and are severe if patient does not receive aggressive antiemesis. Diarrhea commonly occurs in combination with 5-FU/LV. Hepatotoxicity may occur manifested by increases in transaminases and alkaline phosphatase, whereas increases in bilirubin may be related to the concomitant 5-FU/LV as the incidence was similar in the group receiving FOLFOX compared with patients receiving only 5-FU/LV. Liver biopsies showed peliosis, nodular regenerative hyperplasia, or sinusoidal alterations, perisinusoidal fibrosis, and veno-occlusive lesions.

Nursing Implications: Premedicate patient with aggressive combination antiemetics: serotonin antagonist (granisetron or ondansetron) and dexamethasone. Encourage small, frequent feedings of cool, bland foods. Instruct patient to report nausea, and teach self-administration of antiemetics if patient is receiving drug as an outpatient. Teach the patient to report diarrhea that does not respond to usual antidiarrheal medicine and diet modification so that more aggressive management can be instituted and prevent dehydration and electrolyte imbalance. If LFTs are significantly elevated, the drug should be stopped, and hepatic dysfunction, unexplainable by liver metastases, should be evaluated.

V. POTENTIAL FOR INJURY related to DELAYED HYPERSENSITIVITY OR ANAPHYLAXIS REACTIONS (often after 8–12 cycles of therapy)

Defining Characteristics: Delayed hypersensitivity may occur after 10–12 cycles of therapy with symptoms ranging from local rash or vague symptoms such as new onset of vomiting, to anaphylaxis and severe hypersensitivity (characterized by dyspnea, hypotension requiring treatment, angioedema, and generalized urticaria). Anecdotal reports show successful desensitization using carboplatin desensitization regimens.

Nursing Implications: Assess baseline VS and mental status prior to drug administration. If patient has symptoms, discuss premedication using corticosteroid, antihistamine, and H_2 antagonist as ordered. Monitor VS every 15 minutes, and remain with patient during first 15 minutes of drug infusion. Stop drug if signs/symptoms of hypersensitivity or anaphylaxis occur, and notify physician. *Subjective symptoms*: generalized itching, nausea, chest tightness, crampy abdominal pain, difficulty speaking, anxiety, agitation, sense of impending doom, uneasiness, desire to urinate/defecate, dizziness, chills. *Objective signs*: flushed appearance; angioedema of face, neck, eyelids, hands, feet; localized or generalized urticaria; respiratory distress with or without wheezing; hypotension; cyanosis. Provide fluid resuscitation for hypotension per MD order, and maintain a patent airway.

Drug: paclitaxel (Taxol)

Class: Taxoid, mitotic inhibitor.

Mechanism of Action: Promotes early microtubule assembly and prevents depolymerization necessary for normal mitosis and cell division, resulting in cell death in G_2 and M phases of the cell cycle.

Metabolism: Extensively protein-bound, resulting in an initial sharp decline in serum level. Metabolized primarily by hepatic hydroxylation using the P-450 enzyme system. Metabolites are excreted in the bile. Less than 10% of the intact drug is excreted in the urine.

Dosage/Range:
- Dose reduce if hepatic dysfunction.
- Breast cancer.
  - **Adjuvant treatment** of patients with LN-positive breast cancer, administered sequentially to standard doxorubicin containing combination chemotherapy (benefit at 30 months for ER/PR negative tumors): Adjuvant node-positive breast cancer: 175 mg/m^2 IV over 3 hours, every 3 weeks, for 4 courses, administered sequentially to doxorubicin-containing combination chemotherapy.
  - **Advanced breast** cancer after failure of combination therapy for metastatic disease or relapse within 6 months of adjuvant therapy (containing an anthracycline except if not tolerated): 175 mg/m^2 IV over 3 hours, every 3 weeks; if tumor overexpresses HER-2 protein, given in combination with trastuzumab.
- **Ovarian cancer:** First-line (in combination with cisplatin) and subsequent therapy for patients with advanced ovarian cancer.
  - Previously *untreated* ovarian cancer: 135 mg/m^2 IV over 24 hours, followed by cisplatin 75 mg/m^2 every 3 weeks or paclitaxel 175 mg IV over 3 hours followed by cisplatin 75 mg/m^2 q 3 weeks.
  - Previously treated ovarian cancer: 135 mg or 175 mg/m^2 IV over 3 hours every 3 weeks.
- **Non–small-cell lung cancer:** First line (in combination with cisplatin) in patients who are not candidates for surgical or radiation curative therapy: non–small-cell lung cancer (NSCLC): 135 mg/m^2 IV over 24 hours, followed by cisplatin 75 mg/m^2 repeated every 3 weeks.
- **AIDS-related Kaposi's sarcoma:** Second-line treatment: 135 mg/m^2 IV over 3 hours, repeated every 3 weeks, or 100 mg/m^2 IV over 3 hours, repeated every 2 weeks (dose intensity of 45–50 mg/m^2 per week).
- Other doses:
  - Metastatic breast cancer, weekly paclitaxel 80 mg/m^2 IV over 1 hour q wk.
  - Advanced or metastatic NSCLC: weekly paclitaxel 50 mg/m^2 IV over 1 hour in combination with carboplatin AUC 2 with concurrent XRT and after completion of XRT, paclitaxel 200 mg/m^2 and carboplatin AUC 6 q 3 weeks × 2 cycles.
  - Ovarian, intraperitoneal: 60–65 mg/m^2.

- Less myelosuppression with 3-hour vs 24-hour infusion.

Other regimens used/being studied/reported:

- Activity in other tumor types (bladder, head and neck cancers: 250 mg/m^2 IV as 24-hour infusion every 3 weeks; other tumors: esophageal, prostate cancers).

Drug Preparation:

- Drug is poorly soluble in water, so is formulated using polyoxyethylated castor oil (Cremaphor EL) and dehydrated alcohol.
- Further dilute in 5% dextrose or 0.9% sodium chloride.

Drug Administration:

- Glass or polyolefin containers MUST BE USED, and polyethylene-lined administration sets must be used. DO NOT USE polyvinylchloride containers or tubing since the polyoxyethylated castor oil (Cremaphor EL) causes leaching of plasticizer diethylhexlphthalate (DEHP) from polyvinylchloride plastic into the infusion fluid. Do not use Chemo Dispensing Pin device or similar devices since the device may cause the stopper to collapse, sacrificing sterility of the paclitaxel solution.
- Inline filter of < 0.22 microns MUST be used.
- Assess vital signs baseline, and remain with patient during first 15 minutes of infusion. Monitor vital signs every 15 minutes or per hospital policy.
- Assess CBC: Patients with solid tumors: absolute neutrophil count (ANC) must be at least 1500 cells/mm^3 and platelet count at least 100,000/mm^3; patients with AIDS-related Kaposi's sarcoma: ANC at least 1,000 cells/mm^3.

Premedication with corticosteroids:

- Solid tumors: Dexamethasone 20 mg PO 12 and 6 hours prior to treatment. Administer diphenhydramine 50 mg and H2 antagonist (cimetidine 300 mg, famotidine 20 mg, or ranitidine 50 mg) IV 30–60 minutes prior to treatment.
- AIDS-related Kaposi's sarcoma: Dexamethasone 10 mg PO 12 and 6 hours prior to treatment; administer diphenhydramine 50 mg and H_2 antagonist (cimetidine 300 mg, famotidine 20 mg, or ranitidine 50 mg) IV 30–60 minutes prior to treatment.
- Administer paclitaxel IV over 3 hours via infusion controller.
- DO NOT give drug as a bolus, as this may cause bronchospasm and hypotension.
- Assess for hypersensitivity reaction (most often occurs during first 10 minutes of infusion) and for cardiovascular effects (arrhythmia, hypotension).
- Keep resuscitation equipment nearby.
- Administer paclitaxel first when given in combination with cisplatin or carboplatin. There is increased cytotoxic activity when given in this sequence.
- Paclitaxel is being studied as a radiosensitizer, given weekly doses 80–100 mg/m^2 as a 1-hour infusion.
- Intraperitoneal infusion (investigational): Dilute dose into 1–2 liters of 0.9% NS, or as ordered; warm to 37°C and infuse as rapidly as tolerated into peritoneal cavity; assist patient to change position every 15 minutes per protocol × 2 hours to maximize distribution in peritoneal cavity.

Drug Interactions:

- Cisplatin: Myelosuppression is more severe when cisplatin is administered prior to paclitaxel (due to 33% reduction in paclitaxel clearance from the plasma). Therefore, paclitaxel must be given prior to cisplatin when drugs are administered sequentially.
- Carboplatin: Possible increased cytotoxicity when given *after* taxol. Also, combination of paclitaxel and carboplatin results in less thrombocytopenia than would be expected from dose of carboplatin alone (etiology of platelet-sparing effect unknown).
- Paclitaxel is metabolized by P450 cytochrome isoenzymes CYP2C8 and CYP3A4. Potential interactions may occur, including antiretroviral protease inhibitors. Use together cautiously with other drugs metabolized by this system (CYP 2C8 and CYP 3A4 inducers: carbamazine, phenytoin, phenobarbital, rifampin: may decrease serum level of paclitaxel and decrease effect; CYP 2C8 and CYP 3A4 inhibitors: ethinyl estradiol, fluconazole, ketoconazole, sulfonamides, testosterone, tretinoin, ciprofloxacin, clarithromycin, doxycycline, erythromycin, grapefruit juice, isoniazid, protease inhibitors, verapamil: may increase serum level of paclitaxel with increased risk of toxicity). Use together cautiously if at all.
- Doxorubicin and liposomal doxorubicin: Increased incidence of neutropenia and stomatitis when paclitaxel is administered prior to doxorubicin (due to 30–35% decrease in doxorubicin clearance, possibly due to competition for biliary excretion of both agents). Therefore, doxorubicin should be given prior to paclitaxel or sequentially rather than concomitantly.
- Doxorubicin: Increased risk of cardiotoxicity when given in combination with paclitaxel, with sharp increase in risk of congestive heart failure once cumulative dose of doxorubicin is > 380 mg/m^2 (Minotti et al, 2001). Give sequentially rather than concomitantly.
- Cyclophosphamide: increased myelosuppression when cyclophosphamide given before paclitaxel; give sequentially rather than concomitantly.
- Beta-blockers, calcium-channel blockers, digoxin: Additive bradycardia may occur; assess/monitor patients closely.
- Immunosuppressive agents, other antineoplastic agents: Additive immunosuppression may occur; assess toxicity and patient response closely.
- Trastuzumab: increased risk of cardiotoxicity, but studies have shown no increased cardiac events when used together (Dang et al, 2006).
- St. John's wort: may increase paclitaxel serum level; do not use together.

Lab Effects/Interference:

- Decreased CBC.
- Increased LFTs.

Special Considerations:

- Drug has radiosensitizing effects.
- Drug is embryotoxic; avoid use in pregnancy. Women of childbearing age should use effective contraception.

- Drug may be excreted in breast milk, so breast-feeding should be avoided during drug therapy.
- ANC should be = 1500/mm^3 prior to initial or subsequent doses of paclitaxel.
- Dose reductions: 20% dose reduction if severe neuropathy or severe neutropenia (ANC < 500/mm^3 for 7+ days) develop and/or consider addition of colony-stimulating factor support with next cycle; 25–50% dose reduction if hepatic dysfunction (hepatic metastasis > 2 cm) occurs (Chabner and Longo, 2001); 50% or more dose reduction for moderate or severe hyperbilirubinemia or significantly increased serum transferase levels, with dose of paclitaxel not exceeding 50–75 mg/m^2 IV over 24 hours, or 75–100 mg/m^2 IV over 3 hours; if AST > 2 times upper limit of normal, patient dose should not exceed 50 mg/m^2 IV over 24 hours (Venook et al, 1998).
- One-hour infusion of paclitaxel as well as weekly dosing regimens are being studied/used. Lower doses, e.g., 80–100 mg/m^2 IV over 1 hour weekly × 3 with 1 week off per cycle, weekly × 6 with 2 weeks off per cycle, or weekly > 12 weeks, appear to inhibit angiogenesis, and allow for increased dose density.

Potential Toxicities/Side Effects and the Nursing Process

I. POTENTIAL FOR INJURY related to HYPERSENSITIVITY OR ANAPHYLAXIS REACTIONS

Defining Characteristics: Hypersensitivity occurs in 10% of patients, with anaphylaxis and severe hypersensitivity reactions in 2–4% (characterized by dyspnea, hypotension requiring treatment, angioedema, and generalized urticaria). Reaction is to cremaphor in paclitaxel preparation. Signs/symptoms include tachycardia, wheezing, hypotension, facial edema; incidence of supraventricular tachycardia with hypotension and chest pain occurs in 1–2%. Patients who have severe hypersensitivity reaction should not be rechallenged with drug. Those who have less severe reactions have received 24 hours of corticosteroid prophylaxis, and have been successfully rechallenged with drug infused at a slower rate.

Nursing Implications: Assess baseline VS and mental status prior to drug administration. Ensure that patient has taken dexamethasone premedication, and administer diphenhydramine and H_2 antagonist as ordered. Monitor VS every 15 minutes, and remain with patient during first 15 minutes of drug infusion as most reactions occur during the first 10 minutes. Stop drug if cardiac arrhythmia (irregular apical pulse), hypotension, or hypertension occur, and discuss continuance of infusion with physician. Recall signs/symptoms of anaphylaxis, and if these occur, stop drug immediately and notify physician. Subjective symptoms: generalized itching, nausea, chest tightness, crampy abdominal pain, difficulty speaking, anxiety, agitation, sense of impending doom, uneasiness, desire to urinate/defecate, dizziness, chills. *Objective signs*: flushed appearance; angioedema of face, neck, eyelids, hands, feet; localized or generalized urticaria; respiratory distress with or without wheezing; hypotension;

cyanosis. Review standing orders or nursing procedure for patient management of anaphylaxis, and be prepared to stop drug immediately if signs/symptoms occur, keep IV line open with 0.9% sodium chloride, notify physician, monitor VS, and administer ordered medications, which may include epinephrine 1:1000, hydrocortisone sodium succinate, and diphenhydramine. Teach patient the potential of a hypersensitivity or anaphylactic reaction and to immediately report any unusual symptoms.

II. POTENTIAL FOR INFECTION AND BLEEDING related to BONE MARROW DEPRESSION

Defining Characteristics: Neutropenia may be severe, especially when drug is administered via 24-hour infusion. Neutropenia is also more severe when cisplatin precedes paclitaxel in sequential administration, as it reduces paclitaxel clearance by 33%. Neutropenia is also more pronounced in patients who have received prior radiotherapy. Nadir is 7–11 days after dose with recovery in one week. Neutropenia is dose-dependent, with severe neutropenia (ANC $< 500/mm^3$) occurring in 47–67% of patients. Anemia occurs frequently, but thrombocytopenia is uncommon.

Nursing Implications: Assess baseline CBC, WBC, differential, and platelet count prior to chemotherapy, as well as signs/symptoms of infection or bleeding. Teach patient the signs/symptoms of infection or bleeding, and to report these immediately, and teach patient self-care measures to minimize risk of infection and bleeding. This includes avoidance of crowds, proximity to people with infections, and OTC aspirin-containing medications. Administer paclitaxel PRIOR to cisplatin or carboplatin when either is given in combination with paclitaxel. Teach patient self-administration of G-CSF as ordered to prevent severe neutropenia. Transfuse red blood cells and platelets per physician order.

III. SENSORY/PERCEPTUAL ALTERATIONS related to SENSORY NEUROPATHY

Defining Characteristics: Frequency and incidence is dose-dependent but appears not to be influenced by infusion duration. Overall incidence is 60%, with 3% severe neuropathy in women with breast or ovarian cancer treated with single-agent paclitaxel, but severe neuropathy occurred in 8–13% of patients with NSCLC who also received cisplatin. Onset related to cumulative dose, with incidence after first course 27% and remainder occurring after 2–10 courses. Sensory symptoms usually resolve after two or more months following paclitaxel discontinuance. Sensory alterations are paresthesias in a glove-and-stocking distribution, and numbness. There may be a symmetrical loss of sensation,vibration, proprioception, temperature, and pinprick. Sensory and motor neuropathy may occur in patients receiving both paclitaxel and cisplatin. There is an increased risk for motor and autonomic dysfunction in patients with neuropathy from diabetes mellitus or alcohol ingestion prior to treatment with paclitaxel. Arthralgias and myalgias affect 60% of patients, and begin 2–3 days after treatment; they resolve in a few days; may be ameliorated by low-dose dexamethasone.

Nursing Implications: Assess baseline neurologic status. Instruct patient to report signs/symptoms of pins and needle sensation, numbness, pain, increased discomfort with certain sensations, especially in the extremities, or motor weakness. Identify patients at risk: prior cisplatin, or having preexisting neuropathies (ethanol-and diabetes mellitus-related). Assess sensory and motor function prior to each treatment, and if abnormality found, assess impact on patient function, safety, independence, and quality of life. Test patient's ability to button a shirt, or pick up a dime from a flat surface. If severely impacting safety or quality of life, discuss with patient and physician drug reduction (20%) or discontinuance or use of cytoprotective agent. Teach self-care strategies, including maintaining safety when walking, getting up, taking bath or washing dishes and unable to sense temperature, and the need to keep extremities warm in cold weather. See NCI Common Toxicity Criteria, Appendix II: grade 3 motor = objective weakness, interfering with ADLs; grade 3 sensory = sensory loss or paresthesia interfering with ADLs; grade 4 motor = paralysis; grade 4 sensory = permanent sensory loss that interferes with function.

IV. ALTERATION IN SKIN INTEGRITY related to ALOPECIA, ONYCHOLYSIS

Defining Characteristics: Complete alopecia occurs in most patients and is reversible. Onycholysis may occur in patients receiving weekly paclitaxel, and risk increases after the sixth course.

Nursing Implications: Discuss potential impact of hair loss prior to drug administration. Discuss coping strategies and plan to minimize body image distortion (e.g., wig, scarf, cap). Assess patient for signs/symptoms of hair loss. Assess patient's response and use of coping strategies, and help patient to build on effective strategies. If the patient is receiving weekly paclitaxel, teach fingernail care (keep clean and well manicured).

V. ALTERATION IN NUTRITION, LESS THAN BODY REQUIREMENTS, related to NAUSEA AND VOMITING, DIARRHEA, STOMATITIS, HEPATOTOXICITY

Defining Characteristics: Nausea and vomiting occur commonly in 52% of patients and are mild and preventable with antiemetics. Diarrhea occurs in 38% of patients and is mild. Stomatitis occurs in 31% and is mild, appears to be dose- and schedule-dependent, and is more common with 24-hour infusions than 3-hour infusions.

Mild increase in LFTs may occur (7% bilirubin, 22% alk phos, 19% AST). Rarely, hepatic necrosis and hepatic encephalopathy leading to death have been reported. If severe hepatic dysfunction occurs, paclitaxel dose should be reduced (see Special Considerations section).

Nursing Implications: Premedicate patient with antiemetic (either serotonin antagonist or dopamine antagonist). Encourage small, frequent meals of cool, bland foods. Instruct patient to report nausea, and teach self-administration of antiemetics if receiving drug as an outpatient. If nausea/vomiting occur and is severe, assess for signs/symptoms of fluid/electrolyte imbalance. Encourage patient to report onset of diarrhea and to self-administer antidiarrheal medications. Assess baseline oral mucous membranes. Teach patient oral assessment and to report any alterations. Assess LFTs prior to drug administration and periodically during treatment.

VI. POTENTIAL ALTERATION IN CIRCULATION related to HYPOTENSION, ARRYTHMIA

Defining Characteristics: Hypotension during first three hours of infusion in 12% of patients, and transient, asymptomatic bradycardia in 30% of patients have been reported; most often patients did not require intervention. Significant cardiovascular events (syncope, rhythm abnormalities, hypertension, and venous thrombosis) occurred in 1% of patients receiving single-agent paclitaxel, but the incidence was 12–13% in patients with NSCLC receiving cisplatin as well. Of those patients with normal baseline EKGs at the beginning of paclitaxel therapy, 14% of patients developed an abnormal EKG tracing (nonspecific repolarization abnormalities, sinus bradycardia, sinus tachycardia, premature beats). Whether or not the patient received prior anthracycline therapy did not influence these events. Prior anthracycline therapy did influence the rare incidence of CHF. Rarely, patients developed myocardial infarction, atrial fibrillation, and supraventricular tachycardia. For patients receiving doxorubicin in combination with paclitaxel, there is increased risk of CHF once the cumulative dose of doxorubicin is > 380 mg/m^2 (Gianni et al, 1998). Severe conduction abnormalities have been described in < 1% of patients, and required pacemaker insertion in some patients. The drug should be used cautiously in patients with coronary artery disease or prior myocardial infarction within past 6 months, as well as in patients with a history of arrhythmia who are being treated with beta-blockers, calcium-channel blockers, or digoxin.

Nursing Implications: Assess baseline cardiac status, history, and risk for development of CHF. Closely monitor patient during paclitaxel infusion, especially if patient has history of hypertension, or is on cardiac medications (see Drug Interactions section). Teach patient to report any dyspnea, SOB, chest pain, or heart palpitations, or any unusual feeling. If any abnormalities occur, stop infusion as appropriate and discuss further management with physician. If patient is receiving doxorubicin and paclitaxel, discuss with physician stopping combination therapy when cumulative doxorubicin dose is 340–380 mg/m^2, and continuing paclitaxel as a single agent, as this does not increase risk of CHF (Gianni et al, 1998). If the patient develops significant conduction abnormalities, discuss medical management with physician, and expect that patient will have cardiac monitoring during subsequent paclitaxel therapy.

VII. ALTERATION IN COMFORT related to FATIGUE, ARTHRALGIAS AND MYALGIAS

Defining Characteristics: Fatigue occurs commonly, and arthralgias and myalgias affect about 44% of all patients, with 8% experiencing severe symptoms. Arthralgias and myalgias commonly occurred 2–3 days after the drug was given, and resolved within a few days.

Nursing Implications: Teach patient that fatigue may occur, and ways to minimize exertion and energy expenditure by alternating rest and activity, and organizing chores so that they are done as efficiently as possible. Arthralgias and myalgias may be troublesome, and can be managed with NSAIDs, application of warmth, and other comfort measures. Some patients report that swimming is helpful in minimizing discomfort. Studies of gabapentin, glutamine, and steroids have been disappointing. Opioids may be needed if severe.

Drug: paclitaxel protein-bound particles for injectable suspension, albumin-bound (Abraxane, nab paclitaxel)

Class: Taxane; nanoparticle albumin-bound paclitaxel, mitotic inhibitor.

Mechanism of Action: Promotes early microtubule assembly and prevents depolymerization, preventing cells from moving from G_2 to M phase, mitosis, and resulting in cell death. The drug is combined with human albumin in a nanoparticle state and is preferentially taken up by tumors, resulting in increased intratumoral concentrations of paclitaxel, lower drug concentrations in normal tissue, and potentially greater anti-tumor activity as higher doses can be given compared with cremaphor-dissolved paclitaxel.

Metabolism: Distributes extensively in tissue, is highly protein bound, and does not cross the BBB. The half-life is 27 hours. It is metabolized by cytochrome P450 microenzyme system in liver (CYP 2C8, 2C9, 3A4); 20% of the drug is excreted in feces, and little drug excreted in the urine. Lower AUC, slower metabolism of paclitaxel nanoparticles, more rapid and extensive distribution into tissues; and longer half-life than paclitaxel.

Dosage/Range:

- 260 mg/m^2 IV over 30 minutes every 21 days.
- Dose reduce to 220 mg/m^2 if nadir ANC < 500/mm^3 for 1+ weeks or severe neuropathy; further reduce to 180 mg/m^2 if severe neutropenia or neuropathy recur; resume chemotherapy only when neuropathy resolves to grades 1–2, and ANC > 1500 cells/mm^3.
- Also being studied: 100–125 mg/m^2 IV weekly or days 1, 8, and 15 of a 28-day cycle.

Drug Preparation/Administration:

- Available in single use 100 mg vials. Gently dilute in Normal Saline over a minimum of 1 minute, allow to rest, place in IV bag, and administer IV over 30 minutes. If not used immediately after mixing, it may be stored in refrigerator for 8 hours. See package insert. The solution will be milky white.
- Administer only if baseline ANC is > 1500 cells/mm^3.
- Dose reduce for neutropenia and neuropathy.
- DO NOT substitute for other paclitaxel formulations.
- Drug is an irritant; monitor for injection site reactions.

Drug Interactions:

- Paclitaxel is metabolized by P450 cytochrome isoenzymes CYP2C8 and CYP3A4. Potential interactions may occur, including antiretroviral protease inhibitors. Use together cautiously with other drugs metabolized by this system (CYP 2C8 and CYP 3A4 inducers: carbamazine, phenytoin, phenobarbital, rifampin: may decrease serum level of paclitaxel and decrease effect; CYP 2C8 and CYP 3A4 inhibitors: ethinyl estradiol, fluconazole, ketoconazole, sulfonamides, testosterone, tretinoin, ciprofloxacin, clarithromycin, doxycycline, erythromycin, grapefruit juice, isoniazid, protease inhibitors, verapamil: may increase serum level of paclitaxel with increased risk of toxicity). Use together cautiously, if at all.
- Cisplatin: Myelosuppression is more severe when cisplatin is administered prior to paclitaxel (due to 33% reduction in paclitaxel clearance from the plasma). Therefore, paclitaxel must be given prior to cisplatin when drugs are administered sequentially.
- Carboplatin: Possible increased cytotoxicity when given *after* paclitaxel. Also, combination of paclitaxel and carboplatin results in less thrombocytopenia than would be expected from dose of carboplatin alone (etiology of platelet-sparing effect unknown).
- Doxorubicin and liposomal doxorubicin: Increased incidence of neutropenia and stomatitis when paclitaxel is administered prior to doxorubicin (due to significant decrease in doxorubicin clearance, possibly due to competition for biliary excretion of both agents). Administer sequentially rather than concomitantly.
- Doxorubicin: Increased risk of cardiotoxicity when given in combination with paclitaxel, with sharp increase in risk of congestive heart failure once cumulative dose

of doxorubicin is > 380 mg/m^2 (Gianni et al, 1998). Administer sequentially, not concomitantly.
- Beta-blockers, calcium-channel blockers, digoxin: Additive bradycardia may occur; assess/monitor patients closely.
- St. John's wort: may decrease paclitaxel serum level; do not use together.

Lab Effects/Interference:
- Decreased white and red cell counts, neutrophil count, platelet count.
- Increased alkaline phosphatase, AST, ALT, bilirubin.

Special Considerations:
- Indicated for the treatment of breast cancer after failure of combination chemotherapy for metastatic disease or relapse within six months of adjuvant chemotherapy. Prior therapy should have included an anthracycline unless clinically contraindicated.
- Drug is a Cremaphor-free, protein-engineered nanotransporter of paclitaxel. No premedication for hypersensitivity is required.
- Drug needs no special tubing, filter.
- Rarely, pneumothorax, interstitial pneumonia, lung fibrosis, pulmonary embolism have been reported.
- Use cautiously and monitor closely patients with hepatic or renal dysfunction.

Potential Toxicities/Side Effects and the Nursing Process

I. POTENTIAL FOR INFECTION AND BLEEDING related to BONE MARROW DEPRESSION

Defining Characteristics: Neutropenia is dose dependent and reversible, with grade 4 reported as 9% at doses of 260 mg/m^2, without growth factor support. Febrile neutropenia occurred in 2% of patients, compared to 1% in the paclitaxel arm. Neutropenia may be more pronounced in patients who have received prior radiotherapy. Infectious complications occurred in 24% of patients, with oral candidiasis, respiratory tract infection, and pneumonia the most commonly reported. Thrombocytopenia is uncommon, with bleeding reported in 2% of patients. Anemia occurred in 33% of patients, and was severe in 1% of patients (hgb < 8 g/dL).

Nursing Implications: Assess baseline CBC, WBC, differential, and platelet count prior to chemotherapy, as well as signs/symptoms of infection or bleeding. Teach patient the signs/symptoms of infection or bleeding, and to report these immediately, and teach patient self-care measures to minimize risk of infection and bleeding. This includes avoidance of crowds, proximity to people with infections, and OTC aspirin-containing medications. Administer paclitaxel PRIOR to cisplatin or carboplatin when either is given in combination with paclitaxel.

II. SENSORY/PERCEPTUAL ALTERATIONS related to SENSORY NEUROPATHY, OCULAR AND VISUAL DISTURBANCES

Defining Characteristics: Sensory neuropathy is dose related and common, occurring in 71% of patients in clinical studies (10% severe), compared to 56% in patients receiving paclitaxel. Grade 3 neuropathy reversible in many patients, within a mean 22 days. No grade 4 severity have been reported in clinical trials. Rare motor or autonomic neuropathy (e.g., ileus). Ocular/visual disturbances may occur in 13% of the patients, especially at higher doses, and in the literature, persistent optic nerve damage related to paclitaxel has been reported.

Nursing Implications: Assess baseline neurologic status. Instruct patient to report signs/symptoms of pins and needles (paresthesias), numbness, pain, increased discomfort with certain sensations (dysesthesias), especially in the extremities, or motor weakness. Identify patients at risk: prior cisplatin, or having pre-existing neuropathies (ethanol- and diabetes mellitus-related). Assess sensory and motor function prior to each treatment, and if abnormality found, assess impact on patient function, safety, independence, and quality of life. Test patient's ability to button a shirt, or pick up a dime from a flat surface. Teach self-care strategies as needed, including maintaining safety when walking, getting up, taking bath, or washing dishes; explain inability to sense temperature and the need to keep extremities warm in cold weather (see NCI Common Toxicity Criteria, Appendix II). Teach the patient to report any ocular or visual disturbance, and discuss management or need for ophthalmologic consultation with physician.

III. POTENTIAL ALTERATION IN CIRCULATION related to HYPOTENSION, ARRYTHMIA

Defining Characteristics: Hypotension during first three hours of infusion in 5% of patients, and bradycardia in < 1% of patients have been reported; most often patients were asymptomatic, and patients did not require intervention. Significant cardiovascular events (chest pain, cardiac arrest, supraventricular tachycardia, edema, thrombosis, pulmonary embolism, hypertension, cerebral vascular accident) occurred in 3% of patients receiving single-agent paclitaxel albumin-bound particles for injection. Of those patients with normal baseline EKGs at the beginning of single-agent paclitaxel albumin-bound particles for injection therapy, 35% of patients developed an abnormal EKG tracing (nonspecific repolarization abnormalities, sinus bradycardia, sinus tachycardia).

Nursing Implications: Assess baseline cardiac status, history, and risk for development of CHF. Closely monitor patient during paclitaxel infusion, especially if patient has history of hypertension, or is on cardiac medications (see Drug Interactions section). Teach patient to report any dyspnea, SOB, chest pain, or heart palpitations, or any unusual feeling. If any abnormalities occur, stop infusion as appropriate and discuss further management with physician.

IV. ALTERATION IN SKIN INTEGRITY related to ALOPECIA

Defining Characteristics: Alopecia occurs commonly (90% of patients studied).

Nursing Implications: Discuss potential impact of hair loss prior to drug administration. Discuss coping strategies and plan to minimize body image distortion (e.g., wig, scarf, cap). Assess patient for signs/symptoms of hair loss. Assess patient's response and use of coping strategies, and help patient to build on effective strategies.

V. ALTERATION IN NUTRITION, LESS THAN BODY REQUIREMENTS, related to NAUSEA/VOMITING, DIARRHEA, MUCOSITIS, AND HEPATOTOXICITY

Defining Characteristics: Nausea, vomiting, diarrhea, and mucositis were reported in 30%, 18%, 26%, and 7% of patients, respectively. Rarely, hepatic necrosis, hepatic encephalopathy, intestinal obstruction, intestinal perforation, pancreatitis, and ischemic colitis have been reported in patients receiving paclitaxel albumin-bound injection.

Nursing Implications: Premedicate patient with antiemetic (either serotonin antagonist or dopamine antagonist). Encourage small, frequent meals of cool, bland foods. Instruct patient to report nausea, and teach self-administration of antiemetics. If nausea/vomiting occurs and is severe, assess for signs/symptoms of fluid/electrolyte imbalance. Assess bowel elimination pattern and oral mucosa baseline prior to each treatment. Teach patient to report diarrhea unrelieved with self-administered antidiarrheal medications and adequate fluid replacement. Teach patient to assess oral mucosa and to use systematic oral cleansing after meals and at bedtime. Teach patient to report difficulty drinking fluids or ingesting food.

VI. ALTERATION IN COMFORT related to FATIGUE, ARTHRALGIAS AND MYALGIAS

Defining Characteristics: Fatigue occurs commonly, and arthralgias and myalgias affect about 44% of all patients, with 8% experiencing severe symptoms. Arthralgias and myalgias commonly occurred 2–3 days after the drug was given, and resolved within a few days.

Nursing Implications: Teach patient that fatigue may occur, and ways to minimize exertion and energy expenditure by alternating rest and activity, and organizing chores so that they are done as efficiently as possible.

Drug: patupilone (EPO906 investigational)

Class: Epothilone B analogue.

Mechanism of Action: Normally, cells need to have flexibility in making the structures for mitosis, such as tubulin and the microtubules; the tubulin needs to be able to polymerize and then depolymerize. Patupilone binds to the beta-tubulin subunits on microtubules and strongly promotes tubulin polymerization and stabilization, similar to paclitaxel but at a different binding site; the drug causes the cell to stop cycling (mitotic arrest) at the G_2/M phase of the cell cycle and to die (cytotoxicity). The drug avoids multiple tumor resistance mechanisms, so has activity in taxane-resistant tumors.

Metabolism: Unknown.

Dosage/Range:
- Per protocol, 0.3–6 mg/m^2 every 3 weeks, or 0.3–2.5 mg/m^2 weekly × 6 every 9 weeks.

Drug Preparation:
- Per protocol.

Drug Administration:
- Per protocol.

Drug Interactions:
- Unknown.

Lab Effects/Interference:
- Unknown.

Special Considerations:
- DLT is diarrhea, which is different from other epothilones and taxanes where the DLT is neutropenia or peripheral neuropathy.
- Is being studied alone and in combination with other chemotherapy in lung, breast, and other solid tumors.

Potential Toxicities/Side Effects and the Nursing Process

I. POTENTIAL ALTERATION IN NUTRITION, LESS THAN BODY REQUIREMENTS, related to DIARRHEA

Defining Characteristics: Diarrhea is the dose-limiting toxicity.

Nursing Implications: Teach patient that diarrhea may occur and to report it. Teach patient and family to self-administer prescribed antidiarrheal medications per protocol, to drink adequate fluids, and to modify diet to remove insoluble fiber, other nutrients that might promote diarrhea. Teach patient to report diarrhea that does not resolve or worsens.

Drug: pegasparaginase

Class: Miscellaneous agent (enzyme).

Mechanism of Action: Pegasparaginase is a modified form of L-asparaginase, wherein units of monomethoxypolyethylene glycol (PEG) are covalently conjugated to L-asparaginase, forming the active ingredient PEG-L-asparaginase. The enzyme hydrolyzes serum asparagine, a nonessential amino acid for both normal and leukemic cells. Unlike normal cells, leukemic cells are unable to synthesize their own asparagine (lack the enzyme asparagine synthetase and thus require exogenous L-asparagine), resulting in cell death.

Metabolism: Unclear.

Dosage/Range:
- Adults under 21 and adolescents: 2500 international units/m^2 every 14 days.
- Children with BSA = 0.6 m^2: 2500 international units/m^2 every 14 days.
- Children with BSA = 0.6 m^2: 82.5 international units/kg body weight every 14 days.
- NOTE: Safety and efficacy have been established only in patients from 1–21 years of age.

Drug Preparation:
- For intravenous use, reconstitute with sterile water for injection, and dilute further in 100 cc NS or D5W. If giving IM, reconstitute in no more than 2 cc NS for injection. If more than 2 cc of NS is used, more than one injection site must be used.
- IM is the preferred route of administration, because of the lower incidence of hepatotoxicity, coagulopathy, and gastrointestinal and renal disorders as compared with the intravenous route.

Drug Interactions:
- Nonsteroidal anti-inflammatory drugs (NSAIDs), aspirin, dipyridamole, heparin, warfarin, and blood-dyscrasia-causing medications: Pegasparaginase causes imbalances in coagulation factors, predisposing patients to bleeding and/or thrombosis.
- Hepatotoxic medications (increased risk of toxicity).
- Methotrexate: Drug antagonizes antifolate effects of MTX if given before MTX administration. If given 24 hours after MTX, its antifolate activity will be terminated at that point.
- Vaccines, both live and killed virus: Patient's antibody response to the killed vaccine may be reduced for up to one year by the immunosuppression brought on by pegasparaginase. Such immunosuppression may also potentiate the replication of live-virus vaccines, increase the side effects of the vaccine virus, and/or may decrease the patient's antibody response to the vaccine.

Lab Effects/Interference:
- Increased LFTs, serum glucose, BUN, and uric acid.
- Prolonged PT.

Special Considerations:

- Drug should NOT be given in patients with:
  - — Pegasparaginase allergy
  - — Bleeding disorders associated with prior asparaginase therapy
  - — Pancreatitis, or history of
- Hypersensitivity reactions occur more frequently with pegasparaginase than with the vast majority of chemotherapeutic agents. Patients must be closely monitored for signs of allergic/anaphylactic reactions. Ensure immediate access to adverse-reaction kit.

Potential Toxicities/Side Effects and the Nursing Process

I. POTENTIAL FOR INJURY related to HYPERSENSITIVITY OR ANAPHYLACTIC REACTIONS

Defining Characteristics: Occurs less often with IM route of administration. May be life-threatening reaction, but is usually mild.

Nursing Implications: Discuss with physician use of test dose prior to drug administration. Assess baseline VS and mental status prior to drug administration. Review standing orders or nursing procedure for management of anaphylaxis and be prepared to stop drug immediately if signs/symptoms occur; keep IV line open with 0.9% sodium chloride, notify physician, monitor vital signs, and administer ordered medications, which may include epinephrine 1:1000, hydrocortisone sodium succinate, and diphenhydramine. Teach patient the potential of a hypersensitivity or anaphylactic reaction and to immediately report any unusual symptoms. *Escherichia coli* preparation of L-asparaginase and Erwinia carotovora preparation are non-cross-resistant, so if an anaphylactic reaction occurs with one, the other preparation may be used.

II. POTENTIAL FOR INJURY related to HEPATIC DYSFUNCTION OR THROMBOEMBOLISM

Defining Characteristics: Most patients have elevated LFTs starting within first two weeks of treatment, e.g., SGOT, bili, and alk phos. Hepatically derived clotting factors may be depressed, resulting in excessive bleeding or blood clotting. Relatively uncommon.

Nursing Implications: Monitor SGOT, bili, alk phos, albumin, and clotting factors CPT, PTT, fibrinogen. Teach patient of the potential for excessive bleeding or blood clotting, and instruct to report any unusual symptoms. Assess patient for signs/symptoms of bleeding.

III. ALTERED NUTRITION, LESS THAN BODY REQUIREMENTS, related to NAUSEA/VOMITING, ANOREXIA, HYPERGLYCEMIA

Defining Characteristics: Many patients experience mild-to-moderate nausea and vomiting. Anorexia commonly occurs. Hyperglycemia is a transient reaction caused by effects on the pancreas with decreased insulin synthesis. Pancreatitis occurs in some patients.

Nursing Implications: Premedicate with antiemetics and continue prophylactically for 24 hours to prevent nausea and vomiting. Encourage small, frequent meals of cool, bland foods and liquids, as well as favorite foods, especially high-calorie, high-protein foods. Encourage use of spices and do weekly weights. Teach patient about the potential of hyperglycemia and pancreatitis, and instruct to report any unusual symptoms: e.g., increased thirst, urination, and appetite (hyperglycemia) and abdominal or stomach pain, constipation, or nausea and vomiting (pancreatitis). Monitor serum glucose, amylase, and lipase levels periodically during treatment. Report any laboratory elevations to physician. Treat hyperglycemia issues with diet or insulin as ordered by physician. Treat pancreatitis per physician orders.

IV. SENSORY/PERCEPTUAL ALTERATIONS related to NEUROTOXICITY

Defining Characteristics: Neurotoxicity may occur in some patients—commonly, lethargy, drowsiness, and somnolence; rarely coma. Seen more frequently in adults.

Nursing Implications: Teach patient about the potential of CNS toxicity, and instruct to report any unusual symptoms. Obtain baseline neurologic and mental function. Assess patient for any neurologic abnormalities and report changes to physician. Discuss with patient the impact of malaise on his/her general sense of well-being and strategies to minimize the distress.

V. INFECTION, BLEEDING, AND FATIGUE related to BONE MARROW DEPRESSION

Defining Characteristics: Bone marrow depression is not common. Mild anemia may occur. Serious leukopenia and thrombocytopenia are rare.

Nursing Implications: Monitor CBC, platelet count prior to drug administration, as well as signs/symptoms of infection, bleeding, or anemia. Instruct patient in self-assessment of signs/symptoms of infection, bleeding, or anemia and to report immediately.

Drug: pemetrexed (Alimta)

Class: Multi-targeted antifolate (antimetabolite).

Mechanism of Action: Inhibits key metabolic enzymatic steps (Thymidylate synthase [TS], dihydrofolate reductase [DHFR], and glycinamide ribonucleotide formyltransferase [GARFT]) critical to pyrimidine and purine synthesis, thus preventing DNA synthesis and cell division. Drug is carried into tumor cells via reduced folate carriers, metabolized intracellularly to polyglutamated form of pemetrexed that potently inhibits purine and pyrimidine synthesis. Antitumor effect dependent upon size of cellular folate pools, so folic acid must be co-administered to increase drug efficacy and minimize toxicity. Polyglutamates accumulate in the cell, with a long cellular half-life, and increased cytotoxicity. It is active in the S phase of the cell cycle.

Metabolism: Following IV administration, peak plasma levels are achieved within 30 minutes. Drug is widely distributed in body tissues, especially liver, kidneys, small intestines, and colon. Excreted by kidneys (glomerular and tubular) into the urine, with up to 90% of the drug excreted unchanged during the first 24 hours after administration. Plasma half-life is about 3 hours, with prolonged terminal half-life of 20 hours.

Dosage/Range:
- Malignant-pleural mesothelioma: 500 mg/m^2 IV over 10 minutes followed by cisplatin 75 mg/m^2 IV over 2 hours, beginning 30 minutes after the end of the pemetrexed dose, repeated every 21 days.
- Non–small-cell lung cancer: 500 mg/m^2 IV over 10 minutes every 21 days.

Drug Preparation:
- Reconstitute pemetrexed 500 mg vial by adding 20 mL 0.9% sodium chloride for injection, resulting in a concentration of 25 mg/mL.
- Aseptically remove dose and add to 100 mL 0.9% sodium chloride for injection.
- Administer as a 10-minute IV infusion.
- Patient should take dexamethasone 4 mg PO twice daily on the day before, day of, and day after treatment to help prevent skin rash.
- Patient must take daily folic acid supplement (350 to 1000 μg) PO beginning 1 week prior to initial treatment, and continuing throughout treatment and post-treatment.
- Patient must receive vitamin B_{12} (1000 μg) IM injections every 3 cycles, beginning 1 week prior to first treatment, and continuing throughout treatment every 3 cycles thereafter.
- Full dose if ANC > 1500 cells/mm^3, platelets > 100,000 cells/mm^3, AND creatinine clearance > 45 mL/min.

Dose Reduction:
- Hematologic: Nadir ANC < 500 cells/mm^3 and platelet count > 50,000 cells/mm^3 DOSE REDUCE both drugs to 75% of previous doses.

- Hematologic: Nadir platelets < 50,000 cells/mm^3 regardless of ANC nadir DOSE REDUCE both drugs to 50% of previous doses.
- Pemetrexed should be discontinued for any grade 3 or 4 hematologic or non-hematologic toxicity after 2 dose reductions, or immediately if grade 3 or 4 neurologic toxicity.
- If grade 1 neurotoxicity, no dose modifications of either drug. If grade 2 neurotoxicity, 100% pemetrexed dose, but cisplatin is 50% of previous dose.

Drug Interactions:
- Nephrotoxic drugs: Potentially delayed pemetrexed excretion.
- Drugs secreted by renal tubules (e.g., probenecid): potential delayed pemetrexed excretion.
- Thymidine: rescues normal cells.
- Leucovorin: decreases antitumor effect of pemetrexed; do not co-administer.
- 5-FU: may increase antitumor effect of pemetrexed.
- Ibuprofen and other NSAIDs, in people with normal renal function: 20% increase in AUC of pemetrexed, due to 20% reduction in pemetrexed clearance.
  - NSAIDs (short half-lives, e.g., ibuprofen): AVOID if renal compromise (creatinine clearance < 80 mL/min), stop NSAIDs 2 days prior to pemetrexed administration, the day of administration, and for 2 days following pemetrexed administration.
  - NSAIDs (long half-lives): stop NSAID 5 days before, the day of, and for 2 days following pemetrexed administration.
  - If patient must continue NSAIDs, 24-hour creatinine clearance should be > 80 mL/min.

Lab Effects/Interference:
- Transient increase in serum transaminases and bilirubin.

Special Considerations:
- FDA indicated in combination with cisplatin for the treatment of patients with 1) locally advanced or metastatic non-squamous NSCLC OR 2) malignant pleural mesothelioma whose disease is unresectable or who are otherwise not candidates for curative surgery.
- FDA indicated as second-line therapy as a single agent for the treatment of patients with locally advanced or metastatic non–small-cell lung cancer after prior chemotherapy.
- Do not administer drug if creatinine clearance is < 45 mL/min using Cockcroft and Gault formula (estimated creatinine clearance). [140 – age in years] × actual body weight (kg); males = 72 × serum creatinine (mg/dL) = mL/min; females = estimated creatinine clearance for males × 0.85.
- Pemetrexed is fetotoxic and teratogenic. Women of child-bearing age should use effective birth control measures. Women should not breast-feed an infant while receiving pemetrexed.
- Preliminary results of a phase III study suggest that patients with Stage IIIB or IV NSCLC who receive platinum-based induction therapy for four cycles followed

by maintenance therapy with pemetrexate (500 mg/m^2), had significantly longer time to progression (double the time) compared with patients who received placebo (4 vs 2 mo, $p < .0001$). OS was longer, but the difference was not significant (13 vs 10 mo, NS). In subset analysis, patients with nonsquamous cell histology had the best responses (Ciuleanu et al, 2008).

Potential Toxicities/Side Effects and the Nursing Process

I. POTENTIAL INFECTION, BLEEDING, AND FATIGUE related to BONE MARROW DEPRESSION

Defining Characteristics: Bone marrow depression is dose-limiting toxicity. Nadir is day 8 with recovery by day 15 of each cycle. Neutropenia occurred in 58% of patients, with grade 3 (19%), and grade 4 (5%). For grades 3 and 4 neutropenia, the incidence in between patients who were fully supplemented was 24%, in contrast to patients who were never supplemented (38%). The overall incidence of thrombocytopenia is 27%, with grades 3 and 4 (4%/1%, respectively). Anemia occurred in 33% of patients overall.

Nursing Implications: Assess baseline CBC, WBC, differential and ANC, and platelet count prior to chemotherapy as well as for signs and symptoms of infection, bleeding, or anemia. Ensure labs ANC > 1500 cells/mm^3, platelets > 100,000 cells/mm^3, AND creatinine clearance > 45 mL/min prior to drug administration. Ensure that patient has taken vitamin supplements prior to drug administration: low dose oral folic acid or multivitamin with folic acid daily (at least 5 daily doses of folic acid must be taken during the 7-day period prior to the first dose of pemetrexed, and dosing should continue during the full course of therapy, and for 21 days after the last drug dose; Vitamin B_{12} 100 μg IM during the week prior to cycle 1, then every 3 cycles. Subsequent doses can be given on same day as pemetrexed treatment). Discuss dose reductions based on nadir counts with physician as needed. Teach patient signs/symptoms of infection, and bleeding, and instruct to report them right away. Teach measures to minimize infection and bleeding, such as avoidance of crowds, proximity to people with infection, and to avoid aspirin or NSAID-containing medications. Teach patient strategies to minimize fatigue, such as alternating rest with activity, and ways to organize shopping to minimize energy expenditure.

II. POTENTIAL ALTERATION IN NUTRITION, LESS THAN BODY REQUIREMENTS, related to NAUSEA, CONSTIPATION, ANOREXIA, DIARRHEA, STOMATITIS

Defining Characteristics: Nausea occurs in 84% of patients, vomiting 58%, constipation 44%, anorexia 35%, stomatitis/pharyngitis 28%, and diarrhea 26%, in combination with cisplatin.

Nursing Implications: Premedicate with antiemetics, and ensure patient has antiemetics to take to prevent delayed emesis from cisplatin. Teach patient and family delayed emesis regimen. Encourage small, frequent meals of cool, bland foods, and to increase fluid intake. Assess oral mucosa prior to drug administration and instruct patient to report changes. Teach patient oral hygiene measures and self-assessment. Instruct patient to report diarrhea, to self-administer prescribed antidiarrheal medications and to drink adequate fluids. Monitor LFTs baseline and periodically during therapy. Notify physician of any abnormalities and discuss implications as drug studied only in patients with elevated LFTs related to liver metastases.

III. ALTERATION IN SKIN INTEGRITY related to RASH

Defining Characteristics: Incidence of rash with or without desquamation was 22%.

Nursing Implications: Assess baseline skin integrity. Teach patient that this may occur, and to take recommended dexamethasone premedication 4 mg po bid the day before, the day of, and the day after pemetrexed administration. Teach patient potential side effects of corticosteroid administration, including difficulty sleeping, mood alterations, and depression.

IV. POTENTIAL FOR IMPAIRED GAS EXCHANGE related to DYSPNEA

Defining Characteristics: Dyspnea was reported in 66% of patients receiving pemetrexed and cisplatin therapy; 10% had grade 3 dyspnea, and 1% had grade 4 toxicity.

Nursing Implications: Teach patient that this may occur, and to report it right away if severe or worsening. Assess baseline pulmonary status, at rest, and with activity. Assess oxygen saturation with vital signs. Discuss severe or worsening dyspnea with physician.

Drug: pentostatin (Nipent, 2-deoxycoformycin)

Class: Antimetabolite.

Mechanism of Action: Isolated from fermentation cultures of *Streptomyces anti-bioticus*. Drug is a potent inhibitor of adenosine deaminase (ADA), which is found in lymphocytes, with T-cells (and T-cell malignancies) having higher levels of ADA than B-cells (and B-cell malignancies). By blocking ADA, pentostatin is believed to block DNA and RNA synthesis, resulting in cell death. It causes cells to arrest in G_1-S phases of the cell cycle, but also appears to act in a non–cell cycle-specific way.

Metabolism: Is not absorbed orally. After IV administration drug distributes widely in body tissue and water, low protein binding, and crosses blood–brain barrier with up to 12% identified in the CSF within 24 hours of administration. Liver metabolizes minimal amount of drug. More than 90% of drug and metabolites are excreted unchanged in the urine, with half-life of drug about 6 hours unless impaired renal function.

Dosage/Range:

Hairy Cell Leukemia:

- 4 mg/m^2 IV every other week until complete response if tolerated well and then two additional doses. Discontinue after 6 months of treatment if no response or if only partial response after 12 months.
- Check baseline serum creatinine and 24-hour creatinine clearance, and repeat serum creatinine before each dose.
- Dose reduce to 2–3 mg/m^2 IV if creatinine clearance 50–60 mL/min and benefit justifies risk of toxicity.
- Hydration: 500 mL to 1 L of fluid before drug, followed by 1000 mL after drug administration to ensure adequate urine output (and drug excretion).

Drug Preparation:

- Available in single use 10-mg vials, which are reconstituted with 5-mL sterile water (2 mg/mL).
- Stable at room temperature for 8 hours.

Drug Administration:

- IV push over 5 minutes or IV infusion over 20–30 minutes in a 50-mL bag of D5W or 0.9% NS after prehydration and followed by posthydration.
- Hold drug if patient has ANC < 200/mm^3 (when baseline count was > 500/mm^3), active infection, severe reactions to drug, CNS toxicity, or increased serum creatinine.

Drug Interactions:

- Fludarabine: fatal pulmonary toxicity; do not co-administer.
- Bone marrow-suppressing agents: increased bone marrow depression.
- High-dose cyclophosphamide (BMT): possible fatal cardiotoxicity.
- Vidarabine: decreased metabolism, with increased activity and toxicity of vidarabine.
- CNS depressants (sedative, hypnotics): increased CNS toxicity possible.

Lab Effects/Interference:

- Increased AST, ALT, alkaline phosphatase, LDH, uric acid, serum creatinine.
- Decreased WBC (lymphocytes and granulocytes).

Special Considerations:

- Use cautiously with reduced dose, or not at all, in patients with abnormal renal function as > 90% of drug and metabolites excreted intact in urine.
- Rarely, angina, myocardial infarction, CHF, acute arrhythmias, and pulmonary toxicity may occur. Risk highest in patients with prior cardiac dysfunction.

Potential Toxicities/Side Effects and the Nursing Process

I. POTENTIAL FOR INFECTION AND BLEEDING related to BONE MARROW DEPRESSION

Defining Characteristics: Dose-limiting leucopenia, with nadir occurring on days 10–14 and recovery by days 21–27. Profound immunosuppression, with both B and T cells reduced, and increasing risk of viral, bacterial, fungal, and parasitic infections. Less frequent thrombocytopenia. Potent immunosuppressant, with suppressed B, T lymphocytes, and helper T cells during and after treatment for months to years. Immunosuppression increases risk of infection by virus, encapsulated bacteria, fungi, and parasites. In patients with advanced hairy cell leukemia, neutropenia may worsen.

Nursing Implications: Assess 24-hour urine for creatinine clearance to determine whether treatment can be given. Assess CBC with differential, platelet count, and serum creatinine before each drug administration, as well as signs/symptoms of infection or bleeding. Instruct patient in self-assessment of signs/symptoms of infection or bleeding and risk reduction. Teach the patient to call provider immediately for signs/symptoms of infection. Discuss with physician whether prophylactic antimicrobials are indicated. Before each treatment, assess patient tolerance of preceding treatment, especially CNS, gingival bleeding or infection, or other potential sources of infection.

II. ALTERATION IN NUTRITION, LESS THAN BODY REQUIREMENTS, related to NAUSEA/VOMITING, ANOREXIA, AND DIARRHEA

Defining Characteristics: Nausea and vomiting occur commonly but are mild. Diarrhea and anorexia may affect 10–50% of patients.

Nursing Implications: Premedicate with antiemetics, and ensure patient has antiemetics to take at home if needed. Teach patient and family self-administration of antiemetics if needed at home. Encourage small, frequent meals of cool, bland foods and increase in fluid intake. Assess oral mucosa and gums before drug administration and instruct patient to report changes. Teach patient oral hygiene measures and self-assessment. Instruct patient to report diarrhea, to self-administer prescribed antidiarrheal medications, and to drink adequate fluids.

III. SENSORY/PERCEPTUAL ALTERATIONS related to CONFUSION, ACTIVITY INTOLERANCE, FATIGUE

Defining Characteristics: Drug passes through blood–brain barrier into CNS with resulting dose-related headache, lethargy, and fatigue. Less commonly, blurred vision, confusion, depression, dizziness, coma may occur. Conjunctivitis, photophobia, and diplopia, as well as ototoxicity may occur.

Nursing Implications: Assess neurologic, mental status, and intactness of vision and hearing baseline before each treatment. Instruct patient to report any alterations in thinking, behavior, sensation, perception. Develop a plan of care with patient and family if side effects develop to manage distress and promote safety. Drug should be stopped if confusion, hallucinations, and coma occur.

IV. ALTERATION IN COMFORT related to FEVER, CHILLS, MYALGIAS, ARTHRALGIAS

Defining Characteristics: Fever and chills affect 10–50% of patients, whereas myalgias and arthralgias are less common.

Nursing Implications: Assess baseline comfort status. Teach patient these symptoms may occur and self-management techniques, including increased oral fluid intake to at least 1500 mL/24 hours, to call provider if temperature > 100.4°F, warm soaks for arthralgias, and myalgias.

Drug: polifeprosan 20 with carmustine (BCNU) implant (Gliadel®)

Class: Alkylating agent.

Mechanism of Action: Wafer (copolymer) containing carmustine is implanted in the surgical cavity created when brain tumor is resected. In water, the anhydride bonds of the wafer are hydrolyzed, releasing the carmustine into the surgical cavity. The carmustine diffuses into the surrounding brain tissue, reaching any residual tumor cells, and causing cell death by alkylating DNA and RNA.

Metabolism: Unknown. Dime-sized wafer is biodegradable in brain tissue, with a variable rate. More than 70% of the copolymer degrades by three weeks, slowly releasing 7.7 mg of carmustine in concentrations. In some patients, wafer fragments remained up to 232 days after implantation, with almost all drug gone.

Dosage/Range:
- Each wafer contains 7.7 mg of carmustine, and the recommended dose is 8 wafers, or a total dose of 61.6 mg of carmustine.

Drug Preparation:
- Drug must be stored at or below 20°C (–4°F) until time of use.
- Unopened foil packages can stay at room temperature for a maximum of 6 hours at a time. The manufacturer recommends that the treatment box be removed from the freezer and taken to the operating room just prior to surgery.
- The box and pouches should be opened just before the surgeon is ready to implant the wafers. Open the sealed treatment box and remove double foil packages, handling the unsterile outer foil packet by the crimped edge VERY CAREFULLY to

prevent damage to the wafers. See product information for opening the inner foil pouch and removing the wafer with sterile technique.

- Chemotherapy precautions should be used to limit exposure to the chemotherapy: surgical instruments used to remove and implant the wafers should be kept separate from other instruments and sterile fields, and should be cleaned after the procedure according to hospital chemotherapy procedure; all personnel handling the wafers or the inner foil pouches containing the wafers should wear double gloves, which, along with unused wafers or fragments, inner foil packages, and opened outer foil package, should be disposed of as chemotherapeutic waste.

Drug Administration:
- Neurosurgeon places 8 wafers into surgical resection cavity if size and shape appropriate; wafers are placed contiguously or with slight overlapping.
- Wafer may be broken into 2 pieces *only* if needed.

Drug Interactions:
- Unknown but unlikely as drug is probably not systemically absorbed.

Lab Effects/Interference:
- Unknown, but unlikely.

Special Considerations:
- Indicated for the treatment of newly diagnosed patients with high-grade malignant glioma as an adjunct to surgery and radiation.
- Indicated for use as an adjunct to surgery to prolong survival in patients with recurrent glioblastoma multiforme for whom surgical resection is indicated.
- Manufacturer reports that in a study of 222 patients with recurrent glioma who failed initial surgery and radiotherapy, the six-month survival rate after surgery increased from 47% (placebo) to 60%, and in patients with glioblastoma multiforme, the six-month survival for patients receiving placebo was 36% vs 56% for patients receiving polifeprosan 20 with carmustine implant.
- Patients require close monitoring for complications of craniotomy, as intracerebral mass effect has occurred that does not respond to corticosteroid treatment; in one case, this resulted in brain herniation.
- Studies have not been conducted during pregnancy or in nursing mothers. Carmustine is a known teratogen, and is embryotoxic. Use during pregnancy should be avoided, and mothers should stop nursing during use of the drug.

Potential Toxicities/Side Effects and the Nursing Process

I. POTENTIAL SENSORY/PERCEPTUAL ALTERATIONS related to SEIZURES, BRAIN EDEMA, MENTAL STATUS CHANGES

Defining Characteristics: In clinical testing, the incidence of new or worsened seizures was 19% in both the group receiving the implant and those receiving the placebo.

Seizures were mild to moderate in severity. In patients with new or worsened seizures postoperatively, the group receiving the implant had a 56% incidence, with median time to first new or worsened seizure of 3.5 days, versus placebo incidence of 9%, and median time to first new or worsened seizure of 61 days. Incidence of brain edema was 4%, and there were cases of intracerebral mass effect that did not respond to corticosteroids. Other nervous system effects were hydrocephalus (3%), depression (3%), abnormal thinking (2%), ataxia (2%), dizziness (2%), insomnia (2%), visual field defect (2%), monoplegia (2%), eye pain (1%), coma (1%), amnesia (1%), diplopia (1%), and paranoid reaction (1%). Rarely (< 1%), cerebral infarct or hemorrhage may occur.

Nursing Implications: Monitor neurovital signs closely postoperatively, and notify physician of any abnormalities. If intracranial pressure increases, a mass effect is suspected, and if it is nonresponsive to corticosteroids, expect the patient to be taken to surgery, with possible removal of wafer or remnants. Assess baseline mental status and regularly during postoperative care. Validate changes with family members. Discuss abnormalities with physician immediately and continue to monitor closely.

II. POTENTIAL FOR INFECTION related to HEALING ABNORMALITIES

Defining Characteristics: Most abnormalities were mild to moderate, occurred in 14% of patients, and included cerebrospinal leaks, subdural fluid collections, subgaleal or wound effusions, and breakdown. The incidence of intracranial infection (e.g., meningitis or abscess) was 4%. Incidence of deep wound infection was 6% (same as placebo) and included infection of subgaleal space, bone, meninges, and brain tissue.

Nursing Implications: Using aseptic technique, assess postoperative wound/dressing immediately postoperatively, and regularly thereafter. Assess systematically for signs/symptoms of infection or wound breakdown. Notify physician immediately and discuss antimicrobial therapy.

III. ALTERATION IN NUTRITION, LESS THAN BODY REQUIREMENTS, related to GI SIDE EFFECTS, ELECTROLYTE ABNORMALITIES

Defining Characteristics: Rarely, GI disturbances occurred: diarrhea (2%), constipation (2%), dysphagia (1%), gastrointestinal hemorrhage (1%), fecal incontinence (1%). Hyponatremia (3%), hyperglycemia (3%), and hypokalemia (1%) also occurred.

Nursing Implications: Assess baseline nutritional status, including electrolytes. Assess bowel elimination status and monitor nutritional and bowel elimination status closely during postoperative time. Discuss interventions for abnormalities with physician.

IV. ALTERATION IN CIRCULATION, POTENTIAL, related to CHANGES IN BLOOD PRESSURE

Defining Characteristics: Hypertension occurred in 3% of patients, and hypotension in 1%.

Nursing Implications: Assess baseline VS and monitor closely during postoperative phase. Discuss abnormalities with physician.

V. ALTERATION IN COMFORT related to EDEMA, PAIN, ASTHENIA

Defining Characteristics: The following occur rarely: peripheral edema (2%), neck pain (2%), rash (2%), back pain (1%), asthenia (1%), chest pain (1%).

Nursing Implications: Assess baseline comfort level and monitor closely during postoperative phase. Provide comfort measures. If ineffective, discuss symptom-management strategies with physician.

Drug: procarbazine hydrochloride (Matulane)

Class: Miscellaneous agent.

Mechanism of Action: Uncertain but appears to affect preformed DNA, RNA, and protein. It is a methylhydrazine derivative and acts as an alkylating agent. Cell cycle nonspecific.

Metabolism: Metabolized to active metabolites in the liver by the P450 microenzyme system. Rapidly and completely absorbed from the GI tract with peak plasma levels within 1 hour. Procarbazine metabolites taken up by lymph nodes, bone marrow, and cross the BBB, with peak CSF levels occurring in 30–90 minutes. Also metabolized in red blood cells and kidney. Most of the drug (5%) and metabolites (70%) are excreted in the urine. Elimination half-life is 1 hour.

Dosage/Range:
- 100 mg/m^2 orally, daily from 7–14 days every 4 weeks as part of the MOPP regimen.
- Brain tumors: 60 mg/m^2 orally every day × 14 days as part of the PCV regimen.

Drug Preparation:
- None.

Drug Administration:
- Oral.
- Available in 50-mg capsules.

Drug Interactions:

- Procarbazine is synergistic with CNS depressants. Barbiturate, antihistamine, narcotic, and hypotensive agents or phenothiazine antiemetics should be used with caution.
- Disulfiram (Antabuse)-like reaction may result if the patient consumes alcohol. Symptoms include headache, respiratory difficulties, nausea and vomiting, chest pain, hypotension, and mental status changes.
- Exhibits weak MAO (monoamine oxidase) inhibitor activity. Foods containing high amounts of tyramine should be avoided: substances such as beer, wine, cheese, brewer's yeast, chicken livers, and bananas. Consumption of foods high in tyramine in combination with procarbazine may lead to intracranial hemorrhage or hypertensive crisis.
- Levodopa, meperidine: hypertension when either is taken with procarbazine. Avoid co-administration.
- Sympathomimetics, tricyclic antidepressants: CNS excitation, hypertension, palpitations, angina, hypertensive crisis; avoid co-administration.
- Antidiabetic (sulfonylurea, insulin): potentiation of hypoglycemic effect. Monitor blood sugar closely and adjust dose as needed.
- When taken in combination with digoxin, there is a decreased bioavailability of digoxin.

Lab Effects/Interference:

- Decreased CBC.
- Increased LFTs, RFTs.

Special Considerations:

- Discontinue if CNS signs/symptoms (paresthesia, neuropathy, confusion), stomatitis, diarrhea, or hypersensitivity reaction occur.
- Patients with G6PD should be monitored closely for hemolytic anemia.
- Patients may develop hypersensitivity reaction (pruritus, urticaria, maculopapular rash, flushing) responding to steroid therapy and continuation of drug. If pulmonary infiltrates develop, procarbazine should be discontinued.

Potential Toxicities/Side Effects and the Nursing Process

I. POTENTIAL FOR INFECTION AND BLEEDING related to BONE MARROW DEPRESSION

Defining Characteristics: Major dose-limiting toxicity. Thrombocytopenia occurs in 50% of patients, evidenced by a delayed onset (28 days after treatment) and lasting 2–3 weeks. Leukopenia seen in two-thirds of patients, with nadirs occurring after initial thrombocytopenia. Anemias may be due to bone marrow depression or hemolysis.

Nursing Implications: Monitor CBC, platelet count prior to drug administration, as well as signs/symptoms of infection, bleeding, and anemia. Instruct patient in self-assessment of signs/symptoms of infection, bleeding, and anemia and to report this immediately. Dose reduction often necessary (35–50%) if compromised bone marrow function. Platelet and red cell transfusions per physician order.

II. ALTERATION IN NUTRITION, LESS THAN BODY REQUIREMENTS, related to NAUSEA, VOMITING, DIARRHEA

Defining Characteristics: Nausea and vomiting occur in 70% of patients and may be a dose-limiting toxicity. Diarrhea is uncommon, but rarely may be protracted and thus would be an indication for dose reduction.

Nursing Implications: Teach patient to premedicate with antiemetics 30 minutes before taking procarbazine to prevent nausea and vomiting. Encourage small, frequent meals of cool, bland foods and liquids. Minimize nausea and vomiting by dividing the total daily dosage into 3–4 doses. Also, taking the pills at bedtime may decrease the sense of nausea. May administer nonphenothiazine antiemetics. Encourage patients to report onset of diarrhea. Administer, or teach patient to self-administer, antidiarrheal medications.

III. POTENTIAL FOR SENSORY/PERCEPTUAL ALTERATIONS

Defining Characteristics: Symptoms occur in 10–30% of patients and are seen as lethargy, depression, frequent nightmares, insomnia, nervousness, or hallucinations. Tremors, coma, convulsions are less common. Symptoms usually disappear when drug is discontinued. Crosses into CSF.

Nursing Implications: Teach patient the potential for neurotoxicity and provide early counseling about these effects. Assess patients for any symptoms of neurotoxicity. Discuss strategies with patient to preserve general sense of well-being. Obtain baseline neurologic and motor function. CNS toxicity may be manifested as reactions to other drugs, e.g., barbiturates, narcotics, and phenothiazine antiemetics.

IV. ACTIVITY INTOLERANCE related to PERIPHERAL NEUROPATHY

Defining Characteristics: 10% of patients exhibit paresthesias, decrease in deep tendon reflexes. Foot drop and ataxia occasionally reported. Reversible when drug is discontinued.

Nursing Implications: Obtain baseline neurologic and motor function. Assess patient for any changes in motor function, e.g., ability to pick up pencils or buttons.

V. ALTERATION IN COMFORT related to FLU-LIKE SYNDROME

Defining Characteristics: Fever, chills, sweating, lethargy, myalgias, and arthralgias commonly occur at the beginning of therapy.

Nursing Implications: Teach patient the potential for flu-like syndrome and how to distinguish from actual infection. Instruct patient to report any changes in condition.

VI. POTENTIAL FOR IMPAIRED SKIN INTEGRITY related to RARE DERMATITIS REACTIONS

Defining Characteristics: Rarely occurs as alopecia, pruritus, rash, hyperpigmentation.

Nursing Implications: Assess patient for changes in skin, nails, and hair loss. Discuss with patient impact of changes and strategies to minimize distress, e.g., wearing nail polish, long-sleeved tops, wigs, scarfs, caps.

VII. POTENTIAL SEXUAL DYSFUNCTION related to DRUG EFFECTS

Defining Characteristics: Drug is teratogenic. Causes azoospermia. Causes cessation of menses, although may be reversible.

Nursing Implications: As appropriate, explore with patient and partner issues of reproductive and sexuality patterns and the impact chemotherapy may have. Discuss strategies to preserve sexual and reproductive health (e.g., sperm banking, contraception).

Drug: progestational agents: medroxyprogesterone acetate (Provera, Depo-Provera), megestrol acetate (Megace)

Class: Hormone.

Mechanism of Action: Unclear, but progestational agents compete for androgen and progestational receptor sites on the cell. Has potent antiestrogenic properties that disturb estrogen receptor cycle. Also increases synthesis of RNA by interacting with DNA.

Metabolism: Rapidly absorbed from GI tract. Metabolized in the liver. Excreted in the urine. Peak plasma levels reached in 1–3 hours; biological half-life, 3.5 days.

Dosage/Range:

Medroxyprogesterone acetate:

- Provera: 20–80 mg PO daily.

Depo-Provera:
- — 400–800 mg IM every month
- — 100 mg IM three times weekly
- — 1000–1500 mg daily (high dose)

Megestrol acetate:
- Megace, mg PO qid (breast cancer): 80 mg PO qid (endometrial cancer).

Drug Preparation:
- IM preparation is ready to use; shake vial well before drawing up medication.

Drug Administration:
- Give via deep IM injection.

Drug Interactions:
- None.

Lab Effects/Interference:
- Increased LFTs.
- Changes in TFTs.

Special Considerations:
- Patients may become sensitive to oil carrier (oil in which drug is mixed).
- Small risk of hypersensitivity reaction.

Potential Toxicities/Side Effects and the Nursing Process

I. POTENTIAL FOR INJURY related to FLUID RETENTION, THROMBOEMBOLISM

Defining Characteristics: Fluid retention. Thromboembolic complications may occur. Sterile abscess may occur with IM injection.

Nursing Implications: Inform patient of potential for fluid retention and of signs/symptoms to watch for and to report to nurse or physician. Assess for signs/symptoms of fluid overload. Teach patient and family signs/symptoms of thromboembolic events: positive Homan's sign, localized pain, tenderness, erythema, sudden CNS changes, shortness of breath. Instruct patient to notify nurse or physician if any of the above occur. Give drug via deep IM injection: apply pressure to injection site after administering. Inspect used sites; rotate sites systematically.

II. ALTERED NUTRITION, LESS THAN BODY REQUIREMENTS, related to NAUSEA

Defining Characteristics: Nausea is rare.

Nursing Implications: Inform patient that nausea can occur; encourage patient to report nausea. Encourage small, frequent meals of cool, bland foods and liquids.

Drug: raltitrexed (Tomudex, ZD 1694, investigational)

Class: Antimetabolite folate antagonist.

Mechanism of Action: Quinazoline-based folic acid analogue that acts as a folic acid antagonist; by selectively inhibiting the enzyme thymidylate synthase, it blocks purine synthesis. This causes breaks in DNA strands, and thus, DNA, RNA, and protein synthesis cannot proceed and the cell dies.

Metabolism: Drug has triphasic kinetics when administered intravenously over 15 minutes. The drug is rapidly distributed into tissue, with peak plasma levels occurring during or immediately after drug infusion. Cells actively take up drug, which is metabolized intracellularly into polyglutamates (more potent inhibitors of thymidylate synthase than parent drug). Polyglutamates have a long half-life in the cell, simulating continuous infusion therapy, with a terminal elimination half-life 8.2–105+ hours. Except for cellular metabolism, drug is excreted unchanged in the urine and is actively excreted by the renal tubules.

Dosage/Range:
- Per protocol.
- Colorectal cancer: 3 mg/m^2 IV q 3 weeks.

Drug Preparation:
- Available in 2-mg vials, which should be protected from light, and refrigerated at 2–8°C (36–46°F).
- Reconstitute with 4 mL sterile water for injection, producing a concentration of 0.5 mg/mL.
- Withdraw dose, and further dilute in 50–250 mL 0.9% normal saline or 5% dextrose.
- Reconstituted and diluted solutions are stable refrigerated for 24 hours.

Drug Administration:
- IV infusion over 15 minutes.
- Hold if urine creatinine clearance is < 25 mL/min.
- Contraindicated in patients with uncontrolled diarrhea, or hypersensitivity.

Drug Interactions:
- Potential interaction with other drugs that compete for excretion in the renal tubules: penicillin, indomethacin, methotrexate (Taylor, 2000).
- Folate, folic acid: Interferes, decreases cytotoxicity.

Lab Effects/Interference:
- Decreased WBC, neutrophil count, platelet count, Hgb/HCT.
- Increased bili and/or alk phos, liver transaminases (ALT, AST).

Special Considerations:
- Has been used for a long time in Europe; is being studied in the United States in the following tumor types: colorectal, with and without 5-FU/leucovorin and/or irinotecan, oxaliplatin; breast; NSCLC; ovary; pancreas.

- Some U.S. clinical studies in colorectal cancer have shown conflicting results and higher mortality, possibly because dose was not adjusted in renal dysfunction.
- Use cautiously, and monitor closely patients who have previously been heavily pretreated with chemotherapy or radiotherapy, especially if persistent stomatitis, bone marrow depression, hepatic or renal dysfunction; patients with history of gastrointestinal problems (e.g., diarrhea); and patients with hepatic or renal dysfunction.
- Patients should NOT take folate or folate-containing vitamins during therapy, as this interferes with cytotoxicity of drug.
- Drug should not be used during pregnancy or by breast-feeding mothers.
- Dose reduce for myelosuppression, gastrointestinal toxicity, renal dysfunction per protocol; reduced dose should be given only when toxicity resolved.
- Allergic responses (e.g., stridor and wheezing) following first dose are rare, but have been reported.

Potential Toxicities/Side Effects and the Nursing Process

I. POTENTIAL FOR INFECTION, BLEEDING, AND FATIGUE related to BONE MARROW DEPRESSION

Defining Characteristics: Bone marrow depression is one of dose-limiting toxicity. 60% incidence of leukopenia, and severe in 10–22% of patients. Nadir is day 8, but may be delayed to day 21; recovery begins day 10. Thrombocytopenia is less common, occurring in 25% of patients, and is severe in 2%.

Nursing Implications: Assess baseline WBC, differential, platelet and Hgb/HCT prior to chemotherapy, as well as for signs/symptoms of infection or bleeding. Teach patient signs/symptoms of infection and bleeding and to report these immediately; teach patient self-care measures to minimize risk of infection and bleeding. This includes avoidance of crowds, proximity to people with infections, and OTC aspirin-containing medications. Teach patient to report fatigue and teach measures to conserve energy, such as alternating rest and activity periods. Discuss transfusion of red blood cells as needed. Consult protocol for dose reductions if patient has severe bone marrow suppression, renal dysfunction, or severe hepatic dysfunction.

II. ALTERATION IN NUTRITION, LESS THAN BODY REQUIREMENTS, related to DIARRHEA, NAUSEA, VOMITING, STOMATITIS

Defining Characteristics: Diarrhea may be dose-limiting in some studies. Incidence is 11–26%, and drug is contraindicated in patients with uncontrollable diarrhea. Nausea and vomiting are mild to moderate if they occur, with an incidence of 11–19%, and are preventable with antiemetics. Stomatitis may occur, and in some studies had an incidence of 48%. Rarely, patients may experience anorexia or constipation (1–10% incidence).

Nursing Implications: Teach patient that these side effects may occur and to report them. Assess baseline weight and nutritional status, bowel elimination pattern, and oral mucosal integrity, and monitor before each treatment and throughout treatment. Administer premedication to prevent nausea/vomiting. Teach patient to self-administer antiemetics at home, and to report unrelieved or persistent nausea/vomiting. Teach patient to notify provider if diarrhea occurs, to take OTC anti-diarrheal medications if diarrhea develops, and to call nurse/physician if diarrhea persists or recurs. Teach patient self-care of oral mucosa, including assessment, when to notify provider, and oral hygiene regimen. Refer to protocol for dose reductions for gastrointestinal toxicity.

III. ALTERATION IN ACTIVITY related to ASTHENIA, FATIGUE

Defining Characteristics: Asthenia is very common, and may be severe. Appears to be dose-related. Anemia is very common, affecting up to 70% of patients.

Nursing Implications: Assess baseline activity tolerance, and level of fatigue. Teach patient that these side effects may occur and to report them. Teach patient to alternate rest and activity periods. Teach fatigue self-care measures, such as strategies to maximize energy use and conservation while shopping, interacting with friends, and other activities.

IV. POTENTIAL FOR ALTERATION IN COMFORT related to FEVER, RASH, PAIN

Defining Characteristics: Fever occurs in 20% of patients, usually 1–3 days after drug administration. Rash may occur (35% incidence), is papular and pruritic, and commonly affects head and upper trunk. Alopecia and cellulitis have been reported rarely (1–10%). Pain may occur.

Nursing Implications: Assess baseline skin texture, presence of rashes, general comfort level, and also, whether patient commonly has fevers. Teach patient to report fever, pain, or rash. Teach patient to take acetaminophen or other agent to relieve fever or pain. Teach patient to use skin emollient or cream if rash appears to reduce itching. If itching and/or rash persist or are severe, discuss further management with physician.

Drug: rubitecan (9-Nitro-20(S)-Camptothecin, Orathecin, investigational)

Class: Topoisomerase I inhibitor.

Mechanism of Action: Induces protein-linked DNA single-strand breaks and blocks DNA and RNA synthesis in dividing cells, thus preventing cells from entering mitosis. Prevents repair (relegation) of previous, reversible single-strand breaks in DNA by binding to topoisomerase I. Topoisomerase I is an enzyme that relaxes tension in the DNA helix torsion by initially causing this single-strand break in DNA so that

DNA replication can occur. Topoisomerases I and II then work together to bring about replication, transcription, and recombination of DNA material. Topoisomerase I is found in higher-than-normal concentrations in certain malignant cells, such as colon adenocarcinoma cells and non-Hodgkin's lymphoma cells.

Metabolism: Drug is well absorbed after oral administration, with maximal serum levels in 2–4 hours after the first dose, and is converted to 9-aminocamptothecin and other metabolites. Drug is water insoluble, unlike other topoisomerase inhibitors (e.g., irinotecan, topotecan), which are water soluble. Drug is metabolized in the liver, and slowly excreted in the urine, with a terminal half-life of 10.6 hours.

Dosage/Range:
- Studies in solid tumors: 1.5 mg/m^2/d PO on days 1–5, with no therapy on days 6–7, repeated q week.
- Studies in hematologic malignancies: 2 mg/m^2/d on days 1–5, with no therapy on days 6–7, repeated q week.

Drug Preparation:
- Per protocol.

Drug Administration:
- Oral, available in 1.25-mg and 0.5-mg capsules.

Drug Interactions:
- Unknown.

Lab Effects/Interference:
- Unknown.

Special Considerations:
- Drug is a radiosensitizer.
- Being studied in the following cancers: pancreatic (phase III), myelodysplastic syndrome (phase II), refractory ovarian (phase II), advanced colorectal (phase II), metastatic melanoma (phase II), previously treated NSCLC (phase II), sarcoma (phase II), relapsed metastatic breast cancer (phase II), refractory prostate cancer (phase II), recurrent glioma (phase II), chronic phase CML (phase II), refractory/relapsed AML (phase II), refractory lymphoma (phase II).
- Patients should drink 3 L of fluid daily to prevent hemorrhagic cystitis.
- Drug is contraindicated in patients with hypersensitivity to the drug, or to 9-amino-camptothecin.

Potential Toxicities/Side Effects and the Nursing Process

I. POTENTIAL FOR INFECTION, BLEEDING, AND FATIGUE related to BONE MARROW DEPRESSION

Defining Characteristics: Bone marrow depression is the dose-limiting toxicity. 30% of patients in pancreatic clinical trials experienced neutropenia, 11% severe (grades

3/4). Thrombocytopenia in these studies affected 35%, with 21% graded severe (grades 3/4). Finally, anemia was common, with an incidence of 53%, with 16% severe (grades 3/4).

Nursing Implications: Assess baseline WBC, differential, platelet, and Hgb/HCT prior to chemotherapy as well as for signs/symptoms of infection or bleeding. Teach patient signs/symptoms of infection and bleeding and to report these immediately; teach patient self-care measures to minimize risk of infection and bleeding. This includes avoidance of crowds, proximity to people with infections, and OTC aspirin-containing medications. Teach patient to report fatigue and teach measures to conserve energy, such as alternating rest and activity periods. Discuss transfusion of red blood cells as needed.

II. ALTERATION IN NUTRITION, LESS THAN BODY REQUIREMENTS, related to NAUSEA, VOMITING, AND DIARRHEA

Defining Characteristics: Nausea and vomiting are common, but preventable with antiemetics. Incidence in pancreatic studies was 50%, with only 5% having severe (grades 3/4). The incidence of diarrhea in these studies was 28%, with 5% severe (grades 3/4).

Nursing Implications: Teach patient that these side effects may occur and to report them. Teach patients to take ordered antiemetic medications one hour prior to their dose, and to notify provider right away if nausea and/or vomiting persist, or if unable to drink/keep down fluids. Teach patient to take antidiarrheal medications if diarrhea develops, and to notify provider if diarrhea persists or recurs.

III. POTENTIAL FOR ALTERATION IN COMFORT related to FEVER

Defining Characteristics: In the pancreatic studies, 13% of patients reported fever.

Nursing Implications: Teach patient to report fever. Teach patient to take acetaminophen or other agent to relieve fever if it occurs.

IV. ALTERATION IN URINE ELIMINATION, related to CYSTITIS

Defining Characteristics: Interstitial cystitis may occur and be hemorrhagic; in clinical studies, cystoscopy revealed punctate mucosal ulcerations. Histopathologic exam revealed interstitial cystitis, coagulative mucosal necrosis, and little inflammatory infiltrate (Natelson et al, 1996). This is preventable by maintaining hydration. Incidence in patients described in pancreatic studies was 3%.

Nursing Implications: Teach patient that it is imperative to drink 3 L of fluid a day, and to avoid alcoholic beverages, as they may cause diuresis. Teach patient that if nausea and/or vomiting develop, and unable to drink this amount, to notify provider immediately.

Drug: streptozocin (Zanosar)

Class: Alkylating agent (nitrosourea).

Mechanism of Action: A weak alkylating agent (nitrosourea) that causes interstrand cross-linking in DNA and is cell cycle phase nonspecific. Appears to have some specificity for neoplastic pancreatic endocrine cells. Glucose attached to nitrosourea appears to diminish myelotoxicity.

Metabolism: 60–70% of total dose and 10–20% of parent drug appear in urine. Drug is rapidly eliminated from serum in 4 hours, with major concentrations occurring in liver and kidneys. Drug half-life is 35 minutes. Drug metabolized in the liver, and metabolites excreted in the urine.

Dosage/Range:
- 500 mg/m^2 IV daily × 5 days. Repeat every 3–4 weeks; OR
- 1000–1500 mg/m^2 IV every week × 6 followed by observation.
- Dose reduce (DR) based on 24 hour creatinine clearance (10–50 mL/min = 25% reduction; < 10 mL/min = 50% reduction).

Drug Preparation:
- Add sterile water or 0.9% sodium chloride to vial.
- If powder or solution contacts skin, wash immediately with soap and water.
- Solution is stable 48 hours at room temperature, 96 hours if refrigerated.

Drug Administration:
- Assess renal function before each cycle.
- Administer via pump over 1 hour.
- Has also been given as continuous infusion or continuous arterial infusion into the hepatic artery.
- If local pain or burning occurs, slow infusion and apply cool packs above injection site.
- Irritant; avoid extravasation.
- Administer with 1–2 L of hydration to prevent nephrotoxicity.

Drug Interactions:
- Nephrotoxic drugs (cisplatin, aminoglycosides, amphotericin B): additive nephrotoxicity; avoid concurrent use if possible.
- Steroids: increase risk of severe hyperglycemia.
- Phenytoin: antagonism of antitumor effect; do not co-administer.
- Doxorubicin: increased half-life of doxorubicin, resulting in increased myelosuppression.

Lab Effects/Interference:

- Decreased CBC.
- Increased RFTs (especially BUN).
- Increased LFTDH.
- Changes in glucose, phosphorus, albumin serum levels.

Special Considerations:

- Renal function must be monitored closely.
- Drug is an irritant; give IV short infusion over 15–30 minutes or as a 6-hour infusion.

Potential Toxicities/Side Effects and the Nursing Process

I. POTENTIAL FOR ALTERATION IN URINARY ELIMINATION related to RENAL DYSFUNCTION

Defining Characteristics: 60% of patients experience renal dysfunction. Usually transient proteinuria and azotemia, but this may progress to permanent renal failure, especially if other nephrotoxic drugs are given concurrently. Signs/symptoms include proteinuria, increased BUN, hypophosphatemia, glycosuria, renal tubular acidosis, decreased creatinine clearance. Hypophosphatemia is probably earliest sign of renal dysfunction.

Nursing Implications: Closely monitor BUN, creatinine, phosphorus, urine protein, and 24-hour creatinine clearance prior to each treatment. Monitor BUN, creatinine, pH of urine, glucose/protein of urine every shift during therapy. Discuss dose reduction with physician based on creatinine clearance. Strictly monitor I/O during therapy. Hydration per physician, but usually 2–3 L/day. Rarely, renal toxicity may present as glucosuria, hypophosphatemia, and diabetes insipidus.

II. ALTERATION IN NUTRITION, LESS THAN BODY REQUIREMENTS, related to GI SIDE EFFECTS

Defining Characteristics: Nausea and vomiting occur in up to 90% of patients, beginning 1–4 hours after drug dose, and can be significantly reduced when drug is given as continuous infusion. Nausea and vomiting may worsen during 5-consecutive-day therapy; increased severity with doses > 500 mg/m^2. 10% of patients experience diarrhea with abdominal cramping. LFTs may be elevated but normalize with time. Hepatotoxicity occurs in ~50% of patients. Liver enzymes increase 2–3 weeks after therapy, albumin decreases but symptoms rarely occur. May also develop painless jaundice.

Nursing Implications: Premedicate with antiemetics and continue prophylactically for 24 hours; use aggressive antiemetics when drug is given IV over 1 hour (serotonin antagonists effective). Encourage small, frequent feedings of cool, bland foods and liquids.

If patient has nausea or vomiting, discuss with physician more aggressive antiemetics. Monitor I/O closely and replace fluids. Encourage patient to report onset of diarrhea. Administer or teach patient to self-administer antidiarrheal medications. Teach patient diet modifications. Monitor LFTs prior to each treatment (alk phos, SGOT, SGPT, albumin). Assess for signs/symptoms of hepatic dysfunction: jaundice, yellowing of skin, sclera; orange-colored urine; white or clay-colored stools; itchy skin.

III. ALTERATIONS IN GLUCOSE METABOLISM related to HYPOGLYCEMIA

Defining Characteristics: Appears that damage to pancreatic beta cells causes sudden release of insulin, with resulting hypoglycemia in about 20% of patients. Hyperglycemia may occur in patients with insulinomas and decreased glucose tolerance. Increased fasting or postprandial blood levels may occur.

Nursing Implications: Monitor serum glucose levels every day or more frequently as needed; check urine glucose. Assess for, and instruct patient to report, the following signs/symptoms of hypoglycemia: muscle weakness and lethargy, perspiration, flushed feeling, restlessness, headache, confusion, trembling, epigastric hunger pains. If signs/symptoms are found, encourage patient to eat or drink high-glucose food and juice and notify physician. Hypoglycemia can be prevented with nicotinamide. Assess for signs/symptoms of hyperglycemia in patient with insulinomas and instruct patient in self-assessment.

IV. POTENTIAL FOR INFECTION AND BLEEDING related to BONE MARROW DEPRESSION

Defining Characteristics: Bone marrow depression occurs in about 9–20% of patients. Nadir 1–2 weeks after administration. Occasionally, severe leukopenia and thrombocytopenia occur. Mild anemia may occur.

Nursing Implications: Monitor CBC, platelets prior to drug administration, as well as assess for signs/symptoms of infection or bleeding. Instruct patient in self-assessment of signs/symptoms of infection or bleeding.

V. POTENTIAL FOR INJURY related to SECONDARY MALIGNANCIES

Defining Characteristics: Drug is carcinogenic; secondary malignancies are well described.

Nursing Implications: Patients receiving prolonged therapy should be screened periodically.

Drug: tamoxifen citrate (Nolvadex, Soltamox oral solution)

Class: Antiestrogen.

Mechanism of Action: Nonsteroidal antiestrogen that competitively binds to estrogen receptors, forming an abnormal complex that migrates to the cell nucleus and inhibits DNA synthesis. Also, appears to stimulate secretion of transforming growth factor beta, which proceeds to inhibit genes that stimulate cell proliferation. Activity is cell-cycle specific in mid-G_1 phase.

Metabolism: Well absorbed from GI tract with a high degree of protein binding and peak plasma levels in 4–6 hours. Widely distributed in body tissue, especially areas where estrogen receptors are expressed. Metabolized by P450 microenzyme system in liver (CYP 3A4, CYP 2D6). Undergoes enterohepatic circulation, prolonging blood levels. Excreted in feces. Elimination half-life is 7–14 days.

Dosage/Range:
- 20 mg PO daily (most often, 10 mg bid).

Drug Preparation:
- Available in 10-mg tablets or oral liquid solution (10 mg/5 mL).

Drug Administration:
- Oral.

Drug Interactions:
- Anticoagulants: increased PT; monitor PT closely and reduce anticoagulant dose as needed.
- CYP 3A4, 2D6 inducers (carbamazepine, glucocorticoids, phenobarbital, phenytoin, rifamycin, nevirapine): may decrease serum level of tamoxifen.
- CYP 3A4, 2D6 inhibitors (ciprofloxacin, clarithromycin, doxycycline, erythromycin, imatinib, diclofenac, nicardipine, nefazodone, protease inhibitors, verapamil, quinidine, cimetidine, codeine, fluoxetine, haloperidol, paroxetine): may increase tamoxifen serum levels.
- Drugs activated by P450 system: may inhibit metabolic activation of cyclophosphamide.
- Letrozole: decreased letrozole serum levels by 37%; do not give concurrently.
- St. John's wort: decreased tamoxifen serum level; do not give concurrently.

Lab Effects/Interference:
- Decreased CBC.
- Increased LFTs.
- Increased Ca.
- Interference in lab tests such as TFTs and hyperlipidemia.

Special Considerations:
- Measurements of estrogen receptors in tumor are important in predicting tumor response and should be performed at same time as biopsy and before antiestrogen treatment is started.

- Avoid antacids within 2 hours of taking enteric-coated tablets.
- A flare reaction with bone pain and hypercalcemia may occur. Such reactions are short-lived and usually result in a tumor response if therapy is continued.
- No evidence exists that doses > 20 mg/day are more efficacious.
- Indicated for the treatment of (1) adjuvant therapy in lymph node negative breast cancer after surgical resection, (2) adjuvant therapy in lymph node negative breast cancer in postmenopausal women after surgical resection, (3) metastatic breast cancer in men and women, (4) chemoprevention of breast cancer in high risk women (age > 35, Gail model 5 year predicted risk > 1.67%), (5) reduction in the risk of invasive breast cancer in women with ductal carcinoma.
- Tamoxifen resulted in a significant decrease in development of invasive breast cancer in women with atypical hyperplasia (88%).
- Rare side effects include uterine sarcoma, stroke, uterine cancer, blood clot formation.
- Tamoxifen is being studied as an adjunct to in vitro fertilization (IVF) for women with breast cancer who wish to have a child, given with FSH. The addition of either tamoxifen or letrozole with FSH increased the number of ovarian follicles, more mature eggs, and more embryos (Oktay et al, 2005).
- Use cautiously in patients with abnormal liver function or history of thromboembolic disease.
- Patients should be taught to notify physician immediately if patient develops abnormal uterine bleeding, pelvic pain, pain in the legs, or breathing problems.

Potential Toxicities/Side Effects and the Nursing Process

I. POTENTIAL FOR SEXUAL DYSFUNCTION related to CHANGES IN MENSES, HOT FLASHES

Defining Characteristics: May cause menstrual irregularity, hot flashes, milk production in breasts, vaginal discharge, and bleeding. Symptoms occur in about 10% of patients and are usually not severe enough to discontinue therapy. Drug may cause endometrial hyperplasia, polyps, and endometrial cancer.

Nursing Implications: As appropriate, explore with patient and partner issues of reproductive and sexuality patterns and the impact drug may have on them. Discuss strategies to preserve sexual and reproductive health. Teach patient that she should be closely followed by a gynecologist for annual endometrial biopsies and to report immediately abnormal uterine bleeding, or pelvic pain.

II. POTENTIAL FOR ALTERATION IN CIRCULATION related to THROMBOEMBOLISM

Defining Characteristics: Tamoxifen has been associated with thromboembolic events and is associated with antithrombin III deficiency.

Nursing Implications: Teach patient to minimize likelihood of developing DVT such as avoid sitting in the same position for long periods, especially on airplanes and to get up and walk regularly to increase venous return from the lower extremities. Teach patient to report immediately or go to the emergency department if pain in the lower extremities develops or the patient develops abrupt onset of dyspnea, shortness of breath, or any pulmonary symptom.

III. POTENTIAL FOR ALTERATION IN COMFORT related to FLARE REACTION

Defining Characteristics: May cause flare reaction initially (bone and tumor pain, transient increase in tumor size). Nausea, vomiting, and anorexia may occur.

Nursing Implications: Inform patient of possibility of flare reaction, signs/symptoms to be aware of, and encourage patient to report any signs/symptoms. Inform patient of possibility of nausea, vomiting, and anorexia. Encourage small, frequent meals of high-calorie, high-protein foods.

IV. POTENTIAL FOR SENSORY/PERCEPTUAL ALTERATION related to VISUAL CHANGES

Defining Characteristics: Retinopathy has been reported with high doses. Corneal changes, cataracts, decreased visual acuity, and blurred vision have occurred. Headache, dizziness, and light-headedness are rare.

Nursing Implications: Obtain visual assessment prior to starting therapy. Encourage patient to report any visual changes and discuss evaluation by ophthalmologist depending upon symptom(s). Instruct patient to report headache, dizziness, light-headedness.

V. POTENTIAL FOR INFECTION AND BLEEDING related to BONE MARROW DEPRESSION

Defining Characteristics: Mild, transient leukopenia and thrombocytopenia occur rarely.

Nursing Implications: Monitor CBC, platelets prior to drug administration and after therapy has begun. Instruct patient in self-assessment of signs/symptoms of infection or bleeding.

VI. POTENTIAL FOR SKIN INTEGRITY IMPAIRMENT related to RASH, ALOPECIA

Defining Characteristics: Skin rash, alopecia, peripheral edema are rare.

Nursing Implications: Assess patient for signs/symptoms of hair loss, edema, and skin rash. Instruct patient to report any of these symptoms. Discuss with patient the impact of skin changes.

VII. POTENTIAL FOR INJURY related to HYPERCALCEMIA

Defining Characteristics: Hypercalcemia uncommon.

Nursing Implications: Obtain serum calcium levels prior to therapy and at regular intervals during therapy. Instruct patient in signs/symptoms of hypercalcemia: nausea, vomiting, weakness, constipation, loss of muscle tone, malaise, decreased urine output.

Drug: temozolomide (Temodar®)

Class: Alkylating agent.

Mechanism of Action: Drug is a member of the imidazotetrazine class and is the active metabolite of dacarbazine in an oral form. Drug is a prodrug, forming the metabolite monomethyl triazenoimidazole carboxamide (MTIC) when chemically degraded, and is further metabolized to 5-aminoimidazole-4-carboxamide (AIC), the active cytotoxic metabolite. Drug is lipophilic and can pass through the BBB, where it has been shown to be effective against some brain tumors, possibly because of the alkaline pH. MTIC causes alkylation of DNA and RNA strands, and DNA, RNA, and protein synthesis is inhibited.

Metabolism: Well absorbed from the GI tract following oral dose (100% bioavailability), with peak concentrations in 1 hour when taken on empty stomach. The elimination half-life is 1.8 hours. The drug is degraded into MTIC in plasma and tissues. 15% of drug is excreted unchanged in the urine. Differs from dacarbazine in that formation of MTIC does not require liver metabolism. Food decreases the rate and extent of drug absorption.

Dosage/Range:
Refractory anaplastic astrocytoma that has failed prior chemotherapy:
- 150 mg/m^2/day orally × 5 days if patient has received prior chemotherapy, repeated every 28 days.
- Dose should be adjusted to keep ANC 1000–1500/mm^3 and platelet count 50,000–100,000/mm^3.

Newly diagnosed glioblastoma multiforme (GBM) concomitantly with (at the same time as) radiotherapy and then as maintenance treatment.
- 75 mg/m^2 orally, daily starting the first day of RT through the last day of RT, for 42 days (maximum 49 days) as long as ANC > 1500 cells/mm^3, platelet count > 100,000 cells/mm^3, and other toxicity (except alopecia, nausea, vomiting) are less than grade 1 (CTC).

- Prophylaxis for *Pneumocystis carinii* pneumonia while receiving concomitant RT and temozolomide, then 4 weeks after completion of RT.
- Maintenance dose (temozolomide orally daily × 5, then 23 days without treatment, repeated × 6):
- Cycle 1: Temozolomide 150 mg/m^2 orally daily × 5, then 23 days without treatment (as long as ANC > 1500 cells/mm^3, platelet count >100,000 cells/mm^3, and other toxicity [except alopecia, nausea, vomiting] are less than grade 1 [CTC]),
- Cycle 2–6: Temozolomide 200 mg/m^2 orally daily × 5 then 23 days without treatment, repeated for 5 more cycles (as long as ANC > 1500 cells/mm^3, platelet count > 100,000 cells/mm^3, and other toxicity [except alopecia, nausea, vomiting] are < grade 1 [CTC]),
- Monitor CDC on day 22 then weekly until ANC > 1500 cells/mm^3, and platelets > 100,000 cells/mm^3; see package insert for dose reductions based on nadir counts and worst CTC toxicity.

Drug Preparation:
- None.
- Available in 250-mg, 100-mg, 20-mg, and 5-mg strengths.
- Drug is stored at room temperature, protected from light and moisture.

Drug Administration:
- Give orally with full glass of water on an empty stomach. Patient should take medicine at around the same time of day each day, e.g., bedtime.
- Do not crush or dissolve capsule.

Drug Interactions:
- Valproic acid: reduces temozolomide clearance by 5% but may not be clinically significant; monitor drug effect closely if used together.

Lab Effects/Interference:
- Elevated liver function tests (e.g., ALT, AST; occur in up to 40% of patients), increase in alk phos.
- Decreased WBC, Hgb, and platelet count.
- Hyperglycemia.
- Elevated renal function tests.

Special Considerations:
- Drug is indicated for the treatment of adults with (1) refractory anaplastic astrocytoma who have experienced disease progression on a nitrosurea and procarbazine (after first relapse), and (2) newly diagnosed glioblastoma multiforme (GBM) concomitantly with (at the same time as) radiotherapy and then as maintenance treatment.
- Drug has also been used for treatment of glioma after first relapse and advanced metastatic malignant melanoma, high-grade malignant glioma (glioblastoma multiforme, anaplastic astrocytoma) and is being studied in a variety of solid tumors.

- Drug causes severe myelosuppression, and thrombocytopenia is the dose-limiting factor.
- Use with caution, if at all, in the following patients: hypersensitive to dacarbazine; myelosuppressed; have bacterial or viral infection; have renal dysfunction; have received prior chemotherapy or radiation; and women who are pregnant or who are breast-feeding.
- Rarely (1% of patients), hypercalcemia may occur with the 5-day regimen.
- PET (positive emission tomography) scanning showed reduced uptake of fluorodeoxyglucose (FDG) in patients who responded, in 7–14 days following a 5-day course of treatment, as opposed to those patients who did not respond, and who showed increased FDG uptake (Newlands et al, 1997).
- Overall response rate in some studies of patients with malignant glioma that had recurred or progressed after surgery and radiation therapy was 15–25% and 30% in newly diagnosed patients prior to XRT (Bower et al, 1997).

Potential Toxicities/Side Effects and the Nursing Process

I. POTENTIAL FOR INFECTION, BLEEDING, AND FATIGUE related to BONE MARROW DEPRESSION

Defining Characteristics: Thrombocytopenia and leukopenia are dose-limiting factors and occur in grade 2 or higher 40% of the time. This does not usually require administration of G-CSF. Nadir at 21–22 days, unless using 5-day treatment schedule, where nadir is day 28–29. Recovery for platelets is 7–42 days and in shorter time for WBC. Anemia may also occur, but is infrequent and less severe. Severity of bone marrow depression depends on dose and schedule, as well as disease process. In one trial, patients with malignant glioma had severe lymphopenia (41% grade 3 and 15% grade 4).

Nursing Implications: Assess baseline WBC, differential, platelet and Hgb/HCT prior to chemotherapy, as well as for signs/symptoms of infection or bleeding. Teach patient signs/symptoms of infection and bleeding and to report these immediately; teach patient self-care measures to minimize risk of infection and bleeding. This includes avoidance of crowds, proximity to people with infections, and OTC aspirin-containing medications. Teach patient to report fatigue and teach measures to conserve energy, such as alternating rest and activity periods. Discuss transfusion of red blood cells as needed.

II. ALTERED NUTRITION, LESS THAN BODY REQUIREMENTS, related to NAUSEA AND VOMITING, STOMATITIS, AND DIARRHEA

Defining Characteristics: Nausea and vomiting occur in 75% of patients, usually grade 1 or 2, and usually occurring on day 1. In one trial, using a 5-day treatment regimen, 21% had grade 3 nausea, and 23% had grade 4. Stomatitis may occur in up to 20% of patients. Diarrhea, constipation, and/or anorexia may affect up to 40% of patients.

Nursing Implications: Teach patient to self-medicate with antiemetics (serotonin antagonist effective) one hour prior to dose and suggest evening dosing to minimize nausea/vomiting. Encourage small, frequent feedings of cool, bland foods. Teach patient to notify provider right away if nausea/vomiting persists. Assess oral mucosa prior to drug administration and teach patient to report changes. Teach patient oral hygiene measures and self-assessment. Teach patient to report diarrhea, to self-administer prescribed antidiarrheal medications, and to drink adequate fluids. Teach patient to report constipation, and manage with stool softeners or laxatives. If patient has anorexia, teach patient to select acceptable foods and to eat small portions q 2 hours and at bedtime. Teach patient to keep a diary documenting when medications are taken and side effects and to bring in medication bottle for a pill count to evaluate ability to adhere to regimen.

III. ALTERATION IN SKIN INTEGRITY/COMFORT related to RASH, PRURITUS, ALOPECIA

Defining Characteristics: Skin rash, itching, and mild alopecia may occur, and are mild.

Nursing Implications: Teach patient about the possibility of these side effects and to notify the nurse if any develop. Discuss rash with physician if moderate or severe. Teach patient local symptom-management strategies for itch. Reassure patient that hair loss is usually thinning with mild hair loss and will grow back.

IV. ACTIVITY INTOLERANCE POTENTIAL, related to CENTRAL NERVOUS SYSTEM EFFECTS

Defining Characteristics: Lethargy (up to 40% in patients with malignant glioma), fatigue, headache, ataxia, and dizziness may occur, and in clinical testing, it was unclear whether this was due to neurological disease (i.e., malignant glioma), concurrent other drug therapy, or temozolomide.

Nursing Implications: Assess baseline energy and activity level. Teach patients that these side effects may occur, especially if the primary diagnosis is malignant glioma. Teach patient to report them. Teach patient to alternate rest and activity periods, to use supportive device such as a cane if ataxia or dizziness occurs, and other measures to maximize activity tolerance and to prevent injury.

Drug: teniposide (Vumon, VM-26), investigational

Class: Plant alkaloid, a derivative of the mandrake plant (*Mandragora officinarum*).

Mechanism of Action: Cell cycle specific in late S phase, early G_2 phase, causing arrest of cell division in mitosis. Inhibits uptake of thymidine into DNA so DNA synthesis is impaired.

Metabolism: Drug binds extensively to serum protein. Metabolized by the liver and excreted in bile and urine. Half-life is 5 hours.

Dosage/Range:

- 100 mg/m^2 weekly for 6–8 weeks.
- 50 mg/m^2 twice weekly × 4 weeks.

Drug Preparation:

- Available in 50-mg/5-mL glass ampules.
- Add desired 0.9% sodium chloride for injection or 5% dextrose in water to reach final concentration of 0.1 mg/mL–0.4 mg/mL (stable 24 hours) or 1.0 mg/mL (stable 4 hours).
- USE ONLY non-DEHP containers such as glass or polyolefin plastic bags or containers.
- DO NOT USE polyvinylchloride IV bags, as the plasticizer DEHP will leach into the solution.

Drug Administration:

- Assess for presence of precipitate and do not administer solution if precipitate is seen.
- Administer over at least 30–60 minutes.

Drug Interactions:

- Doses of tolbutamide, sodium salicylate, and sulfamethizole will need to be reduced.
- Heparin causes a precipitate.
- Glucosamine: causes tumor resistance to teniposide; DO NOT give together.
- Phenytoin, phenobarbital: increase teniposide serum levels; avoid coadministration or decrease dose.
- Methotrexate: may increase tumor concentration of drug.
- Vincristine: may increase intensity of peripheral neuropathy; do not give together.

Lab Effects/Interference:

- Increased LFTs, RFTs.
- Decreased CBC.

Special Considerations:

- Rapid infusion may cause hypotension and sudden death.
- Chemical phlebitis may occur if drug is not properly diluted, or infused too rapidly.
- Severe myelosuppression may occur.
- Hypersensitivity reactions, including anaphylaxis-like symptoms, may occur with initial or repeated doses.

Potential Toxicities/Side Effects and the Nursing Process

I. POTENTIAL FOR INJURY DURING DRUG ADMINISTRATION related to HYPOTENSION AND HYPERSENSITIVITY REACTION

Defining Characteristics: Hypotension may occur during rapid IV infusion. Hypersensitivity reactions occur in 5% of patients, characterized by fever, chills, tachycardia, dyspnea, flushing, lumbar pain, bronchospasm, and progressive hypotension or hypertension. It is thought that hypersensitivity may be to the drug suspension of castor oil and denatured alcohol, which is used because the drug is poorly water-soluble.

Nursing Implications: Assess baseline temperature (T), VS prior to drug administration, and periodically during infusion. Ensure that drug is properly diluted, and infuse over at least 30–60 minutes. Instruct patient to report untoward signs/symptoms immediately. Have emergency equipment and medications, including epinephrine, diphenhydramine, hydrocortisone nearby. If signs/symptoms develop, stop infusion, keep IV line open, notify physician, monitor VS, and support patient. Be familiar with institution's standing orders or practice guidelines on management of anaphylaxis.

II. POTENTIAL FOR INFECTION AND BLEEDING related to BONE MARROW DEPRESSION

Defining Characteristics: Leukopenia is dose-limiting toxicity but thrombocytopenia may occur; nadir day 7 (3–14 days). Dose reductions need to be made if patient previously received chemotherapy or radiotherapy.

Nursing Implications: Assess CBC, WBC, differential, and platelet count prior to drug administration, as well as for signs/symptoms of infection and bleeding. Teach patient signs/symptoms of infection and bleeding, and instruct to report them immediately. Teach patient self-care measures to minimize infection and bleeding, including avoidance of OTC aspirin-containing medications.

III. ALTERATION IN NUTRITION, LESS THAN BODY REQUIREMENTS, related to NAUSEA AND VOMITING, HEPATIC DYSFUNCTION, MUCOSITIS

Defining Characteristics: Nausea and vomiting occur in 29% of patients but are usually mild; mucositis occurs at high drug doses. Mild elevation of LFTs may occur.

Nursing Implications: Premedicate with antiemetics prior to drug administration, and continue prophylactically for 24 hours, at least for the first cycle. Assess oral mucosa at baseline prior to drug administration; teach patient self-assessment and self-care measures. Monitor LFTs prior to drug administration; discuss dose reduction with physician if results abnormal.

IV. POTENTIAL FOR IMPAIRED SKIN INTEGRITY related to ALOPECIA AND PHLEBITIS

Defining Characteristics: Alopecia is uncommon (9–30% of patients) and is reversible. Phlebitis can occur if drug is improperly diluted or administered too rapidly.

Nursing Implications: If patient develops hair loss, discuss impact of loss and suggest coping strategies, such as wig or cap. Encourage patient to verbalize feelings and provide emotional support. Administer drug only through patent IV, properly diluted, and over at least 30–60 minutes.

V. POTENTIAL FOR SENSORY/PERCEPTUAL ALTERATIONS related to NEUROLOGIC TOXICITY

Defining Characteristics: Peripheral neuropathies may occur and are mild.

Nursing Implications: Assess baseline neurologic status. Teach patient to report any changes in motor or sensory functioning. Encourage patient to verbalize feelings regarding discomfort and sensory loss if these occur.

VI. POTENTIAL FOR ALTERATION IN CARDIAC OUTPUT related to HYPOTENSION AND PALPITATIONS

Defining Characteristics: Hypotension is related to rapid infusion of drug. Palpitations may occur during drug infusion.

Nursing Implications: Assess baseline cardiac status, noting heart rate, rhythm, and monitor heart rate and BP periodically during infusion. Infuse drug over at least 30–60 minutes.

VII. POTENTIAL SEXUAL DYSFUNCTION related to DRUG EFFECT

Defining Characteristics: Drug is carcinogenic, mutagenic, and teratogenic. It is not known if drug is excreted in breast milk.

Nursing Implications: Assess patient's and partner's sexual patterns and reproductive goals. Provide information, supportive counseling, and referral as needed and appropriate. Teach importance of contraception and discuss coping strategies for alterations in fertility (e.g., sperm banking). Mothers receiving drug should not breast-feed.

Drug: thioguanine (Tabloid, 6-Thioguanine, 6-TG)

Class: Thiopurine antimetabolite.

Mechanism of Action: Converts to monophosphate nucleotides and inhibits *de novo* purine synthesis. The nucleotides are also incorporated into DNA. Cell cycle phase specific for S phase. Thioguanine interferes with nucleic acid biosynthesis, resulting in sequential blockage of the synthesis and utilization of the purine nucleotides.

Metabolism: Oral absorption is incomplete (30%) and variable, with a plasma half-life of 11 hours. Food may affect absorption. Drug is metabolized in the liver by deamination and methylation. Metabolites are excreted in the urine and feces.

Dosage/Range:
- Children and adults: 100 mg/m^2 orally every 12 hours for 5–10 days, usually in combination with cytarabine and then 100 mg/m^2 orally every 12 hours for 5 days repeated every 4 weeks for maintenance.
- 1–3 mg/kg orally daily OR 75–200 mg/m^2/day orally in one to two divided doses × 5–7 days or until remission.

Drug Preparation:
- Available in 40-mg tablets.

Drug Administration:
- Given orally between meals; can be given as a single dose.

Drug Interactions:
- Busulfan: increased hepatotoxicity; use caution when used together; monitor patient closely during long-term therapy.
- Other hepatotoxic drugs: increased risk of hepatotoxicity.

Lab Effects/Interference:
- Decreased CBC.
- Increased LFTs.
- Increased uric acid.

Special Considerations:
- Oral dose is to be given on empty stomach to facilitate absorption.
- Dose is titrated to avoid excessive stomatitis and diarrhea.
- Thioguanine can be used in full doses with allopurinol.
- Veno-occlusive disease of the liver can rarely occur; monitor LFTs baseline and during treatment.

Potential Toxicities/Side Effects and the Nursing Process

I. ALTERATION IN NUTRITION, LESS THAN BODY REQUIREMENTS, related to GI SIDE EFFECTS

Defining Characteristics: Nausea and vomiting occur commonly, especially in children, but are dose related; anorexia is rare; stomatitis is rare, but most common with high doses; hepatotoxicity is rare, but may be associated with hepatic veno-occlusive disease or jaundice.

Nursing Implications: Treat symptomatically with antiemetics. Encourage small, frequent feedings of cool, bland foods and liquids. If vomiting occurs, assess for fluid and electrolyte imbalance. Monitor I/O and daily weights if patient is hospitalized. Encourage small, frequent meals of favorite foods, especially high-calorie, high-protein foods. Encourage use of spices; weekly weights. Teach oral assessment and oral hygiene regimen. Encourage patient to report early stomatitis. Provide pain relief measures, if indicated. Monitor LFTs prior to drug dose. Assess patient prior to and during treatment for signs/symptoms of hepatotoxicity. Discuss drug dose reduction if mucositis or diarrhea occurs and is severe.

II. POTENTIAL FOR INFECTION AND BLEEDING related to BONE MARROW DEPRESSION

Defining Characteristics: Bone marrow depression occurs 1–4 weeks after treatment, with nadir 10–14 days and recovery by day 21. Leukopenia and thrombocytopenia are most common. Immunosuppression may occur, with increased risk of bacterial, fungal, and parasitic infections.

Nursing Implications: Monitor CBC, platelet count prior to drug administration as well as for signs/symptoms of infection or bleeding. Instruct patient in self-assessment of signs/symptoms of infection or bleeding. Administer platelet, red cell transfusions per physician's order.

III. POTENTIAL FOR SENSORY/PERCEPTUAL ALTERATION related to LOSS OF VIBRATORY SENSE

Defining Characteristics: Loss of vibratory sensation; unsteady gait may occur.

Nursing Implications: Assess vibratory sensation, gait before each dose and between treatments. Report changes to physician. Encourage patient to report any changes.

Drug: thiotepa (Thioplex, Triethylenethiophosphoramide)

Class: Alkylating agent.

Mechanism of Action: Selectively reacts with DNA phosphate groups to produce chromosome cross-linkage with blocking of nucleoprotein synthesis. Acts as a polyfunctional alkylating agent. Cell cycle phase nonspecific agent. Mimics radiation-induced injury.

Metabolism: Rapidly cleared following IV administration and 40% bound to plasm proteins. Slow onset of action, slowly bound to tissues, extensively metabolized. Metabolized by the P450 microenzyme system in the liver with 63% of dose eliminated in urine within 24–72 hours. When high doses are given in the transplant setting, some of the drug is excreted as perspiration.

Dosage/Range:

Intravenous:

- 8 mg/m^2 (0.2 mg/kg) IV every day × 5 days, repeated every 3–4 weeks, OR
- 0.3–0.4 mg/kg IV, every 1–4 weeks.
- High dose (transplant): 180–1100 mg/m^2 IV.

Intracavitary:

- Bladder: 60 mg in 30- to 60-mL sterile water once a week for 3–4 weeks.

Intracavitary (Effusions):

- 0.6–0.8 mg/kg every 1–4 weeks.

Drug Preparation:

- Add sterile water to vial of lyophilized powder.
- Further dilute with 0.9% sodium chloride or 5% dextrose.
- Do not use solution unless it is clear.
- Refrigerate vial until use (reconstituted solution is stable for 5 days).

Drug Administration:

- IV, IM; intracavitary, intratumor, intra-arterial.

Drug Interactions:

- Myelosuppressive drugs: additive hematologic toxicity.

Lab Effects/Interference:

- Decreased CBC (especially WBC and platelets).
- Increased LFTs and RFTs.

Special Considerations:

- Hypersensitivity reactions have occurred with this drug.
- Is an irritant; should be given IVP via a sidearm of a running IV.
- Increased neuromuscular blockage when given with nondepolarizing muscle relaxants.
- Used intrathecally for leptomeningeal metastases in investigational settings.
- Monitor CBC in patients receiving intravesicular administration of drug, as systemic absorption may occur.

- Second malignancies may occur (e.g., AML, breast and lung cancers).
- High-dose therapy: mucositis, nausea and vomiting, skin changes (skin bronzing, rash, flaking/desquamation of skin).

Potential Toxicities/Side Effects and the Nursing Process

I. POTENTIAL FOR INFECTION AND BLEEDING related to BONE MARROW DEPRESSION

Defining Characteristics: Nadir is 5–30 days after drug administration (WBC 7–10 days, platelets day 21), with recovery of WBC by day 21 and platelets by day 28–35. Thrombocytopenia and leukopenia may occur. Anemia may occur with prolonged use. May be cumulative toxicity with recovery of bone marrow in 40–50 days. Thrombocytopenia is dose limiting.

Nursing Implications: Monitor CBC, platelet count prior to drug administration; monitor for signs/symptoms of infection or bleeding. Instruct patient in self-assessment of signs/symptoms of infection (e.g., temperature > 100.4°F, chills, rigors, colored sputum, burning when urinating, difficulty breathing) or bleeding and to report them immediately. Teach self-care strategies to protect patient from infection (e.g., avoiding crowds, people with colds, handwashing) and bleeding (e.g., wearing gloves when gardening, using electric shaver rather than razor). Administer red cells and platelet transfusions per physician's orders.

II. ALTERATION IN NUTRITION, LESS THAN BODY REQUIREMENTS, related to GI SIDE EFFECTS

Defining Characteristics: Nausea and vomiting occur in 10–15% of patients; dose-dependent; occurs 6–12 hours after drug dose; anorexia occurs occasionally.

Nursing Implications: Premedicate with antiemetics especially with parenteral dosing of high dose. Continue antiemetics at least 12 hours after drug is given. Encourage small, frequent meals of cool, bland, dry foods, and favorite foods, especially high-calorie, high-protein foods. Encourage use of spices; assess weight weekly. Teach patient to report diarrhea that does not resolve in 24 hours and self-administration of antidiarrheals if at home and to increase oral fluids to 2–3 liters a day.

III. POTENTIAL SEXUAL DYSFUNCTION related to DRUG EFFECT

Defining Characteristics: Drug is mutagenic. Sterility may be reversible and incomplete. Amenorrhea often reverses in 6–8 months.

Nursing Implications: As appropriate, explore with patient and partner issues of reproductive and sexuality patterns and the anticipated impact chemotherapy may have. Discuss strategies to preserve sexuality and reproductive health (e.g., sperm banking).

IV. POTENTIAL FOR INJURY related to ALLERGIC REACTION

Defining Characteristics: Allergic responses occur rarely: hives, bronchospasm, skin rash (dermatitis). Secondary malignancies may occur with prolonged therapy.

Nursing Implications: Assess for signs/symptoms of allergic response during drug administration. Stop drug if bronchospasm occurs and notify physician. If symptomatic, institute emergency measures such as bronchodilator, and support other vital signs as needed. Discuss symptomatic treatment with physician. Instruct patient receiving prolonged therapy about importance of regular health maintenance examinations during and after therapy by primary care provider and oncologist.

V. ALTERATION IN COMFORT related to DIZZINESS, FEVER, PAIN

Defining Characteristics: Dizziness, headache, fever, and local pain may occur.

Nursing Implications: Assess for alterations in comfort. Treat symptomatically.

Drug: topotecan hydrochloride for injection (Hycamtin)

Class: Topoisomerase I inhibitor.

Mechanism of Action: Topoisomerase I causes reversible single-strand breaks in DNA, which permits relaxation of DNA helix prior to DNA replication. Topotecan binds to the topoisomerase I-DNA complex thus preventing repair (religation) of the strand breaks. When the cell tries to synthesize DNA, replication enzymes interact with the complex, and this leads to double-strand DNA breaks that cannot be repaired; thus, drug prevents DNA synthesis and replication and leads to cell death.

Metabolism: After IV administration, extensively tissue bound, with about 35% of drug bound to plasma proteins. Crosses BBB. 30% of dose is excreted in the urine. Patients with moderate renal impairment have a 33% decrease in plasma clearance; patients with moderate impairment require a dosage adjustment. Minor metabolism by the liver, so patients with liver dysfunction do not require dose modification. The oral formulation is rapidly absorbed with peak plasma concentration occurring between 1 to 2 hours and 40% bioavailability. Drug demonstrates biexponential pharmacokinetics, and the mean terminal half-life is 3–6 hours. Drug binds to plasma proteins 35%. Fifty-seven percent of the oral dose (five daily doses) was recovered; 20% was excreted in the urine and 33% in the feces.

Dosage/Range:

- IV: Metastatic carcinoma of the ovary after failure of initial or subsequent chemo: 1.5 mg/m^2 IV infusion over 30 minutes for 5 consecutive days every 21 days, but many oncologists use dose of 1.25 mg/m^2, which the manufacturer says has equal efficacy.
- IV: Small-cell lung cancer (SCLC) after failure of first-line chemotherapy: same.
- PO: Relapsed SCLC: 2.3 mg/m^2/d PO × 5 consecutive days, repeated every 21 days. Dose modified for grades 3/4 bone marrow toxicity.

Dose Reduction:

- IV: Ovarian and SCLC:
  - Neutropenia ANC < 1500 cells/mm^3 or platelet count falls to < 25,000 cells/mm^3 during treatment, decrease next dose by 0.25 mg/m^2 or add G-CSF beginning on day 4 (24 hours after the last dose of topotecan) of the next cycle.
  - Counts must be ANC > 1000 cells/mm^3, platelet count > 100,000 cells/mm^3, and Hgb 9.0 g/dL before resuming next cycle.
- IV: Cervical cancer:
  - Severe, febrile neutropenia (ANC < 1000 cells/mm^3 with temperature of 38°C or 100.4°F), reduce dose 20% to 0.60 mg/m^2 for subsequent courses or add G-CSF beginning on day 4 (24 hours after the last dose of topotecan) of the next cycle. If febrile neutropenia again develops despite G-CSF, dose reduce another 20% to 0.45 mg/m^2 for subsequent courses.
  - 20% DR if platelets < 10,000 cells/mm^3.
  - Serum creatinine must be < 1.5 g/dL to administer topotecan with cisplatin.
- Moderate renal impairment (creatinine clearance 20–39 mL/min): 0.75 mg/m^2 should be the starting dose.
  - PO: Relapsed SCLC: bone marrow depression OR grades 3/4. Diarrhea: Reduce dose by 0.4 mg/m^2/day for subsequent doses for the following:
    - ANC must be > 1000 cells/mm^3, platelets > 100,000 cells/mm^3, and hemoglobin level ≥ 9.0 g/dL (with transfusion if necessary).
  - If severe neutropenia (febrile neutropenia lasting 7 or more days with ANC < 500 cells/mm^3), or neutropenia lasting beyond day 21 of treatment course (500–1000 cells/mm^3):
    - Platelet nadir < 25,000 cells/mm^3.
    - Grades 3/4 diarrhea (some patients with grade 2 diarrhea may need this same dose reduction).

Drug Preparation:

- IV formulation available as a 4-mg vial.
- Reconstitute vial with 4 mL sterile water for injection.
- Further dilute in 0.9% sodium chloride or 5% dextrose.
- Use immediately.
- PO formulation: Available as 0.25-mg capsules (opaque white to yellowish white) and 1.0 mg (opaque pink).

Drug Administration:

- Baseline ANC for initial course must be ≥ 1500/mm^3 and platelets > 100,000/mm^3, and for subsequent courses, ANC ≥ 1000/mm^3, platelets 100,000/mm^3, and hemoglobin ≥ 9 mg/dL.
- Ovarian and SCLC: Administer 1.5 mg/m^2 IV over 30 minutes, days 1–5, with cycle repeated q 21 days.
- G-CSF may be required if neutropenia develops.
- Cervical cancer: 0.75 mg/m^2 IV days 1, 2, 3 followed by cisplatin 50 mg/m^2 IV over 1 hour on day 1 of the cycle, and the cycle repeated every 21 days.

Drug Interactions:

- PO: P = glycoprotein inhibitors (e.g., cyclosporine A, elacridar, ketoconazole, ritonavir, and saquinavir): increase topotecan exposure; avoid concurrent use.

Lab Effects/Interference:

- Decreased CBC.
- Increased LFTs, RFTs

Special Considerations:

- Indicated for the treatment of patients with (1) metastatic cancer of the ovary after failure of initial or subsequent chemotherapy; (2) SCLC sensitive disease (response to chemotherapy with progression at least 60–90 days after chemotherapy) and failure of first line chemotherapy; (3) stage IV-B recurrent or persistent carcinoma of the cervix, not amenable to curative surgical treatment and/or radiotherapy. Oral formulation FDA approved for treatment of patients with relapsed SCLC.
- IV: Minimum of 4 courses needed, as clinical responses occur 9–12 weeks after beginning of therapy.
- Contraindicated in patients with history of severe hypersensitivity reactions to topotecan or any of the components; pregnant or breast-feeding mothers; patients with severe bone marrow depression.
- Oral formulation: Teach patient to store pills out of reach of children and pets, at controlled room temperature, and protected from light.

Potential Toxicities/Side Effects and the Nursing Process

I. INFECTION AND BLEEDING related to BONE MARROW DEPRESSION

Defining Characteristics: IV formulation: Myelosuppression is the dose-limiting toxicity. Severe grade 4 neutropenia is seen during the first course of therapy in 60% of patients. Febrile neutropenia or sepsis may occur in up to 26% of patients. Nadir occurs on day 11. Prophylactic G-CSF is needed in 27% of courses after the first cycle. Thrombocytopenia (grade 4 with platelet count < 25,000/mm^3) occurs in 26% of patients. Platelet nadir occurs on day 15. Severe anemia (Hgb < 8 gm/dL) occurs in 40% of patients, and transfusions were needed for 56% of patients. Oral formulation: Grades 3/4 neutropenia occurred in 61% of patients, anemia in 25%, and thrombocytopenia in 37%.

Nursing Implications: Monitor CBC and platelet count prior to drug administration as well as signs/symptoms of infection or bleeding. Assess renal function baseline and prior to each treatment. Discuss dose reductions with physician (see Special Considerations section). Instruct patient in self-assessment of signs/symptoms of infection or bleeding. Administer RBCs and platelet transfusions per physician's orders. Teach patient self-administration of G-CSF as ordered. Discuss dose modification with physician depending on severity of bone marrow depression.

II. ALTERATION IN NUTRITION, LESS THAN BODY REQUIREMENTS, related to NAUSEA AND VOMITING, DIARRHEA, ELEVATED LFTS

Defining Characteristics: IV formulation: Nausea occurs in 77% of patients, and vomiting in 58% without premedication with antiemetics. Diarrhea occurs in 42% of patients, while constipation occurs in 39%. Abdominal pain may occur in 33% of patients. Aspirate aminotransferase (AST, previously SGOT) and alanine aminotransferase (ALT, previously SGPT) elevations occur in 5% of patients. Oral formulation: Grades 3/4 nausea occurred in 27% of patients and vomiting in 19%. Diarrhea occurred in 14%.

Nursing Implications: Premedicate with a serotonin antagonist or dopamine antagonist antiemetic, and continue prophylactically for 24 hours to prevent nausea and vomiting, at least for the first treatment. Teach patient to take oral antiemetics 1 hour before taking oral topotecan. Encourage small, frequent feedings of cool, bland, dry foods. Assess for symptoms of fluid and electrolyte imbalance: monitor I/O and daily weights if administered to an inpatient. Teach patient oral assessment and oral hygiene regimen. Encourage patient to report early stomatitis. Provide pain relief measures if indicated (e.g., topical anesthetics). Encourage patient to report onset of diarrhea. Administer or teach patient to self-administer antidiarrheal medication. Ensure adequate hydration, monitor I/O. Monitor LFTs baseline and periodically during treatment. Discuss dose modification with physician depending on severity of diarrhea in patients receiving oral topotecan.

III. POTENTIAL FOR HEPATOTOXICITY related to HYPOALBUMINEMIA, PREEXISTING HEPATIC INSUFFICIENCY (IV formulation)

Defining Characteristics: Evidence of increased drug toxicity in patients with low protein and hepatic dysfunction. Dose reductions may be necessary.

Nursing Implications: Monitor LFTs prior to drug dose. Assess patient prior to administering drug and during treatment for signs/symptoms of hepatotoxicity.

IV. POTENTIAL FOR SKIN INTEGRITY IMPAIRMENT related to ALOPECIA (oral formulation)

Defining Characteristics: Alopecia occurs in 10–20% of patients.

Nursing Implications: Assess patient for signs/symptoms of hair loss. Instruct patient to report any of these symptoms. Discuss with patient the impact of skin changes.

Drug: toremifene citrate (Fareston)

Class: Synthetic tamoxifen analogue (antiestrogen); selective estrogen receptor modulator (SERM).

Mechanism of Action: Nonsteroidal estrogen antagonist: competitively binds directly to estrogen receptors in breast cancer cells, preventing estrogen from binding. Has four to five times more affinity for estrogen receptor than tamoxifen.

Metabolism: Well absorbed following oral dose. Highly protein bound (99%). Peak serum level after single dose is 3 hours, with terminal half-life of 5–6.2 days. Extensively metabolized in the liver by the P-450 enzyme system. Increased terminal half-life (decreased clearance) in patients with hepatic dysfunction to 10.9 days and 21 days for the principal metabolite. Clearance not significantly changed with renal impairment. Excreted in feces and to a lesser extent urine.

Dosage/Range:
- 60 mg orally, daily.

Drug Preparation/Administration:
- None.

Drug Interactions:
- Warfarin: increased anticoagulation effect; monitor INR and dose accordingly.
- Thiazide diuretics: increases risk of hypercalcemia (decreased calcium excretion).
- CYP3A4 inducers (carbamazepine, phenobarbital, phenytoin, ranitidine, rifampin), and St. John's wort: may decrease toremifene serum level and effect; assess for inadequate dose, and discontinue St. John's wort.
- CYP3A4 inhibitors (ciprofloxacin, clarithromycin, doxycycline, erythromycin, isoniazid, itraconazole, propofol, verapamil, others): may increase toremifene serum level and toxicity; assess for adverse effects.
- Metabolism is inhibited by testosterone and cyclosporin.
- Appears to enhance inhibition of multidrug-resistant cell lines by vinblastine.
- Appears to be cross-resistant with tamoxifen.

Lab Effects/Interference:
- Decreased WBC and platelets (mild).
- Increased alkaline phosphatase, bilirubin, calcium, AST.

Special Considerations:
- Activity, side effects, toxicity in postmenopausal women or women with unknown receptor status appear similar.
- Contraindicated in patients with endometrial hyperplasia as increased risk of endometrial cancer.
- Use cautiously in patients with history of thromboembolic events and patients with brain or vertebral metastases.
- Monitor CBC and LFTs baseline and periodically during treatment.
- Cataracts may develop so patient should be taught to have eye exams by an ophthalmologist baseline and then twice yearly.
- Patients are at risk for endometrial cancer. Teach patient to have a baseline then annual gynecology exam with endometrial biopsy. Teach patient to call right away for a gynecologic exam if vaginal bleeding occurs.

Potential Toxicities/Side Effects and the Nursing Process

I. POTENTIAL FOR SEXUAL DYSFUNCTION related to MENSTRUAL IRREGULARITIES, HOT FLASHES

Defining Characteristics: Similar to tamoxifen toxicity profile. May cause menstrual irregularity, hot flashes (most common), milk production in breasts, and vaginal discharge and bleeding.

Nursing Implications: As appropriate, explore with patient and partner issues of reproductive and sexuality patterns and the impact drug may have on them. Discuss strategies to preserve sexual and reproductive health.

II. POTENTIAL FOR ALTERATION IN COMFORT related to FLARE REACTION

Defining Characteristics: May cause flare reaction initially (bone and tumor pain, transient increase in tumor size). Nausea, vomiting, and anorexia may occur. Tremor may occur and be significant in some patients.

Nursing Implications: Inform patient of flare reaction, signs/symptoms to be aware of, and encourage patient to report any signs/symptoms. Inform patient of possibility of nausea, vomiting, and anorexia. Encourage small, frequent feedings of high-calorie, high-protein foods. Teach patients to report tremor, and discuss impact on self-care ability and comfort. If patient has brain or vertebral metastases, observe closely; any transient increase in tumor size may cause severe neurological symptoms.

III. POTENTIAL FOR INFECTION AND BLEEDING related to BONE MARROW DEPRESSION

Defining Characteristics: Mild, transient leukopenia and thrombocytopenia occur rarely. Lowest WBC count in clinical trials was $2500/mm^3$.

Nursing Implications: Monitor CBC and platelet count prior to drug administration and after therapy has begun. Instruct patient in self-assessment of signs/symptoms of infection or bleeding.

IV. POTENTIAL FOR SKIN INTEGRITY IMPAIRMENT related to RASH, ALOPECIA

Defining Characteristics: Skin rash, alopecia, and peripheral edema are rare.

Nursing Implications: Assess patient for signs/symptoms of hair loss, edema, and skin rash. Instruct patient to report any of these symptoms. Discuss with patient the impact of skin changes.

Drug: trimetrexate (Neutrexin)

Class: Antimetabolite.

Mechanism of Action: Nonclassical folate antagonist; potent inhibitor of dihydrofolate reductase. May be able to overcome mechanism(s) of methotrexate resistance as drug reaches higher concentration within tumor cells. Also, inhibits growth of parasitic infective agents (causing *Pneumocystis carinii* pneumonia [PCP], toxoplasmosis) in patients with immunodeficiency or myelodysplastic disorders.

Metabolism: Significant percentage of drug is protein-bound. Metabolized by liver; 10–20% of dose is excreted by kidneys in 24 hours.

Dosage/Range:

For PCP indication:

- 45 mg/m^2 daily IV infusion over 60–90 minutes × 21 days.
- Leucovorin 20 mg/m^2 IV over 5–10 minutes q 6 hours (80 mg/m^2 24-hour total dose), or 20 mg/m^2 PO qid for days of trimetrexate treatment, extending 72 hours past the last dose of trimetrexate, for a total of 24 days.

Drug Preparation:

- Reconstitute with 2 mL 5% dextrose USP or sterile water for injection (12.5 mg of trimetrexate/mL).
- Filter with 0.22-μ m filter prior to further dilution; observe for cloudiness or precipitate.
- Further dilute in 5% dextrose to a final concentration of 0.25–2.00 mg/mL.
- Stable 24 hours at room temperature or refrigerated.

Drug Administration:
- IV infusion over 60 minutes.
- Incompatible with chloride solutions, as precipitate forms immediately, and leucovorin.
- Leucovorin can be started either before or after first trimetrexate dose, but ensure that IV line is flushed with at least 10 mL of 5% dextrose between drugs.

Drug Interactions:
- Drug is metabolized by P-450 enzyme system, so interactions are possible with erythromycin, fluconazole, ketoconazole, rifabutin, rifampin, protease inhibitors.

Lab Effects/Interference:
- Decreased CBC.
- Increased LFTs, RFTs (especially creatinine).
- Decreased Ca, Na.

Special Considerations:
- Indicated for alternative treatment of moderate-to-severe PCP in patients with immunodeficiency, including AIDS patients who are intolerant or refractory to trimethoprim-sulfamethoxazole (TMP-SMX), or for whom TMP-SMX is contraindicated.
- Increased toxicity is seen in patients with low protein (drug is highly protein bound) and hepatic dysfunction. Dose reduction is indicated.
- Leukopenia is dose-limiting toxicity.
- Other side effects are nausea and vomiting, rash, mucositis, AST elevations, thrombocytopenia.
- Drug is fetotoxic and embryotoxic. Women of childbearing age should use contraceptive measures to prevent pregnancy while receiving the drug.
- Zidovudine (AZT) therapy should be interrupted while receiving trimetrexate.
- Use cautiously in patients with renal, hepatic, or hematologic impairment.
- Transaminase levels or alk phos > 5 times upper limit of normal: HOLD DOSE.
- Serum creatinine ≥ 2.5 mg/dL due to trimetrexate: HOLD DOSE.
- Severe mucosal toxicity (unable to eat): HOLD DOSE, and continue leucovorin.
- Temperature ≥ 40.5°C (105°F) uncontrolled by antipyretics: HOLD DOSE.
- Hematologic toxicity: HOLD DOSE and consult package insert.

Potential Toxicities/Side Effects and the Nursing Process

I. INFECTION AND BLEEDING related to BONE MARROW DEPRESSION

Defining Characteristics: Leukopenia is a dose-limiting toxicity. Thrombocytopenia also occurs commonly.

Nursing Implications: Monitor CBC, platelet count prior to drug administration, as well as for signs/symptoms of infection or bleeding. Instruct patient in self-assessment of signs/symptoms of infection or bleeding. Administer red cells and platelet transfusions per physician's orders.

II. ALTERATION IN NUTRITION, LESS THAN BODY REQUIREMENTS, related to GI SIDE EFFECTS

Defining Characteristics: Nausea and vomiting have been reported in clinical trials; drug has been reported to cause stomatitis; diarrhea may occur also.

Nursing Implications: Premedicate with antiemetics and continue prophylactically for 24 hours to prevent nausea and vomiting, at least for the first treatment. Encourage small, frequent feedings of cool, bland, dry foods. Assess for symptoms of fluid and electrolyte imbalance: monitor I/O, daily weights if administered to an inpatient. Teach patient oral assessment and oral hygiene regimen. Encourage patient to report early stomatitis. Provide pain relief measures if indicated (e.g., topical anesthetics). Encourage patient to report onset of diarrhea. Administer or teach patient to self-administer antidiarrheal medication. Guaiac all stools. Ensure adequate hydration; monitor I/O.

III. POTENTIAL FOR IMPAIRED SKIN INTEGRITY related to ALOPECIA

Defining Characteristics: Alopecia is total in 42% of patients.

Nursing Implications: Discuss with patient the impact of hair loss. As appropriate, suggest wig prior to actual hair loss. Explore patient's response to actual hair loss and plan strategies to minimize distress (e.g., wig, scarf, cap).

IV. ALTERATION IN COMFORT related to HEADACHE

Defining Characteristics: Headache occurs in 21% of patients. Paresthesias may affect 9% of patients.

Nursing Implications: Teach patient that headache may occur and is usually relieved by acetaminophen. Instruct patient to report headache that is not relieved by usual methods.

V. ALTERATION IN OXYGEN POTENTIAL related to DYSPNEA

Defining Characteristics: Dyspnea may occur in 20% of patients, and is severe in 4% of patients.

Nursing Implications: Assess baseline pulmonary status, including presence of dyspnea, and history since last treatment prior to successive drug administrations.

Instruct patient to report new onset or worsening of dyspnea. Discuss occurrences with physician to determine further diagnostic evaluation.

Drug: triptorelin pamoate (Trelstar LA, Trelstar Depot)

Class: Luteinizing hormone-releasing hormone (LHRH) agonist, gonadotropin-releasing hormone (GnRH) agonist.

Mechanism of Action: Potently inhibits gonadotropin secretion, resulting in an initial surge in circulating levels of luteinizing hormone (LH), follicle-stimulating hormone (FSH), testosterone, and estradiol, and then after 2 to 4 weeks of continued drug administration, sustained decreases in LH and FSH secretion, resulting in a reduction of testosterone similar to surgical castration serum levels. This removes the hormonal stimulation from prostate cancer cells, and stops the growth and proliferation of prostate cells. The drug effect is reversible following discontinuance of the drug.

Metabolism: After IM administration, the drug probably undergoes metabolism by the liver, with excretion by liver and kidneys.

Dosage/Range:
- Trelstar depot: 3.75 mg IM once every 28 days.
- Trelstar LA: 11.25 mg IM once every 84 days.

Drug Preparation:
- Using the manufacturer's Clip'n'Ject system, reconstitute drug vial with 2-mL sterile water, shake well, inspect milky solution that results.
- Draw up and administer using the Clip'n'Ject (see package insert).

Drug Administration:
- Administer in large muscle and rotate sites.
- Administer Trelstar LA in buttock.

Lab Effects/Interference:
- Decreased serum testosterone levels.

Special Considerations:
- Indicated for the palliative treatment of patients with advanced prostate cancer for whom orchiectomy or estrogen therapy is unacceptable.
- Monitor drug effectiveness (serum testosterone level, PSA).
- Monitor patients closely after first two treatments, as rarely, anaphylaxis with/without angioedema may occur.
- Monitor patients with bony metastases or disease that could cause ureteral obstruction closely after initial treatment, as flare may cause ureteral obstruction or spinal cord compression depending on location of metastases. In extreme cases, orchiectomy may be required to relieve obstruction of ureters.

- Drug is used off-label for the treatment of patients with endometriosis, in vitro fertilization, and ovarian cancer.
- Contraindicated in pregnant or breast-feeding women.
- Rarely can cause pituitary apoplexy (pituitary infarction) in patients who have an adenoma, characterized by sudden headache, vomiting, visual changes, ophthalmoplegia (paralysis or weakness of the muscles that control eye movement), altered mental status, and sometimes cardiovascular collapse after the first dose (within hours to 2 weeks). Emergency medical care is required.

Potential Toxicities/Side Effects and the Nursing Process

I. ALTERATION IN COMFORT related to HOT FLASHES, TUMOR FLARE, LEG PAIN, EYE PAIN, HEADACHE, EDEMA

Defining Characteristics: Initially, drug causes increased LH secretion, resulting in increased testosterone secretion and tumor flare. Usually disappears after 2 weeks. Headache, dizziness, and hot flashes may occur. Vasodilation most common. Tumor flare may also occur initially (bone and tumor pain, transient increase in tumor size due to transient increase in testosterone levels). Breast tenderness has been reported. Peripheral edema, leg and eye pain, headache may occur.

Nursing Implications: Inform patient that symptoms may occur and that flare reaction will subside after the initial 2 weeks of therapy. Assess and document pain score baseline, and teach patient to report pain, especially if it is new onset of back pain that may be radicular, or pelvic pain, hematuria, or urinary retention. Encourage patient to report symptoms early. Triage symptoms, and discuss emergency management if severe symptoms develop. Develop symptom management plan with patient and physician. Monitor patients with disease near ureters or bony metastases closely after initial treatment, as ureteral obstruction and spinal cord compression have occurred.

II. POTENTIAL SEXUAL DYSFUNCTION related to LIBIDO, IMPOTENCE

Defining Characteristics: Frequently causes decreased libido and erectile impotence in men. Gynecomastia occurs in 1–10% of patients. In women, amenorrhea occurs after 10 weeks of therapy.

Nursing Implications: As appropriate, explore with patient and significant other issues of reproductive and sexual patterns and the impact chemotherapy may have on them. Discuss strategies to preserve sexuality and reproductive health.

III. DEPRESSION, POTENTIAL, related to DRUG EFFECT

Defining Characteristics: Depression may affect up to 5.3% of patients, and less commonly, patients may develop emotional lability, insomnia, nervousness, and anxiety.

Nursing Implications: Assess baseline affect and usual coping strategies. Teach patient to report change in affect. Assess effectiveness of coping strategies. Encourage patient to verbalize feelings, and provide emotional support. Assess need for referral to psychiatric nurse specialist or social worker if supportive efforts ineffective.

IV. ALTERED NUTRITION, LESS THAN BODY REQUIREMENTS, related to GI SIDE EFFECTS

Defining Characteristics: Anorexia, nausea, and vomiting may occur rarely.

Nursing Implications: If patients experience symptoms, encourage small, frequent feedings of favorite foods, especially high-calorie, high-protein foods. Monitor weight weekly. Assess incidence and pattern of nausea, vomiting, or anorexia if they occur. Discuss need for antiemetic with physician and patient.

Drug: valrubicin (Valstar)

Class: Anthracycline antitumor antibiotic.

Mechanism of Action: Semisynthetic analogue of doxorubicin; drug is highly lipophilic and is made soluble in Cremophor EL. Apparently, the drug does not interact with negatively charged molecules, and thus is less irritating to bladder mucosa. Drug metabolites appear to inhibit topoisomerase II so that cellular DNA cannot replicate, thus inhibiting DNA synthesis and causing chromosomal damage and cell death.

Metabolism: Drug is well absorbed by bladder mucosa with little if any systemic absorption unless bladder is injured/perforated. Used for bladder instillation, and excreted unchanged in the urine (98.6%).

Dosage/Range:

- Intravesicular therapy of BCG-refractory carcinoma in situ of the urinary bladder: 800 mg q week × 6 weeks.
- High incidence of metastases in patients receiving drug in clinical trials, probably due to delayed cystectomy. Therefore, therapy should be discontinued in patients not responding to treatment after three months.

Drug Preparation:

- Available as injection form, 200 mg in 5-mL vial, which should be stored in the refrigerator 2–8°C (36–46°F).

- Remove vials from refrigerator and allow to warm to room temperature without heating; dilute by adding 800 mg (20 mL) to 55 mL of 0.9% normal saline injection, USP.

Drug Administration:
- Bladder lavage by intravesicular administration of drug (total volume of 75 mL when diluted as above), allowed to dwell for 2 hours, and then voided out.
- Non-PVC tubing and non-DEHP containers and administration sets should be used to prevent leaching of PVC into drug volume (due to Cremophor EL).

Drug Interactions:
- None known due to limited, if any, systemic absorption.

Lab Effects/Interference:
- Hyperglycemia.

Special Considerations:
- Contraindicated in patients with hypersensitivity to anthracycline antibioticremophor EL, or any drug components, during pregnancy, in breast-feeding mothers, or in patients with urinary tract infection at time treatment is planned or with small bladder unable to hold 75 mL.
- Drug should NOT be given if bladder is injured, inflamed, or perforated, as systemic absorption will occur via loss of mucosal integrity.
- Use with caution in patients with severe irritable bladder symptoms, as drug may cause symptoms of irritable bladder (during instillation and dwell time).
- Teach patients that urine will be red- or pink-tinged for 24 hours.
- Patients with diabetes need to check blood glucose levels, as hyperglycemia may occur with treatment (1% incidence).

Potential Toxicities/Side Effects and the Nursing Process

I. ALTERATION IN URINE ELIMINATION related to DRUG EFFECTS

Defining Characteristics: Intravesicular administration of drug is associated with signs/symptoms of bladder irritation: frequency (61% of patients), dysuria (56%), urgency (57%), bladder spasm (31%), hematuria (29%), pain in bladder (28%), incontinence (22%), cystitis (15%), and urinary tract infection (15%). Less commonly, nocturia (7%), burning on urination (5%), urinary retention (4%), pain in the urethra (3%), pelvic pain (1%).

Nursing Implications: Assess baseline urinary elimination pattern, history of signs/symptoms of bladder irritation. Teach patient that these side effects may occur and to report them. Teach patient to drink 3 L of fluid for at least 2–3 days beginning day of treatment to flush bladder. Reassure patient that signs/symptoms will resolve and to report any persistent symptoms.

II. ALTERATION IN OXYGENATION, POTENTIAL, related to RARE CARDIAC EFFECTS

Defining Characteristics: Rarely, chest pain may occur (2%) as may vasodilation (2%) or peripheral edema (1%).

Nursing Implications: Assess patient's baseline cardiac status, and history of chest pain, peripheral edema. Teach patient to report any pain, or swelling in hands or feet. If this occurs, discuss management with physician. If possible, do EKG while patient is having chest pain to see if ischemia exists. Systemic absorption is possible only if bladder mucosal surfaces are injured, so this should be considered.

III. ALTERATION IN COMFORT, POTENTIAL, related to PAIN, RASH, WEAKNESS, MYALGIA

Defining Characteristics: The following discomfort may occur: headache (4%), malaise (4%), dizziness (3%), fever (2%), rash (3%), abdominal pain (5%), weakness (4%), back pain (3%), myalgia (1%).

Nursing Implications: Assess baseline comfort level, and any pain and the usual pain relief plan. Teach patient that these problems may occur rarely and to report them if they do. Teach patient these symptoms should resolve, and to use local measures to minimize discomfort. Teach patient to report any symptoms that do not resolve or that become worse.

IV. ALTERATION IN NUTRITION, POTENTIAL, related to NAUSEA, DIARRHEA, VOMITING

Defining Characteristics: Rarely, gastrointestinal symptoms may occur: nausea affects approximately 5% of patients, diarrhea 3% of patients, and vomiting 2% of patients.

Nursing Implications: Assess baseline nutritional status, history of nausea, vomiting, or diarrhea. Teach patient that these may occur rarely and to report them if they do. If patient does develop symptoms, teach patient to take antiemetic medication as ordered, and OTC antidiarrheal medicine. Teach patient to call right away if symptoms do not resolve.

Drug: vinblastine (Velban)

Class: Plant alkaloid extracted from the periwinkle plant (*Vinca rosea*).

Mechanism of Action: Drug binds to microtubular proteins, thus arresting mitosis during metaphase; may inhibit RNA, DNA, and protein synthesis. Cell cycle phase specific for M phase and active in S phase.

Metabolism: About 10% of drug is excreted in feces. Vinblastine is partially metabolized by the liver (P450 microenzyme system). Minimal amount of the drug is excreted in urine and bile. Dose modification may be necessary in the presence of hepatic failure.

Dosage/Range:
- 0.1 mg/kg; 6 mg/m^2 IV weekly: continuous infusion 1.5–2.0 mg/m^2/d in 1 L D5W or NS × 5 days.
- Dose reduce (50%) for bilirubin 1.5–3 mg/dL or AST 60–180 units/L; dose reduce 75% if bilirubin 3–5 mg/dL and hold for bilirubin > 5 mg/dL or AST > 180 units/L.

Drug Preparation:
- Available in 10-mg vials. Store in refrigerator until use.

Drug Administration:
- IV: This drug is a vesicant. Give slow IVP over 1–2 min through the sidearm of a running IV so as to avoid extravasation, which can lead to ulceration, pain, and necrosis. Refer to individual hospital policy and procedure for administration of a vesicant.

Drug Interactions:
- CYP3A4 inhibitors (itraconazole, erythromycin, others): increased serum drug level of vinblastine; do not use together or assess possible toxicity and dose reduce vinblastine.
- CYP3A4 inducers (carbamazepine, dexamethasone, phenytoin, others): decreased serum levels of vinblastine; do not use together or assess need to increase dose of vinblastine.
- St. John's wort: may increase vinblastine toxicity; do not administer concomitantly.
- Grapefruit juice: may increase vinblastine toxicity; do not administer concomitantly.
- Decreased pharmacologic effects of phenytoin when given with this drug; check phenytoin levels and dose modify based on levels.
- Increases cellular uptake of methotrexate by certain malignant cells when administered sequentially, but less so than vincristine.
- Antigout medicines: may decrease effect of vinblastine. Do not use together if possible.

Lab Effects/Interference:
- Decreased WBC.

Special Considerations:
- Drug is a vesicant; give through a running IV to avoid extravasation.
- Dose modification may be necessary in the presence of hepatic failure.

Potential Toxicities/Side Effects and the Nursing Process

I. POTENTIAL FOR INFECTION AND BLEEDING related to BONE MARROW DEPRESSION

Defining Characteristics: May cause severe bone marrow depression; nadir 4–10 days. Neutrophils greatly affected. In patients with prior XRT or chemotherapy, thrombocytopenia may be severe.

Nursing Implications: Monitor CBC, platelet count prior to drug administration. Assess for signs/symptoms of infection or bleeding. Instruct patient in self-assessment of signs/symptoms of infection or bleeding. Dose reduction if hepatic dysfunction: 50% if bili > 1.5 mg/dL; 75% if bili > 3.0 mg/dL. Administer red blood cell and platelet transfusions per physician's orders.

II. POTENTIAL FOR SENSORY/PERCEPTUAL ALTERATIONS related to PERIPHERAL OR CENTRAL NEUROPATHY

Defining Characteristics: Occur less frequently than with vincristine. Occur in patients receiving prolonged or high-dose therapy. Symptoms: paresthesias, peripheral neuropathy, depression, headache, malaise, jaw pain, urinary retention, tachycardia, orthostatic hypotension, seizures. Rare ocular changes: diplopia, ptosis, photophobia, oculomotor dysfunction, optic neuropathy.

Nursing Implications: Assess sensory/perceptual changes prior to each drug dose, especially if dose is high (> 10 mg) or patient is receiving prolonged therapy. Notify physician of alterations. Discuss with patient the impact changes have had, as well as strategies to minimize dysfunction and decrease distress.

III. ALTERATION IN BOWEL ELIMINATION related to CONSTIPATION

Defining Characteristics: Constipation results from neurotoxicity (central) and is less common than with vincristine. Risk factor: high dose (> 20 mg). May lead to adynamic ileus, abdominal pain.

Nursing Implications: Assess bowel elimination pattern with each drug dose, especially if dose > 20 mg. Teach patient to promote bowel elimination with fluids (3 L/day), high-fiber, bulky foods, exercise, stool softeners. Suggest laxative if unable to move bowels at least once a day. Instruct patient to report abdominal pain.

IV. ALTERATION IN NUTRITION, LESS THAN BODY REQUIREMENTS, related to GI SIDE EFFECTS

Defining Characteristics: Nausea and vomiting rarely occur. Stomatitis is uncommon but can be severe.

Nursing Implications: Premedicate with antiemetics and continue prophylactically for 24 hours to prevent nausea and vomiting, at least for the first treatment. Encourage small, frequent feedings of cool, bland foods and liquids. Assess for symptoms of fluid and electrolyte imbalance: monitor I/O, daily weights if administered to an inpatient. Teach patient oral assessment. Teach, reinforce teaching, regarding oral hygiene regimen. Encourage patient to report early stomatitis. Provide pain relief measures if indicated (e.g., topical anesthetics).

V. POTENTIAL FOR IMPAIRED SKIN INTEGRITY related to ALOPECIA

Defining Characteristics: Alopecia is reversible and mild and occurs in 45–50% of patients receiving drug. Drug is a potent vesicant and can cause irritation and necrosis if infiltrated.

Nursing Implications: Discuss with patient the impact of hair loss. Suggest wig as appropriate prior to actual hair loss. Explore with patient response to actual hair loss and plan strategies to minimize distress (e.g., wig, scarf, cap). Careful technique is used during venipuncture and intravenous administration. Administer vesicant through freely flowing IV, constantly monitoring IV site and patient response. Nurse should be THOROUGHLY familiar with institutional policy and procedure for administration of a vesicant agent. If vesicant drug is administered as a continuous infusion, drug must be given through a PATENT CENTRAL LINE. If extravasation is suspected, stop drug administration and aspirate any residual drug and blood from IV tubing, IV catheter/needle, and IV site if possible. If drug infiltration is suspected, manufacturer suggests the following after withdrawing any remaining drug from IV: local installation of hyaluronidase; application of moderate heat. Assess site regularly for pain, progression of erythema, induration, and for evidence of necrosis. When in doubt about whether drug is infiltrating, TREAT AS AN INFILTRATION. Teach patient to assess site, and instruct to notify physician if condition worsens. Arrange next clinic visit for assessment of site depending on drug, amount infiltrated, extent of potential injury, and patient variables. Document in patient's record as per institutional policy and procedure.

VI. POTENTIAL FOR SEXUAL DYSFUNCTION related to REPRODUCTIVE HAZARD

Defining Characteristics: Drug is possibly teratogenic. Likely to cause azoospermia in men.

Nursing Implications: As appropriate, explore with patient and partner issues of reproductive and sexuality patterns and the anticipated impact chemotherapy may have. Discuss strategies to preserve sexual health (e.g., sperm banking).

Drug: vincristine (Oncovin)

Class: Plant alkaloid extracted from the periwinkle plant (*Vinca rosea*).

Mechanism of Action: Drug binds to microtubular proteins, thus arresting mitosis during metaphase. Cell cycle phase specific for M phase and active in S phase.

Metabolism: The primary route for excretion is via the liver (P450 microenzyme system) with about 70% of the drug being excreted in feces and bile. These metabolites are a result of hepatic metabolism and biliary excretion. A small amount is excreted in the urine. Dose modification may be necessary in the presence of hepatic failure.

Dosage/Range:
- 0.4–1.4 mg/m^2 weekly (initially limited to 2 mg per dose).

Drug Preparation:
- Supplied in 1-mg, 2-mg, and 5-mg vials. Refrigerate vials until use.

Drug Administration:
- IV: This drug is a vesicant. Give IVP through sidearm of a running IV to avoid extravasation, which can lead to ulceration, pain, and necrosis. Refer to hospital's policy and procedure for administration of a vesicant.

Drug Interactions:
- Neurotoxic drugs: additive neurotoxicity can occur; use cautiously.
- CYP3A4 inhibitors (itraconazole, erythromycin, others): increased serum drug level of vincristine; do not use together or assess possible toxicity and dose reduce vincristine.
- CYP3A4 inducers (carbamazepine, dexamethasone, phenytoin, others): decreased serum levels of vincristine; do not use together or assess need to increase dose of vincristine.
- St. John's wort: may increase vincristine toxicity; do not administer concomitantly.
- Grapefruit juice: may increase vincristine toxicity; do not administer concomitantly.
- Asparaginase: when given prior to vincristine, will decrease vincristine excretion, with resulting increased neurotoxicity; give vincristine 12–24 hours before asparaginase.
- Decreased bioavailability of digoxin when given with this drug.
- Increased cellular uptake of methotrexate by some malignant cells when given sequentially.

Lab Effects/Interference:
- Decreased WBC, platelets.
- Increased uric acid.

Special Considerations:
- Dose is a vesicant; give through a running IV to avoid extravasation.
- Dose modifications may be necessary in the presence of hepatic failure.
- Drug has been given INTRATHECALLY by error, resulting in death. Ensure that vincristine is labeled "For IV use only." In some institutions, vincristine is mixed in a bag to prevent this error; however, this requires administration through a central vein (infusion).

Potential Toxicities/Side Effects and the Nursing Process

I. POTENTIAL FOR SENSORY/PERCEPTUAL ALTERATIONS related to PERIPHERAL CENTRAL NEUROPATHY

Defining Characteristics: Peripheral neuropathies occur as a result of toxicity to nerve fibers: absent deep tendon reflexes, numbness, weakness, myalgias, cramping, and late severe motor difficulties. Reversal or discontinuance of therapy is necessary. Increased risk exists in elderly. Cranial nerve dysfunction may occur (rare), as well as jaw pain (trigeminal neuralgia), diplopia, vocal cord paresis, mental depression, and metallic taste.

Nursing Implications: Assess sensory/perceptual changes prior to each drug dose, e.g., presence of numbness or tingling of fingertips or toes. Assess for loss of tendon reflexes: foot drop, slapping gait. Assess for motor difficulties: clumsiness of hands, difficulty climbing stairs, buttoning shirt, walking on heels. Notify physician of alterations; discuss holding drug if loss of deep tendon reflexes occurs. Discuss with patient the impact alterations have had, and strategies to minimize dysfunction and decrease distress. Discuss with patient type of alteration: memory and sensory/perceptual changes are temporary and reversible when drug is stopped. Assess patient for signs/symptoms of nerve dysfunction before each dose. Notify physician of any changes.

II. ALTERATION IN BOWEL ELIMINATION related to CONSTIPATION

Defining Characteristics: Autonomic neuropathy may lead to constipation and paralytic ileus. A concurrent use of vincristine, narcotic analgesics, or cholinergic medication may increase risk of constipation.

Nursing Implications: Assess bowel elimination pattern prior to each chemotherapy administration. Teach patient to include bulky and high-fiber foods in diet, increase fluids to 3 L/day, and exercise moderately to promote elimination. Suggest stool softeners if needed. Teach patient to use laxative if unable to move bowels at least once every two days. Instruct patient to report abdominal pain.

III. POTENTIAL FOR IMPAIRED SKIN INTEGRITY related to ALOPECIA

Defining Characteristics: Complete hair loss occurs in 12–45% of patients. Both men and women are at risk for body image disturbance. Hair will grow back. Dermatitis is uncommon. Drug is potent vesicant causing irritation and necrosis if infiltrated.

Nursing Implications: Discuss with patient anticipated impact of hair loss. Suggest wig or toupee as appropriate prior to actual hair loss. Explore with patient response to actual hair loss and plan strategies to minimize distress (e.g., wig, scarf, cap). Assess impact on patient: body image, comfort. Careful technique is used during venipuncture and intravenous administration. Administer vesicant through freely flowing IV, constantly monitoring IV site and patient response. Nurse should be THOROUGHLY familiar with institutional policy and procedure for administration of a vesicant agent. If vesicant drug is administered as a continuous infusion, drug must be given THROUGH A PATENT CENTRAL LINE. When administering the drug, if extravasation is suspected, TREAT IT AS AN INFILTRATION. Stop drug administration and aspirate any residual drug and blood from IV tubing, IV catheter/needle, and IV site if possible. Manufacturer suggests the following after withdrawing any remaining drug from IV: local installation of hyaluronidase, application of moderate heat. Assess site regularly for pain, progression of erythema, induration, and evidence of necrosis. Teach patient to assess site and notify physician if condition worsens. Arrange next clinic visit for assessment of site depending on drug, amount infiltrated, extent of potential injury, and patient variables. Document in patient's record as per institutional policy and procedure.

IV. POTENTIAL FOR INFECTION AND BLEEDING related to BONE MARROW DEPRESSION

Defining Characteristics: Rare myelosuppression, mild when it occurs. Nadir 10–14 days after treatment begins.

Nursing Implications: Monitor CBC, HCT, platelet count prior to drug administration. Dose reduction if hepatic dysfunction: 50% reduction if bili > 1.5 mg/dL; 75% reduction if bili > 3.0 mg/dL.

V. POTENTIAL SEXUAL DYSFUNCTION related to IMPOTENCE

Defining Characteristics: Impotence may occur related to neurotoxicity.

Nursing Implications: As appropriate, explore with patient and partner issues of reproductive and sexuality patterns, and impact chemotherapy may have. Discuss strategies to preserve sexual health, e.g., alternative expressions of sexuality. Reassure patient that impotency, if it occurs, is usually temporary, and reversible after drug discontinuance.

Drug: vindesine (Eldisine, Desacetylvinblastine, investigational)

Class: Synthetic derivative of vinblastine; synthetic vinca alkaloid.

Mechanism of Action: Inhibits microtubule formation, causing metaphase arrest during M phase. Causes some cell death during S phase. Cell cycle phase specific.

Metabolism: Short plasma half-life (probably binds to tissue). Prolonged elimination suggesting drug may accumulate with repeated dosing. Excreted primarily by bile.

Dosage/Range:
- 3–4 mg/m^2 every 1–2 weeks.
- 1.0–1.3 mg/m^2/day × 5–7 days, repeated every 3 weeks.
- 1.5–2.0 mg/m^2 twice weekly.

Drug Preparation:
- 10-mg vial of lyophilized powder, reconstituted with provided diluent or 0.9% sodium chloride. Solution is stable for two weeks if refrigerated.

Drug Administration:
- Vesicant precautions: administer slowly as IV push through sidearm of freely running IV; also may be given as continuous infusion.

Drug Interactions:
- Do not give with other vinca alkaloids, such as vincristine or vinblastine, as there is potential for cumulative neurotoxicity.

Lab Effects/Interference:
- Decreased CBC, especially WBC.

Special Considerations:
- Dose reduction may be necessary in patients with abnormal liver function or if patient has received maximal doses of other vinca alkaloids.

Potential Toxicities/Side Effects and the Nursing Process

I. POTENTIAL FOR INFECTION AND BLEEDING related to BONE MARROW DEPRESSION

Defining Characteristics: Dose-limiting side effect. Nadir 5–10 days. Neutropenia is mild to moderate. Thrombocytopenia is mild, rare (may increase on treatment).

Nursing Implications: Monitor CBC, HCT, platelet count prior to drug administration as well as for signs/symptoms of infection or bleeding. Instruct patient in self-assessment of signs/symptoms of infection or bleeding. Dose reduction is often necessary (35–50%) if compromised bone marrow function exists.

II. POTENTIAL FOR SENSORY/PERCEPTUAL ALTERATIONS related to PERIPHERAL, CENTRAL NEUROPATHIES

Defining Characteristics: Neurotoxicity is similar to vincristine. Cumulative toxicity, mild. Begins with distal paresthesias, proximal muscle weakness, loss of deep tendon reflexes. Abdominal cramping is common; constipation and paralytic ileus are less common. Hoarseness, jaw pain (severe and transient) may occur.

Nursing Implications: Obtain visual assessment prior to starting therapy. Encourage patient to report any visual changes. Instruct patient to report headache, dizziness, light-headedness.

III. POTENTIAL FOR IMPAIRED SKIN INTEGRITY related to ALOPECIA

Defining Characteristics: Alopecia affects 80–90%, with 25–50% experiencing complete hair loss. Alopecia may be progressive. Both men and women are at risk for body image disturbance. Hair will grow back. Drug is a vesicant. Inapparent or obvious infiltrations can occur. Presentation is delayed; pain, phlebitis, blister formation occur; may progress to ulceration and necrosis. Management similar to vincristine extravasation.

Nursing Implications: Discuss with patient anticipated impact of hair loss. Suggest wig or toupee as appropriate prior to actual hair loss. Explore with patient response to actual hair loss and plan strategies to minimize distress (e.g., wig, scarf, cap). Assess impact on patient: body image, comfort. Careful technique is used during venipuncture and intravenous administration. Administer vesicant through freely flowing IV, constantly monitoring IV site and patient response. Nurse should be THOROUGHLY familiar with institutional policy and procedure for administration of a vesicant agent. If vesicant drug is administered as a continuous infusion, drug must be given THROUGH A PATENT CENTRAL LINE. If extravasation is suspected, stop drug administration and aspirate any residual drug and blood from IV tubing, IV catheter/needle, and IV site if possible. If drug infiltration is suspected, manufacturer suggests the following after withdrawing any remaining drug from IV: local installation of hyaluronidase, application of moderate heat. Assess site regularly for pain, progression of erythema, induration, and for evidence of necrosis. When in doubt about whether drug is infiltrating, TREAT AS AN INFILTRATION. Teach patient to assess site and instruct to notify physician if condition worsens. Arrange next clinic visit for assessment of site depending on drug, amount infiltrated, extent of potential injury, and patient variables. Document in patient's record as per institutional policy and procedure.

IV. ALTERATION IN BOWEL ELIMINATION related to CONSTIPATION

Defining Characteristics: Autonomic neuropathy may lead to constipation and paralytic ileus.

Nursing Implications: Assess bowel elimination pattern prior to each chemotherapy administration. Teach patient to include bulky and high-fiber foods in diet, increase fluids to 3 L/day, and exercise moderately to promote elimination. Suggest stool softeners if needed. Teach patient to use laxative if unable to move bowels at least once every two days. Instruct patient to report abdominal pain.

V. ALTERATION IN NUTRITION, LESS THAN BODY REQUIREMENTS, related to GI SIDE EFFECTS

Defining Characteristics: Nausea and vomiting typically not severe; occur in 30% of patients. Diarrhea is uncommon but rarely may be protracted and thus would be an indication for dose reduction.

Nursing Implications: Premedicate with antiemetic and continue prophylactically for 24 hours to prevent nausea and vomiting, at least for the first treatment. Encourage small, frequent feedings of cool, bland food and liquids. Encourage patient to report onset of diarrhea. Administer, or teach patient to self-administer, antidiarrheal medications.

Drug: vinorelbine tartrate (Navelbine)

Class: Semisynthetic vinca alkaloid derived from vinblastine.

Mechanism of Action: Inhibits mitosis at metaphase by interfering with microtubule assembly. Specifically, it inhibits tubulin polymerization and binds preferentially to microtubules during mitosis so that mitosis is blocked at G_2-M phase causing cell death. Also appears to interfere with some aspects of cellular metabolism, including cellular respiration and nucleic acid biosynthesis. Cell cycle specific.

Metabolism: Slow elimination; extensive tissue binding (80% bound to plasma proteins); metabolized by the liver (P450 microenzyme system). Terminal half-life is 27–43 hours. Excreted in feces (46%) and urine (18%). The investigational oral form 60–80 mg/m^2 results in comparable serum levels to that of 25- to 30-mg/m^2 IV formulation. The drug is well absorbed following oral administration, T_{max} reached in 1.5 to 3 hours. The drug is significantly taken up by lung tissue, and has an elimination half-life of 35 to 40 hours. Bioavailability of the oral capsules is 33% to 43%, probably because of incomplete absorption and a first-pass effect in the liver. Vomiting 3 hours after swallowing the dose does not reduce the absorption of the drug.

Dosage/Range:

- IV:
  - 30 mg/m^2 IV weekly, OR
  - 25 mg/m^2 IV every week or 30 mg/m^2 IV on days 1 and 29 then every 6 weeks in combination with cisplatin.
- Oral: Investigational: oral vinorelbine (stage III, IV NSCLC; advanced breast cancer).
  - Start at 60 mg/m^2 PO with food once weekly × 3, and then if ANC remains > 1000 cells/mm^3 (except may fall only once), dose increase to 80 mg/m^2. If the ANC falls to < 500 cells/mm^3 once or if the ANC falls to 500–1000 cells/mm^3 more than once, keep dose at 60 mg/m^2.
  - If the ANC falls below 500, or between 500–1000 more than once on the 80 mg/m^2 dose, reduce dose to 60 mg/m^2.
  - Drug dose should be reduced in patients with significant liver impairment due to metastases.
  - Capsules available in 20-, 30-, 40-, and 80-mg strengths.
  - Capsule liquid is an irritant, and thus, patients must not cut or open them.
- Dose modifications
  - Hematologic toxicity: if ANC on day of treatment is 1000–1499/mm^3, use 50% dose (i.e., 15 mg/m^2); drug should be held if ANC < 1000/mm^3. If drug is held for

3 consecutive weeks because ANC < 1000/mm^3, discontinue drug. If patient develops neutropenic fever or sepsis or drug is held for neutropenia for 2 consecutive doses, dose should be reduced 25% (i.e., 22.5 mg/m^2) if ANC < 1500/mm^3; if ANC is 1000–1499/mm^3, drug should be decreased to 11.25 mg/m^2 as per package insert.

- Hepatic dysfunction: if total bili is 2.1–3.0 mg/dL, use 50% dose reduction (i.e., 15 mg/m^2); if total bili is > 3.0 mg/dL, use 75% dose reduction (i.e., 7.5 mg/m^2).

Drug Preparation:

- Drug is available as 10 mg/mL in 1- or 5-mL vials.
- Further dilute drug in syringe or IV bag in 0.9% sodium chloride or 5% dextrose to a final concentration of 1.5–3.0 mg/mL in a syringe, or 0.5–2.0 mg/mL in an IV bag.
- Stable for 24 hours if refrigerated.
- Also available as a 40-mg gelatin capsule.

Drug Administration:

- Infuse diluted drug IV over 6–10 minutes into sidearm port of freely flowing IV infusion, either peripherally or via central line. Use port CLOSEST TO THE IV BAG, not the patient.
- Flush vein with at least 75–125 mL of IV fluid after drug infusion.
- Use vesicant precautions.
- Oral capsule should be taken on an empty stomach at bedtime.

Drug Interactions:

- Increased granulocytopenia occurs when given in combination with cisplatin.
- Possible pulmonary reactions occur when given in combination with mitomycin C, characterized by dyspnea and severe bronchospasm. May require management with bronchodilators, corticosteroids, and/or supplemental oxygen.
- CYP3A4 inhibitors (itraconazole, erythromycin, omeprazole, fluoxetine, others): increased serum drug level of vinorelbine; do not use together or assess possible toxicity and dose reduce vinorelbine.
- CYP3A4 inducers (carbamazepine, dexamethasone, phenytoin, others): decreased serum levels of vinorelbine; do not use together or assess need to increase dose of vinorelbine. Monitor phenytoin levels and dose modify depending upon levels as levels may be low.
- Paclitaxel, docetaxel: give paclitaxel or docetaxel before vinorelbine to reduce myelosuppression (reverse sequence increases toxicity of paclitaxel or docetaxel).
- St. John's wort: may decrease vinorelbine effectiveness, do not give together.
- Grapefruit juice: inhibits CYP3A4 enzymes, which may increase toxicity of vinorelbine; do not use together.

Lab Effects/Interference:

- Decreased CBC (especially WBC).
- Increased LFTs.

Special Considerations:

- Drug indicated as single agent or in combination with cisplatin for the first-line treatment of advanced, unresectable, non–small-cell lung cancer (Stage III, combination therapy; Stage IV, single agent, or in combination with cisplatin).
- Increased nausea, vomiting, and diarrhea with oral administration.
- Drug is embryotoxic and mutagenic, so female patients of childbearing age should use contraception.
- Administer cautiously to patients with hepatic insufficiency. Contraindicated in patients with ANC < $1000/mm^3$.
- Oral drug contraindicated in patients with hepatic insufficiency unrelated to tumor.

Potential Toxicities/Side Effects and the Nursing Process

I. INFECTION AND BLEEDING related to BONE MARROW DEPRESSION

Defining Characteristics: Leukopenia is dose-limiting toxicity; bone marrow depression noncumulative and short-lived (< 7 days), with nadir at 7–10 days. Use with caution in patients with history of prior radiotherapy or chemotherapy. Severe thrombocytopenia and anemia are uncommon.

Nursing Implications: Monitor CBC, ANC, HCT, and platelet count prior to drug administration, as well as for signs/symptoms of infection or bleeding. Instruct patient in self-assessment of signs/symptoms of infection or bleeding. Teach patient self-care measures, including avoidance of OTC aspirin-containing medications. Dose reduction necessary for hematologic toxicity (see Special Considerations section).

II. POTENTIAL FOR SENSORY/PERCEPTUAL ALTERATIONS related to NEUROLOGIC TOXICITY

Defining Characteristics: Incidence of mild-to-moderate neuropathy is 25%. Paresthesias occur in 2–10% of patients, but incidence is increased if patient has received prior chemotherapy with vinca alkaloids or abdominal XRT. Decreased deep tendon reflexes occur in 6–29% of patients. Constipation may occur in 29% of patients. Neuropathy is reversible.

Nursing Implications: Assess baseline neuromuscular function, and reassess prior to drug infusion, especially in the presence of paresthesias; risk is increased if drug is given concurrently with cisplatin. Teach patient to report any changes in sensation or function. Identify strategies to promote comfort and safety.

III. ALTERATION IN NUTRITION, LESS THAN BODY REQUIREMENTS, related to NAUSEA/VOMITING, DIARRHEA, STOMATITIS, HEPATOTOXICITY

Defining Characteristics: Incidence of nausea/vomiting increases with oral dosing; mild in IV dosing, with an incidence of 44%. Vomiting occurs in 20% of patients. Diarrhea increases with oral dosing (17% incidence). Stomatitis is mild to moderate with < 20% incidence. Transient increases in LFTs (AST) occur in 67% of patients, and are without clinical significance.

Nursing Implications: Premedicate with antiemetic, such as a serotonin antagonist, prior to drug administration. Encourage small, frequent meals of cool, bland foods and liquids. Assess for symptoms of fluid/electrolyte imbalance if patient has severe nausea and vomiting. Monitor I/O, daily weights, and lab electrolyte values. Encourage patient to report onset of diarrhea. Administer, or teach patient to self-administer, antidiarrheal medications. Teach patient oral assessment. Teach and reinforce teaching of systemic oral hygiene regimen. Instruct patient to report early stomatitis, and provide pain relief measures as needed. Assess LFTs prior to drug administration baseline and periodically during treatment. Dose modifications may be necessary for hepatic dysfunction (see Special Considerations section).

IV. POTENTIAL FOR ALTERATION IN SKIN INTEGRITY related to ALOPECIA, EXTRAVASATION

Defining Characteristics: Gradual alopecia occurs in 10% of patients, rarely progressing to complete hair loss or requiring a wig. Severity is related to treatment duration. Drug is a moderate vesicant, primarily causing venous irritation and phlebitis; 30% of patients experience injection-site reactions commonly characterized by erythema, vein discoloration, tenderness; rarely, pain and venous irritation at sites proximal to injection site.

Nursing Implications: Discuss potential impact of hair loss prior to drug administration; also assess coping strategies, and plans to minimize body-image distortion (e.g., wig, scarf, cap). Assess patient for signs/symptoms of hair loss. Assess patient's response and use of coping strategies. Scrupulous venipuncture technique is used during venipuncture. Administer vesicant through freely flowing IV via IV port closest to IV fluid bag, not patient, and administer maximally diluted drug over 6–10 minutes (not longer). If extravasation is suspected, TREAT AS AN INFILTRATION and aspirate any remaining drug from IV tubing, locally instill hyaluronidase in area of suspected infiltration, and apply moderate heat. Assess site regularly for pain, progression of erythema, and evidence of necrosis. Document in patient's record. Schedule next clinic visit for assessment of site depending on drug, amount infiltrated, extent of potential injury, and other patient variables.

V. POTENTIAL FOR SEXUAL/REPRODUCTIVE DYSFUNCTION related to TERATOGENICITY

Defining Characteristics: Drug is teratogenic and fetotoxic.

Nursing Implications: As appropriate, explore with patient and partner issues of reproductive and sexuality patterns and the anticipated impact chemotherapy may have. Counsel female patients of childbearing age in contraceptive options.

Chapter 2
Biologic Response Modifier Therapy

Surgery, chemotherapy, and radiation therapy are the three most commonly used treatments against cancer. Biotherapy, or the use of biologic response modifiers (BRMs), comprises the fourth traditional treatment modality for cancer management. BRMs work in a variety of ways to modify the immune response so that cancer cells are injured, killed, or prevented from dividing. This category includes antibodies, cytokines, and other substances that stimulate the immune system (hemopoietic growth factors). It has recently been greatly expanded to include gene therapy and immunomodulating agents, such as vaccines. In this book, Chapter 5 addresses new agents that target specific abnormal molecular events that promote malignant transformation, such as over-expression of cell surface growth factor receptors like epidermal growth factor receptor (EGFR). Inhibitors that target abnormal signal transduction and transcription factors are also included. Monoclonal antibodies are classically targeted against molecular flaws, such as the monoclonal antibody targeting vascular endothelial growth factor (VEGF), bevacizumab (Avastin), an angiogenesis inhibitor, and epidermal growth factor receptor inhibitor cetuximab (Erbitux). Even though they are technically biological agents, for this publication, they appear in Chapter 5, Molecularly Targeted Therapies.

Biological response modifiers can

- Have direct antitumor activity or help cancer cells become recognizable as foreign so that the host immune system can kill the cancer cells.
- Restore, augment, or modulate the host's immune system, such as inhibiting viral infection, and activating natural killer (NK) and lymphocyte-activated killer (LAK) cells.
- Help the host's normal ability to repair or replace damaged cells (e.g., damaged by chemotherapy or radiotherapy).
- Interfere with tumor cell differentiation, transformation, or metastasis.

Cytokines are substances released from activated lymphocytes and include the interferons (IFNs), interleukins (ILs), tumor necrosis factor (TNF), and colony stimulating factors (CSFs). Other BRMs are the monoclonal antibodies (MoAbs or MAbs) and vaccines.

Interferons occur naturally in the body and were the first cytokine to be studied. The interferons can be divided into two types: Type I IFNs bind to cell surface receptors on effector cells. Type I IFNs include IFN-α and IFN-β, which bind to α and β cell surface receptors on effector cells, respectively. Type II IFNs, such as IFN-γ, bind to different cell surface receptors. Interferons of both groups help to regulate the immune system, improve resistance to invading microorganisms, and halt cell proliferation, but each interferon subgroup has specific functions as well (as discussed in this chapter).

IFN-alfa (α) is stimulated by viruses and tumor cells; its antiviral activity is greater than its antiproliferative activity, which is greater than its immunomodulatory effects. There are twenty subtypes of IFN-α. IFN-beta (β) is also stimulated by viruses; it has equal antiviral, antiproliferative, and immunomodulatory effects. There are two subtypes of IFN-β. IFN-gamma (γ) is stimulated by cell-mediated immune response and IL-2; it is released by activated T lymphocytes and natural killer cells. Its immunomodulatory action is greater than its antiproliferative effect, which is greater than its antiviral effect. There is only one type of this interferon. IFN-alfa 2a is used in the treatment of hairy-cell leukemia, acquired immunodeficiency syndrome (AIDS)-related Kaposi's sarcoma, chronic myelogenous leukemia (CML), chronic hepatitis C, and adjuvant therapy of malignant melanoma. IFN-alpha 2b is used for condyloma acuminata, hepatitis B and C, hairy-cell leukemia, high-risk malignant melanoma, and AIDS-related Kaposi's sarcoma. IFN-beta 1a is being studied as to its usefulness in treating AIDS-related Kaposi's sarcoma, metastatic renal cell cancer, malignant melanoma, and cutaneous T-cell lymphoma. IFN-gamma is used for B-cell malignancies, chronic myelogenous leukemia, renal cell cancer, and is being studied in ovarian cancer. Common side effects of interferons include flu-like symptoms, anorexia, and fatigue.

Colony stimulating factors include hematopoietic growth factors. They too occur naturally in the body and help immature blood cell elements develop into mature, effective white blood cells, red blood cells, and platelets. Recombinant DNA techniques have permitted the manufacture of large quantities of these substances. An "r" prefix (e.g., r-IL-2) indicates that it was produced using recombinant technology.

The use of colony-stimulating growth factors has permitted increased doses of chemotherapy to be safely given. Filgrastim, or granulocyte-colony stimulating factor (G-CSF), is approved to prevent infection related to febrile neutropenia following bone marrow suppressive chemotherapy, as well as for other uses, and a sustained-duration pegylated formulation requiring less frequent dosing is available (pegfilgrastim or Neulasta). This is called primary prophylaxis and begins after the first cycle of chemotherapy. Secondary prophylaxis is when the growth factor is used to prevent the recurrence of febrile neutropenia in a patient who has not used growth factor in the past, and therapeutic use is when the growth factor is used at the time of neutropenia or neutropenic fever in high-risk individuals, such as those with sepsis syndrome, pneumonia, or fungal infection (Barbour and Crawford, 2007).

In order to provide guidance and recommendations for evidence-based practice, the American Society of Clinical Oncology (ASCO) published guidelines for the use of colony stimulating factors. In 2006, ASCO updated recommendations for the use of white blood cell growth factors creating an evidence-based practice guideline.

The guideline emphasizes that the reduction of febrile neutropenia is an important clinical outcome justifying the use of colony stimulating factors (CSFs), regardless of the impact on other factors, when the risk of febrile neutropenia is 20% or more, and there is no other equally effective anti-cancer regimen that does not require CSFs available. An example of a common breast cancer regimen with a 20% or greater incidence of febrile neutropenia is Adriamycin Cytoxan followed by Taxol (AC->T). Patient factors and comorbidities can also increase the risk for febrile neutropenia; these include a history of severe neutropenia with similar chemotherapy, extensive prior chemotherapy, poor performance or nutritional status, age of more than 65 years, bone marrow involvement with tumor, open wounds, and liver disease (NCCN, 2007). In addition, CSFs permit the administration of dose-dense chemotherapy regimens as part of a clinical trial or as supported by efficacy data. For example, prophylactic CSF permits patients with diffuse aggressive lymphoma, aged 65 or older who are being treated with curative intent, to have reduced risk of febrile neutropenia and infections (Smith et al, 2006).

Sargramostim, or granulocyte-macrophage colony-stimulating factor (GM-CSF), is approved for myeloid reconstitution after autologous bone marrow transplantation and for other uses. It is now being studied in use with dendritic cell vaccines. Both G-CSF and GM-CSF can be used to mobilize stem cells that will be used to rescue the bone marrow after high-dose chemotherapy.

EPO or rHuEPO (erythropoietin) has become standard therapy as an adjunct to chemotherapy in certain regimens. Together with American Society of Hematology colleagues, ASCO guidelines assert that there is strong evidence to use epoetin as a treatment option for patients with chemotherapy-associated anemia with a hemoglobin concentration below 10 g/dL (Rizzo et al, 2002); however, despite beliefs that increasing the hemoglobin beyond 12 g/dL would improve patient response and quality of life, studies showed the converse, in fact, using erythropoiesis-stimulating agents (ESAs) to target a hemoglobin of 12 g/dL or higher in cancer patients, resulted in shortened time to tumor progression in patients with advanced head and neck cancer receiving radiation therapy, shortened overall survival, and increased deaths related to disease progression in patients with metastatic breast cancer receiving chemotherapy, and increased risk of death in cancer patients not receiving chemotherapy or radiation therapy (FDA, 2007). As a result, the FDA issued an alert (on March 9, 2008) that required all ESA package inserts to add to the black box warning that ESAs be used only on label (e.g., while patients are receiving myelosuppressive chemotherapy). ESAs are *not* indicated when the anticipated outcome is cure. In addition, Medicare revised their guidelines to tighten reimbursement for ESAs. The target hemoglobin has now been changed to 10–<12 g/dL, and the threshold for holding ESAs is the lowest dose necessary to avoid RBC transfusion (NCCN, 2009). In addition, it is imperative to analyze the patient's iron status and replete as necessary. IV iron appears to be superior to oral iron and is being studied (NCCN, 2009). Until additional data about risk versus benefit emerge, these changes have become the standard in guiding

ESA use. In summary, NCCN guidelines for the use of ESAs in cancer patients with chemotherapy-related anemia are as follows:

- Epoetin and darbopoietin are equally safe and effective.
- Cancer treatment goal is noncurative.
- ESAs are recommended when a patient's hgb falls below 10 g/dL.
- Adjusted dose to maintain the lowest hgb level sufficient to avoid RBC transfusion.
- If hgb increases by > 1g/L in a 2-week period, reduce dose by 25–50% of prior dose.
- Monitor the iron levels and provide iron supplements as appropriate.

Platelet growth factor, oprelvekin (Neumega), or IL-11 can be used to prevent and treat thrombocytopenia after myelosuppressive chemotherapy and results in a modest increase in platelets; however, it has side effects that have limited its utility. A new agent, romiplostim (Nplate), is a "peptibody" or peptide antibody that mimics the activity of thrombopoietin to stimulate platelet production. Clinical trials in patients with immune thrombocytopenia purpura (ITP) have shown significant benefit (Kuter et al, 2008). The drug has recently been FDA approved for the treatment of thrombocytopenia in patients with chronic immune (idiopathic) thrombocytopenia purpura (ITP). Research continues on thrombopoietin (TPO), which has a peak effect in 12 days, which often is when the nadir effect of chemotherapy occurs. Common side effects of colony stimulating factors may include bone pain, fatigue, anorexia, and fever.

IL-2 is another naturally occurring cytokine that is made using recombinant technology. It is indicated for the treatment of adults with metastatic renal cell carcinoma and adults with metastatic malignant melanoma; recently, an inhaled high-dose form given together with dacarbazine has been shown to reduce lung metastases from malignant melanoma (Enk et al, 2000). IL-12 is gaining much attention due to its ability to stimulate natural killer (NK) activity and antitumor potential, as well as its synergistic action with IL-2, GM-CSF, and calcium ionophore to enhance dendritic cell function (Bedrosian et al, 2000). IL-12 is being studied in gene therapy (Divino et al, 2000). Side effects of interleukins include flu-like symptoms, fatigue, and anorexia, as well as substance-specific side effects; for example, IL-2 can cause serious side effects, depending upon dose, such as capillary leak syndrome. Research exploring the cytokine IL-7 shows that in the recombinant form given SQ every other day for 2 weeks, patients' immune systems are stimulated to make large numbers of T-helper lymphocytes (CD4+ increased by 300%), and cytotoxic CD8+ cells increased by over 400%; the elevated T-cells remained elevated for 6 weeks after the end of therapy (Sportes et al, 2008).

While many BRMs are still investigational (i.e., being studied in clinical research trials to determine their effectiveness, optimal dose, and method of administration), many are quickly being approved for use. Expected side effects vary according to agent, dose, and patient characteristics. In general, flu-like symptoms (fever, chills, rigor, malaise, arthralgias, headache, myalgias, and anorexia) may occur. Routes of administration include intravenous (IV), intramuscular (IM), intraperitoneal (IP), subcutaneous (SQ), intralesional, inhaled, and topical.

Currently, palifermin or recombinant human keratinocyte growth factor has shown remarkable success in decreasing the oral mucositis associated with bone marrow transplant, and has been approved by the FDA, for use in patients undergoing bone marrow transplantation.

Monoclonal antibodies are produced to target a single foreign antigen, and are designed to attach to specific cancer antigens. Monoclonal antibodies can become targeted therapies and have demonstrated an active role in molecularly targeted therapies. Therefore, further discussion of monoclonal antibodies and specific agents can be found in Chapter 5, Molecularly Targeted Therapies.

References

Barbour SY, Crawford J. Hematopoietic growth factors. In Pazdur R Coia LR Hoskins WJ Wagman LD (eds). *Cancer Management: A Multidisciplinary Approach*, 10th ed. Lawrence, KS: CMP Healthcare Media LLC; 2007

Battiato LA. Biologic and targeted therapy. In Yarbro CH, Frogge MH, Goodman M, eds. *Cancer Nursing: Principles and Practice*, 6th ed. Sudbury, MA: Jones and Bartlett; 2005: 510–559

Bedrosian L, Roras JG, Xu S. Granulocyte-Macrophage Colony-Stimulating Factor, Interleukin-2a and Interleukin-12 Synergize with Calcium Ionophore to Enhance Dendritic Cell Function. *J Immunother* 2000; 23(3) 311–320

Benstein K. Future of Basic/Clinical Hematopoiesis: Research in the Era of Hematopoietic Growth Factor Availability. *Semin Oncol* 1992; 19(4) 441–448

Bronchud MH, Scarffe JH, Thatcher N, et al. Phase I/II Study of Recombinant Human Granulocyte Colony-Stimulating Factor in Patients Receiving Intensive Chemotherapy for SCLC. *Br J Cancer* 1987; 56 809–813

Egrie JC, Dwyer E, Lykos M, et al. Novel Erythropoiesis Stimulating Protein (NESP) Has a Longer Serum Half-life and Greater in vivo Biological Activity than Recombinant Human Erythropoietin (rHuEPO). *Blood* 1997; 90(10) abstract 243 (Suppl 1)

Enk AH, Nashan D, Rubben A, Knop J. High Dose Inhalation Interleukin-2 Therapy for Lung Metastases in Patients with Malignant Melanoma. *Cancer* 2000; 88(9) 2042–2046

Federal Drug Administration (March 9, 2008). Erythropoiesis stimulating agent warning. http://www.fda.gov/cder/drug/infopage/RHE/default.htm. Accessed July 9, 2008

Gabrilove JL, Cleeland CS, Livingston RB. Clinical Evaluation of Once Weekly Dosing of Epoetin Alfa in Chemotherapy Patients: Improvements in Hemoglobin and Quality of Life are Similar to Three Times Weekly Dosing. *J Clin Oncol* 2001; 19 (11) 2875–2882

Genzyme Corporation. Thyrogen [package insert]. Cambridge, MA: Genzyme Corp., Feb 2008

Kammula US, White D, Rosenberg SA. Trends in the Safety of High Dose Bolus Interleukin-2 Administration in Patients with Metastatic Cancer. *Cancer* 1998; 83(4) 797–805

Kuter DJ, Bussel JB, Lyons RM, et al. Efficacy of Romiplostim in Patients With Chronic Immune Thrombocytopenic Purpura: A Double-Blind Randomised Controlled Trial. *Lancet* 2008; 371(9610) 395–403

National Comprehensive Cancer Network (NCCN). *Clinical Practice Guidelines Cancer and Treatment Related Anemia* v3. 2009, http://www.nccn.org. Accessed July 15, 2007

National Comprehensive Cancer Network (NCCN). *Clinical Practice Guidelines Myeloid Growth Factors* v1. 2007, http://www.nccn.org. Accessed July 15, 2007

Pacini F, Molinaro E, Castagna MG, Lippi F, Ceccarelli C, Agate L, Elisei R, Pinchera A. Ablation of Thyroid Residues with 30 mCi 131I: A Comparison in Thyroid Cancer Patients Prepared With

Recombinant Human TSH or Thyroid Hormone Withdrawal. *J Clin Endocrinol Metab* 2002; 87 4063–4068
Rizzo JD, Lichtin AE, Woolf SH, et al. Use of Epoetin in Patients with Cancer: Evidence-based Clinical Practice Guidelines of the American Society of Clinical Oncology and the American Society of Hematology. *Blood* 2002; 100(7) 2303–2320
Simpson C, Seipp CA, Rosenbery SA. The Current Status and Future Applications of Interleukin-2 and Adoptive Immunotherapy in Cancer Treatment. *Semin Oncol Nurs* 1988; 4 132–141
Smith TJ, Khatcheressian J, Lyman GH, 2006 Update of recommendations for the use of white blood cell growth factors: An evidence-based clinical practice guideline. *J Clin Oncol* 2006; 32(10) 3187–3205
Spielberger R, Emmanouilides C, Stiff P, et al. Use of recombinant human keratinocyte growth factor (rHuKGF) can reduce severe oral mucositis in patients with hematologic malignancies undergoing autologous peripheral blood progenitor cell transplantation (auto-PBPCT) after radiation-based conditioning—results of a phase 3 trial. *Proc Am Soc Clin Oncol* 2003; 2(2) 122, abstract 3642
Sportes C, Hakim FT, Memon SA, et al. Administration of rhIL-7 in Humans Increases In Vivo TCR Repertoire Diversity by Preferential Expansion of Naïve T cell Subsets. *J Exp Med 2008*; accessed June 23, 2008
Swanson G, Bergstrom K, Stump E, et al. Growth Factor Usage Patterns and Outcomes in the Community Setting: Collection through a Practice-based Computerized Clinical Information System. *J Clin Oncol* 2000; 18(8) 1764–1770
Timar J, Ladanyi A, Forster-Horvath C, et al. Neoadjuvant immunotherapy of oral squamous cell carcinoma modulates intratumoral CD4/CD8 ratio and tumor microenvironment: A multicenter phase II clinical trial. *J Clin Oncol* 2005; 23(15) 3421–3432

Drug: aldesleukin (Interleukin-2, Proleukin)

Class: Cytokine.

Mechanism of Action: IL-2, previously called T-cell growth factor, is produced by helper T cells following antibody-antigen reaction (processed antigen is mounted on macrophage) and IL-1. IL-2 amplifies the immune response to an antigen by immunomodulation and immunorestoration. IL-2 stimulates T-lymphocyte proliferation, enhances killer T-cell activity, increases antibody production (secondary to increased B-cell proliferation), helps to increase synthesis of other cytokines (IFNs, IL-1, -3, -4, -5, -6, CSFs), and stimulates production and activation of natural killer (NK) cells and other cytotoxic cells (LAK and TIL).

Metabolism: The half-life of distribution is 13 minutes, whereas the elimination half-life is 85 minutes.

Dosage/Range: *Metastatic renal cell carcinoma and metastatic malignant melanoma*:

- 600,000 IUs/kg (0.037 mg/kg) IVB over 15 minutes every 8 hours for a maximum of 14 doses over 5 days and then a 9-day rest, followed by 14 additional doses every 8 hours, for a maximum of 28 doses per course as tolerated. Evaluate for response 4 weeks after completion of a course and before the next treatment course. Tumor shrinkage should be seen before retreatment. Seven-week rest period should separate discharge from the hospital and retreatment. Delay and drug holiday should be used rather than drug dose reduction to manage toxicity.

Contraindications (based on toxicity) *to retreatment*:

- Sustained ventricular tachycardia (≥ 5 beats), uncontrolled cardiac rhythm disturbances, ECG changes showing angina or MI, cardiac tamponade.
- Intubation > 72 hours.
- Renal failure requiring dialysis > 72 hours.
- Coma or toxic psychosis lasting > 48 hours; difficult to control seizures.
- Bowel ischemia or perforation, GI bleeding requiring surgery.

Delay with resumption of dose after resolution of symptoms and condition resolved or ruled out:

- Persistent atrial fibrillation, supraventricular tachycardia, or bradycardia.
- Hypotension (SBP < 90 mmHg with need for pressors).
- ECG change showing MI, ischemia, myocarditis.
- O_2 saturation < 90%.
- Mental status changes (confusion, agitation).
- Sepsis.
- Serum creatinine > 4.5 mg/dL or ≥ 4 mg/dL with severe volume overload, acidosis, or hyperkalemia; persistent oliguria, urine output < 10 mL/hr for 16–24 hours with increasing serum creatinine.
- Signs of hepatic failure (encephalopathy, increasing ascites, liver pain, hypoglycemia): stop this course of treatment and reinitiate new course after at least 7 weeks of rest.
- Stool guaiac repeatedly > 3–4+.
- Bullous dermatitis or marked worsening of preexisting skin condition (do not use topical steroid therapy).

Drug Preparation:

- Vial containing 22 m IUs (1.3 mg) should be reconstituted with 1.2 mL of sterile water for injection, USP so each mL contains 18 million international units of drug. DO NOT SHAKE. Further dilute in 50 mL of 5% dextrose injection, USP. If dose is < 1.5 mg, use a smaller volume. Refrigerate and use within 48 hours of preparation. Bring to room temperature before administration.

Drug Administration:

- Final concentration should be between 30–70 μg/mL.
- Administer IV over 15 minutes.

Drug Interactions:

- Potentiation of CNS effects when given in combination with psychotropic drugs.
- The combination with nephrotoxic, myelotoxic, cardiotoxic, or hepatotoxic will increase toxicity of aldesleukin in these organ systems.
- Increased risk of hypersensitivity reactions when sequential high-dose aldesleukin combined with dacarbazine, cisplatin, tamoxifen, and IFN-α.

- IFN-α and aldesleukin concurrently: increased risk of myocardial injury (MI, myocarditis, severe rhabdomyolysis).
- Glucocorticoid steroids: decreased antitumor effectiveness. Do not use together.
- β-Blockers, antihypertensives: potentiate hypotension of aldesleukin.
- Iodinated contrast medium: increased risk of atypical adverse reaction (12.6% incidence) characterized by fever, chills, nausea, vomiting, pruritus, rash, diarrhea, hypotension, edema, and oliguria and typically happens when contrast is given within 4 weeks of aldesleukin dosing.

Lab Effects/Interference:
- Anemia, leukopenia, thrombocytopenia.
- Elevated LFTs.
- Increased serum creatinine.
- Acidosis.
- Hypomagnesemia.
- Hypocalcemia.

Special Considerations:
- FDA-indicated for treatment of adult patients with metastatic renal cell cancer or metastatic malignant melanoma.
- Patient must have NORMAL cardiac, pulmonary, hepatic, renal (serum creatinine ≤ 1.5 mg/dL) and CNS function before treatment and be free of any known infection.
- Drug may worsen symptoms of patients with unknown/untreated CNS metastases. Thorough evaluation and treatment of CNS metastases should precede the treatment so that the patient has a negative scan before starting aldesleukin.
- Use caution when patient is receiving other drugs that are hepatic or renally toxic.
- Drug may increase rejection in allogeneic transplant patients, exacerbation of autoimmune disease, and inflammatory disorders.
- Contraindicated in male or female patients of child-bearing age/intentionally not using effective contraception; nursing mothers should not nurse while taking the drug unless benefit outweighs unknown risk.

Potential Toxicities/Side Effects (Dose-1 and Schedule-Dependent) and the Nursing Process

I. ALTERATION IN COMFORT related to FLU-LIKE SYNDROME

Defining Characteristics: Chills may occur 2–4 hours after dose; rigors are possible; fever to 39–40°C (102–104°F) and headache. Myalgia and arthralgias may occur at high doses because of accumulation of cytokine deposits/lymphocytes in joint spaces. The incidence of chills is 52%, fever 29%, malaise 27%, asthenia 23%, anorexia 20%.

Nursing Implications: Assess baseline T, VS, neurologic status, and comfort level, and monitor every 4–6 hours if patient is in hospital. Discuss with physician premedication and regular dosing of antipyretic (e.g., acetaminophen ± diphen-hydramine, NSAID). If patient is in hospital and experiences rigor, discuss with physician IV meperidine and monitor BP for hypotension.

II. SENSORY/PERCEPTUAL ALTERATION related to CNS EFFECTS

Defining Characteristics: Confusion, irritability, disorientation, impaired memory, expressive aphasia, sleep disturbances, depression, hallucinations, and psychoses may occur, resolving within 24–48 hours after last drug dose. Mental status abnormalities exaggerated by anxiety and sleep deprivation.

Nursing Implications: Assess baseline mental status and neurologic status before drug administration. Assess patient for changes (impaired memory/attention, disorientation, slow/vague responses to questions, increased lethargy) during treatment. Teach patient to report signs/symptoms. Provide information, emotional support, and interventions to ensure safety if signs/symptoms occur.

III. ALTERATION IN CARDIAC OUTPUT related to HYPOTENSION (HIGH-DOSE THERAPY)

Defining Characteristics: Increased risk with dose > 100,000 IU/kg. Capillary leak syndrome (peripheral edema, CHF, pleural effusions, and pericardial effusions) may occur and is reversible once treatment is stopped. Atrial arrhythmias may occur; occasionally, supraventricular tachycardia, myocarditis, chest pain; and rarely, myocardial infarction. IL-2 causes peripheral vasodilation, decreased systemic vascular resistance, and hypotension that may lead to decreased renal perfusion. A decrease in SBP occurs 2–12 hours after start of therapy and typically will progress to significant hypotension (SBP < 90 mmHg or a 20-mmHg drop from baseline SBP) with hypoperfusion. In addition, protein and fluids will extravasate into the extravascular space forming edema and new effusions.

Nursing Implications: Assess baseline cardiopulmonary status and patients at risk (the older population, those with preexisting cardiac dysfunction). Monitor VS and pulse oximetry frequently, at least q 4 hour (if hypotensive, q 1 hr), noting rate, rhythm of heartbeat, blood pressure, urinary output, fluid status, I/O q 4 hours or more frequent, and daily weights during therapy. Discuss any abnormalities with physician, and revise plan as needed (e.g., diuretics, plasma expanders). Instruct patient to report signs/symptoms of dyspnea, chest pain, edema, or other abnormalities immediately. Hypotension requires fluid replacement, and patient should be monitored with continuous cardiac monitoring if SBP < 90 mmHg. Any ectopy should be documented on EKG. Manufacturer states that early administration of dopamine (1–5 μg/kg/min) to patients with capillary leak syndrome before the onset of hypotension can improve organ perfusion and preserve urinary output. Increased dopamine doses (6–10 μg/kg/min) or the addition of phenylephrine hydrochloride (1–5 μg/kg/min) to low-dose dopamine has been described. After blood pressure is stabilized, the use of diuretics is often effective in relieving edema and pulmonary congestion.

IV. POTENTIAL ALTERATION IN OXYGENATION

Defining Characteristics: Pulmonary symptoms are dose related, such as dyspnea and tachypnea. Pulmonary edema may occur with hypoxia because of fluid shifts.

Nursing Implications: Assess baseline cardiopulmonary status every 4 hours during therapy, noting rate, rhythm, depth of respirations, presence of dyspnea, and breath sounds (presence of wheezes, crackles, rhonchi). Identify patients at risk: those with preexisting cardiac or pulmonary disease, prior treatment with cardio-or pulmonary-toxic drugs or radiation, and smoking history. Instruct the patient to report cough, dyspnea, or change in respiratory status. Strictly monitor I/O, total fluid balance, and daily weight. Discuss abnormalities with physician, as well as the need for oxygen, diuretics, or transfer to ICU.

V. POTENTIAL ALTERATION IN NUTRITION, LESS THAN BODY REQUIREMENTS, related to NAUSEA/VOMITING, DIARRHEA, MUCOSITIS, ANOREXIA

Defining Characteristics: Nausea and vomiting are mild and are effectively controlled by antiemetics. Diarrhea is common and can be severe. Stomatitis is common but mild.

Nursing Implications: Assess the patient's baseline nutritional status. Administer antiemetics as ordered. Teach the patient potential side effects and self-care measures, including oral hygiene, and encourage patient to eat favorite high-calorie, high-protein foods. Teach self-administration of prescribed antiemetics and antidiarrheals as needed. Refer to the dietitian as appropriate.

VI. POTENTIAL ALTERATION IN ELIMINATION related to RENAL DYSFUNCTION, HEPATOTOXICITY

Defining Characteristics: IL-2 causes decreased renal blood flow with cumulative doses. Oliguria, proteinuria, increased serum creatinine and BUN, and increased LFTs (bili, AST, ALT, LDH, alk phos) may occur. Anuria occurs in 5% of patients; renal dysfunction is reversible after drug discontinuance. Hepatomegaly and hypoalbuminemia may occur.

Nursing Implications: Assess baseline renal and hepatic functions and monitor during treatment. Assess fluid and electrolyte balance, urine output hourly, and total body balance. Dipstick urine for protein. Discuss abnormalities with physician and revise plan.

VII. POTENTIAL FOR FATIGUE AND BLEEDING related to ANEMIA, THROMBOCYTOPENIA

Defining Characteristics: Anemia occurs in 29% of patients and may require RBC transfusion. Thrombocytopenia occurs commonly but rarely requires transfusion.

Nursing Implications: Assess baseline CBC and platelet count and signs/symptoms of fatigue, severe anemia, bleeding. Instruct the patient to report signs/symptoms immediately and to manage self-care (alternate rest/activity, minimize bleeding by avoidance of OTC aspirin-containing medicines). Transfuse red cells and platelets as ordered.

VIII. POTENTIAL ALTERATION IN SKIN INTEGRITY related to DIFFUSE RASH

Defining Characteristics: Patients may develop diffuse erythematous rash, which may desquamate (soles of feet, palms of hands, between fingers). Pruritus may occur with or without rash.

Nursing Implications: Assess baseline skin integrity. Teach patient to report signs/symptoms. Discuss/teach symptomatic management, including the use of mild soaps and rinsing skin thoroughly after bathing. Encourage the use of alcohol-free, oil-based moisturizers on skin and the protection of desquamated areas.

Drug: darbepoetin alfa (Aranesp)

Class: Cytokine, CSF.

Mechanism of Action: Recombinant DNA protein that is an erythropoiesis-stimulating protein, closely resembling erythropoietin. Drug is produced in the Chinese hamster ovary. Drug stimulates erythropoiesis in the same way that endogenous erythropoietin does in response to hypoxia. Darbepoetin alfa interacts with progenitor stem cells to stimulate red blood cell production.

Metabolism: Drug is slowly absorbed after subcutaneous injection, with bioavailability of 37%, a peak serum level 34 hours after administration (24–72 hour range), and half-life of 49 hours (27–89 hour range) in patients with chronic renal failure. In patients with cancer, the peak serum concentration occurs at 90 hours with a range of 71–123 hours. When given IV, the drug has a biphasic profile, with a distribution half-life of 1.4 hours, and terminal half-life of 21 hours, which is about 3 times longer than epoetin alfa.

Dosage/Range:

- Use the *lowest dose* of darbepoetin alfa that will gradually increase the hemoglobin concentration to the lowest level sufficient to avoid the need for red blood cell transfusion. Should not be used if goal is cure.
- Cancer patients receiving chemotherapy hgb < 10 g/dL: 2.25 micrograms/kg subcutaneous q week as starting dose.
  - If less than 1.0 g/dL increase in hgb after 6 weeks of therapy, increase the dose to 4.5 μg/kg weekly.
- Cancer patients receiving chemotherapy: 500 micrograms subcutaneous q 3 weeks.
- Modifications:
  - If hgb increases by > 1.0 g/dL in 2-week period or when hgb reaches level to avoid retransfusion, reduce dose by 40% of the prior dose.
  - If hgb > level to avoid RBC retransfusion, hold dose until hgb falls to point where transfusion may be needed and restart at 40% below previous dose.
- Dose increases should not occur more frequently than once a month.
- Adjust dose to maintain target hemoglobin not to exceed 12 g/dL.
- Chronic renal failure patients: 0.45 micrograms/kg IV or SC q week as starting dose.
  - If increase in hgb is < 1.0 g/dL over 4 weeks and iron stores are adequate, increase dose by 25% of the previous dose; dose may be increased at 4-week intervals until hgb is 10–12 g/dL; dose increase no more frequently than once a month.
  - If hgb is increasing and approaching 12 g/dL, reduce the dose by 25%; if the hgb continues to increase, hold the dose until hgb starts to decline, and reinstitute drug at 25% less than prior dose.
  - If hgb increases by > 1 g/dL in 2-week period, decrease dose by 25% as want to maintain the lowest hemoglobin to avoid red blood cell transfusion, not to exceed 12 g/dL.
  - Convert from epoetin alfa to darbepoetin alfa (Special Considerations).
- NCCN alternative regimens (NCCN, 2008).
  - Darbepoetin 100 μg/week fixed dosing—titrate up to 150–200 micrograms fixed dose weekly subcutaneously.
  - Darbepoetin 200 μg every 2 weeks fixed dosing—titrate up to 300 μg fixed dose every 2 weeks subcutaneously.
  - Darbepoetin 300 μg every 3 weeks fixed dosing—titrate up to 500 μg fixed dose every 3 weeks subcutaneously.

Drug Preparation:

- Drug available in single-dose vials or prefilled syringes (SingleJet) containing 25, 40, 60, 100, 150, 200, 300, or 500 micrograms of darbepoetin alfa with either polysorbate or albumin solution; contains no preservative so should not be pooled. Syringe has UltraSafe Needle Guards.

- Available as prefilled SureClick autoinjectors (delivers only full doses) in 25, 40, 60, 100, 150, 200, 300, or 500 μg of darbepoetin alfa with either polysorbate or albumin solution.
- Do not shake drug as it may denature it; keep out of bright light; do not dilute; visually inspect drug for discoloration or particulate matter prior to parenteral administration, and discard if found.
- Store at 2° to 8°C (36° to 46°F). Do not freeze or shake, and protect from light.

Drug Administration:

- Administer subcutaneous or IV weekly to start, and may be able to give every 2 weeks depending upon response to drug.

Drug Interactions:

- No studies have been performed.

Lab Effects/Interference:

- Increased hemoglobin and hematocrit.
- Rare pure red-cell aplasia, severe anemia related to neutralizing antibodies.

Special Considerations:

- New black box warning: Darbepoetin and other erythropoiesis-stimulating agents (ESAs) increased the risk for death and for serious cardiovascular events when given to a target hemoglobin of > 12 g/dL in cancer patients.
  - Shortened the time to tumor progression in patients with advanced head and neck cancer receiving radiation therapy when given to a target hemoglobin > 12 g/dL.
  - Shortened overall survival and increased deaths attributed to disease progression at 4 months in patients with metastatic breast cancer receiving chemotherapy when given to a target hemoglobin > 12 g/dL.
  - Increased risk of death when given to a target hemoglobin > 12 g/dL in patients with active malignant disease receiving neither chemotherapy nor radiation therapy (not indicated for this population).
  - Patients receiving ESAs preoperatively to reduce the need for allogeneic blood cell transfusions had a higher incidence of deep venous thrombosis if not also receiving prophylactic anticoagulation; darbepoetin is not indicated for this condition.
- Contraindicated in patients with uncontrolled hypertension, or known hypersensitivity to any of the active substance or excipients (albumin or polysorbate).
- Drug may increase the risk of cardiovascular events in patients with chronic renal failure (CRF) due to high hemoglobin and risk increased in patients who had a rise of 1 g/dL or more in a 2-week period.
- Once starting drug, weekly hemoglobin should be monitored until stabilized and maintenance dose has been established; once dose has been adjusted, the hemoglobin should be monitored weekly for at least 4 weeks until stabilization occurs; once maintenance established, hemoglobin should be monitored at regular intervals.
- Rarely, patients may develop antibodies that neutralize the effect, and rarely can lead to red cell aplasia. If a patient loses response to darbepoetin alfa, evaluation should

be done to find cause, including presence of binding and neutralizing antibodies to darbepoetin alfa, native erythropoietin, and any other recombinant erythropoietin administered to the patient.

- Overall incidence of thrombotic events 6.2% compared to 4.1% for placebo, characterized by pulmonary embolism, thromboembolism, thrombosis, and thrombophlebitis (deep and/or superficial).
- Target hemoglobin goal is level to avoid RBC transfusion.
- Edema occurred in 21% of patients as compared to 10% with placebo.
- The possibility that darbepoetin alfa can stimulate tumor growth, especially as a growth factor of myeloid malignancies, has not been studied.
- Iron status should be assessed before and during treatment to ensure effective erythropoiesis; supplemental iron is recommended for patients with serum ferritin < 100 mcg/L or whose serum transferring saturation is < 20%. If patient does not respond to darbepoetin alfa, folic acid and vitamin B_{12} levels should also be assessed and deficiencies corrected.
- No studies have been performed on use of the drug in pregnant women. Drug should be used only if potential benefit outweighs risk to the fetus; it is unknown if the drug is excreted in human milk, so caution should be used if used in a nursing mother.
- Rarely, allergic reactions can be severe, including skin rash and urticaria. Drug should be discontinued if serious allergic or anaphylactic reactions occur.
- Patients who have controlled hypertension should have regular assessment of blood pressure. Patients should be encouraged to be compliant with their anti-hypertensive medication regime.
- Dosing in chronic renal failure: Estimated darbepoetin alfa starting doses (mcg/week) based on prior epoetin alfa dose (units/week); darbepoetin should be given less frequently than epoetin alfa (e.g., if patient receiving epoetin alfa weekly, then darbepoetin should be given every 2 weeks via the same route, IV or subcutaneously).

Previous Weekly Epoetin Alfa Dose (units/wk)	**Weekly Darbepoetin Alfa Dose *nl (mcg/week)**
< 1500	6.25
1500–2499	6.25
2500–4999	12.5
5000–10,999	25
11,000–17,999	40
18,000–33,999	60
34,000–89,999	100
≥ 90,000	200

Potential Toxicities/Side Effects and the Nursing Process

I. ACTIVITY INTOLERANCE related to FATIGUE

Defining Characteristics: 33% of cancer patients reported fatigue compared to 30% in the placebo group. Patients had advanced disease, which may explain the high incidence.

Nursing Implications: Assess baseline activity and energy levels. Assess baseline fluid.

II. ALTERATION IN SKIN INTEGRITY, POTENTIAL, related to PERIPHERAL EDEMA, RASH

Defining Characteristics: Peripheral edema occurred in 21% of cancer patients in clinical trials as compared to 10% in the placebo group; rash occurred in 7% of patients receiving darbepoetin alfa compared to 3% in the placebo group.

Nursing Implications: Perform baseline skin assessment, assess baseline weight and presence of edema. Teach patient to report development of peripheral edema. Teach patient self-assessment of skin, weight, and peripheral edema, and to report rash right away. Assess degree of peripheral edema if it develops, and discuss significant edema with physician to determine etiology and management. Teach patient local skin care, including avoidance of tight clothing and shoes, keeping skin moisturized to prevent cracking, and local comfort measures. If rash develops, assess extent, presence of urticaria, and implications regarding allergic reaction and drug discontinuance.

III. ALTERATION IN COMFORT related to HEADACHE, DIZZINESS, FEVER, MYALGIA, ARTHRALGIA

Defining Characteristics: Headache occurred in 12% of cancer patients in the clinical trials compared to 8% in the placebo group; dizziness 14% compared to 8% in placebo group; fever 19% compared to 16% in placebo group; myalgias 13% compared to 6% in placebo group, and myalgias 8% compared to 5% in the placebo group, probably due to bone marrow expansion.

Nursing Implications: Teach patient bone pain may occur and discuss use of nonsteroidal anti-inflammatory drugs with patient and physician for symptom management. Teach patient to remain seated or lying down if feeling dizzy, and when dizziness has resolved, to change position gradually. Monitor hemoglobin weekly during dose determination period, and weekly for at least 4 weeks after each dose adjustment. Teach patient headache, fever, dizziness, myalgia, and arthralgia may occur and to report them if they do not respond to usual management strategies.

IV. ALTERATION IN ELIMINATION related to DIARRHEA

Defining Characteristics: Diarrhea occurred in 22% of cancer patients receiving the drug in clinical trials compared to 12% of placebo group; 18% experienced constipation compared to 17% in the placebo group.

Nursing Implications: Assess baseline patient bowel elimination pattern. Teach patient to report these side effects so that they can be evaluated. Teach patient self-care measures, including dietary modification, local comfort measures, and over-the-counter anti-diarrheal medication. Teach patient to report symptoms that persist, and discuss with physician possible other etiologies and management plan.

V. KNOWLEDGE DEFICIT related to SELF-ADMINISTRATION TECHNIQUE

Defining Characteristics: Drug is administered once weekly, or if response is adequate, may be given once every 2 weeks.

Nursing Implications: Assess baseline psychomotor ability, knowledge, and willingness to learn technique of self-injection. Teach how to refrigerate drug, self-administer using pre-filled syringes, how to activate needle guard, and safely collect used syringes for proper disposal. Drug insert has "Information for Patients and Caregivers." Use written and video supplements to teaching process and have patient correctly demonstrate technique prior to performing at home. Make referral to visiting-nurse agency to reinforce teaching if needed. Teach patient telephone number and who to call if questions or problems arise, and ensure patient can correctly repeat information.

Drug: epoetin alfa (Epogen, Erythropoietin, Procrit)

Class: Cytokine, colony stimulating factor (CSF).

Mechanism of Action: Stimulates the division and differentiation of erythrocyte stem cells in the bone marrow and is a hormone produced by recombinant DNA techniques. Has a naturally occurring counterpart, erythropoietin. Results in the release of reticulocytes into the bloodstream in 7–10 days, where they mature into erythrocytes, taking 2–6 weeks to increase hemoglobin.

Metabolism: Following SC injection, 21–31% of drug is bioavailable, with rapid distribution to tissues. Drug is taken up in the liver, kidneys, and bone marrow. Onset of action in a few days to 2 weeks; peak effect in 2–3 weeks. Half-life is 4–13 h. Eliminated via the liver and urine (10% unchanged drug).

Dosage/Range:

I. 50–150 units/kg TIW; if no increase in HCT within 8 weeks, increase dose by 25–50 units/kg/dose up to 300 units/kg TIW.

II. 40,000 units as a single dose once a week subcutaneous; if HCT does not rise 5–6% in 8 weeks, increase dose to 60,000 units/week; if no response, increase dose to 80,000 units/week (maximum).

- Use the *lowest dose* of darbepoetin alfa that will gradually increase the hemoglobin concentration to the lowest level sufficient to avoid the need for red blood cell transfusion and NOT TO EXCEED 12 g/dL.
- Cancer patients receiving chemotherapy (nonmyeloid, noncurative) with hgb < 10 g/dL:
  - Endogenous erythropoietin levels < 200 U/mL are most likely to respond.
  - Initial dose is 150 U/kg subcutaneous TIW or 40,000 U subcutaneously weekly.
  - Reduce dose by 25% when hgb approaches a level sufficient to avoid RBC transfusion or hgb increases > 1 g/dL in any 2-week period.
  - Hold dose if hgb > level needed to avoid RBC transfusion and resume at 25% below previous dose.
  - Increase dose if inadequate response (no decrease in red blood cell requirement or rise in hgb) after 4 weeks.
    - TIW: increase dose to 300 U/kg TIW.
    - Weekly: increase to 60,000 U weekly.
- Surgery patients (preoperative use for reduction of allogeneic red blood cell transfusion).
  - Assess hgb: must be > 10–13 g/dL.
  - Dose is 300 U/kg/day subcutaneously × 10 days before surgery, on the day of surgery, and for 4 days after surgery.
  - Alternate schedule is 600 U/kg once weekly on days 21, 14, and 7 days before surgery, plus a fourth dose on the day of surgery.
  - All patients should receive adequate iron supplementation to start at least by the beginning of epoetin alfa therapy.
  - Patients should also receive prophylactic anticoagulation to prevent DVT.
- Chronic renal failure:
  - Ensure adequate patient iron stores (transferrin saturation at least 20%, ferritin at least 100 ng/mL).
  - 50–100 U/kg TIW (adult) or 50 U/kg TIW (pediatric) to maintain hgb between 10–12 g/dL.
  - Reduce dose by 25% if hgb approaches 12 g/dL; if hgb continues to increase, hold dose until hgb begins to decline, and then reinstitute drug at dose 25% less than previous dose.
  - Reduce dose by 25% if hgb increases by > 1 g/dL in a 2-week period.
  - Increase dose by 25% if hgb does not increase by 2 g/dL after 8 weeks of therapy, or hgb rise is < 1 g/dL over 4 weeks, and iron stores are adequate (transferrin saturation > 20%); do not increase dose more frequently than once a month; monitor hgb twice weekly for 2–6 weeks after dose increase.
  - Maintain lowest dose to avoid red blood cell transfusion but not to exceed 12 g/dL.
- Zidovudine-treated HIV-infected adult patients:
  - Likely to respond if endogenous serum erythropoietin level ≤ 500 U/mL.
  - If zidovudine dose ≤ 4200 mg/week: epoetin alfa 100 U/kg TIW subcutaneously or IV for 8 weeks; monitor hgb weekly.

- Increase dose if response inadequate, by 50–100 U/kg TIW subcutaneously or IV and evaluate response every 4–8 weeks thereafter, and adjust dose in 50–100 U/kg TIW subcutaneously or IV to a dose of 300 U/kg TIW, as it is unlikely the patient will respond to higher doses.
- Hold drug if hgb > 12 g/dL until hgb < 11 g/dL, and then resume drug with a 25% dose reduction of previous dose.

- Alternative regimens (NCCN, 2007):
  - Epoetin alfa 80,000 Units every 2 weeks subcutaneously.
  - Epoetin alfa 120,000 Units every 3 weeks subcutaneously.

Drug Preparation:

- DO NOT SHAKE vial, as it may denature the glycoprotein.
- Available as preservative-free, single-dose vials for injection in 2000-U/mL, 3000-U/mL, 4000-U/mL, 10,000-U/mL, and 40,000-U/mL vials. These must be refrigerated, and unused portions should be discarded.
- Multidose injection vials, preserved with benzyl alcohol: available as 10,000-U/mL (2 mL) and 20,000-U/mL (1 mL); discard 21 days after initial entry.
- Store at 2°–8°C (36°–46°F).
- Do not dilute or administer with other drugs.
- Subcutaneous administration: At the time of injection, may admix in the syringe, bacteriostatic 0.9% sodium chloride injection USP with benzyl alcohol 0.9% (bacteriostatic saline) to the preservative free epoetin from single use vial to reduce injection site discomfort.

Drug Administration:

- Subcutaneous or IV (chronic renal failure on dialysis at end of dialysis) injection.

Drug Interactions:

- None reported.

Lab Effects/Interference:

- Expect increase in Hgb/HCT in 2–6 weeks.

Special Considerations:

- New black box warning: Darbepoetin and other erythropoiesis-stimulating agents (ESAs) increased the risk for death and for serious cardiovascular events when given to a target hemoglobin of > 12 g/dL in cancer patients.
  - Shortened the time to tumor progression in patients with advanced head and neck cancer receiving radiation therapy when given to a target hemoglobin > 12 g/dL.
  - Shortened overall survival and increased deaths attributed to disease progression at 4 months in patients with metastatic breast cancer receiving chemotherapy when given to a target hemoglobin > 12 g/dL.
  - Increased risk of death when given to a target hemoglobin > 12 g/dL in patients with active malignant disease receiving neither chemotherapy nor radiation therapy (not indicated for this population).

  - Patients receiving ESAs preoperatively to reduce the need for allogeneic blood cell transfusions had a higher incidence of deep venous thrombosis if not also receiving prophylactic anticoagulation; darbepoetin is not indicated for this condition.
- Drug is contraindicated in patients with uncontrolled hypertension.
- Iron stores need to be checked, and replaced to maximize response to therapy.
- Used for management of chemotherapy-related anemia and anemia of chronic disease.

Potential Toxicities/Side Effects (Dose- and Schedule-Dependent) and the Nursing Process

I. ALTERATION IN COMFORT related to PYREXIA, FATIGUE, HEADACHE

Defining Characteristics: May be due to HIV disease, rather than drug, and occurs in 20–25% of patients. Allergic reactions including urticaria may occur. Anaphylaxis has not been reported.

Nursing Implications: Assess baseline temperature (T) and energy level. Instruct patient to report signs/symptoms, and discuss measures to increase comfort.

II. POTENTIAL ALTERATION IN OXYGENATION related to POLYCYTHEMIA

Defining Characteristics: Polycythemia may result if target range is exceeded with consequent complications (Hbg > 12 g/dL).

Nursing Implications: Monitor weekly hgb until stable dose is achieved. Dose should be interrupted if hgb approaches 12 g/dL and then resumed at 75% dose once HCT is < 11 g/dL. When hgb has stabilized, discuss monitoring hgb with physician (e.g., testing).

III. KNOWLEDGE DEFICIT related to SELF-ADMINISTRATION TECHNIQUE

Defining Characteristics: Most often drug is administered subcutaneous three times per week or weekly.

Nursing Implications: Assess baseline psychomotor ability, knowledge, and willingness to learn technique of self-injection. Teach how to prepare drug, self-administer, and safely collect used syringes for proper disposal. Use written and video materials as supplements to teaching process and have patient correctly demonstrate technique prior to performing at home. Make referral to visiting-nurse agency to reinforce teaching.

Drug: filgrastim (Neupogen, G-CSF)

Class: Cytokine, CSF.

Mechanism of Action: Recombinant DNA protein (G-CSF) that regulates the production of neutrophils in the bone marrow (proliferation, differentiation, activation of mature neutrophils). Drug is produced by the insertion of the human G-CSF gene into *Escherichia coli* bacteria.

Metabolism: Elimination half-life is 3.5 hours.

Dosage/Range:
- Starting dose 5 μg/kg/day subcutaneous or IV; dose increase by 5 μg/kg for each chemotherapy cycle, based on duration and severity of neutropenia at nadir.
- BMT: After BMT, 10 μg/kg/day as IV infusion of 4 or 24 hours, or as a continuous subcutaneous, 24-hour infusion, and then titrated based on ANC.
- Mobilization of peripheral blood progenitor cells (PBPC) is 10 mcg/kg/day subcutaneous × at least 4 days until the first leukapheresis procedure, and continued until the last leukapheresis. Modify dose if WBC > 100,000/mm^3.
- Patients with acute myeloid leukemia receiving induction or consolidation: 5 mcg/kg/day subcutaneous beginning 24 hrs after last dose of chemotherapy until ANC > 1000/mm^3 for 3 consecutive days.

Drug Preparation:
- Drug available in refrigerated vials of 300 μg/mL; discard unused portions.
- Unopened vials should be stored in the refrigerator at 2–8°C (36–46°F).
- Avoid shaking.
- Remove from refrigerator 30 minutes prior to injection. Discard if left out > 6 hours.

Drug Administration:
- Subcutaneous or IV, daily, beginning at least 24 hr postadministration of chemotherapy, continuing up to 2 weeks or until ANC > 10,000/mm^3.

Drug Interactions:
- None significant.

Lab Effects/Interference:
- Increased WBC and neutrophil counts.
- Increased LDH, uric acid, alkaline phosphatase.

Special Considerations:
- PEGylated form of filgrastim (sustained duration) is available and is given once a treatment cycle; it is equivalent to daily injections of filgrastim (see pegfilgrastim).
- Indicated for accelerating the recovery of neutrophil counts after myelosuppressive chemotherapy, including BMT and prevention of febrile neutropenia.
- Indicated for the mobilization of hematopoietic progenitor cells into the periphery for collection by leukapheresis, and reinfusion for stem cell rescue.

- Studies showed no statistical difference between Neupogen or placebo group in complete remission rate, disease-free survival, time to disease progression, or overall survival when used in patients with acute myeloid leukemia after induction or consolidation therapy.
- Rarely, drug may exacerbate preexisting psoriasis, Sweet's syndrome (neutrophilic dermatitis), and cutaneous vasculitis.

Potential Toxicities/Side Effects (Dose- and Schedule-Dependent) and the Nursing Process

I. ALTERATION IN COMFORT related to SKELETAL PAIN

Defining Characteristics: Patients (22%) may report transient skeletal pain, believed due to the expansion of cells in the bone marrow in response to G-CSF.

Nursing Implications: Teach patient this may occur and discuss use of nonsteroidal anti-inflammatory drugs (NSAIDs) with patient and physician for symptom management. Monitor WBC and ANC twice weekly during therapy; dose should be discontinued when ANC > $10,000/mm^3$.

II. KNOWLEDGE DEFICIT related to SELF-ADMINISTRATION TECHNIQUE

Defining Characteristics: Drug is administered daily for up to two weeks by subcutaneous injection (outpatients).

Nursing Implications: Assess baseline psychomotor ability, knowledge, and willingness to learn technique of self-injection. Teach how to prepare drug, self-administer, and safely collect used syringes for proper disposal. Use written and video supplements to teaching process and have patient correctly demonstrate technique prior to performing at home. Make referral to visiting-nurse agency to reinforce teaching. Patient instructions in English are on package insert. Video and more detailed patient education are available from Amgen (Thousand Oaks, CA) representative.

Drug: imiquimod 5% topical cream (Aldara®)

Class: Immune response modifier.

Mechanism of Action: Stimulates the immune system to release cytokines, including interferon, which stimulate Langerhans cells to kill skin cancer cells. Has been shown to reduce the expression of Bcl-2 (a protein that causes the cell to avoid apoptosis, or programmed cell death, by preventing the activation of the proapoptotic proteins called capases) and increase apoptosis of basal skin cancer cells.

Metabolism: Unknown.

Dosage/Range:

- Imiquimod 5% topical cream is applied to the superficial basal cell carcinoma (sBCC) lesion (must be 2 cm or less in diameter), including a 1 cm margin around the lesion as shown in the table below.

Target Tumor Diameter	Size of Cream Droplet to be Used (diameter)	Amount of Imiquimod Cream Used
0.5 cm–<1.0 cm	4 mm	10 mg
> 1.0 cm–<1.5 cm	5 mm	25 mg
> 1.5 cm–2.0 cm	7 mm	40 mg

Available in single use packets, supplied 12 per box.

Drug Preparation: Wash hands before and after application of cream, and wear gloves. Wash skin area(s) with mild soap and water, then dry thoroughly before application, and again, after 8 hours application. Apply cream to lesion with an additional 1 cm surrounding the lesion(s), at bedtime leaving the cream on at least 8 hours, 5 nights a week, × 6 weeks.

Drug Interactions:

- Unknown.

Lab Effects/Interference:

- None known.

Special Considerations:

- Indicated for the treatment of sBCC on the body, neck, arms, or legs (not the face, hands, or feet) when surgical removal is not an option.
- Drug is also used for the treatment of external genital and non-genital warts, molluscum contagiosum, solar keratoses.

Potential Toxicities/Side Effects (More Severe with Higher Dosing) and the Nursing Process

I. POTENTIAL ALTERATION IN SKIN INTEGRITY AND COMFORT related to SKIN IRRITATION

Defining Characteristics: Redness, swelling, development of a sore or blister, peeling, itching, and burning are common application site reactions. Response to therapy cannot be determined until the skin reaction resolves, sometimes up to 12 weeks.

Nursing Implications: Explain to the patient that these side effects may occur. Teach patient to wash skin prior to application, and again after 8 hours. Teach patient to assess skin reactions, and to report any symptoms that interfere with activities of daily living, as a rest period of a few days may be necessary if symptoms are severe. In addition, instruct patient to stop cream and report infection in the application area right away.

II. KNOWLEDGE DEFICIT related to SELF-ADMINISTRATION OF CREAM

Defining Characteristics: Treatment is for 6 weeks and must be applied properly for adequate tumor exposure.

Nursing Implications: Teach patient self-administration of the cream, and to keep a diary to keep track of the application schedule. Teach patient to wash hands before and after application. Teach patient verbally and through demonstration to wash treatment area with mild soap and water, then to dry prior to application. Cream should be applied to extend 1 cm beyond the lesion borders, and rubbed into the treatment area until no longer visible. Keep cream away from eyes. Cream should be on for at least 8 hours, and then removed using mild soap and water.

Drug: interferon alfa (α) (Alpha interferon, IFN, Interferon alpha-2a, rIFN-A, Roferon A)

Class: Cytokine.

Mechanism of Action: Antiviral, antiproliferative, and immunomodulatory effects. Activates prenatural killer cells, increases cytotoxicity of NK cells, and enhances immune response.

Metabolism: Well absorbed following subcutaneous or IM injection with 90% bioavailability after subcutaneous injection. Drug peaks at 6–8 hours, and has an elimination half-life of 2 hours (IM/IV) and 3 hours (subcutaneous). Renal filtration and tubular reabsorption as catabolites; minor hepatic metabolism and biliary excretion.

Dosage/Range:

- Hairy-cell leukemia: IFN-α_{2a}: Induction 3 m international units daily for 16–24 weeks (IM, subcutaneous); maintenance 3 million international units three times per week for 6–24 months.
- CML: 9 m international units daily subcutaneous × up to 18 months.
- AIDS-related Kaposi's sarcoma: IFN-α_{2a}: Induction 3 m international units daily for 10–12 weeks (IM, subcutaneous); can escalate dose from 3 m international units → 9 m international units → 18 m international units over 3 days to 36 m international units; maintenance 36 m international units three times per week.
- Malignant melanoma: 3 m international units daily × 8–48 weeks.

Drug Preparation:

- IFN-α_{2a} available as injection solution (3–m international units vial or 18–m international units multidose vial) or powder for injection (3 m international units/0.5 mL in 18–m international units vial). Do not shake or freeze. Store in refrigerator and use reconstituted solution within 30 days.

Drug Administration:
- IM, subcutaneous, or IV.

Drug Interactions:
- May decrease elimination of aminophylline by 33–81% via inhibition of cytochrome P-450 enzyme system.
- Increased effects of CNS depressants.
- Increased bone marrow suppressant effects with zidovudine (AZT).
- Cimetidine may increase antitumor effect in melanoma.
- Vinblastine: may increase incidence of peripheral neuropathy.

Lab Effects/Interference:
- Dose-dependent; leukopenia; elevated liver serum transaminases.

Potential Toxicities/Side Effects (More Severe with Higher Dosing) and the Nursing Process

I. ALTERATION IN COMFORT related to FLU-LIKE SYNDROME

Defining Characteristics: Chills 3–6 hours after dose in 40–60% of patients; fever (74–98% of patients) with onset 30–90 minutes after chill, lasting up to 24 hours. Temperature 39–40°C (102–104°F), tachyphylaxis (decrease in severity/occurrence after successive treatments) common. Fatigue (89–95% of patients) and malaise are cumulative and dose-limiting. Headache, myalgias occur in 60–70% of patients, as well as arthralgias (5–24% of patients).

Nursing Implications: Assess baseline T, vital signs (VS), neurologic status, and comfort level; monitor every 4–6 hours if patient is in hospital. Discuss with physician premedication and regular dosing of antipyretic (e.g., acetaminophen ± diphenhydramine, NSAID). Teach patient self-care measures, including monitoring T, comfort level, self-administration of prescribed medications prior to dose and regularly post-dose, as well as the use of heat or cold for myalgias, arthralgias. Encourage patient to increase oral fluids and alternate rest and activity periods. If patient is in hospital and experiences rigor, discuss with physician IV meperidine (25 mg IV q 15 min to maximum 100 mg in 1 hour) and monitor BP for hypotension. Teach patient to alternate rest and activity periods.

II. POTENTIAL FOR INFECTION AND BLEEDING related to NEUTROPENIA AND THROMBOCYTOPENIA

Defining Characteristics: Although uncommon, increased risk with increased dose; dose-limiting thrombocytopenia; reversible. Onset usually in 7–10 days, nadir at day 14, but may be delayed in hairy-cell leukemia (20–40 days); recovery in 21 days.

Nursing Implications: Assess baseline CBC, WBC, differential, and platelet count, and signs/symptoms of infection or bleeding. Discuss any abnormalities with physician before drug administration. Teach patient signs/symptoms of infection and bleeding, and to report them immediately. Teach patient self-care measures to minimize infection and bleeding, including avoidance of OTC aspirin-containing medications, and oral hygiene regimen.

III. ALTERATION IN NUTRITION, LESS THAN BODY REQUIREMENTS, related to NAUSEA, DIARRHEA, ANOREXIA

Defining Characteristics: Anorexia occurs (46–65% of patients) and is cumulative and dose-limiting. Nausea (32–51% of patients) is mild with tachyphylaxis after one week. Diarrhea (29–42% of patients) is mild, and vomiting is rare (10–17% of patients). Taste alterations and xerostomia may occur.

Nursing Implications: Assess baseline nutritional status. Teach patient potential side effects and self-care measures, including oral hygiene. Encourage patient to prepare favorite high-calorie, high-protein foods ahead of time so can snack when hungry. Teach self-administration of prescribed antiemetics and antidiarrheals as needed. Refer to dietitian as appropriate.

IV. SENSORY/PERCEPTUAL ALTERATION related to CNS EFFECTS

Defining Characteristics: Dizziness (21–41% of patients), confusion (8–10% of patients), decreased mental status (17% of patients), and depression (16% of patients). Somnolence, irritability, poor concentration, seizures, paranoia, hallucinations, psychoses may occur in 70% of patients but are reversible. Use drug cautiously in patients with history of seizures or CNS dysfunction.

Nursing Implications: Assess baseline mental status and neurologic status prior to drug administration. Assess patient for changes (impaired memory/attention, disorientation, slow/vague responses to questions, increased lethargy) during treatment. Instruct patient to report signs/symptoms; provide information and emotional support, as well as interventions to ensure safety if signs/symptoms occur.

V. POTENTIAL ALTERATION IN CARDIAC OUTPUT related to TACHYCARDIA, CHEST PAIN, DYSRHYTHMIAS

Defining Characteristics: Uncommon but dose-related with increased risk in elderly and patients with preexisting cardiac dysfunction: tachycardia, pallor, cyanosis, chest pain, orthostatic hypotension or hypertension arrhythmias, CHF, syncope.

Nursing Implications: Assess baseline cardiopulmonary status and risk (elderly, preexisting cardiac dysfunction). EKG testing is done baseline and during treatment for high-risk individuals. Monitor VS and I/O, every four hours while receiving drug in hospital. Teach patient to report signs/symptoms of dyspnea, chest pain, edema, or other abnormalities immediately.

VI. POTENTIAL ALTERATION IN ELIMINATION related to RENAL AND HEPATIC DYSFUNCTION

Defining Characteristics: Dose-related increased BUN, creatinine, LFTs (increased AST 42–46%) may occur, as well as proteinuria. Patient may develop interstitial nephritis.

Nursing Implications: Assess baseline renal and hepatic function studies and urinalysis prior to drug initiation, and periodically during therapy. Discuss abnormalities with physician.

VII. POTENTIAL FOR SEXUAL DYSFUNCTION related to IMPOTENCE, MENSTRUAL IRREGULARITIES

Defining Characteristics: Impotence and decreased libido, menstrual irregularities, and increased spontaneous abortions have occurred. Drug is excreted in breast milk.

Nursing Implications: Assess patient's baseline sexual patterns and discuss potential alterations. Provide information, emotional support, and referral as appropriate and needed. Encourage patient to use contraceptive measures; mothers receiving the drug should not breast-feed.

VIII. POTENTIAL ALTERATION IN SKIN INTEGRITY related to RASH, PARTIAL ALOPECIA, DRYNESS

Defining Characteristics: Partial alopecia (8–22% of patients), rash (11–18% of patients), throat dryness (15% of patients), as well as skin dryness, flushing, pruritus, and irritation at injection site may occur.

Nursing Implications: Assess baseline skin integrity. Instruct patient to report signs/symptoms. Discuss/teach symptomatic management, including the use of mild soaps and rinsing skin thoroughly after bathing. Encourage patient to use alcohol-free, oil-based moisturizers on skin.

IX. KNOWLEDGE DEFICIT related to SELF-ADMINISTRATION TECHNIQUE

Defining Characteristics: Often patients must receive daily dosing or thrice weekly dosing in the home setting by subcutaneous injection, and they are unfamiliar with technique.

Nursing Implications: Assess baseline psychomotor ability, knowledge, and willingness to learn technique of self-injection. Teach how to prepare drug, self-administer, and safely collect used syringes for proper disposal. Use written and video materials as supplements to teaching process and have patient correctly demonstrate technique prior to performing at home. Make referral to visiting-nurse agency to reinforce teaching.

Drug: interferon alfa-2b (Intron A, IFN-alpha-2b Recombinant, α-2–Interferon, rIFN-α-2)

Class: Cytokine.

Mechanism of Action: Antiviral, antiproliferative, and immunomodulatory effects. Activates prenatural killer cells, increases cytotoxicity of NK cells, and enhances immune response.

Metabolism: Well absorbed following subcutaneous or IM injection with 90% bioavailability after subcutaneous injection. Drug peaks at 6–8 hours, and has an elimination half-life of 2 hours (IM/IV) and 3 hours (subcutaneous). Renal filtration and tubular reabsorption as catabolites; minor hepatic metabolism and biliary excretion.

Dosage/Range:

- Hairy-cell leukemia: IFN-α_{2b}: 2 million international units/m^2 IM or subcutaneous three times per week × 2–6 months.
- AIDS-related Kaposi's sarcoma: IFN-α_{2b}: 30 million international units/m^2 subcutaneous or IM three times per week.
- Malignant melanoma: Induction: 20 million international units/m^2 IV days 1–5/week for 4 weeks; maintenance: 10 million international units/m^2 subcutaneous three times per week for 48 weeks.
- NHL: 5 million international units TIW.

Drug Preparation:

- IFN-α_{2b} (Intron A): Available in powder for injection (3-, 5-, 10-, 25-, 50-million international units vials).
- Albumin free: in 3-, 5-, 10-, 18-, and 25-million international units vials.
- Powder for injection (lyophilized): 3-, 5-, 10-, 18-, 25-, and 50-million international units vials.
- Multidose pens with 6 doses of 3 million international units (18 million international units) or 5 million international units (30 million international units) or 10 million international units (60 million international units).

Drug Administration:

- IM, subcutaneous, or IV (IVB, intermittent or continuous infusion).
- Ensure patient has adequate hydration, especially during treatment for malignant melanoma; this may require IV hydration.

Drug Interactions:

- May decrease elimination of aminophylline by 33–81% via inhibition of cytochrome P-450 enzyme system.
- Increased effects of CNS depressants.
- Increased bone marrow suppressant effects with zidovudine (AZT).
- Increased risk of peripheral neuropathy when combined with vinblastine.

Lab Effects/Interference:

- Dose-dependent; leukopenia; elevated liver serum transaminases.

Potential Toxicities/Side Effects (More Severe with Higher Dosing) and the Nursing Process

I. ALTERATION IN COMFORT related to FLU-LIKE SYNDROME

Defining Characteristics: Chills 3–6 hours after dose in 40–60% of patients; fever (74–98% of patients) with onset 30–90 minutes after chill, lasting up to 24 hours. Temperature 39–40°C (102–104°F); tachyphylaxis (decrease in severity/occurrence after successive treatments) common. Fatigue (89–95% of patients) and malaise are cumulative and dose-limiting. Headache, myalgias occur in 60–70% of patients, as well as arthralgias (5–24% of patients).

Nursing Implications: Assess baseline T, vital signs (VS), neurologic stätus, and comfort level; monitor every 4–6 hours if patient is in hospital. Discuss with physician premedication and regular dosing of antipyretic (e.g., acetaminophen ± diphenhydramine, NSAID). Teach patient self-care measures, including monitoring T, comfort level, self-administration of prescribed medications prior to dose and regularly post-dose, as well as the use of heat or cold for myalgias, arthralgias. Encourage patient to increase oral fluids and alternate rest and activity periods. If patient is in hospital and experiences rigor, discuss with physician IV meperidine (25 mg IV q 15 min to maximum 100 mg in 1 hour) and monitor BP for hypotension. Teach patient to alternate rest and activity.

II. POTENTIAL FOR INFECTION AND BLEEDING related to NEUTROPENIA AND THROMBOCYTOPENIA

Defining Characteristics: Although uncommon, increased risk with increased dose; dose-limiting thrombocytopenia, reversible. Onset in 7–10 days, nadir in 14 days (may be delayed 20–40 days in patients with hairy-cell leukemia), and recovery at day 21.

Nursing Implications: Assess baseline CBC, WBC, differential, and platelet count, and signs/symptoms of infection or bleeding. Discuss any abnormalities with physician before drug administration. Teach patient signs/symptoms of infection and bleeding, and to report them immediately. Teach patient self-care measures to minimize infection and bleeding, including avoidance of OTC aspirin-containing medications, and oral hygiene regimen.

III. ALTERATION IN NUTRITION, LESS THAN BODY REQUIREMENTS, related to NAUSEA, DIARRHEA, ANOREXIA

Defining Characteristics: Anorexia occurs (46–65% of patients) and is cumulative and dose-limiting. Nausea (32–51% of patients) is mild with tachyphylaxis after one week. Diarrhea (29–42% of patients) is mild, and vomiting is rare (10–17% of patients). Taste alterations and xerostomia may occur.

Nursing Implications: Assess baseline nutritional status. Teach patient potential side effects and self-care measures including oral hygiene. Encourage patient to prepare favorite high-calorie, high-protein foods ahead of time so can snack when hungry. Teach self-administration of prescribed antiemetics and antidiarrheals as needed. Refer to dietitian as appropriate.

IV. SENSORY/PERCEPTUAL ALTERATION related to CNS EFFECTS

Defining Characteristics: Dizziness (21–41% of patients), confusion (8–10% of patients), decreased mental status (17% of patients), and depression (16% of patients). Somnolence, irritability, poor concentration, seizures, paranoia, hallucinations, psychoses may occur in 70% of patients but are reversible. Use drug cautiously in patients with history of seizures or CNS dysfunction.

Nursing Implications: Assess baseline mental status and neurologic status prior to drug administration. Assess patient for changes (impaired memory/attention, disorientation, slow/vague responses to questions, increased lethargy) during treatment. Instruct patient to report signs/symptoms; provide information and emotional support, as well as interventions to ensure safety if signs/symptoms occur.

V. POTENTIAL ALTERATION IN CARDIAC OUTPUT related to TACHYCARDIA, CHEST PAIN, DYSRHYTHMIAS

Defining Characteristics: Uncommon but dose-related with increased risk in elderly and patients with preexisting cardiac dysfunction: tachycardia, pallor, cyanosis, chest pain, orthostatic hypotension or hypertension arrhythmias, CHF, syncope.

Nursing Implications: Assess baseline cardiopulmonary status and risk (elderly, preexisting cardiac dysfunction). EKG testing is done baseline and during treatment for high-risk individuals. Monitor VS and I/O, every four hours while receiving drug in hospital. Teach patient to report signs/symptoms of dyspnea, chest pain, edema, or other abnormalities immediately.

VI. POTENTIAL ALTERATION IN ELIMINATION related to RENAL AND HEPATIC DYSFUNCTION

Defining Characteristics: Dose-related increased BUN, creatinine, LFTs (increased AST in 42–46%) may occur, as well as proteinuria. Patient may develop interstitial nephritis.

Nursing Implications: Assess baseline renal and hepatic function studies and urinalysis prior to drug initiation, and periodically during therapy. Discuss abnormalities with physician.

VII. POTENTIAL FOR SEXUAL DYSFUNCTION related to IMPOTENCE, MENSTRUAL IRREGULARITIES

Defining Characteristics: Impotence and decreased libido, menstrual irregularities, and increased spontaneous abortions have occurred. Drug is excreted in breast milk.

Nursing Implications: Assess patient's baseline sexual patterns and discuss potential alterations. Provide information, emotional support, and referral as appropriate and needed. Encourage patient to use contraceptive measures; mothers receiving the drug should not breast-feed.

VIII. POTENTIAL ALTERATION IN SKIN INTEGRITY related to RASH, PARTIAL ALOPECIA, DRYNESS

Defining Characteristics: Partial alopecia (8–22% of patients), rash (11–18% of patients), throat dryness (15% of patients), as well as skin dryness, flushing, pruritus, and irritation at injection site may occur.

Nursing Implications: Assess baseline skin integrity. Instruct patient to report signs/symptoms. Discuss/teach symptomatic management, including the use of mild soaps and rinsing skin thoroughly after bathing. Encourage patient to use alcohol-free, oil-based moisturizers on skin.

IX. KNOWLEDGE DEFICIT related to SELF-ADMINISTRATION TECHNIQUE

Defining Characteristics: Often patients must receive daily dosing or thrice weekly dosing in the home setting by subcutaneous injection, and they are unfamiliar with technique.

Nursing Implications: Assess baseline psychomotor ability, knowledge, and willingness to learn technique of self-injection. Teach how to prepare drug, self-administer, and safely collect used syringes for proper disposal. Use written and video materials as supplements to teaching process and have patient correctly demonstrate technique prior to performing at home. Make referral to visiting-nurse agency to reinforce teaching.

Drug: interferon gamma (Actimmune, IFN-gamma (γ), rIFN-gamma)

Class: Cytokine.

Mechanism of Action: Antiviral, antiproliferative, and immunomodulatory effects. Activates phagocytes and appears to generate toxic oxidative metabolites in phagocytes; interacts with interleukins to orchestrate immune effect, and enhances antibody-dependent cellular cytotoxicity, NK activity, and mounting of antigen on monocytes (Fc expression).

Metabolism: Slowly absorbed following subcutaneous or IM injection, with 89% bioavailability. Peaks in 4–13 hours following IM injection, and 6–7 hours after subcutaneous injection. Elimination half-lives for IV injection are 30–60 minutes, and 2–8 hours for IM or subcutaneous injection. Renal filtration and tubular reabsorption as catabolites; minor hepatic metabolism and biliary excretion.

Dosage/Range:

- Per protocol.
- CML: 0.5–1.5 mg/m^2 IV TIW OR 0.75–1.5 mg/m^2 IV 5 times/week OR 1.5 mg/m^2 IV daily.
- Renal cell carcinoma: 100 micrograms subcutaneous q week OR 0.25 mg IM daily × 8 days q 21–28 days.

Drug Preparation:

- Available in 100-μg (3 million units) vials, which should be refrigerated at 2–8°C (36–46°F); do not freeze. Vials stable at room temperature for up to 12 hours.

Drug Administration:

- IM, subcutaneous, or IV.

Drug Interactions:

- May decrease elimination of aminophylline by 33–81% via inhibition of cytochrome P-450 enzyme system.
- Increased effects of CNS depressants.
- Increased bone marrow suppressant effects with zidovudine (AZT).

Lab Effects/Interference:

- Dose-dependent, leukopenia; elevated liver serum transaminases.
- Increased serum creatinine, BUN, proteinuria.

Potential Toxicities/Side Effects (More Severe with Higher Dosing) and the Nursing Process

I. ALTERATION IN COMFORT related to FLU-LIKE SYNDROME

Defining Characteristics: Chills 3–6 hours after dose in 20% of patients; fever (80% of patients), with onset 30–90 minutes after chill. Tachyphylaxis (decrease in severity/occurrence after successive treatments) common. Fatigue (20% of patients) and myalgia (10%) can occur. Headache occurs in 50% of patients.

Nursing Implications: Assess baseline T, vital signs (VS), neurologic status, and comfort level; monitor every 4–6 hours if patient is in hospital. Discuss with physician premedication and regular dosing of antipyretic (e.g., acetaminophen ± diphenhydramine, NSAID). Teach patient self-care measures, including monitoring T, comfort level, self-administration of prescribed medications prior to dose and regularly postdose, as well as the use of heat or cold for myalgias, arthralgias. Encourage patient to increase oral fluids and alternate rest and activity periods. If patient is in hospital and experiences rigor, discuss with physician IV meperidine (25 mg IV q 15 min to maximum 100 mg in 1 hour) and monitor BP for hypotension. Teach patient to alternate rest and activity.

II. POTENTIAL FOR INFECTION AND BLEEDING related to NEUTROPENIA AND THROMBOCYTOPENIA

Defining Characteristics: Although uncommon, increased risk with increased dose; dose-limiting thrombocytopenia; reversible.

Nursing Implications: Assess baseline CBC, WBC, differential, and platelet count, and signs/symptoms of infection or bleeding. Discuss any abnormalities with physician before drug administration. Teach patient signs/symptoms of infection and bleeding, and to report them immediately. Teach patient self-care measures to minimize infection and bleeding, including avoidance of OTC aspirin-containing medications, and oral hygiene regimen.

III. ALTERATION IN NUTRITION, LESS THAN BODY REQUIREMENTS, related to NAUSEA, DIARRHEA, ANOREXIA

Defining Characteristics: Anorexia occurs (46–65% of patients) and is cumulative and dose-limiting. Nausea (32–51% of patients) is mild with tachyphylaxis after one week. Diarrhea (29–42% of patients) is mild, and vomiting is rare (10–17% of patients). Taste alterations and xerostomia may occur.

Nursing Implications: Assess baseline nutritional status. Teach patient potential side effects and self-care measures, including oral hygiene. Encourage patient to prepare favorite high-calorie, high-protein foods ahead of time so can snack when hungry. Teach self-administration of prescribed antiemetics and antidiarrheals as needed. Refer to dietitian as appropriate.

IV. SENSORY/PERCEPTUAL ALTERATION related to CNS EFFECTS

Defining Characteristics: Incidence 1–10%: dizziness, confusion, seizures, gait instability, and depression (3% of patients). Use drug cautiously in patients with history of seizures or CNS dysfunction.

Nursing Implications: Assess baseline mental status and neurologic status prior to drug administration. Assess patient for changes (impaired memory/attention, disorientation, slow/vague responses to questions, increased lethargy) during treatment. Instruct patient to report signs/symptoms; provide information and emotional support, as well as interventions to ensure safety if signs/symptoms occur.

V. POTENTIAL ALTERATION IN CARDIAC OUTPUT related to TACHYCARDIA, CHEST PAIN, DYSRHYTHMIAS

Defining Characteristics: Uncommon but dose-related with increased risk in elderly and patients with preexisting cardiac dysfunction: tachycardia, pallor, cyanosis, chest pain, orthostatic hypotension or hypertension arrhythmias, CHF, syncope.

Nursing Implications: Assess baseline cardiopulmonary status and risk (elderly, preexisting cardiac dysfunction). EKG testing is done baseline and during treatment for high-risk individuals. Monitor VS and I/O, every four hours while receiving drug in hospital. Teach patient to report signs/symptoms of dyspnea, chest pain, edema, or other abnormalities immediately.

VI. POTENTIAL ALTERATION IN ELIMINATION related to RENAL AND HEPATIC DYSFUNCTION

Defining Characteristics: Dose-related increased BUN, creatinine, LFTs (increased AST in 42–46%) may occur, as well as proteinuria. Patient may develop interstitial nephritis.

Nursing Implications: Assess baseline renal and hepatic function studies and urinalysis prior to drug initiation, and periodically during therapy. Discuss abnormalities with physician.

VII. POTENTIAL FOR SEXUAL DYSFUNCTION related to IMPOTENCE, MENSTRUAL IRREGULARITIES

Defining Characteristics: Impotence and decreased libido, menstrual irregularities, and increased spontaneous abortions have occurred. It is unknown whether drug is excreted in breast milk.

Nursing Implications: Assess patient's baseline sexual patterns and discuss potential alterations. Provide information, emotional support, and referral as appropriate and needed. Encourage patient to use contraceptive measures; mothers receiving the drug should not breast-feed.

VIII. KNOWLEDGE DEFICIT related to SELF-ADMINISTRATION TECHNIQUE

Defining Characteristics: Often patients must receive daily dosing or thrice weekly dosing in the home setting by subcutaneous injection, and they are unfamiliar with technique.

Nursing Implications: Assess baseline psychomotor ability, knowledge, and willingness to learn technique of self-injection. Teach how to prepare drug, self-administer, and safely collect used syringes for proper disposal. Use written and video materials as supplements to teaching process and have patient correctly demonstrate technique prior to performing at home. Make referral to visiting-nurse agency to reinforce teaching.

Drug: levamisole hydrochloride (Ergamisol)

Class: Anthelmintic.

Mechanism of Action: Stimulate immunorestoration in deficient host. Nonspecific immunomodulating agent has antiproliferating action against tumor metastases (with small tumor burdens) rather than primary tumor. Thus, drug is combined with chemotherapy (e.g., 5-FU) and/or surgery (e.g., colon resection).

Metabolism: Rapidly absorbed from GI tract, with elimination half-life of 3–4 hours. Extensively metabolized by liver, and metabolites excreted by kidneys (70% over three days). Unchanged drug is excreted in urine (< 5%) and feces (< 0.2%).

Dosage/Range: *Adjuvant chemotherapy with 5-FU for Duke's Stage C colon cancer*:

- Initial therapy: 50 mg PO q 8 h × 3 days (starting day 7–30 postsurgery); 5-FU 450 mg/m^2/day IV × 5 days (concomitant with levamisole, starting 21–34 days postsurgery).
- Maintenance: 50 mg PO q 8 h × 3 days every 2 weeks for 1 year; 5-FU 450 mg/m^2/day every week beginning 28 days after initiation of 5-day course.
- See package insert for 5-FU dose reductions for stomatitis, diarrhea, leukopenia.

Drug Preparation:

- Available as 50-mg tablets in 36-tablet blister pack.

Drug Administration:

- Oral.

Drug Interactions:

- Alcohol may produce disulfiram-like effect (flushing, throbbing in head and neck, throbbing headaches, respiratory difficulty, nausea and vomiting, sweating, chest pain, dyspnea, hypotension, weakness, blurred vision, confusion, coma, and death).

- Increased phenytoin levels occur when coadministered with levamisole and 5-FU: phenytoin dose may need to be decreased.

Lab Effects/Interference:
- Leukopenia, increased bili when given together with 5-FU.

Special Considerations:
- Indicated for adjuvant treatment in combination with 5-FU after surgical resection of Duke's Stage C colon cancer.
- May be used investigationally with other protocols.

Potential Toxicities/Side Effects (in Combination with 5-fluorouracil) and the Nursing Process

I. ALTERATION IN NUTRITION, LESS THAN BODY REQUIREMENTS, related to NAUSEA/VOMITING, DIARRHEA, STOMATITIS, ANOREXIA

Defining Characteristics: Stomatitis or diarrhea (i.e., 5 stools/day) is an indication to interrupt 5-day course and weekly 5-FU injection; if stomatitis or diarrhea develops during weekly 5-FU, dose-reduce subsequent 5-FU doses. Nausea may occur more commonly than vomiting.

Nursing Implications: Assess baseline oral mucosa, elimination pattern. Inform patient of potential side effects and need to report them if they develop. Premedicate with antiemetic, at least for the first cycle. Assess oral mucosa; ask about incidence of diarrhea during and prior to each course of therapy. Teach patient self-care measures, including diet modifications, self-medication with prescribed antiemetic, and oral hygiene regimen. If stomatitis or diarrhea develops, discuss modification of therapy with physician.

II. POTENTIAL FOR INFECTION AND BLEEDING related to BONE MARROW DEPRESSION

Defining Characteristics: Agranulocytosis may occur and may be preceded by flu-like syndrome (fever, chills). Neutropenia is usually reversible on discontinuance of therapy.

Nursing Implications: Monitor CBC, WBC, differential, platelet count prior to initial drug treatment and then weekly prior to each 5-FU dose. Discuss with physician if abnormalities occur. Manufacturer recommends holding 5-FU dose until WBC > $3500/mm^3$, and holding both 5-FU and levamisole if platelets < $100{,}000/mm^3$. If 5-FU nadir < $2500/mm^3$, next 5-FU dose should be reduced by 20%. Teach patient signs/symptoms of infection and bleeding, and instruct to report these immediately. Teach patient self-care measures to minimize infection and bleeding, including avoidance of OTC aspirin-containing medications.

III. POTENTIAL ALTERATION IN SKIN INTEGRITY related to DERMATITIS, SKIN CHANGES

Defining Characteristics: Dermatitis (23% of patients), alopecia (22% of patients), and pruritus may occur.

Nursing Implications: Assess skin and teach patient about potential side effects. Discuss potential impact hair loss will have, as well as coping strategies (e.g., wig, scarf). Discuss/teach symptom management depending on character of dermatitis.

IV. SENSORY/PERCEPTUAL ALTERATIONS related to NEUROLOGIC CHANGES

Defining Characteristics: Dizziness, headaches, paresthesia, ataxia, taste perversion, and altered sense of smell may occur (4–8% of patients). Less commonly, somnolence, depression, nervousness, insomnia, and anxiety may occur (2% of patients).

Nursing Implications: Assess baseline mental status and neurologic status. Instruct patient to report any abnormalities. Notify physician of any abnormalities and discuss therapy modification depending on severity of side effects.

V. ALTERATION IN COMFORT related to FLU-LIKE SYMPTOMS

Defining Characteristics: Fever, chills, fatigue, chest pain may occur, although they are rare. Fever and chills may precede agranulocytosis.

Nursing Implications: Teach patient that these may occur, and instruct to report fever and chills. Assess CBC, WBC, differential if fever and chills occur. Discuss symptom management with patient, self-administration of prescribed NSAIDs or acetaminophen, and alternation of rest/activity periods.

Drug: megakaryocyte growth and development factor (MGDF)

Class: Cytokine.

Mechanism of Action: Growth-factor-specific for megakaryocyte precursor lineage.

Metabolism: Unknown.

Dosage/Range:
- Per protocol.

Drug Preparation:
- Subcutaneous daily for 5 days, or per protocol.

Drug Interactions:
- None known.

Lab Effects/Interference:
- Expect increase in platelet count.

Special Considerations:
- Minimal toxicity.
- Current studies are exploring platelet recovery after induction therapy for acute myelogenous leukemia (AML), and activity of MGDF as a mobilizing agent for peripheral blood stem cells.
- For further information, contact Amgen (Thousand Oaks, CA).

Potential Toxicities/Side Effects and the Nursing Process

I. POTENTIAL FOR KNOWLEDGE DEFICIT related to INVESTIGATIONAL AGENT

Nursing Diagnosis: Knowledge deficit related to drug's status as an investigational agent.

Defining Characteristics: Clinical studies are defining a toxicity profile, but no toxicity has been reported as yet.

Nursing Interventions: Reinforce teaching about cytokine, including indication, expected benefit, and administration. Instruct patient to report any side effects or unusual occurrences.

Drug: oprelvekin (Neumega)

Class: Biological (interleukin).

Mechanism of Action: IL-11 is a thrombopoietin growth factor that directly stimulates the bone marrow stem cells and megakaryocyte progenitor cells so that the production of platelets is increased. Produced by recombinant DNA technology. Results in higher platelet nadir and accelerates time to platelet recovery postchemotherapy.

Metabolism: Peak serum concentrations reached in approximately 3 ± 2 hours, with a terminal half-life of approximately 7 ± 1 hours. Bioavailability is < 80%. Clearance decreases with age, and drug is rapidly cleared from the serum, distributed to organs with high perfusion, metabolized, and excreted by the kidneys. Little intact drug is found in the urine.

Dosage/Range:
- Adults: 50 μg/kg subcutaneous daily.

Drug Preparation:

- Available as single-use vial containing 5 mg of oprelvekin as a lyophilized, preservative-free powder. This is reconstituted with 1 mL sterile water for injection, USP, gently swirled to mix, and results in a concentration of 5 mg/1 mL in a single-use vial. NOTE: 5 mL of diluent is supplied, but only 1 mL should be withdrawn to reconstitute drug. Drug should be used within 3 hours of reconstitution. If not used immediately, store reconstituted solution in refrigerator or at room temperature, but DO NOT FREEZE OR SHAKE.
- The drug should be administered subcutaneous every day (abdomen, thigh or hip, or upper arm). Begin daily administration 6–24 hours after the completion of chemotherapy, and continue until the postnadir platelet count is equal to or greater than 50,000 cells/mL. Do not give for more than 21 days, and stop at least 2 days before starting the next planned cycle of chemotherapy. Drug has *not* been evaluated in patients receiving chemotherapy regimens longer than 5 days, nor has it been shown to cause delayed myelosuppression (e.g., Mitomycin C, nitrosoureas).

Drug Interactions:

- Unknown.

Lab Effects/Interference:

- Increase in platelet count.
- Anemia associated with increased circulating plasma volume.

Special Considerations:

- Indicated for the prevention of severe thrombocytopenia and to decrease the need for platelet transfusion in patients with nonmyeloid malignancies receiving myelosuppressive chemotherapy.
- Causes fluid retention, so must be used with caution in patients with CHF or in patients receiving chronic diuretic therapy (sudden deaths reported in patients receiving ifosfamide and chronic diuretic therapy due to severe hypokalemia).
- Monitor platelet count frequently during oprelvekin therapy, and at the time of the expected nadir to identify when recovery will begin.
- Contraindicated in pregnant females and nursing mothers.

Potential Toxicities/Side Effects and the Nursing Process

I. ALTERATIONS IN FLUID AND ELECTROLYTE BALANCE related to FLUID RETENTION

Defining Characteristics: Most patients develop mild to moderate fluid retention (peripheral edema, dyspnea on exertion) but without weight gain. Fluid retention is reversible in a few days after drug is stopped. Patients with preexisting pleural effusions, pericardial effusions, or ascites may develop increased fluid, and may require drainage. Patients receiving chronic administration of potassium-excreting diuretics should be monitored extremely closely, as there are reports of sudden death due to severe hypokalemia in patients receiving ifosfamide and chronic diuretic therapy. Capillary leak syndrome has *not* been reported.

Nursing Implications: Assess baseline fluid and electrolyte balance, and weight prior to beginning drug. Assess presence of history of cardiac problems, or CHF, and risk of developing fluid volume overload. If diuretic therapy is ordered, monitor fluid and electrolyte balance very carefully, and replete electrolytes as indicated and ordered. Teach patients that mild-to-moderate peripheral edema and shortness of breath on exertion are likely to occur during the first week of treatment and will disappear after treatment ends. If the patient has CHF or pleural effusions, instruct to report worsening dyspnea to their nurse or physician.

II. ALTERATION IN CIRCULATION related to ATRIAL FIBRILLATION

Defining Characteristics: 10% of patients experience transient arrhythmias, including atrial fibrillation or flutter, after treatment with oprelvekin; it is believed to be due to increased plasma volume rather than the drug itself. Arrhythmias may be symptomatic, are usually brief in duration, and are not clinically significant. Some patients have spontaneous conversion to a normal sinus rhythm, while others require rate-controlling drug therapy. Most patients can receive drug without recurrence of the atrial arrhythmia. Risk factors for developing atrial arrhythmias are: (1) advancing age, (2) use of cardiac medications, (3) history of doxorubicin exposure, (4) history of atrial arrhythmia. Other cardiovascular events include tachycardia, vasodilatation, palpitations, and syncope.

Nursing Implications: Assess baseline risk. If patient has history or presence of atrial arrhythmias, discuss with the physician potential benefit versus risk, and monitor very closely. Monitor baseline heart rate and other VS at each visit. Instruct patient to report immediately palpitations, lightheadedness, dizziness, or any other change in condition, especially if patient has any risk factors.

III. ALTERATION IN SENSORY PERCEPTION related to VISUAL BLURRING

Defining Characteristics: Transient, mild visual blurring has been reported, as has papilledema in 1.5% of patients. Dizziness (38%), insomnia (33%), and injection of conjunctiva (19%) may also occur.

Nursing Implications: Assess risk for papilledema (existing papilledema, CNS tumors); assess for changes in pupillary response in these patients. Teach patients that dizziness and insomnia may occur, and to change positions slowly and to hold onto supportive structures. If insomnia is severe, discuss sleep medications with physician.

IV. ALTERATION IN NUTRITION, LESS THAN FULL BODY REQUIREMENTS, related to GI SYMPTOMS

Defining Characteristics: Nausea, vomiting, mucositis, and diarrhea may occur, although percentage was not significantly greater than placebo control. Oral candidiasis occurred in 14% of patients, and this was significantly greater than control.

Nursing Implications: Instruct patient to report changes, and assess impact on nutrition. Inspect oral mucosa and teach patient to as well. Because patient is receiving myelosuppressive chemotherapy, teaching should include oral hygiene regimen and frequent self-assessment by patient.

V. ALTERATIONS IN BREATHING PATTERN, INEFFECTIVE, POTENTIAL, related to DYSPNEA, COUGH

Defining Characteristics: Dyspnea (48% of patients), rhinitis (42%), increased cough (29%), pharyngitis (25%), and pleural effusions (10%) may occur.

Nursing Implications: Assess baseline pulmonary status and presence of pleural effusions. Instruct patient to report dyspnea and any other changes. Discuss significant changes with physician.

Drug: palifermin (Kepivance)

Class: Keratinocyte Growth Factor.

Mechanism of Action: Palifermin is a keratinocyte growth factor (KGF) produced by recombinant DNA technology, similar to the naturally occurring, endogenous KGF. Once EGF binds to its receptor found on epithelial cells including those of the tongue, buccal mucosa, mammary gland, skin (hair follicles and sebaceous gland), lung, liver, and the lens of the eye, it stimulates proliferation, differentiation, and migration of epithelial cells. KGF decreases the incidence and duration of severe stomatitis in patients with hematologic malignancies who undergo high-dose chemotherapy and radiation therapy with stem cell rescue.

Metabolism: Palifermin has an elimination half-life of 4.5 hours (average).

Dosage/Range:

- 60 mcg/kg/day IV bolus for 3 consecutive days before and 3 consecutive days after myelotoxic therapy for a total of 6 doses.

Drug Preparation:

- Reconstitute Kepivance lyophilized powder with sterile water for injection USP, aseptically, by slowly injecting 1.2 mL Sterile Water for Injection USP to yield final volume of 5 mg/mL. Do not shake or agitate the vial.

- Protect from light.
- Reconstituted solution may be refrigerated in its carton for up to 24 hours at 2°–8°C (36°–46°F); prior to injection, may leave at room temperature for up to 1 hour protected from light. Inspect for discoloration or particulates, and if found, do not use.
- Do not filter drug during reconstitution or administration.

Drug Administration:
- Pre-myelotoxic therapy: The 3rd dose should be 24–48 hours before myelotoxic chemotherapy is administered.
- Post-myelotoxic therapy: The first of the 3 doses should be given after, but on the same day of the hematopoietic stem cell infusion, and at least 4 days after the most recent administration of palifermin.

Drug Interactions:
- Heparin: Palifermin binds to heparin, so drugs should not be used concomitantly; flush central line well with saline prior to administration of palifermin.
- Myelotoxic chemotherapy: If given with chemotherapy, KGF increases the severity and duration of oral mucositis. Palifermin should NOT be administered within 24 hours before, during infusion of, or after the administration of myelotoxic chemotherapy.

Lab Effects/Interference:
- Increase in serum amylase and lipase.

Special Considerations:
- Palifermin is FDA-approved to decrease the incidence and duration of severe oral mucositis in patients with hematologic malignancies receiving myelotoxic therapy requiring hematopoietic stem cell support.
- Drug is being studied in the treatment of patients with solid tumors, but the safety and efficacy has not been established at this time. KFG in laboratory studies can enhance malignant cell growth in tissues with KFG receptors.
- Drug is contraindicated in patients with known hypersensitivity to *E. coli*-derived proteins.
- Drug is embryotoxic to lab animals when given in higher doses; drug should be used in pregnant women only when the potential benefit to the mother exceeds the risk to the fetus.

Potential Toxicities/Side Effects and the Nursing Process

I. POTENTIAL ALTERATION IN SKIN INTEGRITY related to SKIN RASH

Defining Characteristics: Skin rash was the most common serious adverse reaction and occurred in 62% of patients in clinical studies. Skin toxicity was manifested by rash, erythema (32%), edema (28%), pruritus (35%). Median time to onset was 6 days after the first of 3 doses, and lasted a median of 5 days.

Nursing Implications: Teach patient that skin changes may occur and to report them. Teach patient self-care strategies to promote comfort and reduce the risk of infection.

II. ALTERATION IN NUTRITION AND COMFORT related to ORAL TOXICITIES

Defining Characteristics: Dysesthesia, tongue discoloration, tongue thickening, alterations in taste occur related to the increased keratin layer on the lining of the oral cavity.

Nursing Implications: Inform patient that these side effects may occur. Teach patient systematic oral cleansing after meals and at bedtime. Inform patient to report discomfort or inability to chew or swallow, and develop plan with measures to promote comfort and nutrition. Many patients are already receiving TPN. If taste alterations are bothersome, suggest dietitian referral for measures to stimulate taste.

III. ALTERATION IN COMFORT related to PAIN, ARTHRALGIAS, AND DYSESTHESIAS

Defining Characteristics: Dysesthesia, pain, and arthralgias may occur and affect about 12% of patients.

Nursing Implications: Assess baseline comfort, as well as existing arthralgias and dysesthesias. Perform a basic neurologic assessment. Inform patient these side effects may occur and to report them if they occur. Develop a plan of care that includes self-care activities to promote comfort, such as the use of heat or cold for arthralgias. If pain related to stomatitis is severe, then patient-controlled analgesia may be necessary. Teach patient to report any dysesthesias, hyperesthesias, hypoesthesia, or paresthesias that occur. Develop a plan to minimize discomfort, such as keeping sheets off feet if patient has hyperesthesias.

Drug: pegfilgrastim (Neulasta)

Class: Cytokine, CSF.

Mechanism of Action: Recombinant DNA protein (G-CSF) that regulates the production of neutrophils in the bone marrow (proliferation, differentiation, activation of mature neutrophils). Drug is produced by the insertion of the human G-CSF gene into *Escherichia coli* bacteria. Drug has longer half-life and different excretion pattern as compared to the parent drug, filgrastim.

Metabolism: Clearance of drug decreases with increased dose and body weight, and is directly related to the number of neutrophils so that as neutrophil recovery begins after myelosuppressive chemotherapy, serum concentration of pegfilgrastim declines rapidly. In patients with increased body weight, systemic exposure to the drug was higher despite dose normalized for body weight. Pharmacokinetics variable, with a half-life of 15–80 hours after subcutaneous injection. Pharmacokinetics did not vary with age (elderly) or gender.

Dosage/Range:

- 6 mg subcutaneous once per chemotherapy cycle.

Drug Preparation:

- Drug available in refrigerated 6 mg (0.6 mL) prefilled syringes with UltraSafe Needle Guards.
- Unopened vials should be stored in the refrigerator at 2–8°C (36–46°F) in the original carton to protect from light.
- Avoid shaking. Screen for visible particulate matter or discoloration and do not use if found.
- Remove from refrigerator 30 minutes prior to injection, but drug may be left at room temperature for up to 48 hours.
- If drug accidentally freezes, allow to thaw in the refrigerator prior to administration; if frozen a second time, discard.

Drug Administration:

- Subcutaneous × 1 *at least 14 days prior to or more than 24 hours after* chemotherapy administration.
- Following injection, activate UltraSafe Needle Guard by holding hands behind the needle and sliding the guard forward until the needle is completely covered and guard clicks into place. If no click is heard, drop entire syringe/needle into sharps disposal container.

Drug Interactions:

- Lithium: may potentiate the release of neutrophils from the bone marrow: monitor neutrophil count more frequently.

Lab Effects/Interference:

- Increased white blood cell count and neutrophil count.
- Elevated LDH, alkaline phosphatase, uric acid may occur but are reversible and less frequent than with filgrastim.

Special Considerations:

- Indicated to decrease the incidence of infection (febrile neutropenia) in patients with non-myeloid malignancies receiving myelosuppressive anti-cancer therapy associated with a significant incidence of febrile neutropenia.
- Contraindicated in patients with known hypersensitivity to *E. coli*-derived proteins, pegfilgrastim, filgrastim, or any product component; contraindicated in peripheral blood progenitor cell (PBPC) mobilization, as the drug has not been studied in this population.

- Splenic rupture has been reported in patients receiving the parent drug, filgrastim, for PBPC. If a patient receiving pegfilgrastim complains of left upper abdominal or shoulder tip pain, s/he should be evaluated immediately for an enlarged spleen or splenic rupture.
- Adult Respiratory Distress Syndrome (ARDS) has been reported in neutropenic patients with sepsis receiving the parent drug filgrastim, probably related to the influx of neutrophils to inflamed pulmonary sites. Neutropenic patients receiving pegfilgrastim who develop fever, lung infiltrates, or respiratory distress should be immediately evaluated for ARDS. If ARDS is suspected, pegfilgrastim should be stopped until ARDS resolves with appropriate medical care.
- Severe sickle cell crisis, rarely fatal, has been reported in patients with sickle cell disease (homozygous sickle cell anemia, sickle/hemoglobin C disease, sickle/α-thalassemia) who received filgrastim, the parent drug. Pegfilgrastim should be used in this population only when the potential benefit outweighs the risk, and patients should be well hydrated and closely monitored for sickle cell crisis, with immediate intervention.
- Pegfilgrastim should not be administered within *14 days prior to* and *for 24 hours after chemotherapy administration* because of the potential for an increase in sensitivity of rapidly dividing myeloid cells to the chemotherapy.
- Allergic reactions to pegfilgrastim, including anaphylaxis, skin rash, and urticaria, have been reported, most often on initial exposure to the drug but in some instances after the drug was stopped. If a serious allergic reaction occurs, the drug should be discontinued and the patient closely monitored for several days.
- Drug may exacerbate preexisting psoriasis, Sweet's syndrome (neutrophilic dermatitis), and cutaneous vasculitis.
- G-CSF receptor to which drug binds is also found in tumor cell lines (some myeloid, T-lymphoid, lung, head and neck, and bladder cancer), and the potential for the drug to be a tumor growth factor exists.
- Drug should not be used for peripheral blood progenitor cell mobilization.
- Drug should be used in pregnant women only when the potential benefit outweighs risk of fetal harm, as there are no adequate controlled studies in pregnant women, and laboratory animals had increased number of abortions and wavy ribs in fetuses.
- Do not use in infants, children, and smaller adolescents whose weight is < 45 kg.

Potential Toxicities/Side Effects (Dose and Schedule-Dependent) and the Nursing Process

I. ALTERATION IN COMFORT related to SKELETAL PAIN, HEADACHE, MYALGIA, ABDOMINAL PAIN, ARTHRALGIA

Defining Characteristics: Patients (26%) may report transient mild-to-moderate skeletal pain believed due to the expansion of cells in the bone marrow in response to G-CSF. About 12% used non-opioid analgesics, and less than 6% required opioid analgesics. Leukocytosis of more than 100–109/L occurred in < 1% of patients. Other pain related to headache, myalgia and arthralgia, and abdominal pain may occur less commonly, but is easily managed.

Nursing Implications: Teach patient bone pain may occur, and discuss use of nonsteroidal anti-inflammatory drugs with patient and physician for symptom management. Monitor white blood cell count (WBC), hematocrit and platelet count as appropriate prior to each cycle of chemotherapy. Teach patient headache, myalgia, arthralgia, abdominal pain may occur and to report them if they do not respond to usual management strategies.

II. ALTERATION IN NUTRITION, POTENTIAL, related to NAUSEA, VOMITING, CONSTIPATION, DIARRHEA, ANOREXIA, STOMATITIS, MUCOSITIS

Defining Characteristics: Nutritional symptoms are rarely reported and may be related to the underlying malignancy.

Nursing Implications: Perform baseline patient nutritional assessment, history of nausea and vomiting, bowel elimination pattern, oral assessment, and usual appetite. Teach patient to report these side effects so that they can be evaluated. Teach patient self-care measures, including dietary modification, local comfort measures as well as pharmacologic management as determined by the nurse/physician team. Teach patient to report symptoms that persist and do not respond to the planned therapy.

III. ALTERATION IN SKIN INTEGRITY, POTENTIAL, related to PERIPHERAL EDEMA, ALOPECIA

Defining Characteristics: Peripheral edema and alopecia are rarely reported, and may be related to other factors, such as the chemotherapy agents administered.

Nursing Implications: Perform baseline skin and scalp assessment. Teach patient to report development of peripheral edema, hair loss. Discuss with patient acceptable management strategies depending upon impact of hair loss, if it occurs. Assess degree of peripheral edema if it develops, and discuss significant edema with physician to determine etiology and management. Teach patient local skin care, including avoidance of tight clothing and shoes, keeping skin moisturized to prevent cracking, and local comfort measures.

IV. KNOWLEDGE DEFICIT related to SELF-ADMINISTRATION TECHNIQUE

Defining Characteristics: Drug is administered once per chemotherapy cycle, more than 14 days prior to chemotherapy administration or more than 24 hours after chemotherapy is given.

Nursing Implications: Assess baseline psychomotor ability, knowledge, and willingness to learn technique of self-injection. Teach how to refrigerate drug, self-administer using pre-filled syringes, how to activate needle guard, and safely collect used syringes for proper disposal. Drug insert has "Information for Patients and Caregivers." Use written and video supplements in teaching process and have patient correctly demonstrate technique prior to performing at home. Make referral to visiting-nurse agency to reinforce teaching if needed. Teach patient telephone number and whom to call if questions or problems arise, and ensure that patient can correctly repeat information.

Drug: romiplostim (Nplate)

Class: Thrombopoietin stimulating agent (peptibody or peptide antibody); thrombopoeitin receptor agonist.

Mechanism of Action: Drug is an engineered peptibody composed of two parts: an Fc receptor of an antibody and a peptide that is fused to the antibody constant domain (Fc). Binds to and activates the thrombopoietin (TPO) receptor, mimicking natural TPO to stimulate the growth and maturation of megakaryocytes (platelet precursors). This results in increased platelet production in the body.

Metabolism: Peak serum concentration 7–50 hr after the dose with a median time of 15h; half-life 1–34 days, with a median of 3.5 days. Serum concentration does not correlate with the dose. Elimination depends to some degree on the platelet TPO receptors.

Dosage/Range:

- Drug is available only through a restricted distribution program called NPlate NEXUS (Network of Experts Understanding and Supporting Nplate and Patients).
- Initial dose 1 mcg/kg subcutaneously once weekly to achieve/maintain a platelet count ≥ 50,000 cells/mm^3 as needed to reduce bleeding risk.
- Adjust weekly dose by increments of 1 mcg/kg.
- Do not exceed maximum weekly dose of 10 mcg/kg, and do not dose if platelet count is > 400,000 cells/mm^3.
- Discontinue drug if platelet count does not increase after 4 wk at the maximum dose.

Drug Preparation:

- Do not shake during reconstitution; protect reconstituted drug from light, and administer within 24 hr.
- Draw up dose using a syringe with graduations to 0.01 mL. Vial is single use; discard any unused drug.
- Available in 250 mcg and 500 mcg of romiplostim in single-use vials.

Drug Administration:

- Weekly injections.

Drug Interactions:
- Unknown.

Lab Effects/Interference:
- Increased platelet count.
- Decreased platelet count after drug cessation.

Special Considerations:
- Appears effective in patients with ITP who have had their spleen removed, with low toxicity (Kuter et al, 2008). Overall platelet increase occurred in 78.6% of patients receiving romiplostim compared with 0 in the placebo group.
- Drug should only be used in patients with ITP whose degree of thrombocytopenia and clinical condition increase the risk for bleeding. Romiplostim should not be used to normalize platelet count. Indicated in patients who had inadequate response to corticosteroids, IgG, or splenectomy.
- Is being studied in patients with cancer- and treatment-related thrombocytopenia.
- Most common side effects (> 5%) are myalgia, dizziness, pain (extremity, abdomen, shoulder), arthralgia, insomnia, dyspepsia, headache, and paresthesia.
- Rarely, elevation of bone marrow reticulin (reversible with drug discontinuation) and thrombosis occurred. This may result in bone marrow fibrosis with cytopenias; monitor peripheral blood for signs of marrow fibrosis.
- Monitor platelet count for 2 weeks after drug cessation.
- May increase risk of hematologic malignancies.

Potential Toxicities/Side Effects and the Nursing Process

I. ALTERATION IN COMFORT related to MYALGIA, ARTHRALGIA, PAIN, DIZZINESS, INSOMNIA

Defining Characteristics: Transient skeletal pain and headache may occur.

Nursing Implications: Teach patient this may occur and discuss use of NSAIDs with patient and physician for symptom management. Monitor CBC, platelet count, peripheral smear baseline weekly during dose adjustment phase, then monthly when stable.

Drug: sargramostim (Leukine, GM-CSF)

Class: Cytokine.

Mechanism of Action: Granulocyte-macrophage colony-stimulating factor that regulates growth of all levels of granulocytes and stimulates production of monocytes and macrophages; GM-CSF induces synthesis of other cytokines and enhances cytotoxic action. Manufactured using recombinant DNA technology.

Metabolism: Peak serum levels 2–3 hours after injection. Initial half-life 12–17 min, with a terminal half-life of 1.6–2.6 hours.

Dosage/Range:
- 250 μg/m^2/day as a 2–hour infusion for 21 days, beginning 2–4 hours after autologous marrow infusion, > 24 hours after last chemotherapy dose, and > 12 hours after last radiation treatment; administer for 14 days when used for BMT failure.
- Neutrophil recovery after chemotherapy for AML: 250 μg/m^2/day IV over 4 hours beginning on day 11 (4 days after completion of induction chemotherapy if day 10 bone marrow biopsy shows hypoplasia with < 5% blasts).
- Mobilization of peripheral blood progenitor cells (PBPCs): 250 μg/m^2/day IV over 24 hours or subcutaneous daily; continue through PBPC collection.

Drug Preparation:
- Reconstitute per manufacturer's directions. Do *not* filter.
- Further dilute in 0.9% sodium chloride.
- If final concentration is < 10 μg/mL, human albumin (dilute to final concentration of 0.1% human albumin in 0.9% sodium chloride) should be added before adding GM-CSF to prevent absorption of drug in IV container and tubing.

Drug Administration:
- Administer IV over 2 hours, or according to research protocol.

Drug Interactions:
- Corticosteroids, lithium: may ↑ myeloproliferation.
- Sargramostim effect may be ↓ in patients who have received chemotherapy containing alkylating agents, anthracyclines, antibiotics, antimetabolites.

Lab Effects/Interference:
- Increased stem cell, granulocyte, macrophage production.
- Serum glucose, BUN, cholesterol, bili, creatinine, ALT, alk phos; ↓ serum albumin, Ca.
- Leukocytosis, eosinophilia.

Special Considerations:
- Indicated for acceleration of bone marrow recovery (myeloid cells) after autologous or allogeneic BMT; following induction chemotherapy in acute myelogenous leukemia; mobilization and following transplant of autologous PBPCs; and in BMT failure or engraftment delay.
- Produces fever more commonly than G-CSF, and fluid retention.
- Stop drug when WBC > 50,000 cells/mm^3, or ANC > 20,000 cells/mm^3.
- Administer > 24 hours after last chemotherapy, or > 12 hours after radiotherapy.

Potential Toxicities/Side Effects (Dose- and Schedule-Dependent) and the Nursing Process

I. ALTERATION IN COMFORT related to FLU-LIKE SYNDROME

Defining Characteristics: Fever, myalgias, chills, rigors, fatigue, and headache may occur.

Nursing Implications: Assess baseline T, VS, neurologic status, and comfort level, and monitor q 4–6 h if patient in hospital. Discuss with physician premedication and regular dosing of antipyretic (e.g., acetaminophen ± diphenhydramine, NSAID). Teach patient self-care measures, including monitoring T, comfort level, self-administration of prescribed medications prior to dose and regularly postdose, as well as the use of heat or cold for myalgias, arthralgias. Encourage patient to increase oral fluids and alternate rest and activity periods. If patient is in hospital and experiences rigor, discuss with physician IV meperidine (25 mg IV every 15 minutes to maximum 100 mg in 1 hour) and monitor BP for hypotension.

II. ALTERATION IN COMFORT related to SKELETAL PAIN

Defining Characteristics: Transient skeletal pain may occur and is believed to be due to bone marrow expansion in response to GM-CSF.

Nursing Implications: Teach patient this may occur and discuss use of NSAIDs with patient and physician for symptom management. Monitor WBC, ANC twice weekly during therapy; dose reduction or discontinuation depends on purpose of drug.

III. POTENTIAL ALTERATION IN SKIN INTEGRITY related to RASH, FLUSHING, INJECTION SITE REACTION

Defining Characteristics: Facial flushing, generalized rash, and inflammation at injection site may occur.

Nursing Implications: Teach patient that these may occur, and instruct to report rash, inflammation. Teach patient to rotate injection sites. Assess rash, and teach symptomatic management.

IV. POTENTIAL ALTERATION IN OXYGENATION related to DYSPNEA AND FLUID RETENTION

Defining Characteristics: Some patients developed dyspnea during initial 2–6 hours of continuous infusion GM-CSF, thought to be due to migration of neutrophils in the lung. Fluid retention may also occur.

Nursing Implications: Assess baseline pulmonary and fluid status. Teach patient to weigh self daily and instruct to report any changes in weight, breathing (e.g., dyspnea).

Drug: thyrotropin alfa for injection (Thyrogen)

Class: Recombinant hormone (human thyroid stimulating hormone) for tumor remnant ablation.

Mechanism of Action: Patients with thyroid cancer normally have surgery (subtotal or total thyroidectomy) followed by radioactive iodine to remove remaining normal tissue and any malignant cells. In order to stimulate the thyroid to take up the iodine, the TSH level has to be elevated. This drug binds to thyroid stimulating hormone (TSH) receptors on remaining normal thyroid epithelial cells and differentiated thyroid cancer cells, stimulating the uptake of iodine and organification, as well as synthesis and secretion of thyroglobulin (T_g), triiodothyronine (T_3), and thyroxine (T_4). An alternative to increasing the TSH level to destroy tumor remnant is to stop taking thyroid hormone replacement therapy, but this has significant side effects. Thyrotropin alfa for injection allows patients to continue to take their hormone replacement therapy with significantly higher quality of life (Genzyme, 2008; Pacini et al, 2002). This drug is also used as a diagnostic tool in assessment of well-differentiated thyroid cancer recurrence.

Metabolism: After a single 0.9 mg IM dose, mean peak concentrations were reached in 3 to 24 hours (median 10 hours). The mean elimination half-life is 25 ± 10 hours. The drug appears to be metabolized and excreted by the liver and kidneys

Dosage/Range:
- 0.9 mg IM followed by a second injection 24 hours later.
- In dialysis-dependent patients with ESRD, drug elimination is slower, resulting in prolonged TSH level elevation; expect that these patients may have an increased risk for headache and nausea.

Drug Preparation:
- Reconstitute with provided 1.2-mL sterile water for injection, resulting in a 0.9-mg thyrotropin alfa in 1.0 mL-solution immediately prior to administration.
- If necessary, reconstituted solution can be stored for 24 hours, protected from light, at 2–8°C (36–46°F).

Drug Administration:
- Administer IM ONLY, in the buttock.
- Give 0.9-mg thyrotropin alfa for injection IM daily × two doses 24 hours apart.
- Consider pretreatment with glucocorticosteroids in patients who may develop local tumor extension or swelling that could compromise vital structures (trachea, CNS brain or spinal metastases, extensive macroscopic lung metastases).
- Use cautiously and closely monitor older patients with functional thyroid tumors, as they may experience palpitations or cardiac rhythm disturbances (atrial).
- Consider hospitalization for administration and monitoring postdrug dose for patients with known heart disease, extensive metastases, or known serious underlying disease.
- For radioiodine imaging or remnant ablation, give radioiodine 24 hours after the second (final) thyrotropin alfa injection. Diagnostic scanning should be done 48 hours after the radioiodine administration; post-therapy scanning can be delayed additional days (to allow background activity to decline).
- For serum T_g testing, obtain a sample 72 hours after the second (final) injection.

Drug Interactions:

- None known.
- When used for radioiodine imaging in euthyroid patients, clearance of radioiodine is increased 50% compared with hypothyroid patients and should guide selection of the radioiodine used.

Lab Effects/Interference:

- Euthyroid patients for whom the drug is used for diagnostic imaging will have a significant, transient rise in TSH.
- No patients developed antibodies to thyrotropin alfa.

Special Considerations:

- Drug is indicated as an adjunctive.
- Treatment for radioactive ablation of the thyroid tissue remnants in patients who have undergone a near-total or total thyroidectomy for well-differentiated thyroid cancer and who do not have evidence of metastatic thyroid cancer.
- Diagnostic tool for serum thyroglobulin (T_g) testing with or without radioiodine imaging in the follow-up of patients with well-differentiated thyroid cancer.
- Use cautiously in patients who have previously received bovine TSH and those patients who have had hypersensitivity reactions to TSH administration in the past.
- Drug causes a transient but significant rise in serum thyroid hormone when given to patients who still have substantial remaining thyroid tissue; use cautiously, and monitor closely those patients with heart disease.
- It is unknown whether the drug is toxic to a fetus and thus should be given to a pregnant women only when clearly needed; mothers should not breast-feed when receiving the drug.
- Successful ablation can be inferred when Thyrogen-stimulated serum T_g level is < 2 ng/mL.
- Rarely, patient may develop hypersensitivity to the injection, characterized by urticaria, rash, pruritus, flushing, and respiratory symptoms; treat symptomatically.

Potential Toxicities/Side Effects (Dose- and Schedule-Dependent) and the Nursing Process

I. ALTERATION IN COMFORT related to FLU-LIKE SYMPTOMS

Defining Characteristics: Transient flu-like symptoms can occur lasting < 48 hours, characterized by fever, chills, myalgia, arthralgia, fatigue, asthenia, malaise, headache, and chills.

Nursing Implications: Assess baseline T, VS, and comfort level, and teach patient that this may occur and how to manage uncomfortable side effects (e.g., acetaminophen). Teach patient self-care measures, including monitoring T, comfort level, the use of heat or cold for myalgias, arthralgias. Encourage patient to increase oral fluids and alternate rest and activity periods.

II. POTENTIAL ALTERATION IN NUTRITION, LESS THAN BODY REQUIREMENTS, POTENTIAL, related to NAUSEA, VOMITING

Defining Characteristics: Nausea is mild and occurs in 11.9%, with vomiting in 2.3% of patients. Nausea and vomiting were severe when the dose was inadvertently given IV.

Nursing Implications: Assess baseline nutritional status. Teach patient that nausea may occur and that vomiting is rare; self-care measures, including oral hygiene and preparing favorite high-calorie, high-protein foods ahead of time so that the patient can snack when hungry. Teach the patient to report unrelieved nausea and vomiting if it occurs.

III. ALTERATION IN COMFORT related to HEADACHE

Defining Characteristics: Headache occurs in 7.3%.

Nursing Implications: Assess baseline comfort, and teach patient that these side effects may occur. Teach local comfort measures to minimize local injection reactions.

Drug: tumor necrosis factor (TNF)

Class: Cytokine.

Mechanism of Action: Binds to target cell membranes. TNF (cachectin) is produced by activated macrophages. It appears to halt cell growth in G_2 phase of cell cycle (cytostatic), is cytotoxic, and may cause vascular endothelial injury in tumor capillaries, leading to hemorrhage and necrosis of tumor cells. It also activates immune elements: increased NK cytotoxic activity, increased production of NK cells, B cells, and neutrophils.

Metabolism: Half-life is 20 minutes when given as IV bolus but varies with dose and route of administration.

Dosage/Range:
- Per individual protocol.

Drug Preparation:
- Per individual protocol.

Drug Administration:
- IVB or continuous infusion subcutaneous and IM. Refer to protocol for guidelines. When given IV, agent must be administered using a solution of 0.9% sodium chloride containing human serum albumin at a concentration of 2 mg/mL. This albumin prevents TNF from adhering to bag or tubing; prime tubing with solution before adding TNF to bag.

Drug Interactions:

- None reported, but data is being accumulated in clinical trials.

Lab Effects/Interference:

- Granulocytopenia, thrombocytopenia.

Potential Toxicities/Side Effects (Dose- and Schedule-Dependent) and the Nursing Process

I. ALTERATION IN COMFORT related to FLU-LIKE SYMPTOMS

Defining Characteristics: Fever to 39–40°C (102–104°F), and chills occur within 1–6 hours of dose, dependent on administration route; rigor, fatigue, myalgia, arthralgia, headache (dull, aching), and back pain may occur. Gradual disappearance of symptoms with repeated dosing (tachyphylaxis).

Nursing Implications: Assess baseline T, VS, neurologic status, and comfort level, and monitor every 4–6 hours if patient in hospital. Discuss with physician premedication and regular dosing of antipyretic (e.g., acetaminophen ± diphenhydramine, NSAID). Teach patient self-care measures, including monitoring T, comfort level, self-administration of prescribed medications prior to dose and regularly postdose, as well as the use of heat or cold for myalgias, arthralgias. Encourage patient to increase oral fluids and alternate rest and activity periods. If patient is in hospital and experiences rigor, discuss with physician IV meperidine (25 mg IV every 15 minutes to maximum 100 mg in 1 hour) and monitor BP for hypotension.

II. POTENTIAL ALTERATION IN NUTRITION, LESS THAN BODY REQUIREMENTS, related to ANOREXIA, NAUSEA, VOMITING, DIARRHEA

Defining Characteristics: Do not appear dose-dependent. Weight loss is not significant, and nausea/vomiting can be effectively managed.

Nursing Implications: Assess baseline nutritional status. Teach patient potential side effects, and self-care measures, including oral hygiene and preparing favorite high-calorie, high-protein foods ahead of time so patient can snack when hungry. Teach self-administration of prescribed antiemetics and antidiarrheals as needed. Refer to dietitian as appropriate.

III. ALTERATION IN CARDIAC OUTPUT related to ORTHOSTATIC HYPOTENSION

Defining Characteristics: Transient orthostatic hypotension (SBP < 90 mmHg) may occur after IV or subcutaneous injection and resolve with IV saline infusion. Hypertension may occur secondary to rigors.

Nursing Implications: Assess baseline cardiovascular status and orthostatic BP. Teach patient to change position slowly, to report light-headedness, and to increase oral fluids to 3 L/day.

IV. POTENTIAL FOR INFECTION AND BLEEDING related to GRANULOCYTOPENIA, THROMBOCYTOPENIA

Defining Characteristics: Dose-related, especially if > 100 mg/m^2 day, with normalization when treatment terminated.

Nursing Implications: Assess baseline CBC, WBC, differential, and platelet count, and signs/symptoms of infection or bleeding. Discuss any abnormalities with physician before drug administration. Teach patient signs/symptoms of infection, bleeding, and instruct to report them immediately. Teach patient self-care measures to minimize infection and bleeding, including avoidance of OTC aspirin-containing medications, and oral hygiene regimen.

V. POTENTIAL SENSORY/PERCEPTUAL ALTERATIONS related to NEUROLOGIC TOXICITY

Defining Characteristics: Seizures, confusion, aphasia may occur transiently and rarely.

Nursing Implications: Assess baseline mental status and history of seizures. Instruct patient to report any changes and ensure patient safety.

VI. POTENTIAL ALTERATION IN OXYGENATION related to DYSPNEA

Defining Characteristics: Dyspnea may occur, possibly related to alveolar endothelial damage.

Nursing Implications: Assess patient's risk (preexisting pulmonary dysfunction) and baseline pulmonary status. Instruct patient to report any changes.

Drug: zoster vaccine live (Zostavax)

Class: Vaccine.

Mechanism of Action: Initially, varicella zoster virus (VZV) produces chickenpox (varicella). The virus remains dormant in dorsal root or sensory ganglia until reactivation, when zoster occurs. In the body, as the VZV-specific immunity decreases, the virus can become reactivated. The person develops painful, vesicular lesions along a dermatome distribution of the body (on one side). Pain can occur during the prodrome, acute eruptive phase, and the post-herpetic phase, which is called post-herpetic neuralgia. Serious complications of herpes zoster, besides pain, include cranial and motor palsies, encephalitis, visual impairment, hearing loss, and death. The vaccine increases the immune system to prevent the reactivation of VZV.

Metabolism: Unknown.

Dosage/Range: Entire contents (0.65 mL) of reconstituted vaccine lyophilized vial containing at least 19,400 PFU (plaque forming units) of OKA/Merck strain VZV.

Drug Preparation: Remove the lyophilized vaccine powder from the freezer, and immediately and aseptically reconstitute using the provided diluent (stored at room temperature), using a sterile syringe and needle. Inject the entire volume of diluent, and gently agitate the vial to mix thoroughly. When reconstituted, is a semi-hazy to translucent, off-white powder to pale yellow liquid. Use within 30 minutes of reconstitution. Draw up entire contents of vial, and inject subcutaneously into subcutaneous tissue of upper arm (preferable). Vaccine lyophilized powder should be stored in the freezer at −15°C (+5°F) or colder, and protect from light. Diluent can be stored at room temperature or in the refrigerator.

Drug Interactions: None known.

Lab Effects/Interference: None known.

Special Considerations:

- Drug is indicated for the prevention of herpes zoster (shingles) in individuals aged 60 and older; it is not indicated for the treatment of herpes zoster or post-herpetic neuralgia.
- Drug is a live, attenuated virus, which may cause more extensive-vaccine associated rash in patients who are immunosuppressed; the drug's efficacy in patients receiving immunosuppressive drugs, inhaled, oral low dose, or topical corticosteroids, has not been studied.
- Drug is contraindicated in patients with (1) anaphylactoid/anaphylaxis to gelatin, neomycin, or other vaccine components, (2) history of acquired or primary immunodeficiency states, including lymphoma, leukemia or other malignancies that affect the bone marrow or lymphatic system, or AIDS or other infection with HIV, (3) current immunosuppressive therapy, including high-dose corticosteroids, (4) active, untreated TB, (5) patients who are or may become pregnant.
- Most common adverse effects (occurring in < 1% of patients) were injection site reactions and headache.
- Overall vaccine efficacy is 51% (64% in those aged 60–69; 41% in those aged 70–79; and 18% for those patients aged > 80).
- Drug is NOT a substitute for the vaccine VARIVAX (Varicella Virus Live Vaccine).
- Patients should be taught there is a theoretical risk of transmitting the live vaccine to varicella-susceptible individuals.

Potential Toxicities/Side Effects (Dose- and Schedule-Dependent) and the Nursing Process

II. ALTERATION IN COMFORT related to INJECTION SITE REACTIONS, RASH, AND HEADACHE

Defining Characteristics: Injection site reactions included erythema (34%), pain/tenderness (34%), swelling (24%), and pruritus (7%). Headache occurred in 1.4% of patients. Rarely, patients can develop varicella rash.

Nursing Implications: Assess baseline comfort, and teach patient that these side effects may occur. Teach local comfort measures to minimize local injection reactions. Teach patient to report rash right away, and to avoid contact with varicella-sensitive individuals, especially pregnant women.

Chapter 3
Antineoplastic Treatment Agonists: Radiosensitizers, Chemosensitizers, and Chemical Adjuncts

Radiation is the third major cancer treatment modality. Ionizing radiation causes cell damage and death to frequently dividing cells within the radiation port (site being radiated). Damage to DNA in malignant cells depends on the oxygenation of the tumor—cells that are well supplied with oxygen are sensitive to radiation effects, while those that are hypoxic (i.e., large, necrotic tumors) are radioresistant. Oxygen appears to be necessary at the time of radiation because it promotes formation of free radicals, causing DNA damage and preventing DNA repair (Noll, 1992).

Certain drugs called *radiosensitizers* may be administered concurrently with radiation therapy to increase the radiation damage to sensitive cells, thus increasing the tumor response (i.e., tumor reduction) to radiation therapy. Radiosensitizers are classified into three broad groups based on ability to sensitize hypoxic tumor cells and mechanism of action (Noll, 1992).

Hypoxic cell sensitizers mimic oxygen in chemical reactions that occur after ionizing radiotherapy, thus making the hypoxic cells sensitive to radiation damage. Examples are etanidazole, fluosol DA with 100% oxygen breathing, and buthionine, which depletes sulfhydryl-containing compounds from damaged cells so they are unable to repair their DNA.

Nonhypoxic cell sensitizers include the halogenated pyrimidines, which, because they are analogues of the DNA pyrimidine thymidine, are actively taken up by dividing cells and incorporated into DNA. This enhances radiosensitivity of the tumor cells and theoretically increases tumor response to radiotherapy. Drugs undergoing clinical testing include bromodeoxyuridine (BUdR) and iododeoxyuridine (IUdR).

A third group is composed of *chemotherapy agents* that are capable of radiosensitization. They are administered either prior to radiotherapy as part of combined modality therapy or concurrently in low doses to enhance radiosensitivity of tumor cells. These drugs include cisplatin, 5-fluorouracil, carboplatin, paclitaxel, gemcitabine, bleomycin, and mitomycin. Recent research on gemcitabine showed that the radiosensitization mechanism of action is different than when the drug is used as a chemotherapy agent (cytotoxic): When the cancer cells start to move through the synthesis phase of the cell cycle and the DNA strands are damaged by radiation, the cell undergoes programmed cell death (apoptosis) (Symon et al, 2002).

Finally, a fourth group called *molecular targeted agents* can also produce radiosensitization, thus increasing the therapeutic index (so cancer cells are killed rather than normal cells). These include the epidermal growth factor receptor (EGFR) tyrosine kinase inhibitor cetuximab (Erbitux), the EGFR tyrosine kinase inhibitor gefitinib (Iressa), and farnesyl transferase inhibitors (Lawrence and Nyati, 2002).

This is a promising frontier in cancer treatment, and the next decade will bring greater understanding and options in radiotherapy, chemosensitization, and new adjuncts.

References

Brown JM. Therapeutic Targets in Radiotherapy. *Int J Radiat Oncol Biol Phys* 2001; 49(2) 319–326

Bunn PA. Triplet Combination Chemotherapy and Targeted Therapy Regimens. *Oncology* 2001; 15 (3 Suppl 6) 26–32

Choy H, Nabid A, Stea B, et al. Phase II Multicenter Study of Induction Chemotherapy Followed by Concurrent Efaproxiral (RSR13) and Thoracic Radiotherapy for Patients With Locally Advanced Non-Small-Cell Lung Cancer. *J Clin Oncol* 2005; 23 5918–5928

Coleman CN. Radiation and Chemotherapy Sensitizers and Protectors. In Chabner BA, Longo DL, (eds), *Cancer Chemotherapy and Biotherapy*, 2nd ed. Philadelphia: Lippincott Raven; 1996; 553–584

Coleman CN, Bump EA, Kramer RA. Chemical Modifiers of Cancer Treatment. *J Clin Oncol* 1989; 6 709–733

Craighead PS, Pearcey R, Stuart G. A Phase I/II Evaluation of Tirapazamine Administered Intravenously Concurrent with Cisplatin and Radiotherapy in Women with Locally Advanced Cervical Cancer. *Int J Radiat Oncol Biol Phys* 2000; 48(3) 791–795

Denny WA, Wilson WR. Tirapazamine: A Bioreductive Anticancer Drug that Exploits Tumour Hypoxia. *Expert Opin Investig Drugs* 2000; 9(12) 2889–2901

Dische S. Chemical Sensitizers for Hypoxic Cells: A Decade of Experience in Clinical Radiotherapy. *Radiother Oncol* 1985; 3 97–111

Fowler JF. Chemical Modifiers of Radiosensitivity: Theory and Reality: A Review. *Int J Radiat Oncol Biol Phys* 1985; 11 665–674

Goldberg Z, Evans J, Birrell G, Brown JM. An Investigation of the Molecular Basis for the Synergistic Interaction of Tirapazamine and Cisplatin. *Int J Radiat Oncol Biol Phys* 2001; 49(1) 175–182

Kinsella TJ, Mitchell JB, Russo A, et al. The Use of Halogenated Thymidine Analogues as Clinical Radiosensitizers: Rationale, Current Status, and Future Prospects. *Int J of Radiat Oncol Biol Phys* 1984; 10 1399–1406

Lawrence TS, Nyati MK. Small-molecule Tyrosine Kinase Inhibitors as Radiosensitizers. *Semin Radiat Oncol* 2002; 12 (suppl 2) 33–36

Mallinkckrodt Phosphocol P32 Package Insert. St. Louis: Mallinkckrodt Inc.; 1997

Noll L. Chemical Modifiers of Radiation Therapy. In Hassey-Dow K Hilderly LJ (eds.), *Nursing Care in Radiation Oncology*. Philadelphia: WB Saunders; 1992

Novartis Pharmaceuticals Corp (2005). Exjade. East Hanover, NJ: Novartis Pharmaceuticals Corporation

Rischin D, Peters L, Hicks et al. R, Phase I Trial of Concurrent Tirapazamine, Cisplatin, and Radiotherapy in Patients with Advanced Head and Neck Cancer. *J Clin Oncol* 2000; 19(2) 535–545

Symon Z, Davis M, McGinn CJ, Concurrent Chemoradiotherapy with Gemcitabine and Cisplatin for Pancreatic Cancer: From Laboratory to the Clinic. *Int J Radiat Oncol Biol Phys* 2002; 53 140–145

Drug: chromic phosphate P32 suspension (Phosphocol™ P32)

Class: Radiopharmaceutical agent.

Mechanism of Action: Provides local irradiation by beta emission and is administered into cavities for the treatment of peritoneal or pleural effusions due to metastatic cancer; it may also be given interstitially to treat cancer.

Metabolism: Phosphorus P32 decays by beta emission with a physical half-life of 14.3 days, with a residence time of 495 hours. The mean energy of the beta particle is 695 keV. Distribution in the pleural or peritoneal space is nonuniform, with extremes of local dosage.

Dosage/Range:
- Intraperitoneal: 370–740 megabecquerels (10–20 millicuries).
- Intrapleural: 222–444 megabecquerels (6–12 millicuries).
- Interstitial (e.g., prostate): based on estimated gram weight of tumor, about 3.7–18.5 megabecquerels/gm (0.2–0.5 millicuries/gm).
- 37 kilobecquerels = 1 millicurie (mCi) = 7.3 grays = 730 rads.

Drug Preparation:
- None.
- Available as chromic phosphate P32 suspension in 10 mL vials containing 555 megabecquerels (15 mCi) with a concentration of up to 185 megabecquerels (5 mCi)/mL.

Drug Administration:
- Always given into pleural or peritoneal cavity, or may be given interstitially (e.g., prostate), but NEVER intravenously.

For pleural effusions:
- Interventional radiologist visualizes pleural space with ultrasound to ensure that it is open without adhesions.
- Interventional radiologist places a thoracentesis catheter in the pleural space, having a three-way stopcock, and verifies position by ultrasound; removes pleural fluid by opening ports 1 and 2.
- Port 2 is closed and port 3 is opened for a qualified MD to administer chromic phosphate P32 suspension (injecting 6–12 mCi into the port, then rinses with 10 mL 0.9% NS).
- Close ports and ensure that they are closed to prevent leakage of radionucleotide and radiation contamination. The catheter is then removed. If there is leakage or contamination, refer to institutional policy/procedure for radiation spill.
- Reposition patient from supine to prone, onto the right side, and onto the left side, and lastly, have the patient stand and bend over.
- CXR is done to make certain there is no pneumothorax.
- Patient is given one-month follow-up appointment for a CXR, and is asked to return if shortness of breath occurs, as this may signify reaccumulation of effusion.

Drug Interaction:
- Unknown.

Lab Effects/Interference:
- Unknown.

Special Considerations:
Eligible candidates for treatment of pleural effusion:
- History of prior pleurodesis with talc.
- Evidence of pleural plaques.
- Prior treatment using a chest tube.
- Emphysema.
- History of pleural asbestos exposure.

Contraindications:
- Presence of ulcerative tumors.
- Pregnant or nursing mothers, unless benefit outweighs risks.
- Presence of large tumor masses.
- Risk of improper placement: intestinal fibrosis or necrosis, and chronic fibrosis of body wall have been described.
- Radiation damage may occur if injected interstitially or into a loculation.
- Treatment may be less effective if effusion bloody.

Potential Toxicities/Side Effects and the Nursing Process

I. POTENTIAL FOR INFECTION, BLEEDING, AND FATIGUE related to BONE MARROW DEPRESSION

Defining Characteristics: Bone marrow suppression, if it occurs, is transitory.

Nursing Implications: Assess baseline WBC, differential, platelet and Hgb/HCT prior to treatment, as well as for signs/symptoms of infection or bleeding. Teach patient signs/symptoms of infection and bleeding and to report these immediately; teach patient self-care measures to minimize risk of infection and bleeding. This includes avoidance of crowds, proximity to people with infections, and avoidance of OTC aspirin-containing medications. Teach patient to report fatigue, and teach measures to conserve energy, such as alternating rest and activity periods. Discuss transfusion of red blood cells as needed.

II. PAIN related to PLEURITIS, PERITONITIS, AND ABDOMINAL CRAMPING

Defining Characteristics: Symptoms depend upon area treated, with pleuritis arising from treatment of pleural effusion, and peritonitis, abdominal cramping, and nausea arising from treatment of peritoneal effusion.

Nursing Implications: Assess baseline pain level. Teach patient of potential side effects and to report them. Teach patient symptom-management techniques and discuss with physician medications for analgesia and nausea. Teach patient to report if symptoms do not subside or improve.

III. ALTERATION IN COMFORT related to RADIATION SICKNESS

Defining Characteristics: Exposure to ionizing radiation causes symptoms, the severity of which are dependent upon the volume of radiation, the length of time of exposure, and the area of the body affected. Moderate symptoms may occur from treatment with chromic phosphate P32 suspension, and these include headache, nausea, vomiting, anorexia, and diarrhea. Long-term exposure may result in sterility, malformation of the fetus in a pregnant woman, and cancer.

Nursing Implications: Assess baseline comfort level. Teach patient that moderate symptoms may arise. Teach patient to report symptoms as soon as possible, and discuss management strategies. Discuss pharmacologic management of nausea/vomiting and diarrhea with physician, and give patient prescriptions for antiemetic and antidiarrheal medications for PRN use.

Drug: deferasirox tablets for oral suspension (Exjade)

Class: Iron chelating agent.

Mechanism of Action: Orally active chelator that binds iron, thus preventing iron overload resulting from multiple red blood cell transfusions (transfusional hemosiderosis).

Metabolism: Drug is absorbed after oral ingestion with 70% bioavailability (compared to an IV dose), achieving maximum plasma concentrations at a median of 1.5–4 hours. Area Under the Curve (AUC) was increased when drug is taken with food. Drug is highly (~99%) protein bound, primarily to serum albumin. Deferasirox is metabolized via the glucuronidation pathway, and excreted in the bile. Although UGT1A1 and, to a lesser extent, UGT1A3 are involved, there is no apparent induction or inhibition of metabolic enzymes. Drug and metabolites are primarily excreted in the feces (84%), and to a lesser extent via the kidneys (8%). Mean elimination half-life is 8–16 hours. In children < 6 years of age, systemic exposure was 50% lower than adults.

Dosage/Range:

- Therapy is recommended when a patient has evidence of chronic iron overload (transfusion of ~100 mL/kg of packed red blood cells or 20 units for a 40 kg patient, and a serum ferritin consistently > 1000 mcg/L).
- Initial daily dose: 20 mg/kg daily.

- Maintenance: Adjust dose of deferasirox tablets for oral suspension every 3–6 months, based on trends of monthly serum ferritin levels. Dose adjustments should be made in increments of 5–10 mg/kg based on response and therapeutic goals (e.g., maintenance or reduction of iron burden). Dose should not exceed 30 mg/kg per day. Dose should be interrupted if serum ferritin falls consistently < 500 mcg/L.

Dose Adjustments

- Increased serum creatinine (reduction, interruption, or discontinuation): in adults, dose reduce by 10 mg/kg if serum creatinine increases by > 33% above the average of the pretreatment measurements on two consecutive measures and cannot be attributed to other causes. A similar dose reduction was used in clinical studies for patients > 15 years old and if serum creatinine increases in children < 15 years old was > 33% above the age-appropriate upper limit of normal.
- Increased liver function tests (LFTs): dose reduction, interruption, or discontinuation if increase in LFTs severe or persistent.
- Severe rash: drug may be interrupted and reintroduced at a lower dose with escalation in combination with a short period of oral steroids.
- Auditory or ocular disturbances: dose reduction or interruption.
- The decision to remove accumulated iron should be individualized based on risk–benefit discussions.

Drug Preparation:

- Drug is available in 125 mg, 250 mg, and 500 mg tablets for oral suspension.
- Teach patient:
  - Patient should have the following tests prior to starting drug, and then regularly during therapy:
    - Auditory and ophthalmic testing baseline and every 12 months.
    - Serum creatinine and liver function tests baseline and monthly; urine protein baseline and regularly.
  - Take drug as follows on an empty stomach, 30 minutes before eating:
    - Disperse tablet for oral suspension in water, orange juice, or apple juice until a fine suspension results. Dose should be calculated to the nearest whole tablet size. If dose is < 1 g, use 3.5 oz of liquid, and if > 1 g, use 7 oz of liquid.
    - Once the suspension is swallowed, ensure the entire dose is ingested by filling the glass again with a small amount of liquid to resuspend the residue, and swallow this as well.
  - DO NOT chew or swallow tablets whole.
  - DO NOT take with aluminum-containing antacid products.
  - DO NOT drive or operate machinery if experiencing dizziness.

Drug Interactions:

- Aluminum-containing antacids: potential interactions, as formal studies have not been done; deferasirox should not be taken with aluminum-containing antacids.
- Other iron chelating agents: safety has not been determined; do not take in combination.

Lab Effects/Interference:

- Serum ferritin: decrease in serum ferritin. Monitor baseline and monthly.
- Serum creatinine: increased (dose-dependent) in 11% of patients. Monitor serum creatinine baseline × 2, and at least monthly.
- Urine protein: intermittent proteinuria occurred in 18.6% patients on clinical trials. Assess baseline and monthly. Monitor patients at risk closely.
- Liver function studies: increased in some patients. Monitor baseline and monthly.
- Liver iron concentration (LIC): decreased; however, correlation coefficient between serum ferritin and LIC is 0.63, so serum ferritin levels may not always reflect changes in LIC.

Special Considerations:

- Drug is indicated for the treatment of chronic iron overload due to blood transfusions in patients aged 2 and older.
- Drug is contraindicated in patients with hypersensitivity to deferasirox or to any other drug component.
- Hepatic failure, sometimes fatal, has been reported. Risk factors appear to include age greater than 55. Most patients with hepatic failure had significant comorbidities, including liver cirrhosis and multiorgan failure. Consider dose interruption for severe or persistent elevation of LFTs. Monitor LFTs monthly.
- Acute renal failure has been reported, and fatal outcomes have occurred in patients with multiple comorbidities with advanced hematologic dysfunction. Monitor patients very carefully who have preexisting renal conditions, are older, have comorbid conditions, or are receiving medicines that depress renal function.
- Patients should have baseline complete blood count, serum ferritin, creatinine, liver function tests, urine protein, and auditory and ophthalmic (slit lamp and dilated funduscopy) testing. Baseline serum creatinine should be repeated so that two tests are done before starting the drug. Serum lab tests and urine protein should be repeated monthly, and auditory and ocular testing yearly during treatment. The older patients or patients with preexisting renal conditions or other risk factors noted previously here should be monitored weekly during the first month after drug initiation or any dose modification and then monthly thereafter.
- In postmarketing reports, neutropenia, thrombocytopenia, agranulocytosis, and serious hypersensitivity reactions (anaphylaxis and angioedema) have occurred. Monitor blood counts regularly and drug dose modified or stopped if the patient develops unexplained cytopenias. Teach patient to call an ambulance if the patient develops signs/symptoms of hypersensitivity or angioedema, usually within the first month of treatment.
- Drug is not carcinogenic, mutagenic, and has no adverse effects on fertility or reproductive performance in laboratory animals.
- Although drug was not teratogenic in lab animals, drug should be used in pregnancy only if clearly needed (Pregnancy Category B).

- Drug is excreted in breast milk of lab animals, so caution should be exercised when drug is administered to a nursing woman.
- During the 1 year clinical trial, safety and efficacy of pediatric patients was similar to that of adults, so recommended starting dose and dosing modifications are the same. During this time, the growth and development of the children were within normal limits.
- Use drug cautiously in elderly patients due to the greater frequency of decreased hepatic, renal, or cardiac function, and polypharmacy.

Potential Toxicities/Side Effects and the Nursing Process

I. POTENTIAL FOR SENSORY/PERCEPTUAL ALTERATIONS related to AUDITORY AND OCULAR DISTURBANCES

Defining Characteristics: Auditory disturbances (high frequency hearing loss, decreased hearing), and ocular disturbances (lens opacities, cataracts, elevated intraocular pressure, retinal disorders) were reported rarely (< 1%).

Nursing Implications: Ensure that patient has had baseline auditory and ophthalmic (slit lamp and full funduscopy) examinations prior to beginning therapy and then annually (every 12 months). Teach patient to report any changes in hearing or vision right away; discuss need to modify dose or stop the drug with the physician. Ensure that patient has 12-month follow-up auditory and ophthalmic examinations during therapy.

II. ALTERATION IN URINARY ELIMINATION, POTENTIAL, related to RENAL DYSFUNCTION

Defining Characteristics: Acute renal failure, sometimes fatal, has occurred in postmarketing reports. Patients at risk are older, those with preexisting renal impairment, receiving medicines that depress renal function, or who have comorbidities. Increased serum creatinine occurred in 38% of patients and appeared to be dose-related. These increases were WNL in 94% of patients. Intermittent proteinuria (urine protein/creatinine ration > 0.6 mg/mg) occurred in 18.6% of patients treated compared with 7.2% in the deferoxamine arm.

Nursing Implications: Assess baseline renal function in terms of serum creatinine and urine protein; serum creatinine should be repeated × 2 baseline to confirm finding. If patients are at risk for renal dysfunction (history of renal dysfunction, older, comorbidities, other renally depressing drugs), monitor serum creatinine weekly during the first month of treatment or after any dose adjustments and then monthly. Monitor serum creatinine and urine protein monthly during treatment. If increased, discuss dose adjustment (interruption, reduction, or discontinuance) with physician.

III. ALTERATION IN NUTRITION, LESS THAN BODY REQUIREMENTS, related to NAUSEA/VOMITING, DIARRHEA, HEPATOTOXICITY

Defining Characteristics: Nausea occurred in 10.5%, vomiting 10%, and diarrhea in 11.8% of patients. These gastrointestinal side effects appear dose related. Hepatotoxicity, occasionally fatal, has been described after marketing. Patients at risk are those aged > 55 years old, who have comorbidities that may include hepatic cirrhosis and multiorgan failure.

Nursing Implications: Reinforce teaching to administer drug on an empty stomach 30 minutes before a meal. Teach patient to report nausea, vomiting, and/or diarrhea. If nausea and/or vomiting occur, discuss premedication with an antiemetic with physician. Encourage small, frequent feedings of favorite foods. Ensure that the patient can repeat hydration schedule (one glass of fluid every hour when awake, or as appropriate) if patient experiences diarrhea or vomiting. If diarrhea occurs, teach patient to self-administer antidiarrheal medication. Monitor LFTs baseline and then monthly; if there is an unexplained, persistent, or progressive increase in serum transaminases, hold or dose reduce drug. Monitor patients closely, and repeat testing frequently if dose is reduced.

IV. ALTERATION IN SKIN INTEGRITY related to RASH

Defining Characteristics: Rash affected 8.4% of patients and appears dose-related. Rash can be mild to moderate or severe, and often resolves spontaneously. Leukocytoclastic vasculitis and urticaria have been reported in the postmarketing period.

Nursing Implications: Assess skin integrity and presence of rash baseline and periodically during treatment. Teach patient to report skin rash, and explain that rash often resolves spontaneously. If rash is severe, discuss dose interruption with physician. Teach patient that once rash resolves, drug can be reintroduced at lower dose with escalation in combination with a short course of oral steroids.

V. ALTERATION IN COMFORT related to ABDOMINAL PAIN, HEADACHE, FEVER, ARTHRALGIA, FATIGUE

Defining Characteristics: Abdominal pain occurred in about 14% of patients in 1 study, compared to about 10% in the comparator group who received deferoxamine IV. Arthralgia occurred in 7.4% of patients and fatigue in 6.1%.

Nursing Implications: Teach patient that abdominal pain may occur, and to report it. Teach patient to report fevers. Teach local measures to improve comfort. If abdominal pain persists or worsens, discuss further testing and drug interruption with physician.

Liver function tests should be monitored baseline and monthly; chemical hepatitis occurred in 2 patients, and should be ruled out. Teach patient that fatigue and arthralgias are uncommon, but may occur. Teach local comfort measures, and teach patient to report symptoms that worsen.

Drug: efaproxiral (investigational)

Class: Radiosensitizing agent.

Mechanism of Action: Drug is a small molecule, which enhances the diffusion of oxygen from hemoglobin to hypoxic tissue. Drug binds centrally to hemoglobin core, modifying its structure and weakening the bond between oxygen and hemoglobin. This makes more oxygen available for diffusion into hypoxic tissues, increases the partial pressure of oxygen in the area, and reduces the number of hypoxic areas. RT works by damaging cells and creating free radicals in the target cells. The efficacy of RT is a function of having intracellular oxygen that stabilizes and extends the half life of these free radicals so that cancer cells can not repair their damaged cells. Cells in hypoxic areas are resistant to RT, and the protected cells can continue to divide and grow. Radiosensitizers remove the areas of hypoxia thus reducing the likelihood that cancer cells can escape.

Metabolism: Works quickly and has a short half life of 4–5 hours. Metabolism is unknown.

Dosage/Range:
Per protocol.

Drug Preparation/Administration:
- IV via central line, given 30 minutes prior to RT treatment, along with supplemental oxygen; monitor VS including O_2 sat, BP per protocol; discharge home from clinic if O_2 saturation > 90% and BP WNL.

Drug Interactions:
- Yes, hold interfering medications during clinical trial. See protocol.

Lab Effects/Interference:
- Rare ↑ renal function studies.
- ↓ oxygen saturation in blood.
- Anemia.

Special Considerations:
- Drug is being studied in patients receiving RT for (1) brain metastases from breast cancer, (2) NSCLC, (3) cervical cancer, (4) glioblastoma multiforme.
- Side effect profile mild, with low O_2 saturation/hypoxemia, fatigue, and radiation-induced lung disease being the most severe (Choy et al, 2005); other acute effects are nausea, vomiting, headache, dizziness, hypertension, tingling around the mouth.

Potential Toxicities/Side Effects and the Nursing Process

I. POTENTIAL ALTERATION IN NUTRITION, LESS THAN BODY REQUIREMENTS, related to NAUSEA, VOMITING

Defining Characteristics: Nausea/vomiting can be effectively managed.

Nursing Implications: Assess baseline nutritional status. Teach patient potential side effects, and self-care measures, including oral hygiene and preparing favorite high-calorie, high-protein foods ahead of time so patient can snack when hungry. Teach self-administration of prescribed antiemetics as needed. Refer to dietitian as appropriate.

II. ALTERATION IN COMFORT related to HEADACHE, DIZZINESS, TINGLING AROUND THE MOUTH

Defining Characteristics: Headache, dizziness, and tingling may occur.

Nursing Implications: Teach patient these side effects may occur and to report them. Assess comfort level baseline and prior to each administration of drug and RT. Establish plan for symptom management, and discuss severe or persistent symptoms with physician or NP.

Drug: etanidazole (investigational)

Class: Nitroimidazole, hypoxic radiosensitizer.

Mechanism of Action: Sensitizes hypoxic tumor cells to the effects of ionizing radiotherapy by mimicking oxygen. This enhances formation of free radicals, which damage cellular DNA and prevent DNA repair so that tumor cell kill is enhanced.

Metabolism: Metabolized by liver.

Dosage/Range:
- Per protocol.

Drug Preparation:
- Per protocol, but may be administered as a rapid intravenous infusion three times per week, immediately prior to radiotherapy.

Drug Interactions:
- Unknown.

Special Considerations:
- Peripheral neuropathy is dose-limiting toxicity.
- Less toxic than nitroimidazole, with less nerve tissue penetration.

Potential Toxicities/Side Effects and the Nursing Process

I. SENSORY PERCEPTUAL ALTERATION related to PERIPHERAL NEUROPATHY

Defining Characteristics: Peripheral neuropathy occurs, with sensory loss and paresthesias of feet, toes, hands. May have decreased sensitivity to pinprick, decreased vibratory sense. May resolve over days, while severe neuropathies may be permanent. Related to cumulative drug exposure.

Nursing Implications: Assess baseline neurologic status. Assess for numbness, tingling, burning, loss of temperature sensation, and ache at each visit. Instruct patient to report these or other changes immediately. Discuss drug discontinuance with physician as appropriate to prevent permanent severe neuropathy.

II. ALTERATION IN NUTRITION, LESS THAN BODY REQUIREMENTS, related to GI SIDE EFFECTS

Defining Characteristics: Nausea and vomiting may occur.

Nursing Implications: Assess baseline nutritional status and signs/symptoms of nausea, vomiting. Instruct patient to report occurrence of nausea, vomiting. Discuss premedication with physician and administer prescribed antiemetic prior to drug. Teach patient to self-administer prescribed antiemetic at home.

III. ALTERATION IN COMFORT related to RASH, ARTHRALGIAS

Defining Characteristics: Rash, transient arthralgias may occur.

Nursing Implications: Assess baseline comfort level. Assess for rash, arthralgias, and instruct patient to report these side effects. If they occur, provide and teach patient symptomatic measures to reduce discomfort.

Drug: fluosol DA (20%) (investigational)

Class: Perfluorocarbon emulsion, hypoxic radiosensitizer.

Mechanism of Action: Hydrocarbon with hydrogen atom replaced by fluorine, so acts as artificial oxygen carrier. Thus, it decreases cell hypoxia and enhances formation of free radicals, which damage tumor cell DNA and prevent DNA repair.

Metabolism: By liver.

Dosage/Range:
- Per protocol.

Drug Preparation:
- Per protocol.

Drug Interactions:
- None known.

Special Considerations:
- Administer prior to radiation with patient breathing 100% oxygen before and during radiation.
- Increases solid tumor response to radiotherapy without increased damage to normal cells.
- Mild myelosuppression may be due to radiotherapy rather than drug.

Potential Toxicities/Side Effects and the Nursing Process

I. ALTERATION IN COMFORT related to DRUG ALLERGY

Defining Characteristics: Allergic-type reaction may occur with first dose, characterized by facial flushing, chest pressure, and/or chills and fever. Premedication with antihistamines and corticosteroids prevents further episodes.

Nursing Implications: Assess baseline drug allergies, temperature, VS. Teach patient to report sensation of warmth, chest pressure, chills, facial flushing. Discuss with physician premedication with antihistamines and corticosteroids.

II. ALTERATION IN NUTRITION, LESS THAN BODY REQUIREMENTS, related to HEPATOTOXICITY

Defining Characteristics: Transient, self-limited increases in LFTs may occur (AST, ALT, alk phos).

Nursing Implications: Assess baseline LFTs and monitor throughout treatment. Discuss abnormalities with physician.

Drug: leucovorin calcium (Folinic Acid, Citrovorum Factor)

Class: Water-soluble vitamin in the folate group (folinic acid).

Mechanism of Action: Potentiates antitumor activity of 5-FU when given prior to or concurrently with 5-FU, ± XRT. Acts as an antidote for methotrexate and other folic acid antagonists. Circumvents the biochemical block of the enzyme inhibitors (e.g., dihydrofolate reductase [DHFR]) to permit DNA and RNA synthesis.

Metabolism: Leucovorin is metabolized to polyglutamates that are more effective in potentiating 5-FU tumor cell kill. Metabolized primarily in the liver; 50% of the single dose is excreted in 6 hours in the urine (80–90% of the dose) and stool (8% of the dose).

Dosage/Range:

Antidote for methotrexate:

- Dose of drug and duration of rescue is dependent on serum methotrexate levels:

Methotrexate Level	Leucovorin
< 5.0 $(10)^{-7}$M	10 mg/m^2 q 6 h
5 $(10)^{-7}$M$(10)^{-6}$M	30–40 mg/m^2 q 6 h
> 5 $(10)^{-6}$M	100 mg/m^2 q 3–6 h

- Potentiation of 5-FU ± XRT: dose varies leucovorin 20 mg/m^2/d–2.5 g/m^2 CI.

Drug Preparation:

- Drug is supplied in ampules or vials.
- Reconstitute vials with sterile water for injection.
- Dilute reconstituted vials or ampules further with 5% dextrose or 0.9% sodium chloride.

Drug Administration:

- With 5-FU, in a variety of combinations; e.g., leucovorin: 500 mg/m^2/week for 6 weeks as a 2-hour infusion; 5-FU: 500–600 mg/m^2/week for 6 weeks, IVB midway through leucovorin infusion, then 2-week rest, then repeat 6-week cycle.
- Administered 24 hours after first methotrexate dose is begun. Dose every 6 hours for up to 12 doses.
- First dose is given IV; others can be given IM or PO when given as methotrexate "rescue."
- IV doses are given via bolus over 15 minutes unless otherwise specified.
- When given as a rescue dose, must be given exactly on time in order to rescue normal cells from methotrexate toxicity.

Drug Interactions:

- 5-FU: potentiation.
- Folic acid: provides folinic acid so cells can make DNA (antagonizes drug effect).
- Phenobarbital, phenytoin, primidone: decreases anticonvulsant action (when leucovorin given in large doses); monitor patient closely and increase anticonvulsant as needed.

Lab Effects/Interference:

- None.

Special Considerations:

- It is imperative that the patient receive the leucovorin on schedule to avoid fatal methotrexate toxicity. Notify the physician if the patient is unable to take the dose orally, as it must then be given IV.
- Usually free of side effects, but allergic reaction and local pain may occur.

Potential Toxicities/Side Effects and the Nursing Process

I. POTENTIAL FOR INJURY related to HYPERSENSITIVITY, DRUG INTERACTIONS

Defining Characteristics: Allergic sensitization has been reported: facial flushing, itching. Leucovorin in large amounts may counteract the antiepileptic effects of phenobarbital, phenytoin, and primidone.

Nursing Implications: Monitor patient for signs/symptoms of allergic reaction. Diphenhydramine is effective for relieving symptoms of allergic reaction. Monitor patient for symptoms of increased seizure activity (if on antiepileptic drugs); monitor antiepileptic drug levels.

II. ALTERED NUTRITION, LESS THAN BODY REQUIREMENTS, related to NAUSEA, VOMITING

Defining Characteristics: Oral leucovorin rarely causes nausea or vomiting.

Nursing Implications: Administer oral leucovorin with antacids, milk, or juice.

Drug: levoleucovorin (Fusilev, d,1-leucovorin)

Class: Folate analogue.

Mechanism of Action: Drug is the pharmacologically active isomer of 5-formyl tetrahydrofolic acid that does not require further reduction by the enzyme dihydrofolate reductase in order to use folates. Acts as an antidote for methotrexate and other folic acid antagonists. Circumvents the biochemical block of the enzyme inhibitors (e.g., dihydrofolate reductase [DHFR]) to permit DNA and RNA synthesis. Potentiates antitumor activity of 5-FU when given before or concurrently with 5-FU.

Metabolism: After an IV dose of 15 mg, peak serum levels were reached in 0.9 hr. Mean terminal half-life was 5–6.8 hr.

Dosage/Range:

- Based on a methotrexate dose of 12 g/m^2 administered IV over 4 hours: 7.5 mg (5 mg/m^2) every 6 hr × 10 doses starting exactly 24 hours after the beginning of the methotrexate.
- Determine serum creatinine and methotrexate (MTX) levels at least once daily.
- Continue levoleucovorin administration, hydration, and urinary alkalinization (pH ≥ 7.0) until MTX level $< 5 \times 10^{-8}$ (0.05 micromolar).

- The levoleucovorin dose may need to be adjusted:

Clinical Situation	Laboratory Findings	Levoleucovorin dosage/duration
Normal MTX Elimination	Serum MTX level 10 micromolar at 24 hr after administration, 1 micromolar at 48 hr, and < 0.2 micromolar at 72 hr	7.5 mg IV q 6 hr × 60 hr (10 doses starting at 24 hr after start of MTX infusion)
Delayed late MTX elimination	Serum MTX level > 0.2 micromolar at 72 hr, and > 0.05 micromolar at 96 hr after administration	Continue 7.5 mg IV q 6 hr until MTX level is < 0.05 micromolar
Delayed Early MTX Elimination and/or evidence of acute renal injury	Serum MTX level at ≥ 50 micromolar at 24 hr, or ≥ 5 micromolar at 48 hr after MTX administration, OR ≥ 100% increase in serum creatinine level at 24 hr after MTX administration (e.g., an increase from 0.5 mg/dL to a level of 1 mg/dL or more)	75 mg IV q 3 hr until MTX level is < 1 micromolar; then 7.5 mg IV q 3 hr until MTX level is less than 0.05 micromolar

Drug Preparation:
- Drug available in 50-mg single-use vial as a lyophilized powder with 50 mg mannitol.
- Reconstitute with 5.3 mL of sterile 0.9% sodium chloride for injection USP, resulting in a 10 gm/mL solution.
- May further dilute to concentrations of 0.5 mg/mL to 5 mg/mL in 0.9% sodium chloride injection USP (stable for 12 hours at room temperature) or 5% dextrose injection USP (stable for 4 hours at room temperature).

Drug Administration:
- Administer IVP (not faster than 16 mL [160 mg] per minute because Ca^{2+} content limits speed of injection) or as short IV infusion.

Lab Effects/Interference:
- None known.

Drug Interactions:
- 5-Fluourouracil (5-FU): increased toxicity.
- Trimethoprim-sulfamethoxazole (used to treat *Pneumocystis carinii* pneumonia in HIV patients): Combination increased rates of treatment failure in one study.

Special Considerations:
- Indicated as (1) a rescue after high-dose methotrexate therapy in osteosarcoma and (2) to diminish the toxicity and counteract the effects of impaired methotrexate elimination and of inadvertent overdosage of folic acid antagonists.
- Do not administer intrathecally.
- Dosed at one-half the usual dose of leucovorin calcium (folinic acid citrovorum factor).

- Contraindicated in patients who have had a previous allergic reaction to folic acid or folinic acid.
- When given with 5-FU weekly in older patients, severe enterocolitis, diarrhea, and dehydration resulting in death have occurred.
- Not approved for treatment of pernicious anemia or megaloblastic anemias.

Potential Toxicities/Side Effects and the Nursing Process

I. POTENTIAL FOR INJURY related to HYPERSENSITIVITY, DRUG INTERACTIONS

Defining Characteristics: Allergic reactions have been reported: facial flushing, itching.

Nursing Implications: Monitor patient for signs/symptoms of allergic reaction. Diphenhydramine is effective for relieving symptoms of allergic reaction.

II. ALTERATION IN NUTRITION, LESS THAN BODY REQUIREMENTS, related to NAUSEA, VOMITING

Defining Characteristics: Levoleucovorin causes vomiting in 38% of patients, stomatitis in 38%, and nausea in 19% after high-dose MTX therapy.

Nursing Implications: Discuss need to continue antiemetics after high-dose MTX therapy with physician. Assess oral mucosa, teach patient self-assessment and to report any abnormalities. Teach patient to rinse oral mucosa after meals and at bedtime with oral rinse, such as salt water or sodium bicarbonate solution, as per institution guidelines for chemotherapy.

Drug: porfirmer sodium (Photofrin)

Class: Photosensitizing agent.

Mechanism of Action: Porfirmer sodium is selectively distributed and maintained in tumor tissue. When exposed to 630 nanometer laser light, porfirmer is activated and a chain reaction ensues, resulting in damage to tumor cell mitochondria and intracellular membranes. The therapy also causes the release of thromboxane A, resulting in vasoconstriction, activation and aggregation of platelets, and increased clotting. Ischemic necrosis ensues, causing tissue and tumor death.

Metabolism: Distributed through a variety of tissues, but is selectively retained by tumors, skin, and organs of the reticuloendothelial system (liver, spleen). Drug is not dialyzable.

Dosage/Range:
- 2 mg/kg body weight, injected over 3–5 minutes.
- May be given for a total of 3 courses of therapy, each separated by at least 30 days.

Drug Preparation:
- Add 31.8 mL D5W or NS to the 75-mg vial, producing a concentration of 2.5 mg/ml.
- Protect reconstituted solution from bright light and use immediately.

Drug Interactions:
- The following drugs may decrease the effectiveness of profirmer sodium therapy: allopurinol, corticosteroids (glucocorticoid), calcium channel blockers, prostaglandin synthesis inhibitors, Thromboxane A inhibitors, beta-carotene, DMSO, ethanol, formate, and mannitol.
- Some drugs may increase photosensitivity, including griseofulvin, phenothiazines, sulfonamides, sulfonylurea hypoglycemia agents, tetracyclines, and thiazide diuretics.

Lab Effects/Interference:
- None.

Special Considerations:
- Drug is for use in esophageal and non-small-cell lung carcinoma (NSCLC).
- Photodynamic therapy should NOT be used in patients with:
  - porphyria
  - tumor erosion into a major blood vessel
  - bronchoesophageal fistula
  - tracheoesophageal fistula
  - tumor erosion into the trachea or bronchial tree
- Extreme caution should be exercised when deciding candidacy for therapy, as it can cause an initial inflammation at the site and can cause fistulas as tumors shrink.
- When photodynamic therapy is preceded or followed by local radiation therapy, sufficient time should be allowed between treatments for inflammation to subside (e.g., radiation therapy should not be given to the site until at least 2–4 weeks after photodynamic therapy).
- If extravasation occurs during IV administration, the area should be protected from light for 30 days.

Potential Toxicities/Side Effects and the Nursing Process

I. POTENTIAL FOR INJURY related to ANEMIA, INFLAMMATION AT SITE OF THERAPY

Defining Characteristics: Photodynamic therapy can cause significant tumor bleeding at the site of treatment, sometimes resulting in anemia. Inflammation at the site can cause narrowing and/or obstruction of vital structures and pulmonary and cardiovascular changes (pleural effusion or edema, atrial fibrillation, and angina), particularly since much of this therapy occurs in the mediastinal area.

Nursing Implications: Monitor respiratory, cardiovascular systems during treatment. Instruct patient to contact physician immediately for dyspnea, excessive coughing, abdominal pain, fever, dysphagia, bleeding/hemoptysis, chest pain, etc. Substernal chest pain in esophageal cancer patients can be treated with opioids.

II. POTENTIAL FOR INJURY related to PHOTOSENSITIVITY

Defining Characteristics: May cause photosensitivity reactions for 30 days after administration, both to sunlight and bright indoor light. Skin around the eyes may be particularly sensitive. Sunscreens are not protective, as phototherapy causes sensitivity to visible light. Porfirmer is slowly inactivated by ambient light.

Nursing Implications: Patients should test skin (do not use facial skin) by exposing a small area to sunlight for 10 minutes. If area is free of erythema, blistering, and edema 24 hours later, patient may gradually increase exposure. Patients should wear dark glasses that transmit less than 4% of white light for 30 days after treatment.

Drug: tirapazamine (investigational)

Class: Hypoxic cell cytoxin (benzotriazine bioreductive compound).

Mechanism of Action: When given concurrently with radiotherapy, increases damage to aerobic malignant cells throughout different oxygen levels, probably due to the fact that in hypoxic conditions, tirapazamine is reduced to a free radical form, which produces DNA strand breaks. Drug also shows marked potentiation of cisplatin, probably by preventing repair of cisplatin-induced DNA cross-linkages in hypoxic cells. Additive effect when given with cisplatin, and synergy when given before cisplatin. It is possible that under hypoxic conditions, tirapazamine may act as a topoisomerase II inhibitor.

Metabolism: Is metabolized by reductases to form a transient oxidizing radical, which is scavenged by molecular oxygen. In hypoxic conditions, the oxidizing radical removes a proton from DNA to form DNA radicals (at the C4' position on the ribose ring). The radicals are then oxidized, forming DNA strand breaks, preventing cell division, and causing cell death.

Dosage/Range:

- Maximum tolerated dose is 290 mg/m^2 IV on days 1, 15, and 29, and 220 mg/m^2 on days 8, 10, 12, 22, 24, and 26 concurrent with cisplatin and radiotherapy (Craighead et al, 2000).

Drug Preparation:
- Administer IV over 2 hours followed 1 hour later by cisplatin IV given over 1 hour, followed immediately by radiotherapy. When given without cisplatin, radiotherapy follows 30–120 minutes after tirapazamine infusion.

Drug Interactions:
- Additive cytotoxicity when given concurrently with cisplatin.
- Synergy with increased cell kill when given prior to cisplatin.

Lab Effects/Interference:
- Unknown.

Special Considerations:
- Administer prior to cisplatin chemotherapy.
- Is being studied in treatment of head and neck, advanced cervical and ovarian cancers.

Potential Toxicities/Side Effects and the Nursing Process

I. ALTERATION IN NUTRITION, LESS THAN BODY REQUIREMENTS, related to NAUSEA, VOMITING, DIARRHEA

Defining Characteristics: Nausea and vomiting can be severe, especially when drug is given in combination with cisplatin. Diarrhea can also occur, but is usually mild.

Nursing Implications: Ensure aggressive antiemesis, with serotonin antagonists and dexamethasone recommended to prevent nausea and vomiting. Assess efficacy of regimen, and modify as needed. Explain to patient that this may occur, and teach dietary modifications, including the avoidance of greasy, spicy foods.

II. POTENTIAL FOR INFECTION AND BLEEDING related to NEUTROPENIA AND THROMBOCYTOPENIA

Defining Characteristics: In one study, febrile neutropenia necessitated decreasing the dose and frequency of tirapazamine. Thrombocytopenia was uncommon.

Nursing Implications: Assess baseline CBC and differential prior to therapy, and at least weekly during therapy. Teach patient to report signs and symptoms of infection and bleeding right away. Teach patient to check temperature during treatment, and to report T > 100.5°F. If infection occurs, discuss antibiotic treatment, and teach patient self-care strategies.

III. ALTERATION IN COMFORT related to MUSCLE CRAMPS

Defining Characteristics: Muscle cramps can occur, especially during the first 2 weeks of treatment, generally resolving by the third week of treatment.

Nursing Implications: Teach patient that muscle cramps may occur, and to report them. Teach patient self-care measures to minimize discomfort. Discuss alternative approaches with physician if plan is ineffective. Refer to protocol for other management strategies.

IV. POTENTIAL ALTERATION IN SKIN INTEGRITY related to RASH

Defining Characteristics: Rash that is transient may occur.

Nursing Implications: Teach patient that rash may occur, and to report it. Discuss local management with physician.

Chapter 4
Cytoprotective Agents

Advances in the development of effective, new chemotherapeutic agents have been slow, although a number of excellent agents have recently been approved for use. All traditional chemotherapeutic agents work by interfering with DNA and RNA replication, and protein synthesis, causing cell death or stasis. Unfortunately, the chemotherapy, unless attached to a targeted vehicle, such as a monoclonal antibody, is nonselective, and normal cells are damaged by the chemotherapy. Often, the dose-limiting toxicity is myelosuppression, but organ toxicity specific to the chemotherapy agent may limit the drug's usefulness. Specific organ toxicity that can occur includes neurotoxicity (e.g., cisplatin, oxaliplatin, the taxanes), cardiotoxicity (e.g., anthracyclines, alone or together with trastuzumab), bladder toxicity (e.g., high-dose cyclophosphamide, ifosfamide), and nephrotoxicity (e.g., cisplatin). Thus, both doses and duration of therapy of treatment are often limited by these organ toxicities. This can compromise optimal treatment, as well as compromise quality of life. Similarly, radiation therapy causes cell damage (e.g., ionization causes the formation of free radicals, which, in the presence of oxygen, cause damage to DNA, leading to cell death when the cell tries to replicate). Again, normal tissue in the radiation port also are damaged, such as the bone marrow in the skull, sternum, and heads of long bones, and can lead to side effects such as bone marrow depression, which results in the need for treatment breaks and less-than-optimal radiotherapy.

In an effort to protect normal cells from treatment toxicity and to limit organ toxicities, a number of agents have been developed that offer cyto (cell) or organ protection, and even more are being studied (investigational agents). Agents that are currently approved for use are amifostine (Ethyol), mesna, and dexrazoxane (Zinecard, a chelating agent). Amifostine has shown "broad spectrum" activity in protecting multiple organ systems, such as the kidneys, bone marrow, and nerves. In addition, it protects the parotid glands from radiation damage. Amifostine is indicated for the reduction of cumulative nephrotoxicity from cisplatin in patients with advanced ovarian and NSCLC, as well as for reducing the incidence of moderate-to-severe xerostomia in patients with head and neck cancer whose radiation port covers the parotid glands. Mesna is included in this chapter because it provides bladder protection from the toxic effects of high-dose cyclophosphamide and ifosfamide. Leucovorin is also a classic cytoprotectant in that it "rescues" normal cells from methotrexate toxicity (bone marrow and mucosal cells). This drug appears in Chapter 3. A new addition to this chapter is dexrazoxane (Totect), which has been FDA approved to neutralize potential damage from anthracycline extravasation. In an effort to help establish a practice standard for the use of currently available cytoprotectants in patients not enrolled on clinical trials, the American Society of Clinical Oncology (ASCO) has developed guidelines (ASCO, 1999).

One organ toxicity that is receiving increased attention is neurotoxicity. Many highly effective agents are limited in both dose and duration of treatment by the development of peripheral neuropathy, such as the taxanes (paclitaxel causes axonal degeneration and demyelination), oxaliplatin, and cisplatin (segmental demyelination). This side effect can be one of the most clinically challenging problems for oncology nurses. See Table 4.1 for a list of antitumor agents that cause neurotoxicity.

Table 4.1 Chemotherapy Agents Likely to Cause Neurotoxicity

High Incidence (very common > 80% incidence)	
Cisplatin	Interferon (especially at HD)
Interleukin-2 (if patient develops capillary leak syndrome)	
Moderate Incidence (common, 20–80% incidence)	
Arsenic trioxide	Methotrexate (IT, HD)
Carmustine (intra-arterial)	Oxaliplatin, ormaplatin
Cytosine arabinoside (HD)	Paclitaxel
Docetaxel	Procarbazine
Hexamethylmelamine	Suramin
Ifosfamide	Tretinoin
l-asparaginase	Vincristine, vinblastine, vinorelbine
Uncommon (< 20% incidence)	
Busulfan	Fludarabine
Capecitabine	5-fluorouracil
Cladrabine	Pentostatin
Etoposide	Teniposide

IT = intrathecal; HD = high dose

Data from: Armstrong T, Rust D, and Kohtz JR (1997); Cheson BD, Vena DA, Foss FM, and Sorensen JM (1994); Furlong TG (1993); Weiss RB (2001).

Peripheral neuropathy is defined as the injury, inflammation, or degeneration of any nerve outside the central nervous system. Chemotherapy may cause damage to the sensory and motor axons. Symptoms of sensory damage include tingling, pricking or numbness of the extremities, a sensation of wearing an invisible glove or sock and thus the term *glove and stocking distribution*; burning or freezing pain; sharp, stabbing, or electric shock-like pain; and extreme sensitivity to touch. Patients, in some cases, will be reluctant to admit to these symptoms because they believe that if they do, their chemotherapy drug will be stopped. If the motor neurons are affected, then symptoms include muscle weakness and loss of balance or coordination. If myelinated nerves are injured, then there is a reduction in conduction velocity of the nerve impulse, and on examination, the patient has depressed or absent deep tendon reflexes (Wilkes, 2004). Although in many instances, peripheral neuropathy may be reversible, it may take many months for this to occur. Unfortunately, damage to peripheral nerves can have long-term effects on quality of life and cause much discomfort, injury, and distress. In addition, while the exact percentage of patients with cancer who experience peripheral neuropathy is unknown, the economic impact is considerable. It has been estimated that it costs $5,507 per patient to treat neuropathy (both medical and indirect costs) (Calhoun et al, 1999). Nurses have been pivotal in performing assessments of sensory and motor function, and assessing the impact of peripheral neuropathy on the patient's safety and quality of life, making them strong advocates for patients. Nurses monitor patients' neurological status prior to each treatment and between treatment cycles. A simple six-step neurosensory exam should be performed throughout the course of chemotherapy to identify any potential deficits. The exam should include a history, such as the questionnaire developed by Berghorn and shown in Figure 4.1, as well as a physical exam of gait, motor and sensory systems, and testing of reflexes. Grading of neurotoxicity is based on a neurosensory exam that includes assessment of gait, motor and sensory system, functional ability, and reflexes, and is scored from 0–4 according to the National Cancer Institute (NCI) Common Toxicity Criteria (see Appendix II). In obtaining the history, since it is imperative to involve patients in the assessment of function and ability to perform activities of daily living, an excellent patient neurotoxicity questionnaire has been developed by Berghorn et al (2000) and incorporated in one clinical trial evaluating neuroprotectants (see Figure 4.1). Patients are asked if they have difficulties in performing their normal activities of daily living, such as buttoning a shirt or holding a fork to eat (fine motor movement), mobility in terms of difficulty going up or down stairs, and communicating. Currently, in clinical practice, the offending drug is usually stopped if the patient develops grade 3 or 4 toxicity. Fortunately, clinical studies are being conducted to find effective neuroprotectants that have little or no toxicity. Agents being studied include amifostine, BNP7787, and glutamine. These agents are included in this chapter.

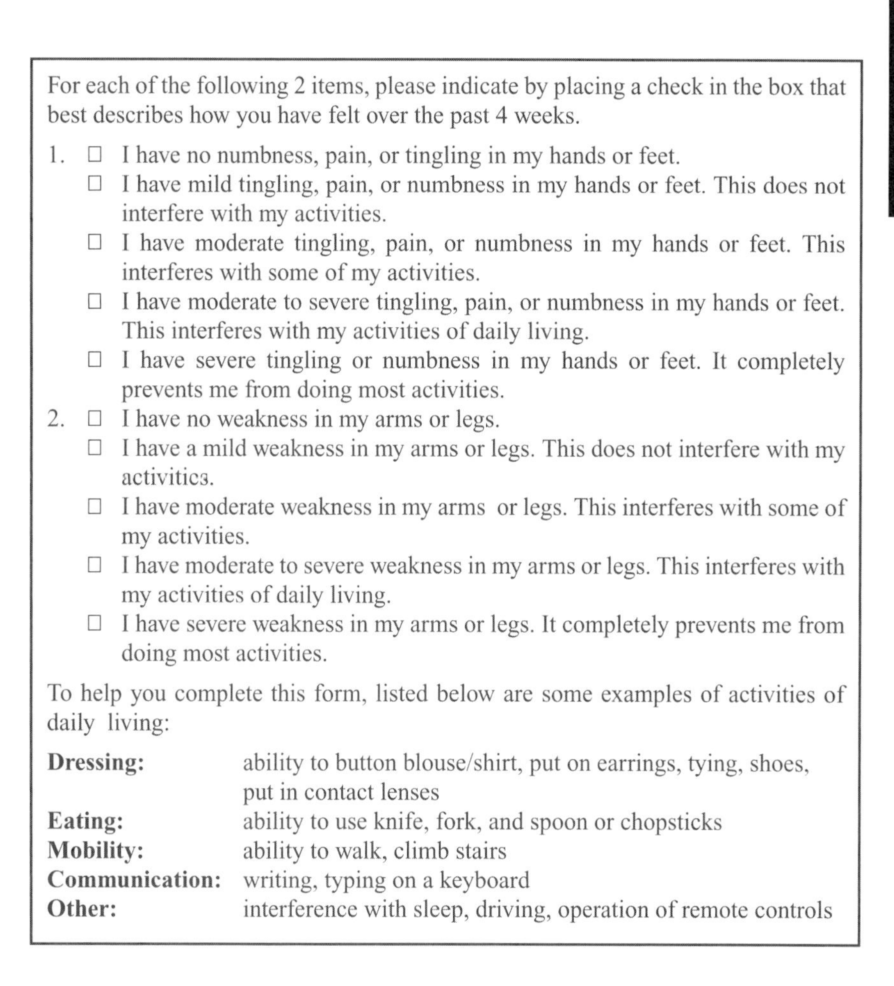

For each of the following 2 items, please indicate by placing a check in the box that best describes how you have felt over the past 4 weeks.

1. ☐ I have no numbness, pain, or tingling in my hands or feet.
   ☐ I have mild tingling, pain, or numbness in my hands or feet. This does not interfere with my activities.
   ☐ I have moderate tingling, pain, or numbness in my hands or feet. This interferes with some of my activities.
   ☐ I have moderate to severe tingling, pain, or numbness in my hands or feet. This interferes with my activities of daily living.
   ☐ I have severe tingling or numbness in my hands or feet. It completely prevents me from doing most activities.
2. ☐ I have no weakness in my arms or legs.
   ☐ I have a mild weakness in my arms or legs. This does not interfere with my activitics.
   ☐ I have moderate weakness in my arms or legs. This interferes with some of my activities.
   ☐ I have moderate to severe weakness in my arms or legs. This interferes with my activities of daily living.
   ☐ I have severe weakness in my arms or legs. It completely prevents me from doing most activities.

To help you complete this form, listed below are some examples of activities of daily living:

Dressing: ability to button blouse/shirt, put on earrings, tying, shoes, put in contact lenses
Eating: ability to use knife, fork, and spoon or chopsticks
Mobility: ability to walk, climb stairs
Communication: writing, typing on a keyboard
Other: interference with sleep, driving, operation of remote controls

Figure 4.1 Patient Neurotoxicity Questionnaire
Source: Berghorn E and Hausheer F (2000) Bionumerik Patient Neurotoxicity Questionnaire. San Antonio, TX, Bionumerik Pharmaceuticals, Inc.

References

Armstrong T, Rust D, Kohtz JR. Neurologic, Pulmonary, and Cutaneous Toxicities of High-Dose Chemotherapy. *Oncology Nursing Forum* 1997; 24(Suppl 1) 23–33

Berghorn E, Hausheer F. Bionumerik Patient Neurotoxicity Questionnaire. San Antonio, TX: Bionumerick Pharmaceuticals, Inc.; 2000

Boyle FM, Wheeler HR, Shenfield GM. Glutamine Ameliorates Experimental Vincristine Neuropathy. *J Pharmacol Exp Ther* 1996; 279(1) 410–415

Boyle FM, Wheeler HR, Shenfield GM. Amelioration of Experimental Cisplatin and Paclitaxel Neuropathy with Glutamate. *J Neuro-Oncol* 1999; 41 107–116

Calhoun EA, Fishman DA, Roland PY, Lurain JR, Bennett CL. Total Cost of Chemotherapy-induced Hematologic and Neurologic Toxicity. *Proc Am Soc Clin Oncol* 1999; 18A 1606

Cassidy J, Bjarnason GA, Hickish T, Randomized Double Blind (DB) Placebo (Plcb) Controlled Phase III Study Assessing the Efficacy of Xaliproden (X) in Reducing the Cumulative Peripheral Sensory Neuropathy (PSN) Induced by the Oxaplatin (Ox) and 5-FU/LV Combination (FOLFOX4) in First-Line Treatment of Patients (pts) with Metastatic Colorectal Cancer (MCRC). *Proceedings from the 42nd annual meeting of the American Society of Clinical Oncology. Atlanta, GA.* June 2006; Abstract #3507

Cheson BD, Vena DA, Foss FM, Sorensen JM. Neurotoxicity of Purine Analogues: A Review. *J Clin Oncology* 1994; 12(10) 2216–2228

Furlong TG. Neurologic Complications of Immunosuppressive Cancer Therapy. *Oncology Nursing Forum* 1993; 20(9) 1337–1352

Hensley ML, Schuchter LM, Lindley C. American Society of Clinical Oncology Clinical Practice Guidelines for the Use of Chemotherapy and Radiotherapy Protectants. *J Clin Oncol* 1999; 17(10) 3333–3355

Liu T, Liu Y, He S, et al. Use of Radiation with or without WR-2721 in Advanced Rectal Cancer. *Cancer* 1992; 69(11) 2820–2825

Mouridsen HT, Langer SW, Buter J, et al. Treatment of Anthracycline Extravasation with Savene (dexrazoxane): Results from Two Prospective Clinical Multicentre Studies. *Annals of Oncology* 2007; 18 546–550

Savarese D, Boucher J, Corey B. Glutamine Treatment of Paclitaxel-induced Myalgias and Arthralgias [letter]. *J Clin Oncol* 1998; 16(12) 3918–3939

Schuchter LM, Luginbuhl WE, Meropol NJ. The Current Status of Toxicity Protectants in Cancer Therapy. *Semin Oncol* 1992; 19(6) 742–751

Schulmeister L. Totect: A New Agent for Treating Anthracycline Extravasation. *Clin J Oncol Nurs* 2007; 11(3) 387–395

Susman E. Xaliproden lessens oxaliplatin-mediated neurotoxicity. *Lancet Oncology* 2006; 7(4) 288

Viele CS, Holmes BC. Amifostine: Drug Profile and Nursing Implications of the First Pancytoprotectant. *Oncol Nurs Forum* 1998; 25(3) 515–523

Weiss RB. Miscellaneous Toxicities. In DeVita VT -Jr Hellman S Rosenberg SA (eds). *Principles and Practice of Oncology*, 5th ed. New York, NY: Lippincott-Raven Publishers; 1997; 2802

Weiss RB. Miscellaneous Toxicities, Adverse Effects of Treatment. In DeVita VT -Jr Hellman S Rosenberg SA (eds). *Principles and Practice of Oncology*, 6th ed. New York, NY: Lippincott-Raven Publishers; 2001: Chapter 55

Wilkes GM. Peripheral Neuropathy. In Yarbro CH Frogge MH Goodman M (eds). *Cancer Symptom Management*, 3rd ed. Sudbury, MA: Jones and Bartlett Publishers; 2004; 362–367

Drug: allopurinol sodium (Aloprim, Zyloprim, Zurinol)

Class: Xanthine oxidase inhibitor.

Mechanism of Action: Drug inhibits xanthine oxidase, the enzyme necessary for conversion of hypoxanthine (natural purine base) to xanthine, and then xanthine to uric acid, without affecting biosynthesis of purines. This lowers serum and urinary uric acid levels.

Metabolism: Well absorbed orally and IV with comparable oxypurinol (major pharmacologic component) serum levels with the relative bioavailability of oxypurinol 100%.

Time to peak serum concentration is 30–120 minutes, with half-life of allopurinol 1–3 hours, and of oxypurinol 18–30 hours. Drug metabolized in liver to active metabolite oxypurinol, and excreted by kidneys and enterohepatic circulation.

Dosage/Range:

- Oral: 600 mg–800 mg/day for 2–3 days with hydration (dose-reduce if creatinine clearance is < 60 mg/mL).
- IV: in management of patients with leukemia, lymphoma, and solid tumors receiving cancer therapy expected to cause elevated serum and urinary uric acid levels and who can not tolerate oral therapy.
- Adults: 200–400 mg/m^2/day, maximum 600 mg/day as a single dose or in divided doses every 6, 8, or 12 hours; optimally begin allopurinol 24–48 hours prior to chemotherapy.
- Dose-reduce for renal dysfunction based on creatinine clearance (10–20 mL/min = 200 mg/day; 3–10 mL/min = 100 mg/day).

Drug Preparation:

- Oral: available in 100-mg and 300-mg tablets.
- IV: available as 30-mL vial containing 500 mg allopurinol lyophilized powder, which is stable at room temperature (25°C, 77°F).
- Reconstitute by adding 25 mL Sterile Water for Injection.
- The ordered dose should be withdrawn, and further diluted in 0.9% NS Injection or 5% Dextrose for Injection to achieve a final concentration of no greater than 6 mg/mL.
- Store at 20–25°C (68–77°F) for up to 10 hours after reconstitution.
- Do not refrigerate reconstituted or diluted product.

Drug Administration:

- Oral: give with food or immediately after meals to decrease gastric irritation.
- IV: administer over appropriate period of time given volume of diluted drug.

Drug Interactions:

- Dicoumarol: PT may be prolonged due to prolonged half-life; monitor PT closely and adjust dose as needed.
- Mercaptopurine/azathioprine: allopurinol decreased drug metabolism so dose of mercaptopurine or azathioprine must be reduced to 1/3 or 1/4 the usual dose, and then subsequent dose adjusted based on clinical response.
- Uricosuric agents: decrease the inhibition of xanthine oxidase by oxypurinol and increase the urinary excretion of uric acid. Avoid concomitant use.
- Ampicillin/amoxicillin: increased frequency of skin rash; use together cautiously.
- Chlorpropamide: allopurinol may prolong half-life of drug, as both drugs compete for excretion in renal tubule; monitor closely for hypoglycemia if drugs used concomitantly in a patient with renal dysfunction.
- Cyclosporin: cyclosporine levels may be increased, so drug levels should be monitored closely, and dose of cyclosporine adjusted accordingly.

- Theophylline: prolonged half-life when used together; monitor theophylline levels closely and adjust dose accordingly.

Physical incompatibilities with IV allopurinol:

- Amikacin sulfate, amphotericin B, carmustine, cefotaxime sodium, chlorpromazine HCl, cimetidine HCl, clindamycin phosphate, cytarabine, dacarbazine, daunorubicin HCl, diphenhydramine HCl, doxorubicin HCl, doxycycline hyclate, droperidol, floxuridine, gentamicin sulfate, haloperidol lactate, hydroxyzine HCl, idarubicin HCl, imipenem-cilastin sodium, mechlorethamine HCl, meperidine HCl, metoclopramide HCl, methylprednisolone sodium succinate, minocycline HCl, nalbuphine HCl, netilmicin sulfate, ondansetron HCl, prochlor perazine edisylate, promethazine HCl, sodium bicarbonate, streptozocin, tobramycin sulfate, vinorelbine tartrate.

Lab Effects/Interference:

- Increased alk phos, AST, ALT, bili.

Special Considerations:

- Dose reduction necessary in renal dysfunction.
- Contraindicated in patients hypersensitive to drug (even mild allergic reaction).
- Discontinue at first sign of a rash.
- Use cautiously with patients on diuretics, as may decrease renal function and increase serum levels of allopurinol.
- Allopurinol hypersensitivity syndrome may occur rarely and is characterized by fever, chills, leukopenia or leukocytosis, eosinophilia, arthralgias, rash, pruritus, nausea, vomiting, renal and hepatic compromise.
- Drug MUST be discontinued immediately if rash develops.
- To prevent tumor lysis syndrome, patient should receive aggressive IV hydration and alkalinization of urine, together with allopurinol.

Potential Toxicities/Side Effects and the Nursing Process

I. POTENTIAL SENSORY/PERCEPTUAL ALTERATIONS related to CNS EFFECTS

Defining Characteristics: Drowsiness, chills, and fever have been reported in > 10% of patients. Headaches, and somnolence occur in 1–10% of patients. Rarely, seizure, myoclonus, twitching, agitation, mental status changes, cerebral infarction, coma, paralysis, and tremor can occur. If fever and chills are associated with rash, eosinophilia, nausea, vomiting, they are most likely related to rare allopurinol hypersensitivity reaction.

Nursing Implications: Assess baseline neurological status, including mental status, and periodically during treatment. If any abnormalities, discuss with physician right away. Teach patient to report chills, fever, drowsiness, or any changes, if they occur. If they do, teach patient self-management strategies, and to report if they are ineffective.

If so, discuss management strategies with physician. If fever and chills are associated with rash, eosinophilia, nausea, vomiting, they are most likely related to rare allopurinol hypersensitivity reaction and should be discussed with the physician immediately, and drug discontinued.

II. ALTERATION IN SKIN INTEGRITY, POTENTIAL, related to RASH, STEVENS-JOHNSON SYNDROME

Defining Characteristics: More than 10% of patients develop maculopapular rash, often associated with urticaria and pruritus; may be exfoliative. Less common but more severe, 1–10% of patients develop Stevens-Johnson syndrome or toxic epidermal necrolysis, which may be fatal. For IV administration, local injection site reactions may occur. Alopecia has been reported in 1–10% of patients.

Nursing Implications: Assess baseline skin integrity and intactness of scalp hair. Teach patient that rash may occur, and to report it right away, as drug must be discontinued. Teach patient self-care strategies, including skin cream to moisturize the skin and to prevent itching. Discuss drug discontinuance and management with physician. Teach patient to report any hair loss. If it occurs, discuss impact on patient, self-care strategies, and if severe, discuss drug discontinuance with physician.

Drug: amifostine for injection (Ethyol, WR-2721)

Class: Cytoprotectant; free-radical scavenger, metabolized to a free thiol.

Mechanism of Action: Drug is phosphorylated by alkaline phosphatase bound in tissue membranes, producing free thiol. Inside the cell, free thiol binds to and detoxifies reactive metabolites of cisplatin and other chemotherapeutic agents, thus neutralizing the chemotherapy drug in normal tissues so that cellular DNA and RNA are not damaged. Normal cells are protected because of differences in cell physiology (higher alkaline phosphatase concentrations and tissue pH, as well as more effective vascularity in normal cells as compared to malignant cells) and transport mechanisms that promote the preferential uptake of free thiol into normal tissues. Free thiol may also scavenge reactive free-radical reactive oxygen molecules resulting from chemotherapy or radiotherapy. Free thiol may also upregulate p53 expression, so that cells accumulate in the G_1-S cell cycle phase, enabling DNA repair.

Metabolism: Drug is rapidly metabolized to an active free-thiol metabolite and cleared from the plasma, so the drug should be administered 30 minutes prior to drug dose.

Dosage/Range:

- Chemoprotectant: 740 mg/m^2 in 50 mL 0.9% NS administered intravenously (IV) over 5 minutes, 30 minutes prior to beginning chemotherapy.

- Radioprotectant: 200 mg/m^2/day IVP over 3 minutes, 15–30 minutes prior to standard fraction radiation therapy (1.8–2.0 Gy).
- Clinical studies: myelodysplastic syndrome: 200 mg/m^2 IV 3d/week × 3 weeks, then 2 weeks off, q 5 weeks; evaluate response after 2 cycles (10 weeks).
- Clinical studies: reversal of neurotoxicity: 500 mg/m^2 IV daily × 5, q 21 days × 3 cycles (evaluate response after 2 cycles).

Drug Preparation:
- Available in 10-mL vials containing 500 mg of drug; store at room temperature.
- Use only 0.9% Sodium Chloride.
- Reconstitute vial with 9.7 mL of sterile 0.9% Sodium Chloride.
- Further dilute with sterile 0.9% Sodium Chloride to total 50 mL.
- Stable at 5 mg/mL to 40 mg/mL for 5 hours at room temperature, and for 24 hours if refrigerated.

Drug Administration:
- Hypertension medicines should be stopped 24 hours prior to drug administration.
- Place patient in supine position.
- Administer combination antiemetics.
- Infuse amifostine IV over 15 minutes, beginning 30 minutes prior to chemotherapy or IVP 15–30 minutes prior to radiotherapy.
- Administer IV antiemetic medication 1 hour prior, and oral antiemetic 2 hours prior to amifostine administration.
- Generally, patients should be hydrated with 1 L 0.9% NS prior to amifostine when used as a chemoprotectant.
- Monitor BP baseline, immediately after amifostine infusion and as needed until BP returns to baseline.
- Resume diuretic(s) and/or antihypertensive medications 30 minutes after amifostine infusion is complete as long as patient is normotensive.

Drug Interactions:
- Antihypertensive and diuretic medications may potentiate hypotension.

Lab Effects/Interference:
- May cause hypocalcemia.

Special Considerations:
- Patients unable to tolerate cessation of antihypertensive medications are not candidates for the drug.
- Drug is indicated to reduce the cumulative renal toxicity from cisplatin in patients with advanced ovarian cancer or non-small-cell lung cancer.
- Studies have shown no decrease in drug efficacy when given with first-line therapy in ovarian cancer.
- No evidence exists that drug interferes with tumor response from chemotherapy in other cancers, but research is ongoing.

- Offers significant protection of kidneys.
- Offers protection of bone marrow and nerves.
- Drug has been shown to protect skin, mucous membranes, and bladder and pelvic structures against late moderate-to-severe radiation reactions.

Potential Toxicities/Side Effects and the Nursing Process

I. ALTERATION IN NUTRITION, LESS THAN BODY REQUIREMENTS, related to NAUSEA AND VOMITING, HYPOCALCEMIA

Defining Characteristics: Incidence is frequent, and nausea and vomiting may be severe. These are preventable by using serotonin antagonist and dexamethasone. Hypocalcemia noted in trials using higher doses.

Nursing Implications: Administer serotonin antagonist (e.g., granisetron, ondansetron, or dolasetron) and dexamethasone 20 mg IV prior to amifostine. Encourage small, frequent meals of cool, bland foods and liquids. Teach patient self-management tips and to avoid greasy or heavy foods. Instruct patient to report nausea and/or vomiting that is not resolved by antiemetics. Teach patient to maintain oral hydration as tolerated. Identify patients at risk for hypocalcemia, i.e., nephrotic syndrome and depletion from many courses of cisplatin. Check baseline calcium and albumin, and monitor during therapy. Assess for signs/symptoms of hypocalcemia. Patients may receive calcium supplements as needed.

II. ALTERATION IN OXYGENATION related to HYPOTENSION, POTENTIAL

Defining Characteristics: Drug causes transient, reversible hypotension in 62% of patients at a dose of 910 mg/m^2. Hypotension is usually manifested by a 5- to 15-minute transient decrease in systolic BP of ≥ 20 mm Hg. Incidence is less when dose is 740 mg/m^2, and infused over 5 minutes.

Nursing Implications: Assess patient's medication profile. Antihypertensives should be stopped 24 hours prior to drug administration. Assess baseline BP, heart rate, and hydration status. Ensure that patient is well hydrated, and per physician, administer 1 L of 0.9% NS IV prior to amifostine if needed to assure euhydration; if dehydrated, patient may require 2 L. Place patient in supine position during administration of drug, and monitor BP q 5 min during administration, immediately after administration, and as needed postinfusion. If the BP falls below threshold (see following table), interrupt infusion and give an IVB of 0.9% NS per physician order. If BP comes back above threshold (returns to threshold within minutes and patient is asymptomatic), then resume infusion and give full dose. If BP does not return to threshold within

5 minutes, infusion should be terminated and IV hydration fluids administered per physician, and patient placed in Trendelenburg position, if symptomatic. If BP does not return to normal in 5 minutes, dose should be reduced in next cycle. Manufacturer recommends the following thresholds for supine BP:

Systolic BP (SBP)	Threshold SBP in mm Hg
< 100	< 80
100–119	75–94
120–139	90–109
140–179	100–139
≥ 180	≥ 130

III. ALTERATION IN COMFORT related to FLUSHING CHILLS, DIZZINESS, SOMNOLENCE, HICCUPS, AND SNEEZING

Defining Characteristics: These effects may occur during or after drug infusion and are mild. Allergic reactions are rare, ranging from skin rash to rigors, but anaphylaxis has not been reported.

Nursing Implications: Assess comfort level, and ask patient to report these symptoms. Discuss comfort measures with patient.

Drug: dexrazoxane for injection (Totect)

Class: Anthracycline extravasation neutralizer

Mechanism of Action: Drug is a derivative of edetic acid (EDTA) and is a metal ion chelator that protects against free radical tissue damage from extravasated anthracycline chemotherapy. It appears that by binding iron it is unavailable for oxygen; most likely it is due to the drug's activity as a free radical scavenger. Theoretically, it may antagonize the chemotherapeutic effect of previously administered drug.

Metabolism: Biphasic elimination with mean initial elimination half-life of 30 minutes and a mean terminal half-life of 2.8 hours; 42% of the dose is excreted in the urine. No plasma protein binding of drug. Dose reduce in patients with renal dysfunction.

Dosage/Range:
- Given IV infusion for 3 consecutive days beginning as soon as possible after anthracycline extravasation but within 6 hours of the extravasation.
- Days 1 and 2: 1000 mg/m^2 IV infusion (max 2000 mg).

- Day 3: 500 mg/m^2 IV infusion (max 1000 mg).
- Dose reduce by 50% in patients with creatinine clearances < 40 mL/min.

Drug Preparation:

- Available as a Totect kit with ten 500-mg vials of dexrazoxane HCl.
- Reconstitute drug with provided diluent (50-mL vials), forming a solution of drug 10 mg/mL. Use immediately.
- Stable 4 hours after reconstitution refrigerated.
- Store unopened vials of drug powder and diluent at room temperature and protected from light and heat.
- USE SAFE CHEMOTHERAPEUTIC AGENT HANDLING PRECAUTIONS!

Drug Administration:

- Give as soon as possible following anthracycline extravasation but within 6 hours of the extravasation. Give at approximately the same time each day (e.g., 24 hours apart).
- Administer IV infusion over 1 to 2 hours in an area or extremity other than that with the extravasation.
- DO NOT use with other extravasation management strategies (e.g., topical dimethyl sulfoxide application), as this may worsen tissue injury.
- Remove topical cooling applications at least 15 minutes before and during drug administration.
- USE CHEMOTHERAPY personal protective equipment when preparing and administering drug.

Drug Interactions:

- None known.

Lab Effects/Interference:

- Neutropenia and thrombocytopenia.
- Increased LFTs.

Special Considerations:

- Drug is indicated for the treatment of adults who have an anthracycline extravasation (e.g., doxorubicin, daunorubicin, epirubicin, idarubicin).
- In two prospective European studies, dexrazoxane proved to be effective and well tolerated and prevented the need for surgical resection in 53 of 54 patients.
- When used as a cardioprotectant, drug may reduce the response from 5-FU, doxorubicin, and cyclophosphamide (FAC) chemotherapy when given concurrently on the first cycle of therapy (48% response rate vs. 63% without the drug, and shorter time to disease progression).
- DRUG REQUIRES SAFE CHEMOTHERAPEUTIC AGENT HANDLING PRECAUTIONS!
- Most common side effects are neutropenia, thrombocytopenia, fever, infusion site reactions, nausea, and vomiting.

Potential Toxicities/Side Effects and the Nursing Process

I. POTENTIAL FOR INJURY related to BONE MARROW DEPRESSION

Defining Characteristics: Drug may cause neutropenia and thrombocytopenia.

Nursing Implications: Monitor WBC, HCT/Hgb, and platelets baseline and monitor after injections. Instruct patient in self-assessment for signs/symptoms of infection and bleeding and how to report them. Teach patient self-care measures to minimize risk.

II. POTENTIAL ALTERATION IN METABOLISM related to HEPATIC AND RENAL ALTERATIONS

Defining Characteristics: Possible elevations in liver function studies are reversible.

Nursing Implications: Assess hepatic and renal function tests (bili, BUN, creatinine, and alk phos), baseline and before each treatment. Notify physician of any abnormalities. Dose should be reduced 50% if 24-hour creatinine clearance is < 40 mL/min.

III. ALTERATION IN COMFORT related to PAIN AT INJECTION SITE, FEVER

Defining Characteristics: Pain at the injection site may occur, as may fever.

Nursing Implications: Assess site during and after infusion. Instruct patient to notify nurse if discomfort arises. Apply local measures to reduce discomfort. Teach patient that fever may occur, to check temperature, and if necessary to take acetaminophen and report if the fever does not resolve.

IV. ALTERATION IN NUTRITION, LESS THAN BODY REQUIREMENTS, related to NAUSEA/VOMITING

Defining Characteristics: Nausea and vomiting may occur. Drug is an antineoplastic agent.

Nursing Implications: Assess baseline nutritional status. Premedicate before initial treatment and then give as needed for days 2 and 3. Encourage small, frequent meals and liquids. Teach patient to avoid greasy, fried, or fatty foods. Encourage patient to report onset of nausea/vomiting.

Drug: dexrazoxane for injection (Zinecard)

Class: Cardioprotector.

Mechanism of Action: Enters easily through cell membranes, but the exact mechanism of cardiac cell protection is unclear. A possible mechanism is that the drug becomes a chelating agent within the cell and interferes with iron-mediated free-radical formation that otherwise would cause cardiotoxicity from anthracyclines. Drug is a derivative of edetic acid (EDTA).

Metabolism: 42% of the dose is excreted in the urine. No plasma protein binding of drug.

Dosage/Range:

- 10:1 ratio of dexrazoxane to doxorubicin (i.e., 500 mg/m^2 of dexrazoxane to 50 mg/m^2 of doxorubicin).

Drug Preparation:

- Available in 250- or 500-mg vials.
- Reconstitute drug with provided diluent.
- Drug may be further diluted in 0.9% Sodium Chloride or 5% Dextrose to a concentration of 1.3–5 mg/mL.
- Stable 6 hours at room temperature or refrigerated.
- USE SAFE CHEMOTHERAPEUTIC AGENT HANDLING PRECAUTIONS!

Drug Administration:

- Give slow IV push or IVB < 30 minutes prior to beginning doxorubicin.

Drug Interactions:

- None known.

Lab Effects/Interference:

- May increase myelosuppression of concomitant doxorubicin, with leukopenia, neutropenia, and thrombocytopenia.

Special Considerations:

- Drug is indicated for reduction of the incidence and severity of cardiomyopathy associated with doxorubicin in women with metastatic breast cancer who have received a cumulative doxorubicin dose of 300 mg/m^2 and who would benefit from continuing doxorubicin.
- Drug may reduce the response from 5-FU, doxorubicin, and cyclophosphamide (FAC) chemotherapy when given concurrently on the first cycle of therapy (48% response rate vs. 63% without the drug, and shorter time to disease progression).
- DRUG REQUIRES SAFE CHEMOTHERAPEUTIC AGENT HANDLING PRECAUTIONS!

Potential Toxicities/Side Effects and the Nursing Process

I. POTENTIAL FOR INJURY related to ENHANCED BONE MARROW DEPRESSION

Defining Characteristics: Drug may increase doxorubicin-induced bone marrow depression.

Nursing Implications: Monitor WBC, HCT/Hgb, and platelets baseline and prior to each dose. Instruct patient in self-assessment for signs/symptoms of infection and bleeding, and how to report them. Teach patient self-care measures to minimize risk.

II. POTENTIAL ALTERATION IN METABOLISM related to HEPATIC AND RENAL ALTERATIONS

Defining Characteristics: Possible elevations in liver and renal function studies may occur. Incidence did not differ from patients who received same chemotherapy (FAC) without the protector.

Nursing Implications: Assess hepatic and renal function tests (bili, BUN, creatinine, and alk phos), baseline and prior to each treatment. Notify physician of any abnormalities.

III. ALTERATION IN COMFORT related to PAIN AT INJECTION SITE

Defining Characteristics: Pain at the injection site may occur.

Nursing Implications: Assess site during and after infusion. Instruct patient to notify nurse if discomfort arises. Apply local measures to reduce discomfort.

Drug: glutamine (investigational)

Class: Nutrient (amino acid).

Mechanism of Action: Glutamine is the most abundant amino acid in blood and human tissues. It is a precursor of neurotransmitters and necessary in nucleic acid and nucleotide synthesis. Deficiency can occur during metabolic stress or catabolic periods. It is unclear how glutamine may protect or reduce neurotoxicity related to taxanes, or how it may reduce the arthralgias and myalgias related to paclitaxel administration.

Metabolism: Unknown.

Dosage/Range:
- Per research protocol.
- Neuroprotectant: glutamine 10 g PO tid beginning 24 hours after HD paclitaxel × 3–4 days prior to autologous BM.

- Prevention of arthralgias and myalgias: paclitaxel dose > 135 mg/m^2: glutamine 10 g tid starting on day 2 × 4 days; paclitaxel plus radiotherapy: glutamine 10 g tid 24 hours after paclitaxel × 3 days.

Drug Preparation:
- Oral, available in packets of 10 g per envelope; mix powder with water or preferred beverage.

Drug Administration:
- Per research protocol; drink immediately after mixing; tid.

Drug Interaction:
- None known.

Lab Effects/Interference:
- None known.

Special Considerations:
- In laboratory animals, glutamine was shown to improve neuropathy associated with vincristine, cisplatin, and paclitaxel.
- Anecdotal reports have shown prevention of arthralgias and myalgias in patients receiving paclitaxel who were their own controls.
- Numerous clinical research studies are ongoing to determine effectiveness, mechanism of action, pharmacokinetics.
- Glutamine available from health food stores.

Potential Toxicities/Side Effects and the Nursing Process

I. LACK OF KNOWLEDGE ABOUT DRUG, SELF-ADMINISTRATION, related to NEW PRODUCT

Defining Characteristics: Unclear how nutrient may work, but there are published reports suggesting its effectiveness. Randomized clinical trials are being undertaken to determine effectiveness, pharmacokinetics, and mechanism of action. There are no known side effects.

Nursing Implications: Assess baseline knowledge of nutrient and its use. Teach patient dosing and self-administration per protocol.

Drug: mesna for injection (Mesnex)

Class: Sulfhydryl.

Mechanism of Action: Used to prevent ifosfamide-induced hemorrhagic cystitis. Drug is rapidly metabolized to the metabolite dimesna. In the kidney, dimesna is reduced to mesna, which binds to the urotoxic ifosfamide and cyclophosphamide metabolites acrolein and 4-hydroxyfosfamide, resulting in their detoxification.

Metabolism: Rapidly metabolized, remains in the intravascular compartment, and is rapidly eliminated by the kidneys. The drug is eliminated in 24 hours as mesna (32%) and dimesna (33%). Majority of the dose is eliminated within 4 hours. Oral mesna has 50% bioavailability of IV dose.

Dosage/Range:

- Initial dose should be given IV; subsequent doses can be given PO or IV.
- Recommended IV-IV-IV: clinical dose 20% of the mesna dose IV bolus 15 minutes before (or at the same time as the ifosfamide), 4 hours and 8 hours after ifosfamide or cyclophosphamide dose. Mesna dose is 20% of ifosfamide or cyclophosphamide dose, with total daily dose 60% of the ifosfamide or cyclophosphamide dose.
- IV-oral-oral: Mesna is given as an IV bolus injection in a dosage equal to 20% of the ifosfamide dosage at the time of ifosfamide administration. Mesna tablets are given orally in a dosage equal to 40% of the ifosfamide dose at 2 and 6 hours after each dose of ifosfamide. The total daily dose of mesna is 100% of the ifosfamide dose.
- Patients who vomit within two hours of taking oral mesna should repeat the dose or receive IV mesna. The efficacy and safety of this ratio of IV-oral-oral mesna has not been established as being effective for daily doses of ifosfamide higher than 2.0 gm/m^2 for 3–5 days.
- For continuous ifosfamide infusions, mesna is mixed with ifosfamide in equal amounts (1:1 mix). Prior to initiating continuous infusion, mesna is given IVB (10% of total ifosfamide dose). Following completion of the infusion, mesna alone should be infused for 12–24 hours to protect against delayed drug excretion activity against the bladder.
- Oral mesna: dose is 40% of ifosfamide or cyclophosphamide dose (not recommended for initial dose if the patient experiences nausea and vomiting).

Drug Preparation:

- Dilute mesna with 5% Dextrose, 5% Dextrose/0.9% Sodium Chloride, or 0.9% Sodium Chloride to create a designated fluid concentration.
- For continuous ifosfamide infusion, mesna should be mixed together with the ifosfamide.

Drug Administration:

- Diluted solution is stable for 24 hours at room temperature.
- Refrigerate and use reconstituted solution within 6 hours.
- Oral preparation can be diluted from 1:1–1:10 in cola, chilled fruit juice, or plain or chocolate milk (if patient vomits within 1 hour, patient should receive repeated IV dose).

Drug Interactions:

- Ifosfamide: mesna binds to drug metabolites; is given concurrently for bladder protection.

Lab Effects/Interference:

- None.

Special Considerations:

- At clinical doses, mild nausea, vomiting, and diarrhea are the only side effects expected.
- Can cause false-positive result on urinalysis for ketones.

Potential Toxicities/Side Effects and the Nursing Process

I. POTENTIAL FOR INJURY related to MAINTENANCE OF BLADDER MUCOSAL INTEGRITY

Defining Characteristics: Mesna uniquely concentrates in the bladder and has a very low degree of toxicity, making it the uroprotector of choice against ifosfamide-related urotoxicity.

Nursing Implications: Assess daily urinalysis. Assess for hematuria per hospital policy and procedure. Hydrate vigorously.

II. ALTERATION IN NUTRITION, LESS THAN BODY REQUIREMENTS, related to NAUSEA/VOMITING, DIARRHEA

Defining Characteristics: Nausea and vomiting are minor in incidence and severity. Diarrhea is mild if it occurs.

Nursing Implications: Assess baseline nutritional status. Usual antiemetics for ifosfamide or cyclophosphamide-induced nausea/vomiting protect against mesna contribution. Encourage small, frequent meals and liquids. Teach patient to avoid greasy, fried, or fatty foods. Encourage patient to report onset of nausea/vomiting or diarrhea.

Drug: xaliproden (Xenon, SR57746A)

Class: Neuroprotectant.

Mechanism of Action: Drug is a non-peptide agent with neurotrophin properties (nerve cell growth factor), as well as a serotonin (5-HT1A) agonist. Mechanism not well understood, but thought to be related to the drug's ability to mimic neurotrophic activity such as NGF and BDNF, or to stimulate endogenous production of these short-lived growth factors. These neurotrophic growth factors are necessary for neural cell survival. Drug also protects neurons.

Metabolism: Unknown.

Dosage/Range:

- Per protocol, but may be 1–2 mg PO daily, beginning the day of oxaliplatin chemotherapy, and continuing 15 days after the last chemotherapy treatment.

Drug Preparation:

- Oral, per protocol. Teach patients to keep medicine out of the reach of children and pets.

Drug Interactions:

- Unknown.

Lab Effects/Interference:

- Unknown.

Special Considerations:

- Being studied in preventing chemotherapy-induced peripheral neuropathy (e.g., oxaliplatin), and also ALS (amyotrophic lateral sclerosis).
- In the Xenon study, xaliproden significantly decreased the neurotoxicity of oxaliplatin by 39% (grade 3 peripheral neuropathy), and fewer patients discontinued oxaliplatin due to neurotoxicity. In addition, the drug did not affect tumor response to oxaliplatin (Cassidy et al, 2006; Sussman, 2006). Side effects that increased as a result of the 5-HT1A agonist properties were diarrhea (62.3% vs 56.1%), dizziness (13.3% vs 8.7%), insomnia (18.5% vs 12.8%), anxiety (6.8% vs 3.4%), tinnitus (3.7% vs 0.6%).

Potential Toxicities/Side Effects and the Nursing Process

I. ALTERATION IN COMFORT related to SEROTONIN-INDUCED SIDE EFFECTS

Defining Characteristics: Drug may cause increased serotonin-related side effects such as diarrhea, dizziness, insomnia, anxiety, tinnitus.

Nursing Implications: Teach patient that these side effects may occur, and to report them if they do not resolve with symptomatic treatment.

Chapter 5
Molecularly Targeted Therapies

The new millennium has brought exciting promise to patients with cancer and to their nurses. As a better understanding of the process of carcinogenesis and metastases has emerged, with it has come identified molecular flaws that can be therapeutically targeted. For the past decades, systemic and local therapies have provided cure, disease stabilization, and palliation for many patients with cancer. However, the physical cost of these benefits was often significant, and included bone marrow depression with increased risk of infection and bleeding, nausea, and vomiting. The "magic bullet" was always sought so that benefit could be achieved with minimal toxicity. Today, a number of molecularly targeted agents have been FDA approved and thousands more are undergoing clinical testing. This chapter lays the groundwork for a sound understanding of the molecular basis of cancer, the identified and potential molecular flaws and targets, and the agents that target them. In addition, the question arises why the immune system is unable to mount a sustained attack against the tumor-expressed antigens. In some way, malignant transformation is able to also suppress the immune response. This chapter begins a discussion about today's understanding as well as agents currently being studied to augment the immune response. This chapter's presentation is simplified, and if the reader wishes more in-depth discussion of the material covered, please consult the references for more advanced readings.

Dr. Andrew von Eschenbach, MD, former NCI Director, described the future of cancer care (2003):

"Today we understand cancer as both a genetic disease and a cell signaling failure. Genes that control orderly replication become damaged, allowing the cells to reproduce without restraint. A single cell's progress from normal, to malignant, to metastatic, appears to involve a series of interactive processes, each controlled by a different gene or set of genes. These altered genes produce defective protein signals, which are, in turn, mishandled by the cell. This understanding of the biology of cancer is enabling us to design interventions to preempt the cancer's progression to uncontrolled growth."

In order to better understand the molecular basis of cancer, it is important to recall early courses in biology and genetics. The following will be reviewed: basic cell biology, genetic mutations, malignant transformation, communication within the cell (signal transduction), mutations in proto-oncogene, suppressor and DNA repair genes, cell cycle regulation, loss of apoptosis, loss of telomerase activity, invasion, angiogenesis, and metastases.

Basic Cell Biology

Cancer is a disease of the cell. The nucleus of the cell is where the genetic material, or deoxyribonucleic acid (DNA), is located. DNA is the building block of life, an incredibly simple yet complex double helix in which each strand is made up of millions of chemical bases, and each chemical base attaches to its complementary partner to pair in a specific way (cytosine with guanine, thymine with adenosine). See Figure 5.1.

Genes are a subunit of DNA, and each gene contains a code or recipe for a specific product, such as a protein or enzyme. Scientists have now identified all the 35,000 or so genes in the human genome. Genes carry the blueprint of who we are. All cells have the genetic blueprint, but only the genes we need are "turned on," such as the color for blue eyes. The genes we don't need at the moment are turned off. In early fetal growth, many genes are turned on, and then when the embryo develops into a baby, these genes are no longer necessary and the genes are "turned off." Genes code for specific proteins and are contained in a chromosome. Humans have 46 chromosomes: 22 autosomal pairs and 1 pair of sex chromosomes. When the body needs to make a specific protein or enzyme, or to make more cells, this requirement message comes to the cell, attaches to a receptor, such as a growth factor receptor, on the outside of the cell membrane. Once complexed at the growth factor receptor site, the receptor asks a neighbor receptor to pair up with it (dimerize), or the receptor can activate itself (autostimulation); this begins the journey of the message, which is now sent through the membrane to tyrosine kinase molecules right inside the cell membrane, which exchange the currency of a phosphate group (phosphorylation) to send the message from one molecule to another (signal transduction), like a bucket brigade. The information ultimately arrives at the cell nucleus, the DNA strands separate exposing the gene that codes for the requested enzyme or protein, and information from the gene is copied onto a special type of RNA or ribonucleic acid, called messenger RNA (m-RNA).

The sequence of chemical bases in the gene is copied base by base onto a new strand of m-RNA so that the complementary recipe is shown on the m-RNA. This piece of m-RNA then travels out of the nucleus into the cytoplasm of the cell to the ribosomes, which are the cell's "protein factory." Here the complementary copy of the protein recipe is recopied onto a ribosome by transfer RNA (t-RNA) so that now it is exactly like the DNA copy. Now the ribosome is being told to make the specific protein. Amino acids are then assembled into a completed protein molecule. See Figure 5.2.

The body is very careful that cell birth always equals cell death so that no cell can divide unless the body needs it. When a cell needs to divide to make another cell (proliferation) to replace another cell, such as a cell lining the gastrointestinal tract, the cell's nucleus receives a message from a growth factor to divide. Recall the process of cell division in terms of the cell cycle, as discussed in Chapter 1. When each cell prepares to divide, the DNA is copied during the Synthesis (S) Phase to make a duplicate set of DNA so that each of the daughter cells will have identical DNA. Millions of coded genes are copied during cell division, or when the necessary protein or enzyme recipes are being copied and manufactured. Occasionally a mistake is made, such

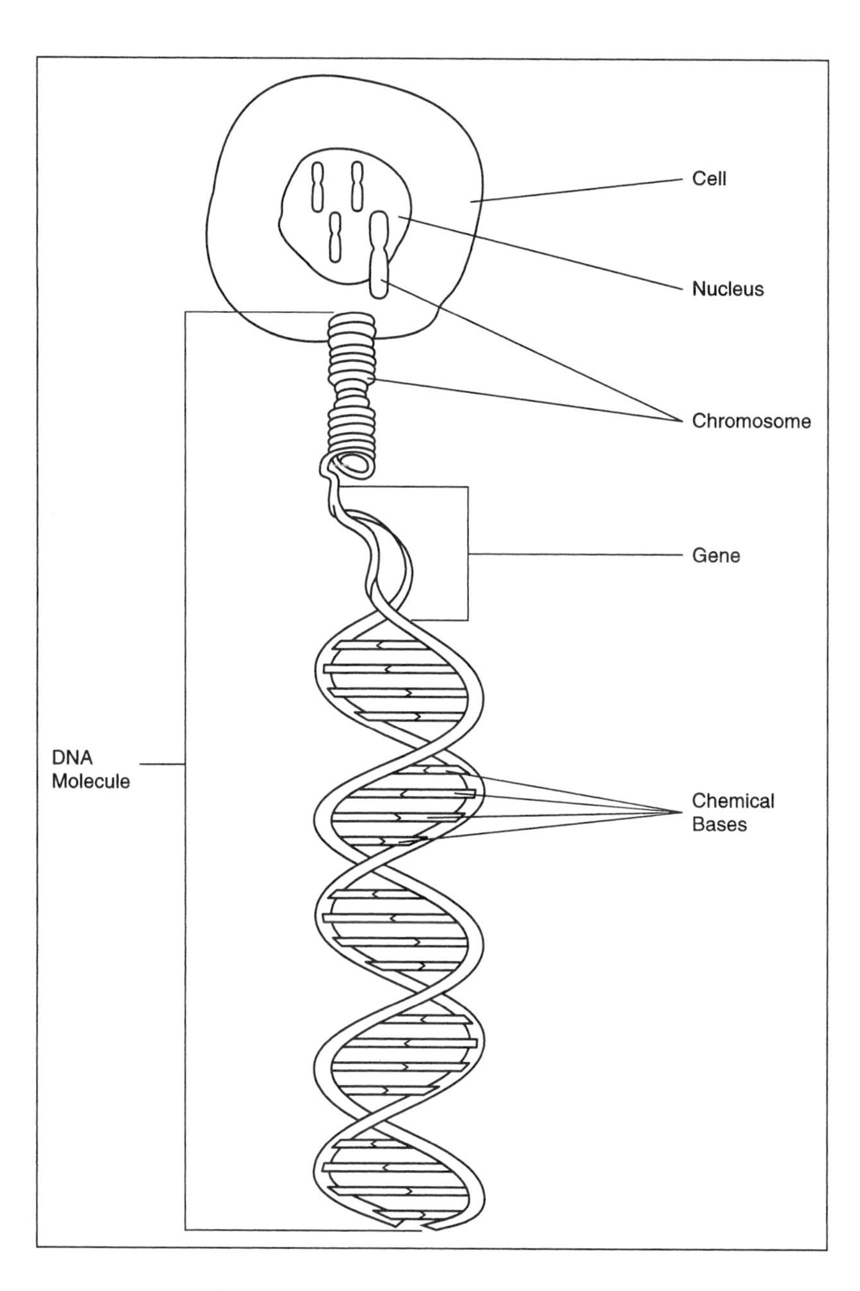

Figure 5.1 DNA: base pairs and double helix (NCI, Understanding Gene Testing, p ii, 1997)

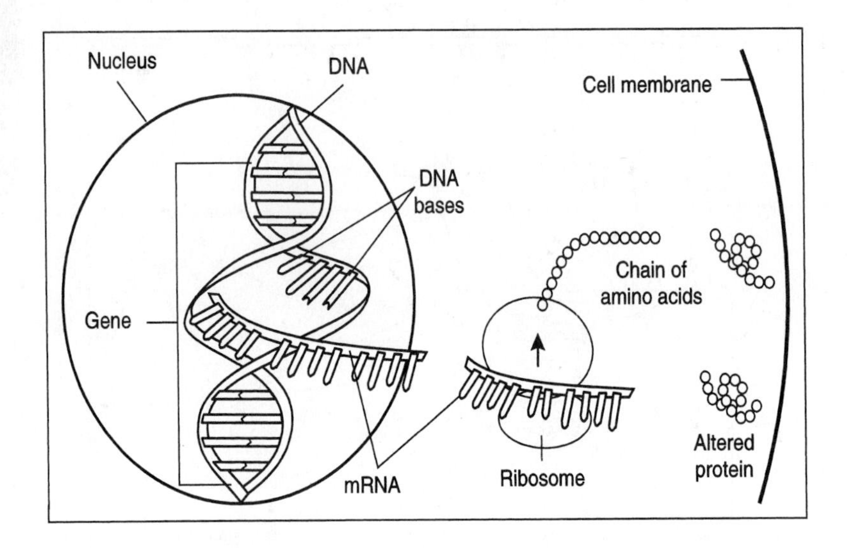

Figure 5.2 Protein synthesis (NCI, Understanding Gene Testing p 2, 1995)

as when one chemical base is not correctly copied. Often this is quickly fixed, but sometimes a mutation can result in the production of an abnormal protein, enzyme, or product. Figure 5.3 shows how a mutation can lead to the production of an abnormal protein. Different types of mutations are shown in Figure 5.4. If the mutation occurs near or on a proto-oncogene or a tumor suppressor gene, then it can potentially turn

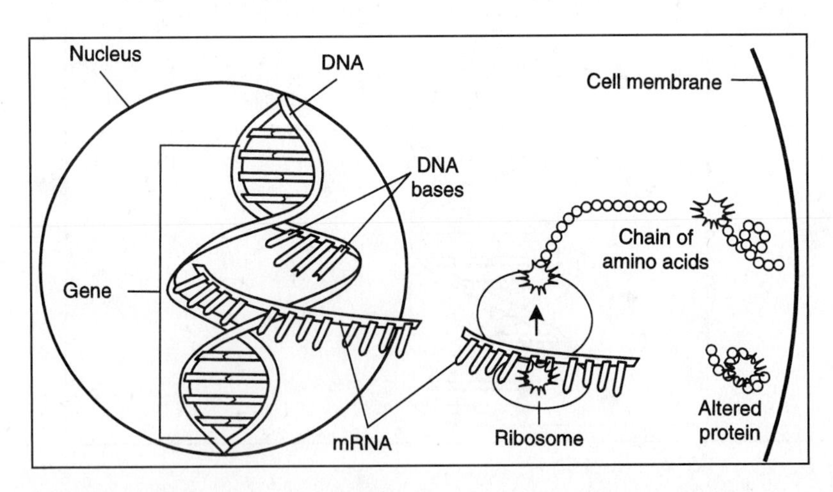

Figure 5.3 Mutation Leading to Abnormal Protein Production (NCI, Understanding Gene Testing p 4, 1995)

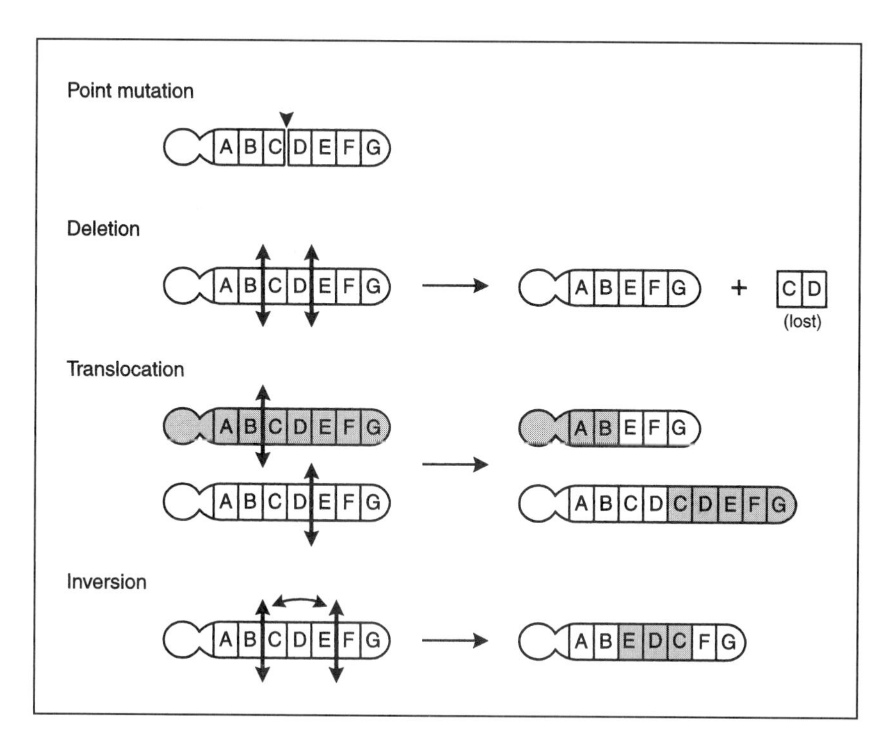

Figure 5.4 Types of Chromosomal Mutations

on cell division when the body does not need more cells (oncogene) or silence tumor suppressor genes so that they do not stop uncontrolled cell division. In other words, the oncogene is like the accelerator of a car, driving cell division, whereas the tumor suppressor genes when silenced are like the brakes of a car that are failing and unable to stop the car.

One example of a serious mutation is the reciprocal translocation between chromosome 9 and 22, forming an extra-long chromosome 9. The other chromosome is short, called the Philadelphia chromosome (Ph^1) which contains the fused ABL-BCR gene, and is shown in Figure 5.5. This genetic abnormality occurs in 90% of patients with Chronic Myelogenous Leukemia (CML), and results in the formation of an abnormal receptor tyrosine kinase, which can turn on continually and tell the cell nucleus to make more (leukemic) cells. Imatinib mesylate (Gleevec), a receptor tyrosine kinase inhibitor that selectively targets this flaw, has been FDA approved due to its extraordinary ability to block this mutation.

It appears that all malignancies are caused by mutations in DNA. However, it usually takes at least four mutations to cause malignant transformation. This is shown in Figure 5.6.

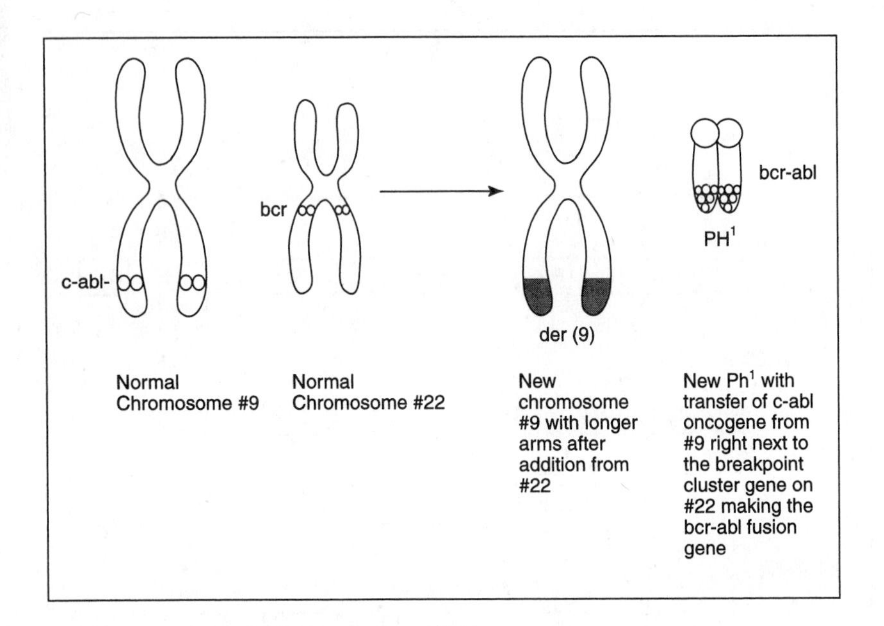

Figure 5.5 Philadelphia Chromosome

Approximately 10% of these mutations are inherited or carried in the DNA of reproductive cells in individuals whose parents carry the gene, while 90% of mutations are acquired and considered sporadic. Usually, an inherited mutation does not result in cancer; rather, it increases the risk the person will develop cancer in the course of their lifetime. Sporadic mutations develop during the course of one's life, due to exposure to carcinogens and are related to relationships among and between genes and the environment. Most cancers are not inherited, although two examples of inherited vulnerability to cancer are:

- Women who carry the BRCA-1 gene represent 5% or so of women who develop breast cancer, and
- Individuals with hereditary polyposis in which one allele of the APC tumor suppressor gene is silenced. This gene is located in the intraepithelial cells of the intestines. When the second allele becomes mutated, the gene no longer functions as a tumor suppressor gene. Thousands of polyps are formed, and many can progress to malignancy. Fortunately, COX-2 inhibitors appear to prevent many polyps from forming. This also suggests that cyclo-oxygenase 2 (COX-2) is an important mediator of not only inflammation, but also of malignant transformation. Scientists are studying the process of inflammation to see how it is such an essential part of malignant transformation. COX-2 is overexpressed in many premalignant and malignant tumors, in addition to colorectal adenomas and cancer, such as pancreatic cancer,

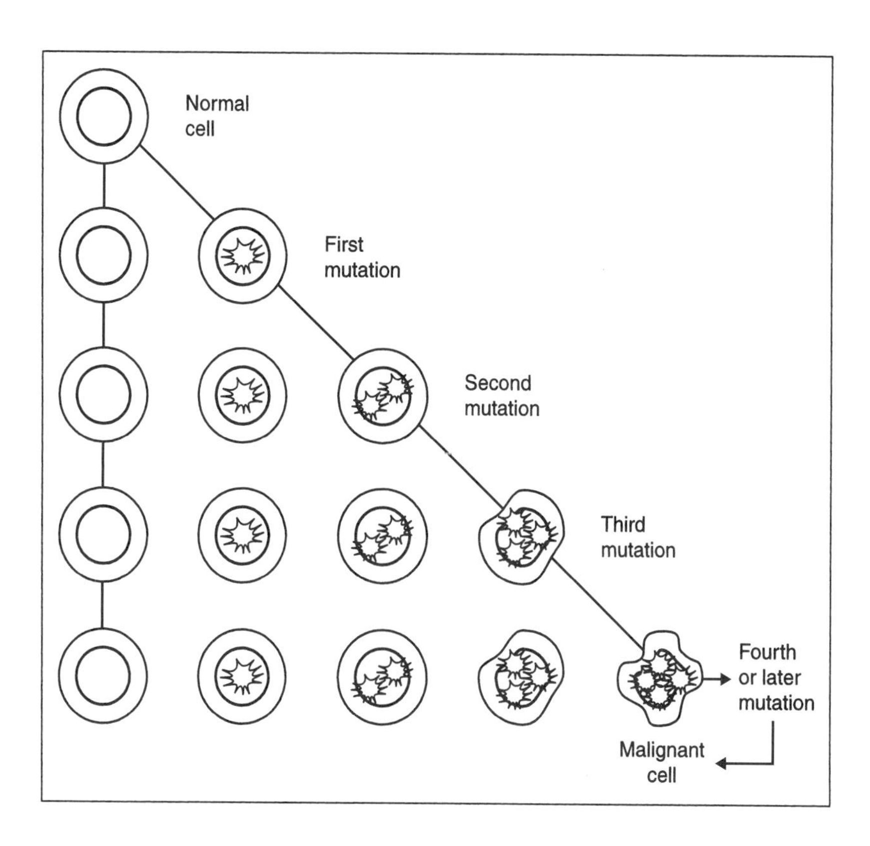

Figure 5.6 Mutations and Malignant Transformation (NCI, Understanding Gene Testing, p 13, 1995)

oral leucoplakia and head and neck cancer, prostate intraepithelial neoplasia and prostate cancer, ductal carcinoma in situ, and breast cancer. Specifically, it appears that COX-2 plays a role in angiogenesis, apoptosis, inflammation, immunosuppression, and invasiveness (Dannenberg et al, 2001).

Thus, people who have a genetic mutation start with one mutation. Most cancers, however, are related to acquired mutations, occurring when the genes become damaged during one's lifetime by factors in the environment or chemicals made in the cells. Genetic errors may be added during cell division when enzymes are copying DNA so that the mutation is copied into permanent DNA. Usually the body's DNA repair mechanism (DNA repair genes) catches the mistake, and if unable to repair it, causes the cell to die (programmed cell death or apoptosis). Sometimes, the system fails; the error becomes permanent and is passed on to successive generations of cells.

According to Lippman (2000) mutations in DNA can result from:

- **Gain of function:** The mutation activates one or more genes that lead to malignant transformation, such as with the *Ras, Myc, Epidermal Growth Factor Receptor* family. This results in the speeding up of cell growth and division, which makes more cells than the body needs.
- **Loss of function:** The mutation(s) inactivate genes that control cell growth, such as the tumor suppressor gene p53. In this case, there are no "mutation police" so that the genetic mutation is not caught, the DNA is not repaired or the cell destroyed if unable to repair the mutation, and the genetic flaw is perpetuated with each further cell division.

Cell Communication (Signal Transduction)

How does a cell know when it needs to divide or make proteins or other cellular products? Signal transduction is the communication link between and among cells. It depends on signals that often originate on the cell surface, such as the growth factors or hormones that attach to cell surface receptors. The growth factor or hormone is called a *ligand*. Once the growth factor attaches to the receptor, the receptor dimerizes with another receptor, and a message is generated. The receptor has three domains: one that sticks outside the cell (external), one that is transmembrane, and one that is internal. The message from a growth factor telling the cell to divide starts when it attaches to the receptor's external domain or "docking station." The message passes through the transmembrane domain into the internal domain, which changes in shape to allow it to interact with the receptor tyrosine kinases or "information-relaying molecules" in the cytoplasm (Scott and Pawson, 2000). Receptor tyrosine kinases pick the message up from the internal end of the receptor and pass it along from one molecule to another until it gets to the cell nucleus. The name *kinase* means enzyme, and this group adds a specific phosphate group to the amino acid tyrosine, called phosphorylation. This transfer of chemical energy activates the tyrosine kinase and it passes the message along from one molecule to another, like a "bucket brigade" or "signal cascade" (Weinberg, 1996). This way, the message is relayed "downstream" to the cell nucleus or down specific signaling pathways to get the desired effect, such as normal cell growth, cell division, differentiation (specialization), or cell death (apoptosis). It is a precise system and has many redundant parallel pathways. As the understanding of the complexity of cell signal transduction has grown, the many potential targets for anticancer therapy have skyrocketed. Figures 5.7 and 5.8 show schemas of cell signals resulting in important cell functions.

Important growth factors that initiate the message for a cell to divide are the epidermal growth factor family (EGF or erb-1, erb-2 or HER-2-neu, erb-3, and erb-4), platelet derived growth factor (PDGF), vascular endothelial growth factor (VEGF), transforming growth factor α (TGF-α), and fibroblast growth factor (FGF). The EGF family of receptors is very important for cell growth, differentiation, and survival.

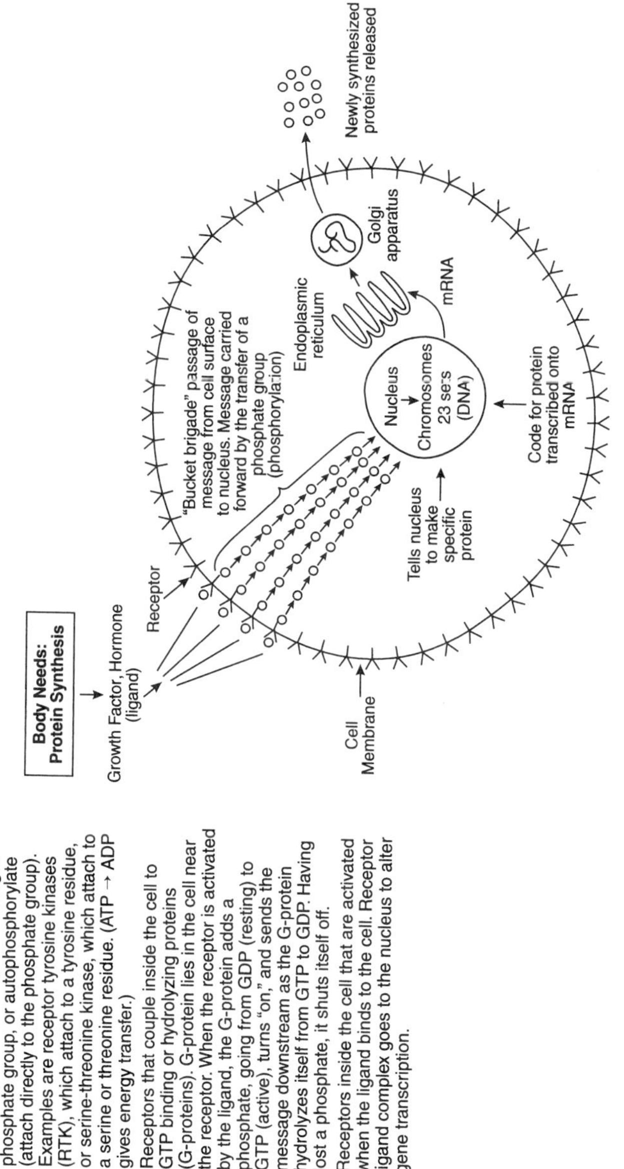

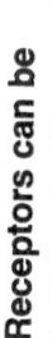

Figure 5.7 Signal Transduction (Figure modified and redrawn from "Cell Communication: The Inside Story," Scott JD and Pawson T. *Scientific American*, June 2000)

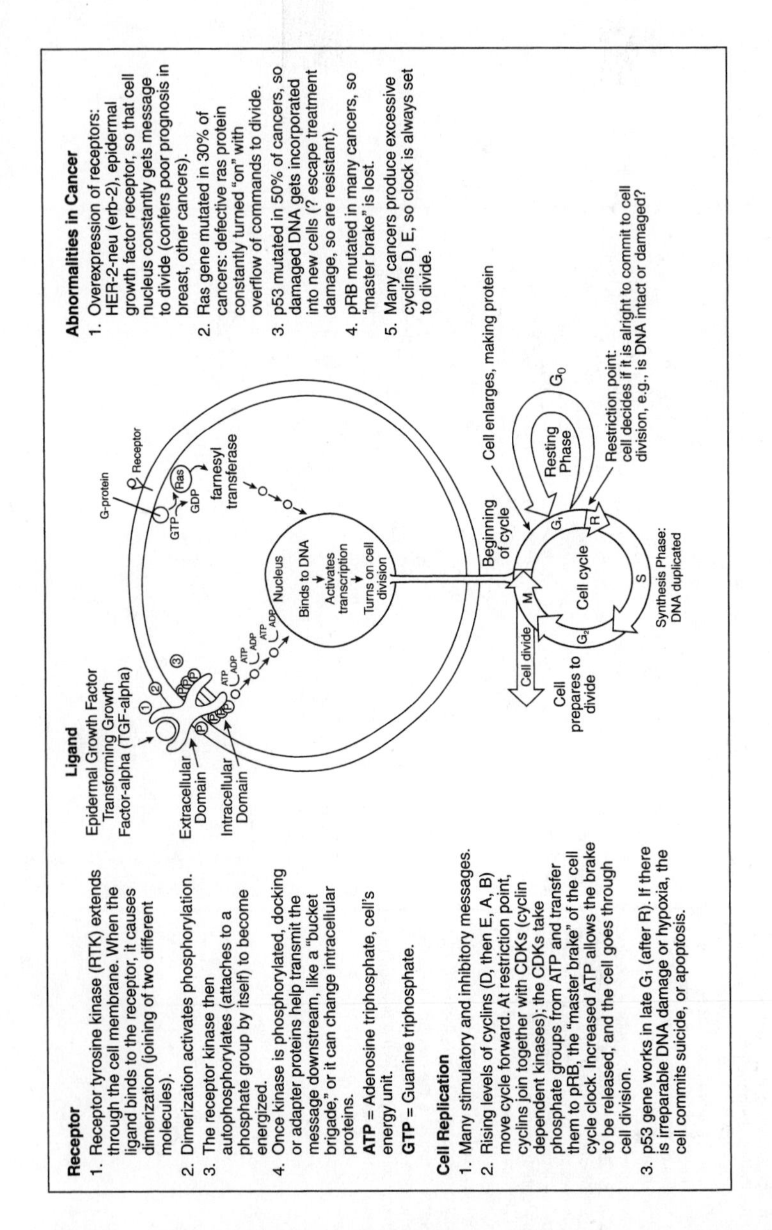

Figure 5.8 Epidermal Growth Factor Receptor and Its Role in Signal Transduction and Tumor Progression (Modified from Huang SM and Harari PM. Epidermal growth factor receptor inhibition in cancer therapy: Biology, rationale and preliminary clinical results. *Invest New Drugs*. 2000 17 259–269.)

Many cancers overexpress this receptor resulting in a more aggressive tumor behavior with increased tendency for invasion and metastases and shorter patient survival. HER-2-neu has become well known because it is overexpressed in about 20% of patients with breast cancer, again conferring a poor prognosis. A number of monoclonal antibodies have been developed to block the external domain of the EGF-1 receptor (cetuximab or Erbitux, panitumumab or Vectibix), and the EGF-2 receptor (trastuzumab or Herceptin); and the internal domain by receptor tyrosine kinase inhibitors such as erlotinib (Tarceva) and gefitinib (Iressa). Today, many tyrosine kinase inhibitors are multitargeted, inhibiting more than one receptor or pathway, such as lapatinib (Tykerb), which blocks both EGFR-1 and 2 receptor kinases. It may be beneficial to combine a monoclonal antibody from outside of the cell, such as trastuzumab, with a small molecule that blocks the tyrosine kinase portion inside the cell, such as lapatinib (Tykerb), which can cross the blood–brain barrier, and trials in HER-2-neu positive women with breast cancer are ongoing.

Class effects of drugs that inhibit EGFR-1 are a sterile, inflammatory skin rash, changes in the skin appendages like hair and nails caused by the high expression of EGFR1 in these tissues, rare risk of pulmonary interstitial lung disease (which depend on EGFR1 to repair pulmonary injury), and diarrhea (caused by blockade of the EGFR in the gut cells). The monoclonal antibodies cetuximab and panitumumab also cause hypomagnesemia and subsequent hypocalcemia related to blockade of the distal renal tubules that depend on EGFR to function and that normally reabsorb magnesium.

Malignant Transformation

How exactly does malignant transformation occur? Hallmarks of cancer include (Hanahan and Weinberg, 2001): (1) self-sufficiency in growth signals, (2) insensitivity to antigrowth signals, (3) evasion of apoptosis, (4) sustained angiogenesis, (5) tissue invasion and metastases, and (6) limitless replication potential.

Normally, cell division occurs only when the tissue needs to replace lost or dead cells and the body has many mechanisms to make sure that cell birth equals cell death. Proto-oncogenes are normal cells that encourage cell growth. They are kept in check by tumor suppressor genes that not only tell the cell nucleus not to divide if cells are not needed, but they also prevent injured or mutated cells from going through cell division and then passing on genetic errors to their progeny. Mutations must occur in both proto-oncogenes and suppressor genes to get malignant transformation, as well as DNA repair genes that normally repair the mutations in DNA, or direct the damaged cell to undergo apoptosis or programmed cell death.

For example, a mutation in a proto-oncogene can start the process. This is because proto-oncogenes often produce the protein molecules in the bucket brigade. As a result, when the proto-oncogene is mutated to form an oncogene, the oncogene keeps sending the message to the nucleus for the cell to divide over and over again, leading to uncontrolled cell division. Other oncogenes can also lead to the overproduction of growth factors. PDGF or TGF-α can repeatedly tell the cell to divide, while HER-2-neu overexpression causes proliferation of cell surface receptors that flood the cell with signals to divide, again leading to uncontrolled cell division.

Proto-oncogenes code for other molecules in the signal cascade, such as the *ras* family of proto-oncogenes that include the H-ras gene, the K-ras-gene, and the N-ras gene (Weinberg, 1996). Normally, the *ras* gene, a proto-oncogene, codes for proteins that bring the message from the cell surface growth factor receptors to other protein messengers further down the signal cascade as part of the bucket brigade, activating downstream effectors such as the Raf-1/mitogen-activating protein kinase (MAPK) pathway, and the Rac/Rho pathway (Rowinsky et al, 1999). Once the message is sent to the nucleus, the ras protein is turned "off" and remains off until recruited again to the cell membrane to bring another message from the extracellular growth factor to inside the cell, and down to the cell nucleus. If the ras proto-oncogene is mutated and then activated, it becomes locked in an "on" position, and keeps sending the message to divide even when there is no growth factor binding to the surface receptor, and no message was actually generated. In order to become activated and to attach to the inner surface of the cell membrane, ras has a molecule added called farnesyl isoprenoid; it depends upon an enzyme called farnesyltransferase (FTase) to catalyze this addition. If the enzyme is inhibited, then the ras protein is blocked, and in many tumors, causes cells to undergo programmed cell death (apoptosis). Tipifarnib (R115777, Zarnestra) is a farnesyltransferase inhibitor (FTI) that is being studied. If farnesylation is not blocked, and the ras protein goes to the cell membrane, then Raf-1 kinase is activated and phosphorylates two MAPK kinases (MEK_1 and MEK_2 that are also known as extracellular signal-regulated kinases 1 and 2). Once activated, phosphorylated, the MAPKs move to the nucleus, where they start a chain reaction leading to cell proliferation (Rowinsky et al, 1999). Sorafenib (Nexavar, BAY 43-9006) is a multi-targeted protein kinase inhibitor that inhibits Raf-kinase, as well as two kinases involved in angiogenesis (VEGF-2, PDGF-β). It is now approved for the treatment of metastatic renal cell and unresectable hepatocellular cancers. It is estimated that 33% of all cancers have a mutated *ras* proto-oncogene (forming the ras oncogene), especially cancers of the colon, pancreas, and lungs (Weinberg, 1996). These oncogenes, or their products, are therapeutic targets being studied in clinical trials to block their function so that, for example, the abnormal *ras* proteins are not produced.

Another key pathway that appears to play an important role in cancer is the STAT (Signal Transducers and Activators of Transcription) pathway. This pathway is made up of proteins in the cytoplasm of the cell that join together (dimerize) when activated by tyrosine phosphorylation (Haura et al, 2005). This causes the activated STAT proteins to move into the cell nucleus, then into the DNA where they bind to gene promoters and regulate the expression of certain genes involved in malignancy. The STAT proteins that are activated by themselves (constitutively) without normal growth regulation, during malignant transformation, regulate pathways such as cell-cycle progression, programmed cell death (apoptosis), angiogenesis, invasion, metastases, and evasion of the immune system by tumor (Haura et al, 2005). Many tumors have dysregulation of Stat 3, Stat 4, and loss of Stat 1 function. Agents are being studied to target the flaws in the STAT signaling pathway.

Via an analogous bucket brigade of inhibitory signals from the cell surface to the nucleus, the normal cell nucleus also receives messages from tumor suppressor genes telling it not to divide unless the body tissues need more cells. This normally prevents the oncogene from causing uncontrolled cell growth, and can be thought of as "putting brakes on" the cell division process. However, tumor suppressor genes also become mutated, effectively silencing them, and this must occur in order for the malignant transformation to happen. The most famous of these tumor suppressor genes is p53; it appears to be mutated in over 50% of human cancers.

Once there are mutations in both the proto-oncogene and tumor suppressor genes, then there is no longer balance between cell growth and division. Instead, there is uncontrolled cell growth. How does this happen? Again, recall the cell cycle as shown in Figures 5.8 and 5.9. Normally, the nucleus activates the cell cycle by putting the cell into cell division mode only when the stimulatory signals are greater than the inhibitory

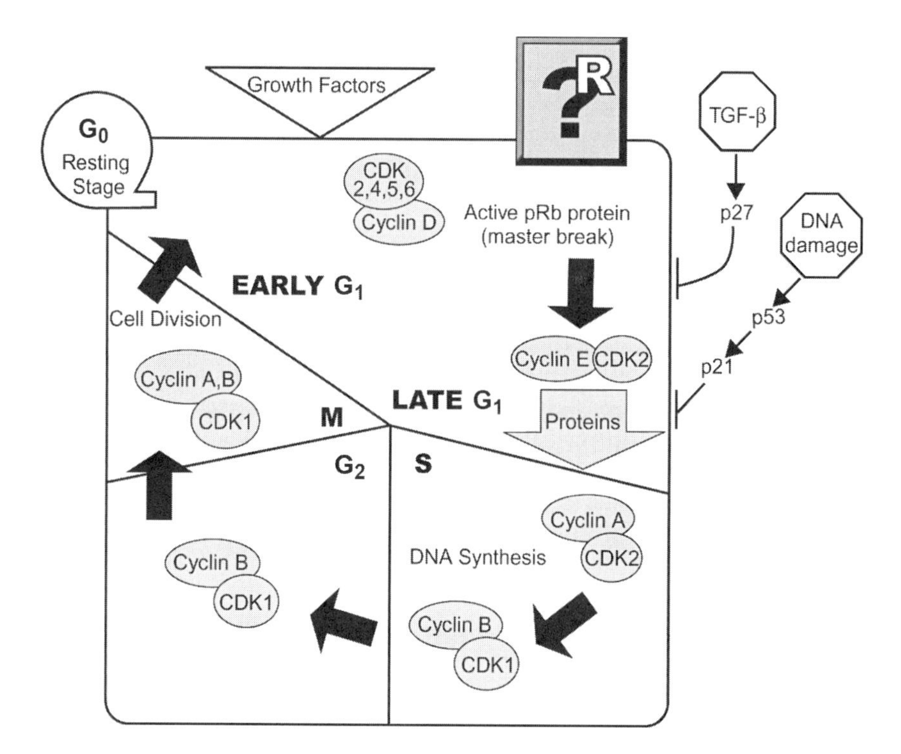

Figure 5.9 The Cell Cycle (Merkle CJ, Loescher LJ. The Biology of Cancer. In Yarbro CH, Frogge MH and Goodman M, (eds). *Cancer Nursing: Principles and Practice*, 6th ed. Sudbury, MA: Jones and Bartlett Inc; 2005;15)

signals. When this happens, levels of cyclins rise (cyclin D, followed by E, A, and B) as the cell moves through the phases of the cell cycle. This causes the cell to start moving through the cell cycle, starting in the G_1 phase. During this phase, the cell produces new proteins that will make DNA in preparation for cell division. The cell enlarges, and the time spent in this phase is highly variable. If division is not needed or if the cellular conditions are not right (the cell is too small or there is not enough nutrition), then the cell goes into a resting phase called G_0. Near the end of G_1, the cell decides whether to commit to cell division, and this is called a *restriction point*. Weinberg (1996) describes this as a time when the molecular switch needs to be moved from the "off" mode to "on mode," as follows: Cyclins D then E combine/activate cyclin-dependent kinases, enzymes which then transfer phosphate groups from adenosine triphosphate (ATP), the energy molecule, to the retinoblastoma protein (pRB) which is the "master brake" of the cell cycle. If no phosphate groups are added to pRB, the brake keeps the cell cycle in the "off" position; however, the brake is lifted when sufficient phosphate groups are added. When the brake is lifted, transcription factors are released which interact with genes (turns them on or off) so that proteins are actively synthesized for progression through the cell cycle. Studies have helped us better understand the role of cyclin D1 in breast cancer. Normally, the BRCA 1 gene is a tumor suppressor gene that acts to protect against cancer by making a protein that binds to the BRCA1 docking site on the estrogen receptor. Cyclin D1 binds to the same estrogen receptor alpha as the BRCA-1 protein, and antagonizes or competes with the BCRA-1 protein. Unfortunately, in 30–40% of breast cancer patients, cyclin D1 is overexpressed. This overexpression takes over the ER-alpha binding, thus negating BRCA-1's repression of estrogen-responsive genes (Pestell et al, 2005). Thus, overexpression of cyclin D1 correlates with resistance to tamoxifen in post-menopausal women with breast cancer (Stendahl et al, 2004), and to a poor prognosis in ER-alpha positive breast cancer. This makes cyclin D1 an excellent therapeutic target.

Mutations can also occur in the genes that make important inhibitory proteins that would otherwise stop the cell cycle from progressing forward, specifically p53, pRB, p16, and p15. This is important because the cell's DNA is examined by DNA repair genes to see whether there are any mutations or mistakes and if so whether they can be repaired. If the DNA cannot be repaired, p53 causes the cell to go into "programmed cell death," or apoptosis. This normally eliminates any abnormal cells from the body so that the cells undergoing cell division all have intact DNA. There are often mutations in the DNA repair genes as well. Unfortunately, in over 50% of cancers p53 is inactive. In some cancers, such as cervical cancer, both p53 and pRB are both inactivated (Weinberg, 1996), and in small cell lung cancer and retinoblastoma, pRB is lost. Other proteins such as the cyclins or cyclin-dependent kinases (CDK), which can be synthesized in greater number, or loss of CDK inhibitors, can move the cell through the cell cycle relentlessly. Most cancers have some abnormalities in the cell cycle machinery, and each of these becomes a molecular flaw that can be targeted.

As discussed, protein kinases are key regulators of a cell's communication system, passing messages along the signaling cascade. They are enzymes that attach phosphate groups to serine/threonine proteins or tyrosine proteins in the cell, which then effectively passes the message like a bucket brigade. According to Adjei and Hidalgo (2005), most of these are *tyrosine protein kinases* and are called small molecules. They can be *receptor* tyrosine kinases, and then they include the extracellular portion of the receptor outside the cell to which the ligand binds to start the message and which leads to the phosphorylation of the intracellular tyrosine kinase portion inside the cell membrane. There are 19 families of receptor tyrosine kinases, including the epidermal growth factor receptor family (EGFR), VEGF, platelet-derived growth factor (PDGF), insulin and insulin-like growth factor (IGF1) receptors, and stem factor receptor (c-KIT). The tyrosine protein kinases that do not have the outside receptor portion or the transmembrane portion are called nonreceptor tyrosine kinases. They work to relay the message in the cytoplasm of the cell to the nucleus (downstream signaling). There are 10 families, such as the Jak, abl, and src. The other type of protein kinase is called the *serine/threonine protein kinase*. One example of a serine/threonine protein kinase is the mammalian target of rapamycin (mTOR), which plays a central role in cell proliferation (turning on the cell cycle) and cell metabolism and in regulating cell growth and angiogenesis. mTOR was named as such because Rapamycin, an immunosuppressant, was able to inhibit this kinase in organ transplant patients.

Many of the genes mutated during malignant transformation are those responsible for control of the mTOR pathway; for example, a loss of PTEN, a tumor suppressor gene, activates mTOR signaling. mTOR signaling is downregulated by rapamycin, which binds to a specific (FK506) binding protein domain in mTOR but not the ATP pocket of the catalytic domain (McMahon et al, 2002). mTOR is a member of the phosphatidylinositide kinase (PIK) subgroup of serine/threonine protein kinases. The other members of this family act as checkpoints in controlling DNA damage repair while mTOR controls nutrient and energy signaling and exists as two distinct complexes. mTOR Complex 1 is sensitive to rapamycin and has three proteins: regulatory associate protein of mTOR (raptor), G-protein β-subunit-like protein (GβL), and praline-rich PKB/Akt substrate 40 kDa (PRAS40); whereas mTOR Complex 2 is not rapamycin sensitive and has four proteins: GβL, rapamycin-insensitive companion of mTOR (rictor), mammalian stress-activated protein kinase (SAPK)–interacting protein-1 (mSin1), and protein observed with rictor (protor) (Dann et al, 2007). While the two pathways are controlled by growth factors (VEGFs, PDGF, EGF, IGF-1) and hormones (such as insulin, estrogen, progesterone), mTOR Complex 1 is also under the control of input about nutrients (glucose, amino acids, oxygen) and available energy (Shaw and Canthley, 2006). Many tumors make ATP using inefficient anaerobic glycolysis rather than aerobic or oxidative phosphorylation in the mitochondria (Warburg effect) (Dennis et al, 2001).

Activation of mTOR Complex 1 is often involved in malignant transformation (e.g., breast, colon, kidney, lung, neuroendocrine, lymphoma, sarcoma, and glioblastoma) and is activated by oncogene stimulated pathways P13K, PKB/Akt, and Ras. A number of tumor suppressor genes are located upstream of mTOR Complex 1 to turn down signaling to mTOR such as PTEN, and some are also located downstream of mTOR Complex 1. mTOR signaling is necessary for estrogen-induced breast cancer cellular proliferation (Boulay et al, 2005). As discussed, one of the characteristics of cancer is uncontrolled cell proliferation. The cell cycle is responsible for cell proliferation, and cyclin-dependent kinases (CDKs) regulate cells moving through the cell cycle. Cyclins regulate the activity of CDKs. mTOR controls cell proliferation by controlling cyclin D1, which in turn controls key CDKs (4 & 6) that are responsible for moving the cell through the G_1-S restriction point. Cyclin D1 is involved in transcribing genes, cell metabolism, and cell migration (Fu et al, 2004). Thus, malignant transformation and mutations in upstream signaling proteins can "turn on" mTOR, resulting in overexpression of Cyclin D1 and cell proliferation in a number of cancers (breast, colon, prostate, and melanoma). Cancer cells damaged by chemotherapy are either able to repair the damaged DNA or are able to tell the cell to ignore the fact that the DNA is damaged, as otherwise the cell with damaged DNA that cannot be repaired undergoes programmed cell death (apoptosis). Activated mTOR controls p21, a gene product that stops the cell cycle so that the damaged DNA can be repaired. Theoretically, by combining a mTOR inhibitor with chemotherapy, the tumor cells will not be able to repair their DNA or fool the cell, as p21 will be inactivated (Shaw et al, 2006).

Additionally, mTOR plays a central role in angiogenesis, as it controls production of hypoxia-inducible factor (HIF) proteins HIF1-ά and HIF1-β. HIF is a critical transcription factor that allows the expression of genes whose products (proteins) are involved in angiogenesis, as well as cell proliferation, motility, adhesion, and survival—all qualities necessary for tumor progression (Semenza, 2003). HIF induces gene expression to produce VEGF (which stimulates endothelial cells to proliferate and migrate toward the tumor in a new tube) and angiopoietin-2 (destabilizes existing blood vessels so they can develop the tube extension in concert with VEGF and then will grow toward the tumor). Angiogenesis is tightly controlled. Hypoxia tips the balance toward angiogenesis to increase the oxygen delivered to tissues and is mediated by hypoxia inducible factor (HIF), which is controlled by the von Hippel-Linday (VHL) protein, a tumor suppressor. During hypoxia, HIF is released so new blood vessels can be stimulated, and when tissue is oxygenated, HIF is rapidly broken down. In the presence of very high levels of HIF, apoptosis occurs (Semenza, 2003). When tumors subvert the upstream signaling pathways, mTOR is activated, and high levels of HIF are produced; if HVL protein is mutated or lost, HIF is not broken down, and high levels persist. This way the tumor can get the proteins and essential nutrients it needs to continue to proliferate and have adequate energy even in hypoxic conditions, such as aerobic glycolysis (Shaw, 2006). Activated mTOR also upregulates VEGF-C, which is associated with lymphangiogenesis (Kobayashi et al, 2007).

Clearly, if mTOR Complex 1 can be blocked, this theoretically will turn off cell proliferation and survival. Analogues (or "rapalogues") of rapamycin (sirolimus) are temsirolimus and everolimus. Temsirolimus (Torisel) is the first FDA-approved mTOR inhibitor and is indicated for the treatment of patients with advanced renal cell cancer, as its study endpoint of increased survival was met. Many of these patients had poor prognostic features. Another drug being studied is everolimus (RAD001), which is being studied in a variety of tumors, as well as in combination with letrozole as preoperative therapy of primary breast cancer in postmenopausal women (Chollet et al, 2006). This is especially interesting because inhibition of mTOR Complex 1 primarily results in a cytostatic response rather than a cytotoxic one. It is expected that these agents may be combined with cytotoxic chemotherapy or other agents. Another interesting potential application is in the treatment of patients with CML, to overcome imatinib resistance due to secondary mutations in BCR/ABL-kinase (mediated by activation of P13K and mTOR) (Burchert et al, 2005).

The genes that produce p53 and pRB are also active in regulating normal cell senescence, leading to programmed cell death. All somatic cells have a finite life of 50–60 doublings, after which the cell dies. At the end of the chromosomes, caps called *telomeres* count each of the cell divisions, and snip off a piece of the chromosome with each division. After 50–60 divisions, the chromosome is too short to divide again. In a developing embryo, where there is rapid cell division, the chromosome is protected from being snipped off with each division by the enzyme telomerase, which replaces each snipped piece. This enzyme is not found in normal cells after the embryo develops into a fetus but is found in all tumor cells. If there is a mutation that inactivates either of these genes, the cells can use telomerase to replace each of the snipped off pieces of chromosome, to become immortal. Again, telomerase becomes a molecular target.

The relationship between cancer and chronic inflammation has been widely publicized. For example, *Helicobacter pylori* and chronic gastritis are causal agents of adenocarcinoma of the stomach, Human papilloma virus has been found to cause cervical cancer, and Hepatitis B virus to cause hepatocellular carcinoma. As more is learned about this relationship, it appears that recurrent or persistent inflammation may induce or promote cancer through DNA damage leading to cell proliferation in an effort to heal the area, as well as creating a stromal "soil" rich in cytokines and growth factors ideal for a malignant cell to flourish (Schottenfeld and Beebe-Dimmer, 2006).

Recently, the FDA approved a vaccine for the prevention of cervical cancer that kills millions of women worldwide each year. In the last 5 years we have seen many new targeted agents. Bortezomib (Velcade) is the first of the proteasome inhibitor class that is FDA approved for cancer therapy, specifically multiple myeloma as it interferes with the interaction of the myeloma cells with the bone marrow micro-environment. Proteasomes are enzyme complexes that are the housekeeping enzymes which degrade or breakdown proteins in the cell nucleus that are no longer needed. The proteins are recycled and used again. They are found in every cell of the body. The proteasomes know which proteins to degrade because they are tagged with ubiquitin, a small protein. The ubiquitin-proteasome pathway regulates protein homeostasis within the cell (Kemple, 2003). Proteasome inhibitors block this process from occurring, so the cell gets conflicting signals about cell regulation. The high volume of the conflicting messages the cell nucleus receives causes malignant cells to go into apoptosis or programmed cell death, while normal cells are less sensitive to this overload and can recover. Specifically, 3 pathways are affected by proteasome inhibition: the cell cycle (proteins active in the cell cycle such as cyclins, cyclin-dependent kinase inhibitors, and the tumor suppressor p53), apoptosis (proteins which inhibit apoptosis like XIAP, cIAP, and Bcl-2 proteins), and Nuclear Factor-kappa B dependent signaling (inhibitor of this pathway is I kappa B-alpha) [Glickman and Ciechanover, 2002]. Nuclear Factor (NF)-kappa B is a transcription factor that has been found to regulate a number of genes that control malignant transformation and metastases. Inactive proteins p50, p65, I kappa B-alpha, and NF-kappa B are found in the cytoplasm of the cell (outside the nucleus). When NF-kappa B is activated by carcinogens, tumor promoter factors, inflammatory cytokines, and some chemotherapy agents, I kappa B-alpha is broken down and the other two proteins move into the nucleus. They attach to DNA in the nucleus at a promoter region and activate the gene. Once NF-kappa B is activated, it can stop apoptosis, which leads to tumor formation and resistance to chemotherapy. There is much excitement about using chemoprevention strategies to block activation of the NF-kappa B by inhibiting its signaling pathway, much as the proteasome does. In addition, it theoretically increases tumor sensitivity to chemotherapy (Bharti and Aggarwal, 2002). One such preventative approach is with non-steroidal anti-inflammatory drugs (NSAIDs) such as aspirin. Aspirin appears to induce signal-specific IK-Bα degradation, followed by NF-kappa B nuclear translocation, leading to apoptosis, in colorectal cancer cells (Din et al, 2004).

A number of agents are being investigated that target Bcl-2 or other proteins that may suppress apoptosis. Since Bcl-2 protein inhibits apoptosis and makes the cells resistant to treatment with standard chemotherapy, drugs such as antisense oligonucleotides theoretically can disable Bcl-2 and restore responsiveness to chemotherapy. Oblimersen sodium is an anti-sense oligonucleotide that binds to Bcl-2 messenger RNA (mRNA), leading to the degradation of Bcl-2 mRNA, which then results in decreased Bcl-2 protein translation or downregulation of Bcl-2. Apoptosis is now possible, and the cancer cells should be more responsive to chemotherapy.

As more is known about the pathophysiology of apoptosis, new drugs will emerge. Two agents being studied are Apo2L/TRAIL (activates two cell-death pathways) and YM155, which causes the cancer cell to undergo apoptosis.

Well, what other factors can turn a gene on or off besides transcription factors, which can mutate? Most mutations as discussed involve changes in DNA which silence (tumor suppressor) or activate (oncogene) genes. However, epigenetics can help explain how the environment can influence gene expression. Epigenetics refers to the fact that there is an extra layer of instructions in the chromosome that influences which genes get turned off or silenced without altering DNA sequence. This silencing of genes without mutational changes in DNA (that occur during cell division or mitosis) is becoming more important, and has been linked to the silencing of tumor suppressor genes in a number of malignancies. This can occur through DNA methylation and histone deacetylation (Claus and Lubbert, 2003). These two exciting areas offer new targets, and we have already seen the success of low-dose azacytidine (Vidaza) in the treatment of myelodysplastic disease (MDS). Let's take a moment to look at this.

DNA methylation: Whether the DNA is methylated or not influences gene transcription. DNA methylation means that a methyl group is added to part of the chemical structure (cytosine ring), and this methyl group sticks out into a major groove of the DNA helix so it inhibits or stops transcription of the gene located on that part of the DNA (Herman and Baylen, 2003). This occurs mostly in what are called CpG rich islands located near promoter regions of genes. At least 50% of the human genes, including housekeeping genes, have these CpG island-containing promoter regions, but they are generally unmethylated (Jones, 2005). Hypermethylation occurs in myelodysplastic syndrome and acute leukemia, and the activity of two hypomethylating agents has led to their FDA approval for treating MDS: 5-azacitidine and decitabine, found in Chapter 1. These agents get into the DNA and trap methyltransferases (enzymes which help put the methyl into the DNA) on the DNA strand so that there can be no further methylation when the cell goes to divide again. However, they do not remove methyl groups from existing genes. As expected, unlike chemotherapy, which kills or stops the growth of cancer cells right away, hypomethylating agents probably require prolonged therapy to get the optimal efficacy.

Histone deacetylation: Another exciting group of agents being explored is the histone deacetylase (HDAC) inhibitor class. The chromosomal DNA is wrapped around histones, a specific type of protein. The histones determine how tightly the chromatin or DNA is wrapped: If it is tightly wrapped, the gene is turned off or silenced; if it is loosely wrapped, the gene is turned on. Normally, HDACs complex with cell regulatory proteins to regulate gene transcription (copying the recipe for that gene's protein onto mRNA to be taken outside of the nucleus to the protein synthesis factory of ribosome) and are key components of cell proliferation, angiogenesis, apoptosis, and cell differentiation. Histone deacetylators remove the acetyl groups from proteins such as histones and transcription factors, causing the tightly wrapped chromatin and shutting off the genes. Some cancer cells have overexpression of HDACs, or they recruit extra HDACs to oncogene transcription factors, causing hypoacetylation, tightening of the chromatin structure, and gene silencing. HDAC inhibitors cause hyperacetylation, which decreases expression of oncogenes such as Bcr-Abl and HER-2, stops the cell cycle, induces apoptosis, and stops angiogenesis and cell motility (George et al, 2005). HDAC inhibitors are intended to help malignant cells become normal again, since they target and accumulate in malignant cells. One example is vorinostat (Zolinza), recently FDA approved for the treatment of progressive or recurrent symptoms of cutaneous T-cell lymphoma (CTCL). Other examples include (1) suberoylanilide hydroxamic acid (SAHA), which has demonstrated activity in cutaneous T-cell lymphoma, diffuse large B-cell lymphoma, and mesothelioma. SAHA is synergistic with radiation, tyrosine kinase inhibitors, and cytotoxic agents (NCI, 2004), and (2) LBH589, a drug being studied in chronic myelogenous leukemia, may be able to overcome resistance to tyrosine kinase inhibitors (George et al, 2005).

Invasion and Metastases

Once mutation of an epithelial cell occurs, further development and transformation into malignancy occurs in stages. For example, the first mutation causes hyperplasia or increased proliferation of normal-appearing cells, and the second leads to dysplasia. The cells now appear abnormal. A third mutation may cause a change to carcinoma in situ, in which the cells remain within normal tissue boundaries. If allowed to continue, the cells may again mutate and develop invasiveness, allowing them to invade underlying tissue and enter blood and lymphatic vessels. As cells are shed, they travel via the blood or lymph system to distant sites. This is called *metastases*. It initially seemed that metastases begins after the development of a detectable tumor, but it is now clear that, in some tumors, metastases can begin even before the primary tumor is detectable. In general, a tumor can not grow beyond a size of 2 mm (the head of a pin) unless it forms new blood vessels (angiogenesis) as the diffusion distance of oxygen, a critical cell nutrient, is only 1–2 mm.

However, not all cancers are invasive or metastasize. The explosion of scientific discovery about cell function and the molecular processes of metastases have led to clinical trials of numerous molecularly targeted therapies, including agents that interrupt different steps in the metastases process. Fortunately, it appears that the metastatic process is highly inefficient, especially in late disease, and, in addition, each of the steps is "rate limiting," so that if one step is not achieved, the process cannot move forward (Stetler-Stevenson and Kleiner, 2001).

Stetler-Stevenson and Kleiner (2001) identify eight steps in the "metastatic cascade," each controlled by a number of gene products in the malignant cell. Some aggressively permit invasion and others subvert the normal body's defenses against metastases. These steps include the detachment of cells from the primary tumor, invasion of the underlying basement membrane and extracellular tissue, movement of cells into blood vessels, and survival in the venous or lymphatic circulation until reaching a capillary bed. There the malignant cell must attach to the basement membrane of the blood vessel, enter the tissue of the organ fed by the capillary bed, respond to local growth factors, begin cell division to form a small tumor, and begin the formation of local blood vessels to support growth beyond 2 mm.

As seen, a cell undergoes multiple mutations during malignant transformation. A single cell (clone) that goes through multiple mutations usually results in cells that are not all alike (heterogenous). Some of the cells are more likely to metastasize than others. Activation of the *ras* oncogene turns a malignant cell into one that invades and metastasizes, and there appears to be a survival advantage for more aggressive cells that respond to local growth factors. The new, tiny tumor gets nourishment by simple diffusion. However, once the tumor reaches 2 mm, it can grow no larger until it gets its own blood supply to increase the delivery of nutrients and remove waste products. The microenvironment helps give the necessary growth factors and nourishment.

As the tumor grows, the cells on the outside get nourishment (e.g., oxygen), but the cells in the inside (core) become hypoxic. This causes the activation of an "angiogenic switch," involving secretion of angiogenic growth factors (e.g., Vascular Endothelial

Growth Factor, VEGF) and suppressing normal inhibitors of angiogenesis (e.g., angiostatin). The blood vessels that form are leaky but have an invasiveness not seen in normal new blood vessels. If the tumor grows near an existing vessel, it may invade and use existing vessels before making its own. Unfortunately, studies have shown that turning on the angiogenic switch is associated with increased frequency of metastases, disease recurrence, and shorter patient survival (Weidner, 1998).

Cells continue to mutate in the primary tumor, and a clone of cells emerges that is superior in growth and is highly invasive. This clone of cells turns down (down regulates) the activity of substances that keep normal cells sticking to their neighboring cells (cell-cell adhesion molecules called *cadherins*, and in epithelial cells, *E-cadherin*) and to the extracellular matrix (integrins). Thus, the tumor cells become mobile and can separate from the rest of the primary tumor. Stromolysin-1 is a matrix metalloproteinase (MMP) that can degrade E-cadherin, and is associated with tumor progression.

More and more, the microenvironment has taken center stage in our understanding of invasion and metastases. The microenvironment is composed of the extracellular matrix, growth factors, fibroblasts, and immune and endothelial cells, and begins a critical interaction with premalignant cells. This interaction is necessary in malignant transformation, as well as invasion and metastases.

The tumor cell then uses enzymes (e.g., MMPs) to destroy the integrity of the basement membrane that the tumor lies on, as well as the extracellular matrix. Imagine it like a tank destroying the area ahead so that the invading army can move forward. Now the malignant cells can invade neighboring normal tissue and the newly made leaky blood vessels or nearby thin-walled lymph vessels. Normal epithelial cells must remain attached to the extracellular matrix or they die. It is unclear how malignant cells can overcome this. It is believed that the microenvironment or stroma surrounding the tumor sends signals telling the tumor cells on the outer edges of the epithelial mass to undergo a change from epithelial cells to mesenchymal cells, called the epithelial mesenchymal transition (EMT). Mesenchymal cells are less tightly woven together so that they can separate easily; in the embryo, they also have the ability to migrate. TGF-β helps transmit these stromal signals, as do TNF-α, EGF, HGF or scatter factor, and IGF-1. In addition, if the ras oncogene is mutated, this also helps activate EMT. Once activated, these cells make their own TGF-β, which helps to keep the mesenchymal phenotype.

Integrins are critical molecules in the extracellular matrix and also have a role in cell signal transduction and cell growth. Changes in integrin-mediated signaling allow the malignant cell to become invasive and to migrate. Integrin attached to the extracellular matrix gives the malignant cell adhesive traction. As the actin filaments in the cell's cytoskeleton contract, the cell body is propelled forward. Proportionate to the age and size of the primary tumor, huge numbers and clumps of malignant cells can be shed into the bloodstream. The clinical effect depends on whether the embolized cells reach a favorable environment and can achieve the steps in metastases. The role of the micro-environment of this metastatic site is critical in the establishment of a metastatic site.

Individual cells or clumps of cells are carried in the blood or lymph circulation, and many do not survive. The cells need to survive the turbulence of blood flow as well as the circulating cell-mediated and humoral immune cell elements (e.g., cytotoxic and killer lymphocytes). Most die.

Cells that survive the ride to distant organs or lymph nodes either get stuck in the microcirculation or attach to specific endothelial cells in capillaries or lymph vessels. In addition, they may attach to an exposed basement membrane of the organ or lymph node.

The cells "extravasate" from the blood or lymph vessel into the extracellular tissue and either grow in response to growth factors or stay dormant in this secondary site. Malignant cells migrate to find a "favorable" site. Many die. In order to respond to the growth signals from this microenvironment or stroma, the tumor cells must revert back to epithelial cells, and thus, they undergo a mesenchyme-to-epithelial transition, or MET (Weinberg, 2007).

If successful in finding a hospitable local environment, after some growth to 2 mm, the tumor cells release angiogenic growth factors to build blood vessels in this secondary site. This increases the ability of the metastatic cells to metastasize again.

How the metastatic cells evade the body's host immune responses is not well known.

Angiogenesis

Many similarities exist between angiogenesis and tumor invasion and, as a result, they may have similar molecular targets. The body normally needs the ability to make new blood vessels for processes such as wound healing, female menstruation, rebuilding the endometrial lining, or making the placenta during pregnancy. The body maintains a fine balance between turning angiogenesis on and turning it off. When there are more factors favoring angiogenesis than opposing it (inhibitors), angiogenesis occurs. Angiogenic growth factors are shown in Table 5.1. When cells are hypoxic or lacking oxygen, they release vascular endothelial growth factor (VEGF), also known as vascular permeability factor. VEGF initiates new blood vessel growth and causes the release of nitric oxide (NO) from the endothelial cells lining the blood vessel, which causes them to dilate. Malignant blood vessels are flawed: they are leaky, they are disorganized and may have blind channels that do not connect with other vessels, and they have many different diameters so that parts of the tumor fed by narrow vessels with low blood flow remain hypoxic and resistant to chemotherapy as chemotherapy does not reach that area.

VEGF and its receptor on the endothelial cell are essential for angiogenesis. VEGF is a family of glycoproteins: VEGF-A is essential for blood vessel formation, and it is commonly referred to as VEGF (Takahashi and Shibuy, 2005). VEGF-B may be a redundant ligand; VEGF-C and VEGF-D appear to be involved with lymphangiogenesis. The VEGF ligands bind to VEGFR (receptors) 1, 2, and 3 (Flt-4), which then stimulate a signal cascade, resulting in endothelial cell (vascular or lymphangenic) proliferation, migration, and survival. VEGFR2 is most commonly associated with VEGF-A, but

Table 5.1 Natural Factors That Stimulate or Inhibit Angiogenesis

Factors Stimulating Angiogenesis	Factors Inhibiting Angiogenesis
• Angiopoietin-1	• Cartilage derived inhibitor (CDI)
• Fibroblast growth factor	• Herparinases
• Interleukin-8	• Human chorionic gonadotropin (hCG)
• Tumor Necrosis Factor (TNF) alpha	• Interferon (alpha, beta, gamma)
• Transforming Growth Factor (TGF) alpha and beta	• Interleukin-12
• Plasminogen activator inhibitor retinoids	• Plasminogen activator inhibitor retinoids
• Platelet derived growth factor (PDGF) BB	• Tissue inhibitors of metalloproteinases called TIMPs
• Granulocyte-Colony Stimulating Factor (G-CSF)	• Thrombospondin-1
• VEGF, also known as vascular permeability factor (VPF)	• Vasculostatin
	• Platelet factor-4

VEGFR-1 also may be linked to VEGF-A. In developing agents to target VEGF or VEGFR, some agents are selective for VEGF, like the monoclonal antibody bevacizumab (Avastin), whereas others are oral, small molecule tyrosine kinase inhibitors that target VEGF receptors, such as axinitinib (VEGFR-1, 2, 3) and cediranib (pan-VEGFR). Other agents are multitargeted for VEGFR as well as other related or unrelated targets such as the more well known sorafenib (Nexavar), that inhibits VEGFR-2, PDGFR-β, and Raf-kinase, and sunitinib (Sutent), which inhibits (VEGFR-1, 2, 3), stem cell factor receptor (KIT), fms-like tyrosine kinase-3 (FLT-3), colony stimulating factor receptor type 1 (CSF-1R), and the glial cell-line-derived neurotrophic factor receptor (RET). It is becoming clear that angiogenesis occurs earlier in the malignant process, as it is necessary in the microenvironment to help the transformed cells invade and metastasize.

The most important VEGFR appears to be VEGFR-2. When the ligand VEGF attaches to the VEGF receptor on the endothelial cell, the receptor dimerizes (come together as partners with another cell surface receptor, which activates the message sending), and the message for proliferation and migration of endothelial cells is sent via a tyrosine kinase system. Neuropilin, a nontyrosine kinase receptor, is hypothesized to be a survival factor for tumors (Parikh et al, 2004). Bevacizumab (Avastin) prevents VEGF (the ligand) from binding to VEGFR-2. Two multitargeted tyrosine kinase inhibitors that block the message in the endothelial cell (initiated by the VEGF-receptor 2) are sunitinib (Sutent) and sorafinib (Nexavar). Integrins, specifically $\alpha 5\beta 1$ integrin, are proteins on the proliferating endothelial cell. The sprouting endothelial tube has to migrate or move toward the tumor, and it does this by having the integrin on the endothelial cell attach to fibronectin in the extracellular matrix. The integrins then act like grappling hooks to move the new blood vessel tube to the tumor. New agents are being developed to block integrin binding so that the new blood vessel sprout cannot move toward the tumor; the proliferating endothelial cell cannot bind to fibronectin, and thus, it undergoes apoptosis (programmed cell death). One agent currently being studied in Phase II clinical trials is volociximab (M200) (Bhaskar et al, 2008).

Of interest, clinical trials with bevacizumab (Avastin) showed not only the cessation of tumor angiogenesis and growth, but also tumor regression suggesting that when combined with chemotherapy, anti-angiogenesis agents alter the tumor blood flow so that the chemotherapy is more effective in killing tumor cells. Thus, the mechanism of bevacizumab is thought to be two-fold: (1) blocking development of new blood vessels and (2) blocking VEGF, which is necessary for the maintenance of existing malignant blood vessels, so existing blood vessels actually normalize; this then increases blood flow within the tumor so that concomitantly administered chemotherapy can now enter the tumor more uniformly. In addition, it is now believed that there are VEGF-receptors on tumor cells which are involved in tumor cell migration and invasion; thus, anti-angiogenesis agents appear to directly affect tumor cells (Fan et al, 2005). Mancuso et al (2006) have shown in the laboratory that antiangiogenesis agents reduce the tumor blood vessels by 50–60%, but the empty sleeves of the blood vessels in the basement membrane remain, along with nonmalignant appearing pericytes (provide strength to the new blood vessel, but can also differentiate into a fibroblast, smooth muscle cell, or macrophage if needed). One day after the antiangiogenesis drug was stopped, new blood vessels sprouted in the empty sleeves in the basement membrane, connected to nearby capillaries, and by 7 days after the drug was stopped, tumors were fully revascularized and protected with tumor-related pericytes. However, when the tumor was again retreated with an antiangiogenesis drug, the regrown vasculature regressed as much as it did the first time. This suggests that the empty sleeves of the basement membrane, as well as the pericytes, should be targeted by anticancer therapies and also suggests that perhaps antiangiogenic drugs should be continued after tumor progression with just a change in the chemotherapy. New agents with ability to target multiple receptors are being developed.

Platelet-derived growth factor is necessary for the pericytes, which give the newly formed blood vessel stability, much like the shingles of a house give a house protection. Sorafenib (Nexavar, BAY 43-9006), a multiple targeted protein tyrosine kinase inhibitor, appears to block the Raf kinase step in the ras pathway, VEGFR-2 and PDGF-β.

Drugs such as bevacizumab (Avastin) neutralize Vascular Endothelial Growth Factor (VEGF), which is released by tumors to start the process of angiogenesis. This drug, in combination with chemotherapy, has produced statistically significant increased response rates, increased time to progression, and overall survival in patients with metastatic colon, rectal, breast, and lung cancers. It is also being studied in patients with curable stage II/III colon cancer in the adjuvant setting, and it is hoped that it may prevent metastases and increase the cure rate.

Some substances in the extracellular matrix components undergo proteolysis and release angiogenesis inhibitors such as endostatin and others (Stetler-Stevenson and Kleiner, 2001). On their Web site, http://www.angio.org/understanding/understanding.html, the Angiogenesis Foundation describes the process of angiogenesis (see also Figure 5.10) as follows:

- Angiogenic growth factors are released, normally by injured tissue, and in the case of malignancy, by tumor cells that require blood vessels to grow beyond their current size. The growth factors diffuse into the neighboring tissue.

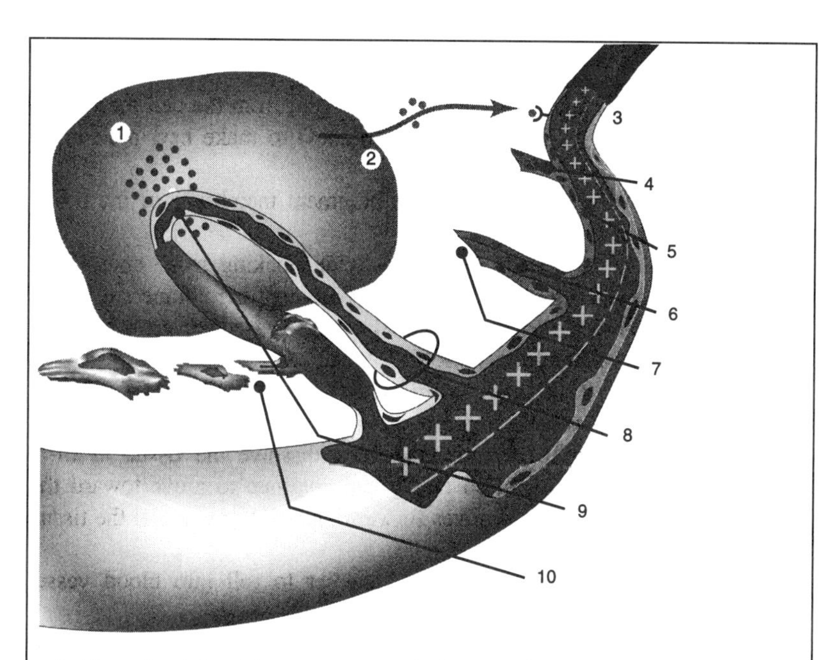

1. Hypoxic or injured tissues produce and release angiogenic growth factors (proteins) that diffuse into the nearby tissues.
2. The angiogenic growth factors bind to endothelial receptors located on the endothelial cells (EC) of nearby preexisting blood vessels.
3. Once growth factors bind to their receptors, the endothelial cells become activated. Signals are sent from the cell's surface to the nucleus. The endothelial cell's machinery begins to produce new molecules, including enzymes.
4. Enzymes dissolve tiny holes in the sheath-like covering (basement membrane) surrounding all existing blood vessels.
5. The endothelial cells begin to divide (proliferate), and they migrate out through the dissolved holes of the existing vessels towards the diseased tissue (tumor).
6. Specialized molecules called adhesion molecules, or integrins (avb3, avb5), serve as grappling hooks to help pull the sprouting new blood vessel forward.
7. Additional enzymes (matrix metalloproteinases, or MMP) are produced to dissolve the tissue in front of the sprouting vessel tip in order to accommodate it. As the vessel extends, the tissue is remolded around the vessel.
8. Sprouting endothelial cells roll up to form a blood vessel tube.
9. Individual blood vessel tubes connect to form blood vessel loops that can circulate blood.
10. Finally, newly formed blood vessel tubes are stabilized by specialized muscle cells (smooth muscle cells, pericytes) that provide structural support. Blood flow then begins.

Figure 5.10 The Angiogenesis Cascade (Modified from the Angiogenesis Foundation, 2000, Angiogenesis Cascade)

- The growth factors bind to receptors on the endothelial cells of a nearby blood vessel, activating the endothelial cells.
- Once activated, the endothelial cells send a signal from the cell membrane into the cell nucleus telling the nucleus (genes) to make new molecules, including enzymes.
- The enzymes dissolve tiny holes in the basement membrane of the blood vessels in the area.
- The endothelial cells are stimulated to divide, making more endothelial cells that migrate through the holes in the basement membrane and move toward the injured tissue or malignant cells that released the growth factor, like tiny sprouting new blood vessels.
- Adhesion molecules (integrins) act like little grappling hooks and pull the sprouting new blood vessels forward toward the tumor.
- Additional enzymes (MMPs) are made and dissolve the tissue in front of the sprouting blood vessel so that it can continue to move toward the tumor. After the blood vessel moves forward, the MMPs remodel the tissue to anchor the blood vessel.
- The sprouting endothelial cells come together to roll into blood vessel tubes.
- The individual blood vessel tubes connect to form blood vessel loops.
- Smooth muscle cells stabilize the blood vessels, and blood begins to flow from the parent blood vessel to the new blood vessel loops.

Table 5.2 lists agents currently being tested to inhibit angiogenesis. These are only some of the many agents undergoing clinical testing. In addition, altering the dose and administration schedule of some standard chemotherapy agents appears to change the mechanism of action. As illustrated in the complex steps of metastases, there are innumerable opportunities for interruption, causing the arrest of the metastatic cascade.

Table 5.2 Selected Agents Currently Being Tested to Inhibit Angiogenesis

Block Matrix Breakdown Inhibit Integrin/Survival	Inhibitors of Endothelial Cells Directly	Blockade of Activators of Angiogenesis
• Dalteparin (Fragmin)[1] • Neovastat (AE-941) • ATN-161 • EMD-121974 (Cilenigtide) • Celecoxib (Celebrex) (nonspecific mechanism of action)	• ABT-510 • Combretastatin (causes programmed cell death of proliferating endothelial cells) • Lenalidomide • LY317615 (Enzastaurin) • Soy isoflavone (Genistein) • Thalidomide	• ADH-1 (Exherin) • AG-013736 • AMG-706 • AZD 2171 (Cediranib, Recentin) • GW786034 (Pazopanib) • PTK/ZK (Vatalanib, multi-targeted VEGFR) • RAD001 (Everolimus) • ZD 6474 (vandetanib, Zactima)

Source: NCI (http://www.cancer.gov/clinical trials/developments/anti-angio-table). Accessed June 11, 2007.

Drugs that inhibit angiogenesis, either by neutralizing VEGF (e.g., bevacizumab) or blocking signaling within the endothelial cell (e.g., sunitinib or sorafinib), cause class-related effects. These include hypertension, believed related to the blockade of nitric oxide, which is necessary for the walls of arterioles and other resistance vessels to relax; rare gastrointestinal perforation with unknown relationship; and bleeding events (epistaxis) with rare hemorrhage. In addition, with the tyrosine protein kinases sunitinib and sorafinib, left ventricular ejection fraction can be decreased.

Finding and Establishing a Metastatic Site

Ruoslahti (1996) describes the "area code" hypothesis first developed by Dreyer and Sperry in the late 1960s. The theory may help to explain how certain malignancies develop metastases in preferential areas given that, as we have seen, metastatic cells are blindly embolized into the bloodstream.

First, in order to be embolized, malignant epithelial cells must overcome two types of adhesion which keep normal cells adhering to one another and attached to the protein meshwork (extracellular matrix), especially in epithelial tissue. This is important because most cancers are epithelial, arising from the epithelial covering of the outer layer of skin and outer layer and lining of many organs, such as the gut and lungs.

Cell-to-cell adhesion molecules keep normal cells orderly. One molecule is especially important, E-cadherin, which ensures intercellular adhesion. Early studies show that when this molecule is manipulated in cancer cells, it changes a cell from a non-invasive cell to an invasive cell capable of forming tumors. When functional E-cadherin is restored, this tendency can be reversed. Malignant cells are able to inactivate E-cadherin and are released from this requirement of cell-to-cell adhesion.

In addition, for cell survival and reproduction, normal cells must adhere to the extracellular matrix. In laboratory tests, cells in culture can not grow unless they attach to a surface, or achieve *anchorage dependence* (Ruoslahti and Reed, 1994). The molecules on the cell surface that actually do the attachment are *integrins*. Integrins must be intact for cell growth and cell division. It appears that integrins influence a protein in the cell nucleus called cyclin E-CDK2 complex (cyclin dependent kinase [CDK]), which is necessary for the cell cycle (division) clock to move toward cell growth and division. When cells do not adhere to the extracellular matrix, the lack of integrin adherence causes inhibition of cyclin E-CDK2 in the cell nucleus; the cell cycle clock stops; and the cell commits suicide (programmed cell death, or apoptosis). Unfortunately, cancer cells are able to circumvent this process, to become *anchorage independent* so cyclin E-CDK2 stays active whether or not the cell is attached, and cells keep growing and dividing, thus avoiding programmed death. In addition, with only a few exceptions (e.g., neutrophils), normal cells can not penetrate through the underlying basement membrane on which they rest, or through basement membranes of blood vessels (endothelial lining). Like neutrophils, malignant cells release the enzymes called *matrix metalloproteinases* (*MMPs*) that dissolve parts of the basement membrane as well as the extracellular matrix, so that like a military tank, the cells can migrate away from the primary tumor and into the blood vessels for the process of metastases.

Once in the blood vessel, it is estimated that only one cell in 10,000 is successful in setting up a new metastatic site distant from the primary tumor. As stated, it must attach to the inner lining of capillaries and dissolve holes in the blood vessel basement membrane to escape into the extravascular tissue. It appears that most cells get trapped in the nearest capillary bed they encounter after leaving the primary tumor. Metastatic cells tend to be large and easily trapped, and many secrete clotting factors that cause platelets to aggregate around them. The primary destination for venous blood from most organs is the lungs, thus this is the most common metastatic site. Venous blood leaves the gut and goes to the liver first; the liver is the most common metastatic site for intestinal tumors. While this is true, it appears that, in addition, the cell surface adhesion molecules are directed to specific organ locations, via a code much like telephone area codes, so that malignant cells migrate to specific areas, such as prostate cancer to bone. This was further defined by Muller et al (2001). It also appears that there is "metastatic inefficiency"; some cells go to places without "area codes," or cells from a primary tumor that lack metastatic qualities undergo apoptosis (Wong et al, 2001). The micro-environment of the metastatic site is critical, and it releases growth factors to help the newly arrived metastatic cell survive.

By studying neutrophils, normal cells that migrate where needed to fight infection, Muller et al (2001) were able to demonstrate that chemokines, soluble substances that carry messages between cells, are responsible for directing breast cancer cells to the primary organs where breast cancer metastasizes: lymph nodes, bone marrow, lung, and liver. Chemokines are small molecules that resemble cytokines and connect with specific receptors on the cell surface causing rearrangement of the cell's cytoskeleton. This allows cells to adhere firmly to endothelial cells (lining blood vessels) and migrate in a specific direction. Chemokines work with integrins and other proteins on the surface of the cell to direct the breast cancer cells to specific organs. The authors found that breast cancer cells have functionally active chemokine receptors. When these receptors are activated by binding with a ligand (a substance that binds to a receptor on the cell surface and that turns on signal transduction within a cell), the cell activates actin (which gives structure to a cell) polymerization with the formation of pseudopods (fake feet) that allow the cell to migrate and invade tissue. The tissues in which these ligands are overexpressed are the primary metastatic sites in breast cancer. Further, in studies, by neutralizing interactions between the chemokines and their receptors, metastases to lymph nodes and lung could be inhibited. As more is learned about the process of metastases, new agents can be developed to inhibit each of the critical steps, thus preventing the process.

As more is understood about the complexity of the immune response (innate and adaptive including, humoral, and cell mediated), it is more surprising that the immune system cannot be mobilized to attack and kill malignant cells in the body. The innate immune system is an intrinsic system we are born with and includes antibodies in our saliva and other cells that provide protection against pathogens that we encounter in our daily lives. In contrast, the adaptive immune system is made up of humoral (B-lymphocyte or antibody, complement) and cell-mediated (T-lymphocyte) immune components and protects a person from invading foreign antigens. In the adaptive immune system, the immune cells are able to distinguish self from non-self, to remember the "foreign" antigens to which they have been exposed (memory T and B cells), and to mount an immune attack to eliminate the "foreign" antigen. When the antigen is encountered again, the immune system will mount a rapid and increasingly more potent defense against the antigen. Once an antigen is recognized as not belonging to self, dendritic cells (a type of B-lymphocyte) take the antigen and present it on itself (antigen presenting cell, or APC) to T-lymphocytes. Three key immune fighters can be activated by the dendritic cells: cytotoxic T-lymphocytes, B-lymphocytes, and natural killer (NK) cells. First, the dendritic cell activates helper T-lymphocytes cells, which produce cytokines that activate the appropriate B-lymphocyte and/or T-lymphocyte to seek and destroy the antigen(s) marked for destruction. These helper T-lymphocytes may be activated to differentiate into cytotoxic T-lymphocytes, which proliferate rapidly against the specific antigen(s). Second, B-lymphocytes can recognize APCs, and then seek and destroy the cells with this cell surface antigen. Third, NK cells can recognize self from non-self and attack and destroy cells with foreign antigen(s).

Tumor cell antigens should be able to be recognized as foreign; however, tumors are able to evade the immune system, possibly because some of the antigens are indented and thus not recognizable; tumors often have more than one tumor antigen on their cell surface, and tumors may minimize or eliminate MHC expression so that they cannot be seen by cytotoxic T-lymphocytes. Other possible causes are that the tumor inhibits the maturation of the dendritic cell, or blocks signaling between the co-stimulatory molecule B7 and CD28, which is required for maturation of activated T-lymphocytes. Without this signaling, cytokines are not produced, such as IL-2, which is necessary for full activation of T-lymphocytes, and the proliferating T-lymphocytes are not fully activated (Scandella and Ludewig, 2005).

Dendritic cells have great potential in recognizing and orchestrating an immune attack against tumor cell antigens; however, they must mature before they can activate T-lymphocytes. After the dendritic cell recognizes the foreign antigen on the surface of the tumor cell, it infiltrates into the tumor, processes intracellular proteins and/or antigens, and matures so that it can express the antigens on its surface to present to the T-lymphocytes. The mature dendritic cell uses the major histocompatibility complex (MHC) to present the foreign antigen, and when bound to the T-lymphocyte, a signal is sent to make more T-lymphocytes: the B7 co-stimulatory molecule on the dendritic cells binds to the CD 28 receptor on the T-lymphocyte, which then signals T-lymphocyte replication. The resulting activated T-lymphocytes should be able to seek and destroy tumor cells expressing that particular antigen.

For decades, different clinical trials explored ways to stimulate and/or augment immune function; however, although very promising, none have significantly impacted malignant progression. Today, one group of agents is monoclonal antibodies directed against cytotoxic T-lymphocyte-associated antigen 4 (CTLA-4) designed to augment cytotoxic T-cell function. CTLA-4 is a protein that turns off T-lymphocyte proliferation and activation when the immune response has destroyed the foreign antigen by sending an inhibitory protein that shuts down or downregulates T-lymphocyte proliferation and IL-2 production. By blocking CTLA-4, no inhibitory protein is sent so that T-cell proliferation and IL-2 production continues.

Ipilimumab (MTX-010), a fully human monoclonal antibody directed against CTLA-4, is being studied in patients with malignant melanoma, renal cell cancer, and adenocarcinoma of the pancreas. The second is tremelimumab. The isotype (reflects Ig skeleton of the MAb) of a monoclonal antibody (MAb) is a deliberate design element. IgG1 MAb's stimulate host immune response and complement activation, as well as stimulating antibody-dependent cell-mediated cytotoxicity (ADCC) when the MAb attaches to an antigen. ADCC mobilizes immune elements that can destroy cancer cells, such as Natural Killer (NK) cells and macrophages. Examples of MAbs that are isotype IgG1 are bevacizumab, trastuzumab, cetuximab, and ipilimumab. IgG2 MAbs mildly if at all activate host defenses, do activate complement, but do not activate ADCC. Examples of IgG2 MAbs are panitumumab and tremelimumab. Ipilimumab has been successful in two of three clinical trials of patient with malignant melanoma, showing at least 10% tumor shrinkage and overall disease control in about 19% of patients; however, it may take 12 weeks or longer for patients to respond. In subset analysis, when studied at a dose of 10 mg/kg, disease control was 39%, which lasted at least 6 months in most patients (ASCO 2007 #8523). Toxicities included immune mediated rash, diarrhea, adrenal insufficiency, and hepatitis. Tremelimumab was evaluated and not approved by the FDA in 2008, as the drug failed to meet its endpoint in a phase III trial (improvement in overall survival in first-line treatment of patients with unresectable stage III or IV malignant melanoma).

As the twenty-first century unfolds, there is tremendous momentum in transforming cancer care. The human genome project and other molecular research have given great insight into the process of carcinogenesis, metastases, and molecular flaws that can be targeted to provide cytostatic and cytocidal effects. In addition, genomics has enabled the identification of molecular signatures of different cancers, and this will lead to individualized therapy tailored to the individual tumors of patients. Also, pharmacogenomics has helped to identify which tumor types are responsive to which drugs or therapies, as well as which patients have difficulty metabolizing certain drug(s). This chapter presents investigational as well as FDA approved agents in which an agent targets one or more molecular flaw(s), thus interrupting the malignant process.

As targets are identified, often they can be directly attacked, as with the fusion protein denileukin diftitox (Ontak) which carries the diphtheria toxin directly to high-affinity IL-2 receptors containing a CD25 component, such as activated T- and B-cell lymphocytes. The drug is indicated in the treatment of persistent or recurrent cutaneous

T-cell lymphoma (CTCL or mycoses fungoides). The uses of monoclonal antibodies include:

- Blocking a receptor so that the ligand can not bind to it, such as Erb-B1 or EGFR [Cetuximab (Erbitux) or panitumumab (Vectibix), or Erb-B2 or HER-2-neu (trastuzumab (Herceptin)], which prevent over-expressed growth factor receptors from sending the signal for cell division.
- Attaching to a cell receptor to bring the body's immune system to kill the cell, such as rituximab (Rituxan), which targets B-lymphocytes that express the CD20 antigen.
- Carrying chemotherapy or radioisotopes like a Trojan Horse, which, when internalized into the cell, cause cell death, such as gemtuzumab ozogamicin (Mylotarg) and 90Y ibritumomab (Zevalin).

Figure 5.11 shows mechanisms of monoclonal antibody therapy. As can be seen, chimeric monoclonal antibodies contain more mouse than humanized or human monoclonal antibodies, so premedication is usually required to prevent infusion reactions.

Table 5.3 shows current agents in clinical trials that target molecular flaws. *Matrix metalloproteases* (*MMPs*) have been shown to be overexpressed in breast, lung, and prostate cancers, and it appears that certain MMPs are necessary for the formation of new capillaries (angiogenesis), movement of the cancer cells into neighboring tissue (invasion), and metastases. Normally, the extracellular matrix provides structure between cells, with basement membranes that separate subdivisions within tissues. This matrix prevents aberrant cells from invading other tissues or moving into the bloodstream to go elsewhere in the body. MMPs are zinc-dependent enzymes that maintain the extracellular matrix of tissues by breaking down different parts of the matrix as needed for ongoing remodeling (synthesis and breakdown of these proteins) over time. There are five main subcategories, based on their site of action: collagenases (MMP-1, MMP-8, MMP-13); gelatinases (MMP-2, MMP-9); stromelysins (MMP-3, MMP-7, MMP-10); membrane-type MMPs or MT-MMPs (MMP-14, MMP-15, MMP-16, MMP-17); and others (MMP-11, MMP-12, MMP-18) (Agouron Pharmaceuticals, 1999; Chambers and Matrisian, 1997). The principal MMPs that appear to be involved in tumor angiogenesis, invasion, and metastases are gelatinase A (MMP-2), gelatinase B (MMP-9), and MT-MMP-1 (MMP-14). It is known that tumors larger than 2 mm require new blood vessels to nourish the tumor cells and support tumor growth. As the tumor grows, it releases MMPs to enable cells to break from the tumor and attach to pieces of the extracellular matrix, then to break down the extracellular matrix so the cells can move through the tissue compartments, and, finally, to move through the created openings to invade blood and lymphatic vessels and travel to distant sites. It is hoped that through inhibiting the MMPs, new blood vessel growth (angiogenesis), invasion, and metastases can be prevented. Currently, MMP inhibitors (MMPIs) can be specific, such as inhibiting MMP-2 and MMP-9, or broad spectrum, and are being clinically tested either alone as a single agent, or together with chemotherapy, and then continued as a maintenance agent. Clinical studies with MMPIs have been disappointing, and this book will be updated as more promising agents appear.

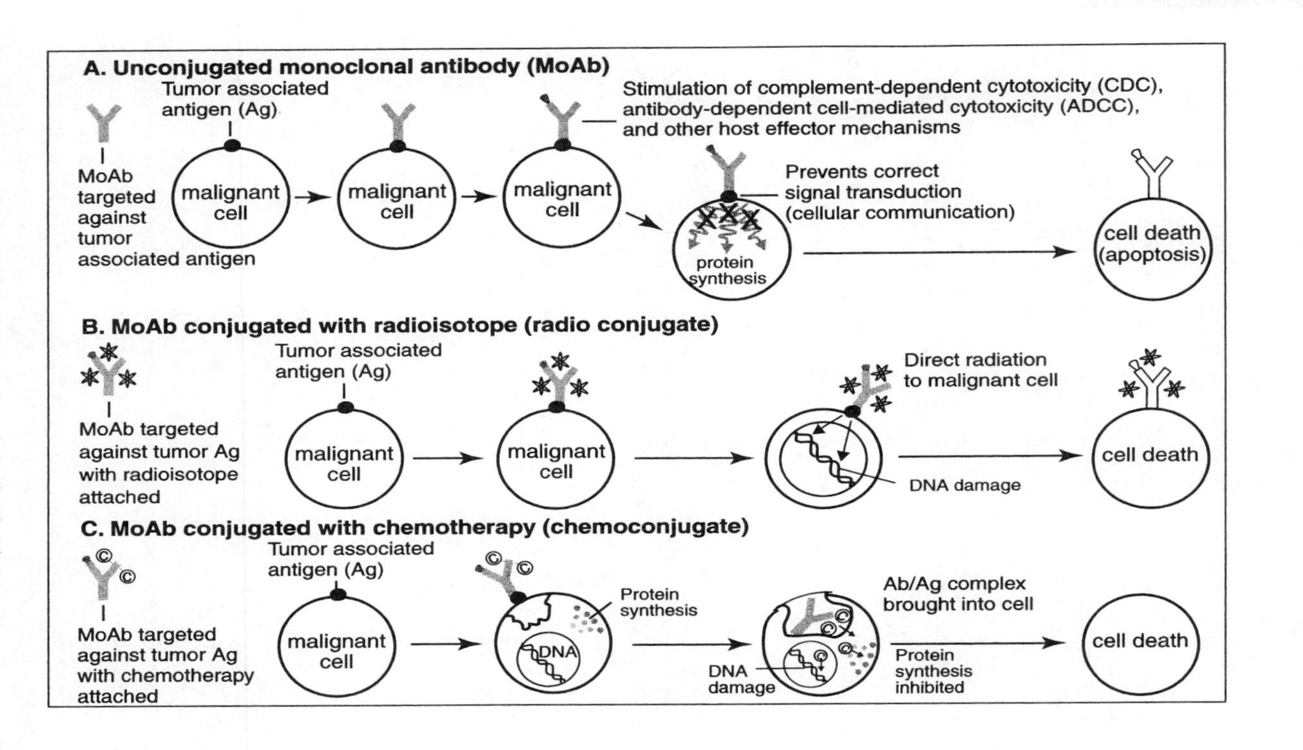

Figure 5.11 Mechanisms of Monoclonal Antibody Therapy
Source: Modified from Wyeth-Ayerest Laboratories (1999) *Antibody-Targeted Chemotherapy*. Philadelphia, PA: Wyeth-Ayerest Laboratories, p. 3

Table 5.3 Quick Tips on Understanding Monoclonal Antibody Names

1st syllable	Name unique to the product	Tras
2nd syllable	Target, e.g., tumor = tu	Tu
3rd syllable	Identifies the source, where	U
	0 = mouse	
	u = human	
	I = chimeric (mouse and human)	
4th syllable	mab = monoclonal antibody	Mab
X and z	Consonants to link syllables	Tras tu z u mab

Retinoids appear to function by interfering with tumor differentiation. They are believed to have a role in cancer prevention as well as therapy. There are receptors in the cell nucleus that are retinoid-dependent and function in the transcription of proteins. When retinoids bind to the receptors, it is believed that they dimerize nuclear proteins, the complex then binds to DNA, and then there is transcription of a number of target genes. Thus, these activated retinoid receptors regulate the expression of genes responsible for differentiation and replication of cells. Retinoids have been effective in treating superficial Kaposi's sarcoma lesions (alitretinoin) and acute promyelocytic leukemia (tretinoin).

In acute promyelocytic leukemia (APL), there is a translocation of a gene called retinoic-receptor alpha (RAR-alpha) on chromosome 17 that is switched with a gene called PML on chromosome 15. It appears that this translocation of RAR-alpha is part of the etiology of APL. Treatment with all-trans retinoic acid induces the primitive leukemic blast cells to differentiate, with replacement by normal myelocyte cells. This drug is now indicated for induction remission in patients with APL with subtype 3, including the M3 variant of AML. Other cancers that appear sensitive to 13-*cis* retinoic acid in combination with interferon alpha are squamous cell cancers of the skin and cervix. Alitretinoin (9-*cis*-retinoic acid) occurs naturally in the body and is able to bind and activate intracellular retinoid receptors. It has been shown to inhibit the growth of Kaposi's sarcoma when used topically and is now indicated for topical treatment of cutaneous lesions in patients with AIDS-related Kaposi's sarcoma who do not require systemic therapy.

As more is learned about the pathways involved in malignant transformation, targets are selected and agents developed to target these molecularly flawed pathways. Many patients do well. It is very humbling to realize the plethora of pathways involved, the interrelatedness, and the redundant pathways. As more patients are studied, it is becoming clear that cancer is a dynamic process, and initial responses may over time give way to loss of control as tumor cells mutate and find different pathways to communicate the demands of cancer: proliferation, blood vessels, invasiveness, and immortality. This has led to studies that combine agents that block different pathways, such as bevacizumab (VEGF inhibitor) and cetuximab (EGFR inhibitor). In addition, it raises the question about anticipating the emergence of resistance and adding that drug to the regime. For example, Batchelor et al (2007) in a phase II study of the investigational drug cediranib (AZD2171) also combined biomarker and imaging; the investigators were able to visualize impressive normalization of blood vessels in patients with recurrent glioblastoma, leading to reduced cerebral edema, a steroid-sparing effect, as well as almost a doubling of PFS compared with historical controls. However, as most of these patients eventually progressed, biomarkers revealed that the tumor now was using fibroblast growth factor (bFGF) and a new growth factor, chemokines-stroma-cell-derived factor I α (SDF1α) to build new blood vessels. The authors stated that this underscores the need for multitargeted agents to treat the multiple pathways.

Similarly, patients who respond to erlotinib (Tarceva) or gefitinib (Iressa) in the treatment of lung cancer have specific mutations in the EGFR gene, but ultimately, the tumor becomes resistant to the drug. Pao et al (2005) described the finding of a new, second mutation that prevented the drug from binding to the EGFR in the same way. Engleman (2007) identified that a subset of patients who did not develop the second mutation developed resistance because the tumor cells found a different pathway to go around the drug-inhibited tyrosine protein kinase—they sent the message via the *MET* oncogene, which now became amplified, and it reactivated the same, mutated signaling pathway that had been shut off by the drug by going through ERBB3. *MET* tyrosine kinases are normally activated by hepatocyte growth factor, but in cancer, they are associated with metastases.

Another exciting advance accompanying the understanding of different signaling pathways and tumor signature mutational pathways is the use of proteinomics and genomics to guide individualized treatment planning. For example, it is now clear that the EGFRI Mabs cetuximab and panitumumab are only effective in patients with tumors that have the wild-type or normal k-ras gene (about 55% of patients with colon cancer) and ineffective in patients with a mutant gene, as k-ras is downstream from the EGFR receptor (Benvenuti et al, 2007; Finocchiaro et al, 2007). We are learning more and more about the importance of specific mutational sequences in breast cancer, which correspond to different types of breast cancer that can be used to guide individualized treatment plans (Chaitlanya et al, 2008). Similarly, with K-RAS in CRC, we see that there are at least two different diseases, one with a mutation in K-RAS, an important oncogene. K-RAS is also mutated in about 20% of patients with lung cancer who have a mutated K-RAS gene. This can be used to guide the use of cetuximab and panitumumab.

Yet, it is still a very exciting time in cancer care as the paradigms of care change. Genetic microarrays are being perfected, thus improving diagnosis and treatment and promising to pave the way for individualized multidimensional therapy. It may be possible in the near future to prevent tumors from enlarging beyond 2 mm, prevent metastases, and if patients are not cured of their cancer, contain cancer as a chronic disease much like diabetes, since most patients die from metastasis, not the primary tumor. Given world politics and individual lifestyle choices, it is probably not possible to eliminate environmental carcinogens. However, the future looks promising that cancer, if not cured, will soon be a chronic, not terminal, disease.

New Targeted Therapy: New Toxicities

The tremendous growth in oral agents has helped nurses to refocus on concordance or patient adherence to a prescribed regimen and to identify strategies to help patients manage self-administration, calling the provider when specific signs and symptoms of toxicity occur, and to be knowledgeable about insurance coverage of oral agents. Now, as new categories of targeted therapies emerge, many class effects are common denominators for agents in that class, in addition to some drug specific potential toxicities that relate to other signaling pathways affected. Specific classes of drugs and their class effects include: EGFR inhibitors (EGFRI): sterile inflammatory rash and related skin changes, ILD, diarrhea, and with the MAbs, hypomagnesemia; VEGF inhibitors: HTN, bleeding, gastrointestinal perforation; and mTOR inhibitors. This chapter reviews two patient problems that nurses encounter most frequently: EGFRI rash and risk of cardiotoxicity from TKIs. There are few evidence-based interventions in the care of patients with new toxicities from targeted therapy; however, nurses across the country share anecdotal successes that may lead to prospective clinical trials. In addition, evidence based interventions used to manage chemotherapy-related toxicities have been found successful in the management of similar toxicities resulting from targeted therapy, such as diarrhea. As a class, tyrosine kinase inhibitors affect signaling pathways and, as the heart cannot be spared, have some degree of cardiotoxicity, which is discussed later here.

Rash and Related Skin Problems

With the success and promise of epidermal growth factor receptor inhibitors (EGFRIs), the dose-limiting toxicities of skin rash and diarrhea are clearly within the domain of nursing practice. As responding patients need to consider this treatment as chronic therapy, the challenge to nurses is to help patients minimize and manage symptoms and to maximize quality of life. A number of authors have described effective approaches, including Perez-Soler et al (2005) followed by Lynch et al (2007) who reported the results of a consensus group, Lacouture (2006), Fox (2006), and Segaert and Van Cutsem (2005, 2007). The following describes the evolution and etiology of EGFR toxicity.

EGFRs are located in the epidermis (skin keratinocytes, hair follicles, and sweat and sebaceous glands) and lining of the gastrointestinal tract where EGF is important in stimulating replacement cells and repair of gut mucosal injury. Blockade of EGF pathways in skin results in an inflammatory, sterile rash that then crusts and looks like acne but is pathologically quite distinct. Pathophysiology and key nursing assessment and management are discussed in the following paragraph. Skin rash is more intense with MoAbs such as cetuximab and panitumumab, whereas the rash with small molecular TKIs (erlotinib, gefitinib) may last longer, and dark-skinned patients such as African Americans may have less rash than their white counterparts. In addition, rash does not appear in previously irradiated skin, thought to be due to depletion of the EGFRs, but EGFRIs are radiosensitizers (Lynch et al, 2007). Blockade of EGFR in the gut results in diarrhea. EGFRs are also located in the ascending limb of the loop of Henle in the glomerulus (kidney) (Schrag et al, 2005), where 70% of magnesium is resorbed; EGFR blockade most likely causes the hypomagnesemia associated with monoclonal antibody EGFRIs.

Normally, when skin epidermis is damaged or aged, it is replaced by underlying keratinocytes that have differentiated and migrated to the skin surface. The skin is the primary protective barrier for the body and helps to keep in moisture. Lacouture (2006) describes the pathophysiology. Thinking of the pathophysiology in phases can help understand the skin toxicity related to EGFRIs (Wilkes, 2007).

Phase I: EGFR inhibition in the skin stops the keratinocytes from differentiating and migrating, and thus, they are arrested. The body senses that they should not be there and thus causes them to undergo apoptosis. The dead keratinocytes cause the release of chemokines, which recruit neutrophils to the area as part of the sterile, inflammatory response. The patient feels a sunburn-like reaction (erythema, tenderness, slight swelling) on the face and areas that have previously been exposed to the sun. The goal is to preserve skin integrity, minimize discomfort, and prevent infection. Key patient teaching includes (1) use skin cream with emollients to keep the skin from drying out; (2) avoid sun exposure using a sunblock of SPF 30 or higher, with a zinc base; (3) use a mild soap with active ingredients that reduce skin drying such as pyrithione zinc (Head and Shoulders); (4) consider aloe gel to red, tender areas; (5) report distressing tenderness as pramoxine (lidocaine topical anesthetic) may help; (6) keep fingernails clean and trimmed; and (7) apply zinc ointment to rectal mucosa after washing (Walker and Lacouture ME, 2006).

Phase II: This sterile inflammatory process results in death of the keratinocytes (undergo apoptosis) and the formation of debris, which causes a papular rash on the skin. At the same time, the skin is no longer fortified by healthy keratinocytes, and thus, it thins and is unable to preserve water in the body, leading to skin dryness (xerosis) and itching. The rash begins within 7–10 days of starting therapy and peaks in intensity in 2–3 weeks and then gradually gets better. The goal is to prevent infection, promote healing, and maximize comfort and coping. Management: Grade 1/mild rash, which is localized, does not interfere with ADLs and is not infected (Lynch et al, 2007): maintain current drug dose, observe or give topical hydrocortisone 1% or 2.5% or clindamycin 1% gel (anti-inflammatory benefit); reassess in 2 weeks. For grade 2/moderate, which is generalized, mild symptoms, and has minimal effect on ADLs, and no infection: continue EGFRI dose; use topicals (hydrocortisone 2.5% or clindamycin 1% gel or consider pimecrolimus cream (immunomodulator) and add doxycycline 100 mg PO twice daily or minocycline 100 mg PO twice daily (give antimicrobial and anti-inflammatory effect) and reassess after 2 weeks. For grade 3/4 or severe rash (generalized, severe, has a significant impact on ADLs, and increased risk of infection): Dose reduce EGFRI drug based on manufacture's recommendation, and treat rash with topicals (hydrocortisone 2.5% or clindamycin 1% gel or pimecrolimus cream, doxycycline 100 mg PO twice daily or minocycline 100 mg PO twice daily, and methylprednisolone (Medrol dose pack); reassess after 2 weeks, and interrupt or discontinue drug if rash worsens (Lynch et al, 2007). If the rash appears infected (exudate, vesicular formation, different appearance), obtain C+S, treat empirically until sensitivity received, and/or obtain dermatology consult.

Phase III: The rash develops into pustules with crusting related to the drying of the cellular debris (keratinocytes, neutrophils, fibrin, serum) in about 4–6 weeks after the initial EGFRI drug dose; the skin tenderness goes away. Use the same algorithm for management as in phase II.

Phase IV: The skin becomes drier (xerosis) with pruritus and the formation of telangiectasias (dilated capillaries in the skin). The skin flakes and itches. For flaking skin, keratolytics such as lactic acid, salicylic acid, or urea-containing topicals such as 12% Lac-Hydrin or other exfoliating lotions can be helpful. Topical agents for itch include Sarna Ultra Anti-Itch Cream, Aveeno Anti-Itch Concentrated Cream, and Regenecare gel for the body and for the scalp, Clobetasol propionate (Olux foam™) or fluocinolone acetonide) Topical Shampoo, 0.01% (Capex shampoo) (O'Keefe et al, 2006; Walker and Lacouture, 2006). Itching may require pharmacologic management: diphenhydramine 25–50 mg PO and cetirizine 10–20 mg PO daily, and for resistant itch, pregabalin (Porzio et al, 2006) and doxepin (Greene et al, 1985) have shown impressive results.

Phase V: EGFR blockade of the hair follicles and nail beds results in hair changes (hair thinning or alopecia on scalp but increased hair growth on the eyelids) (trichomegaly), face (hypertrichosis). The hair texture can change (changes in texture and strength). Paronychia (periungual inflammation) can develop with crusted lesions on nail folds and tenderness. Painful skin fissures on the fingers can develop. For paronychia, treat with emollients, and consider flurandrenolone (Cordran) for wrapping around the finger. Consider flurandrenolone as well for fissures (O'Keefe et al, 2006). It is important to assess eyelashes, and if they are long, they can fold back and irritate the conjunctiva; refer to an ophthalmologist for trimming as needed.

Skin-related problems from sunitinib and sorafinib are a bit different, as their targets are different from EGFR. Sorafinib can cause facial erythema, splinter subungual hemorrhage, with or without alopecia, whereas sunitinib can cause hair depigmentation (white when on therapy, and dark during treatment break), splinter subungual hemorrhage, with or without periorbital edema (Widakowich et al, 2007). Both agents can cause hand–foot syndrome (acral erythema) involving the palms of the hands and soles of the feet and are characterized by symmetrical red, swollen skin that may have dysesthesia or paresthesia and may progress to pain and desquamation. Specific nursing interventions are discussed under the specific drug.

Cardiotoxicity

Tyrosine kinases (TKs) transduce signals from the outside of the cell to the cell nucleus to stimulate or inhibit cell functions. Tyrosine kinase inhibitors (TKIs) can block receptor TKs or their ligands (MAbs) outside the cell or inside the cell by small molecule TKIs, which prevent phosphylation, and thus, this message, which is the intent in malignant cells to turn off proliferation or other survival functions, never reaches the cell nucleus. TKs in the heart are blocked as well, however, which leads to damage to myocytes and in some individuals altered heart function. Because cardiac function is not a clinical endpoint of the drug trials and many of the drugs are nonselective in some of their targets, it is difficult to know the exact risk and incidence of cardiotoxicity except for the well studied trastuzumab and lapatinib. Force et al (2007) describe our understanding of the TKI-specific cardiotoxicity. The authors point out that cardiac myocytes have a very high demand for energy (ATP) and are thus especially susceptible to agents that alter mitochondrial function. The first and most widely studied drug is trastuzumab (Herceptin), a MAb directed against EGFR2 (HER2), which had an incidence of cardiotoxicity of 4–7% as a single agent, increasing to 27% when combined with an anthracycline, and manifested first as a decrease in LVEF (left ventricle pumping ability) and later as symptomatic CHF. Lapatinib blocks both EGFR1 and EGFR2 but in contrast only has a small risk of lowering LVEF below normal values of 50–70%. EGFR2 (HER2) is an important pathway in cardiomyocyte development and function. In addition, HER2 dimerizes with EGFR3 and EGFR4 receptor tyrosine kinases and is a co-receptor for their ligands the neuregulins, which are all expressed in cardiac tissue. HER2 (EGFR2)–EGFR4 signaling is essential to myocardial contractility in the adult. The authors hypothesize that by blocking the HER2 receptor dimerization does not occur, with loss of signaling leading to changes in mitochondrial membrane polarization, ATP depletion, and loss of contractility. Mitochondria are the energy factory and storehouse of ATP, the energy currency of the cell. Other factors enhancing cardiotoxicity might be mediated by ADCC as trastuzumab is an IgG1 MAb.

Force et al (2007) also discuss cardiotoxicity related to TKIs. Imatinib (Gleevec) has rarely caused CHF, and in those patients, electron microscopy of the heart has shown nonspecific mitochondrial abnormalities. When cardiomyocytes are studied in culture with imatinib, there is significant damage to the mitochondria resulting in cell death and declines in ATP stores. The active myocardium uses tremendous amounts of energy in the form of ATP to contract, and if these are inadequate, the heart fails. Other hypotheses include the fact that this drug and others like the related dasatinib inhibit ABL, which may be protecting the heart from oxidant stress. Dasatinib has an incidence of 4% LVEF dysfunction or CHF when taken for 6 months or longer. The multitargeted TKIs sorafinib and sunitinib may cause myocardial injury as collateral effects. Patients receiving sunitinib reportedly have an 11% incidence of declines in LVEF $< 50\%$ when taken for 6 months, which may have been compounded by possible drug induced hypothyroidism. The drug inhibits PDGFα/β, which are also expressed on cardiomyocytes and believed important in cardiomyocyte survival; however, the exact cause is unknown. Patients taking sorafinib have a 2.9% incidence of acute coronary syndrome (compared to 0.4% in the placebo arm). Sorafinib inhibits PDGFRs as well as RAF1 and BRAF, which are important in oxidant stress-induced injury. In addition, when Raf1 is deleted in a mouse heart, it develops a dilated, hypocontractile heart with fibrosed and dead cardiomyocytes; however, the actual mechanisms of cardiotoxicity with these drugs is still unclear. Although there is some provocative evidence that statins may provide not only some degree of cardioprotection, but also specific antitumor effects, focused research on this and other agents needs to be done to define any potential benefit or interaction (Popat and Smith, 2008). Future targeted therapy studies need to consider possible influences on the heart cells, either directly or indirectly.

Nursing care focuses on minimizing symptoms and helping patients maximize their quality of life. Specifically, nursing priorities have been highlighted in each of the phases, and treatment options may overlap as symptoms occur earlier or later. Patient educational materials are available, including Herbst et al (Managing Rash and Other Skin Reactions to Targeted Treatments, found at http://www.cancercare.org/pdf/booklets/ccc_managing_rash.pdf) and American Society of Clinical Oncology (Skin Reactions to Targeted Therapy, found at http://www.asco.org). All patients should be taught to keep their skin well moisturized using a water-based emollient, avoiding sun exposure and using a sunblock (at least SPF 30, and zinc based), and staying well hydrated (Lynch et al, 2007). There is much opportunity for nurses to become involved in nursing research to test different approaches to minimizing rash and optimizing quality of life. For example, Hetherington et al (2007) reported a case report of a patient receiving cetuximab 500 mg/m^2 every other week. She developed a grade 2 rash on her face and thorax, but when she received local cooling before and during her treatment, she has only developed a grade 1 rash. Studies are beginning to look at quality of life. Zachariae et al (2003) found that dermatological disease-related impairment of quality of life predicted psychological symptoms. Molinari et al (2005) found that 5 of 13 patients in a study of cetuximab-induced rash felt the rash significantly impacted on their quality of life. Wagner et al (2007) reported that the most commonly distressing aspects of skin toxicity on patients receiving EGFRIs are pain, irritation, pruritus, dryness, hair changes, interference with activities (work or hobbies), and the emotional impact (feeling depressed, frustrated, isolated). Fortunately, in a study by Humblet (2007), patients with the most severe rash also tended to have the highest response rate; patients who were most bothered by skin toxicity also had the highest quality of life scores and less symptoms from cancer. Nurses need to assess the impact of skin changes on patients in terms of function, emotion, social, and physical, such as pain or tenderness.

However, monoclonal antibodies (MoAbs) continue to have a role in targeted therapy. The nurse should be cognizant of the drug risk for causing infusion reactions (cytokine release syndrome or grades 1/2 hypersensitivity), should premedicate the patient before infusion as ordered, and should monitor the patient closely during treatment. Other MoAbs may cause severe hypersensitivity reactions (HSRs), either anaphylactoid (nonimmune mediations, no prior sensitization) or hypersensitivity (IgG E mediated, prior sensitization) reactions, and the reader is referred to Chapter 1 for a review of assessment and management of HSRs.

Class-related toxicities have been identified and are highlighted with each drug. For example, the EGFRIs all cause skin toxicity to some degree, diarrhea, and risk of interstitial lung disease as the function of EGFRs is blocked. EGFRI MoAbs block the EGFRs in the distal loop of Henle responsible for reabsorption of magnesium, and thus, these drugs are associated with significant hypomagnesemia. Angiogenic inhibitors block the action of VEGF to stimulate VEGFRs. VEGF appears to be necessary for nitric oxide, a vasodilator, and thus, all angiogenic inhibitors are associated with hypertension. As more experience is gained in the treatment of patients, more class-related side effects will be identified, helping the nurse to anticipate side effects.

References

Acharya CR, Hsu DS, Anders CK, et al. Gene Expression Signatures, Clinicopathological Features and Individualized Therapy in Breast Cancer. *J Am Med Assoc* 2008; 299(13) 1574–1587

Adjei AA, Hidalgo M. Intracellular Signal Transduction Pathway Proteins as Targets for Cancer Therapy. *J Clin Oncol* 2005; 23 5386–5403

Agus DB, Gordon MS, Taylor C. Phase I Clinical Study of Pertuzumab, a Novel HER Dimerization Inhibitor, in Patients with Advanced Cancer. *J Clin Oncol* 2005; 23(11) 2534–2543

Agus DB, Sweeny CJ, Morris M, Efficacy and Safety of Single Agent Pertuzumab (rhuMAb 2C4), a HER Dimerization Inhibitor, in Hormone Refractory Prostate Cancer after Failure of Taxane-based Therapy. *J Clin Oncol* 2005; 23(16s) 408s, abstract 4624

Ault P. Overview of Second-Generation Tyrosine Kinase Inhibitors for Patients With Imatinib-Resistant Chronic Myelogenous Leukemia. *Clin J Oncol Nurs* 2007; 11(1) 125–129

Ault P, Kaled S, Rios MB. Management of Molecular-Targeted Therapy for Chronic Myelogenous Leukemia. *J Am Acad Nurse Pract* 2003; 15 292–296

Bartlett JB, Dredge K, Dalgleish AG. The Evolution of Thalidomide and its IMiD Derivatives as Anticancer Agents. *Nat Rev Cancer* 2004; 4(4) 314–322

Batchelor TT, Sorensen AG, di Tomaso E. AZD2171, a Pan-VEGF Receptor Tyrosine Kinase Inhibitor, Normalizes Tumor Vasculature and Alleviates Edema In Glioblastoma Patients. *Cancer Cell* 2007; 11(1) 83–95

Beck KE, Blansfield JA, Tran KQ, et al. Enterococolitis in Patients With Cancer After Antibody Blockade of Cytotoxic T-Lymphocyte–Associated Antigen 4. *J Clin Oncol* 2006; 24 2283–2289

Benvenuti S, Sartore-Bianchi A, Di Nicolantonio F, et al. Oncogenic Activation of RAS/RAF Signaling Pathway Impairs the Response of Metastatic Colorectal Cancers to Anti-Epidermal Growth Factor Receptor Antibody Therapies. *Cancer Res* 2007; 67 2643–2648

Bernier J, Bonner J, Vermorken JB, et al. Consensus Guidelines for the Management of Radiation Dermatitis and Coexisting Acne-Like Rash In Patients Receiving Radiotherapy Plus EGFR Inhibitors for the Treatment of Squamous Cell Carcinoma of the Head and Neck. *Ann Oncol* 2008; 19(1) 142–149

Bharti AC, Aggarwal BB. Nuclear Factor-kappa B and Cancer: Its Role in Prevention and Therapy. *Biochem Pharmacol* Sept 2002; 64(5-6) 883–888

Bhaskar V, Fox M, Breinberg D, et al. Volociximab, a Chimeric Integrin Alpha5beta1 Antibody, Inhibits the Growth of VX2 Tumors in Rabbits. *Invest New Drugs* 2008; 26(1) 7–12

Blansfield JA, Beck KE, Tran K, et al. Cytotoxic T-lymphocyte–Associated Antigen-4 Blockage Can Induce Autoimmune Hypophysitis in Patients With Metastatic Melanoma and Renal Cancer. *J Immunotherapy* 2005; 28 593–598

Boulay A, Rudloff J, Ye J. Dual Inhibition of mTOR and Estrogen Receptor Signaling In Vitro Induces Cell Death in Models of Breast Cancer. *Clin Cancer Res* 2005; 11(14) 5319–5328

Burchert A, Wang Y, Cai D, et al. Compensatory P13-Kinase/Akt/mTOR Activation Regulates Imatinib Resistance Development. *Leukemia* 2005; 19 1774–1782

Cemeus C, Zhao TT, Barrett GM, Lorimer IA, Dimitroulakos J. Lovastatin Enhances Gefitinib Activity in Glioblastoma Cells Irrespective of EGFRvIII and PTEN Status. *J Neuro-Oncology* published online at 10.1007/s11060-008-9627-0. Accessed on June 20, 2008

Chan S, Scheulen ME, Johnston S. Phase II Study of Temsirolimus (CCI-779), a Novel Inhibitor of mTOR, in Heavily Pretreated Patients with Locally Advanced or Metastatic Breast Cancer. *J Clin Oncol* 2005; 23 1–9

Chollet P, Abrial C, Tacca O, et al. Mammalian Target of Rapamycin Inhibitors in Combination With Letrozole in Breast Cancer. *Clin Breast Cancer* 2006; 7 336–338

Claus R, Lubbert M. Epigenetic Targets in Hematopoietic Malignancies. *Oncogene* 2003; 22 6489–6496

Cortes J, Baselga J, Kellokumpu-Lehtinen P. Open Label, Randomized Phase II Study of Pertuzumab (P) in Patients (pat) with Metastatic Breast Cancer with Low Expression of HER-2. *Proc Am Soc Clin Oncol* 2005; abstract 3068

Cunningham D, Humblet Y, Siena S. Cetuximab (C225) Alone or in Combination with Irinotecan (CPT-11) in Patients with Epidermal Growth Factor Receptor (EGFR)-Positive, Irinotecan Refractory Metastatic Colorectal Cancer (MCRC). *Proc Am Soc Clin Oncol* 2003; 22 252, abstract 1012

Dann SG, Selvaraj A, Thomas G. mTOR Complex-1-S6K1 Signaling: At the Crossroads of Obesity, Diabetes and Cancer. *Trends Mol Med* 2007; 13 252–259

Dannenberg AJ, Altorki NK, Boyle JO. Cyclo-oxygenase 2: A Pharmacological Target for the Prevention of Cancer. *Lancet Oncology* 2001; 2(9) 544–551

Deininger M, Buchdunger E, Druker BJ. The Development of Imatinib as a Therapeutic Agent for Chronic Myeloid Leukemia. *Blood* 2005; 105 2640–2653

Dennis PB, Jaeschke A, Saitoh M, Fowler B, Kozma SC, Thomas G. Mammalian TOR: A Homeostatic ATP Sensor. *Science* 2001; 294 1102–1105

Department of Health and Human Services. Understanding Gene Testing. Washington, DC, National Cancer Institute, NIH Publication. 1995; 96–3905

Digel W, Lubbert M. DNA Methylation Disturbances as Novel Therapeutic Target in Lung Cancer and Clinical Results. *Crit Rev Oncol Hematol* 2005; 55 1–11

Dimopoulous M, Weber D, Chen C. Evaluating Oral Lenalidomide (Revlimid) and Dexamethasone Versus Placebo and Dexamethasone in Patients with Relapsed or Refractory Multiple Myeloma. *European Hematology Assoc 10th Conference* June 2–5 2005, Stockholm, Sweden, abstract 0402

Din FNV, Dunlop MG, Stark LA. Evidence for Colorectal Cancer Cell Specificity of Aspirin Effects on NF Kappa B Signaling and Apoptosis. *Br J Cancer* 2004; 91 381–388

Divino CM, Chen SH, Yang W. Anti-tumor Immunity Induced by Interleukin-12 Gene Therapy in a Metastatic Model of Breast Cancer Is Mediated by Natural Killer Cells. *Breast Cancer Res Treat* 2000; 60(2) 129–134

Duvic M. Optimizing Denileukin Diftitox (Ontak®) Therapy. *Hematologic Rep* 2006; 2(13) 57–60

Engleman JA, Zejnullaha K, Mitsudomi T. MET Amplification Leads to Gefitinib Resistance in Lung Cancer by Activating ERBB3 Signaling. *Science* 2007; 316 1039–1043

Fakih M. Management of anti-EGFR-targeting monoclonal antibody-induced hypomagnesemia. *Oncology* 2008; 22(1): Accessed at http://cancernetwork.com/showArticle.jhtml?articleId=205900749, 14 July 2008

Fan F, Wey JS, McCarty MF. Expression and Function of Vascular Endothelial Growth Factor Receptor 1 on Human Colorectal Cancer Cells. *Oncogene* 2005; 24 2647–2653

Ferrara N, Alitalo K. Clinical Applications of Angiogenic Growth Factors and Their Inhibitors. *Nature Medicine* 1999; 5 1359–1364

Finocchiaro G, Cappuzzo F, Janne PA, et al. EGFR, HER2 and Kras as Predictive Factors for Cetuximab Sensitivity in Colorectal Cancer. Program and abstracts of the 43rd *American Society of Clinical Oncology* Annual Meeting; June 1–5, 2007; Chicago, IL. Abstract 4021

Folkman J. Pharmacology of Cancer Biotherapeutics: Antiangiogenesis Agents. In DeVita VT Hellman S Rosenberg SA *Principles and Practice of Oncology*, 6th ed. Philadelphia, PA: Lippincott, Williams and Wilkins 2001; 509–521

Fox LP. Pathology and Management of Dermatologic Toxicities Associated with Anti-EGFR Therapy. *Oncology* 2006; 20 26–34

Francois B, Jourdes P, Benabid A. AE-941 (Neovastat) Induces the Expression of Angiostatin in Experimental Glioma. *Proc Am Soc Clin Oncol* 2001; 20(Part 1) 100a. Abstract 395. 37th Annual Meeting: San Francisco

Fruehauf JP, Lutzky J, McDermott DF, et al. Axinitib (AG-013736) in Patients With Metastatic Melanoma: A Phase II Study. *J Clin Oncol* 2008; 26 (May 20 suppl: abstr 9006)

Fu M, Wang C, Li Z, Sakamaki T, Pestell RG. Minireview: Cyclin D1: Normal and abnormal functions. *Endocrinology* 2004; 145 5439–5447

Giles FJ, Cortes JE, Halliburton TAF. Intravenous Corticosteroids to Reduce Gemtuzumab Ozogamicin Infusion Reactions. *Ann Pharmacother* 37(9) 1182–1185

Glickman MH, Ciechanover A. The Ubiquitin-Proteasome Proteolytic Pathway: Destruction for the Sake of Construction. *Physiology Review* 2002; 82 373–428

Greene SL, Reed CE, Schroeter AL. Double Blind Crossover Study Comparing Doxepin With Diphenhydramine for the Treatment of Chronic Urticaria. *J Am Acad Derm* 1985; 12 669–675

Grothey A, Sugrue M, Hedrick E, et al. Association Between Exposure to Bevacizumab (BV) Beyond First Progression and Overall Survival (OS) in Patients (pts) With Metastatic Colorectal Cancer (mCRC): Results From a Large Observational Study (BriTE). *J Clin Oncol* 2007 ASCO Annual Meeting Proceedings Part I. Vol 25, No. 18S, (June 20 Supplement), 4036

Hanahan D, Folkman J. Patterns and Emerging Mechanisms of the Angiogenic Switch During Tumorigenesis. *Cell* 1996; 86 353–358

Hanahan D, Weinberg RA. The Hallmarks of Cancer. *Cell* 2000; 100 57–100

Harari PM, Huang SM. Modulation of Molecular Targets to Enhance Radiation. *Clin Cancer Res* 2000; 6 323–325

Harris AL, Zhang H, Moghaddam A. Breast Cancer Angiogenesis. New Approaches to Therapy Via Antiangiogenesis, Hypoxic Activated Drugs, and Vascular Targeting. *Breast Cancer Research Treatment* 1996; 38 97–108

Haura EB, Turkson J, Jove R. Mechanisms of Disease: Insights into the Emerging Role of Signal Transducers and Activators of Transcription in Cancer. *Nature Clinical Practice Oncology* 2005; 2(6) 315–324

Herman JG, Baylin SB. Gene Silencing in Cancer in Association with Promoter Hypermethylation. *New England J Med* 2003; 349 2042–2054

Hetherington J, Andrews C, Vaynshteyn Y, Fishel R. Managing Follicular Rash Related to Chemotherapy and Monoclonal Antibodies. *Commun Oncol* 2007; 4(3) 157–162

Hidalgo M, Siu LL, Neumanitis J, Phase I and Pharmacologic Study of OSI-774, an Epidermal Growth Factor Receptor Tyrosine Kinase Inhibitor, in Patients with Advanced Solid Malignancies. *J Clin Oncol* 2001; 19(13) 3267–3279

Humblet Y, Peeters M, Siena S, Association of Skin Toxicity (ST) Severity With Clinical Outcomes and Health-Related Quality of Life (HRQoL) With Panitumumab. *J Clin Oncol* 2007 ASCO Annual Meeting Proceedings Part I. Vol 25, No. 18S (June 20 Supplement), 2007; 4038

Hurwitz H, Fehrenbacher L, Novotny W. Bevacizumab plus Irinotecan, Fluorouracil, and Leucovorin for Metastatic Colorectal Cancer. *N Engl J Med* 2004; im350(23) 2335–2342

Jones P. DNA methylation and cancer. Presented at: *Breakthroughs in Therapeutic Epigenetics: An Emerging Clinical Approach,* symposium held in conjunction with the 41st Annual Meeting of the American Society of Clinical Oncology, Orlando, FL, May 2005

Jonker DJ, O'Callaghan CJ, Karapetis CS, et al. Cetuximab for the Treatment of Colorectal Cancer. *N Engl J Med* 2007; 357 2040–2048

Kabbinavar FF, Schulz J, McCleod M, et al. Addition of Bevacizumab to Bolus Fluorouracil and Leucovorin in First-Line Metastatic Colorectal Cancer: Results of a Randomized Phase II Trial. *J Clin Oncol* 2005; 23(16) 3697–3705

Kamba T, McDonald DM. Mechanisms of Adverse Effects of Anti-VEGF Therapy for Cancer. *Br J Cancer* 2007; 96 1788–1795

Keating M, Byrd J, Rai K, Multicenter Study of Campath-1H in Patients with CLL Refractory to Fludarabine. *Blood* 1999; 94 3118 (abstract)

Keefe DL. Trastuzumab-associated Cardiotoxicity. *Cancer* 2002; 95(7) 1592–1600

Kemple SN. *The proteasome: A novel target in multiple myeloma.* Cambridge, MA: Millennium Pharma; 2003

Kobayashi S, Kishimoto T, Kamata S, Otsuka M, Miyazaki M, Ishikura H. Rapamycin, a Specific Inhibitor of the Mammalian Target of Rapamycin, Suppresses Lymphangiogenesis and Lymphatic Metastasis. *Cancer Sci* 2007; 98 726–733

Lacouture ME. Mechanisms of Cutaneous Toxicities to EGFR Inhibitors. *Nat Rev Cancer* 2006; 6 803–812

Lacouture ME, Basti S, Patel J, Benson A. The SERIES Clinic: An Interdisciplinary Approach to the Management of Toxicities of EGFR Inhibitors. *J Support Oncol* 2006; 4 236–238

Lacouture ME, Lai SE. The PRIDE (Papulopustules And/Or Paronychia, Regulatory Abnormalities of Hair Growth, Itching and Dryness Due to Epidermal Growth Factor Receptor Inhibitors) Syndrome. *Br J Dermatol* 2006; 155 852–854

Lancet JE, Gotlib J, Gojo I. Tipifarnib (ZARNESTRA™) in Previously Untreated Poor-Risk AML of the Elderly: Updated Results of a Multicenter Phase 2 Trial. *Blood (ASH Annual Meeting Abstracts)*, November 2004; 104 874

Levy C. Detect and Manage Adverse Events Associated With Ipilimumab. *Targeted and Biological Therapies SIG Newsletter* May 2007. Accessed 14 July, 2008, at http://onsopcontent.ons.org/Publications/SIGNewsletters/tbt/tbt18.1.html

Li F. Angiogenesis. The Angiogenesis Foundation. 2000; (http://www.angioorg)

Liekens S, DeClercq E, Neyts J. Angiogenesis: Regulators and Clinical Applications. *Biochem Pharmacol* 2001; 61(3) 253–270

Linderholm B, Grankvist K, Wilking N. Correlation of Vascular Endothelial Growth Factor Content with Recurrences, Survival, and First Relapse Site in Primary Node-positive Breast Carcinoma after Adjuvant Treatment. *J Clin Oncology* 2000; 18 1423–1431

Lippman ME. New Approaches to the Treatment of Breast Cancer in the Next Century. *Clinical Dialogues in Oncology*, Kingston, NJ: Medicom; 2000

List A, Kurtin S, Roe DJ. Efficacy of Lenalidomide in Myelodysplastic Syndromes. *N Eng J Med* 2005; 352 549–557

Liu ET. Tumor Suppressor Genes: Changing Concepts. ASCO Educational Book. 35th Annual Meeting, Atlanta, GA: 1999

Llovet J, Ricci R, Mazzaferro V. Sorafinib Improves Survival in Advanced Hepatocellular Carcinoma (HCC): Results of a Phase III Randomized, Placebo-Controlled Trial (SHARP Trial). *J Clin Oncol* 2007 ASCO Annual Meeting Proceedings Part I; 25(18S) LBA1

Lundin J, Kimby E, Bjorkholm M, Phase II Trial of Subcutaneous Anti-CD52 Monoclonal Antibody Alemtuzumab (Campath-1H) as First-Line Treatment for Patients With B-Cell Chronic Lymphocytic Leukemia (B-CLL). *Blood* 2002; 100(3) 768–773

Lynch TJ, Bell DW, Sordella R. Activating Mutations in the Epidermal Growth Factor Receptor Underlying Responsiveness of Non-Small-Cell Lung Cancer to Gefitinib. *N Eng J Med* 2004; 350(21) 2129–2139

Lynch TJ, Kim ES, Eaby B, Garey J, West DP, Lacouture ME. Epidermal Growth Factor Receptor Inhibitor-Associated Cutaneous Toxicities: An Evolving Paradigm in Clinical Management. *The Oncologist* 2007; 12(5) 610–621

Mancuso MR, Davis R, Norberg SM. Rapid Vascular Regrowth in Tumors After Reversal of VEGF Inhibition. *J Clin Invest* 2006; 116 2610–2621

Marks PA, Richon VM, Miller T. Histone deacetylase inhibitors. *Adv Cancer Res* 2004; 91 137–168

Mavragani CP, Vlachoyiannopoulos PG, Kosmas N, et al. A Case of Reversible Posterior Leucoencephalopathy Syndrome After Rituximab Infusion: Letter to the Editor. *Rheumatology* 2004; 43(11) 1450–1451

McMahon G. VEGF Receptor Signaling in Tumor Angiogenesis. *The Oncologist* 2000; 5(suppl 1) 3–10

McMahon LP, Choi KM, Lin TA, Abraham RT, Lawrence JC Jr. The Rapamycin-Binding Domain Governs Substrate Selectivity by the Mammalian Target of Rapamycin. *Mol Cell Biol* 2002; 22 7428–7438

Merkle CJ, Loescher LJ. The Biology of Cancer. In Yarbro CH Frogge MH Goodman M *Cancer Nursing: Principles and Practice*, 6th ed. Sudbury, MA: Jones and Bartlett Publishers; 2005; 15

Miller KD, Wang M, Gralow J. E2100: A Randomized, Phase III trial of Paclitaxel Compared with Bevacizumab and Paclitaxel as First Line Therapy for Locally Recurrent or Metastatic Breast Cancer. Paper presented at 41st Annual Meeting of the American Society of Clinical Oncology, May 13–17, 2005; Orlando FL, available at http://www.asco.org. Accessed 11 June 2007

Molinari E, De Quatrebarbes J, Andre T, Aractingi S. Cetuximab-Induced Acne. *Dermatology* 2005; 211(4) 330–333

Motzer RJ, Rini BL, Michaelson MD. SU 11248, a Novel Tyrosine Kinase Inhibitor, Shows Antitumor Activity in Second-Line Therapy for Patients with Metastatic Renal Cell Carcinoma: Results of a Phase II Trial. *Proc Am Soc Clin Oncol* 2004; 23 381, abstract 4500

Motzer RJ, Escudier B, Oudard S, et al. RAD001 Vs Placebo in Patients With Metastatic Renal Cell Carcinoma(RCC) After Progression on VEGFr-TKI Therapy: Results From a Randomized, Double-Blind, Multi-Center Phase III Study. *J Clin Oncol* 2008; 26 (May 20 suppl; abstr LBA5026)

Muller A, Homey B, Soto H. Involvement of Chemokine Receptors in Breast Cancer Metastases. *Nature* 2001; 410 50–56

Murray JL, Witzig TE, Wiseman GA. Zevalin Therapy Can Convert Peripheral Blood bcl-2 Status from Positive to Negative in Patients with Low-grade, Follicular or Transformed Non-Hodgkin's Lymphoma (NHL). *Proc ASCO 2000* 19 22a (77) New Orleans, LA: May 20–23, 2000

National Cancer Comprehensive Network (NCCN). Clinical Practice Guidelines in Colon Cancer, Rectal Cancer, Version 2, 2007, http://www.nccn.org. Accessed 30 June, 2007

National Cancer Institute. *Histone Deacetylase Inhibitors. Also Everolimus*. Available at http://cancer.gov/clinicaltrials. Accessed 11 June 2007

Niu G, Carter WB. Human Epidermal Growth Factor Receptor 2 Regulates Angiopoietin-2 Expression in Breast Cancer Via AKT and Mitogen-Activated Protein Kinase Pathways. *Cancer Res* 2007; 67 1487–1493

O'Keefe P, Parrilli M, Lacouture ME. Toxicity of Targeted Therapy: Focus on Rash and Other Dermatologic Side Effects. *ONCOLOGY Nurse Ed* 2006(Suppl 13) 1–6

O'Shaughnessy J, et al. A Randomized Study of Lapatinib +/– Trastuzumab in Patients With Heavily Pretreated HER2+ Metastatic Breast Cancer Progressing on Trastuzumab Therapy. *J Clin Oncol* 2008; 26 (May 20 suppl; abstr 1015)

Paik S, Bryant J, Tan-Chiu E, et al. Real-World Performance of HER2 Testing: National Surgical Adjuvant Breast and Bowel Project Experience. *J Natl Cancer Inst* 2002; 94 852–854

Pao W, Miller VA, Politi KA. Acquired Resistance of Lung Adenocarcinomas to Gefitinib or Erlotinib Is Associated with a Second Mutation in the EGFR Kinase Domain. *PLoS Medicine* 2005; 2(3) 225–235, http://www.plosmedicine.org. Accessed 11 June 2007

Perez EA. Interim Cardiac Safety Analysis of NCCTG N9831. *Proc Am Soc Clin Oncol* 2005; Scientific Session presented May 16, 2005, 41st Am Soc Clin Oncol Meeting, Orlando, FL

Pestell Cyclin D1 Nullifies BRCA1' Tumor Suppressive Function. *Cancer Res* 2005; 65 6557–6566

Piccart-Gebhart MJ. First Results of the HERA Trial. *Proc Am Soc Clin Oncol* 2005; Scientific Session presented May 16, 2005, 41st Am Soc Clin Oncol Meeting, Orlando, FL

Piccart-Gebhart MJ, Procter M, Leyland-Jones B, et al. Trastuzumab After Adjuvant Chemotherapy in HER2-Positive Breast Cancer. *N Engl J Med* 2005; 353(16) 1659–1672

Pirker R, Szczesna A, von Pawel J, et al. A Randomized, Multi-Center, Phase III Study of Cetuximab in Combination With Cisplatin/Vinorelbine (CV) Versus CV Alone in the First-Line Treatment of Patients With Advanced Non-Small Cell Lung Cancer (NSCLC). Presented at the 44th American Society of Clinical Oncology Annual Meeting. May 30–June 3, 2008. Chicago, IL.

Popat S, Smith IE. Therapy Insight: Anthracyclines and Trastuzumab: The Optimal Management of Cardiotoxic Side Effects. *Nat Clin Pract Oncol* 2008; 5(6) 324–335

Porzio G, Aielli F, Verna L, Efficacy of Pregabalin in the Management of Cetuximab-Related Itch. *J Pain Symptom Manage* 2006; 32(5) 397–398

Prince G, Bali P, Annavarapu S. LBH589 and 17-AGG Are Highly Active Against Human CML-BC and AML cells. *Blood* 2005; 105(4) 1768–1776

Punt CJ, Nagy A, Douillard JY. Edrecolomab Alone or in Combination with Fluorouracil and Folinic Acid in the Adjuvant Treatment of Stage III Colon Cancer: A Randomized Study. *Lancet* 2002; 360 671–677

Raponi M, Lowenberg R, Lancet JE. Identification of Molecular Predictors of Response to ZARNESTRA™ (Tipifarnib, R115777) in Relapsed and Refractory Acute Myeloid Leukemia. *Blood* (ASH Annual Meeting Abstracts) November, 2004; 104 861

Reidy DL, Chung KY, Imoney JP, et al. Bevacizumab 5 mg/kg Can Be Infused Safely Over 10 Minutes. *J Clin Oncol* 2007; 28(19) 2691–2695

Robert F, Ezekiel MP, Spencer SA. Phase I Study of Anti-epidermal Growth Factor Receptor Antibody Cetuximab in Combination with Radiation Therapy in Patients with Advanced Head and Neck Cancer. *J Clin Oncol* 2001; 19(13) 3234–3243

Romond EH, Perez EA, Bryant J, et al. Trastuzumab Plus Adjuvant Chemotherapy for Operable HER2-Positive Breast Cancer. *N Engl J Med* 2005; 353(16) 1673–1684

Rowinsky EK, Schwartz GH, Gollob JA. Safety, Pharmakinetics, and Activity of ABX-EGF, a Fully Human Anti-epidermal Growth Factor Receptor Monoclonal Antibody in Patients with Metastatic Renal Cell Cancer. *J Clin Onco* 2004; 22(15) 3003–3015

Rowinsky EK, Windle JJ, Von Hoff DD. Ras Protein Farnesyltransferase: A Strategic Target for Anticancer Therapeutic Development. *J Clin Oncol* 1999; 17(11) 3631–3652

Ruoslahti E. How Cancer Spreads. *Scientific American (Sept 1996)*. 1996; 275(3) 72–77

Ruoslahti E, Reed JC. Anchorage Dependence, Integrins, and Apoptosis. *Cell* 1994; 77(4) 477–478

Sandler AB, Blumenschein GR, Henderson T. Phase I/II Trial Evaluating the Anti-VEGF MAb Bevacizumab in Combination with Erlotinib, a HER1/EGFR-TK Inhibitor, for Patients with Recurrent Non-small Cell Lung Cancer. 2004 ASCO Annual Meeting Proceedings, Post Meeting Edition. *J Clin Oncol* 2004; 22(14S) 2000

Sandler AB, Gray R, Bhramer J. Randomized Phase II/III Trial of Paclitaxel (P) Plus Carboplatin with or without Bevacizumab (NSC 704865) in Patients with Advanced Non-Squamous Non-small Cell Lung Cancer: An Eastern Cooperative Oncology Group (ECOG) Trial-E4599. *Proc Am Soc Clin Oncol* 2005; abstract LBA4

Sausville EA. Cyclin Dependent Kinases: Novel Targets for Cancer Development. ASCO 1999 Educational Book 35th Annual Meeting, Atlanta: 1999

Scandella E, Ludewig B. Dendridic Cells and Autoimmunity. *Transfusion Medicine and Hemotherapy* 2005; 32(6) 363–368.

Schlom J, Gulley JL, Arlen PM. Paradigm Shifts in Vaccine Therapy. *Exp Biol Med* 2008; 233(5) 522–534

Schottenfeld D, Beebe-Dimmer J. Chronic Inflammation: A Common and Important Factor in the Pathogenesis of Neoplasia. *CA Cancer J Clin* 2006; 56 69–83

Schrag D, Chung KY, Flombaum C, Saltz L. Cetuximab Therapy and Symptomatic Hypomagnesemia. *J Natl Cancer Inst* 97(16) 1221–1224

Segaert S, Van Cutsem E. Clinical Management of EGFRI Dermatological Toxicities: The European Perspective. *Oncology* (Williston Park) 2007; 21(11 Suppl 5) 22–26

Segaert S, Van Cutsem E. Clinical Signs, Pathophysiology and Management of Skin Toxicity During Therapy with Epidermal Growth Factor Receptor Inhibitors. *Ann Oncol* 2005; 16 1425–1433

Semenza GL. Targeting HIF-1 for Cancer Therapy. *Nat Rev Cancer* 2003; 3 721–731

Shaw RJ, Cantley LC. Ras, PI(3)K and mTOR Signaling Controls Tumour Cell Growth. *Nature* 2006; 441 424–430

Shaw RJ. Glucose Metabolism in Cancer. *Curr Opin Cell Biol* 2006; 18 598–608

Siegel JA. Revised Nuclear Regulatory Commission Regulation for Release of Patients Administered Radioactive Materials: Outpatient Iodine-131 Anti-B1 Therapy. *J Nucl Med* 1998; 39(8) 285–335

Slamon D, Eiermann W, Robert N, et al. BCIRG 006: 2nd Interim Analysis Phase III Randomized Trial Comparing Doxorubicin and Cyclophosphamide Followed by Docetaxel (AC∅T) With Doxorubicin and Cyclophosphamide Followed by Docetaxel and Trastuzumab (AC∅TH) With Docetaxel, Carboplatin and Trastuzumab (TCH) in Her2neu Positive Early Breast Cancer Patients. Paper presented at: 29th Annual San Antonio Breast Cancer Symposium; December 14–17, 2006; San Antonio, TX. Abstract 52. Available at http://www.abstracts2view.com/sabcs06/view.php?nu=SABCS06L_78. Accessed June 21, 2008

Stendahl M, Kronblad A, Ryden L. Cyclin D1 Overexpression Is a Negative Predictive Factor for Tamoxifen Response in Postmenopausal Breast Cancer Patients. *Br J of Cancer* 2004; 90 1942–1948

Stetler-Stevenson WG, Kleiner DE. Molecular Biology of Cancer: Invasion and Metastases. In DeVita VT Hellman S Rosenberg SA. *Principles and Practice of Oncology*, 6th ed. Philadelphia, PA: Lippincott Williams and Wilkins; 2001: 123–137

Takahashi H, Shibuy M. The Vascular Endothelial Growth Factor (VEGF)/VEGF Receptor System and Its Role Under Physiologic and Pathologic Conditions. *Clin Sci* 2005; 109 227–241

Tan-Chiu E, Yothers G, Romond E, et al. Assessment of Cardiac Dysfunction in a Randomized Trial Comparing Doxorubicin and Cyclophosphamide Followed by Paclitaxel, With or Without Trastuzumab as Adjuvant Therapy in Node-Positive, Human Epidermal Growth Factor Receptor 2-Overexpressing Breast Cancer: NSABP B-31. *J Clin Oncol* 2005; 23 7811–7819

Tasigna package insert. East Hanover, NJ: Novartis Pharmaceuticals Corporation, October 2007

Tejpar S, Peeters M, Humblet Y, et al. Relationship of Efficacy With KRAS Status (Wild Type Versus Mutant) in Patients With Irinotecan-Refractory Metastatic Colorectal Cancer (mCRC), Treated With Irinotecan (q2 wk) and Escalating Doses of Cetuximab (q 1 wk): The EVEREST Experience (Preliminary Data). *J Clin Oncol* 2008; 26 (May 20 suppl: abstract 4001)

Van Cutsem E, Lang I, D'haens G, et al. KRAS Status and Efficacy in the First-Line Treatment of Patients With Metastatic Colorectal Cancer (mCRC) Treated With FOLFIRI With or Without Cetuximab: The CRYSTAL Experience. *J Clin Oncol* 2008; 26 (May 20 suppl: abstr 2)

von Eschenbach keynote presentation: Summit series on cancer clinical trials. Executive Summary VIII: Retooling the System: Implementing Solutions. September 29–October 1, 2003

Vose J, Saleh M, Lister A. Iodine-131 Anti-B1 Antibody for Non-Hodgkin's Lymphoma (NHL): Overall Clinical Trial Experience. *Proc Am Soc Clin Oncol* 1998; 17 38, abstract 38

Wagner LI. Psychological Impact and Quality of Life Issues Associated with Therapy-Induced Rash. Presentation ONS Ancillary Event April 25, 2007, Las Vegas, NV

Wahl RL, Tidmarsh G, Krolls. Successful Retreatment of Non-Hodgkin's Lymphoma (NHL) with Iodine-131 Anti-B1 Antibody. *Proc Am Soc Clin Oncol* 1998; 17 40, abstract 156

Walker S, Lacouture ME. Wall Chart Featuring Skin-Related Toxicities of Targeted Therapies. *Oncology* 2006; 20(suppl 7)

Weber J. Review: Anti-CTLA-4 Antibody Ipilimumab: Case Studies of Clinical Response and Immune-Related Adverse Events. *Oncologist* 2007; 12 864–872

Weber JS, Berman D, Siegel J, et al. Safety and Efficacy of Ipilimumab With or Without Prophylactic Budesonide in Treatment-Naïve Previously Treated Patients With Advanced Melanoma. *J Clin Oncol* 2008; 26 2008 (May 20 suppl; abstr 9010)

Weidner N. Tumoral Vascularity as a Prognostic Factor in Cancer Patients: The Evidence Continues to Grow. *J Pathol* 1998; 184 119–120

Weinberg RA. Fundamental Understandings: How Cancer Arises. *Scientific American*. Sept 1996; 275(3) 62–72

Weinberg RA. *The Biology of Cancer*. London, UK: Garland Science. Taylor and Francis Group LLC; 2007

Weiner LM. Phase 1 Open-Label Dose Escalation Trial, poster presented at the 41st Annual American Society of Clinical Oncologists (ASCO), Orlando, FL, May 2005, abstract K4, 3509

Widakowich C, De Castro G, Azanbuja E, Dinh P, Awada A. Review: Side effects of Approved Molecular Targeted Therapies in Solid Cancers. *Oncologist* 2007; 12 1443–1455

Wilkes G. Maximizing Treatment Benefit for Colorectal Cancer Patients Through Evidence-Based Toxicity Management Strategies: Focus on Skin Toxicity and Peripheral Neuropathy. *Colorectal Cancer Nurs Index Rev* 2007; 1(1) 4–6

Wilkes GM, Barton-Burke M. *Oncology Nursing Drug Handbook*. Sudbury, MA: Jones and Bartlett; 2008

Williamson TS. Alemtuzumab. *Clin J Oncol Nurs* 2001; 5(6) 287–288

Wiseman GA, Leigh BR, Gordon LI. Zevalin Radioimmunotherapy (RIT) for B-Cell Non-Hodgkin's Lymphoma (NHL): Biodistribution and Dosimetry Result. *Proc ASCO 2000* 19 10a (29) New Orleans, LA: May 20–23, 2000

Wong CW, Lee A, Shientag L. Apoptosis: An Early Event in Metastatic Inefficiency. *Cancer Res* 2001; 61(1) 333–338

Wood LS. Managing the Side Effects of Sorafenib and Sunitinib. *Commun Oncol* 2006; 3(9) 558–562

Wyeth-Ayerst Laboratories. Antibody-Targeted Chemotherapy: Coming of Age. Philadelphia, PA: Wyeth-Ayerest Laboratories; 1999

Zachariae R, Zachariae C, Ibsen HHW, Psychological Symptoms and Quality of Life of Dermatology Outpatients and Hospitalized Dermatology Patients. *Acta Dermatol-Venereol* 2003; 84(3) 205–212

Drug: alemtuzumab (campath-1H anti-CD52 Monoclonal Antibody, Humanized IgG1 MoAb)

Class: Monoclonal antibody.

Mechanism of Action: Humanized monoclonal antibody, which targets the CD52 antigen present on the surface of most normal human lymphocyte cells, as well as malignant T-cell and B-cell malignant lymphocytes (lymphomas). Once the monoclonal antibody binds with the CD52 antigen, it initiates antibody dependent cellular cytotoxicity

(ADCC) and complement binding, which then lead to apoptosis, or programmed cell death, and activation of normal T-cell cytotoxicity against the malignant cells.

Metabolism: When given subcutaneously or intravenously, pharmacokinetics appears similar, but the absorption is much slower with subcutaneous administration. It takes a higher cumulative dose (an additional 6 weeks) to achieve a therapeutic level. The mean half-life is 11 hours after the first 30-mg dose, but steady-state plasma levels are not reached until week 6. Levels appear to correlate with the number of circulating CD52-positive cells. Drug clearance decreases with repeated dosing as more leukemic cells are killed. Given subcutaneously, CLL cells were cleared from the blood in 95% of patients in a median time of 21 days (Lundin et al, 2002). Host antibodies may develop 14–21 days after the first dose and theoretically can decrease lymphocyte killing.

Drug Preparation:
- Available in single use vials containing 30 mg alemtuzumab in 1 mL of diluent. Draw up ordered dose, and dilute in 100 mL sterile 0.9% sodium chloride USP or 5% dextrose in water. Gently invert IV bag to mix. Use within 8 hours. Store at room temperature or refrigerated.

Dosage/Range:
- Initial dose is 3 mg IV infusion over 2 hours, daily, with dose escalated to 10 mg daily when well tolerated (side effects are grade 2 or less)
- When dose of 10 mg is well tolerated, the dose is increased to 30 mg and becomes the maintenance dose given three times a week (e.g., Monday, Wednesday, and Friday) for up to 12 weeks. Dose escalation to 30 mg usually takes 3–7 days.
- Subcutaneous administration is better tolerated and results in similar efficacy (Lundin et al, 2002).

Drug Administration:
- Stop drug immediately if a reaction develops during the infusion.
- Premedicate with acetaminophen 650 mg and diphenhydramine 50 mg 30 min prior to beginning infusion. Severe reactions may require hydrocortisone 200 mg. If drug requires slower infusion, repeat premedications at 4 hours.
- Subsequent dosing: 30 mg IV over 2 h 3-times-a-week, for a minimum of 4 weeks, but may continue up to 12 weeks. Give on Monday, Wednesday, and Friday.
- If dose held more than 7 days, reinstitute gradually with dose escalation.
- Give IV hydration (at least 500 mL D5W or 0.9% NS) before and after drug dose (Williamson, 2001).
- Anti-infective prophylaxis recommended, starting on day 8 and continuing for 2 months after treatment completed or stopped, or CD4 count ≥ 200 cells/μL, e.g., with trimethoprim and sulfamethoxazole (Bactrim) DS/twice a day, three times weekly, an antiviral such as famciclovir 250 mg twice daily, and an antifungal, such as fluconazole. Stop the drug immediately if a serious infection occurs.
- Monitor CBC/differential weekly; dose reduce ANC < 250/μL and /or platelet count ≤ 25,000/μL. See package insert.

Drug Interactions:

- Unknown.

Lab Effects/Interference:

- An immune response to the drug may interfere with subsequent serum laboratory tests using antibodies.
- Decreased WBC, lymphocyte, red blood cell, and platelet counts.

Special Considerations:

- Indicated for the treatment of B-cell chronic lymphocytic leukemia (B-CLL) in patients who have received alkylating agents and failed fludarabine.
- The drug may cause serious infusion reactions, including adult respiratory distress syndrome, cardiopulmonary arrest, and death. The drug must be gradually increased at the initiation of therapy or if therapy is interrupted for 7 or more days.
- Patients who have received multiple courses of chemotherapy prior to campath-1H are at increased risk for bacterial, viral, and other opportunistic infections.
- Immunosuppression related to drug may reactivate herpes simplex infections, septicemia.
- Subcutaneous and intravenous have similar efficacy and effect.
- Following 3-times-a-week therapy, destruction of CLL cells takes about 14 days before being removed from the peripheral blood, with no cells detectable at 5 weeks (Solimandro et al, 2000). Bone marrow clearance takes 6–12 weeks, and bulky lymphadenopathy takes considerably longer.
- Is being studied in the treatment of chronic lymphocytic leukemia, low-grade lymphoma, graft-versus-host disease, multiple sclerosis, and rheumatoid arthritis.

Potential Toxicities/Side Effects (Dose- and Schedule-Dependent) and the Nursing Process

I. POTENTIAL FOR INJURY related to HYPERSENSITIVITY REACTION DURING INFUSION

Defining Characteristics: Infusion reactions are common and require premedication to prevent them. Hypotension occurs in 15%, rash in 30%, nausea in 47%, vomiting in 33%, drug-related fever 83%, and rigors in 89% of patients. Infusion reactions usually resolve after 1 week of therapy. Subcutaneous dosing significantly reduces the risk of allergic reactions.

Nursing Implications: Assess vital signs baseline and frequently during infusion, especially during dose escalation. Teach patient that reactions may occur and to tell nurse or physician immediately. Administer premedication as ordered, usually acetaminophen and diphenhydramine. Provide adequate hydration, as this seems to decrease the incidence of infusion reactions (e.g., at least 500 mL before and after dose). Dose is begun low at 3 mg, then gradually increased based on patient tolerance to 10-mg dose, then to a 30-mg dose. If the patient has a treatment break of seven days or more, then it is necessary to reintroduce drug at the lower dose and gradually escalate dose. If reaction happens, stop infusion but keep main IV line open, notify physician, and, if rigors, give meperidine and any other medications ordered by physician. Expect reaction to resolve in 20 minutes or so, and gradually resume infusion per physician order. Assess skin for integrity and presence of rash. Teach patient to report this, and discuss management with physician. Teach patient that nausea may develop, and to report it right away. Discuss antiemetic agent with physician, and administer as ordered.

II. POTENTIAL FOR INFECTION AND BLEEDING related to BONE MARROW DEPRESSION

Defining Characteristics: All patients develop leukopenia, with approximately 85% of patients developing neutropenia. There is a dramatic fall in WBC during the first week. As both T and B cell lymphocytes are injured, patients are at an increased risk for bacterial, viral, and other opportunistic infections. Most patients require prophylactic antimicrobials with/without antiviral therapy, especially heavily pretreated patients. Most common pulmonary infections are opportunistic: *Pneumocystis carinii* pneumonia, cytomegalus virus (CMV) pneumonia, and pulmonary aspergillosis. Commonly, there is reactivation of herpes simplex infections and development of oral candidiasis. Thrombocytopenia affects 72%, with platelet recovery weeks 7 to 12. Incidence of anemia is 80%. Rarely, pancytopenia, and marrow aplasia occurs and may be fatal.

Nursing Implications: Assess baseline leukocyte, platelet, and Hgb/HCT and monitor before each treatment, during therapy, and more often as needed. Hold drug for ANC $< 250/\mu L$ or platelets $\leq 25,000/\mu L$. See package insert for dose modifications. Assess risk for infection and integrity of skin and mucous membranes, pulmonary status, and ability to clear secretions, as well as history of past infections, baseline and prior to each treatment. Teach patient to self-administer prophylactic antibiotics, antiviral, and antifungal agents as ordered by physician. Ensure that patient has coverage or can purchase antimicrobial medications. Teach patient to self-administer oral antifungal agent if oral candidiasis develops. Teach patient to self-assess for signs/symptoms of infection, and to call provider immediately or come to the emergency room if temperature > 100.5°F, shaking chills, or rash, productive cough, burning on urination, or any signs/symptoms of infection or bleeding. Teach self-care strategies to minimize risk of infection and bleeding, including avoidance of OTC aspirin-containing medications.

III. ALTERATION IN COMFORT related to PAIN, ASTHENIA, PERIPHERAL EDEMA, HEADACHE, DYSTHESIAS, DIZZINESS

Defining Characteristics: Pain is common, and in clinical studies 24% of patients experienced skeletal pain, 13% asthenia, 13% peripheral edema, 10% back or chest pain, 9% malaise, 24% headache, 15% dysthesias, and 12% dizziness.

Nursing Implications: Assess comfort and presence of peripheral edema, baseline and prior to each treatment. Teach patient that these side effects may occur and to report them. Teach patient local comfort measures, and discuss management plan with physician if ineffective.

IV. ALTERATION IN OXYGENATION, POTENTIAL, related to HYPOTENSION, HYPERTENSION, TACHYCARDIA

Defining Characteristics: Hypotension is common, affecting 32% of patients in clinical studies, while 11% had hypertension. 11% of patients also had sinus or supraventricular tachycardia.

Nursing Implications: Assess baseline cardiac status, including blood pressure and heart rate, noting rhythm and rate. Assess past medical history for arrhythmia, hypertension. If heart rate irregular, document rhythm on EKG, monitor blood pressure for evidence of decompensation, and discuss management with physician. If hypertension noted, discuss management with physician. If hypotension noted, assess patient tolerance and need for intervention; discuss management with physician.

Drug: alitretinoin gel 0.1% (Panretin®)

Class: Retinoid.

Mechanism of Action: A9-*cis*-retinoic acid, alitretinoin is a naturally occurring, endogenous retinoid necessary for regulation of gene expression responsible for cell differentiation and replication. 9-*cis*-retinoic acid binds to and activates intracellular retinoid receptors that enable transcription of these genes. Alitretinoin has been found to inhibit the growth of Kaposi's sarcoma (KS) cells directly.

Metabolism: Drug is used topically, without any detectable plasma concentrations or metabolites.

Dosage/Range:
- Sufficient gel applied to cover the lesion with "generous" coating.
- Available in 60-gram tube.

Drug Preparation:
- None.
- Gel tube should be stored at room temperature.

Drug Administration:
- Use glove to apply generous coating of gel to lesions bid, avoiding surrounding skin.
- DO NOT APPLY on or near mucosal surfaces.
- Allow to dry for 3–5 minutes before covering with clothing.

- Gradually increase applications to 3–4 per day.
- If severe skin irritation develops, stop application for a few days until irritation resolves.
- DO NOT USE an occlusive dressing over gel.

Drug Interactions:
- DEET (*N*, *N*-diethyl-*m*-toluamide) insect repellent or products containing DEET, as gel increases DEET toxicity.
- No testing has been done to assess possible interactions between systemic antiretroviral agents, or other agents used in the systemic management of HIV infection.

Lab Effects/Interference:
- None known.

Special Considerations:
- Responses may be seen in 2 weeks, but most often take longer, rarely 14 weeks. Gel should be used as long as there is clinical benefit.
- Indicated for TOPICAL treatment of cutaneous KS lesions in patients with AIDS. It should not be used when systemic therapy for KS is necessary (> 10 KS lesions in prior month, or symptomatic lymphedema, pulmonary KS, or visceral involvement).
- Contraindicated in patients having hypersensitivity to retinoids.
- Women of childbearing age should use contraception to prevent pregnancy, as it is unknown whether topical gel can modulate endogenous 9-*cis*-retinoic levels. 9-*Cis*-retinoic acid is teratogenic.
- Drug SHOULD NOT BE USED by nursing mothers; mothers must discontinue nursing prior to using the drug.
- Drug may increase photosensitivity, so patients should be taught to AVOID sunlamps and to minimize sunlight exposure.
- Safety testing has not been done in pediatric or geriatric (> 65 yr) populations.
- Toxicity almost exclusively related to skin reactions at the application site.

Potential Toxicities/Side Effects and the Nursing Process

I. ALTERATION IN COMFORT AND SKIN INTEGRITY, POTENTIAL, related to APPLICATION SITE REACTIONS

Defining Characteristics: Toxicity begins as erythema. This may increase, and edema may develop with continued application. Most of reactions are mild to moderate, but in some patients (10%), severe reactions may occur with intense erythema, edema, and formation of vesicles. Other skin reactions occurring in > 5% of patients are rash, pain, pruritus, exfoliative dermatitis, cracking, crusting, drainage, oozing, stinging, or tingling.

Nursing Implications: Assess baseline skin integrity and condition of KS cutaneous lesions. Teach patient to apply gel only to lesions and AVOID surrounding skin, as irritation will occur. Teach patient to assess and report any changes in the lesions, such as erythema, and edema. Teach patient to reduce frequency of application if skin reaction occurs, to stop use of the gel if severe reactions occur, and to report this as soon as possible.

Drug: axitinib (AG-013736, investigational)

Class: Angiogenesis inhibitor (VEGFRs inhibitor).

Mechanism of Action: Potent, and selective inhibitor of vascular endothelial growth factor receptors 1, 2, 3 on the endothelial cells lining blood vessels, as well as platelet derived growth factor (PDGFR)-β and cKIT (CD117). VEGFR inhibition prevents the blood vessel from sending capillary tubes to the tumor so angiogenesis does not occur.

Metabolism:
- Unknown.

Dosage/Range:
- Per protocol (e.g., starting dose 5 mg PO bid).

Drug Preparation:
- None, oral.

Drug Administration:
- Oral, per protocol.

Drug Interactions:
- Unknown.

Lab Effects/Interference:
- Decreased soluble VEGFR-2 and VEGFR-3 and increased VEGF in blood.

Special Considerations:
- Most common toxicities were fatigue (62.5%), hypertension (43.8%), hoarseness (34.4%), diarrhea (31.3%). Bowel perforation may occur.
- Interestingly, in this study of 32 patients with stage IV melanoma, those with diastolic elevation > 90 mm Hg had a median OS of 13.0 mo compared with 6.2 mo in patients with diastolic BP < 90 mm Hg (Fruehauf et al, 2008).
- Drug is being studied in patients with metastatic melanoma, metastatic renal cell cancer, NSCLC, pancreatic, breast, colorectal and thyroid cancers, alone or in combination with chemotherapy.
- Drug can cause hoarseness: assess impact on patient, communication ability, and need for assistance.

Potential Toxicities/Side Effects and the Nursing Process

I. ALTERATION IN COMFORT AND ACTIVITY INTOLERANCE, POTENTIAL, related to FATIGUE

Defining Characteristics: Fatigue occurs in 62% of patients with metastatic melanoma receiving axitinib.

Nursing Implications: Assess comfort and presence of discomfort, fatigue, inability to do ADLs baseline and before each treatment. Teach patient that these side effects may occur and to report them. Teach patient local comfort measures as well as energy conservation, calling in other members of the family to assist with performing energy draining functions, and discuss management plan with physician if ineffective.

II. POTENTIAL ALTERATION IN CIRCULATION related to HYPERTENSION

Defining Characteristics: Axitinib increases the incidence and severity of hypertension, a class effect of all angiogenesis inhibitors believed caused by the influence of VEGF on nitric oxide and blood vessel dilation. Overall incidence of hypertension was 60%, with 12% grade 3/4. Patients who had diastolic hypertension had higher median overall survival.

Nursing Implications: Assess baseline BP prior to and during treatment, at least for the first treatment and then prior to each drug administration. If the patient has a history of hypertension, monitor BP more closely, although hypertension develops over time rather than during the drug infusion. Blood pressure should continue to be monitored after patient has stopped the drug. Teach patient drug administration, potential side effects, and self-care measures if prescribed antihypertensive medication, such as angiotensin-converting enzyme inhibitors, beta-blockers, diuretics, and calcium-channel blockers. Drug should be permanently discontinued if the patient develops hypertensive crisis (diastolic blood pressure > 120 mm Hg). Drug can be temporarily suspended in patients with severe hypertension until BP can be controlled with medical management.

III. ALTERATION IN NUTRITION, LESS THAN BODY REQUIREMENTS, related to DIARRHEA

Defining Characteristics: 34.4% of patients in clinical studies developed diarrhea.

Nursing Implications: Assess baseline weight, nutritional status, elimination status, and monitor at each visit. Teach patient that these side effects may occur and to report them. Develop symptom management plan, including dietary modification, increased fluids, self-administration of antidiarrheal medicines, and to call if diarrhea persists > 24 hours.

Drug: bevacizumab (Avastin)

Class: Recombinant humanized Monoclonal Antibody targeted against Vascular Endothelial Growth Factor (VEGF); Angiogenesis inhibitor.

Mechanism of Action: VEGF binds to receptors on endothelial cells, turning on the cell surface receptors KDR and Flt-1, which then function as tyrosine kinases sending the message to the cells to proliferate and migrate. This leads to the establishment of new blood vessels (neovascularization) in tumors. Studies show that tumors that express VEGF tend to be more aggressive, more invasive, and more likely to metastasize. Bevacizumab binds to all human forms of VEGF-A, thus preventing it from binding to its receptors on the endothelial cells. This theoretically prevents one step in the process of angiogenesis from occurring. In addition, it appears that VEGF is necessary to maintain existing tumor blood vessels, and when blocked by bevacizumab, these blood vessels normalize, reducing tumor interstitial pressure, and allowing normal blood flow throughout the tumor. When given with chemotherapy, this theoretically results in increased chemotherapy penetrating the tumor, and cell kill. Bevacizumab may augment the body's antitumor immune response by helping dendritic cells function more effectively. Finally, bevacizumab is an IgG1 monoclonal antibody that theoretically recruits immune effector cells such as natural killer cells and macrophages, which attack tumor cells (antibody-dependent cellular cytotoxicity), as well as stimulating complement-mediated killing of tumor cells.

Metabolism: Humanized via recombinant technologies resulting in a 93% human monoclonal antibody. It is widely distributed throughout the body and has a terminal half-life of approximately 20 days (range 11–50 days). It appears to reach steady state in 100 days. Drug clearance varies by body weight, gender, and tumor burden: men and patients with a large tumor burden have higher clearances than females, but this does not appear to decrease drug efficiency. Drug clearance has not been studied in patients with either renal or hepatic impairment, but it appears that there is minimal drug clearance by these organs. Concurrent administration of 5-fluourouracil, carboplatin, doxorubicin, cisplatin, or paclitaxel does not affect pharmacokinetics of the drug.

Dosage/Range:

- 5 mg/kg IV every 2 weeks when combined with IFL (CRC).
- 10 mg/kg IV every 2 weeks when combined with FOLFOX (CRC).
- 15 mg IV every 3 weeks when combined with carboplatin and paclitaxel (non-squamous cell NSCLC).
- 10 mg/kg IV every 2 weeks when combined with paclitaxel (breast cancer).

Drug Preparation:

- Single use vials contain 4 mL to deliver 100 mg, and 16 mL to deliver 400 mg per vial. Use within 8 hours of opening. Store at 2–8°C (36–46°F). Protect from light. Do not freeze or shake.
- Further dilute in 100 mL 0.9% normal saline for injection.

Drug Administration:

- Administer IV over 90 minutes as an infusion. If tolerated well without fever and/or chills, may give second dose over 60 minutes; if this is well tolerated, administer all subsequent doses as a 30 minute infusion.
- Bevacizumab 5 mg/kg has been shown to be safely infused over 10 minutes (Reidy et al, 2007).

Drug Interactions:

- SN-38 (the active metabolite of irinotecan) concentration is 33% higher when bevacizumab is given concurrently; monitor for increased diarrhea and neutropenia.
- Paclitaxel/carboplatin combination: may decrease paclitaxel exposure after four cycles of treatment (day 63).
- Incompatible with dextrose solutions.

Lab Effects/Interference:

- Thrombocytopenia.
- Proteinuria.
- Leukopenia and neutropenia.
- Hypokalemia.
- Bilirubinemia.

Special Considerations:

- FDA approved for (1) first- and second-line treatment of patients with metastatic colon or rectal cancer in combination with a fluorouracil-based regimen. Is being studied in adjuvant treatment of patients with stage III colon cancer. (2) First-line treatment of patients with unresectable, locally advanced, recurrent or metastatic, nonsquamous NSCLC in combination with carboplatin and paclitaxel, and (3) treatment, in combination with paclitaxel, of patients, who have not received chemotherapy for metastatic HER-2 negative breast cancer.
- The addition of bevacizumab appears to improve survival significantly in first-line regimens.
  - BRiTE study suggests continuing bevacizumab after first line progression in patients with advanced CRC significantly improves OS (Grothey et al, 2007).
  - Bevacizumab as a second- and third-line treatment in patients with metastatic breast cancer who had previously received anthracycline and taxane therapy was studied in a single open-label randomized trial (AVF2119) and did not show a clinically significant improvement in DFS or OS and thus is not recommended.
  - Bevacizumab improved OS in patients with metastatic colorectal cancer when given with IFL (irinotecan, 5-fluorouracil or 5-FU, leucovorin or LV) chemotherapy by 4.7 months as compared with IFL alone (Hurwitz et al, 2004), and by 4.1 months in combination with 5-FU/LV as compared with 5-FU/LV alone (Kabbinavar et al, 2004).
  - Patients with advanced NSCLC with carboplatin/paclitaxel plus bevacizumab had a survival of 12.3 months versus 10.3 months in patients who received chemotherapy alone. Subset analysis showed less robust response in women, patients more than 65 years old, and patients with a more than 5% weight loss before entering the study (Sandler et al, 2005).
  - Patients with advanced breast cancer (E2100): patients receiving paclitaxel plus bevacizumab had a PFS of 11.3 months compared with patients receiving chemotherapy alone of 5.8 months ($P < .001$), as well as twice the RR. Overall

survival was 1.7 mo longer, but this was not statistically significant (p = 0.14) (Miller et al, 2005).

- Increased neutropenia and infection when combined with chemotherapy.
- Black box warnings discuss risk of (1) gastrointestinal perforations (incidence in patients with CRC was 2.4%, NSCLC 0.9%) breast cancer (0.5%), sometimes associated with intra-abdominal abscesses, and fistula formation; (2) complications of wound healing; and (3) hemorrhage (fatal hemoptysis occurred in 5 patients with NSCLC—incidence was 31% in patients with squamous cell and 2.3% in patients with adenocarcinoma histology).
- Warnings include:

  1) Gastrointestinal perforation (GI perforation, intra-abdominal abscesses and/or fistula formation); permanently discontinue drug if this occurs.
  2) Non-GI fistula formation (tracheoesophageal, bronchopleural, biliary, vagina, bladder); permanently discontinue drug if fistula forms involving an internal organ.
  3) Wound healing: discontinue drug if wound healing complications require medical intervention.
  4) Hemorrhage: discontinue drug if serious hemorrhage requiring medical intervention.
  5) Arterial thromboembolic events (ATE) with risk of stroke, myocardial infarction, transient ischemic attacks, and angina: permanently discontinue drug if a severe ATE occurs.
  6) Hypertension (HTN): permanently discontinue drug if hypertensive crisis or encephalopathy occurs; temporarily suspend drug if patient develops severe, uncontrolled HTN until it can be controlled.
  7) Reversible posterior leukoencephalopathy syndrome (RPLS) has an incidence of < 0.1%, with signs and symptoms of headache, seizure, lethargy, confusion, blindness, and other visual changes and may be associated with uncontrolled HTN: discontinue drug and treat HTN.
  8) Neutropenia and infection: increased risk of severe neutropenia and febrile neutropenia when combined with myelosuppressive chemotherapy.
  9) Proteinuria and rare nephrotic syndrome: discontinue drug if nephrotic syndrome develops.
  10) Congestive heart failure: in patients receiving paclitaxel (incidence 2.2% vs 0.3% in control) or receiving anthracyclines (3.8% vs 0.6% in control).

- Temporarily suspend drug in patients who require elective surgery for a period of time prior to surgery, as the drug half-life is about 20 days. Drug should not be initiated for at least 28 days after major surgery, and the incision should be fully healed.
- Patients with active hemoptysis (> ½ tsp of red blood) should not receive the drug.
- Drug may impair fertility, and is teratogenic. Women of childbearing age taking drug should use contraceptive measures during treatment, and for the expected time of drug elimination from the body (half-life is 20 days, with a range of 11–50 days)

after the drug is stopped. Nursing mothers should discontinue nursing during treatment with bevacizumab and for the expected time of drug elimination after the drug is stopped.

- Drug toxicities that occur more commonly in the elderly (> 2%) were asthenia, sepsis, deep thrombophlebitis, hypertension, hypotension, myocardial infarction, congestive heart failure, diarrhea, constipation, anorexia, leukopenia, anemia, dehydration, hypokalemia, and hyponatremia. In those aged 75 or older, in addition, dyspepsia, gastrointestinal hemorrhage, edema, epistaxis, increased cough, and voice alteration occurred more commonly than those under age 65.
- In a subset analysis of phase III AVF2107 study, bevacizumab was shown to have high activity in patients with the normal (wild-type) K-Ras gene with a PFS of 13.5 mo compared with 7.4 mo with chemotherapy alone. Overall survival was significantly longer at 27.7 mo compared with 17.6 mo with chemotherapy alone. In addition, patients with mutations in K-Ras also had a benefit: PFS was 9.4 mo with the addition of bevacizumab compared to 5.5 mo in the group receiving chemotherapy alone.

Potential Toxicities/Side Effects and the Nursing Process

I. ALTERATION IN INTESTINAL AND SKIN INTEGRITY related to GASTROINTESTINAL PERFORATION AND WOUND DEHISCENCE

Defining Characteristics: Rarely, patients may develop gastrointestinal perforation, sometimes fatal. It may be associated with intra-abdominal abscesses, or fistula, and occur at variable times during the treatment. Incidence across all studies was 0–3.7%. In patients with mCRC receiving bevacizumab plus chemotherapy, the incidence was 2.4% compared with 0.3% in the bolus IFL-only arm. In patients with NSCLC receiving bevacizumab plus chemotherapy, the incidence was 0.9% compared with 0% in the chemotherapy only arm. In study 7 (metastatic breast cancer), two fatal GI perforations occurred.

Presenting symptoms were abdominal pain associated with nausea and constipation. Colonoscopy has a similar risk of GI perforation, so drug should be stopped 28 days before a planned colonoscopy. Also in clinical testing, 1% of patients receiving bevacizumab plus either IFL or 5-FU/LV developed wound dehiscence, compared to 0.5% in the IFL arm alone. It is unknown how long the interval between surgery and treatment with bevacizumab should be, but it may be greater than 2 months and the surgical incision should be completely healed; similarly, it is not known how long the interval should be between treatment with bevacizumab and elective surgery, but it certainly should be longer than the elimination time of the drug (half-life 20 days). In one small clinical study, 15% of patients who had surgery following bevacizumab treatment had wound healing or bleeding complications (Genentech, 2004). Exfoliative dermatitis occurred in 19% of patients receiving 5-FU/LV plus bevacizumab. GI perforation has occurred in patients with NSCLC and advanced breast cancer receiving bevacizumab.

Nursing Implications: Assess baseline bowel, skin integrity, and healing of any wounds or incisions; assess for dehiscence, and integrity of skin or wound at each visit. Teach patient that very rarely GI perforation or wound dehiscence may occur and to report or come to the emergency room for severe abdominal pain associated with nausea, vomiting, constipation, or other symptoms; or problems with wound healing right away for immediate evaluation. Bevacizumab should be discontinued if perforation or wound dehiscence occurs. Bevacizumab should be held prior to elective surgery based on the drug half-life of 20 days (range, 10–50 days) and not started until at least 28 days after major surgery; the surgical incision must be fully healed. For patients who are undergoing metastectomy, the drug may be stopped 2 months before and not resumed for at least 60 days after hepatectomy. Teach patient to self-assess changes in skin or wound integrity and to report it right away.

II. ALTERATION IN HEMOSTASIS related to BLEEDING and THROMBOSIS

Defining Characteristics: Two patterns of bleeding may rarely occur: minor hemorrhage such as mild epistaxis, and serious hemorrhage. Of note, hemorrhage (pulmonary) occurred when drug was being studied in patients with lung cancer, with a higher incidence (31% in a small study) in patients with squamous cell histology. Many of these patients bled from a cavitation or area of necrosis in the pulmonary tumor. CNS bleeding was not evaluated, as patients with CRC and brain metastases were excluded from clinical trials. It is being studied now in a NSCLC patient population. Rarely, the following other events were described in clinical trials: gastrointestinal hemorrhage (24% in patients receiving bevacizumab and IFL compared to 6% In IFL alone patients), subarachnoid hemorrhage, hemorrhagic stroke, thrombosis (grade 3–4 incidence 3% compared to 1% in IFL only group), embolism, epistaxis, hematemesis, hemoptysis, and bleeding at tumor sites. Epistaxis occurred in 35% of patients receiving bevacizumab + IFL, compared to 10% in IFL-alone arm. Thrombocytopenia may occur in 5% of patients. Deep vein thrombosis may occur in 6–9%, and epistaxis in 32–35% of patients. Epistaxis is easily controlled with pressure application. Patients on low-dose Coumadin for implanted port patency had no increased risk of bleeding. There was no increased venous thromboembolism in a review of clinical studies when bevacizumab was added to chemotherapy, but was a significant increase in arterial thromboembolic events (incidence 4.4% compared with 1.9% receiving chemotherapy alone). Risk factors for development of arterial thromboembolic events: history of arterial thromboembolism and age of more than 65 years.

Nursing Implications: Assess baseline hematologic parameters and monitor during therapy. Teach patient that bleeding may occur and is most commonly epistaxis; but may also rarely occur as bleeding in the gastrointestinal tract, vagina in women, or elsewhere, and to report signs/symptoms of bleeding, changes in mental status, mobility, vision, weakness, or any new sign or symptom right away. Teach patient to assess for and report right away signs/symptoms of thrombosis: new swelling, pain, skin warmth and/or change in color (e.g., erythema, mottling) on the legs or thighs; new onset pain in the abdomen; dyspnea or shortness of breath, rapid heartbeat, chest pain, or pressure that may signal a pulmonary embolism; and any changes in vision, new onset of severe headache, lightheadedness, or dizziness. Assess baseline mental status and neurological signs and monitor during therapy, especially in patients with brain metastases. Teach patients to apply pressure if epistaxis occurs. Discuss any abnormalities with physician. Bevacizumab should be discontinued if the patient develops serious hemorrhage, and is should not be given to patients with recent hemoptysis (> ½ tsp bright red blood).

III. POTENTIAL ALTERATION IN CIRCULATION related to HYPERTENSION and CONGESTIVE HEART FAILURE

Defining Characteristics: Bevacizumab increases the incidence and severity of hypertension, a class effect of all angiogenesis inhibitors believed caused by the influence of VEGF on nitric oxide and blood vessel dilation, which is now blocked. The incidence of hypertension (> 150/100 mm Hg) was 60% in the clinical study arm IFL + bevacizumab and 67% in the arm 5-FU/LV + bevacizumab arm, compared to 43% in the IFL arm. Severe hypertension defined as > 200/110 mm Hg occurred in 7% of patients in the clinical study arm IFL + bevacizumab and 10% in the arm 5-FU/LV + bevacizumab arm, compared with 2% in the IFL-only arm. Hypertension may persist following drug cessation, as shown in clinical studies: 69% in patients receiving IFL + bevacizumab, and 80% in the IFL-only arm. Grade 3–4 hypertension occurred in 12% of patients in clinical trials, compared to 2% in the IFL group. Severe hypertension necessitated hospitalization or drug discontinuation, and was rarely complicated by hypertensive encephalopathy or subarachnoid hemorrhage in some patients. Overall incidence of hypertension is 23–34%, with 12% grade 3/4. Rarely, 2% of patients may develop grade 2–4 congestive heart failure (CHF). Incidence is higher in combination with, or if a past history of, receiving anthracycline chemotherapy with or without left chest wall irradiation.

Nursing Implications: Assess baseline BP prior to and during treatment, at least for the first treatment, then prior to each drug administration. If the patient has a history of hypertension, monitor BP more closely, although hypertension develops over time rather than during the drug infusion. Blood pressure should continue to be monitored after patient has stopped the drug. Teach patient drug administration, potential side-effects, and self care measures if prescribed antihypertensive medication, such as angiotensin-converting enzyme inhibitors, beta-blockers, diuretics, and calcium-channel blockers. Drug should be temporarily suspended in patients with severe hypertension until BP can be controlled with medical management. Drug should be permanently discontinued if the patient develops hypertensive crisis (diastolic blood pressure > 120 mm Hg).

IV. ALTERATION IN RENAL FUNCTION related to NEPHROTIC SYNDROME

Defining Characteristics: Nephrotic syndrome and proteinuria may occur. 17–28% of patients receiving bevacizumab in combination with IFL or 5-FU/LV had 2+ proteinuria compared to 14% of patients on IFL alone. 2–4% had grade 3 proteinuria (> 3.5 g protein/24 h), as compared to 0% in the IFL arm. Nephrotic syndrome is rare, occurring in 0.5% of patients, but 1 of the 5 affected patients required dialysis and 1 patient died. Although there may be an improvement in renal function, no patient had normalization following drug discontinuation.

Nursing Implications: Assess baseline renal function and presence of protein in urine (1+ or greater by dipstick), and monitor prior to each treatment. Discuss any abnormalities with the physician. Patients with 2+ or higher proteinuria by urine dipstick should be asked to collect a 24 hour urine sample for protein. Drug should be held for proteinuria > 2 g/24 h, and resume when proteinuria < 2 g/24 h. Monitor patients closely if moderate to severe proteinuria until improved or resolved. Drug should be discontinued if the patient develops nephrotic syndrome.

V. ALTERATION IN COMFORT related to ARTHRALGIA, ASTHENIA, PAIN, HEADACHE

Defining Characteristics: Discomfort may occur when drug is given with paclitaxel, related to arthralgias, asthenia, myalgia. The incidence of grade 3/4 bone pain was 3.9% in breast cancer patients compared with 1.7% in the control. The incidence of headache occurs in 3–3.6% in patients. Sensory neuropathy was higher in the bevacizumab/paclitaxel arm: 24.2% compared with 17.5% in the control.

Nursing Implications: Assess baseline comfort, and teach patient to report any changes. Assess peripheral nervous system for signs/symptoms of peripheral neuropathy (e.g., paresthesias, dysesthesias) prior to each treatment. Discuss further evaluation of symptoms with physician. Develop symptom management plan with patient and implement. If discomfort continues, discuss management with physician, nurse practitioner, and physician assistant. Revise plan as appropriate.

VI. POTENTIAL FOR INFECTION related to NEUTROPENIA

Defining Characteristics: In patients with NSCLC, febrile neutropenia occurred in 5% (compared with 2% in control), infection with neutropenia 4% (vs. 2%), and infection without neutropenia in 7% (vs. 3%).

Nursing Implications: Assess baseline white blood cell count, differential, and absolute neutrophil count, and monitor closely prior to each treatment when given in combination with irinotecan. Teach patient to avoid opportunities for infection (crowds, people with colds), and to report signs/symptoms of infection right away. Ensure that patient has a thermometer and knows how to use it; alternatively, a family member can monitor patient's temperature at home. Teach patient to monitor temperature, and report temperature > 100.5°F. If patient develops febrile neutropenia, discuss immediate antibiotics and hospitalization as needed.

Drug: bexarotene (Targretin oral capsules and topical gel)

Class: Retinoid.

Mechanism of Action: Retinoid that selectively binds to and activates retinoid × receptors, which have biologic activity distinct from retinoic acid receptors. The activated receptors can partner with receptor partners (e.g., retinoic acid receptors), and then function as transcription factors that regulate the expression of genes which control cellular differentiation and proliferation. The exact mechanism of action in cutaneous T-cell lymphoma is unknown.

Metabolism: Drug is well absorbed after oral administration, especially after a fat-containing meal, with a terminal half-life of seven hours. Drug is highly protein-bound (> 99%). Drug appears to be metabolized by the cytochrome P450 CYP3A4 isoenzyme system in the liver, forming glucuronidated oxidative metabolites. Four metabolites are formed and are active, but it is unclear which metabolites or whether the parent drug is responsible for the efficacy of the drug. Probably excreted via the hepatobiliary system.

Dosage/Range: *Oral capsules*:

- Indicated for the treatment of cutaneous manifestations of cutaneous T-cell lymphoma in patients who are refractory to at least one prior systemic therapy.
- Initial dose of 300 mg/m^2 PO per day for up to 97 weeks (maximum in clinical trials).
- Dose-reduce for toxicity to 200 mg/m^2 PO daily, then down to 100 mg/m^2 PO daily, or stop temporarily until toxicity resolves. After resolution, gradually titrate dose upward.
- Evaluate treatment efficacy at 8 weeks, and if no tumor response but the drug is well tolerated, increase dose to 400 mg/m^2 PO daily and monitor closely.

Topical gel:

- 1% gel indicated for the topical treatment of skin lesions in patients with early stage cutaneous T-cell lymphoma who have failed other therapies.

Drug Preparation:

- Available as 75-mg gelatin capsules in bottles of 100 capsules. The contents of the bottle should be protected from light, high temperatures, and humidity once opened.
- Store at 2–25°C (36–77°F).
- 1% gel available in tube. Store at 2–25°C (36–77°F).

Drug Administration:
- Oral: single daily oral dose with a meal.
- Topical gel: apply to affected areas only (NOT entire body) as needed.

Drug Interactions: *Oral capsules*:
- Presumed to be related to P450 CYP3A4 isoenzyme system metabolism.
- Inhibitors of cytochrome P450 CYP3A4 enzyme system (e.g., ketoconazole, itraconazole, erythromycin, gemfibrozil, grapefruit juice) theoretically can increase serum levels of bexarotene; DO NOT GIVE GEMFIBROZIL concomitantly with bexarotene.
- Inducers of cytochrome P450 CYP3A4 enzyme system (e.g., rifampin, phenytoin, Phenobarbital, St. John's wort) may cause a decrease in serum bexarotene concentrations. If used concomitantly, assess response, and increase bexarotene accordingly. Do not give together with St. John's wort.
- Theoretically, as drug is highly protein bound, it is possible that bexarotene can displace drugs or be displaced by drugs which bind to plasma proteins (e.g., methotrexate); use together cautiously.
- Insulin, sulfonylureas, or insulin-sensitizers: may increase action with resultant hypoglycemia; use together cautiously.
- Tamoxifen: may increase effect of tamoxifen.
- Vitamin A: avoid high doses (>15,000 IU/day), as it may increase retinoid toxicity.
- DEET (N,N-diethyl-m-toluamide): bexarotene gel will increase DEET toxicity.

Lab Effects/Interference: *Oral capsules*:
- CA 125 assay values in patients with ovarian cancer may be increased.
- Significantly increased serum triglycerides, total cholesterol, and decreased HDL.
- Increased LFTs.
- Decreased TSH and total T4.
- Leukopenia and neutropenia.
- Increased LDH.

Special Considerations: *Oral capsules*:
- Baseline serum lipid levels must be assessed prior to initiation of therapy, and any abnormalities treated so that fasting triglycerides are normal before starting therapy.
- Drug is contraindicated during pregnancy and nursing mothers, as it is teratogenic. Women of childbearing age should use effective contraception—optimally, two forms unless abstinence is chosen. This should continue during therapy and for one month after the completion of therapy. A pregnancy test should be done one week prior to beginning therapy, and repeated monthly during therapy. If pregnancy occurs, the drug must be stopped immediately and the woman counseled.
- Drug should be used cautiously in patients who have hypersensitivity to other retinoids.
- Male patients with sexual partners who are pregnant, possibly pregnant, or who could become pregnant, should use condoms during therapy, and for one month after therapy is ended.
- Most patients have major lipid abnormalities, and one patient died of pancreatitis. In general, patients with risk factors for pancreatitis should not take the drug

(e.g., history of pancreatitis, uncontrolled hyperlipidemia, uncontrolled diabetes mellitus, biliary tract disease, or medications known to increase triglyceride levels or to be associated with pancreatic toxicity).
- Drug may cause cataracts; patients who experience visual difficulties should have an ophthalmologic exam.
- Baseline laboratory assessment prior to starting drug should include WBC with differential, thyroid function tests, fasting blood lipid profile, and liver function tests.
- Patients should limit vitamin A intake to ≤ 15,000 international units/day to avoid possible additive toxicity.
- Patients should avoid direct sunlight and artificial ultraviolet light while taking bexarotene pills or gel as severe sunburn and skin sensitivity reactions may occur due to photosensitization; patients should also wear SPF 30 or higher.
- No studies have been done with patients having hepatic dysfunction, but theoretically, hepatic dysfunction would greatly reduce metabolism/excretion and increase serum drug levels. Use cautiously if at all in this setting.
- Response rate in patients with cutaneous T-cell lymphoma who were refractory to one prior systemic therapy was 32%.
- Drug being studied in clinical trials of patients with advanced breast cancer or moderate/severe psoriasis.

1% gel:
- Main side effects are rash, itching, and pain at application site.

Potential Toxicities/Side Effects and the Nursing Process

I. ALTERATION IN NUTRITION, POTENTIAL, related to ABNORMAL LIPID LEVELS, PANCREATITIS, ELEVATED LFTs, AND NAUSEA (oral capsules)

Defining Characteristics: Almost all patients experience major lipid abnormalities, including elevated fasting triglycerides (70% receiving doses of ≥ 300 mg/m^2/day had elevations of more than 2.5 times upper limits of normal (ULN), and 55% had values over 800 mg/dL with a median of 1200 mg/dL), elevated cholesterol (60% of patients receiving 300 mg/m^2/day, and 75% of patients receiving doses of ≥ 300 mg/m^2/day), and decreased levels of the protective high-density lipoproteins (HDL) to < 25 mg/dL (55% of patients receiving a dose of 300 mg/m^2/day, and 90% of patients receiving a dose of > 300 mg/m^2/day). These values normalize after bexarotene is stopped. In most patients, either antilipemic medication or dose reduction of bexarotene allowed control over elevated levels. Rarely, patients with markedly elevated triglycerides (lowest level 770 mg/dL) can develop pancreatitis, which can be fatal. Patients with risk factors for pancreatitis should not receive the drug (e.g., history of pancreatitis, uncontrolled hyperlipidemia, uncontrolled diabetes mellitus, biliary tract disease, or medications known to increase triglyceride levels or to be associated with pancreatic toxicity). Uncommonly, patients may have elevated LFTs (5% of patients receiving an initial dose of 300 mg/m^2/day and 7% when doses of > 300 mg/m^2/day were used), but one patient developed cholestasis and died of liver failure in clinical trials. Nausea/vomiting occurs in 15%/3% of patients receiving a dose of 300 mg/m^2/day and 7%/13% of patients receiving doses of > 300 mg/m^2/day. Anorexia affects 2% of patients receiving a dose of 300 mg/m^2/day, and 22% of patients receiving higher doses.

Nursing Implications: Assess baseline triglyceride, cholesterol, and HDL levels. If abnormal, discuss pharmacological management plan, e.g., atorvastatin, as fasting triglyceride level should be normal before patient begins therapy. Gemfibrozil should NOT be used. Fasting triglyceride level should then be monitored weekly until the lipid response to bexarotene is known (2–4 weeks), then at 8-week intervals. Goal is to keep fasting triglyceride level < 400 mg/dL to prevent pancreatitis. If fasting triglyceride level becomes elevated during treatment, discuss with physician antilipemic medication, e.g., atorvastatin, and if no response, discuss with physician bexarotene dose reduction or drug holiday. Teach patient about importance of testing fasting triglycerides, and monitoring level throughout treatment. LFTs should be assessed baseline, and after 1, 2, and 4 weeks of starting treatment; if stable, then assess every 8 weeks during treatment. Monitor serum LFTs, HDL, and discuss any abnormalities with physician (manufacturer recommends suspension or discontinuance of bexarotene if LFTs [SGOT/AST, SGPT/ALT, and bilirubin] > 3 times ULN). Assess baseline nutritional status, teach patient that nausea, vomiting, and anorexia may occur and to report them. If these occur, teach strategies to minimize occurrence, and if ineffective or symptoms are severe, discuss pharmacologic management with physician.

II. ALTERATION IN ACTIVITY, POTENTIAL, related to HYPOTHYROIDISM (oral capsules)

Defining Characteristics: Bexarotene binds and activates retinoid × receptors, and can partner with thyroid receptor; once activated, the receptor functions as a transcription factor that regulates gene expression controlling cellular differentiation and proliferation. Drug induces reversible clinical hypothyroidism in about 50% of patients (decrease in TSH in 60% of patients, and total T4 in 45% of patients at a dose of 300 mg/m^2/day), and hypothyroidism was reported in 29% of patients. Asthenia occurs in 29.8% of patients at a dose of 300 mg/m^2/day and in 45% of patients at higher doses.

Nursing Implications: Assess baseline thyroid function tests (TFTs), and discuss pharmacologic replacement of thyroid hormone with physician if values indicate hypothyroidism. Monitor TFTs during treatment. Teach patient that this may occur, importance of laboratory testing, fact that hypothyroidism induced by drug is reversible following discontinuance of drug, and to report signs/symptoms of hypothyroidism (e.g., weight gain, lethargy, slowed thinking, skin dryness, constipation, joint pain/stiffness). Teach patient to alternate rest and activity periods, and other measures to conserve energy.

III. POTENTIAL FOR INFECTION related to LEUKOPENIA (oral capsules)

Defining Characteristics: Reversible leukopenia (WBC/mm^3 1000–3000) occurred in 18% of patients receiving dose of 300 mg/m^2/day, and in 43% of patients receiving higher doses. Patients receiving 300 mg/m^2/day had grade 3 (12%) and grade 4 (4%) neutropenia. Incidence of bacterial infection was 1.2% in patients receiving dose of 300 mg/m^2/day (overall body infection was 13%), and bacterial infection was 13% (overall infections 22%) in patients receiving higher doses. Onset of leukopenia was 4–8 weeks. Resolution of leukopenia/neutropenia occurred in 30 days with drug dose reduction or discontinuance in most patients (82–93%). There were rare serious adverse events associated with leukopenia/neutropenia.

Nursing Implications: Assess baseline WBC, ANC and periodically during therapy. Teach patient that leukopenia may occur, and teach self-care measures, including self-assessment for infection, minimizing risk of infection, and when to notify provider. Teach patient/family signs/symptoms of infection, and how to take temperature if this is not known.

IV. ALTERATION IN BOWEL ELIMINATION related to DIARRHEA (oral capsules)

Defining Characteristics: Diarrhea is uncommon in patients receiving dose of 300 mg/m^2/day, but is more common (41%) when dose is increased.

Nursing Implications: Assess baseline elimination status, and monitor throughout treatment. Teach patient that diarrhea may occur, especially if dose is > 300 mg/m^2/day, and to report it. Teach patient self-care measures, including dietary modification (decreased insoluble fiber, increased soluble fiber, and increased fluid) and self-administration of OTC medicines to manage diarrhea. Teach patient to report diarrhea that does not resolve in 24 hours, or is severe, and discuss management with physician.

V. ALTERATION IN COMFORT related to HEADACHE, ABDOMINAL PAIN, CHILLS, FEVER, FLU SYNDROME, BACK PAIN, INSOMNIA (oral capsules)

Defining Characteristics: Symptoms occur with the following incidence (300 mg/m^2/day dose vs higher dose): headache (30% vs 42%), abdominal pain (11% vs 4%), chills (9% vs 13%), fever (5% vs 17%), insomnia (5% vs 11%), flu-like symptoms (3% vs 13%), back pain (2% vs 11%).

Nursing Implications: Assess baseline comfort status. Teach patient that these symptoms may occur and teach self-management measures. Teach patient to report fever > 100.5°F, chills, or symptoms that persist or are severe. Discuss management with physician if these occur.

VI. POTENTIAL ALTERATION IN SKIN INTEGRITY related to RASH, DRY SKIN, ALOPECIA, PERIPHERAL EDEMA (oral capsules), and RASH, PRURITUS, PAIN AT GEL APPLICATION SITE (topical gel)

Defining Characteristics: Oral capsules: Symptoms occur with the following incidence (300 mg/m^2/day vs higher dose): rash (17% vs 23%), exfoliative dermatitis (10.7% vs 9%), alopecia (3.6% vs 11%), and peripheral edema (13% vs 11%). Topical gel: Commonly, rash, pruritus, and pain at application site occur.

Nursing Implications: Oral capsules: Assess baseline skin integrity and extent of cutaneous lesions, and teach patient to report rash right away after taking capsules, especially if peeling. Discuss drug continuance with physician if this occurs. Teach patient to use skin cream to keep skin moist, to prevent cracking and peeling, and to prevent itching as directed by the physician. Teach patient to report any hair thinning, and if it occurs, assess impact on patient's body image. Discuss measures to enhance coping, such as use of scarf, measures to protect hair follicles (e.g., gentle shampoo, avoidance of hair perms or use of curling iron), encourage patient to verbalize feelings, and provide emotional support. Teach patient to report swelling of feet or hands, to keep skin moisturized to prevent cracking or dryness, and to report skin changes that persist or are severe. Discuss management with physician. Topical gel: Assess integrity/extent of cutaneous lesions prior to patient starting therapy. Teach patient application of topical gel on areas of lesions only. Teach patient to report rash, persistent itching, or pain at application site. Teach patient self-care measures to manage itching, or pain at application site if they occur. Discuss with physician management of rash, and if severe, discontinuance of gel.

Drug: bortezomib (Velcade)

Class: Proteasome inhibitor.

Mechanism of Action: A reversible inhibitor of the 26S proteasome; inhibits the breakdown of ubiquinated intracellular proteins and disrupts the ubiquitin-proteasome pathway. This pathway normally regulates the intracellular concentration of specific proteins, thus controlling homeostasis. Cancer cells depend on the proteins that are available from this process to turn on the cell cycle and to make the apparatus of mitosis. When the ubiquitin–proteasome pathway is disrupted, the proteins are not available, and multiple signaling pathways within the cell are disrupted, encouraging the cell to undergo apoptosis. Cell cycle movement (cell division) stops. Cells are unable to migrate, and sensitivity to chemotherapy is increased. In addition, the drug appears to downregulate the NF-κB pathway, which is necessary for cell growth, avoidance of apoptosis, and adhesion. This may restore chemosensitivity. In multiple myeloma, it interferes with cellular adhesion molecules so that tumor cells can not bind to the bone marrow.

Metabolism: After IV administration, the drug is rapidly cleared from the plasma, with a mean elimination half-life range of 40–193 hours after multiple dosing. Drug undergoes oxidative metabolism via cytochrome P450 enzymes 3A4, 2D6, 2C19, 2C9, and 1A2. Drug is deboronated into 2 metabolites that are then hydroxylated into several metabolites. Unknown elimination path.

Dosage/Range:

- Newly diagnosed multiple myeloma (9–6 week treatment cycles, given with melphalan 9 mg/m^2 and prednisone 60 mg/m^2): Cycles 1–4: 1.3 mg/m^2 per dose IVB twice weekly × 2 weeks (days 1, 4, 8, 11) followed by a 10-day rest period, then resume on days 22, 25, 29 and 32. Cycle repeated q 6 weeks. Cycle 5–9: bortezomib is given weekly on days 1, 8, 22, 29. Doses should be separated by at least 72 hours (to give normal cells a chance to recover).
- Relapsed multiple myeloma or mantle cell lymphoma: 1.3 mg/m^2 IV twice weekly × 2 weeks (days 1, 4, 8, 11) followed by a 10-day rest period (days 12–21).
- For extended therapy of > 8 cycles, bortezomib is given on standard schedule or maintenance (once weekly × 4 weeks (days 1, 8, 15, and 22 followed by a 13 day rest period days 23–35) every 35 days.

Dose Reduction:

- *Newly diagnosed multiple myeloma*: (1) prolonged grade 4 neutropenia or thrombocytopenia, or bleeding: consider 25% dose reduction of melphalan next cycle; (2) platelet count ≤ 30,000 cells/mm^3 or ANC ≤ 750 cells/mm^3 on a bortezomib dosing day, hold bortezomib; (3) If several bortezomib doses are held, decrease dose of bortezomib by 1 dose level, e.g., from 1.3 mg/m^2 to 1.0 mg/m^2, (4) Hold drug at onset any grade 3 non-hematologic toxicity or grade 4 hematologic toxicity, and when resolved to grade 1 or less, resume at dose reduced by 1 dose level. If neuropathic pain or neuropathy, see dose reduction in Nursing Considerations.
- *Relapsed multiple myeloma or mantle cell lymphoma*: Hold drug at onset any grade 3 non-hematologic toxicity or grade 4 hematologic toxicity, and when resolved to grade 1 or less, resume at dose reduced by 1 dose level. If neuropathic pain or neuropathy, see dose reduction in Nursing section.
- Recalculate dose if weight loss of > 8% between cycles.
- Drug dose is not modified for renal impairment, including patients requiring renal dialysis.

Drug Preparation:

- Available in 10 mL vials containing 3.5 mg of bortezomib powder; store unopened vials at room temperature 25°C (77°F), and protect from light.

- Reconstitute each vial with 3.5 mL 0.9% sodium chloride injection USP, forming a colorless and clear solution (stable for 8 hours at controlled room temperature).
- Draw up prescribed amount (stable in syringe for 3 hours).

Drug Administration:

- Administer IVP over 3–5 seconds, followed by saline flush.
- Local skin irritation reported in 5% of patients, but drug is not a vesicant.
- Bortezomib, melphalan, prednisone regimen: at the beginning of each cycle, platelet count must be > 70,000 cells/mm^3 and ANC > 1000 cells/mm^3. In addition, non-hematologic toxicities must have resolved to grade 1 or less.

Drug Interactions:

- Potent CYP3A4 inhibitors (eg, ketoconazole, ritonavir): increased bortezomib exposure; monitor closely for toxicity.
- Drugs which either induce or inhibit Cytochrome P450 CYP3A4: monitor patients closely for efficacy or toxicity of bortezomib.
- In clinical trials, the addition of dexamethasone 20 mg PO given the day of and day after bortezomib resulted in increased response rate in patients with stable disease or progressive disease on bortezomib alone.

Lab Effects/Interference:

- Decreased neutrophil, platelet and red blood cell counts.
- Rare hyponatremia.
- Increased LFTs.

Special Considerations:

- Indicated for the treatment of patients with (1) multiple myeloma, including initial treatment, and (2) mantle cell lymphoma who have received at least one prior therapy.
- Contraindicated in patients with hypersensitivity to bortezomib, boron, or mannitol; avoid use in pregnancy and do not breast-feed while receiving the drug.
- Use cautiously in patients with hepatic dysfunction and monitor closely; in patients with a history of CHF, peripheral neuropathy, or syncope; in patients receiving antihypertensive medications (additive hypotension); and in patients who are dehydrated.
- Additive/synergistic antitumor effect when given with chemotherapy.
- No studies have been conducted with patients having hepatic dysfunction, renal dysfunction, pediatric patients, or to determine whether age, gender, or race affect the drug pharmacokinetics.
- Clinical studies conducted in patients with creatinine clearances ranging from 13.8 to 220 mL/min.
- Studies showed 28% response to bortezomib, with median response 1 year.
- Rarely, CHF may worsen, and the onset of decreased LVEF has been reported. In addition, there have been rare reports of cases of QT-interval prolongation. Monitor patients with preexisting cardiac disease closely.

- Rarely, reversible posterior leukoencephalopathy syndrome (RPLS) has occurred, characterized by seizure, hypertension, headache, lethargy, confusion, blindness, and/or other visual or other neurological disturbance. Diagnosis is confirmed with brain imaging, preferably MRI. Discontinue bortezomib.
- Carefully consider risk–benefit ratio in patients with pre-existing peripheral neuropathy, and monitor closely; dose modify or discontinue drug as needed.
- Hypotension may occur in up to 13% of patients; monitor patients receiving antihypertensive therapy, those with a history of syncope, and dehydrated patients closely.
- There are rare reports of pulmonary hypertension in the absence of left heart failure or significant pulmonary disease. If patient develops new or worsening cardiopulmonary symptoms, a comprehensive diagnostic evaluation should be done.
- Tumor lysis syndrome and acute hepatic failure have been reported; consider allopurinol and hydration for newly diagnosed patients with high tumor burden.

Potential Toxicities/Side Effects and the Nursing Process

I. POTENTIAL SENSORY/PERCEPTUAL ALTERATIONS related to SENSORY PERIPHERAL NEUROPATHY

Defining Characteristics: 80% of patients on clinical trials had a preexisting baseline peripheral neuropathy. 37% of patients had new onset or aggravation of existing peripheral neuropathy (PN). 14% developed grade 3 PN overall, with 5% occurring in patients without baseline PN symptoms. There were no patients with grade 4 PN. Peripheral neuropathy improved/resolved in 51% of patients who underwent a dose adjustment for ≥ grade 2 PN and in 73% of patients who discontinued the drug.

Nursing Implications: Teach patient to report new onset or worsening of PN symptoms (paresthesias, dysesthesias), any changes in sensory function (temperature sensation, knowing where body parts are in relation to the whole, etc.), functional ability (e.g., especially senses of smell and taste), and ability to carry out activities of daily living (ADLs). Assess severity of symptom(s) if they arise and potential for injury. If moderate, consult protocol and discuss medical intervention with physician. Teach patient measures to minimize symptoms and ensure safety. Discuss coadministered medication profile with physician as concomitant administration of the following drugs increases risk of PN: amiodarone, antivirals, isoniazid, nitrofurantoin, or statins. Discuss adding agents that may decrease development or worsening of PN, such as glutamine.
Dose Reductions:

- Grade 1 (paresthesias +/or loss of reflexes) without pain or loss of function: no action.
- Grade 1 with pain or Grade 2 (interfering with function but not ADLs): ↓ dose to 1.0 mg/m^2/dose.
- Grade 2 with pain or Grade 3 (interfering with ADLs): hold drug until toxicity resolves, then reinitiate with dose reduced to 0.7 mg/m^2 and change treatment schedule to once a week.
- Grade 4 (permanent sensory loss that interferes with function): discontinue drug.

II. POTENTIAL FOR INFECTION AND BLEEDING related to BONE MARROW DEPRESSION

Defining Characteristics: Thrombocytopenia occurred in 43% of patients (27% gr 3, 3% gr 4, with nadir day 11, and recovery by day 21) and neutropenia in 24% of patients (13% gr 3 and 3% gr 4; incidence higher in patients with multiple myeloma than mantle cell lymphoma). Febrile neutropenia occurred in < 1% of patients. Anemia incidence was 32%. Fever is common and higher in patients with multiple myeloma (37%) compared with mantle cell (19%).

Nursing Implications: Assess baseline leukocyte, platelet, and Hgb/HCT and monitor before each treatment, during therapy, and more often as needed. Hold drug for Grade 4 hematologic toxicity (NCI, see Appendix 1) and dose reduce 25%. Assess risk for infection and integrity of skin and mucous membranes, pulmonary status, and ability to clear secretions, as well as history of past infections, baseline and prior to each treatment. Teach patient to self-assess for signs/symptoms of infection, and to call provider immediately or come to the emergency room if temperature < 100.5°F, shaking chills, or rash, productive cough, burning on urination, or any signs/symptoms of infection or bleeding. Teach self-care strategies to minimize risk of infection and bleeding, including avoidance of OTC aspirin-containing medications.

III. ALTERATION IN NUTRITION, LESS THAN BODY REQUIREMENTS, related to NAUSEA, DIARRHEA, DECREASED APPETITE, CONSTIPATION, VOMITING, AND DEHYDRATION

Defining Characteristics: Patients on clinical studies developed these symptoms with the following incidence: nausea (64%), diarrhea (51%), decreased appetite (43%), constipation (43%), vomiting (36%), dehydration (18%). Diarrhea, nausea, and vomiting occur 6–24 hours after infusion. Nausea is more common in patients with multiple myeloma. Diarrhea and constipation may occur during cycles 1 and 2, and then disappear. Patients with diabetes require close monitoring of their blood glucose and may require adjustments in their antidiabetic medication.

Nursing Implications: Assess baseline weight and nutritional status, and monitor prior to each treatment. Assess glucose, electrolytes prior to each treatment to weekly, especially serum sodium and potassium; replete as necessary and teach diet high in sodium and potassium. Teach patient that serum electrolytes may be decreased and to assess for s/s: hyponatremia (confusion, weakness, seizures), hypokalemia (muscle weakness, confusion, irregular heartbeats), hypercalcemia (constipation, thirst, confusion, muscle cramps, sleepiness), and hypomagnesemia (muscle cramps, headache, weakness). Teach patient that side effects may occur, self-care strategies, and to report them if symptoms do not resolve. Use aggressive antiemetics to prevent nausea and vomiting: serotonin antagonist IV prior to bortezomib dose, and for 36 hours after each drug dose, if needed. If diarrhea develops after 1st treatment, teach patient to take loperamide prior to next dose of bortezomib and after every loose stool × 36 hours (not to exceed 8 tablets a day), as well as to use the BRAT diet (bananas, rice, applesauce, toast). If patient develops constipation, teach preventative self-care (stool softener, flax seed oil, MOM, prunes or prune juice every A.M. to ensure BM at least every other day). Teach patient to drink 2 quarts of fluid daily, drinking 1 glass an hour while awake to prevent dehydration. Teach patient to report dizziness, lightheadedness, or fainting spells, and to avoid operating heavy machinery or driving a car if these occur. Develop symptom management plan with physician. Make referral to dietitian as appropriate. Teach diabetic patients to monitor their blood glucose closely, and discuss abnormalities and changes in their antidiabetic dose with their NP, PA, or physician.

IV. ALTERATION IN OXYGENATION, POTENTIAL, related to HYPOTENSION

Defining Characteristics: Orthostatic hypotension/postural hypotension can affect up to 13% of patients throughout therapy.

Nursing Implications: Identify patients at risk: patients with history of syncope, dehydration, or taking medications associated with hypotension. Assess baseline cardiac status, including blood pressure and heart rate, noting rhythm and rate. Teach patient to prevent injury by gradual change in position, and to report any dizziness. Teach patients to avoid dehydration, especially in warm climates. If hypotension noted, assess patient tolerance and need for intervention; discuss management with physician. Manage orthostatic/postural hypotension with adjustment of antihypertensive doses (if patient is on them), hydration, and administration of mineralocorticoids and/or sympathomimetics.

V. ALTERATION IN COMFORT related to ASTHENIA, PYREXIA, HEADACHE, INSOMNIA, EDEMA, DIZZINESS, RASH, MYALGIA, MUSCLE CRAMPS, BLURRED VISION

Defining Characteristics: Asthenia (characterized by fatigue, malaise, and weakness) was most common, affecting 65% of patients in clinical trials. Other symptoms included pyrexia (36%), headache (28%), insomnia (27%), arthralgias (26%), edema (26%), dyspnea (22%), dizziness (21%), myalgia (14%), pruritus (11%), and blurred vision (11%).

Nursing Implications: Assess comfort and presence of discomfort, fatigue, peripheral edema, baseline and prior to each treatment. Teach patient that these side effects may occur and to report them. Teach patient local comfort measures as well as energy conservation, and discuss management plan with physician if ineffective.

Drug: cediranib (Recentin, AZD2171, investigational)

Class: Pan VEGF-receptor tyrosine kinase inhibitor.

Mechanism of Action: Drug is an oral, highly selective vascular endothelial growth factor (VEGF) signaling inhibitor and blocks VEGFR-1, -2, -3, all of which are implicated in tumor growth. It appears to stabilize tumor vasculature and reduce cerebral swelling in patients with glioblastoma (Batchelor, 2007).

Metabolism:
- Half-life of drug is 20 hours, compatible with daily dosing.

Dosage/Range:
- Oral, per protocol.

Drug Interactions:
- Unknown.

Lab Effects/Interference:
- Unknown.

Special Considerations:
- Most common side effects are diarrhea, voice change (hoarseness), headache, hypertension.
- Radiation sensitizer.
- Drug had steroid-sparing effect by shrinking cerebral edema in patients with recurrent glioblastoma; there were no serious bleeding events (Batchelor et al, 2007).
- Appears to cross the blood–brain barrier.

Potential Toxicities/Side Effects (Dose and Schedule Dependent) and the Nursing Process

I. POTENTIAL ALTERATION IN CIRCULATION related to HYPERTENSION

Defining Characteristics: Drug may increase the incidence and severity of hypertension. Headache may also occur.

Nursing Implications: Assess baseline BP before and during treatment, and manage according to protocol. If the patient has a history of hypertension, monitor BP more closely, although hypertension develops over time rather than during the drug infusion. Blood pressure should continue to be monitored after patient has stopped the drug. Teach patient drug administration, potential side effects, and self-care measures if prescribed antihypertensive medication, such as angiotensin-converting enzyme inhibitors, β-blockers, diuretics, and calcium-channel blockers. Drug should be permanently discontinued if the patient develops hypertensive crisis (diastolic blood pressure of more than 120 mm Hg) or per protocol. Drug can be temporarily suspended in patients with severe hypertension until BP can be controlled with medical management.

II. ALTERATION IN COMFORT related to FATIGUE, ASTHENIA

Defining Characteristics: Asthenia (characterized by fatigue, malaise, and weakness) was common.

Nursing Implications: Assess comfort and presence of discomfort, fatigue, baseline and at each visit. Teach patient that these side effects may occur and to report them. Teach patient local comfort measures as well as energy conservation, and discuss management plan with physician if ineffective.

III. ALTERATION IN NUTRITION, LESS THAN BODY REQUIREMENTS, related to DIARRHEA

Defining Characteristics: Diarrhea occurs commonly.

Nursing Implications: Assess baseline weight and nutritional status. Teach patient that diarrhea may occur and to report it if uncontrolled by self-care measures or per protocol. Monitor serum electrolytes before each dose, and replete as needed. Teach patient dietary modifications for diarrhea (small feedings with low fat or nonspicy foods, BRAT diet: bananas, rice, applesauce, and toast). Assess efficacy of intervention, and revise plan as needed.

IV. POTENTIAL ALTERATION IN BODY IMAGE related to VOICE CHANGE

Defining Characteristics: Patients may develop hoarseness.

Nursing Implications: Teach patient that hoarseness may occur. Teach patient to report any distress. Refer to protocol for management.

Drug: cetuximab (Erbitux)

Class: Chimeric (mouse/human) monoclonal antibody targeted against epidermal growth factor receptor (EGFR).

Mechanism of Action: Blocks growth factor (ligand, such as epidermal growth factor and transforming growth factor-alpha) from binding to EGFR, thus preventing dimerization and initiation of cell signaling via receptor tyrosine kinase phosphorylation; thus, the message telling the cell to divide does not occur. In addition to cell growth inhibition, there is induction of apoptosis, and decreased matrix metalloproteinase and vascular endothelial growth factor production. As an IgG_1 MoAb, it may also recruit immune effector cells via antibody-dependent cellular cytotoxicity (ADCC), as well as complement activation. Drug is synergistic with chemotherapy and radiotherapy, as it appears to prevent the malignant cell from repairing DNA damage.

Metabolism: Drug is an IgG_1 chimerized antibody, and it is postulated that clearance is via binding of the antibody to EGFR of hepatocytes with internalization of the cetuximab-EGFR complex. Mean elimination half-life is approximately 97 hours (range, 41–213 h). Steady state reached by 3rd weekly infusion. Mean half-life is 112 hours. Females have a 25% lower clearance of drug than males, but there was no difference in efficacy. No differences were found related to race, age, and hepatic and renal functional impairment.

Dosage/Range:

- Metastatic Colorectal Cancer: Loading dose of 400 mg/m^2 IV over 2 hours, followed by a weekly maintenance dose of 250 mg/m^2 IV over 1 hour (alone or in combination with irinotecan).
- Squamous Cell Cancer of the Head and Neck: Loading dose of 400 mg/m^2 IV over 2 hours one week prior to the initiation of RT, followed by weekly maintenance dose of 250 mg/m^2 IV over 1 hour given 1 hour prior to RT for the duration of RT (6–7 weeks).
- Recurrent or Metastatic Squamous Cell Cancer of the Head and Neck: Loading dose of 400 mg/m^2 IV over 2 hours, followed by a weekly maintenance dose of 250 mg/m^2 IV over 1 hour until disease progression or unacceptable toxicity.
- Premedicate with an H_1 antagonist such as diphenhydramine 50 mg IV.

Drug Preparation: Available in 50 mL vials containing 100 mg of drug, with a concentration of 2 mg/mL. Do not shake or dilute. Solution should be clear and colorless, and may contain small, white particles of cetuximab that are easily visible.

- Store vials under refrigeration at 2–8°C (36–46°F). Do not freeze. Increased particulate formation may occur at temperatures at or below 0°C. Drug contains no preservatives. Drug prepared in infusion containers are chemically and physically stable for 12 hours at 2–8°C (36–46°F), and for 8 hours at controlled room temperature (20–25°C or 68–77°F). Discard any remaining solution in the infusion container after 8 hours at room temperature, or 12 hours at 2–8°C (36–46°F). Discard any unused portion of the vial.

Drug Administration:

- Drug must be filtered using a low protein-binding 0.22 μm filter prior to infusion.
- Administer as an IV infusion over 2 hours for a loading dose, and 1 hour for a maintenance dose, using an infusion or syringe pump. Premedicate with an antihistamine before administration, and administer at a maximum of 5 mL/min. Observe patient for 1 hour following infusion, or longer if an infusion reaction develops as needed.

- Infusion pump: draw up calculated volume of cetuximab from vials using sterile syringe and needle or transfer device, using a new needle for each vial, and inject into sterile, evacuated container or infusion bag.
  - Prime infusion tubing and attach 0.22 μm in-line filter closest to patient.
  - Piggyback cetuximab line into mainline.
  - Maximum infusion rate is 5 mL/min.
  - Flush with 0.9% saline solution at the end of the infusion.
- Syringe pump: draw up calculated volume of cetuximab from vials using sterile syringe and needle, using a new needle for each vial, and place in syringe driver of syringe pump; set rate.
  - Administer through a low protein binding 0.22 μm in-line filter rated for syringe pump, placed closest to patient; piggyback cetuximab line into mainline
  - Connect infusion line, prime line, and start the infusion.
  - Repeat procedure until the calculated volume has been infused, using a new needle and filter for each vial.
  - Maximum infusion rate is 5 mL/min.
  - Flush with 0.9% saline solution at the end of the infusion.
- Dose modification for infusion reactions:
  - Mild to moderate infusion reactions (grade 1–2): reduce infusion rate by 50% for all subsequent infusions.
  - Severe (grade 3 [symptomatic bronchospasm], grade 4 [anaphylaxis]): stop drug.
- Dose reductions for severe acneform rash:
  - 1st occurrence: delay infusion 1–2 weeks; if improvement, continue at 250 mg/m^2; if no improvement, discontinue cetuximab.
  - 2nd occurrence: delay infusion 1–2 weeks; if improvement, decrease dose to 200 mg/m^2; if no improvement, discontinue cetuximab.
  - 3rd occurrence: delay infusion 1–2 weeks; if improvement, reduce dose to 150 mg/m^2; if no improvement, discontinue cetuximab.
  - 4th occurrence: discontinue cetuximab.
- Irinotecan doses and scheduling when used in combination: 350 mg/m^2 q 3 weeks, 180 mg/m^2 q 2 weeks, or 125 mg/m^2 q week × 4 q 6 weeks with dose modifications as needed.

Drug Interactions:

- Synergy with cytotoxic chemotherapy (e.g., irinotecan, cisplatin) or radiotherapy; bevacizumab (Avastin).
- Radiation sensitizer.

Lab Effects/Interference:

- Hypomagnesemia; also related hypocalcemia, hypokalemia.

Special Considerations:

- Indicated for the treatment of EGFR-expressing, metastatic colorectal carcinoma in combination with irinotecan in patients refractory to irinotecan-based chemotherapy; indicated as a single agent in patients who are intolerant to irinotecan-based chemotherapy.

- Indicated for the treatment of patients.
- Indicated in combination with Radiation Therapy (RT) for the treatment of locally or regionally advanced squamous cell carcinoma of the head and neck; also indicated as a single agent for the treatment of patients with recurrent or metastatic squamous cell carcinoma of the head and neck for whom prior platinum-based therapy has failed.
- In clinical trials of patients refractory to irinotecan, cetuximab in combination with irinotecan was shown to have a 23.8% response rate, and in oxaliplatin-irinotecan refractory patients, a 25.8% response rate. Median duration of response was 5.7 months. Response rate to monotherapy was 10.8% overall, with a median duration of 4.2 months (Cunningham et al, 2003).
- EGFR overexpression is associated with more aggressive tumors (poor prognosis, increased risk of metastases, and decreased survival).
- High EGFR copy number and wild-type K-ras (normal, unmutated) associated with response (Finocchiaro et al, 2007).
- Tumors with mutated K-Ras genes did not respond to cetuximab in subset analyses of two clinical trials, EVEREST and CRYSTAL (Tejpar et al, 2008; Van Cutsem et al, 2008).
- Tumors likely to overexpress EGFR are cancers of the colon and rectum, head and neck, pancreas, lung (NSCLC), breast, and bladder.
- Incidence of severe infusion reactions low (3%) but may be fatal (1/1000). 90% occur during 1st infusion, and are characterized by rapid onset of airway obstruction (stridor, hoarseness, bronchospasm), urticaria, and/or hypotension. Treat with epinephrine, corticosteroids, antihistamines, bronchodilators, oxygen as needed, and keep available. Drug should be discontinued if severe reaction occurs. Mild to moderate reactions require infusion rate reduction and prophylactic diphenhydramine.
- In one clinical trial of patients with squamous cell cancer of the head and neck receiving RT and cetuximab, 2% of patients experienced cardiopulmonary arrest. Drug should be used cautiously in combination with RT in patients with coronary artery disease, congestive heart failure, and arrhythmia. In addition, electrolytes including magnesium, calcium, and potassium should be closely monitored during and after cetuximab therapy, as low serum magnesium, calcium, and potassium increase risk of development of torsades de pointes, with subsequent ventricular fibrillation and sudden death.
- NCCN Guidelines (2008) for Patient with Colon and Rectal Cancers states that EGFR testing for overexpression should not be routinely done as EGFR testing has not demonstrated predictive value. No patient should be denied access to cetuximab on the basis of EGFR expression results.
- Responses have been shown in irinotecan refractory colorectal cancer when adding cetuximab to irinotecan; cisplatin refractory squamous cell cancer of the head and neck when adding cetuximab to cisplatin; and when added to radiotherapy in the treatment of patients with unresectable squamous cell cancer of the head and neck.

- Studies show similar pharmacokinetics when drug is administered weekly or as a 500-mg/m^2 biweekly regimen.
- Very rarely (< 0.5%), interstitial lung disease may occur, which may be complicated with non cardiogenic pulmonary edema and death. Onset is between 4–11th cycle of cetuximab, and is more likely in patients with preexisting fibrotic lung disease. Hold drug and evaluate patients who develop acute or worsening pulmonary symptoms. Discontinue the drug if interstitial lung disease is found.
- Skin toxicity (acneform rash) is major toxicity; patients should be taught to wear sunscreen and hats, as well as to limit sun exposure. Rash is not acne (see Chapter 5 introduction for a complete discussion).
- Pretreatment assessment for EGFR expression is not required for patients with squamous cell cancer of the head and neck. Patients with colorectal cancer in clinical trials were required to have evidence of EGFR overexpression. If EGFR overexpression is tested, it is important to use a laboratory with demonstrated proficiency.
- Women of childbearing age should use effective contraception, and for 60 days from the last dose of cetuximab; nursing mothers should not nurse during cetuximab and for 60 days from the last dose of the drug.
- Cetuximab improved overall survival when compared with best supportive care (BSC), which led to its second indication in treatment of patients with advanced CRC: patients receiving cetuximab had a 23% improvement in OS and a 32% reduction in risk of disease progression. OS was 6 mo in the cetuximab arm compared with 4.5 mo in the BSC arm (Jonker et al, 2007).
- Cetuximab was studied in patients with Stage IIIB or IV NSCLC with cisplatin/vinorelbine compared with chemotherapy alone. Patients receiving cetuximab had a significantly higher median OS (10.5 mo vs. 9.1 mo) and higher 1 year survival (45% vs. 37%). Patients of Asian descent had significantly longer OS of 19.5 mo (Pirker et al, 2008).

Potential Toxicities/Side Effects and the Nursing Process

I. POTENTIAL FOR INJURY related to HYPERSENSITIVITY/ ANAPHYLAXIS and INFUSION REACTION

Defining Characteristics: 19–25% of patients experience an infusion reaction. Rarely it is severe (3% of patients receiving drug in combination with Irinotecan, and 2% in patients receiving monotherapy), characterized by rapid onset of airway obstruction (bronchospasm, stridor, hoarseness), urticaria, and/or hypotension. In some cases this may be fatal. Most (90%) occur during the 1st infusion. Mild-to-moderate infusion reactions characterized by chills, fever, dyspnea usually occur during the 1st infusion in 16% of patients receiving combination therapy, and 23% of patients receiving monotherapy. In addition, 73% of patients who received the combination reported asthenia vs 49% who received monotherapy; 33% fever, 9% chills, and 7% headache.

Nursing Implications: Ensure patient receives premedication with diphenhydramine as ordered. Assess baseline VS and mental status prior to drug administration, at 15 minutes, and periodically during infusion, as needed. Remain with patient during first 15 minutes of first infusions. Recall signs/symptoms of anaphylaxis, and if these occur, stop drug immediately, notify physician, and assess patient's vital signs. Subjective symptoms are generalized itching, nausea, chest tightness, crampy abdominal pain, difficulty speaking, anxiety, agitation, sense of impending doom, uneasiness, desire to urinate/defecate, dizziness, and chills. Objective signs are flushed appearance; angioedema of face, neck, eyelids, hands, and feet; localized or generalized urticaria; respiratory distress with or without wheezing; hypotension; and cyanosis. Review standing orders or nursing procedures for patient management of anaphylaxis, and be prepared to stop drug immediately, notify physician, monitor VS, and administer ordered medications, which may include epinephrine 1:1000, hydrocortisone sodium succinate, and diphenhydramine. Teach patient to report any unusual symptoms. For mild-to-moderate infusion reactions (grade 1–2), decrease infusion rate permanently by 50%. Patient should be observed for 1 hour after each treatment, and longer periods may be required if the patient experiences an infusion reaction. Drug should be discontinued in patients who experience severe infusion reactions (grade 3/4).

II. POTENTIAL ALTERATION IN BODY IMAGE, SKIN INTEGRITY, COMFORT related to SKIN RASH

Defining Characteristics: Drug inhibits epidermal growth factor receptor, so major toxicity is manifested in the skin. Most patients (88%–90%) develop a mild-to-moderate acne-like rash that is self-limiting. 14% report a grade 3 rash, and in clinical studies 1.6% of patients discontinued treatment due to skin rash. Rash is a sterile, suppurative rash with multiple follicular or pustular lesions that appear during the first 2 weeks of therapy on the face, upper chest, and back, but in some cases, extended to the arms. Rash maximizes within 4 weeks, and then improves. Rash also resolves when treatment is stopped. However, in 50% of patients, it takes longer than 28 days to resolve. 7% of patients reported dry skin, which may be associated with fissures and in some cases, inflammation and infection such as blepharitis and cellulitis. Infection can be treated with topical clindamycin, or oral antibiotics. It appears that patients who have significant rash, also have a tumor response.

Nursing Implications: Teach patient that rash most likely will occur due to mechanism of drug action. Assess baseline skin integrity on areas of face, neck, and trunk; assess baseline comfort and satisfaction with body image, and monitor at each treatment. Teach patient to report any distress and assess extent of rash. For severe rash, first occurrence, hold drug for 1–2 weeks, and if improvement, continue drug at usual dose. For second occurrence, hold for 1–2 weeks, and then if improved, reduce dose to 200 mg/m^2. If third occurrence of severe rash, hold drug for 1–2 weeks, and if improvement, dose reduce to 150 mg/m^2. For the fourth occurrence or if there is no improvement after holding drug for 2 weeks in prior occurrences, drug is stopped. If skin appears to be infected, (exudate, vesicle formation, abnormal appearance), obtain C+S and discuss empiric treatment with physician. *For rash management, refer to introduction in Chapter 5.* Teach all patients to (1) use a water-based emollient frequently during the day to prevent dryness, (2) stay hydrated, (3) avoid sun exposure and wear SPF 30 (zinc based). Do not use antiacne medications. Tetracycline analogues provide anti-inflammatory benefit. **Grade 1/mild rash (localized, does not interfere with ADLs, and is not infected):** Goal is to preserve skin integrity, minimize discomfort, and prevent infection. Key patient teaching includes (1) use a mild soap with active ingredients that reduce skin drying such as pyrithione zinc (Head and Shoulders), (2) consider aloe gel to red, tender areas, (3) report distressing tenderness as pramoxine (lidocaine topical anesthetic) may help, (4) keep fingernails clean and trimmed, and (5) apply zinc ointment to rectal mucosa after washing. Management: maintain current drug dose, observe or give topical hydrocortisone 1% or 2.5% or clindamycin 1% gel (anti-inflammatory benefit), reassess in 2 weeks. **For grade 2/moderate, which is generalized, mild symptoms, and has minimal effect on ADLs, and no infection:** Goal is to prevent infection and promote comfort. Continue EGFRI dose; use topicals (hydrocortisone 2.5% or clindamycin 1% gel or consider pimecrolimus cream (immunomodulator) and add doxycycline 100 mg PO twice daily or minocycline 100 mg PO twice daily (give antimicrobial and anti-inflammatory effect) and reassess after 2 weeks. **For grade 3/4 or severe rash (generalized, severe, has a significant impact on ADLs, and increased risk of infection):** The goal is to prevent infection or identify it early to minimize complications and to promote effective coping. Dose reduce EGFRI drug based on manufacturer's recommendation, and treat rash with topicals (hydrocortisone 2.5% or clindamycin 1% gel or pimecrolimus cream), doxycycline 100 mg PO twice daily or minocycline 100 mg PO twice daily, and methylprednisolone (Medrol dose pack); reassess after 2 weeks, and interrupt or discontinue drug if rash worsens (Lynch et al, 2007). If rash appears infected (exudate, vesicular formation, different appearance), obtain C+S, treat empirically until sensitivity received, and/or obtain dermatology consult.

III. ALTERATION IN ELECTROLYTE BALANCE related to HYPOMAGNESEMIA, potential

Defining Characteristics: Magnesium wasting appears related to EGFR inhibition in the renal tubular epithelial cells so that excreted magnesium is not resorbed in the distal convoluted tubules. This leads to initial magnesium wasting, followed by losses of calcium and potassium. Hypomagnesemia occurs in about 55% of patients receiving the drug and is severe in 10–15% of patients. It begins within days to months of receiving the drug, and there is much interpatient variability. There appears to be a direct relationship between the duration of cetuximab treatment and severe hypomagnesemia (Fakih, 2007). Symptoms of grade 3/4 hypomagnesemia include fatigue, cramps, and somnolence.

Nursing Implications: Assess baseline electrolyte balance before initial treatment and before each successive weekly treatments. Grade 1 is a serum level of 1.0 mg/dL LLN, grade 2 is 0.9–1.0 mg/dL, grade 3 is 0.7–0.8 mg/dL, and grade 4 is ≤ 0.6 mg/dL. Replete magnesium, calcium, and potassium as needed. Oral magnesium may be ineffective and result in diarrhea (Tejpar et al, 2007). Magnesium repletion regimens include weekly IV replacement of 4-g magnesium sulfate for grade 2. For grade 3/4, patients may be symptomatic and magnesium replacement may involve once to twice weekly IV infusions of 6–10 grams. Provide support for patients, as magnesium replacement infusions require lengthy time in clinic, as an 8-gram infusion requires 4 hours. Post-IV replacement with every other day serum magnesium monitoring is important until the patient develops a steady state (Fakih, 2007). Continue to monitor after drug has been discontinued (half-life of the drug and time drug persists, e.g., 8 weeks). Magnesium replacement in IV hydration starting when a patient has grade 1 hypomagnesemia may be effective in preventing worsening hypomagnesemia. For patients who have refractory grade 4 hypomagnesemia, a stop-and-go approach has been effective where cetuximab is held for 4–8 weeks until the magnesium corrects; it is reported that grade 4 hypomagnesemia does not recur when cetuximab is then reintroduced (Fakih, 2007).

IV. ALTERATION IN NUTRITION, LESS THAN BODY REQUIREMENTS, related to NAUSEA, VOMITING, DIARRHEA, STOMATITIS/ MUCOUS MEMBRANE DISORDER, CONSTIPATION, WEIGHT LOSS

Defining Characteristics: Incidence of mild-to-moderate digestive symptoms include nausea (55% for combination patients, and 29% for monotherapy), diarrhea (72% vs 28%), vomiting (41% vs 25%), stomatitis/mucous membrane disorder (26% vs 11%), weight loss (21% vs 9%), anorexia (36% vs 25%), and constipation 504(30%). Seven percent of patients develop mucous membrane disorder (MMD); 86% of patients with squamous cell cancer of the head and neck receiving concurrent RT experienced mucositis.

Nursing Implications: Assess baseline weight and nutritional status. Teach patient that these symptoms may occur, and to report them. Administer antiemetic and other symptom management medications as ordered. Teach patient self-administration of these medications at home. Monitor serum electrolytes (magnesium, calcium) prior to each dose, and replete magnesium as needed. Teach patient dietary modifications to address symptoms such as anorexia (small, frequent high-calorie, high-protein foods, stimulants as permitted by protocol); constipation (high-fiber, high-fluid, high-roughage foods, stool softeners); diarrhea (bananas, rice, applesauce, and toast); nausea (avoid food preparation odors by cooking in zipped plastic bag, or having someone else cook; choose cool, soft, non-spicy, or fatty foods); mucositis (blenderized high calorie, high protein dense foods, cold or cool soft foods, avoidance of spicy or acidic foods; or Percutaneous Endoscopically placed Gastrostomy tube [PEG] feedings when unable to swallow, local anesthetics to reduce oral and esophageal discomfort/pain). Assess efficacy of intervention, and revise plan as needed.

V. POTENTIAL FOR INFECTION AND FATIGUE related to LEUKOPENIA AND ANEMIA

Defining Characteristics: Leukopenia occurs in about 25% of patients (combination vs 1% monotherapy) with 17% grade 3–4 (combination) and anemia in 16% (combination vs 10% monotherapy (4–5% grade 3–4).

Nursing Implications: Assess baseline WBC, hematocrit and hemoglobin, and monitor prior to each treatment, especially if drug is given in combination with irinotecan Teach patient to monitor temperature, and report temperature > 100.5°F. Assess level of fatigue and teach energy baseline and prior to each treatment. Teach patient that fatigue may occur due to anemia, and teach energy conserving strategies such as alternating rest and activity periods.

Drug: dasatinib (Sprycel, BMS354825)

Class: Multi-targeted tyrosine kinase inhibitor.

Mechanism of Action: Inhibits the following kinases: BCR-Abl, SRC-family (SRC, LCK, YES, FYN), c-KIT, EPHA2, and PDGFR-β. Drug forms a tighter bond with BCR-Abl kinase (300–1000 times more potently) than imatinib mesylate (Gleevec) and binds to both active and inactive forms.

Metabolism: Drug is rapidly absorbed after oral ingestion with peak serum levels in 0.5–6 hours and an overall mean half-life of 3–5 hours. If ingested with a high fat meal, there was a 14% increase in the mean area under the curve exposure, but this is not felt to be clinically relevant. Drug and its active metabolite bind to plasma proteins 96 and 93%, respectively. Drug is extensively metabolized by the P450 microenzyme CYP3A4. Drug is excreted in the feces (85%), and to a lesser degree the urine (4%).

Dosage/Range:
- Chronic phase CML: 100 mg PO once daily.
- Accelerated phase CML, myeloid or lymphoid blast phase CML or Ph+ ALL: 70 mg PO BID daily.
- Dose may be increased or decreased in 20 mg increments based on individual patient response, or co-administration with drugs that either increase or decrease dasatinib serum levels (see drug interactions).
- In clinical studies, adult patients with CML and Ph+ ALL, dose escalations were permitted to 90 mg BID (chronic phase CML) or 100 mg BID (advanced phase CML

and Ph+ ALL) if patients did not achieve a hematologic or cytogenetic response on usual doses.
- Dose modifications for hematologic toxicity. Monitor CBC weekly for the initial 2 months and then periodically.

Drug Preparation: None, oral. Available in 20-mg, 50-mg, and 70-mg tablets, each in 60 tablet bottles.

Drug Administration: Oral, once in the morning and once in the evening, with or without food; do not crush or cut.

Drug Interactions:
- **CYP3A4 inhibitors:** (e.g., ketoconazole, itraconazole, erythromycin, clarithromycin, atazanavir, indinavir, nefazodone, nelfinavir, ritonavir, saquinavir, telithromycin) May decrease metabolism of dasatinib, thus increasing serum concentrations of dasatinib; avoid co-administration, and if they must be given together, decrease dose of dasatinib.
- **CYP3A4 inducers:** Rifampin: decreased dasatinib serum concentrations by 81%; others: dexamethasone, phenytoin, carbamazepine, Phenobarbital, St. John's wort; avoid co-administration and if they must be given together, increase dose of dasatinib. Patients receiving dasatinib should NOT take St. John's wort.
- **Antacids (aluminum hydroxide/magnesium hydroxide):** Decreases dasatinib AUC by 55% as drug requires acid pH; avoid concurrent administration or administer 2 hours prior to or 2 hours after dasantinib dose.
- **H2 blockers/Proton Pump Inhibitors:** Famotidine decreases dasatinib AUC 61%; avoid concurrent administration.
- **Simvastatin, CYP3A4 substrates:** Dasatinib is a time-dependent inhibitor of CYP3A4, and may decrease the metabolism of drugs primarily metabolized by CYP3A4, such as alfentanil, astemizole, terfenadine, cisapride, cyclosporine, fentanyl, pimozide, quinidine, sirolimus, tacrolimus, or ergot alkaloids; decreases simvastatin AUC 37%; avoid concurrent administration or administer cautiously.

Lab Effects/Interference:
- Grade 3–4 neutropenia, thrombocytopenia, and anemia.
- Hypophosphatemia, hypocalcemia.
- Elevated ALT, AST, bilirubin.
- Elevated creatinine.

Special Considerations:
- Drug is indicated for the treatment of adults with chronic, accelerated, or myeloid or lymphoid blast phase chronic myeloid leukemia with resistance or intolerance of prior therapy, including imatinib. There are no controlled trials demonstrating a clinical benefit, such as improvement in disease-related symptoms or increased survival.
- Drug is indicated for the treatment of adults with Philadelphia chromosome positive acute lymphoblastic leukemia with resistance or intolerance to prior therapy.

- Drug is teratogenic and embryo-fetal toxic. Women of childbearing age should be advised to avoid pregnancy, or if the patient becomes pregnant while receiving the drug, patient should be apprised of potential hazard to the fetus. Women should not breast-feed while receiving the drug.
- Drug has the potential to impair reproductive function and fertility in both men and women.
- Use cautiously, if at all, in patients with hepatic dysfunction.
- Drug causes severe myelosuppression, especially in patients with advanced CML or Ph+ ALL than in chronic phase CML. This is reversible and manageable with dose interruption or reduction.
- Drug can cause bleeding events, most commonly related to thrombocytopenia, which can be severe (e.g., CNS hemorrhage). Use cautiously in patients requiring drugs that inhibit platelet function or anticoagulants.
- Drug is associated with fluid retention (including pleural and pericardial effusions), which can be severe in up to 9% of patients. If a patient develops dyspnea, dry cough, suggestive of pleural effusions, evaluate by CXR. Pleural effusions may require thoracentesis and patients may require oxygen therapy. Fluid retention is manageable with supportive measures including diuretics and a short course of steroids.
- Drug can cause QT interval prolongation (cardiac ventricular repolarization). Administer cautiously to patients who may develop prolongation of the QTc interval (hypokalemia, hypomagnesemia, congenital long QT syndrome), patients taking anti-arrhythmic medications, cumulative high-dose anthracycline therapy. Monitor and correct deficits in magnesium and potassium prior to administering dasatinib.
- Assess patient drug profile; teach patient possible interacting drugs, and instruct to tell nurse or physician before starting any over-the-counter or herbal medications.

Potential Toxicities/Side Effects and the Nursing Process

I. POTENTIAL FOR INFECTION AND BLEEDING related to BONE MARROW DEPRESSION

Defining Characteristics: Grades 3–4 neutropenia, thrombocytopenia, and anemia are common, especially severe in patients with advanced CML or Ph+ ALL, as compared to those in chronic phase CML. Drug can cause platelet dysfunction, resulting in rare CNS or GI hemorrhage, and are most often associated with severe thrombocytopenia. Use caution if patients are also taking medications that inhibit platelet function, or anti-coagulants, and monitor very closely. Infection (bacterial, viral, fungal) occurred in 34% of patients. Hemorrhage occurred in 40% of patients (GI and CNS bleeds).

Nursing Implications: Assess baseline CBC, including WBC, differential, and platelet count prior to dosing, as well as at least weekly during first month of treatment, at least every other week for the second month of treatment, and then as clinically indicated and ordered. Discuss dose interruption and reduction as above for neutropenia and thrombocytopenia. Teach patient self-assessment of signs/symptoms of infection and bleeding (including epistaxis and development of petechiae), and instruct patient to report them right away. Teach patient self-care measures to minimize risk of infection and bleeding, including avoidance of OTC aspirin-containing medications. Discuss dose reductions as needed:

Chronic Phase CML (starting dose 100 mg once daily)	ANC $< 0.5 \times 10^9$/L and/or platelets $< 50 \times 10^9$/L	1. Stop dasatinib until ANC $\geq 1.0 \times 10^9$/L and platelets $\geq 50 \times 10^9$/L. 2. Resume dasatinib at original starting dose if recovery in < 7 da. 3. If plt $< 25 \times 10^9$/L and/or recurrence of ANC $< 0.5 \times 10^9$/L for > 7 da, repeat step 1 and resume at reduced dose of 80 mg once a day (2nd episode) or discontinue if third episode.
Accelerated Phase CML, Blast Phase CML and Ph+ ALL (starting dose 70 mg BID)	ANC $< 0.5 \times 10^9$/L and/or platelets $< 10 \times 10^9$/L ANC: Absolute neutrophil count	1. Check if cytopenia is related to leukemia (marrow aspirate or biopsy). 2. If cytopenia is unrelated to leukemia, stop drug until ANC $\geq 1.0 \times 10^9$/L and platelets $\geq 20 \times 10^9$/L, and resume at original starting dose. 3. If recurrence of cytopenia, repeat step 1 and resume drug at a reduced dose of 50 mg BID (2nd episode) or 40 mg BID if 3rd episode. 4. If cytopenia is related to leukemia, consider dose escalation to 100 mg BID.

Bristol-Myers Squibb Company. Sprycel (dasatinib) package insert. Princeton, NJ: Bristol-Myers Squibb Company; November 2007.

II. ALTERATION IN FLUID AND ELECTROLYTE BALANCE related to FLUID RETENTION, EDEMA

Defining Characteristics: Fluid retention is common (50%). Superficial edema most common, but pleural effusion may occur in 22% of patients. However, ascites, rapid weight gain, and pulmonary edema may develop, and in some cases, be life-threatening (pleural effusion, congestive heart failure, pulmonary hypertension, pericardial effusion, anasarca).

Nursing Implications: Assess baseline parameters of weight, presence of edema, pulmonary function, and monitor closely during therapy. Teach patient to monitor weight daily at home, and to report weight gain of 2 pounds in one week, development of edema, or dyspnea. Develop a plan to protect skin and maintain skin integrity, and discuss the prescription of diuretics with physician or NP.

III. ALTERATION IN NUTRITION, POTENTIAL, LESS THAN BODY REQUIREMENTS, related to NAUSEA, VOMITING, DIARRHEA

Defining Characteristics: Nausea affected 34% of patients; vomiting affected 22%. Diarrhea affected 50%, while constipation affected 14%.

Nursing Implications: Assess baseline nutritional status and bowel elimination status. If patient develops nausea and/or vomiting, teach patient to self-administer antiemetics one hour prior to each dose, and to call if nausea/vomiting persist. Discuss with physician more effective antiemetic regime if nausea/vomiting persist. Encourage small, frequent intake of cool, bland foods as tolerated if nausea develops. Refer to dietitian as needed for meal planning. Teach patient to report diarrhea that does not respond to OTC anti-diarrheal medication. Teach self-care measures of diet modification and increased oral fluids to 2–3 L during the waking hours. If constipation, teach patient self-care measures to prevent constipation.

IV. ALTERATION IN COMFORT related to PAIN, HEADACHE, FATIGUE, ARTHRALGIA, AND FATIGUE

Defining Characteristics: Headache affected 40% of patients, musculoskeletal pain affected 39% of patients, fatigue 39% of patients, myalgias/arthralgias 19% of patients, and abdominal pain affected 25% of patients.

Nursing Implications: Teach patient that these events may occur and to report them. Assess baseline comfort, and monitor closely during treatment. Develop plan to assure comfort depending on symptoms reported. Discuss ineffective strategies with physician, and revise plan as needed.

Drug: denileukin diftitox (ONTAK®)

Class: Fusion protein.

Mechanism of Action: Agent is recombinant DNA-derived cytotoxic protein containing diphtheria toxin fragments, and IL-2. It targets cells with high affinity for IL-2 receptors containing a CD25 component, such as activated T and B lymphocytes, and activated macrophages. The IL-2 portion of the fusion protein binds to the IL-2 receptor on malignant cells, which contain a CD25 component. The diphtheria toxin fragments are brought into the cell through the receptor (receptor-mediated endocytosis) and into the endosomal vesicles. Acidification cleaves the active fragment of diphtheria toxin, which is then actively transported into the cytoplasm. There, it catalyzes a reaction that inhibits protein synthesis and causes cell death within hours.

Metabolism: Distribution phase has half-life of 2–5 minutes, and terminal phase half-life of 70–80 minutes; the development of antibodies to denileukin diftitox significantly increases clearance 2–3 times, with a consequent decrease in mean systemic exposure of about 75%. Metabolized by proteolytic degradation and primarily excreted via the liver and kidneys; excreted material is < 25% of total dose.

Dosage/Range:
- 9 or 18 micrograms/kg/day IV daily × 5 days, repeated every 3 weeks × at least 3 cycles.

Drug Preparation:
- Bring ONTAK vial to room temperature (25°C, or 77°F); may thaw in refrigerator at 2–8°C (36–46°F) over less than 24 hours, or at room temperature for 1–2 hours. DO NOT HEAT.
- Mix by gentle swirling. DO NOT SHAKE VIGOROUSLY.
- DO NOT REFREEZE DRUG.
- Inspect solution for clarity and discard if it remains hazy (will be hazy after thawing, but becomes clear when at room temperature).
- Withdraw ordered dose from vial and inject into an empty IV infusion bag; add up to 9 mL of sterile saline without preservative for each 1 mL of ONTAK to the IV bag, for a final concentration of at least 15 mcg/mL.
- Discard any unused portion of the drug.

Drug Administration:
- Give by IV infusion over at least 15 minutes, but less than 80 minutes.
- Slow or stop infusion if infusion reaction occurs, depending upon severity of symptoms.
- DO NOT administer with other drugs, or give through an inline filter.
- Administer prepared IV solution within 6 hours, using a syringe pump or infusion bag.

- Administer at least 500-mL 0.9% normal saline IV hydration to reduce risk of vascular leak syndrome.
- Premedicate with acetaminophen, corticosteroids, and antihistamine to minimize the risk of infusion reaction.

Drug Interactions:
- Unknown.

Lab Effects/Interference:
- Hypoalbuminemia may occur in up to 83% of patients, with nadir 1–2 weeks after drug administration.
- Increased serum transaminases (temporary).

Special Considerations:
- ONTAK is indicated for the treatment of patients with persistent or recurrent cutaneous T-cell lymphoma (CTCL, or mycosis fungoides) whose malignant cells express the CD25 component of the IL-2 receptor.
- Hypoalbuminemia increases risk of capillary leak syndrome. Delay administration of drug until serum albumin is ≥ 3.0 g/dL.
- Avoid use during pregnancy unless benefit outweighs risk.
- Nursing mothers should not breast-feed while receiving the drug.
- Adverse reactions tend to be more frequent and/or more severe in the elderly (anorexia, hypotension, anemia, confusion, rash, nausea and/or vomiting).
- The frequency of adverse effects decreases after the second course of therapy.
- CBC, chemistries, including albumin, liver, and renal function studies, should be done baseline and weekly during therapy. Hepatotoxicity may occur in 15–20% of patients, often together with hypoalbinemia during the first course of treatment, and resolve within 2 weeks.

Potential Toxicities/Side Effects and the Nursing Process

I. POTENTIAL FOR INJURY related to HYPERSENSITIVITY OR ANAPHYLAXIS REACTIONS

Defining Characteristics: Acute hypersensitivity reactions occurred in 69% of patients during clinical trials during or within 24 hours of the ONTAK infusion, with 50% occurring during the first day of dosing of each cycle. Reactions were characterized by hypotension (50%), back pain (30%), dyspnea (28%), vasodilation (28%), rash (25%), chest pain/tightness (24%), tachycardia (12%), dysphagia or laryngismus (5%), syncope (3%), allergic reaction (1%), anaphylaxis (1%). Infusion reaction (fever, chills, asthenia, myalgias, arthralgias, headache) is easily managed. Risk of reaction decreases with premedication with acetaminophen, antihistamines, and corticosteroids (dexamethasone or prednisone 10–20 mg). Steroid premedication may also increase response rates.

Nursing Implications: Assess baseline VS and mental status prior to drug administration, at 15 minutes, and periodically during infusion. Remain with patient during first 15 minutes of infusion. Recall signs/symptoms of anaphylaxis and, if these occur, stop drug immediately and notify physician. Subjective symptoms are generalized itching, nausea, chest tightness, crampy abdominal pain, difficulty speaking, anxiety, agitation, sense of impending doom, uneasiness, desire to urinate/defecate, dizziness, chills. Objective signs are flushed appearance; angioedema of face, neck, eyelids, hands, feet; localized or generalized urticaria; respiratory distress with or without wheezing, hypotension, cyanosis. Review standing orders or nursing procedure for patient management of anaphylaxis and be prepared to stop drug immediately, notify physician, monitor VS, and administer ordered medications, which may include epinephrine 1:1000, hydrocortisone sodium succinate, and diphenhydramine. Teach patient to report any unusual symptoms.

II. POTENTIAL FOR INJURY related to VASCULAR LEAK SYNDROME (VLS)

Defining Characteristics: 27% of patients in clinical trial testing developed VLS about 10 days after the first infusion, characterized by hypotension, edema, and hypoalbuminemia. Onset of symptoms occurs within the first two weeks of infusion and may persist or become more severe after the drug has been stopped. Patients with preexisting cardiac problems are at risk for developing myocardial infarctions. Syndrome is usually self-limiting, but may rarely require management of edema or hypotension. Low serum albumin is a predictor of development of syndrome. The incidence of VLS can be decreased by saline hydration after drug infusion (Duvic, 2006).

Nursing Implications: Monitor weight, BP, and serum albumin levels baseline and throughout treatment; assess for presence of edema baseline and throughout treatment. Notify physician if edema, hypotension, or serum albumin < 3.0 g/dL. Treatment should be delayed until serum albumin is ≥ 3.0 g/dL. Hydrate with at least 500-mL 0.9% NS after drug dose.

III. POTENTIAL FOR INFECTION related to LYMPHOPENIA, IMMUNE SUPPRESSION OF MACROPHAGES

Defining Characteristics: Cutaneous T-cell lymphoma increases risk of cutaneous infection, together with drug-induced lymphopenia, and impaired immune function further increases risk. During clinical trials, 48% of patients developed infections (23% severe). Lymphocyte counts < 900 cells/μl occurred in 34% of patients. Counts decreased during days 1–5 (dosing period) with recovery by day 15; subsequent cycles had less lymphopenia and more rapid recovery.

Nursing Implications: Assess baseline WBC, lymphocyte count, and monitor weekly during therapy. Assess skin integrity, potential for infection, and teach patient measures to prevent infection (e.g., keeping skin intact, avoiding sources of infection, good handwashing). Teach patient to report any signs/symptoms of infection (e.g., redness, heat, exudate on skin, T > 100.5, sputum production, dysuria). Assess for signs/symptoms of infection during therapy and at each visit.

IV. ALTERATION IN COMFORT related to FLU-LIKE SYMPTOMS

Defining Characteristics: 91% of patients developed flu-like symptom complex during clinical trials, consisting of fever and chills (81%), asthenia (66%), nausea/vomiting (64%), myalgias (18%), arthralgias (8%). Dehydration occurred in 9% of patients. Symptoms developed within hours to days after having received drug infusion. Symptoms are generally mild to moderate and are responsive to symptom management.

Nursing Implications: Teach patient that flu-like symptoms may occur commonly following treatment, and teach symptom management with antipyretics (e.g., acetaminophen) and dietary modification if nausea experienced. Discuss with physician giving patient prescription for antiemetic agent in case nausea is severe or vomiting develops. Discuss use of meperidine, diphenhydramine if patient develops rigors. Teach patient to call nurse or physician if symptoms do not respond, become worse, if unable to take at least 1 qt of fluid orally per day, or new symptoms develop.

V. ALTERATION IN NUTRITION related to DIARRHEA, ANOREXIA, NAUSEA/VOMITING, HYPOALBUMINEMIA

Defining Characteristics: Nausea/vomiting occurs in 64% of patients as part of flu-like syndrome, anorexia occurs in 36% of patients, and diarrhea occurs in 29%. Hypoalbuminemia occurs in 83%, weight loss in 14%, and elevated transaminases 61%. Elevation of serum transaminases occurred during first cycle of therapy, and resolved within two weeks. Hypocalcemia (17%) and hypokalemia (6%) have also been reported. Constipation occurred in 9%, dyspepsia 7%, and dysphagia 6%. Rarely, pancreatitis, hyperthyroidism, and hypothyroidism may occur.

Nursing Implications: Assess baseline nutritional status, as well as baseline LFTs and serum albumin, and monitor weekly during therapy. Teach patient to eat high-calorie, high-protein foods. Assess for occurrence of symptoms of nausea, vomiting, diarrhea, anorexia, other problems, and teach patient to report them. Teach patient self-administration of prescribed medications to manage symptoms.

VI. ALTERATION IN COMFORT related to SKIN RASHES, PAIN AT TUMOR SITES

Defining Characteristics: During clinical trials, rash occurred in 34%, pruritus 20%, and sweating 10%. Rashes occurred during/after treatment or were delayed. They were varied, as generalized maculopapular, petechial, vesicular bullous, urticarial, or as eczema.

Nursing Implications: Assess baseline skin integrity and presence of rashes. Assess daily during treatment and weekly thereafter; teach patient to report any skin changes. Assess need for diphenhydramine or other antihistamines for pruritus, and use of topical and/or oral corticosteroids for moderate to severe rashes and discomfort.

VII. POTENTIAL ALTERATION IN CARDIAC OUTPUT related to HYPOTENSION, TACHYCARDIA, THROMBOTIC EVENTS

Defining Characteristics: The following cardiovascular side effects occurred in clinical testing: hypotension (36%), vasodilation (22%), tachycardia (12%), thrombotic events (7%), hypertension (6%), and arrhythmia (6%). Two patients with preexisting coronary artery disease developed myocardial infarctions while receiving the drug. Thrombotic events included deep vein thrombosis, pulmonary embolus, arterial thrombosis, and superficial thrombophlebitis.

Nursing Implications: Assess baseline cardiovascular status and presence of risk factor of coronary artery disease. Teach patient to report any chest pain or discomfort, palpitations, pain in calf, heat/redness of calf immediately, or to come to the emergency room if at home. Discuss onset of hypotension, tachycardia with physician, relationship to drug administration, and management strategies. If symptoms are severe, stop drug infusion and discuss use of saline hydration to raise BP and decrease HR.

VIII. POTENTIAL FOR FATIGUE AND BLEEDING related to BONE MARROW SUPPRESSION

Defining Characteristics: Anemia occurs in about 18% (6% grades 3 or 4), thrombocytopenia in 8% (2% grades 3 or 4), and leukopenia in 6% (3% grades 3 or 4).

Nursing Implications: Monitor CBC/differential, HCT, and platelet count and assess for signs/symptoms of infection, fatigue, and bleeding baseline prior to treatment, and weekly during treatment. Instruct patient in self-assessment of signs/symptoms of infection, fatigue, bleeding. Transfuse platelet, red cell transfusions per physician's order.

IX. POTENTIAL ALTERATION IN OXYGENATION related to DYSPNEA, COUGH

Defining Characteristics: In clinical trials, 29% of patients reported dyspnea, 26% increased cough, 17% pharyngitis, 13% rhinitis, and 8% "lung disorder."

Nursing Implications: Assess VS, pulmonary exam, and weight prior to each treatment, and at each weekly visit. Teach patient to do daily weights, and to report any SOB, weight gain, increased cough, or other problems. If this occurs, notify physician and discuss obtaining CXR and focused exam. Discuss chest X-ray findings with physician.

X. POTENTIAL SENSORY/PERCEPTUAL ALTERATIONS related to NERVOUSNESS, CONFUSION, INSOMNIA

Defining Characteristics: Nervousness may affect 11%, confusion 8%, and insomnia 9%.

Nursing Implications: Teach patient that these symptoms may occur and to report them. Assess baseline mental status, affect, and sleep pattern prior to each treatment cycle, and weekly during treatment. Discuss need for pharmacologic symptom management if symptoms are severe.

XI. POTENTIAL ALTERATION IN URINE ELIMINATION related to HEMATURIA, ALBUMINURIA, PYURIA

Defining Characteristics: Patients in clinical trials experienced hematuria (10%), albuminuria (10%), and pyuria (10%). 7% had increases in serum creatinine. Rarely, acute renal insufficiency occurs.

Nursing Implications: Assess baseline urinary elimination status, urinalysis, as well as serum renal function studies. Teach patient to report blood in urine, and dysuria, or any problems in voiding. Discuss abnormalities with physician.

Drug: elesclomol (STA-4783; investigational)

Class: Oxidative stress inducer.

Mechanism of Action: Small molecule that induces metabolic oxidative stress in malignant cells, leading to selective, malignant, cell death. It does this by increasing the amount of reactive oxygen species (ROS) in the cell, and when these exceed the cell's antioxidant ability to neutralize the ROS, the resulting oxidative stress kills the cell. Normal cells have a low level of ROS, but cancer cells have higher level of ROS and oxidative stress so that this additional oxidative stress exceeds the survival thres-hold for malignant cells. In combination with chemotherapy, the drug may also lower the threshold for apoptosis so that the chemotherapy is more efficient in killing cells.

Metabolism:
- Unknown.

Dosage/Range:
- Per protocol.

Drug Preparation:
- Per protocol.

Drug Administration:
- Per protocol, given in combination with paclitaxel.

Drug Interactions:
- Unknown.

Lab Effects/Interference:
- Unknown.

Special Considerations:
- Showed increased median progression-free survival for patients with Stage IV metastatic melanoma in combination with paclitaxel compared with paclitaxel alone (3.7 mo vs 1.8 mo, $p = 0.035$).
- Most common side effects in combination with paclitaxel were fatigue, alopecia, constipation, nausea, hypoesthesia, arthralgia, insomnia, diarrhea, and anemia.

Potential Toxicities/Side Effects (Dose- and Schedule-Dependent) and the Nursing Process (in Combination with Paclitaxel)

I. POTENTIAL FOR INFECTION AND FATIGUE related to BONE MARROW DEPRESSION

Defining Characteristics: Grade 3/4 neutropenia occurred in 6–7.7% of patients, compared to 0% in patients receiving paclitaxel alone. Anemia was common.

Nursing Implications: Assess baseline leukocyte, platelet, and Hgb/HCT and monitor before each treatment, during therapy, and more often as needed. See protocol for dose modifications. Assess risk for infection and integrity of skin and mucous membranes, pulmonary status, and ability to clear secretions, as well as history of past infections baseline and prior to each treatment. Teach patient to self-administer prophylactic antibiotics and antiviral agents as ordered by physician. Teach patient to self-administer oral antifungal agent if oral candidiasis develops. Teach patient to self-assess for signs/symptoms of infection and to call provider immediately or come to the emergency room if temperature > 100.5°F, shaking chills, rash, productive cough, burning on urination, or any signs/symptoms of infection or bleeding. Teach self-care strategies to minimize risk of infection and bleeding, including avoidance of OTC aspirin-containing medications. Teach patient self-care strategies to manage fatigue.

II. ALTERATION IN COMFORT related to BACK PAIN, HYPOESTHESIA, ARTHRALGIAS, INSOMNIA

Defining Characteristics: Back pain, hypoesthesia, arthralgias, and insomnia occurred less commonly than in the control paclitaxel arm. Grade 3/4 back pain occurred in 2% of patients, compared to 7% of patients receiving paclitaxel alone.

Nursing Implications: Teach patients these side effects may occur, and to discuss them with study nurse and physician. Discuss self-care strategies and symptom management agents permitted by protocol.

Drug: erlotinib (OSI-774, Tarceva™)

Class: Epidermal Growth Factor Receptor (HER1/EGFR) tyrosine kinase inhibitor (quinazoline type).

Mechanism of Action: Mechanism of anti-tumor activity not fully characterized. Inhibits the phosphorylation of the intracellular portion of the EGFR or tyrosine kinase domain of the EGFR. This inhibits the activation of cell signaling telling the nucleus of the cell to divide, to avoid programmed cell death, and to release VEGF.

Metabolism: Drug bioavailability is about 60% after oral administration with peak plasma concentration occurring 4 hours after ingestion. Drug is highly protein-bound (90–95%). It is primarily metabolized by the cytochrome P450 hepatic microsomal enzyme system (CYP3A4). Food can increase drug bioavailability by 100%.

Dosage/Range:
- 150 mg PO q day.

Drug Preparation:
- Oral, available in 150-, 100-, and 25-mg tablets.
- Dose should be taken on an empty stomach, either 1 hour before meals or 2 hours after meals.

Drug Interactions:
- *Inducers of the CYP3A4* (may increase metabolism of erlotinib and decrease its plasma concentration): rifampin, phenytoin, phenobarbital, St. John's wort, carbamazepine, rifapentine, rifabutin. May need to increase dose of erlotinib.
- *Inhibitors of the CYP3A4* (may increase metabolism of erlotinib and increase its plasma concentration): ketoconazole, itraconazole, grapefruit (fruit or juice), clarithromycin, ritonavir, indinavir, atanazavir, nelfinavir, saquinavir, metronidazole, isoniazid, telithromycin, troleandomycin, voriconazole. May need to decrease dose of erlotinib.
- *Warfarin* increases INR and bleeding possible; monitor INR, patient bleeding, and decrease warfarin dose as needed.

Lab Effects/Interference:

- May increase liver function tests (serum transaminases).

Special Considerations:

- Drug is FDA approved for the treatment of patients with locally advanced or metastatic non-small cell lung cancer after failure of at least one prior chemotherapy regimen.
- Drug is FDA approved in combination with gemcitabine for the treatment of patients with locally advanced, unresectable, or metastatic pancreatic carcinoma. In this combination, principle toxicities were fatigue, rash, nausea, anorexia, and diarrhea. Rare but severe toxicities of the combination included stroke, syncope, microangiopathic anemia with thrombocytopenia, myocardial infarction/ischemia, arrhythmias, renal insufficiency, ileus, pancreatitis, and neuropathy.
- Infrequently, drug can cause interstitial lung disease (ILD) (< 1% of patients), which can be serious. This is a class effect, and similar to that of gelfitinib. Drug should be stopped immediately in patients who develop worsening or unexplained pulmonary symptoms, and appropriate diagnostic work-up begun to establish the cause. If ILD is diagnosed, erlotinib should be discontinued.
- Drug can cause keratitis and conjunctivitis with drying of eyes, ameliorated by artificial tears.
- Patients may require temporary interruption or dose reduction for severe diarrhea that does not resolve with anti-diarrheals, or for severe and intolerable rash; dose modification if refractory or intolerable. Also, consider if patient has severe liver dysfunction.
- Rarely, drug may cause interstitial lung disease (ILD); if the patients develops pulmonary symptoms, hold drug until ILD can be ruled out.
- Appears to cross the blood–brain barrier, as some patients with brain metastases have demonstrated responses.
- Rare hepatotoxicity and renal failure, as well as deaths in patients with moderate hepatic impairment receiving erlotinib reported.

Potential Toxicities/Side Effects and the Nursing Process

I. ALTERATION IN SKIN INTEGRITY related to RASH

Defining Characteristics: As expected, because EGFR is important in skin function, this is the area of major toxicity. Rash ranges from maculopapular to pustular on the face, neck, chest, back, and arms, affecting up to 75% of patients. Most rashes are mild to moderate (Sandler et al, 2004). Typically, rash begins on days 8–10 of therapy, maximizing in intensity by week 2, and resolving gradually on therapy (often by week 4). Use of skin treatments (corticosteroids, topical clindamycin, or minocycline) have been used with varying results.

Nursing Implications: Assess skin integrity of face, neck, arms, and upper trunk baseline, and regularly during treatment. Teach patient that rash may occur, its usual course, and self-care measures for comfort. Emphasize the need to keep skin with rash clean to prevent infection, and to continue taking erlotinib until told to stop by nurse or physician. Teach patient that skin may become dry, and to use skin emollients or moisturizers. Assess body image intactness, and if rash develops, its threat to body image. Encourage patient to verbalize feelings; provide emotional support, and individualize care plan to patient response. For rash management, refer to the introduction in Chapter 5. Teach all patients to (1) use a water-based emollient frequently during the day to prevent dryness, (2) stay hydrated, (3) avoid sun exposure and wear SPF 30 (zinc based). Do not use anti-acne medications. Tetracycline analogues provide anti-inflammatory benefit. **Grade 1/mild rash (localized, does not interfere with ADLs, and is not infected):** The goal is to preserve skin integrity, minimize discomfort, and prevent infection. Key patient teaching includes (1) use a mild soap with active ingredients that reduce skin drying such as pyrithione zinc (Head and Shoulders), (2) consider aloe gel to red, tender areas, (3) report distressing tenderness as pramoxine (lidocaine topical anesthetic may help), (4) keep fingernails clean and trimmed, and (5) apply zinc ointment to rectal mucosa after washing. Management: maintain current drug dose, observe or give topical hydrocortisone 1% or 2.5% or clindamycin 1% gel (anti-inflammatory benefit); reassess in 2 weeks. **For grade 2/moderate rash, which is generalized, mild symptoms, and has minimal effect on ADLs, and no infection:** Goal is to prevent infection and promote comfort. Continue EGFRI dose; use topicals (hydrocortisone 2.5% or clindamycin 1% gel or consider pimecrolimus cream [immunomodulator]) and add doxycycline 100 mg PO twice daily or minocycline 100 mg PO twice daily (give antimicrobial and anti-inflammatory effect) and reassess after 2 weeks. **For grade 3/4 or severe rash (generalized, severe, has a significant impact on ADLs, and increased risk of infection):** The goal is to prevent infection or to identify it early to minimize complications and to promote effective coping. Dose reduce erlotinib in 50-mg increments as needed, and treat rash with topicals (hydrocortisone 2.5% or clindamycin 1% gel or pimecrolimus cream), doxycycline 100 mg PO twice daily or minocycline 100 mg PO twice daily, and methylprednisolone (Medrol dose pack); reassess after 2 weeks, and interrupt or discontinue drug if rash worsens (Lynch et al, 2007). If rash appears infected (exudate, vesicular formation, different appearance), obtain C+S, treat empirically until sensitivity received, and/or obtain dermatology consult.

II. ALTERATION IN ELIMINATION PATTERN related to DIARRHEA

Defining Characteristics: Affects approximately 54% of patients, and is mild to moderate with only 6% of patients experiencing grade 3 diarrhea. Diarrhea usually beginning weeks 3–4. Symptoms may be self-limited or require an anti-diarrheal agent, such as loperamide. Severe diarrhea not responsive to anti-diarrheal medication may require temporary dose-interruption or adjustment if refractory.

Nursing Implications: Assess bowel elimination pattern baseline, and regularly during therapy. Teach patient to report diarrhea; teach patient self-care strategies to manage diarrhea such as dietary modification and self-administration of loperamide;

teach patient to minimize potential complications such as dehydration and electrolyte depletion. Identify patients at risk for dehydration and follow closely, such as patients with renal insufficiency, diabetes, CHF, or the older population. If diarrhea does not resolve or is severe, discuss with physician dose interruption, as well as fluid and electrolyte replacement. If dose needs to be reduced, reduce in 50-mg increments.

III. SENSORY/PERCEPTUAL ALTERATION, POTENTIAL related to CONJUNCTIVITIS AND EYE DRYNESS

Defining Characteristics: Conjunctivitis and eye dryness may occur, and are generally mild to moderate (grades 1–2).

Nursing Implications: Teach patient to report any eye irritation or change in visual acuity. Teach patient to use artificial tears to keep eyes lubricated.

IV. POTENTIONAL ALTERATION IN NUTRITION, LESS THAN BODY REQUIREMENTS, related to MUCOSITIS and ANOREXIA

Defining Characteristics: Stomatitis is uncommon, occurring in 17% of patients receiving erlotinib, compared to 3% receiving placebo. Grade 3/4 occurs in < 1% of patients. It is usually mild to moderate and is generally self-limited. Anorexia affects about 52% of patients with 8% experiencing grade 3.

Nursing Implications: Assess oral hygiene practices, and status of oral mucosa, gums, and teeth baseline, and regularly throughout therapy. Teach patient to report stomatitis, and to use a systematic cleansing regimen as determined by institutional policy.

Drug: everolimus (RAD001, investigational)

Class: mTOR inhibitor.

Mechanism of Action: mTOR is an intracellular kinase protein that regulates cell proliferation and angiogenesis. It is found in the cytoplasm and turns on and off the translation of signals that tell the cell's protein factory (ribosomes) to make proteins. Proteins control all the cell functions. Proteins that activate mTOR are growth signals from EGF, insulin-like growth factor (IGF), and VEGFs. Proteins that stop mTOR activity are tuberous sclerosis complex (TSC) 1 and 2, and if there are not enough nutrients to support more cells, mTOR activity is blocked. As an mTOR inhibitor, everolimus interferes with the central regulation of tumor cell division, metabolism, and angiogenesis. Blocking this important protein results in cell cycle arrest and cell death.

Drug is currently used as an immunosuppressant to prevent transplanted organ rejection; it reduces incidence of chronic allograft vasculopathy in heart transplant patients (drug name Certican). Drug is a proliferation signal inhibitor and inhibits the proliferation and clonal expansion of antigen-activated T-cells, which are stimulated by cytokines IL-2 and IL-5. Cells are arrested in the G_1 phase of the cell cycle.

Metabolism: In the transplant setting: after an oral dose, peak levels reached in 1–2 hr after the dose, and steady state reached in 4 days. Area under the curve was reduced by 16% when taken with a high-fat diet. Plasma binding about 74%. Everolimus is mainly metabolized by CYP3A4 in the liver and to some extent in the intestinal wall and is a substrate for the multidrug efflux pump P-glycoprotein. Drug is excreted in the feces (80%) and urine (5%).

Dosage/Range:
- Per protocol, or for example, in one study, 10 mg PO daily.

Drug Preparation:
- Oral.

Drug Administration:
- Orally, once daily per protocol.

Drug Interactions:
- Co-administration with strong CYP3A4-inhibitors (e.g., ketoconazole, itraconazole, voriconazole, clarithromycin, telithromycin, ritonavir) and inducers (e.g., rifampicin, rifabutin) is not recommended unless the benefit outweighs the risk.
- Grapefruit and grapefruit juice can interfere with the CYP3A4 metabolic pathway; do not take while receiving everolimus.
- St. John's Wort can increase the metabolism of everolimus and thus lower drug serum levels; do not use together.
- Inhibitors of P-glycoprotein may decrease the efflux of everolimus from intestinal cells and increase everolimus blood concentrations.
- Everolimus is a competitive inhibitor of CYP3A4 and of CYP2D6 microsomal pathways so that drugs metabolized via these pathways may have higher serum levels; if the drug has a narrow therapeutic window, monitor for side effects or decrease dose of interacting drug.

Lab Effects/Interference:
- Increased serum lipid profile.
- Hyperglycemia.
- Anemia.
- Decreased serum phosphate level.

Special Considerations:
- Phase III clinical trial in renal cell cancer was stopped early as study endpoints met (at 6 mo, patients receiving this drug had superior progression-free survival [26%] compared with those on placebo [2%]). The difference in median progression-free survival was 4 mo in the everolimus group compared with 1.9 mo in placebo group. Patients in the study included those who had progressed on sorafinib,

sunitinib, both agents, and bevacizumab and interferon (RECORD-1 trial; Motzer et al, 2008).

- Being studied in renal cell cancer, carcinoid neuroendocrine tumors, lymphoma, other solid tumors, alone or in combination with other anti-cancers drugs, and tuberous sclerosis.
- Common toxicities included stomatitis (36% vs 7% control), anemia (28% vs 15%), weakness (28% vs 20%). Other side effects that occurred were high blood lipids, hyperglycemia, skin rash, hypophosphatemia, interstitial lung disease, which responds to drug discontinuance and/or corticosteroids.

Potential Toxicities/Side Effects and the Nursing Process

I. POTENTIAL ALTERATION IN NUTRITION, LESS THAN BODY REQUIREMENTS, related to STOMATITIS, HYPERGLYCEMIA, HYPERTRIGLYCERIDEMIA

Defining Characteristics: In clinical studies, mucositis affected 36% of patients (compared with 7% placebo). Hyperglycemia, hypercholesteremia, and hypophosphatemia have been reported. mTOR is involved in insulin signaling, which possibly explains the hypertriglyceridemia and hyperglycemia.

Nursing Implications: Assess serum triglycerides, cholesterol, phosphate, glucose, baseline and during treatment with the drug. Teach the patient to report signs/symptoms of hyperglycemia (polyuria, polydipsia, polyphagia). Assess oral mucosa prior to drug administration, and instruct patient to self-assess and report changes. Teach patient oral hygiene measures and self-assessment. Teach patient to notify physician/nurse if excessive thirst or any increase in volume or frequency of urination. Notify physician of any abnormalities and discuss implications and management.

II. ALTERATION IN SKIN INTEGRITY, POTENTIAL, related to RASH

Defining Characteristics: Rash has been reported.

Nursing Implications: Assess patient skin integrity, including nails baseline and regularly during treatment. Teach patient self-assessment and local comfort measures, including the use of water-based emollients. Teach patient to report skin changes and if self-care is ineffective to discuss plan with physician, especially if severe.

III. ALTERATION IN COMFORT AND ACTIVITY TOLERANCE, POTENTIAL, related to ASTHENIA, ANEMIA

Defining Characteristics: Asthenia, weakness (affects 36% vs. 7%) and anemia (28% vs. 15%) have been reported in clinical studies.

Nursing Implications: Assess baseline CBC, hgb, comfort, and activity tolerance, and reassess during treatment, asking patient to identify what activities now unable to do, sleep habits, and also feeling state. Discuss alternating rest and activity periods and also possibility of other family members or friends assisting with energy-consuming responsibilities to increase energy reserve. Teach patient to report increasing fatigue, signs of severe anemia (shortness of breath, chest pain/angina, headaches). Monitor hemoglobin/hematocrit; discuss transfusion with physician if signs/symptoms develop or hematocrit falls < 25 mg/dL. Teach patient about diet high in iron.

Drug: gefitinib (Iressa)

Class: Tyrosine kinase inhibitor.

Mechanism of Action: Drug inhibits the intracellular phosphorylation of a number of tyrosine kinases associated with transmembrane cell surface receptors, including the epidermal growth factor receptor (EGFR-TK). This prevents the message for cell division from being sent to the nucleus. Thus cell division, growth, and angiogenesis do not occur. Drug resistance develops with the tumor using alternate pathways to stimulate the cell nucleus (MET oncogene is stimulated and message sent via ERB3; Engleman et al, 2007).

Metabolism: Absorbed slowly from the gastrointestinal tract following oral administration with peak plasma levels occurring 3–7 hours after dosing. Bioavailability 60%, and unaffected by food. Drug is 90% protein bound (serum albumin). Drug is metabolized via the P450 microenzyme system, primarily the CYP 3A4 subsystem, and excreted in the feces (86%). Elimination half-life 48 hours with steady state plasma level achieved within 10 days.

Dosage/Range:

- 250 mg PO daily. As of 9/15/05, the manufacturer, Astra Zeneca, is limiting availability of the drug to patients who have previously taken the drug and are benefiting, or who have benefited. The drug will be available through the IRESSA access program only. In clinical trials, the drug will be available to patients who are enrolled. If new study data shows an improvement in survival, then the labeling will change.

Drug Preparation:

- Available as 250 mg tablets in a bottle of 30 tablets.

Drug Administration:

- Administer with or without food at about the same time each day: If severe diarrhea or skin reaction, briefly interrupt therapy for up to 14 days, and then resume at same dose.
- If new onset or worsening of pulmonary symptoms (dyspnea, cough, fever), interrupt therapy until pulmonary evaluation can rule out interstitial lung disease. IF interstitial lung disease confirmed, STOP gefitinib and treat pulmonary toxicity.

- If new onset eye pain or other eye symptoms, interrupt therapy and evaluate cause.
- Inducers of CYP3A4 (increase metabolism of gefitinib and decrease its plasma concentrations or AUC by 85%): rifamycin, phenytoin; consider increasing gefitinib dose to 500 mg/d. St. John's wort: teach patient to discontinue herbal.

Drug Interactions:
- Inhibitors of CYP 3A4 (decrease metabolism of gefitinib and increase its plasma concentration or AUC by 88%): Itraconazole; consider another antifungal or decrease gefitinib if increased toxicity.
- High gastric pH > 5.0 (e.g., ranitidine with sodium bicarbonate): decreases gefitinib AUC by 44%; do not give together.
- Warfarin: increased INR and bleeding; monitor INR frequently and patient for s/s bleeding and decrease warfarin dose accordingly.
- Lovastatin enhances gefitinib activity in glioblastoma cells irrespective of EGFRvIII and PTEN status (Cemeus et al, 2008).

Lab Effects/Interference:
- Asymptomatic elevations in liver function tests (transaminases, bilirubin, and alkaline phosphatase).

Special Considerations:
- Indicated as monotherapy for the treatment of patients with locally advanced or metastatic non-small cell lung cancer (NSCLC) after failure of both platinum-based and docetaxel chemotherapies. For the following reasons, the drug is restricted to prior responders: (1) response rate of 10%, (2) no survival advantage together, and (3) erlotinib (Tarceva) has since been FDA approved. The drug is only available to (1) patients who are currently or who have previously taken the drug and are benefiting, or who have benefited and (2) previously enrolled patients or new patients in noninvestigational new drug (IND) clinical trials approved by an IRB prior to 6/17/05. The drug will be available through the IRESSA access program only.
- Specific point or deletion mutations in the EGFR gene (around the ATP pocket of the tyrosine kinase domain of the EGFR gene) predict response, as about 10% of patients have a rapid and dramatic response. More patients in Japan have these mutations than in the United States. The mutations increase the tyrosine kinase activity to EGFR stimulation, and also to gefitinib blockade (Lynch et al, 2004). These mutations do not explain the approximate 30% of patients that have disease stabilization.
- Results from two large controlled, randomized clinical trials in first-line treatment of NSCLC showed no benefit from gefitinib added to platinum-based chemotherapy.
- Interstitial lung disease occurs in about 1% of patients. In Japan the incidence was 2%, but in the prospective first-line studies, incidence of interstitial lung disease was equal in treatment and placebo groups. Patients with concurrent idiopathic pulmonary fibrosis whose condition worsens during therapy have an increased mortality compared to those without pulmonary fibrosis.

- Primary side effects are diarrhea, rash, acne, dry skin, nausea, and vomiting.
- No dose reduction necessary for hepatic (related to metastases) or renal dysfunction. No studies have been done in non-cancer-related liver impairment.
- Contraindications: allergy to gefitinib or its components; avoid administration in pregnant women or women who are breast-feeding.
- Drug is associated RARELY with pancreatitis, and allergic reactions including angioedema, urticaria, toxic epidermal necrolysis, and erythema multiforme.
- Patients with specific gene mutations in the EGFR are most likely to respond to the drug (Lynch et al, 2004), and for those patients, ultimately they develop resistance due to a 2nd mutation that develops in this receptor.

Potential Toxicities/Side Effects and the Nursing Process

I. ALTERATION IN OXYGENATION related to INTERSTITIAL LUNG DISEASE (ILD)

Defining Characteristics: Rarely (1%) patients develop interstitial lung disease, with a 33% mortality. In some studies, incidence was similar in treatment and placebo groups. This toxicity has been reported as interstitial pneumonia, pneumonitis, and alveolitis. Onset characterized by dyspnea, sometimes with cough or low-grade fever, and rapidly becoming severe. Incidence increased in patients with prior radiotherapy, prior chemotherapy. Mortality was increased in patients with concurrent pulmonary fibrosis who developed ILD.

Nursing Implications: Assess baseline pulmonary status, and periodically during treatment. Teach patient to report cough, low-grade fever, and shortness of breath (or worsening of pulmonary status). If it develops, discuss with physician pulmonary function tests, and further pulmonary work-up as ordered.

II. ALTERATION IN BOWEL ELIMINATION related to DIARRHEA

Defining Characteristics: Mild to moderate diarrhea occurred in 48% of patients, and in a few patients was severe and associated with dehydration. Drug may be interrupted for up to 14 days if patient develops severe diarrhea, and then restarted when diarrhea resolves.

Nursing Implications: Assess bowel elimination pattern baseline, and regularly during therapy. Teach patient to report diarrhea that does not resolve with anti-diarrheal medication right away. Teach patient self-care strategies to manage diarrhea, including increased oral fluids to 2–3 liters a day, dietary modification and use of anti-diarrheal medications such as loperamide. Identify patients at risk for diarrhea and dehydration, and monitor them closely. Discuss with physician dose interruption for up to 2 weeks, or dose reduction for severe diarrhea, as well as fluid and electrolyte replacement and aggressive anti-diarrheal medication.

III. ALTERATION IN SKIN INTEGRITY, POTENTIAL, related to RASH, DRY SKIN, PRURITUS

Defining Characteristics: As expected, because EGFR is important in skin function, this is the area of major toxicity. Rash occurred in 43% of patients in clinical trials, with acne occurring in 25%, dry skin 13%, pruritus 8% of patients. Rash is manifested as patches of erythema/acneiform (pustular) lesions on the face; with higher doses, it affects the upper torso. Rash resolves quickly after drug discontinuance. Drug may be interrupted for up to 14 days if patient develops severe rash, and then restarted. Ensure that rash is not allergic, and rule out urticaria, toxic epidermal necrolysis, and erythema multiforme that may occur rarely.

Nursing Implications: Assess skin integrity of face, neck, arms, and upper trunk baseline, and regularly during treatment. Teach patient that rash may occur, its usual course, and self-care measures for comfort. Assess body image intactness, and if rash develops, its threat to body image. Encourage patient to verbalize feelings; provide emotional support, and individualize care plan to patient response. For rash management, refer to the introduction in Chapter 5. Teach all patients to (1) use a water-based emollient frequently during the day to prevent dryness, (2) stay hydrated, (3) avoid sun exposure and wear SPF 30 (zinc based). Do not use antiacne medications. Tetracycline analogues provide an anti-inflammatory benefit. **Grade 1/mild rash (localized, does not interfere with ADLs, and is not infected):** The goal is to preserve skin integrity, minimize discomfort, and prevent infection. Key patient teaching includes (1) use a mild soap with active ingredients that reduce skin drying such as pyrithione zinc (Head and Shoulders), (2) consider aloe gel to red, tender areas, (3) report distressing tenderness as pramoxine (lidocaine topical anesthetic may help), (4) keep fingernails clean and trimmed, and (5) apply zinc ointment to rectal mucosa after washing. Management: maintain current drug dose, observe or give topical hydrocortisone 1% or 2.5% or clindamycin 1% gel (anti-inflammatory benefit); reassess in 2 weeks. **For grade 2/moderate rash, which is generalized, mild symptoms, and has minimal effect on ADLs, and no infection:** The goal is to prevent infection and promote comfort. Continue EGFRI dose; use topicals (hydrocortisone 2.5% or clindamycin 1% gel) or consider pimecrolimus cream (immunomodulator) and add doxycycline 100 mg PO twice daily or minocycline 100 mg PO twice daily (give antimicrobial and anti-inflammatory effect) and reassess after 2 weeks. **For grade 3/4 or severe rash (generalized, severe, has a significant impact on ADLs, and increased risk of infection):** The goal is to prevent infection or to identify it early to prevent complications and to promote effective coping. Rarely described. Hold drug for up to 2 weeks, and restart at prior dose, and treat rash with topicals (hydrocortisone 2.5% or clindamycin 1% gel or pimecrolimus cream), doxycycline 100 mg PO twice daily or minocycline 100 mg PO twice daily, and methylprednisolone (Medrol dose pack); reassess after 2 weeks, and interrupt or discontinue drug if rash worsens (Lynch et al, 2007). If rash appears infected (exudate, vesicular formation, different appearance), obtain C+S, treat empirically until sensitivity received, and/or obtain a dermatology consult.

IV. ALTERATION IN NUTRITION, LESS THAN BODY REQUIREMENTS, related to NAUSEA, VOMITING, ANOREXIA, WEIGHT LOSS

Defining Characteristics: Nausea affects 13% and vomiting 12% of patients.

Nursing Implications: Assess baseline nutritional status risk of nausea and vomiting. Teach patient to self-administer antiemetic medications 1 hour prior to taking drug if nausea or vomiting develops. Teach patient to report persistent or continued nausea and/or vomiting. Assess efficacy and discuss change in antiemetic drug with physician if regimen ineffective.

V. ALTERATION IN COMFORT AND ACTIVITY TOLERANCE related to ASTHENIA

Defining Characteristics: Asthenia affects approximately 6% of patients.

Nursing Implications: Assess baseline comfort, energy/activity level, and ability to do self-care. Teach patient that these side effects may occur, and energy conservation strategies to manage them. If patient is unable to do ADLs, assess need for home support from outside agency.

VI. SENSORY/PERCEPTUAL ALTERATIONS, POTENTIAL, related to VISUAL AND OCULAR CHANGES

Defining Characteristics: Amblyopia occurred in 2% of patients, and conjunctivitis 1%. There are reports of patients with eye pain and corneal erosion/ulceration, sometimes associated with abnormal eyelash growth. In addition, rarely, corneal membrane sloughing and ocular ischemia/hemorrhage occurred.

Nursing Implications: Teach patient to stop drug and report any eye discomfort or visual changes immediately. For irritation of conjunctiva due to dryness, teach patient to use an over-the-counter lubricant such as Artificial Tears. Discuss a referral of the patient to ophthalmologist for evaluation, trimming of eyelashes, and advice. Discuss drug continuance with physician depending on the cause of problem.

Drug: gemtuzumab ozogamicin for injection (Mylotarg)

Class: Monoclonal antibody conjugated to a cytotoxic antibiotic.

Mechanism of Action: Drug is composed of a recombinant humanized Ig4 kappa antibody conjugated with a cytotoxic antitumor antibiotic, calicheamicin. The antibody portion of the drug binds to the CD33 antigen found on the cell surface of leukemic blast and immature normal cells in the myeloid cell line but not the pluripotent stem cell. The CD33 antigen is expressed on more than 80% of patients with acute myeloid leukemia. 98.3% of the amino acids used are of human origin, while the remainder are derived from murine antibody. Once the MoAb binds to the CD33 antibody, the complex is brought inside the cell, calicheamicin is released inside lysosomes within the myeloid cell and then binds to DNA, resulting in DNA double-strand breaks and cell death.

Metabolism: Rapidly bound to CD33-positive tumor cells in the peripheral blood (within 30 minutes of dose). Following first dose, terminal half-lives of total and unconjugated calicheamicin were 45 and 100 hours, while after the second dose 14 days later, the terminal half-life of total calicheamicin was 60 hours, and the area under the concentration-time curve was double that following the first treatment. The cytotoxic drug calicheamicin derivative is hydrolyzed to release it from the monoclonal antibody and forms many metabolites.

Dosage/Range:
- 9 mg/m^2 given as a 2-hour IV infusion q 14 days × 2.
- Premedicate 1 hour before the drug is given with diphenhydramine 50 mg PO and acetaminophen 650–1000 mg PO, with acetaminophen repeated q 4 h × 2 PRN.
- WBC should be < 30,000 cells/mm^3 to minimize infusion reaction; the patient may need to be leukapheresed or cytoreduced with other chemotherapy (e.g., hydroxyurea).

Drug Preparation:
- Protect from direct and indirect sunlight and unshielded fluorescent light during preparation and administration of drug (fluorescent light must be turned off in biological safety cabinet during preparation).
- Allow refrigerated vials to come to room temperature.
- Reconstitute 5 mg vial with 5 mL sterile water for injection, USP, using sterile syringes. Gently swirl the vial to dissolve. Final concentration is 1 mg/mL. While in the amber vial, the reconstituted solution can be refrigerated (2–8°C, 36–36°F) and protected from light for up to 8 hours.
- Withdraw ordered dose and inject into 100 mL bag of 0.9% normal saline injection, and then place the bag inside an UV-protectant bag. Use the medication immediately.

Drug Administration:
- Premedicate 1 hour before the drug is given with diphenhydramine 50 mg PO and acetaminophen 650–1000 mg PO, with acetaminophen repeated q 4 h × 2 PRN; the addition of a corticosteroid (e.g., methylprednisolone sodium succinate 50 mg) reduces the incidence of infusion reactions (Giles, 2003).
- Administer in light-protected bag IV over 2 hours via separate IV tubing containing a 1.2 micron terminal filter.
- Can be given via peripheral or central IV line.
- DO NOT administer by IVP or bolus.

Drug Interactions:

- Unknown.

Lab Effects/Interference:

- Increased LFTs.
- Hyperglycemia (part of post-infusion syndrome).
- Significant decrease in WBC, Hgb/HCT, platelet count.
- Increased LDH.
- Decreased serum K, Mg.

Special Considerations:

- Drug is indicated for the treatment of patients with CD33 positive acute myeloid leukemia in first relapse who are 60 years or older, and who are not considered candidates for cytotoxic chemotherapy.
- Drug is contraindicated in patients with known hypersensitivity to gemtuzumab ozogamicin or its components (anti-CD33 antibody), calicheamicin derivatives, or inactive ingredients and in pregnant or nursing women.
- Give premedication to prevent post-infusion symptom complex, and monitor closely. Consider the risk for tumor lysis syndrome and the need for hydration and allopurinol.
- Severe myelosuppression will occur in all patients, and systemic infections must be treated.
- Use cautiously in patients with renal or hepatic dysfunction.
- Women of childbearing age should use effective contraception measures.
- Tumor lysis syndrome may occur commonly in leukemic patients, so patients should be well hydrated, receive allopurinol, and receive alkalinization if at risk (high tumor burden).

Potential Toxicities/Side Effects and the Nursing Process

I. POTENTIAL FOR INJURY related to ACUTE INFUSION-RELATED EVENTS

Defining Characteristics: Patients often experience an infusion syndrome during or after the infusion characterized by chills (62%), fever (61%), nausea (38%), vomiting (32%), headache (12%), hypotension (11%), hypertension (6%), hypoxia (6%), dyspnea (4%), and hyperglycemia (2%). Rarely, severe pulmonary complications can occur, including ARDS. Syndrome may occur any time within 24 hours after administration, and resolves about 2–4 hours later with supportive therapy of acetaminophen, diphenhydramine, and IV fluids. Hypotension can be severe especially if WBC > 30,000 cells/mm^3 before treatment. Patients are less likely to experience this syndrome when receiving the second treatment.

Nursing Implications: Premedicate patient as ordered with acetaminophen and diphenhydramine and consider corticosteroids 1 hour before drug therapy. If tumor lysis syndrome is possible, give hydration and allopurinol as ordered. Monitor VS and oxygen saturation every 15–30 minutes during the infusion and for at least 2 hours but up to 24 hours depending on the patient's response after the infusion has finished. Ensure that medications necessary for the management of hypersensitivity/anaphylaxis are readily available (e.g., epinephrine, antihistamines, corticosteroids). Assess baseline VS and monitor frequently during the infusion, and for 4 hours post infusion; keep IV line patent. Monitor VS, and notify physician of abnormalities. Be prepared to provide emergency support as necessary (including IV saline, epinephrine, antihistamines, bronchodilators).

II. POTENTIAL FOR INFECTION, BLEEDING, AND FATIGUE related to BONE MARROW DEPRESSION

Defining Characteristics: Severe (grade 3 or 4) neutropenia occurs in 98% of patients, with recovery of an ANC of 500 cells/micro liter by day 40 (after first dose) in those patients who respond. During treatment phase, 28% developed grades 3 and 4 infections, with 16% experiencing sepsis and 7% pneumonia. 22% of patients developed herpes simplex infection. Thrombocytopenia is common, with 99% of patients developing grades 3 and 4. For those responding to treatment, platelet recovery (25,000/microliter) occurs by day 39 after first day of drug. 23% of patients required platelet transfusions. During treatment phase, bleeding occurred in 15% of patients (grades 3 and 4). These episodes included epistaxis (3%), cerebral hemorrhage (2%), disseminated intravascular coagulation (2%), intracranial hemorrhage (2%) and hematuria (1%). Anemia also was common, with 47% of patients developing grades 3 and 4 anemia, and 26% of patients requiring transfusions.

Nursing Implications: Monitor CBC, platelets baseline and regularly during treatment. Assess for signs/symptoms of infection, bleeding, and fatigue baseline, between treatment, and prior to each treatment. Teach patient to self-assess for these, including taking temperature, and instruct to report them immediately. Teach patient measures to minimize infection, bleeding, and fatigue, including avoidance of crowds, and not taking OTC medications containing aspirin. Transfuse red blood cells and platelets as ordered. Teach patient strategies to conserve energy and minimize fatigue.

III. ALTERATION IN NUTRITION, POTENTIAL, related to NAUSEA, MUCOSITIS, VOMITING, HEPATOTOXICITY

Defining Characteristics: Nausea is common, affecting 70% of patients, with 63% developing vomiting. Stomatitis affected 35% of patients, with 4% having grades 3 or 4 toxicity. Transient increases in LFTs occurred, and were usually reversible. In clinical studies, 23% of patients developed grades 3 or 4 hyperbilirubinemia, 9% in levels of ALT, and 17% in levels of AST. In clinical studies, there were deaths reported: one patient died with liver failure as part of multisystem failure related to tumor lysis syndrome, another patient died of persistent jaundice and hepatosplenomegaly five months after treatment, and finally, 4 (of 27) patients died of veno-occlusive disease following stem cell transplantation after Mylotarg administration.

Nursing Implications: Assess baseline nutritional status, integrity of oral mucosa, and liver function studies and regularly after treatment. Administer antiemetic medications prior to chemotherapy to prevent nausea/vomiting, and teach patient self-administration of antiemetics after discharge if drug is given on an outpatient basis. Teach patient to report persistent or continued nausea and/or vomiting. Assess efficacy and discuss change in antiemetic drug with physician if regimen ineffective. Teach patient to assess oral mucosa regularly, use oral hygiene regimen, and report signs/symptoms of stomatitis. If patient develops stomatitis, teach patient self-administration of oral analgesics, antifungals, as ordered and appropriate. Monitor liver function tests, and discuss any abnormalities with physician.

IV. ALTERATION IN BOWEL ELIMINATION related to CONSTIPATION OR DIARRHEA

Defining Characteristics: Diarrhea affects 38% of patients, and constipation 25%.

Nursing Implications: Assess baseline bowel elimination status, and teach patient that alterations may occur. Teach patient self-care measures to manage constipation or diarrhea, and to report persistent or recurrent episodes. Discuss management with physician for refractory constipation or diarrhea. Teach patient dietary modifications such as increased fluid and fiber to prevent constipation, and the BRAT (bananas, rice, applesauce, toast) diet as well as increased hydration to manage diarrhea.

V. ALTERATION IN SKIN INTEGRITY, POTENTIAL, related to RASH, EDEMA, INFECTION

Defining Characteristics: Nonspecific rash affects approximately 22% of patients. 25% of patients had a local reaction, while 16% developed peripheral edema. 22% developed herpes simplex infections.

Nursing Implications: Assess baseline skin integrity, presence of rash or peripheral edema, and history of herpes simplex infections. Teach patient that these side effects may occur and to report them. Discuss with physician prophylactic use of antiviral agent if patient has a history of herpes simplex infections. If patient develops rash, local reaction, or peripheral edema, teach patient local strategies to maintain skin integrity, and use of skin moisturizers to prevent itching or scratching.

Drug: ^{90}Y ibritumomab tiuxetan (Zevalin, IDEC-Y2B8)

Class: Monoclonal antibody chelated to radioisotope ^{90}Y yttrium.

Mechanism of Action: Ibritumomab tiuxetan is a monoclonal antibody that targets the cell surface antigen CD_{20}, which is found on the surface of normal and malignant B-cell lymphocytes. The CD_{20} antigen is also present (expressed) on more than 90% of B-cell non-Hodgkin's lymphoma (NHL) cells but fortunately is not found on normal bone marrow stem cells, pre-B cells, or other normal tissues. The complex is made up of a murine anti-CD_{20} monoclonal antibody conjugate to the linker chelator tiuxetan, which then securely chelates the radioisotope ^{90}Y yttrium. The complex attaches to the CD_{20} receptor, and then the radioisotope delivers high beta energy waves to the malignant cell, causing cell death. The isotope delivers high energy with a short half-life of 64 hours. It appears that if the malignant cells are pretreated with an anti-CD_{20} antibody (e.g., Rituximab), this clears malignant and normal B lymphocytes from the blood, and ^{90}Y ibritumomab tiuxetan is better able to target the lymphoma B-lymphocytes.

Metabolism: ^{90}Y yttrium has a half-life of 64 hours, and effective half-life in the blood of 28 hours, median biological half-life of 47 hours, and median area under the curve (AUC) of 25 hours (Wiseman et al, 1996).

Dosage/Range:

- Indium III (gamma emitter) is used to determine biodistribution. (1) Indium III: 5.0 mCi day 1, (2) Rituximab 250 mg/m^2 dl, d 7 or 9: 250 mg/m^2; (3) Y-90 dose 0.4 mCi/Kg with maximal total dose of 32.0 mCi, dose reduce to 0.3 mCi/Kg platelet count 100K–149K.

Drug Preparation:

- See package insert.

Drug Administration:

- Day 1: In-111 IV over 10 min using 0.22 micron filter, followed by rituximab IV within 4 hours, initially at 50mg/hr, and gradually increasing the rate in 50 mg/hr increments if no infusion reaction, to a maximum of 400 mg/hr. Premedicate with acetaminophen and antihistamine prior to rituximab.
- Biodistribution imaging 1: 2–24 hr after In-111 injection; image 2: 48–72 hr later; optional image 3; at 90–120 hr.
- If biodistribution acceptable, on day 7–9, rituxan 250 mg/m^2, and within 4 hours, Y-90 Zevalin IV over 10 min. Avoid extravasation.

Drug Interactions:

- Increased bone marrow suppression if combined with other myelosuppressive drugs, or drugs interfering with blood clotting.

Lab Effects/Interference:

- Decreased WBC and neutrophil, platelet count, and Hgb/HCT.

Special Considerations:

- FDA indicated for the treatment of patients with relapsed or refractory low-grade, follicular, or transformed B-cell non-Hodgkin's lymphoma, including patients with refractory to rituximab.
- Documented fatal infusion reaction within 24 hours of rituximab dose characterized by hypoxemia, pulmonary infiltrates, ARDS, MI, VF, and shock.
- Agent has been shown to clear circulating lymphoma cells with the bcl-2 translocation (bcl-2 [t(14:18)]) (Murray et al, 2000) and predicted response to therapy (80% response rate if these cells were cleared from circulation vs. 20% if the cells were not cleared).
- After treatment, there is rapid reduction in malignant and normal B-cell lymphocytes, with circulating B-cells undetectable for the first 12 weeks, followed by recovery of normal B cells starting in the sixth month after therapy.
- Patient's own circulating antibodies stay within normal range after therapy.
- Rarely, patient may develop an antiantibody response (human antichimeric antibody/human antimouse antibody). Contraindicated in patients with altered biodistribution of Indium-111 Zevalin, patients with ≥ 25% lymphoma marrow involvement or impaired bone marrow reserve.
- 2% incidence of development of secondary malignancy (acute myeloid leukemia, myelodysplastic syndrome). Radiation is a potent carcinogen and mutagen.

Potential Toxicities/Side Effects and the Nursing Process

I. POTENTIAL FOR INJURY related to ANAPHYLAXIS

Defining Characteristics: Rare but potentially life-threatening reaction may occur. Mouse antibodies are used that are foreign and may stimulate anaphylaxis. Rare, fatal anaphylactic reactions have occurred within 24 hours of rituximab dose. Of the reactions, 80% occur during the first rituximab infusion, and within 30–120 minutes of the infusion. Severe infusion reactions include pulmonary infiltrates, acute respiratory distress syndrome, myocardial infarction, ventricular fibrillation, and cardiogenic shock.

Nursing Implications: Assess baseline T, VS. Administer premedications prior to rituximab as ordered, usually acetaminophen and diphenhydramine. Initiate infusion at 50 mg/hr, and increase in 50mg/hr increments q 30 min to a maximum of 400 mg/hr. If patient develops discomfort, slow infusion; stop infusion if reaction is severe. Once symptoms have improved, resume rate at 50% of previous rate. Have emergency equipment and medications nearby, including epinephrine and corticosteroids. Assess patient for signs/symptoms, including generalized flushing andurticaria leading to pallor, cyanosis, bronchospasm, hypotension, unconsciousness. Teach patient to report signs/symptoms, including sense of doom, tickle in throat. If signs/symptoms occur, stop infusion immediately, assess VS, notify physician. Physician may prescribe epinephrine 0.3 mL (1:1000) subcutaneous if hypotensive. Oxygen, antihistamines, corticosteroids may also be used.

II. POTENTIAL FOR INFECTION, BLEEDING, AND FATIGUE related to BONE MARROW SUPPRESSION

Defining Characteristics: Neutropenia common, with 77% incidence, and 25–32% of patients experiencing grade 4 neutropenia, with a median nadir of 900/mm^3–1100/mm^3; Thrombocytopenia incidence 95% with median platelet nadir of 49,500/mm^3; Anemia incidence 61% with median nadir for red blood cells 9.9 g/dL hemoglobin. Nadir occurred around 7–9 weeks after treatment, and duration of cytopenias was 22–35d. Chills and fever were common, affecting 27.5% and 21.6% of patients in one study. There appears to be increased hematologic toxicity in patients with bone marrow involvement by tumor, as expected. Rare fatal cerebral hemorrhage, severe infections.

Nursing Implications: Drug contraindicated in patients with > 25% bone marrow hypocellular bone marrow, or history of failed stem cell collection. Assess baseline CBC, platelet count, and monitor closely during and after therapy at least weekly for the first 12 weeks after treatment. Assess risk for increased hematological toxicity, e.g., whether bone marrow involvement by tumor. Teach patient that blood counts will fall and potential signs/symptoms of infection, bleeding, and fatigue. Teach patient self-care measures including self-assessment for signs/symptoms of infection, bleeding, and anemia; self-care strategies to minimize risk for infection (e.g., avoiding crowds, proximity to people with colds), bleeding (e.g., avoid aspirin-containing OTC medicines), and fatigue (e.g., alternating rest and activity periods), and what/where to report fever, bleeding, signs/symptoms of infection. Most studies show that few patients developed severe infections, and there were few if any deaths from treatment-related infections. Transfuse red blood cells and platelets as ordered.

III. ALTERATION IN COMFORT related to ASTHENIA, NAUSEA, ABDOMINAL PAIN, HEADACHE

Defining Characteristics: Asthenia commonly affects 21.6%, nausea (grades 1 or 2) 21.6%, and abdominal pain and headache 9.8%. Nausea, vomiting, diarrhea, increased cough, dizziness, arthralgia, anxiety may occur.

Nursing Implications: Assess baseline comfort and energy level. Teach patient that these side effects may occur, and strategies to manage them. If the symptom persists or is unresolved, teach patient to report it, and discuss with physician other management strategies.

IV. POTENTIAL FOR INJURY related to RADIATION EXPOSURE

Defining Characteristics: Y-90 Zevalin is a beta-emitter so that patients should protect others from exposure to their body secretions (saliva, stool, blood, urine).

Nursing Implications: Teach patient importance of specific radiation precautions, beginning at the start of treatment, and continuing for 1 week after treatment is completed: use condom during sexual intercourse, refrain from deep kissing; avoid transfer of body fluids; wash hands thoroughly after using the toilet; and continue effective contraception for 12 months following completion of treatment.

Drug: imatinib mesylate (Gleevec, STI 571)

Class: Protein tyrosine kinase inhibitor.

Mechanism of Action: Inhibits abnormal tyrosine kinase encoded by the Philadelphia chromosome (Bcr-Abl) in Chronic Myelocytic Leukemia (CML), thus preventing cell proliferation. Drug also inhibits receptor tyrosine kinases for platelet-derived growth factor (PDGF). Inhibits c-Kit receptor called stem cell factor receptor (SCFR) tyrosine kinases as well, which has resulted in marked responses in GIST (gastrointestinal stromal tumors). 15–85% of GISTs have Kit mutations that result in constitutively active kinases; imatinib mesylate selectively inhibits this mutated tyrosine kinase.

Metabolism: Well absorbed after oral administration with 98% bioavailability and Cmax in 2–4 hours after dosing. Elimination half-life of imatinib is 18 hours, and 40 hours for primary active metabolite N-desmethyl derivative. Drug is 95% protein bound. It is metabolized via CYP3A4 hepatic cytochrome P450 enzyme system, with 81% of the dose eliminated in 7 days, primarily via fecal route (68%) and, to a lesser degree, urinary (13%). 25% of drug dose is excreted unchanged in feces and urine.

Dosage/Range:
- 400 mg/day orally (single dose) for patients in chronic phase of CML.
- 600 mg/day orally (single dose) for patients in accelerated phase or blast crisis.
- Treatment continued as long as patient derives benefit from drug.
- In case of disease progression at any time, failure to achieve a satisfactory hematologic response after 3 months of treatment, failure to achieve a cytogenetic response after 6–12 months of treatment, or loss of a hematologic or cytogenetic response: increase dose to 600 mg/day (chronic CML), or to 800 mg/day given as 400 mg twice daily (accelerated or blast crisis) if no severe adverse drug reactions occur.
- GIST dosing: 400 mg/day or 600 mg/day orally.
- MDS, MPD: 400 mg/day orally.
- Pediatric dosing (newly diagnosed): 340 $mg/m^2/day$ (not to exceed 600 mg/day).
- Pediatric dosing (recurrence after stem cell transplant or who are intolerant of interferon-α therapy): 260 $mg/m^2/day$.

Drug Preparation:

- Available in hard gelatin 100 mg capsules or scored 100 mg tablets, in bottles of 120.
- Administer dose orally, once daily (unless the total dose is 800 mg, which is given as 400 mg twice daily), with a meal and a large glass of water.

Drug Interactions:

- CYP3A4 inhibitors (ketoconazole, itraconazole, erythromycin, clarithromycin, voriconazole, aprepitant) may increase imatinib plasma concentrations; do not coadminister, or monitor closely for imatinib adverse effects.
- CYP3A4 substrates (simvastatin): imatinib decreases simvastatin metabolism with simvastatin serum levels increased 2–3.5 times. Use together cautiously, if at all, and monitor BP and dose reduce of simvastatin if needed.
- CYP3A4 inducers (dexamethasone, phenytoin, carbamazepine, rifampicin, phenobarbital, St. John's wort) may increase metabolism of imatinib so imatinib serum levels are reduced. Use together cautiously, if at all. When used with dexamethasone, phenytoin, carbamazepine, phenobarbital, rifabutin or rifampin, increase imatinib dose by 50%. Do not take St. John's wort if taking imatinib.
- Other CYP3A4 substrates (Cyclosporine, pimozide) increased plasma concentrations if co-administered with imatinib. Do not administer together because drug has a narrow therapeutic window.
- Other CYP3A4 substrates (Triazolo-benzadiazepines, dihydropyridine calcium-channel blockers, HMG-CoA reductase inhibitors) may have increased serum levels when given together with imatinib. Use together cautiously, and monitor patient closely.
- Other CYP3A4 substrates: eletriptan (Relpax). Do not administer eletriptan within 72 hours of imatinib. Monitor vital signs closely.
- Warfarin: Do not give together with imatinib because imatinib inhibits warfarin metabolism by CYP2C9 enzymes. Use low molecular heparin or standard heparin instead.

Lab Effects/Interference:

- Neutropenia, thrombocytopenia.
- Elevated hepatic transaminases (SGOT/AST, SGPT/ALT) and bilirubin.

Special Considerations:

- Imatinib mesylate is indicated for the treatment of patients with CML: (1) initial treatment of newly diagnosed adult and pediatric patients with Ph+ chromosome CML in chronic phase, (2) Ph+ CML in blast crisis, in accelerated phase, or in chronic phase after failure of interferon alpha therapy, (3) pediatric patients with Ph+ chronic phase CML whose disease has recurred after stem cell transplant or who are resistant to interferon-α therapy, (4) adult patients with relapsed or refractory Ph+ acute lymphoblastic leukemia (ALL), (5) adult patients with myelodysplastic/myeloproliferative diseases (MDS/MPD) associated with PDGFR gene rearrangements, (6) patients with Kit (CD117)-positive unresectable and/or metastatic malignant gastrointestinal stromal tumors (GIST), (7) adult patients with aggressive systemic mastocytosis (ASM) without the D816V c-Kit mutation or unknown, (8) adult patients with hypereosinophilic syndrome (HES) and/or chronic eosinophilic leukemia (CEL) who have FIP1L1-PDGFRα fusion kinase, as well as those who do not, (9) adult patients with unresectable, recurrent, and/or metastatic dermatofibrosarcoma protuberans (DFSP).

- Clinical trials results were remarkable: Chronic phase (n > 500 patients): hematologic complete response (88%), complete cytogenic response (genetic correction) (30%); Accelerated phase (n = 235): hematologic (28%), complete cytogenic response (14%); Blast crisis: hematologic complete response (4%), cytogenic complete response (5%).
- Emerging evidence indicates that resistance can develop with reactivation of the Bcr-Abl signal transduction, and, in some patients, amplification of the *bcr-abl* fusion gene occurs (Gorre et al, 2001).
- Drug is teratogenetic. Women should avoid pregnancy or breast-feeding while taking the drug.
- Drug often causes edema that may be serious in some patients. There is increased risk in patients at higher drug doses and in the elderly (> 65 years).
- Drug is associated with neutropenia and thrombocytopenia. Blood counts should be checked weekly for the first month, biweekly for the second month, and then every 2–3 months as clinically indicated. Patients with accelerated phase CML or blast crisis require closer monitoring.
- Liver function tests (LFTs) should be monitored baseline and monthly or as clinically indicated. Drug should be stopped if bilirubin is increased to 3 times institutional upper limit of normal (IULN), or if liver transaminases is > 5 times IULN and held until these tests have returned to bilirubin < 1.5 times IULN or transaminase levels to < 2.5 times IULN. Drug should then be resumed at a reduced dose (400 mg dose reduced to 300 mg daily, and 600 mg dose reduced to 400 mg daily).
- Use cautiously in patients with liver impairment, and monitor liver function tests closely prior to and throughout treatment.
- Drug modifications for hematologic toxicity: *Chronic phase CML at initial dose of 400 mg/da or GIST at initial dose of 400–600 mg/da*: ANC < 1000/mm^3 and/or platelets < 50,000/mm^3: stop drug until ANC ≥ 1500/mm^3 and/or platelets > 75,000/mm^3 and then resume at usual dose; if recurrence of ANC < 1000/mm^3, and/or platelets < 50,000/mm^3, hold until recovered, and reduce dose to 300 mg daily if initial dose 400 mg/da, and 400 mg/da if initial dose was 600 mg/da.
- *Accelerated phase and Blast Crisis:* ANC < 500/mm^3 and/or platelets < 10,000/mm^3: determine if related to leukemia by bone marrow aspirate/biopsy; if unrelated to leukemia, reduce dose to 400 mg daily; if cytopenia persists 2 weeks, reduce again to 300 mg daily; if cytopenia persists 4 weeks and is still unrelated to leukemia, stop imatinib until ANC ≥ 1000/mm^3 and platelets ≥ 20/mm^3, and then resume at 300 mg/da.

Potential Toxicities/Side Effects and the Nursing Process

I. POTENTIAL FOR INFECTION AND BLEEDING related to BONE MARROW DEPRESSION

Defining Characteristics: Neutropenia and thrombocytopenia were common, especially in patients who received higher doses, and in patients with advanced stages of disease (blast crisis and accelerated phase). Median duration of neutropenia was 2–3 weeks, and thrombocytopenia from 3–4 weeks. Dose needs to be held and reduced as noted in *Special Considerations*. Fever affected 14% (chronic phase) to 38% (accelerated phase) of patients. Hemorrhage (CNS and GI) was treated in 13% (chronic phase) to 48% (accelerated phase) of patients.

Nursing Implications: Assess baseline CBC, including WBC and differential and platelet count prior to dosing, as well as at least weekly during first month of treatment, at least every other week for the second month of treatment, and then as clinically indicated and ordered. Discuss dose interruption and reduction as above for neutropenia and thrombocytopenia (hold for ANC < 500, platelets < 40 K). Teach patient self-assessment of signs/symptoms of infection and bleeding (including epistaxis and development of petechiae), and instruct patient to report them right away. Teach patient self-care measures to minimize risk of infection and bleeding, including avoidance of OTC aspirin-containing medications.

II. POTENTIAL ALTERATION IN CIRCULATION related to CONGESTIVE HEART FAILURE

Defining Characteristics: The Abelson tyrosine kinase (ABL) protein is necessary for the general health and maintenance of cardiac muscles, especially the mitochondria (Kerkela et al, 2006). Kerkela et al reported that 10 patients developed CHF between 1–14 months after starting the drug, and although patients had an average LVEF of 56%, on repeat testing, the average LVEF was 25%.

Nursing Implications: Patients should have determination of their LVEF baseline and periodically while receiving the drug. Assess baseline cardiac status, history, and risk for development of CHF. Closely monitor patient while receiving imatinib mesylate, especially if patient has history of hypertension, or is on cardiac medications. Teach patient to report any dyspnea, SOB, chest pain, or heart palpitations, or any unusual feeling. If any abnormalities occur, teach patient to stop drug and to call the physician or nurse immediately.

III. ALTERATION IN FLUID AND ELECTROLYTE BALANCE related to FLUID RETENTION, EDEMA, AND HYPOKALEMIA

Defining Characteristics: Fluid retention is common (52% chronic phase and 67% accelerated phase patients), especially in the elderly, and primarily reflects periorbital and lower extremity edema. However, pleural effusions, ascites, rapid weight gain, and pulmonary edema may develop, and in some cases, be life-threatening (pleural effusion, congestive heart failure, renal failure, pericardial effusion, anasarca). Hypokalemia was reported to occur in 2–12% of patients.

Nursing Implications: Assess baseline parameters of weight, presence of edema, pulmonary function, and monitor closely during therapy. Teach patient to monitor weight daily at home, and to report weight gain of 2 pounds in one week, development of edema, or dyspnea. Teach the patient comfort measures for periorbital edema, such as ice packs, and self-administration of diuretics as ordered. Discuss with physician drug dose modification or interruption if severe fluid retention occurs.

IV. ALTERATION IN NUTRITION, POTENTIAL, LESS THAN BODY REQUIREMENTS, related to NAUSEA, VOMITING, DIARRHEA, HEPATOTOXICITY

Defining Characteristics: Nausea affected 68% of patients with accelerated phase, and 55% with chronic phase; vomiting affected 54% and 28%, respectively. Diarrhea affected 54%, while constipation affected 13%. Dyspepsia affected about 19%.

Nursing Implications: Teach patient to self-administer antiemetics one hour prior to each dose, and to call if nausea/vomiting develop. Discuss with physician more effective antiemetic regime if nausea/vomiting develop. Encourage small, frequent intake of cool, bland foods as tolerated if nausea develops. Refer to dietitian as needed for meal planning. Assess bowel-elimination pattern baseline and at each visit. Teach patient to report diarrhea or constipation that does not respond to antidiarrheal or anticonstipation medications. Teach dietary modifications as appropriate. Monitor LFTs baseline and periodically during therapy. Hold therapy if LFTs become abnormal (see Special Considerations).

V. ALTERATION IN COMFORT related to MUSCLE CRAMPS, MUSCULOSKELETAL (BONE) PAIN, HEADACHE, FATIGUE, ARTHRALGIA, AND ABDOMINAL PAIN

Defining Characteristics: Muscle cramps are common, affecting 25–46% of patients. Musculoskeletal pain affects 27–37% of patients, headache 24–29% of patients, fatigue 33% of patients, rash 32% of patients, and arthralgias 26% of patients. In clinical studies, abdominal pain affected 20% of patients with chronic phase, and 26% of patients in blast crisis.

Nursing Implications: Teach patient that these events may occur and to report them. Assess baseline comfort, and monitor closely during treatment. Develop plan to assure comfort depending on symptoms reported. For cramps, suggest drinking tonic water and taking calcium gluconate, and if ineffective, discuss with physician the prescription of quinine; for the management of bone pain, suggest NSAIDs as appropriate (Ault et al, 2003). Discuss ineffective strategies with physician, and revise plan as needed.

VI. ALTERATION IN SKIN INTEGRITY, related to RASH

Defining Characteristics: Rash may occur. In clinical studies, 32% of patients with accelerated phase, and 36% of patients in chronic phase CML reported rash. 10% of patients complained of pruritus.

Nursing Implications: Teach patient that rash may occur and to report it. Assess patient skin integrity baseline and regularly during treatment. Teach patient local comfort measures. Teach patient self-application of topical steroids to rash or, if prescribed, systemic steroids (Ault, 2007). Discuss rash and management plan with physician, especially if severe.

Drug: ipilimumab (investigational)

Class: Anti cytotoxic T-lymphocyte antigen-4 (CTLA-4); human monoclonal antibody.

Mechanism of Action: CTLA-4 is an antigen that is expressed on human activated T-lymphocytes that is believed to be very important in regulating the body's immune response; it has an affinity for B7 co-stimulatory molecules, which determine how the T-lymphocyte will interact with antigen-presenting cells. T-lymphocytes are important in immune surveillance to distinguish between self and non-self-antigens. CTLA-4 downregulates (turns off) T-lymphocytes after the invading antigen has been removed so that the immune system does not injure normal tissue. Ipilimumab is a fully human monoclonal antibody that binds (blocks) the antigen (CTLA-4) so that it enhances the activation of the cytotoxic T-lymphocytes (sustaining an active attack against cancer cells, and allowing T-cell replication and differentiation) and at the same time blocks B7-1 and B7-2 co-stimulatory pathways (blocks the activity of this off switch so the activated T-lymphocytes keep working).

Metabolism: Unknown. Long half-life of 2–4 weeks.

Dosage/Range:
- Per protocol, for example, in treatment of metastatic melanoma, 10 mg/kg IV infusion, and in the adjuvant setting 3 mg/kg every 8 weeks for 12 months.

Drug Preparation:
- Per protocol.

Drug Administration:
- Per protocol. IV infusion may be associated with infusion reactions, such as chest pain, flushed/red face, back pain. Stop infusion, and assess response. Administer ordered antihistamines (H_1 and H_2) and corticosteroid.

Drug Interactions:

- Unknown.

Lab Effects/Interference:

- Elevated LFTs (must distinguish between liver metastases and immune hepatitis).
- Alterations in cortisol, ACTH, testosterone, TSH, free T_4 levels.

Special Considerations:

- Increased T-lymphocyte activation and resulting inflammation are responsible for the major toxicities: dermatitis, enterocolitis and hypophysitis (rare). Rarely, inflammation of the eyes (uveitis), pituitary, thyroid, kidneys (nephritis), lungs (alveolitis), adrenal glands can occur, as can aseptic meningitis, and arthritis. Grade III/IV events are largely reversible with high dose steroids therapy (Weber, 2007).
- Drug is being studied in the treatment of patients with malignant melanoma, renal cell, ovarian, prostate, and pancreatic cancers. Also being studied alone and in combination with cytokines (e.g., IL-2), chemotherapy (e.g., dacarbazine), or vaccines.
- May take 12 weeks or longer of treatment before a response is shown, and responses have been documented up to 3 months after drug is stopped. Patients may have short-term progression followed by delayed regression with a prolonged duration of clinical response or stable disease (Weber, 2007).
- Concurrent administration of budesonide to prevent diarrhea was ineffective (Weber et al, 2008).

Potential Toxicities/Side Effects and the Nursing Process

I. ALTERATION IN SKIN INTEGRITY, POTENTIAL, related to DERMATITIS

Defining Characteristics: Dermatitis is most common side effect, often associated with pruritus. Biopsy may show T-lymphocyte infiltrates.

Nursing Interventions: Assess baseline skin integrity, presence of abnormalities, and monitor during therapy. Teach patient that dermatitis may occur and to manage it with nonsteroidal topical lotions. Assess need for antipruritic medications such as diphenhydramine and hydroxyzine and oral steroids.

II. ALTERATION IN ELIMINATION, POTENTIAL, related to ENTEROCOLITIS

Defining Characteristics: Incidence is approximately 17% and manifests initially as diarrhea. Rarely, enterocolitis can result in bowel perforation.

Nursing Interventions: Check protocol for guidance. Diarrhea grade 1–2 is generally treated with diphen. Most protocols require patient admission for more than three diarrhea stools in 24 hours and treated with IV fluids and NPO status. Expect endoscopy and colonoscopy to be performed, with biopsies. If enterocolitis is found, high-dose IV corticosteroids are initiated. Once symptoms have resolved, patient resumes nutrition with a progressive graft-vs-host diet (low fat, fiber, lactulose) and IV steroids converted to oral. Patients are discharged home on an oral steroid, dose taper over at least 1 month (Weber, 2007). If the patient is refractory to high-dose parenteral steroids, infliximab (Remicade, a chimeric MAb targeting TNF-α) as a single dose may be prescribed (Beck et al, 2005). This requires TB testing, as it can reactivate dormant TB. Teach patient to report signs and symptoms of diarrhea, both when three episodes occur in 24 hours, and if fewer than three episodes per 24 hours do not resolve. Teach patient to go to the ED or call 911 if severe abdominal pain, with or without vomiting and constipation, occurs, as the patient needs to be evaluated for bowel perforation right away, although this is a rare event. If bowel perforation occurs, anticipate and prepare patient for immediate surgical intervention.

III. ALTERATION IN FLUID, ELECTROLYTES, AND METABOLISM related to HYPOPHYSITIS

Defining Characteristics: Uncommon but significant because symptoms are vague initially (e.g., fatigue, headaches, low TSH and serum cortisol levels), and if untreated, dysfunction of the hypophysis (such as pituitary enlargement) is far reaching (e.g., severe headaches, severe fatigue, memory loss, loss of libido) (Blansfield et al, 2005).

Nursing Interventions: Monitor baseline and periodic blood tests for TSH and cortisol levels during treatment. Ensure that patient has a baseline MRI to evaluate any increased size of the pituitary gland. Assess baseline activity and comfort levels and at each visit. Teach patient to report onset of worsening fatigue, headaches, changes in mental status. If hypophysitis is suspected, discuss evaluation with physician or NP/PA: MRI to compare size of pituitary baseline, cortisol, ACTH, TSH, and free T_4 levels. If the diagnosis of hypophysitis is confirmed, teach patient about, and administer ordered high-dose steroids and hormonal replacement as needed (e.g., thyroid hormone, testosterone for male patients). Expect that most patients will continue on low dose hydrocortisone to protect the pituitary gland (Blansfield et al, 2005).

IV. ALTERATION IN NUTRITION related to IMMUNE HEPATITIS

Defining Characteristics: Uncommon, but may occur characterized by increasing LFTs.

Nursing Interventions: Assess baseline LFTs and monitor during therapy as ordered. If increasing LFTs and/or BR, check labs every 3 days or per protocol until stable or decreasing and then weekly. Hold drug per protocol. If LFTs continue to rise and immune hepatitis suspected, follow protocol, or anticipate physician will admit patient with daily lab assessment, and order IV steroids to reduce inflammation. If this is ineffective, mycophenolate mofetil, tacrolimus, or infliximab may be tried (Weber, 2007).

Drug: lapatinib ditosylate (Tykerb, GW572016)

Class: Tyrosine kinase inhibitor.

Mechanism of Action: Drug inhibits tyrosine kinases of both Human Epidermal growth factor Receptor (EGFR or HER)-1 and (EGFR or) HER-2-neu, leading to arrest of cell growth and/or apoptosis in tumor cells that depend upon ErbB1 and ErbB2 cell signaling. Normally, HER-2 dimerizes with other members of the HER family, including HER-1. The message is then sent repeatedly via the tyrosine kinases to the cell nucleus telling the cell to divide. In 20% of patients with breast cancer, HER-2-neu is overexpressed, leading to increased cell proliferation, invasiveness, and conferring a poor prognosis associated with reduced survival. By blockading the tyrosine kinases, the message for repeated cell division is halted. Crosses the blood–brain barrier.

Metabolism: After oral ingestion, drug undergoes incomplete and variable absorption. Initial serum concentration identifiable in 15 minutes (median). Peak concentrations achieved in 4 hours, with steady state reached in 6–7 days of single daily dosing. Dividing the dose results in a twofold higher exposure at steady state. When given with food, systemic exposure is increased threefold higher (low fat diet) or fourfold higher (high fat). Drug is highly protein bound (> 99%). Drug is a substrate for the transporter proteins breast cancer-resistance protein and P-glycoprotein, and yet, lapatinib is also able to inhibit these efflux transporters. Drug is extensively metabolized by the CYP3A4 and CYP 3A5 microenzyme system. Terminal half-life of the drug is 14.2 hours and with daily dosing is 24 hours. Drug is eliminated by the liver (P450 system) with about 27% recoverable from feces and less than 2% from the urine.

Dosage/Range:

- 1250 mg orally once daily × 21 days, in combination with capecitabine, 2000 mg/m^2/day days 1–14, repeated every 21 days.
- Dose modify for
  - Decrease in LVEF: hold drug for grade 2 or higher (NCI CTCAE), or if LVEF drops below LLN, wait a minimum of 2 weeks until LVEF returns to normal and the patient is asymptomatic before restarting the dose at 1000 mg/day.
  - Pre-existing severe hepatic impairment: reduce dose as systemic exposure to lapatinib (AUC) increased 14% in patients with moderate, and 63% in patients with severe pre-existing hepatic dysfunction.
  - Discontinue drug if patient develops severe hepatotoxicity while receiving lapatinib.

- Drug interactions: *strong CYP3A4 inhibitors*: reduce lapatinib dose to 500 mg orally a day and when interacting drug discontinued, allow 1 week washout period before adjusting lapatinib dose up to 1250 mg a day.
- Drug interactions: *strong CYP3A4 inducers*: if must give both together, gradually titrate dose of lapatinib up to 4500 mg/day based on tolerability; if interacting drug is discontinued, resume 1250-mg/day dose.
- Other toxicities: hold drug if grade 2 or higher toxicities (NCI CTCAE). Resume at full dose when improvement to grade 1 or less; for recurrent toxicity, restart at 1000 mg/day.

Drug Preparation:

- Oral. Available in 250-mg tablets.

Drug Administration:

- Give lapatinib in a single dose 1 hour before or 2 hours after meals; capecitabine is given in two divided doses about 12 hours apart with food or within 30 minutes of a meal.

Drug Interactions:

- Capecitabine: additive benefits.
- Drugs metabolized by the CYP3A4 and CYP2C8 microenzyme system: lapatinib inhibits CYP3A4 and CYP2C8; monitor for toxicity of drug coadministered with lapatinib.
- Inhibitors of CYP3A4 (ketoconazole, itraconazole, clarithromycin, atazanavir, indinavir, nefazodone, nelfinavir, ritonavir, saquinavir, telithromycin, voriconazole, grapefruit juice); do not coadminister.
- Inducers of CYP3A4 (dexamethasone, phenytoin, carbamazepine, rifampin, rifabutin, rifapentine, phenobarbital, St. John's wort): do not coadminister.
- Lapatinib inhibits p-glycoprotein (transport system), if given with drugs that are substrates of p-glycoprotein, assess for toxicity resulting from increased substrate concentration.

Lab Effects/Interference:

- Unknown.
- Increased BR, AST, ALT.

Special Considerations:

- Drug is indicated in combination with capecitabine in patients with advanced or metastatic breast cancer whose tumors overexpress HER-2-neu and have received prior therapy, including an anthracycline, a taxane, and trastuzumab.
- Rarely, severe hepatotoxicity can occur (ALT or AST > 3 times ULN and total bilirubin > 1.5 ULN), occurring days to months after start of therapy, and may be fatal. Monitor LFTs baseline and every 4–6 weeks during treatment, and as clinically indicated.
- Drug should be avoided in pregnancy; if the patient becomes pregnant while on the drug, the patient should be told of potential hazard to the fetus.
- The most common side effects (> 20%) of lapatinib together with capecitabine were diarrhea, nausea, vomiting, palmar-plantar erythrodysesthesia, rash, and fatigue.

- The most common grade 3 and grade 4 side effects were diarrhea and palmar-plantar erythrodysesthesia.
- Diarrhea can be severe: proactive treatment with anti-diarrheal agents should be instituted, and aggressive support as needed with oral or IV hydration and electrolytes; drug should be interrupted until diarrhea resolves (or discontinued).
- Is also being studied in combination with the monoclonal antibody trastuzumab, which blocks the external domain of the HER-2 receptor, while lapatinib blocks the internal domain of this receptor, as well as that of EGFR1. In addition, patients on trastuzumab often progress in the brain, and lapatinib crosses the blood–brain barrier and thus may prevent brain metastases.

Potential Toxicities/Side Effects and the Nursing Process

I. ALTERATION IN CIRCULATION, POTENTIAL, related to LEFT VENTRICULAR DYSFUNCTION, QT PROLONGATION, HEMORRHAGE

Defining Characteristics: Rarely, patients may develop a decrease in left ventricular ejection fraction (LVEF) to below the institutional lower limit of normal (ILLN). Sixty percent of the time this occurs within the first 9 weeks of treatment. QT prolongation may occur; administer with caution in patients with prolonged or who may develop prolonged QTc (hypokalemia, hypomagnesemia, other drugs that prolong the QTc, cumulative high-dose anthracycline therapy). Bleeding may occur, primarily epistaxis.

Nursing Implications: Assess baseline and periodic LVEF tests, as well as assess patients for any signs or symptoms of congestive heart failure. Identify patients at risk for further decrease in LVEF or development of prolonged QTc. Correct electrolyte abnormalities (e.g., magnesium, potassium) before starting lapatinib, and monitor periodically during therapy. If LVEF falls below ILLN, the drug should be stopped for at least 2 weeks until the LVEF is above the ILLN. Discuss any abnormalities with physician or NP. Teach patient bleeding may occur and to come to ED/notify physician/NP right away if bleeding (e.g., epistaxis) does not resolve in 15 minutes with local pressure and cooling. Ensure that major surgery is planned with adequate time for drug elimination from body, and that it is not resumed until after adequate wound healing.

II. ALTERATION IN NUTRITION, LESS THAN BODY REQUIREMENTS, related to DIARRHEA, NAUSEA, VOMITING, STOMATITIS, DYSPEPSIA, INCREASED LFTS

Defining Characteristics: Diarrhea occurs in 65% of patients, 13% grade 3, and 1% grade 4. Nausea occurs in 44% with 2% grade 3, whereas vomiting affected

26% of patients, with 2% grade 3. Capecitabine primary side effects include diarrhea, nausea, and vomiting. Stomatitis affected 14% and dyspepsia 11%. In combination with capecitabine, which causes some elevation of LFTs, BR was elevated in 45% of patients (4% grade 3), AST in 49% of patients, and ALT in 37% of patients. 1% of patients may develop severe hepatotoxicity, which was fatal in some instances.

Nursing Implications: Assess nutritional status, bowel elimination pattern, and appetite, including LFTs, at baseline and repeated periodically during treatment. LFTs should be repeated every 4–6 weeks during treatment. Inform patient these side effects may occur. Teach self-administration of antinausea and antidiarrheal medications (e.g., loperamide) according to protocol and to notify provider if symptoms persist so that the dose can be interrupted per protocol. Teach the patient dietary modification if nausea and vomiting or diarrhea occur (e.g., for diarrhea, bananas, rice, applesauce, and toast) and to increase oral fluids to prevent dehydration. Consult dietitian to see patient for dietary counseling for anorexia. Discuss any abnormalities with physician or NP.

III. ALTERATION IN COMFORT related to PALMAR-PLANTAR ERYTHRODYSESTHESIA (PPE), RASH, FATIGUE

Defining Characteristics: PPE is a dose-limiting side effect of capecitabine. The incidence is 53% with 12% grade 3. Acneform rash is characteristic of EGFRIs and is usually mild to moderate. A rash occurred in 28% of patients and dry skin in 10%. Fatigue is common.

Nursing Implications: Assess patient's baseline comfort, and teach that these symptoms may occur. Assess skin integrity (especially sun-exposed skin and palms of hands, soles of feet) baseline, and during therapy. Teach symptom management strategies to minimize discomfort. Teach patient to notify nurse or physician if fatigue or rash is severe, or does not resolve with local management. Discuss dose interruption or delay with physician or NP.

Teach patient about PPE: this side effect may occur, and instruct patient to stop drug and call physician/nurse immediately should it occur. If patient has pain, expect dose interruption, with dose reduction if this is the second or subsequent episode at current dose. Teach patient self-assessment of soles of feet and palms of hands daily for erythema, pain, and dry desquamation and to report pain right away. Teach patients to avoid hot showers, whirlpools, paraffin treatments of nails, vigorous repetitive movements of hands and feet, as well as other body areas; avoid tight-fitting shoes and clothes. Teach patients to take cool showers and keep skin surfaces intact and soft with skin emollients. Studies ongoing establishing evidence base for prophylaxis or treatment: vitamin B6, urea moisturizers, nicotine patch.

Teach patient about EGFRI rash: (Refer also to the introduction in Chapter 5.) Do not use antiacne medications. Tetracycline analogues provide an anti-inflammatory benefit. Teach all patients to (1) use a water-based emollient frequently during the day to prevent dryness, (2) stay hydrated, (3) avoid sun exposure and wear SPF 30 (zinc based). **Grade 1/mild rash (localized, does not interfere with ADLs, and is not infected):** The goal is to preserve skin integrity, minimize discomfort, and prevent infection. Key patient teaching includes to (1) use of a mild soap with active ingredients that reduce skin drying such as pyrithione zinc (Head and Shoulders), (2) consider aloe gel to red, tender areas, (3) report distressing tenderness as pramoxine (lidocaine topical anesthetic may help), (4) keep fingernails clean and trimmed, and (5) apply zinc ointment to rectal mucosa after washing. Management: maintain current drug dose; observe or give topical hydrocortisone 1% or 2.5% or clindamycin 1% gel (anti-inflammatory benefit); reassess in 2 weeks. **For grade 2/ moderate rash which is generalized, mild symptoms, and has minimal effect on ADLs, and no infection:** The goal is to prevent infection and promote comfort. Continue EGFRI dose; use topicals (hydrocortisone 2.5% or clindamycin 1% gel) or consider pimecrolimus cream (immunomodulator) and add doxycycline 100 mg PO twice daily or minocycline 100 mg PO twice daily (give antimicrobial and anti-inflammatory effect) and reassess after 2 weeks. **For grade 3/4 or severe rash (generalized, severe, has a significant impact on ADLs, and increased risk of infection):** The goal is to prevent infection or identify it early to minimize complications and maximize patient coping with side effects Hold drug for until rash improves, and treat rash with topicals (hydrocortisone 2.5% or clindamycin 1% gel or pimecrolimus cream, doxycycline 100 mg PO twice daily or minocycline 100 mg PO twice daily, and methylprednisolone, Medrol dose pack); reassess after 2 weeks, and interrupt or discontinue drug if rash worsens (Lynch et al, 2007). If rash appears infected (exudate, vesicular formation, different appearance), obtain C+S, treat empirically until sensitivity received, and/or obtain dermatology consult. Discuss dose modification with a physician.

Drug: lenalidomide (Revlimid)

Class: Immunomodulator with anti-angiogenesis properties.

Mechanism of Action: Exact mechanisms not fully known. Drug has antineoplastic, immunomodulatory, and antiangiogenic properties. Induces G0/G1 growth arrest and apoptosis, increases expression of genes found on 5q locus including genes involved in cell adhesion. Inhibits COX-2 expression, stimulates T-cell proliferation, as well as the anti-inflammatory cytokines Interleukin-2, Interleukin-10, and Interferon-gamma. Decreases the secretion of proinflammatory cytokines that mediate cell growth and survival (TNF-α, Interleukin-1β, and Interleukin-6); stimulates host natural killer cell immunity (Bartlett et al, 2004).

When Blood Counts	Recommended Course
MDS	
If thrombocytopenia develops within 4 weeks of starting at 10 mg daily	
1) Plt < 50,000/mcL. 2) Plt returns to > 50,000/mcL.	1) Interrupt lenalidomide. 2) Resume lenalidomide at 5 mg daily.
1) Plt ↓ to 50% of baseline value. 2) If baseline > 60,000/mcL and returns to > 50,000/mcL.	1) Interrupt lenalidomide. 2) Resume lenalidomide at 5 mg daily.
If thrombocytopenia develops AFTER 4 weeks of starting treatment at 10 mg daily	
1) Plt < 30,000/mcL or < 50,000/mcL and plt transfusions. 2) Plt return to > 30,000/mcL without hemostatic failure.	1) Interrupt lenalidomide. 2) Resume lenalidomide at 5 mg daily.
If thrombocytopenia develops during treatment at 5 mg daily	
1) Plt < 30,000/mcL or < 50,000/mcL and plt transfusions. 2) Plt return to > 30,000/mcL without hemostatic failure.	1) Interrupt lenalidomide. 2) Resume lenalidomide at 5 mg daily.
If neutropenia develops within 4 weeks of starting treatment at 10 mg daily	
1) ANC < 750/mcL. 2) Return to > 1,000/mcL.	1) Interrupt lenalidomide. 2) Resume lenalidomide at 5 mg daily.
If neutropenia develops within 4 weeks at 10 mg daily dose	
1) ANC < 500/mcL for > 7 days or < 500/mcL with fever (> 38.5°C). 2) Return to > 500/mcL	1) Interrupt lenalidomide. 2) Resume lenalidomide at 5 mg daily.
If neutropenia develops during treatment at 5 mg daily	
1) ANC < 500/mcL for > 7 days or < 500/mcL with fever (> 38.5°C). 2) Return to > 500/mcL	1) Interrupt lenalidomide. 2) Resume lenalidomide at 5 mg daily.

(continued)

Multiple Myeloma: for grades 3/4 toxicity	
1) Plt < 30,000/mcL. 2) Return to > 30,000/mcL. 3) For each subsequent drop < 30,000/mcL. 4) Plt return to > 30,000/mcL.	1) Interrupt lenalidomide, follow CBC weekly. 2) Restart lenalidomide at 15 mg daily. 3) Interrupt lenalidomide. 4) Resume lenalidomide at 5 mg less than previous dose (do not dose below 5 mg daily).
1) ANC < 1,000/mcL. 2) ANC Returns to > 1,000/mcL and neutropenia is the only toxicity. 3) ANC returns to > 1,000/mcL and there is other toxicity. 4) For each subsequent drop ANC < 1,000/mcL. 5) ANC returns to > 1,000/mcL.	1) Interrupt lenalidomide and add G-CSF, follow CBC weekly. 2) Resume lenalidomide at 25 mg daily. 3) Resume lenalidomide at 15 mg daily. 4) Interrupt lenalidomide. 5) Resume lenalidomide at 5 mg less than the previous dose. Do not dose below 5 mg daily.
Other Grade 3/4 toxicities related to lenalidomide	Hold treatment and restart at next lower dose level when toxicity has resolved to < Grade 2.

Source: Celgene Corp. Revlimid package insert. Celgene Corp: Summit, NJ; June 29, 2006.

Metabolism: Rapidly absorbed after oral administration, with maximal plasma concentrations occurring .6–1.5 hours after dose in normal subjects. Co-administration with food reduces maximal plasma concentration by 36%. In patients with multiple myeloma, area under the curve (AUC) exposure was 57% higher than in healthy volunteers, due to mild renal impairment. Drug has 30% protein binding. Two-thirds of the drug is excreted unchanged in the urine. Elimination half-life of the drug is 3 hours.

Dosage/Range:

- Myelodysplastic Syndrome (MDS): 10 mg PO with water daily with dose adjustment based on ANC and platelet count;
- Multiple Myeloma: 25 mg/day PO with water d1–21 of repeated 28 day cycles, together with dexamethasone 40 mg/day on days 1–4, 9–12, and 17–20 of each 28-day cycle for the first 4 cycles of therapy, and then 40 mg/day PO on days 1–4 every 28 days.

Drug Preparation:

- Oral available in 5, 10, 15, and 25 mg capsules, in bottles of (5 and 10 mg caps) 30 or 100; (15 mg) 21 or 100; (25 mg) 25 or 100, under a restricted distribution

program, RevAssist, similar to the STEPS program for Thalidomide; prescribers and pharmacists must be registered with the program.
- Patients must meet all the conditions of the RevAssist program (see Potential Toxicity 4).
- Pregnancy test results must be verified by the prescriber and the pharmacist prior to dispensing the prescription.

Drug Interactions:
- Bone marrow suppressive agents: additive bone marrow suppression.
- Additive anti-tumor effect when combined with dexamethasone in the treatment of multiple myeloma.

Lab Effects/Interference:
- Decreased neutrophil, platelet, and red blood cell count.
- Decreased potassium and magnesium (uncommon).
- Decreased alanine aminotransferase increased (uncommon).

Special Considerations:
- Selectively designed to be more potent (10,000 times) and to have a different adverse event profile than thalidomide; drug is not teratogenic at similar doses, but has been found embryotoxic in animal studies.
- Drug is indicated for the treatment of patients with transfusion-dependent anemia due to low or intermediate 1-risk myelodysplastic syndromes associated with a deletion 5 q cytogenetic abnormality, with or without additional cytogenetic abnormalities; drug is also indicated in combination with dexamethasone for the treatment of patients with multiple myeloma who have received at least one prior therapy.
- Drug is associated with significant neutropenia and thrombocytopenia in patients with del 5 q MDS; 80% of patients required a dose delay/reduction during the major study for the indication.
- Drug significantly increases the risk of deep vein thrombosis (DVT) and pulmonary embolism (PE) in patients with multiple myeloma treated with lenalidomide combination therapy.
- ABSOLUTE CONTRAINDICATION IS PREGNANCY. Pregnancy tests must be routinely negative prior to beginning therapy in women of childbearing age. Contraception is mandatory in men and women.
- Drug is largely excreted by the kidneys; use cautiously in patients with renal impairment, and dose reduce as needed.
- Overall frequency of adverse events was equivalent between elderly and other patients studied; the elderly (aged > 65 years old) had more serious adverse events, possibly because more elder patients have renal impairment.
- Drug does not cause sleepiness, constipation, or peripheral neuropathy like thalidomide.
- Drug may cause tumor lysis syndrome in newly diagnosed multiple myeloma patients with large tumor burdens that lyse quickly when lenalidomide is given.

- Drug is being studied in the treatment of type-1 Complex Regional Pain Syndrome.
- In the treatment of patients with relapsed or refractory multiple myeloma, patients receiving lenalidomide plus dexamethasone had significantly longer TTP (40 to > 60 weeks vs about 20 weeks) and ORR (51.3% vs 22.9%; Dimopoulous et al, 2004); and more mature results reported by Fonseca et al (2005) showed a 61% RR compared to 24% with dexamethasone alone, and a 26% CR.
- Drug has hematologic activity in patients with low risk myelodysplastic syndromes who have no response to erythropoietin (List et al, 2005).

Potential Toxicities/Side Effects and the Nursing Process

I. POTENTIAL FOR INFECTION AND BLEEDING related to BONE MARROW SUPPRESSION

Defining Characteristics: Significant neutropenia and thrombocytopenia, requiring dose adjustments in 80% of patients in initial dose, and 34% required second dose adjustment in the pivotal study of MDS patients. 48% of patients developed grade neutropenia with a median time to onset of 42 days, and recovery in 17 days. 54% of patients developed grade thrombocytopenia with a median time of onset of 28 days, and recovery in 22 days. Anemia occurred 11% of patients.

Nursing Implications: Assess baseline CBC, WBC, differential, and platelet count prior to chemotherapy, then weekly for the first 8 weeks of treatment, then monthly. Assess for signs/symptoms of infection or bleeding. Teach patient the signs/symptoms of infection or bleeding, and to report these immediately, and teach patient self-care measures to minimize risk of infection and bleeding. This includes avoidance of crowds, proximity to people with infections, and OTC aspirin-containing medications. Discuss need for blood product support or growth factors with physician or NP. Drug should be used in combination with another agent that does not cause bone marrow suppression, like bortezomib (Velcade) rather than chemotherapy.

II. ALTERATION IN COMFORT related to RASH, FATIGUE, LIGHT-HEADEDNESS, AND LEG CRAMPS

Defining Characteristics: 42% of patients develop itching, 36% rash, and 14% dry skin. Pruritus may be limited to the scalp and occur within 1 week of treatment. 31% of patients experience fatigue, 20% peripheral edema, 21% arthralgias, 21% back pain, and 18% muscle cramps. About 20% of patients reported dizziness or headache.

Nursing Implications: Assess patient's baseline comfort, and teach patient that these symptoms may occur. Assess skin integrity baseline and during therapy. Teach symptom management strategies to minimize discomfort. Teach patient to notify nurse or physician if fatigue, rash, itching, or leg cramps are severe, or do not resolve with local management. Teach patient to change position slowly and to report severe dizziness. Teach patient to report leg cramps or new onset of shortness of breath or chest pain, and evaluate for DVT or PE.

III. ALTERATION IN NUTRITION, LESS THAN BODY REQUIREMENTS, related to DIARRHEA, CONSTIPATION OR NAUSEA, ELECTROLYTE DISTURBANCE

Defining Characteristics: Diarrhea occurs in about 49% of patients, while constipation affects about 23%. Nausea affects about 23% of patients, and vomiting 10%. 6% of patients have dysgeusia, 10% have hypokalemia, 10% anorexia, and 6% hypomagnesemia.

Nursing Implications: Assess baseline nutrition, electrolytes, and bowel elimination pattern. Teach patient that nausea, rarely vomiting, diarrhea, or less commonly, constipation, may occur. Teach patient self-care strategies to minimize symptoms and to report them if they do not resolve. Teach patient self-administration of antiemetics or anti-diarrheals as prescribed, and to notify provider if diarrhea persists for dose interruption. Teach patient dietary modification if diarrhea, constipation, nausea, or vomiting occur, (e.g., the BRAT diet for diarrhea: bananas, rice, applesauce, and toast), and to increase oral fluids to prevent dehydration. Assess baseline electrolytes and periodically during treatment.

IV. KNOWLEDGE DEFICIT, POTENTIAL, related to PATIENT INSTRUCTIONS (RevAssist), CONTRACEPTION AND PREGNANCY TESTING

Defining Characteristics: Drug is a potent teratogen. Patients must be able to understand the risk of teratogenicity and be able to safeguard the drug in the home.

Nursing Implications: Assess patient's ability to understand rationale and importance of pregnancy testing in women of childbearing age prior to drug prescription, and during treatment, treatment holidays, and for 4 weeks following drug discontinuance. Assess the understanding and ability to comply of patients with childbearing potential with contraception requirement and other self-care strategies:

- Female patients of childbearing age must use effective (one highly effective and one additional effective method at the same time) contraception for at least 4 weeks before beginning lenalidomide, during therapy and dose interruptions, and for 4 weeks following drug discontinuation. Patient must have two negative pregnancy tests before the drug is prescribed (UNLESS the woman completely abstains form heterosexual sexual contact).
- Male patients must always use a latex condom during any sexual contact with females of childbearing potential.

- Once treatment has started and during dose interruptions, pregnancy testing should be repeated every 4 weeks in women with regular menstrual cycles.
- If menses are irregular, pregnancy tests should be done every 2 weeks. If a patient misses her period, if there is an abnormal pregnancy test or menstrual bleeding, the woman should have a pregnancy test and counseling.
- Notify the physician immediately:
  - If the woman is able to become pregnant, she must stop the drug and notify the physician immediately for emergency contraception if she becomes pregnant or thinks she might be pregnant, misses her menses, has unusual menstrual bleeding, or stops birth control.
  - If a male patient has had unprotected sex with a woman who can become pregnant, or if he thinks his sexual partner may be pregnant.

• Participate in a telephone survey and patient registry as part of the RevAssist program. Assess ability of patient to keep drug/drug supply out of the reach of children and pets, and NEVER to share drug with anyone else, even if they have similar symptoms. Discuss any concerns with the physician.

Drug: neovastat (investigational)

Class: Angiogenesis inhibitor made from cartilaginous spine of dogfish shark.

Mechanism of Action: Appears to inhibit vascular endothelial growth factor (VEGD) signaling, to inhibit matrix metalloproteinases (MMPs), and to induce apoptosis (programmed cell death).

Dosage/Range:
- Per protocol.

Drug Preparation:
- Available orally in liquid form, taken bid, per protocol.

Drug Interactions:
- Unknown.

Lab Effects/Interference:
- Unknown.

Special Consideration:
- Differs from OTC shark cartilage, which is made primarily from shark fins.
- In a small study of patients with renal cell cancer, patients receiving a higher dose of neovastat survived 16.3 months compared to those receiving a lower dose whose survival was 7.1 months (Bukowski, 2001).
- Well tolerated without reported side effects.
- Clinical trials in patients with lung or ovarian cancer, multiple myeloma, with or without chemotherapy, are ongoing (NCI, others).

Potential Toxicities/Side Effects and Nursing Implications

I. KNOWLEDGE DEFICIT relating to LACK OF KNOWLEDGE, MEDIA MISINFORMATION

Defining Characteristics: Media about shark cartilage has been rife with misinformation, because there is no distinction between the cartilage-derived drug and that sold as an OTC miracle drug. Neovastat is made from shark spine cartilage, and the active substance is found in all animal cartilage. Shark is used because there is a high percentage of cartilage per body weight, and it is abundantly available. OTC shark cartilage is made from shark fins.

Nursing Implications: Assess basic understanding of drug and its mechanism of action, and explain how it differs from OTC shark cartilage. Teach the patient self-administration of the drug. Provide information, and answer questions. Ensure patient makes an informed consent prior to entering the study.

Drug: Nilotinib (Tasigna)

Class: Tyrosine kinase inhibitor (second generation).

Mechanism of Action: Ph+ CML and ALL are caused by a reciprocal mutation involving two chromosomes in the bone marrow (genetic material is exchanged between chromosomes 9;22), creating the Philadelphia chromosome, the fusion gene (bcr-abl) and Bcr-Abl, the oncogenic fusion protein encoded by bcr-abl (Deininger et al, 2005). Bcr-Abl causes cell proliferation, decreased adhesion/increased migration, inhibition of apoptosis, and degradation of regulatory proteins, and prevents DNA repair. The Bcr portion of the Bcr-Abl fusion protein is a tyrosine kinase that turns on cell proliferation signals that create the excessive production of white blood cells (leukemia); however, the binding site is sometimes blocked (inactive) and sometimes active and able to bind to ATP. When a patient progresses on imatinib, it is because Bcr-Abl is reactivated through a number of processes, such as amplification of bcr-abl gene expression, or over 30 point mutations in the Bcr-Abl kinase domain so that the drug cannot bind (Deininger et al, 2005). Nilotinib is a designer drug that is highly specific for and binds very tightly to the ATP binding site of ABL (more selective and 30 times more potent an inhibitor than imatinib mesylate). The drug is active against 32 of the 33 most common Bcr-Abl mutations causing imatinib resistance. The drug also inhibits the KIT and PDGFR-A proteins found in patients with GIST.

Metabolism: The drug is metabolized via the cytochrome P450 microenzyme system in the liver (CYP3A4). A high-fat diet greatly increases drug bioavailability (82%), and thus, the drug must be given on an empty stomach. Peak concentrations reached 3 hours after drug administration. Serum protein binding is 98%. Elimination half-life with daily dosing is 17 hours, and steady state is reached by day 8. Metabolism occurs by oxidation and hydroxylation. Metabolites are not pharmacologically active. More than 90% of administered dose is eliminated within 7 days primarily via the feces. Age, weight, gender, and ethnicity do not significantly affect pharmacokinetics.

Dosage/Range: 400 mg orally twice daily to start, approximately 12 hours apart on an empty stomach (no food 2 hours before or 1 hour after the dose).
Dose reduce for QTc interval prolongation > 480 msec, hematologic (ANC < 1.0 $\times 10^9$/L and/or platelet count < 50 $\times 10^9$/L [see package insert]).

Preparation/Administration:
- Oral.
- Available in 200-mg capsules.
- Administer two capsules on an empty stomach (2 hours after a meal or 1 hour before a meal) with a glass of water. Drink only water for the 1 hour after drug administration. This is a critical point of patient education.
- Therapy is continued until disease progression or unacceptable toxicity.

Drug Interactions:
- CYP3A4 (strong) inhibitors (ketoconazole, itraconazole, clarithromycin, atazanavir, indinavir, nefazodone, nelfinavir, ritonavir, saquinavir, telithromycin, voriconazole, grapefruit juice) may increase imatinib plasma concentrations; do not coadminister. IF their administration is necessary, interrupt nilotinib therapy; if continued co-administration is necessary, adjust nilotinib dose to 400 mg qd (by 50%), and monitor QTc interval closely for any prolongation. If then the strong inhibitor is discontinued, a washout period should be allowed before increasing the dose of nilotinib back to 400 mg every 12 hours.
- CYP3A4 substrates (simvastatin): nilotinib decreases simvastatin metabolism with simvastatin serum levels increased 2 to 3.5 times. Use together cautiously, if at all, and monitor BP and dose reduce simvastatin if needed.
- CYP3A4 (strong) inducers (dexamethasone, phenytoin, carbamazepine, rifampicin, phenobarbital, St. John's wort) may increase metabolism of nilotinib so that nilotinib serum levels are reduced. Use together cautiously, if at all. When used with dexamethasone, phenytoin, carbamazepine, phenobarbital, rifabutin, or rifampin, increase nilotinib dose by 50%. Teach patient to not take St. John's wort if taking nilotinib.
- Other CYP3A4 substrates (cyclosporine, pimozide) increased plasma concentrations if coadministered with nilotinib. Do not administer together because drug has a narrow therapeutic window.
- Other CYP3A4 substrates (triazolo-benzadiazepines, dihydropyridine calcium-channel blockers, HMG-CoA reductase inhibitors) may have increased serum levels when given together with nilotinib. Use together cautiously, and monitor patient closely.
- Other CYP3A4 substrates: eletriptan (Relpax). Do not administer eletriptan within 72 hours of nilotinib. Monitor vital signs closely.

- Warfarin: nilotinib is a competitive substrate, and thus, INR must be monitored closely and warfarin dose adjusted frequently.
- Drugs prolonging QTc (e.g., serotonin antagonists, other tyrosine kinase inhibitors): do not use together, as will increase risk of prolonged QTc and sudden death.

Lab Effects/Interference:

- Increased LFTs—AST, ALT, alkaline phosphatase, BR (total)—transient
- Increased serum creatinine, lipase (transient), glucose
- Decreased serum calcium, magnesium, phosphate, potassium, sodium
- Decreased neutrophils, platelet count

Special Considerations:

- FDA indicated for the treatment of patients with chronic phase and accelerated phase Philadelphia chromosome positive chronic myelogenous leukemia (CML) in adult patients resistant or intolerant to prior therapy that included imatinib.
- Imatinib is successful in treating patients with Ph+ CML (chronic, accelerated, and blast phases) and inducing a complete cytogenic response in 80%; however, 10% will develop resistance by amplification, mutations, additional chromosomal mutations (Ault, 2007). Nilotinib able to induce major cytogenetic response in 52% of patients after 6 months in imatinib-resistant or -intolerant patients.
- Patient teaching about self-administration on an empty stomach critical to prevent increased toxicity.
- Drug can increase QTc interval, and sudden deaths have been reported.
- Contraindicated in patients with:
  - Congenital long QT syndrome.
  - Prolonged QT interval (> 450 msec).
  - Receiving medications known to prolong the QT interval.
  - Hypokalemia and/or hypomagnesemia.
- Not recommended for patients who have galactose intolerance, severe lactase deficiency, or glucose–galactose malabsorption, as the capsule contains lactose.
- Use cautiously in patients with hepatic impairment.
- Minimal cross-intolerance in imatinib-intolerant patients.
- Fluid retention uncommon and rare hepatotoxicity.
- Rare grade 3/4 myelosuppression.
- Teach women of child-bearing age to use effective contraception while receiving the drug; mothers should not breast-feed.
- Lab monitoring: **CBC/diff** baseline and then every 2 weeks for the first 2 months and then monthly; ECG to monitor **QTc** baseline, 7 days after first dose, and then periodically as well as after any dose adjustments; monitor QTc closely in patients with liver impairment or receiving strong CYP3A4 inhibitors; **electrolytes**: baseline and correct prior to starting drug, especially magnesium and potassium; monitor magnesium, potassium, calcium, phosphorus, sodium; monitor **serum lipase and glucose** baseline in patients with a history of pancreatitis; monitor **LFTs** baseline and periodically.

- Teach patient self-administration of drug: Take drug at least 2 hours after eating, and then wait at least 1 hour before eating food; avoid grapefruit juice, the fruit, or any supplement containing grapefruit. Tell nurse or physician before taking ANY over-the-counter medicine, vitamin, or mineral; be sure to tell nurse or physician all medications that patient is taking and whether he or she has had any trouble digesting lactose in the past.

Potential Toxicities/Side Effects and the Nursing Process

I. POTENTIAL FOR INFECTION AND BLEEDING related to NEUTROPENIA AND THROMBOCYTOPENIA

Defining Characteristics: Grade 3/4 neutropenia occurred in 28% of patients in chronic phase and 37% of patients with accelerated phase; thrombocytopenia in 28–37% of patients; anemia in 8–23% of patients. Febrile neutropenia occurred in < 10% of patients with accelerated phase CML.

Nursing Implications: Assess baseline CBC, WBC, differential, and platelet count before initiating therapy and then weekly for the first 8 weeks of treatment and then monthly. Assess for signs/symptoms of infection or bleeding. Teach patient the signs/symptoms of infection or bleeding and to report these immediately, and teach patient self-care measures to minimize risk of infection and bleeding. This includes avoidance of crowds, proximity to people with infections, and OTC aspirin-containing medications. Discuss need for blood product support or growth factors with physician or NP.

II. ALTERATION IN CIRCULATION, POTENTIAL, related to QTc PROLONGATION

Defining Characteristics: Rarely, patients may develop QT prolongation on ECG. Administer with caution in patients with prolonged or who may develop prolonged QTc (hypokalemia, hypomagnesemia, other drugs which prolong the QTc, cumulative high-dose anthracycline therapy). Prolonged QTc in the setting of low magnesium and hypokalemia sets the stage for torsades de pointes, with ventricular tachycardia and fibrillation possible.

Nursing Implications: Assess baseline and periodic QTc interval. Identify patients at risk for development of prolonged QTc (congenital long QTc syndrome, prolonged QTc > 450 msec, taking antiarrhythmics or other drugs that can prolong the QTc interval, hypokalemia, hypomagnesemia). Correct electrolyte abnormalities (e.g., magnesium, potassium) before starting nilotinib, and monitor periodically during therapy. Hypokalemia and hypomagnesemia in the setting of prolonged QTc may lead to torsades de pointes and ventricular fibrillation.

III. ALTERATION IN SKIN INTEGRITY related to RASH, PRURITUS, EDEMA

Defining Characteristics: Rash may occur. In clinical studies, 33% of patients reported rash (2% grades 3/4); 29% of patients complained of pruritus. Peripheral edema occurred in 11% of patients.

Nursing Implications: Teach patient that rash may occur and to report it. Assess patient skin integrity baseline and regularly during treatment. Teach patient local comfort measures. Teach patient self-application of topical steroids to rash or, if prescribed, systemic steroids (Ault, 2007). Discuss rash and management plan with physician, especially if severe. Teach patient to report any weight increase, swelling of the ankles, feet, or face, and any difficulty breathing or shortness of breath.

IV. POTENTIAL ALTERATION IN NUTRITION related to NAUSEA, DIARRHEA, VOMITING, CONSTIPATION, HEPATOTOXICITY, PANCREATITIS

Defining Characteristics: Nausea affected 31% of patients (1% grades 3/4), and vomiting affected 21% (<1% grades 3/4). Diarrhea affected 22% (3% grades 3/4), whereas constipation affected 20%. Hepatotoxicity characterized by transient and reversible increase in LFTs. Grade 3/4 lipase increased in 15–17% of patients and glucose in 11% of patients. The largest increase in bilirubin was found in patients with $(TA)^7(TA)^7$ genotype (UGT1A1*28).

Nursing Implications: Teach patient to self-administer antiemetic 1 hour before each dose if needed and to call if nausea/vomiting develop. Discuss with physician more effective antiemetic regime if nausea/vomiting develop despite antiemetics. Encourage small, frequent intake of cool, bland foods as tolerated if nausea develops. Refer to dietitian as needed for meal planning. Assess bowel elimination pattern baseline and at each visit. Teach patient to report diarrhea or constipation that does not respond to antidiarrheal or anticonstipation medications. Teach dietary modifications as appropriate. Monitor LFTs, serum, lipase, and glucose baseline and periodically during therapy. Discuss abnormalities with physician. Teach patient to report any abdominal pain with nausea or vomiting.

V. POTENTIAL ALTERATION IN COMFORT related to HEADACHE, FATIGUE, ARTHRALGIA, MYALGIA

Defining Characteristics: In clinical studies, headache affected 30% of patients, 3% grades 3/4. Arthralgias affected 18% of patients (2% grades 3/4) and myalgias 14% (2% grades 3/4). Bone pain and muscle spasms affected 11% of patients.

Nursing Implications: Teach patient that these events may occur and to report them. Assess baseline comfort, and monitor closely during treatment. Develop plan to assure comfort depending on symptoms reported. If appropriate, suggest NSAIDs, the application of heat or cold, for control of myalgias and arthralgias. Discuss ineffective strategies with physician, and revise plan as needed.

Drug: panitumumab (Vectibix, ABX-EGF)

Class: IgG_2 Human monoclonal antibody targeted against epidermal growth factor receptor (EGFR).

Mechanism of Action: Drug is a human IgG_2 monoclonal antibody. It blocks growth factor (ligand, such as epidermal growth factor and transforming growth factor-alpha) from binding to EGFR, thus preventing dimerization and initiation of cell signaling via receptor tyrosine kinase phosphorylation; thus, the message telling the cell to divide does not occur. The drug competes with natural ligands but has a higher affinity for the EGFR than the ligands. In addition to cell growth inhibition, there is induction of apoptosis, and decreased matrix metalloproteinase and vascular endothelial growth factor production. This decreases angiogenesis.

Metabolism: Steady-state reached by 3rd infusion. Elimination half-life is approximately 7.5 days.

Dosage/Range: 6.0 mg/kg q 2 weeks as a 1 hour infusion.

Drug Preparation:
- Available as single use 20 mg/mL vials (100 mg, 200 mg, 400 mg).
- Inspect drug (should be colorless; do not shake) and withdrawal ordered dose; add to 0.9% NS USP final concentration is ≤10 mg/mL.
- Mix diluted solution by gentle inversion.

Drug Administration:
- Administer IV using low-protein binding 0.2 μm or 0.22 μm inline filter using infusion pump over 60 minutes (90 minutes for dose ≥ 1000 mg).
- Does not require premedication to prevent hypersensitivity reactions as drug is a humanized monoclonal antibody.
- Reduce the infusion rate by 50% if patient experiences a mild or moderate (grades 1/2) infusion reaction for the remainder of the infusion.
- Stop and discontinue drug for grade 3/4 infusion reactions (symptomatic bronchospasm or anaphylaxis).

Drug Interactions:
- IFL: Severe diarrhea (1 fatality). DO NOT COADMINSTER.

Lab Effects/Interference:
- ↓ magnesium 6 weeks after beginning therapy.
- ↓ calcium in some patients.

Special Considerations:

- FDA indicated for the treatment of EGFR-expressing MCRC with disease progression on or following fluoropyrimidine-, oxaliplatin-, and irinotecan-containing chemotherapy regimens. It is NOT indicated for use in combination with chemotherapy with or without bevacizumab, as interim analysis of the PACCE trial showed the addition of panitumumab to the combination of bevacizumab and chemotherapy resulted in decreased PFS and increased grade 3–5 toxicity (87% vs. 72%).
- Severe hypersensitivity occurred in 1% of patients (NCI grade 3–4) and 3% experienced infusion reactions.
- Tumors over-expressing epidermal growth factor receptors are colorectal, lung, breast, bladder, pancreas, kidney, head and neck cancers. Principal study is in patients with metastatic colorectal cancer.
- Drug exposure and tolerability similar between weekly, every-other-week, and every-three-week dosing schedules (Weiner LM, 2005).
- In patients studied who developed HAHA formation, it did not appear to change pharmacokinetic profile.
- Interstitial lung disease, a class effect, may occur in <1% of patients, but caution should be used when treating patients with a history of interstitial pneumonitis, pulmonary fibrosis, as after the first fatality, these patients were excluded from clinical trials.
- Drug may cause grade 3–4 hypomagnesemia in 2% of patients.
- Drug can cause diarrhea; in combination with bolus-irinotecan (IFL) grade 3–4 diarrhea occurred in 58% of patients (1 fatality) while in combination with FOLFIRI (infusional) the grade 3–4 incidence of diarrhea was 25%. DO NOT administer with IFL chemotherapy.
- Patient should use birth control measures; mothers should not breast-feed while receiving the drug.
- Compared with best supportive care (BSC), panitumumab significantly improved PFS, but there was no significant difference in OS between groups.

Potential Toxicities/Side Effects and the Nursing Process

I. POTENTIAL ALTERATION IN BODY IMAGE, SKIN INTEGRITY, COMFORT related to SKIN RASH, PARONYCHIA, SKIN FISSURES, PRURITUS

Defining Characteristics: Drug inhibits epidermal growth factor receptor, so major toxicity is manifested in the skin with 90% of patients experiencing some type of skin toxicity. Most patients develop a mild-to-moderate acne-like rash that is self-limiting. 16% report a grade 3–4 rash. Rash is a sterile, suppurative rash with multiple follicular or pustular lesions that appear during the first 2 weeks of therapy on the face, upper chest, and back, but in some cases, extended to the arms. Rash resolves when treatment is stopped, without scar formation. Pruritus affects 57%, dry-skin 10%, acneiform dermatitis 57%, skin desquamation 25%, erythema 65%, paronychia 25%, macular rash 22%, skin fissures 20%, stomatitis 7%, oral mucositis 6%. Fissures can become infected; infection can be treated with topical clindamycin, or oral antibiotics. However, severe dermatologic toxicities result in infectious complications including sepsis, death, and abscesses requiring incision and drainage. Eye-related toxicities occurred in 15% of patients (conjunctivitis 4%, hyperemia 3%, lacrimation 2%, eyelid irritation 1%), median time to most severe toxicity 15 days from starting drug, median time to solution was 84 days.

Nursing Implications: Teach patient that rash most likely will occur due to mechanism of drug action. Assess baseline skin integrity on areas of face, neck, and trunk; assess baseline comfort and satisfaction with body image, and monitor at each treatment. Teach patient to report any distress and assess extent of rash. For severe rash (grade 3/4 or intolerable), hold drug for up to 1 month until it resolves to grade 2 or less; if it does not, discontinue drug. When rash resolves to grade 2 and the patient is symptomatically improved and no more than two doses have been held, resume drug at 50% of the original dose. If skin toxicity recurs, discontinue drug. If skin appears to be infected (exudate, vesicle formation, abnormal appearance), obtain C+S and discuss empiric treatment with physician. *For ras, fissure, and paronychia management, refer to the introduction in Chapter 5.* Teach all patients to (1) use a water-based emollient frequently during the day to prevent dryness, (2) stay hydrated, (3) avoid sun exposure and wear SPF 30 (zinc based). Do not use antiacne medications. Tetracycline analogues provide anti-inflammatory benefit. **Grade 1/mild rash (localized, does not interfere with ADLs, and is not infected):** The goal is to preserve skin integrity, minimize discomfort, and prevent infection. Key patient teaching includes (1) use a mild soap with active ingredients that reduce skin drying such as pyrithione zinc (Head and Shoulders), (2) consider aloe gel to red, tender areas, (3) report distressing tenderness as pramoxine (lidocaine topical anesthetic may help), (4) keep fingernails clean and trimmed, and (5) apply zinc ointment to rectal mucosa after washing. Management: maintain current drug dose, observe or give topical hydrocortisone 1% or 2.5% or clindamycin 1% gel (anti-inflammatory benefit); reassess in 2 weeks. **For grade 2/moderate rash which is generalized, mild symptoms, and has minimal effect on ADLs, and no infection:** The goal is to prevent infection and promote comfort. Continue EGFRI dose; use topicals (hydrocortisone 2.5% or clindamycin 1% gel) or consider pimecrolimus cream (immunomodulator) and add doxycycline 100 mg PO twice daily or minocycline 100 mg PO twice daily (give antimicrobial and anti-inflammatory effect) and reassess after 2 weeks. **For grade 3/4 or severe rash (generalized, severe, has a significant impact on ADLs, and increased risk of infection):** The goal is to prevent infection or to identify it early to minimize complications and to promote effective coping. Dose reduce EGFRI drug based on manufacture's recommendation, and treat rash with topicals (hydrocortisone 2.5% or clindamycin 1% gel or pimecrolimus cream, doxycycline 100 mg PO twice daily or minocycline 100 mg PO twice daily, and methylprednisolone) (Medrol dose pack);

reassess after 2 weeks, and interrupt or discontinue drug if rash worsens (Lynch et al, 2007). If rash appears infected (exudate, vesicular formation, different appearance), obtain C+S, treat empirically until sensitivity received, and/or obtain dermatology consult.

II. ALTERATION IN NUTRITION, LESS THAN BODY REQUIREMENTS, related to NAUSEA, VOMITING, DIARRHEA, STOMATITIS, CONSTIPATION, ANOREXIA, ABDOMINAL PAIN

Defining Characteristics: Incidence of mild-to-moderate digestive symptoms include nausea (23%), diarrhea (21%), abdominal pain (25%), vomiting (19%), constipation (21%), stomatitis (7%) hypomagnesia (39%), and oral mucositis (6%) in patients on clinical trials.

Nursing Implications: Assess baseline weight and nutritional status. Inform patient that these symptoms may occur, and to report them. Administer antiemetic and other symptom management medications as ordered. Teach patient self-administration of these medications at home. Monitor serum electrolytes (magnesium, calcium) prior to each dose, and replete magnesium as needed. Teach patient dietary modifications to address symptoms such as anorexia (small, frequent high-calorie, high-protein foods, stimulants as permitted by protocol); constipation (high-fiber, high-fluid, high-roughage foods, stool softeners); diarrhea (bananas, rice, applesauce, and toast); nausea (avoid food preparation odors by cooking in zipped plastic bag, or having someone else cook; choose cool, soft, non-spicy, or fatty foods). Teach patient to report any symptoms that do not resolve or improve on the plan. Assess efficacy of intervention, and revise plan as needed.

III. POTENTIAL FOR ALTERATION IN COMFORT related to FATIGUE, DYSPNEA, PERIPHERAL EDEMA, PYREXIA, ARTHRALGIA

Defining Characteristics: In clinical trials, the following symptoms were reported in patients with advanced colorectal cancer: fatigue (51%), cough (18%), dyspnea (14%), peripheral edema (14%), pyrexia (14%), arthralgia (14%), back pain (12%), headache (12%), dizziness (11%), insomnia (11%).

Nursing Implications: Assess patient comfort level, self-care measures baseline and periodically during therapy. Teach patient that these symptoms may arise, either from the drug and/or the treatment. Develop a plan for symptom management, assess efficacy and revise as needed. Assess level of fatigue and teach energy baseline and prior to each treatment. Inform patient that fatigue may occur due to anemia, and teach energy conserving strategies such as alternating rest and activity periods.

IV. ALTERATION IN ELECTROLYTE BALANCE related to HYPOMAGNESEMIA, POTENTIAL

Defining Characteristics: Magnesium wasting appears related to EGFR inhibition in the renal tubular epithelial cells so that excreted magnesium is not resorbed in the distal convoluted tubules. This leads to initial magnesium wasting, followed by losses of calcium and potassium. Hypomagnesemia occurs in about 38% of patients receiving the drug and is severe in 2–4% of patients. It begins within days to months of receiving the drug, and there is much interpatient variability. There appears to be a direct relationship between duration of EGFRI MAb treatment and severe hypomagnesemia (Fakih, 2007). Symptoms of grade 3/4 hypomagnesemia include fatigue, cramps, and somnolence.

Nursing Implications: Assess baseline electrolyte balance prior to initial treatment and prior to each successive weekly treatments. Grade of hypomagnesemia: Grade 1 is a serum level of < LLN-1.2 mg/dL, grade 2 is 0.9–1.2 mg/dL. Grade 3 is 0.7–0.9 mg/dL, and grade 4 is ≤ 0.7 mg/dL. Replete magnesium, calcium, and potassium as needed. Oral magnesium may be ineffective and may result in diarrhea (Tejpar et al, 2007). Magnesium repletion regimens include weekly IV replacement of 4-g magnesium sulfate for grade 2. For grade 3/4, patients may be symptomatic and magnesium replacement may involve once to twice weekly IV infusions of 6–10 grams. Provide support for patients as magnesium replacement infusions require lengthy time in clinic, as an 8-gram infusion requires 4 hours. Post-IV replacement with every other day serum magnesium monitoring is important until the patient develops a steady state (Fakih, 2007). Continue to monitor after drug has been discontinued (half-life of the drug and time drug persists, e.g., 8 weeks). Magnesium replacement in IV hydration starting when a patient has grade 1 hypomagnesemia may be effective in preventing worsening hypomagnesemia. For patients who have refractory grade 4 hypomagnesemia, a stop-and-go approach has been effective where EGFRI MAb is held for 4–8 weeks until the magnesium corrects; it is reported that grade 4 hypomagnesemia does not recur when cetuximab is then reintroduced (Fakih, 2007).

Drug: pertuzumab (Omnitarg, rhuMab 2C4)

Class: First of a new class called Human Epidermal (Growth Factor) Receptor dimerization inhibitors (HDI). Multiple targeted Tyrosine kinase inhibitor blocking multiple HER-mediated pathways, anti-angiogenesis agent.

Mechanism of Action: In order for a growth signal to be sent to the cell nucleus, a growth factor (ligand) attaches to the Human Epidermal Growth Factor Receptor, or HER. The growth factor receptor now needs to dimerize or pair with another growth factor receptor to activate the receptor tyrosine kinase; for example, HER-2 receptor needs to dimerize or pair with another HER receptor, such as HER-1. Pertuzumab is an IgG1 monoclonal antibody that binds to the dimerization domain of HER so the binding of the antibody directly inhibits the ability of HER-2 to dimerize with other HER (EGFR) proteins. This disrupts the activation of downstream effectors so that the growth signal is not sent, notably the AKT pathway (cell survival). Drug is a recombinant, humanized monoclonal antibody.

Metabolism: Unknown.

Dosage/Range: Per protocol; studies have included doses 0.5–15 mg/kg every 3 weeks.

Drug Preparation: Per protocol; IV infusion.

Drug Interactions: Unknown.

Lab Effects/Interference: Unknown.

Special Considerations:
- Drug is being investigated in prostate, NSCLC, metastatic breast, ovarian cancers, but may need to be given with chemotherapy to improve response.
- Drug is targeted against tumors that do not over-express HER-2.
- Side effects varied according to patient population with diarrhea and rash most common in prostate cancer patients studied, and diarrhea, fatigue, nausea, vomiting, and uncommon drop in LVEF in patients with metastatic breast cancer who previously had received anthracyclines (Cortes et al, 2005).
- Currently being studied in a phase III CLEOPATRA study.

Potential Toxicities/Side Effects and the Nursing Process

I. POTENTIAL ALTERATION IN NUTRITION related to DIARRHEA, NAUSEA, VOMITING

Defining Characteristics: Diarrhea was most common, affecting about 50–59% of patients, and ranging in severity from grade 1–3; nausea and vomiting affected patients with metastatic breast cancer, affecting 32% and 23% of women, respectively.

Nursing Implications: Assess bowel elimination patterns and nutritional status baseline prior to each treatment. Teach patient to take antidiarrheal medication per protocol. Administer anti-emetics prior to drug administration per protocol, and teach patient to self-administer anti-emetics as permitted on protocol. Teach patient to report any symptoms that do not resolve or improve with the established plan.

II. ACTIVITY INTOLERANCE, POTENTIAL, related to FATIGUE

Defining Characteristics: Fatigue occurs commonly in patients with advanced cancer who were studied.

Nursing Implications: Assess baseline activity and energy level, and teach patient that this symptom may occur. Assess patient's activity patterns, and suggest ways to conserve energy.

Drug: quadrivalent human papillomavirus (HPV) (Types 6, 11, 16, 18) recombinant vaccine (Gardasil)

Class: Vaccine.

Mechanism of Action: Appears to be mediated by the development of humoral immune responses.

Metabolism: Vaccine is prepared from highly purified virus like particles (VLP) of the major capsid protein of HPV types 6, 11, 16, 18. The vaccine is a sterile liquid suspension prepared by combining the adsorbed VLPs of each HPV type and additional amounts of aluminum containing adjuvant and buffer.

Dosage/Range:
- 0.5 mL of vaccine administered.
- 1st dose at elected date.
- 2nd dose 2 months after the 1st dose.
- 3rd dose 6 months after the 1st dose.

Drug Preparation:
- Drug is available as single dose vials (1 or 10 vial cartons, each containing 0.5 mL single dose vials) or pre-filled syringes (cartons of 1 or 6 prefilled 0.5 mL single dose syringes). Drug should be stored at 2–8°C (36–46°F); do not freeze and protect from light. Thoroughly shake or agitate vaccine well before use to maintain suspension of vaccine. Vaccine is a white, cloudy liquid. Draw up 0.5 mL dose from the single use vial or place included luer needle on prefilled syringe.
- Vaccine is administered IM into the deltoid muscle of the upper arm or in the higher anterolateral area of the thigh, as 3 separate 0.5 mL doses using standard IM injection protocol. Administer entire dose. Activate needle guard device. If using prefilled syringe, depress plunger while grasping the finger lance until the entire dose has been given. Remove needle from patient, release plunger, and allow syringe to move up until the entire needle is guarded. Remove detachable label and use in documentation of vaccination. Discard guarded syringe in an approved sharps container.

Drug Interactions: Immunosuppressants of any type (e.g., corticosteroids, chemotherapy) may reduce immune responses to vaccine.

Lab Effects/Interference: Unknown.

Special Considerations:
- Indicated for the vaccination of females aged 9–26 years of age for the prevention of the following diseases caused by HPV 6, 11, 16, 18: cervical cancer, genital warts

(condyloma acuminate), cervical adenocarcinoma in situ (AIS), cervical intraepithelial neoplasia (CIN) grades 2 and 3, vulvar intraepithelial neoplasia (VIN) grades 2 and 3, vaginal intraepithelial neoplasia (VaIN) grade 2 and 3, and cervical intraepithelial neoplasia (CIN) grade 1.

- Contraindicated in patients hypersensitive to any of the excipients of the drug.
- Drug does not protect against diseases not caused by HPV or to non-vaccine HPV types.
- As with any drug or vaccine, be prepared for rare anaphylaxis.
- Individuals with impaired immune responsiveness may have reduced antibody response to active immunization.
- Drug may be co-administered (at separate injection sites) with hepatitis B vaccine (recombinant), but co-administration with other vaccines has not been done.
- Safety and efficacy in individuals < 9 years or older than 26 years have not been studied.
- Drug is effective in reducing the incidence of CIN (any grade), AIS, genital warts, VIN (any grade), and VaIN (any grade) in women who were seronegative and PCR negative at baseline. Drug is 100% effective in preventing HPV 16/18 related disease for CIN3 or AIS, VIN 2/3, and VaIN 2/3. Efficacy against HPV 6, 11, 16, 18-related VIN 1 or VaIN 1 was 100%.

Potential Toxicities/Side Effects and the Nursing Process

I. ALTERATION IN COMFORT related to INJECTION SITE DISCOMFORT, FEVER

Defining Characteristics: Of the patients experiencing injection site reactions, 94% said the reaction was mild or moderate in intensity. Pain occurred in 84% (saline placebo 49%), swelling 25% (saline placebo 7%), erythema 25% (saline placebo 12%), and itching 3% (1%) within 1–5 days of the vaccination, largely due to aluminum in the preparation. Fever occurred in 10% of patients receiving the vaccine, compared to 9% receiving placebo.

Nursing Implications: Teach patient that this may occur, and local strategies to minimize this, such as distraction, warm compresses.

Drug: rituximab (Rituxan)

Class: Monoclonal antibody (anti-CD_{20} antibody).

Mechanism of Action: Anti-CD_{20} antibody that is genetically engineered (chimeric monoclonal antibody, or part mouse part human) directed against the CD_{20} antigen found on the surface of normal and malignant B-cell lymphocytes. The CD_{20} antigen is also present (expressed) on more than 90% of B-cell non-Hodgkin's lymphoma (NHL) cells, but fortunately is not found on normal bone marrow stem cells, pre-B cells, normal plasma cells, or other normal tissues. A section of the rituximab (Fab domain) CD_{20} binds to the CD_{20} antigen on B lymphocytes; another section of the rituximab (Fc domain) calls together other immune effectors, resulting in lysis of the B lymphocyte.

Metabolism: Serum and half-life of drug varies with dose and sequence, and at 375 mg/m^2, the median serum half-life was 76.3 hours after the first infusion, as compared to 205 hours after the fourth infusion. Drug was detected in patient serum up to 3–6 months after completion of treatment.

Dosage/Range: Relapsed or refractory, low grade or follicular, CD_{20} positive, B-cell NHL.

- 375 mg/m^2 given as IV infusion weekly for 4 weeks or 8 doses.
- Retreatment: 375 mg/m^2 once weekly for 4 doses in responding patients who develop progressive disease after previous rituximab therapy.

Diffuse Large B-cell NHL in combination with CHOP chemotherapy.

- 375 mg/m^2 IV day 1 of each cycle of CHOP chemotherapy for up to 8 infusions.

Previously untreated, low-grade, CD20-positive, B-cell NHL.

- The recommended dose of Rituxan in patients who have not progressed following 6–8 cycles of CVP chemotherapy is 375 mg/m^2 IV infusion, once weekly for 4 doses every 6 months for up to 16 doses.

Rheumatoid Arthritis in combination with methotrexate.

- 1000 mg **(NOT per meter squared)** IV q 2 weeks × a total of 2 treatments; administer glucocorticoids (Methylprednisolone 100 mg IV or equivalent) 30 minutes prior to each infusion to reduce incidence and severity of infusion reactions.

As a component of Zevalin (Ibritumomab Tiuxetan) Therapeutic regimen.

- Rituximab 250 mg/m^2 IV within 4 hours prior to the administration of Indium-111 (In-111) Zevalin, and within 4 hours prior to the administration of Yttrium-90 (Y-90) Zevalin.
- Rituximab and In-111-Zevalin administration should precede rituximab and Y-90-Zevalin by 7–9 days.

Drug Preparation:

- Do not mix with or dilute with other drugs.
- Store at 2–8°C (36–46°F) and protect vials from direct sunlight.
- Available as 100-mg (10-mL) and 500-mg (50-mL) single-use preservative-free vials.
- Add ordered dose to 0.9% sodium chloride USP or 5% dextrose, resulting in a final concentration of 1–4 mg/mL; gently invert to mix, and inspect for presence of any particulate matter or discoloration.
- Drug is stable in infusion solution at 2–8°C (36–46°F) for 24 hours, and at room temperature for another 24 hours.
- DO NOT GIVE AS AN INTRAVENOUS PUSH OR BOLUS.
- First infusion: initial infusion rate should be 50 mg/hr; if no infusion-related problems occur, increase the infusion rate in 50 mg/hr increments every 30 minutes to

a maximum of 400 mg/hr. If infusion reaction occurs, slow or stop the infusion depending on severity. May continue the infusion at half the previous rate once symptoms resolve.

- Second, third, fourth infusions: If the patient tolerated the first infusion well, administer at initial rate of 100 mg/hr, and increase by 100 mg/hr increments every 30 minutes, to a maximum of 400 mg/hr as tolerated.
- Fatal infusion reactions have rarely occurred within 24 hours of rituximab dose, characterized by hypoxemia, pulmonary infiltrates, ARDS, MI, VF, and shock.
- Drug has been associated with progressive leukoencephalopathy when used off-label in the treatment of patients with SLE.

Drug Interactions:

- There have been no formal drug interaction studies performed with rituximab. However, renal toxicity was seen with this drug in combination with Cisplatin in clinical trials.

Lab Effects/Interference:

- Decreased lymphocyte count (B cells); decreased IgM and IgG serum levels.

Special Considerations:

- Drug is indicated for the treatment of patients with (1) low-grade or follicular, CD_{20}-positive, B-cell non-Hodgkin's lymphoma who have relapsed or who are refractory to standard therapy, (2) as initial (1st line) therapy for diffuse, large B-cell CD_{20}-positive, NHL (DLBCL) in combination with CHOP or other anthracycline-based chemotherapy regimens, (3) low-grade, CD_{20}-positive, NHL in patients with stable disease or who achieve a partial or complete response after first-line therapy with CVP chemotherapy, (4) first-line treatment of follicular, CD_{20}-positive, NHL in combination with CVP chemotherapy.
- Drug is indicated for treatment of moderate to severe rheumatoid arthritis in combination with methotrexate, in patients who have had an inadequate response to one or more TNF antagonist therapies, in order to reduce signs and symptoms of RA.
- US Pharmacopeia-Drug Information off-label use in chronic lymphocytic leukemia (CLL), in combination with fludarabine, and with fludarabine and cyclophosphamide in the 1st line treatment of CLL.
- Severe mucocutaneous reactions may occur, resulting in death. Drug should be stopped if a reaction develops and a skin biopsy performed.
- Infusion reactions are common (fever, chills) during the first infusion. Hypotension, bronchospasm, and angioedema may occur. STOP infusion for severe reactions, and manage symptoms with diphenhydramine and acetaminophen, and additional treatment with bronchodilators, epinephrine, or IV saline as indicated. Infusion may be resumed at 50% of the previous rate once symptoms have resolved.
- Emergency medications should be readily available: epinephrine, antihistamines, and corticosteroids.

- STOP infusion if serious cardiac arrhythmias develop; patient should receive cardiac monitoring during and after subsequent infusions of the drug. Patients with a history of arrhythmias and angina should be cardiac monitored during infusion and immediately post-infusion for evidence of recurrence of these problems.
- Monitor CBC, platelet count regularly during therapy.
- In clinical studies of patients with low-grade or follicular NHL receiving single-agent Rituxan, human antichimeric antibody (HACA) was detected in 4 of 356 (1.1%) patients, and 3 had an objective clinical response.
- Birth control practices during and for 12 months following therapy should be used by individuals of childbearing potential.
- Women should not breast-feed infants while drug is detectable in the serum.
- Reversible posterior leukoencephalopathy syndrome after rituximab infusion has been reported in a patient receiving the drug off-label (Mavragani et al, 2004).

Potential Toxicities/Side Effects and the Nursing Process

I. POTENTIAL FOR INJURY related to INFUSION-RELATED REACTIONS

Defining Characteristics: Infusion-related reactions occurred within 30 minutes to 2 hours of the beginning of the first infusion. Fever and chills/rigors affect most patients during the initial infusion. Other infusion-related symptoms include: nausea; urticaria; fatigue; headache; pruritus; bronchospasm; dyspnea; sensation of swelling of tongue, throat; hypotension; flushing; and pain at disease site. Infusion-related reactions generally resolve with slowing or interrupting the drug infusion, and/or symptomatic treatment (IV saline, acetaminophen, diphenhydramine). Premedications often reduce the severity and/or occurrence of these reactions. In patients who receive retreatment after having completed at least one course of drug therapy, reactions that were reported include: fever, chills, asthenia, pruritus, and infusion-related events (fever, chills, pain, and throat irritation). The incidence of abdominal pain, anemia, dyspnea, hypotension, and neutropenia is higher in patients with bulky tumors > 10 cm.

Nursing Implications: Discuss with physician the use of premedications such as acetaminophen and an antihistamine before drug therapy. Ensure that medications necessary for the management of **severe infusion reactions** are readily available (e.g., epinephrine, antihistamines, corticosteroids). Assess baseline VS and monitor frequently during the infusion. Follow infusion rate guide (see Drug Administration section) for first and subsequent infusions. Slow or stop the infusion if severe infusion-related reactions occur. Monitor VS, and notify physician. Be prepared to provide emergency support as necessary (including IV saline, epinephrine, antihistamines, bronchodilators). If/when symptoms resolve, resume the infusion at 50% of the rate of the previous infusion, as directed by the physician.

II. ALTERATION IN ELIMINATION, RENAL, related to TUMOR LYSIS SYNDROME

Defining Characteristics: Patients with high tumor burden receiving rituximab for the first time are at risk for rapid tumor lysis. Tumor lysis syndrome (TLS) occurs as a result of rapid release of intracellular contents into the bloodstream. The risk of TLS appears higher in patients with a high number of circulating lymphocytes, e.g., > 25,000/mm^3.

Nursing Implications: For first infusion, expect patient orders to include: Hydration at 150 mL/hr with or without alkalinization, oral allopurinol, strict monitoring of I/O, daily weight and body balance determination. Monitor baseline and daily BUN, creatinine, K+, phosphorus, uric acid, and calcium. Monitor for renal, cardiac, neuromuscular signs/symptoms hyperkalemia, hyperphosphatemia, hypomagnesemia, hypocalcemia, and elevated uric acid.

III. POTENTIAL FOR INFECTION related to LYMPHOPENIA AND BONE MARROW DEPRESSION

Defining Characteristics: B-cell lymphocytes are reduced in 70–80% of patients, together with a decrease in immunoglobulins in some patients. Bacterial infections that occurred in these patients were not associated with neutropenia, and 9% were severe, involving sepsis due to *Listeria, Staphylococcus*, and polymicrobials; post-treatment infections included rare sepsis, and viral infections (herpes simplex and herpes zoster). Leukopenia occurs in 11% of patients, thrombocytopenia 8%, and neutropenia 7%. Serious bone marrow suppression was uncommon and may occur up to 30 days following treatment. These include severe neutropenia, thrombocytopenia, and severe anemia. Rarely, transient aplastic anemia or hemolytic anemia may occur. Incidence of neutropenia, anemia, and abdominal pain was higher, as was the severity, in patients with bulky tumors > 10 cm.

Nursing Implications: Monitor CBC, platelets baseline and regularly during treatment. If the patient develops cytopenia, monitor more frequently. Assess for signs/symptoms of infection, bleeding, fatigue, and chest pain prior to each treatment. Teach patient to self-assess for these, including taking temperature, and instruct to report them immediately. Transfuse red cells and platelets as ordered.

IV. LOSS OF SKIN INTEGRITY, POTENTIAL, related to SEVERE MUCOCUTANEOUS REACTIONS

Defining Characteristics: Severe skin reactions have rarely occurred and, in some cases, ended in death of patient. Skin abnormalities include paraneoplastic pemphigus (uncommon autoimmune disorder, may be related to underlying malignancy), Stevens-Johnson syndrome (may be caused by HSV or other infectious disorder), lichenoid dermatitis, vesiculobullous dermatitis, and toxic epidermal necrolysis. Onset is 1–13 weeks following rituximab exposure.

Nursing Implications: Assess baseline skin and mucous membrane integrity. Teach patient that rarely skin and mucous membrane reactions may occur, and to report any changes right away. Manufacturer recommends stopping rituximab therapy and obtaining skin biopsy to determine cause. Discuss with physician. Teach patient local care strategies depending upon symptoms.

V. ALTERATION IN COMFORT related to ASTHENIA, HEADACHE, NAUSEA, VOMITING, PRURITUS, MYALGIA, AND DIZZINESS

Defining Characteristics: From single-agent Rituxan studies for relapsed or refractory, low-grade or follicular NHL, the incidence of asthenia was 26%. Headache (19%), nausea (23%), pruritus (14%), vomiting (14%), myalgia (10%), and dizziness (10%) may also occur.

Nursing Implications: Assess baseline comfort prior to each infusion, and tolerance of past infusion. Discuss strategies to manage symptoms. If symptoms are severe, discuss management with physician.

Drug: sorafenib (Nexavar, BAY 43-9006)

Class: Multiple targeted Tyrosine kinase inhibitor, anti-angiogenesis agent.

Mechanism of Action: Drug inhibits a number of tyrosine kinases, including Raf kinase, an enzyme in the RAS pathway (RAS is mutated in about 20–30% of solid tumors), as well as receptor tyrosine kinases VEGFR-2 and PDGFR-β, thus preventing cell proliferation and angiogenesis. First, sorafenib inhibits the signaling cascade in the RAS pathway, blocking uncontrolled cell growth from either excessive stimulation of the RAS pathway, or through mutations of RAS and RAF proteins. In addition, sorafenib inhibits angiogenesis by preventing the message from Vascular Endothelial Growth Factor (VEGF), telling endothelial cells to proliferate and migrate, from reaching the cell nucleus (signal transduction) and angiogenesis is prevented. It also inhibits the message that would be sent to the cell nucleus when the ligand Platelet Derived Growth Factor (PDGF) attaches to its receptor PDGFR-β; PDGF is necessary for pericytes around the blood vessels to provide external structure during angiogenesis, and when they are not available, angiogenesis is stopped (Onyx, 2005).

Metabolism: After oral administration, mean relative bioavailability is 38–49%, peak plasma levels in 3 hours, and mean elimination half-life of 25–48 hours. Steady state plasma concentrations reached in 7 days with multiple doses. When drug is given with a high-fat meal, bioavailability is reduced 29% compared to that in a fasted state. Drug is highly protein bound (99.5%). Drug is metabolized by liver P450 microenzyme system, mediated by CYP3A4, with glucuronidation mediated by UGT1A9. There are 8 metabolites of the drug. Following oral dose, 96% of the drug was recovered in 14 days, with 77% of the dose excreted in the feces, and 19% in the urine. Japanese patients may have a 45% lower systemic exposure. Patients with mild to moderate hepatic dysfunction may have sorafinib AUC 23–65% lower than those with normal hepatic function.

Dosage/Range:

- 400 mg PO bid (total daily dose of 800 mg) taken 1 hour before or 2 hours after a meal, until patient is no longer clinically benefiting from drug or toxicity is unacceptable.
- When dose reduction is indicated, reduce to a single 400-mg PO dose daily; if further reduction needed, change to 400 mg PO every other day.
- Dose reduce for skin toxicity grade 2 without improvement (painful erythema and swelling of hands or feet and/or affecting ADLs) or grade 3 (moist desquamation, blistering, discomfort, cannot do ADLs or work).
- No dose reduction for renal dysfunction (mild, moderate, or severe not requiring dialysis).
- Hepatic dysfunction may reduce serum levels of sorafinib.

Drug Preparation:

- None, oral.
- Drug is available in 200 mg tablets.

Drug Interactions:

- CYP3A4 inhibitors (e.g., ketoconazole): none.
- CYP Isoform-selective substrates (e.g., midazolam, omeprazole, dextromethorphan): none.
- CYP2C9 substrates (e.g., warfarin): monitor INR regularly.
- CYP3A4 inducers (e.g., rifampin, St. John's wort, phenytoin, carbamazepine, Phenobarbital, dexamethasone): are expected to increase the metabolism of sorafenib and decrease sorafenib serum concentration. If they must be co-administered, consider an increase in sorafinib dose, and monitor closely for toxicity.
- Antineoplastic agents: 21% increase in doxorubicin area under the curve; 67–120% increase in irinotecan active metabolite SN-38 (UGT1A1 and UGT1A9 substrates), and 26–42% increase in irinotecan serum concentrations; increase in docetaxel AUC by 36–80%; increase (21–47%) or decrease (10%) in 5-FU AUC: do not give concomitantly or dose reduce, and monitor patient closely.
- CYP 2B6 and CYP 2C 8 substrates: sorafinib inhibits the metabolism of these substrates, thus increasing serum levels. Avoid concomitant administration.

Lab Effects/Interference:
- Increased lipase (41%), amylase (30%).
- Decreased phosphate (45%).
- Lymphopenia (23%), neutropenia (5%), anemia (44%), thrombocytopenia (12%).

Special Considerations:
- Indicated for the treatment of patients with advanced renal cell cancer, as well as patients with unresectable hepatocellular carcinoma.
- Drug is well tolerated with principal side effects being hypertension (11% vs 1% placebo), rash (34% vs 13%), hand-foot syndrome (27% vs 5%), and diarrhea (33% vs 10%).
- In patients with malignant melanoma, a specific RAS kinase, BRAF, is mutated in 66% of patients and some patients with colorectal cancer (Onyx Pharmaceuticals, 2005).
- Drug is teratogenic and embryo-fetal toxic. Women of childbearing age should be advised to avoid pregnancy, or if the patient becomes pregnant while receiving the drug, patient should be apprised of potential hazard to the fetus. Women should not breast-feed while receiving the drug.
- Peripheral sensory neuropathy occurs in 11% of patients.
- Drug should be temporarily interrupted prior to undergoing major surgical procedures, and resumed after the wound has healed.
- Drug may rarely cause gastrointestinal perforation. Patients should be taught to go to the ED immediately if they develop severe abdominal pain, with or without nausea, vomiting, or constipation, and the provider should be notified.
- Sorafinib has been shown to increase overall survival of patients with hepatocellular carcinoma by 44% (SHARP trial; Llovet et al, 2007).

Potential Toxicities/Side Effects and the Nursing Process

I. POTENTIAL ALTERATION IN CIRCULATION related to HYPERTENSION, CARDIAC ISCHEMIA, OR MYOCARDIAL INFARCTION

Defining Characteristics: Hypertension occurred in 17% of renal cell cancer patients being studied, compared to 2% receiving placebo. Rarely, hypertensive crisis, myocardial ischemia and/or infarction occurred. In the HCC group receiving sorafinib, the incidence of cardiac ischemia/infarction was 2.7% (1.3% in placebo group), and in the RCC group receiving sorafinib, the incidence was 2.9% (0.4% in placebo group).

Nursing Implications: Assess baseline blood pressure, and monitor weekly during the first 6 weeks of treatment. Discuss anti-hypertensive therapy with physician or NP. If hypertension is severe and refractory to maximal anti-hypertensive therapy, drug should be interrupted or discontinued. If a patient develops cardiac ischemia and/or infarction while receiving the drug, discuss drug interruption or discontinuance with the physician. If the patient has cardiac ischemia or has had an infarction, discuss the risks and benefits before beginning therapy.

II. ALTERATION IN SKIN INTEGRITY AND COMFORT related to HAND-FOOT SYNDROME, RASH, POTENTIAL

Defining Characteristics: Erythema is common. Rash or skin desquamation occurred in 40% of patients, and hand-foot syndrome (acral erythema) in 30% of patients compared to 16% and 7% of patients, respectively, receiving placebo. Hand-foot syndrome is generally grade 1–2, and appears during the first 6 weeks of treatment. Alopecia occurred in 27% of patients, pruritus in 19% and dry skin in 11%. Areas of hyperkeratosis may occur on the soles of the feet, forming calluses (Wood, 2006). Rarely, folliculitis, eczema, erythema multiforme occurs.

Nursing Implications: Assess baseline skin integrity, including soles of feet and palms of hands, and teach patient that these symptoms may occur. If the patient develops calluses on the feet, suggest applying topical exfoliating agents such as Kerasal (over the counter) or Keralac (prescription) on the calluses ONLY. Teach patient to self assess all skin areas, and to report rash, as well as redness, swelling, and/or pain anywhere, particularly the soles of feet and palms of hands. Teach patient to avoid activities that increase blood flow in the hands and feet, such as hot showers and baths, and to take tepid showers to reduce likelihood and severity of hand-foot syndrome. Teach patient to avoid constrictive clothing and repetitive movements that can irritate the opposing skin. Teach patient to use skin emollients to prevent skin from drying and cracking. Discuss dose modification with physician or NP if grade 2 (PAIN) or 3, as follows (per manufacturer):

Grade 1: numbness, dysesthesia, paresthesia, tingling, painless swelling, erythema, or discomfort of the hands or feet which does not disrupt ADLs; no change, use topical therapy for symptomatic relief.

Grade 2: painful erythema and swelling of the hands or feet and/or discomfort affecting ADLs: 1st occurrence, continue therapy and use local symptomatic treatment; if no improvement within 7 days, or 2nd or 3rd occurrence, interrupt therapy until grade 0–1, then resume with dose reduction by one dose level, either 400 mg daily or every other day; if 4th occurrence, discontinue drug.

Grade 3: moist desquamation, ulceration, blistering or severe pain of the hands or feet, or severe discomfort that causes the patient to be unable to work or do ADLs: 1st or 2nd occurrence, interrupt until toxicity resolves to grade 0–1; then decrease dose by one dose level (400 mg daily or every other day); 3rd occurrence: discontinue drug.

III. ALTERATION IN NUTRITION, LESS THAN BODY REQUIREMENTS, related to DIARRHEA, NAUSEA, ANOREXIA, VOMITING, CONSTIPATION

Defining Characteristics: Diarrhea occurs in 43% of patients, constipation 15%, nausea 23%, vomiting 16%, and anorexia 16%.

Nursing Implications: Assess nutrition status, bowel elimination status baseline and periodically during treatment. Involve nutritionist as needed to minimize symptoms, such as BRAT diet for patient with diarrhea (e.g., bananas, rice, applesauce, and toast); increase dose-dense calories and fluid in the diet, and strategies to increase appetite. Teach patient how to manage nausea, vomiting, diarrhea, and constipation, including self-administration of OTC medications or prescribed medications, dietary modifications, and increased hydration. Teach patient to report symptoms that do not improve or that persist despite interventions.

IV. ALTERATION IN CIRCULATION related to HEMORRHAGE, POTENTIAL

Defining Characteristics: Hemorrhage occurred in 15% of patients as compared to 8% in the placebo arm.

Nursing implications: Teach patient to report any episodes of bleeding right away. If bleeding requires medical intervention, discuss drug discontinuation with the physician.

V. POTENTIAL FOR INFECTION AND BLEEDING related to NEUTROPENIA AND THROMBOCYTOPENIA

Defining Characteristics: Neutropenia occurred in 5% of patients, anemia 44% of patients, and thrombocytopenia 12% of patients in clinical trials.

Nursing Implications: Assess baseline blood counts and platelets. Teach patient to report fever, and signs/symptoms of infection or bleeding right away. Assess medication profile and OTC medications taken. Teach patient to avoid OTC medications containing NSAIDs or aspirin. Teach patient to talk to nurse or physician before beginning any OTC medications.

Drug: sunitinib malate (Sutent, U-11248)

Class: Multi-targeted tyrosine kinase inhibitor.

Mechanism of Action: Drug has both anti-tumor and anti-angiogenesis activity, and inhibits multiple receptor tyrosine kinases which are involved in tumor growth, angiogenesis, and metastatic cancer progression. It inhibits platelet derived growth factor receptors (alpha and beta), vascular endothelial growth factor receptors (VEGFR-1, -2, -3), stem cell factor receptor (KIT), fms-like tyrosine kinase-3 (FLT-3), colony stimulating factor receptor Type 1 (CSF-1R), and the glial cell-line derived neurotrophic factor receptor (RET).

Metabolism: After oral ingestion, maximal plasma concentrations are reached within 6–12 hours, regardless of food intake. Drug and primary metabolite bind to plasma protein 90–95%. Drug is metabolized by the cytochrome P450 enzyme CYP3A4, to produce its primary metabolite, which is then itself metabolized by CYP3A4. Terminal half-life of sunitinib and its primary metabolite are 40–60 hours and 80–110 hours, respectively. Drug is primarily excreted via the feces.

Dosage/Range:

- 50 mg PO daily × 4 weeks, followed by 2 weeks off, in a 6-week cycle. Dose escalation or reduction in 12.5 mg increments.

Drug Preparation:

- None, oral tablet.
- Available as 12.5 mg (orange/orange), and 25 mg (caramel/orange) capsules.

Drug Interactions:

- CYP3A4 inhibitors: (e.g., ketoconazole, itraconazole, clarithromycin, atazanavir, indinavir, nefazodone, nelfinavir, ritonavir, saquinavir, telithromycin, voriconazole, grapefruit or grapefruit juice): increases plasma level of sunitinib; do not give together, or dose reduce sunitinib if used concurrently.
- CYP3A4 inducers: (e.g., rifampin, dexamethasone, phenytoin, carbamazepine, rifabutin, rifapentine, phenobarbital, St. John's wort): decreases plasma level of sunitinib by 23–46%; do not give together, or increase dose of sunitinib if given concurrently.

Lab Effects/Interference:

- Decreased lymphocyte (38%), neutrophil (53%), red blood cell (26%), and platelet counts (38%). Elevated serum lipase (25%) and amylase (17%).
- Elevated AST/ALT (39%), alkaline phosphatase (24%), total bilirubin (16%), indirect bilirubin (10%).
- Elevated serum creatinine (12%), uric acid (15%).
- Decreased phosphate (9%), increased or decreased potassium (6%, 12%), increased or decreased sodium (10%, 6%).
- Decreased thyroid function (acquired hypothyroidism).

Special Considerations:

- Drug is FDA approved for the treatment of gastrointestinal stromal tumor (GIST) after disease progression on imatinib mesylate, and advanced renal cell carcinoma (based on response rate and response duration).
- Drug is teratogenic and embryo-fetal toxic. Women of childbearing age should be advised to avoid pregnancy, or if the patient becomes pregnant while receiving the drug, patient should be apprised of potential hazard to the fetus. Women should not breast-feed while receiving the drug.
- Patient should have CBC with platelet count, serum chemistries, including phosphate and liver function tests at the beginning of each treatment cycle; check baseline thyroid function, as acquired hypothyroidism may occur.
- Drug may cause adrenal insufficiency, so patients who are experiencing stress (e.g., surgery, trauma, severe infection) should be monitored closely.

- Drug may cause bleeding, hypertension, and reduction of left ventricular ejection fraction with increased risk of CHF.
- Drug may prolong QTc interval (inhibit the cardiac action potential repolarization process in the heart).
- 2% of patients receiving sunitinib developed DVT.
- Patients with brain metastases receiving the drug may rarely develop seizures.
- Patients on sunitinib may rarely develop pancreatitis (1%); if this occurs, the drug should be discontinued.
- There are no randomized trials of sunitinib demonstrating clinical benefit such as increased survival or improvement in disease-related symptoms in renal cell carcinoma.

Potential Toxicities/Side Effects and the Nursing Process

I. ALTERATION IN CIRCULATION, POTENTIAL, related to LEFT VENTRICULAR DYSFUNCTION, HEMORRHAGE

Defining Characteristics: 15% of patients had a decrease in left ventricular ejection fraction (LVEF) to below the lower limit of normal (LLN). 18–26% of patients developed bleeding events: epistaxis was most common. Less commonly, patients experienced rectal, gingival, upper GI, genital, wound bleeding, and tumor hemorrhage (NSCLC, squamous histology). Rarely, patients on clinical trials had myocardial ischemia, and one patient experienced a fatal myocardial infarction while on treatment.

Nursing Implications: Assess baseline and periodic LVEF tests, as well as assess patients for any signs or symptoms of congestive heart failure. Discuss any abnormalities with physician or NP. Teach patient to report any signs or symptoms of dyspnea or bleeding right away. Teach patient that nosebleeds may occur, and to apply pressure and hold the head down. If nosebleed does not stop within 15 minutes, to go to ED and call physician.

II. POTENTIAL ALTERATION IN CIRCULATION related to HYPERTENSION

Defining Characteristics: Hypertension occurred in 15–28% of patients being studied, compared to 11% receiving placebo. Rarely, hypertensive crisis, myocardial ischemia and/or infarction occurred. Rarely on clinical trials, patients presented with seizures and radiological evidence of reversible posterior leukoencephalopathy syndrome RPLS (hypertension, headache, decreased alertness, altered mental functioning, and visual loss).

Nursing Implications: Assess baseline blood pressure, and monitor weekly during the first treatment cycle. Discuss anti-hypertensive therapy with physician or NP. If hypertension is severe (SBP > 200 mmHg, DBP > 100 mmHg), or refractory to maximal anti-hypertensive therapy, drug should be interrupted until BP controlled, or discontinued. If RPLS occurs, the drug should be interrupted.

III. ALTERATION IN SKIN INTEGRITY AND COMFORT related to SKIN DISCOLORATION, HAND-FOOT SYNDROME, RASH, DEPIGMENTATION OF HAIR

Defining Characteristics: Rash affected 14% of patients, skin discoloration (yellow color) 30%, and hand-foot syndrome 14%. Hair color changes occurred in 7% of patients: when on the drug for 4 weeks, the hair is depigmented (white), while pigment returns on the 2 week break off treatment, giving the hair a zebra appearance. Alopecia occurred in 5% of patients.

Nursing Implications: Assess baseline skin integrity, including soles of feet and palms of hands, and teach patient that these symptoms may occur. Teach patient to self-assess all skin areas, and to report rash, as well as redness, swelling, and/or pain anywhere, particularly the soles of feet and palms of hands. Teach patient to avoid activities that increase blood flow in the hands and feet, such as hot showers and baths, and to take tepid showers to reduce likelihood and severity of hand-foot syndrome. Teach patient to avoid constrictive clothing and repetitive movements that can irritate the opposing skin. Teach patient to use skin emollients to prevent skin from drying and cracking.

IV. ALTERATION IN BOWEL ELIMINATION STATUS related to DIARRHEA, CONSTIPATION

Defining Characteristics: Diarrhea occurs in 40% of patients, constipation 20%.

Nursing Implications: Assess bowel elimination status, baseline and periodically during treatment. Teach patient how to manage diarrhea including self-administration of OTC medications or prescribed medications, dietary modifications 572 (avoid spicy, fatty foods, caffeine, fruit), and increased hydration. Involve nutritionist as needed to minimize symptoms, such as BRAT diet for patient with diarrhea (e.g., bananas, rice, applesauce, and toast); increase dose-dense calories and fluid in the diet, and strategies to increase appetite. If patient develops constipation, teach self-care strategies to prevent it (stool softeners, increased fluids, fruits, and vegetables). Teach patient to report symptoms that do not improve or that persist despite treatment.

V. POTENTIAL FOR INFECTION AND BLEEDING related to NEUTROPENIA AND THROMBOCYTOPENIA

Defining Characteristics: Neutropenia occurred in 39–45% of patients, anemia 25–37% of patients, and thrombocytopenia 18–19% of patients in clinical trials.

Nursing Implications: Assess baseline blood counts and platelets. Teach patient to report fever, and signs/symptoms of infection or bleeding right away. Assess medication profile and OTC medications taken. Teach patient to avoid OTC medications containing NSAIDs or aspirin. Teach patient to talk to nurse or physician before beginning any OTC medications.

VI. ALTERATION IN NUTRITION, LESS THAN BODY REQUIREMENTS, related to NAUSEA, STOMATITIS

Defining Characteristics: Patients developed nausea (31%), vomiting (24%), stomatitis (29%), and anorexia (33%).

Nursing Implications: Assess nutritional status, integrity of oral mucosa baseline and periodically during treatment. Teach patient that these side effects may occur and to report them. Teach patient self-administration of antiemetics prior to administration of drug if nausea or vomiting has occurred. Teach patient other self-care strategies such as to eat small, frequent meals; avoid foods that are sweet, fried, or fatty; avoid bad smells; and drink small amounts of fluids frequently. Teach patient to report persistent or continued nausea and/or vomiting. Assess efficacy and discuss change in antiemetic drug with physician if regimen ineffective. Teach patient to assess oral mucosa regularly, use oral hygiene regimen such as sodium bicarbonate in water after meals and at bedtime, and report signs/symptoms of stomatitis. Teach patient diet modification to minimize oral discomfort, such as avoiding hot, spicy, or acidic foods; eating small pieces of cool or cold foods; using a straw for drinking liquids.

Drug: temsirolimus (Torisel, CCI-779)

Class: mTOR inhibitor.

Mechanism of Action: Drug binds to the intracellular protein FKBP-12, and the protein-drug complex inhibits mTOR (mammalian Target of Rapamycin or FKBP 12) kinase that is responsible for cell division. mTOR is also responsible for sensing the nutrients in the cell's environment and also for organizing actin, trafficking of the membrane, insulin secretion, protein degradation, protein kinase C signaling, and tRNA synthesis. Inhibition of the kinase makes the cell think it is starving and it stops growing (arrests cell growth in G_1 phase of the cell cycle). This reduces the levels of hypoxia-inducible factors (HIF) and VEGF. As more is learned about the function of this pathway, it appears that rapamycin and mTOR inhibitors affect only some of mTOR functioning.

Metabolism: The drug is metabolized by the P450 microenzyme system in the liver (CYP3A4) into five metabolites. Sirolimus is the active metabolite. Metabolites are primarily excreted in the feces (82% within 14 days). Mean half-lives of temsirolimus and sirolimus were 17.3 hours and 54.6 hours, respectively.

Dosage/Range:

- 25 mg IV over 30–60 minutes weekly until tumor progression or intolerable toxicity.
- Premedicate with 25- to 50-mg diphenhydramine 30 minutes before temsirolimus dose.
- Hold for ANC < 1000 cells/mm^3, platelet count < 75,000 cells/mm^3, or grade 3 or higher toxicity (NCI CTCAE).

Drug Interactions:

- Strong CYP3A4 inhibitors: decrease temsirolimus dose to 12.5 mg weekly; when interacting drug discontinued, allow a 1-week washout period, and then resume dose prior to giving interacting drug.
- Strong CYP3A4 inducers: increase temsirolimus dose to 50 mg weekly; when interacting drug is discontinued, resume dose before giving interacting drug.

Drug Preparation:

- Before preparation, store in the refrigerator at 2–8° C (36–46°F) and protect from light.
- During preparation, protect from excessive room light and sunlight. Inspect product for particulate matter and decolorization before administration.
- Step 1: Inject 1.8-mL diluent into vial that together with an overfill of 0.2 mL results in a 10-mg/mL solution. Withdraw 3 mL (including overfill).
- Invert vial to mix, and allow air bubbles to subside. This vial is stable for 24 hours at controlled room temperature.
- Step 2: Withdraw ordered drug amount from vial (prepared in step 1), and inject rapidly into a 250-mL container (glass, polyolefin, polyethylene) of 0.9% sodium chloride injection. Invert bag or bottle to mix but do not shake, as this will cause foaming.
- Drug must be used within 6 hours.

Drug Administration:

- Check CBC weekly, and chemistries every other week.
- Drug should be stored in bottles (glass, polypropylene) or plastic IV bags (polypropylene, polyolefin) and administer through a polyethylene-lined administration set with an in-line polyether sulfone filter with a pore size *less than* 5 microns.
- After premedication, administer IV over 30–60 minutes once a week via an infusion pump if possible.
- Do not use bags or tubing containerizing the plasticizer DEHP (di-2-ethylhexyl phthalate), which may leach from the PVC infusion bags or sets into IV solution and be administered into the patient.

Drug Interactions:

- Strong CYP3A4 inhibitors (e.g., ketoconazole, itraconazole, clarithromycin, atazanavir, indinavir, nefazodone, nelfinavir, ritonavir, saquinavir, telithromycin, voriconazole, grapefruit juice); do not coadminister.

- Strong CYP3A4 inducers (dexamethasone, phenytoin, carbamazepine, rifampin, rifabutin, rifapentine, phenobarbital, St. John's wort): do not coadminister.
- Sunitinib: dose-limiting toxicity when coadministered is grade 3/4 erythematous papular rash, gout/cellulites requiring hospitalization; use together at lower doses cautiously if at all.

Lab Effects/Interference:

- Hyperglycemia, hypertriglyceridemia, hypophosphatemia; elevated AST, alkaline phosphatase, and serum creatinine; decreased potassium.
- Neutropenia, thrombocytopenia, anemia, lymphopenia.

Special Considerations:

- Indicated for the treatment of advanced renal cell cancer.
- Use with caution if at all in patients with hypersensitivity to drug, sirolimus, or polysorbate 80.
- Warnings:
  - Bowel perforation occurred rarely and may be fatal. Teach patients to report worsening abdominal pain and bloody stools right away and to come to the emergency department for immediate evaluation.
  - Drug may cause interstitial lung disease, which may be fatal. Patient may be asymptomatic with ILD seen on CT or CXR, or patient may be symptomatic with dyspnea, cough, hypoxia, and fever. Stopping drug and treatment with corticosteroids and/or antibiotics was beneficial for some patients; others continued treatment or discontinued therapy. Teach patients to report new or worsening pulmonary symptoms.
  - Abnormal wound healing: ensure that wound is well healed before giving drug.
  - Hyperglycemia/glucose intolerance, infections, ILD, hyperlipidemia, renal failure, and intracerebral hemorrhage may occur rarely.
- Most common (> 30%) side effects are rash, asthenia, mucositis, nausea, edema, anorexia.
- Women should avoid becoming pregnant or breast-feeding while receiving the drug, and men should not father a child. Men with partners of childbearing potential should use reliable birth control throughout treatment and for 3 months after the last drug dose.
- Drug has shown anti-tumor activity in patients with advanced renal cell and advanced breast cancer. In the treatment of glioblastoma multiforme, the drug is called a "smart drug," because it targets molecular changes in the malignant cell related to its unfortunate aggressiveness (Galanis et al, 2005).
- Vaccinations may be less effective while receiving this drug, and live vaccines should be avoided.
- FDA approval based on significant improvement in overall survival in poor risk patients with advanced renal cell cancer who received daily temsirolimus (10.9 months) compared with interferon (7.3 months), $P = .0078$. Temsirolimus plus interferon actually resulted in increased toxicity without any survival benefit.

Potential Toxicities/Side Effects and the Nursing Process

I. POTENTIAL FOR INJURY related to INFUSION-RELATED REACTIONS AND HYPERSENSITIVITY

Defining Characteristics: The incidence of hypersensitivity is uncommon, as most patients received premedication with diphenhydramine (Chan et al, 2005).

Nursing Implications: Administer premedication with diphenhydramine. Stop the infusion right away if the patient has a reaction, monitor VS and O_2 saturation for at least 30–60 minutes depending on the severity of the reaction. Discuss the addition of an H_2 antagonist 30 minutes prior to resuming the infusion to prevent further hypersensitivity with physician. Ensure that medications necessary for the management of hypersensitivity/anaphylaxis are readily available (e.g., epinephrine, antihistamines, corticosteroids). Assess baseline VS and monitor frequently during the infusion, as specified by the infusion. Be prepared to provide emergency support as necessary (including IV saline, epinephrine, antihistamines, bronchodilators). If/when symptoms resolve, resume the infusion at 50% of the rate of the previous infusion, as directed by the physician.

II. POTENTIAL FOR INFECTION AND BLEEDING related to NEUTROPENIA AND THROMBOCYTOPENIA

Defining Characteristics: Incidence of decreased neutrophils was 19% (grade 3/4 5%), platelets 40% (1%), hemoglobin 94% (20%), and lymphocytes 53% (16%). Grade 3 or 4 neutropenia occurred in 7% of patients, thrombocytopenia in 5%, and anemia in 9% of patients in clinical trials comparing doses 75–250 mg weekly. Drug is immunosuppressive, and thus, patients are at risk for opportunistic infections.

Nursing Implications: Assess baseline blood counts and platelets. Teach patient to report fever, and signs/symptoms of infection or bleeding right away. Assess medication profile and OTC medications taken. Teach patient to avoid OTC medications containing NSAIDs or aspirin. Teach patient to talk to nurse or physician before beginning any OTC medications.

III. POTENTIAL ALTERATION IN NUTRITION, LESS THAN BODY REQUIREMENTS, related to MUCOSITIS, NAUSEA, ANOREXIA, DIARRHEA, HYPERGLYCEMIA, HYPERTRIGLYCERIDEMIA, BOWEL PERFORATION

Defining Characteristics: In clinical studies, mucositis affected 70% of patients, nausea 43%, diarrhea 27%, and anorexia 40% of patients. Bowel perforation occurs rarely but may be fatal. Presentation includes fever, abdominal pain, metabolic acidosis, bloody stools, diarrhea, and/or acute abdomen. The incidence of hypercholesteremia is 87%, triglyceridemia 83%, and hyperglycemia was 89%; in terms of grade 3 and 4 toxicities, hyperglycemia occurred in 17% of patients, hypophosphatemia 13%, and hypertriglyceridemia in 6% of patients. mTOR is involved in insulin signaling, which possibly explains the hypertriglyceridemia and hyperglycemia.

Nursing Implications: Assess serum triglycerides, cholesterol, glucose baseline and during treatment with the drug. Teach the patient to report any new or worsening abdominal pain or bloody stools right away and to come to the emergency department for immediate evaluation. Premedicate with antiemetics. Encourage small, frequent meals of cool, bland foods, and increase fluid intake. Assess oral mucosa prior to drug administration and instruct patient to report changes. Teach patient oral hygiene measures and self-assessment. Teach patient to notify physician/nurse if excessive thirst or any increase in volume or frequency of urination. Notify physician of any abnormalities and discuss implications and management.

IV. ALTERATION IN SKIN INTEGRITY, POTENTIAL, related to RASH

Defining Characteristics: Maculopapular rash is the most common toxicity, affecting 47%; 10% had acne, 14% had a nail disorder, 11% had dry skin, and 19% pruritus.

Nursing Implications: Assess patient skin integrity, including nails baseline and regularly during treatment. Teach patient self-assessment and local comfort measures, including the use of water-based emollients. Teach patient to report skin changes and if self-care ineffective, discuss plan with physician, especially if severe.

V. ALTERATION IN COMFORT AND ACTIVITY TOLERANCE, POTENTIAL, related to ASTHENIA

Defining Characteristics: Asthenia affects 51% of patients in clinical studies, depression 4%, but at the higher dose of 250 mg q week, 5% had grade 3 and 4 depression.

Nursing Implications: Assess baseline comfort, mental status, and activity tolerance, and reassess during treatment, asking patient to identify what activities now unable to do, sleep habits, and also feeling state. Discuss alternating rest and activity periods, and also possibility of other family members or friends assisting with energy consuming responsibilities to increase energy reserve. Assess baseline alertness, sleep patterns. Assess other drugs taken, especially those with sedating qualities, and alcohol ingestion. Instruct patient to avoid alcohol and to take drug at bedtime. Assess degree of drowsiness and dizziness for safety of patient. If significant, teach measures to ensure safety.

Drug: thalidomide (Thalomid)

Class: Inhibitor of TNF-alpha, antiangiogenesis agent.

Mechanism of Action: Drug has immunomodulatory, anti-inflammatory, and anti-angiogenic properties. Drug probably decreases TNF alpha production, and modifies some cell surface adhesion molecules involved in leukocyte migration. It is hypothesized that drug may modulate VEGF (vascular epithelial growth factor) by inhibiting neovasculature and thus have an antiangiogenesis effect in malignant tumors.

Metabolism: Well absorbed after oral administration. Mean peak serum level reached at 4–5 hours. Elimination half-life is 4–12 hours, with drug found in the plasma after 24 hours. NOT metabolized using P450 hepatic enzyme system, and has low renal excretion.

Dosage/Range:

- Multiple myeloma: in combination with dexamethasone in 28-day treatment cycles. Thalidomide 200 mg PO daily with water, preferably at bedtime, at least 1 hour after a meal. Give dexamethasone 40 mg PO days 1–4, 9–12, 17–20, every 28 days.
- Dose modification: if constipation, oversedation, or peripheral neuropathy, patient may benefit by either temporary discontinuation of the drug, or continuing at a lower dose and then readjusting once side effects abate.

Drug Preparation:

- Oral, give at bedtime.
- Available as 50-mg, 100-mg, 150-mg, and 200-mg capsules.

Drug Interactions:

- Barbiturates, alcohol, chlorpromazine, reserpine: increased sedation.

Lab Effects/Interference:

- Rare neutropenia.
- HIV mRNA levels may be increased (monitor levels after the first and third months of treatment and then every 3 months).

Special Considerations:

- Drug is indicated for the treatment of newly diagnosed multiple myeloma in combination with dexamethasone and for the treatment of patients with erythema nodosum leprosum (ENL) (acute treatment of moderate to severe cutaneous manifestations and maintenance and suppression of cutaneous recurrence).
- ABSOLUTE CONTRAINDICATION IS PREGNANCY. Pregnancy tests must be routinely negative prior to beginning therapy in women of childbearing age. Contraception is mandatory in men and women.
- Women taking hormonal contraception as well as any of the following drugs—barbiturates, glucocorticoids, phenytoin, carbamazepine—have decreased efficacy of the hormonal contraception and must use barrier contraception as well.
- Most common side effects are dry skin, occasional tingling of extremities, somnolence, fatigue, constipation, and neutropenia, followed by rash, peripheral neuropathy, lightheadedness, dizziness and edema. Uncommonly, severe rash, DVT, PE, URI and pneumonia, renal insufficiency, severe neutropenia and bradycardia may occur.

Potential Toxicities/Side Effects and the Nursing Process

I. ALTERATION IN SEXUALITY/REPRODUCTION related to POTENTIAL TERATOGENICITY

Defining Characteristics: Drug is teratogenic and a single dose can cause birth defects. Unclear if drug is excreted in semen.

Nursing Implications: Assess reproductive status, sexual activity, and birth control measures used for both men and women. Instruct male patients to use barrier contraception, and women to use both barrier and hormonal contraception. Women of childbearing age must have a negative pregnancy test baseline to begin the drug, and pregnancy test should be repeated every two weeks for two months, then every month. Instruct patient to continue contraception one month after drug is discontinued. Physicians, patients, and pharmacists must participate in drug manufacturer (Celgene, Warren, NJ) STEPS program (System for Thalidomide Education and Prescription Safety).

II. ALTERATION IN SENSORY/PERCEPTUAL PATTERNS related to PERIPHERAL NEUROPATHY

Defining Characteristics: Peripheral neuropathy occurs in about 25% of patients (range, 10–50%). If drug is discontinued at the first sign of neuropathy, symptoms are reversible. Neuropathy is a distal axonal degeneration affecting long and large-diameter motor and sensory axons in hands and feet. Initially, there is numbness of toes/feet, described often as a "tightness around the feet." There may be decreased sensitivity to light touch, pinprick (sensory loss) in hands and feet, muscle cramps, symmetrical sensorimotor neuropathy, painful paresthesias in hands and feet, distal hypoesthesia, proximal weakness in lower limbs, slight postural tremor, leg cramps, absent ankle jerks. If treatment is continued, there is permanent paresthesias of feet and hands, which progresses proximally. Increased risk of occurrence with increased age (> 70 years old) and high total doses > 14 g (40–50 g).

Nursing Implications: Assess baseline neurologic status, especially presence of peripheral neuropathy. Teach patient to stop drug and report immediately dysesthesias, numbness, and/or muscle cramps. Perform assessment for peripheral neuropathy at every visit.

III. ALTERATION IN SENSORY/PERCEPTUAL PATTERNS related to DROWSINESS

Defining Characteristics: Drug has nonbarbiturate sedative qualities, and drowsiness is the most frequent side effect. Tolerance to daytime drowsiness occurs over several weeks of use. Drowsiness and dizziness are more frequent at doses of 20–400 mg/day than at lower doses. HIV-infected patient studies reported drowsiness, dizziness, and mood changes 33–100% of the time.

Nursing Implications: Assess baseline alertness, sleep patterns. Assess other drugs taken, especially those with sedating qualities, and alcohol ingestion. Instruct patient to avoid alcohol and to take drug at bedtime. Assess degree of drowsiness and dizziness and safety of patient. If significant, teach measures to ensure safety. Tell patient that tolerance develops over 2–3 weeks.

IV. ALTERATION IN SKIN INTEGRITY, POTENTIAL, related to RASH

Defining Characteristics: Pruritic, erythematous macular rash may appear over trunk and back 2–13 days after initiation of therapy. Increased incidence in patients with HIV infection with low CD4 counts. Drug rechallenge often results in immediate reaction of rash, tachycardia, and fever. Rash resolves with drug discontinuation.

Nursing Implications: Teach patient to self-assess for rash, and instruct to discontinue drug and report rash to nurse or physician immediately. If necessary, manage symptomatic itching with antihistamines.

V. ALTERATION IN ELIMINATION related to CONSTIPATION

Defining Characteristics: Mild constipation occurs in 3–30% of patients.

Nursing Implications: Instruct patient to prevent constipation by using stool softeners, mild laxatives if needed (e.g., milk of magnesia), and to use bulk (e.g., psyllium). In addition, teach dietary interventions (e.g., increased fiber, fluids of 3 quarts/day), and mild exercise. Instruct patient to report constipation unresponsive to these interventions.

VI. POTENTIAL FOR INFECTION related to NEUTROPENIA

Defining Characteristics: Rare (< 1%) in most patients, but increased incidence of 2–20% in HIV-infected patients. Average onset 6–7 weeks after initiation of treatment (range, 3–12 weeks).

Nursing Implications: Determine baseline WBC and absolute neutrophil count (ANC). Do not initiate therapy if ANC < 750/mm^3. If on treatment, ANC < 750/mm^3, consider drug discontinuance, but drug definitely should be discontinued if ANC < 500/mm^3. Drug may be reinstituted after neutrophil recovery (e.g., G-CSF). WBC and ANC should be monitored closely in HIV-infected patients (e.g., every other week for three months), and then at least every month. If non-HIV-infected patients, monitor baseline and monthly.

Drug: tipifarnib (R115777, Zarnestra)

Class: Farnesyl transferase inhibitor.

Mechanism of Action: Inhibits farnesyl transferase, which activates a cell growth promoting a gene called Ras. Ras acts like a "switch," that, when turned on, allows growth signals from outside to be passed along to other pathways to reach the cell nucleus, resulting in uncontrolled cell division. It is estimated that 30% of all cancers have a mutated form of the Ras protein, permitting uncontrolled cell growth. Tipifarnib blocks the action of farnesyl transferase, theoretically stopping uncontrolled cell division. As it has effect in tumors that do not have a mutation in the ras gene, it appears to interrupt other signaling pathways involved in cell survival and growth as well.

Metabolism: P450 microenzyme system involved in the drug's metabolism, CYP3A4 and CYP3A5, as well as UDP glucuronosyltransferase isoenzyme UGT1A1. Peak plasma concentration reached after 2 hours.

Dosage/Range:
- Per clinical trial protocol. Acute myelocytic leukemia (aged 65+ with newly diagnosed AML): 300–600 mg PO bid × 3 weeks, 1–3 weeks of recovery.

Drug Preparation:
- None, oral.

Drug Interactions:
- Unknown.

Lab Effects/Interference:
- Decreased white blood cell, red blood cell, and platelet count.
- Hypokalemia.
- Rare increased LFTs.

Special Considerations:
- Being studied in AML, multiple myeloma, CML, breast cancer, glioma, and myelodysplastic syndrome.
- Phase II trial of newly diagnosed patients aged 65+ with AML presented at ASH 2004: Overall response rate 34%, CR 18%, mean duration of CR 6.4 months (Lancet et al, 2004); appears 3 gene sequence predicts response (Raponi et al, 2004).
- Contraindicated in patients with CHF, unstable angina, cardiac arrhythmias, psychiatric problems, allergies to imidazoles, and active infections.

Potential Toxicities/Side Effects and the Nursing Process

I. POTENTIAL FOR BLEEDING AND FATIGUE related to BONE MARROW DEPRESSION

Defining Characteristics: In clinical trials, the following occurred: bone marrow depression 78%, fatigue 54%.

Nursing Implications: Monitor CBC, platelet count baseline and periodically during therapy per protocol. Assess for signs and symptoms of bleeding, fatigue, and anemia. Teach patient to self-assess for signs and symptoms of bleeding, anemia, and to call if they occur. Assess patient medication profile, and any OTC medications such as those containing aspirin or NSAIDs that would increase risk of bleeding. Instruct patient to avoid these drugs, and not to begin any OTC medications without first discussing with nurse or physician. Teach patient to alternate rest and activity periods if feeling fatigued and to organize shopping and chores in a way to minimize energy expenditures.

II. ALTERATION IN NUTRITION, LESS THAN BODY REQUIREMENTS, related to NAUSEA, DIARRHEA, ANOREXIA, DEHYDRATION, HYPOKALEMIA, AND RARE HEPATOTOXICITY

Defining Characteristics: In clinical trials, nausea occurred in 61% of patients, anorexia 21%, diarrhea 32%, hypokalemia 9%, and hepatotoxicity 5%.

Nursing Implications: Assess weight, bowel elimination status, baseline nutritional status, as well as serum electrolytes and LFTs. Teach patient that nausea, anorexia, and diarrhea can occur; ways to minimize this effect, such as self-administration of anti-nausea and anti-diarrheal medications; and to report symptoms that do not resolve with established plan. Teach patient to identify nutritionally-dense (high calories and protein in the smallest amount) foods and to keep them handy in the refrigerator. Teach patient to eat small, frequent meals and to have a bedtime snack. Teach patient to drink a glass of fluid every hour while awake if patient is at risk for developing dehydration (elderly, forgetful). Monitor electrolytes and LFTs during treatment and discuss abnormalities with the physician.

III. ALTERATION IN SENSORY/PERCEPTUAL PATTERNS related to CENTRAL NEUROTOXICITY, NEUROPATHY, OPTIC NEURITIS

Defining Characteristics: Central neurotoxicity may occur, as well as neuropathy and optic neuritis.

Nursing Implications: Assess baseline neurologic status, especially presence of peripheral neuropathy. Teach patient to stop drug and report immediately dysesthesias, numbness, and/or muscle cramps. Perform assessment for peripheral neuropathy at every visit.

Drug: tositumomab, I^{131} tositumomab (Bexxar™)

Class: Radioimmunotherapeutic agent.

Mechanism of Action: Iodine-I^{131}-labeled anti-B1 murine monoclonal antibody directed against the CD_{20} B-lymphocyte antigen found on the surface of some normal lympho-cytes, and lymphocytes in non-Hodgkin's lymphoma (NHL). The agent contains two parts: an IgG_2 murine (mouse) monoclonal antibody directed against the CD_{20} surface antigen, and antibody labeled with iodine-131. The antibody attaches to the CD_{20} surface antigen on the lymphocytes, directly killing the cells by inducing apoptosis, and mediating antibody-dependent cell killing, plus delivering ionizing radiation directly to the cell. Radiation is delivered directly to the tumor cells, as well as some normal cells with CD_{20} antigens.

Metabolism: The median clearance of tositumomab (the monoclonal antibody) is about 68.2 mg/hr but clearance rate increases in patients with a higher tumor burden. Patient specific dosing is based on total body clearance. Radioactive I-131 decays and is excreted in the urine, with 67% of the injected dose excreted after 5 days. At 7 weeks after the therapeutic dose, the median number of circulating CD_{20} positive lymphocytes was zero, and lymphocyte recovery began about 12 weeks after treatment.

Dosage/Range:
- Total body dose of 65–75 cGy based on platelet count.

Drug Preparation:
- See package insert for preparation and radioactivity calibration.

Drug Administration:
- Regimen consists of 4 components administered in 2 steps using the same IV tubing set with in-line 0.22 micron filter throughout the entire dosimetric or therapeutic step. Otherwise, changing the filter can result in loss of drug:
  - **Day 1: At least 24 hours prior to dosimetric dose:**
    - Start saturated solution of potassium iodide (SSKI) 4 drops PO tid, Lugol's solution 20 drops PO tid, or potassium iodide tablets 130 mg PO daily; and continue until 2 weeks after administration of the I-131 tositumomab therapeutic dose.
    - Patient must receive at least 3 doses of SSKI, or 3 doses of Lugol's solution, or 1 dose of potassium iodide 24 hours prior to day 0. Refer to *Workbook for Dosimetry Methodology and Administration* set-up for configuration of tubing using a 3-way stopcock, and shielding.
  - **Day 0: Dosimetric dose**
    - Premedicate patient with acetaminophen 650 mg PO and diphenhydramine 50 mg PO 30 minutes prior to initial tositumomab.
    - Tositumomab 450 mg in 50 mL 0.9% sodium chloride IV infusion over 60 min. Then give iodine I-131 (containing 5.0 mCi I-131 and 35 mg tositumomab) in 30 mL 0.9% sodium chloride IV over 20 min. During either infusion: reduce infusion rate by 50% for mild to moderate infusional reactions; stop if reactions severe. After complete resolution of severe symptoms, resume infusion at 50% slower rate.
    - Post-infusion gamma camera scan is done to determine whole body counts, and then this is repeated over the next week. The whole body counts are used to determine the therapeutic dose.

- **Day 7–14: Therapeutic dose** (about 1–2 weeks after dosimetric dose):
  - Premedicate patient with acetaminophen 650 mg PO and diphenhydramine 50 mg PO 30 minutes prior to initial tositumomab.
  - Tositumomab 450 mg in 50 mL 0.9% sodium chloride IV over 60 min. Then give calculated I-131 tositumomab IV over 20 min. During either infusion: reduce infusion rate by 50% for mild to moderate infusional reactions; stop if reactions severe. After complete resolution of severe symptoms, resume infusion at 50% slower rate.
  - Dosing: patients with platelet count $\geq$ 150,000/mm^3: dose is activity of I-131 calculated to deliver 75 cGy total body irradiation and 35 mg tositumomab; patients with platelet count 100,000/mm^3 but $<$ 150,000/mm^3: dose is activity of I-131 that will deliver 65 cGy total body irradiation and 35 mg tositumomab.

Drug Interactions:
- Unknown.

Lab Effects/Interference:
- Bone marrow suppressive agents: further depression of red blood cells, white blood cells, and platelets.
- If human anti-murine antibodies (HAMA) develop: interference with accuracy and results of diagnostic tests relying on murine antibody technology may occur.

Special Considerations:
- Indicated for the treatment of patients with CD_{20} positive, follicular, non-Hodgkin's lymphoma, whose disease is refractory to rituximab and has relapsed following chemotherapy.
- In rituximab-resistant patients, 63% responded with a median duration of 25 months.
- Therapeutic regimen should be prescribed by a physician certified or in the process of being certified by Corixa Corporation in dose calculation and administration of BEXXAR.
- Bexxar should be administered only once.
- Contraindicated in patients with known hypersensitivity to murine (mouse) proteins, patients with > 25% lymphoma marrow involvement and/or impaired bone marrow reserve.
- Drug causes fetal harm so avoid use in pregnant women; women who are breast-feeding should discontinue nursing.
- Delayed adverse reactions that can develop are hypothyroidism, HAMA, myelodysplasia/leukemia, and secondary malignancies.
- Oral iodine supplements are given one day prior to dosimetric dose, and continued for 2 weeks after the therapeutic dose (to block the thyroid uptake of I-131).
- Overall summary of responses in 116 patients with low-grade or transformed low-grade NHL showed 78% responses (11.7-month median duration of response), with 46% complete responses (36.5-month median duration of response). 24 patients

with no prior chemotherapy had a 100% response, with 71% having a complete response (Vose, 1998).
- The development of human antimouse antibodies (HAMA) was related to extent of prior chemotherapy: in chemonaïve patients, 38% developed HAMA, while only 4% did who received more than one prior chemotherapy regimen.
- Response rate and duration of response were lower in patients aged 65 and older, and duration of severe hematologic toxicity was longer.

Potential Toxicities/Side Effects and the Nursing Process

I. POTENTIAL FOR INJURY related to ANAPHYLAXIS

Defining Characteristics: Rare but potentially life-threatening reaction may occur. Mouse antibodies are used that are foreign and may stimulate anaphylaxis. No grade 4 adverse experiences have been reported. Approximately 8% of patients in clinical trials require slowing of the infusion to manage symptoms.

Nursing Implications: Assess baseline T, VS. If patient develops discomfort, slow infusion per protocol. Have emergency equipment and medications nearby. Assess patient for signs/symptoms, including generalized flushing and urticaria leading to pallor, cyanosis, bronchospasm, hypotension, unconsciousness. Teach patient to report signs/symptoms, including sense of doom, tickle in throat. If signs/symptoms occur, stop infusion immediately, assess VS, notify physician. Physician may prescribe epinephrine 0.3 mL (1:1000) subcutaneous if hypotensive. Oxygen, antihistamines, corticosteroids may also be used.

II. POTENTIAL FOR INFECTION, BLEEDING, AND FATIGUE related to NEUTROPENIA, THROMBOCYTOPENIA, AND ANEMIA

Defining Characteristics: Prolonged Bone marrow suppression is the dose-limiting toxicity. Patients at risk are patients who have been heavily pretreated with minimal bone marrow reserve, who have lower nadir counts with longer times to recovery. The maximum tolerated total body dose is 75 cGy to avoid severe myelosuppression. Nadir counts occur approximately six weeks post-therapy. Median nadirs were ANC 1,000 cells/m^3, platelets 62,000 cells/m^3, and hemoglobin 11.1 gm/dL. Grade 4 toxicity occurred in < 5% of patients: absolute neutropenia < 100 cells/mm^3 (3%), platelet count < 10,000 cells/mm^3 (5%), and Hgb < 6.5% (4%). Supportive use of growth factors and transfusions was 18%, especially in patients heavily pretreated.

Nursing Implications: Assess prior bone marrow suppressive therapy and risk for toxicity. Assess baseline WBC, differential, Hgb/HCT and platelet count, and signs/symptoms of infection, bleeding, or fatigue. Discuss any abnormalities with physician before drug administration. Teach patient signs/symptoms of infection and bleeding, and to report them immediately. Teach patient self-care measures to minimize infection and bleeding, including avoidance of aspirin-containing OTC medication, and oral hygiene regimen. Teach patient signs/symptoms of fatigue, and self-care measures to maximize energy, and to minimize fatigue (e.g., alternate rest and activity periods, organize activities).

III. ALTERATION IN COMFORT related to INFUSION REACTION

Defining Characteristics: Approximately 29% of patients have infusion-related reactions, despite premedication with acetaminophen and diphenhydramine. Symptoms include fever, rigors or chills, sweating, hypotension, dyspnea, bronchospasm and nausea either during or up to 48 hours after the infusion.

Nursing Implications: Assess baseline T, VS, neurological status, and comfort level; monitor q 4–6 h if patient is in hospital. Assure patient receives premedication and regular dosing of antipyretic (e.g., acetaminophen ± diphenhydramine, nonsteroidal anti-inflammatory drug [NSAID]), and antiemetic as ordered by physician. Teach patient self-care measures, including monitoring T, comfort level, self-administration of prescribed medications prior to dose and regularly postdose, as well as the use of heat or cold for myalgias, arthralgias. Encourage patient to increase oral fluids and alternate rest and activity periods. If patient is in hospital and experiences rigor, discuss with physician IV meperidine (25 mg IV q 15 min to maximum 100 mg in 1 hour) and monitor BP for hypotension.

IV. KNOWLEDGE DEFICIT, POTENTIAL, related to RADIATION PRECAUTIONS

Defining Characteristics: The Nuclear Regulatory Commission recommends that patients receiving outpatient I-131 anti-B1 therapy follow measures to prevent radiation contamination of others. Patients may receive outpatient treatment as long as total dose to an individual at 1 meter is < 500 millirem.

Nursing Implications: Teach patient rules of time and distance, and review protocol patient discharge instructions. If in doubt, discuss with radiotherapist or radiation physicist. Patients are advised to sleep alone for at least the first night. Discuss need for longer separation based on dose received. Other teaching is based on dose and should include (1) remain at distances of > 3 feet from other people, except for brief periods as necessary, for at least two days; (2) infants, young children, and pregnant women should not visit the patient; if necessary, visits should be brief, and a distance of at least 9 feet from the patients should be maintained; (3) do not travel by commercial transportation or go on a prolonged automobile trip with others for at least the first two days; (4) have sole use of the bathroom for at least two days; and (5) drink "plenty" of fluids for at least the first two days, e.g., 3+ quarts per day.

Drug: trastuzumab (Humanized anti-*Her*-2 Antibody, rhuMAbHER2, Herceptin)

Mechanism of Action: Recombinant humanized monoclonal antibody targeted against the human epidermal growth factor receptor 2 (*HER*-2). *HER*-2 is an oncogene that is overexpressed in a number of cancers, including 25–30% of breast cancers. The drug binds to HER-2 tightly, thus inhibiting cell signaling and cell proliferation. This monoclonal antibody is believed to act through three different mechanisms: (1) the antagonizing function of the growth-signaling properties of *HER*-2, (2) signaling immune cells to attack and kill malignant cells with this receptor (ADCC), and (3) synergistic and/or additive effects seen with many chemotherapeutic agents.

Metabolism: Initial studies using a loading dose of 4 mg/kg followed by a weekly maintenance dose of 2 mg/kg, a mean half-life of 5.8 days, with a range of 1–32 days was seen. The mean half-life is 16 days (range, 11–23 days) when a loading dose of 8 mg/kg followed by a three-weekly 6 mg/kg dose is used. Steady state is reached between weeks 6–37.

Dosage/Range:
Adjuvant (for a total of 52 weeks):
When given after completion of AC chemotherapy in combination with paclitaxel or docetaxel or docetaxel/carboplatin, during and after as a single agent:
- Loading dose: 4 mg/kg IV infusion over 90 minutes week 1.
- Maintenance dose: 2 mg/kg IV infusion over 30 minutes weekly beginning at week 2 during paclitaxel or docetaxel chemotherapy for 12 weeks or 18 weeks (docetaxel/carboplatin).
- One week after the last weekly dose, give as 6 mg/kg IV infusion over 30–60 minutes every 3 weeks for a total trastuzumab treatment of 52 weeks.
- As a single agent within 3 weeks after completion of multimodality, anthracycline-based chemotherapy regimens.
- Loading dose 8 mg/kg IV infusion IV over 90 minutes.
- Maintenance dose: 6 mg/kg IV infusion over 30–60 minutes every 3 weeks.

Metastatic breast cancer:
- Alone or in combination with paclitaxel, initial dose of 4 mg/kg IV over 90 minutes followed by subsequent once-weekly doses of 2 mg/kg IV over 30 minutes until disease progression.

Dose modifications:
- Decrease rate of infusion for mild or moderate infusion reactions.
- Interrupt infusion if patient develops dyspnea or clinically significant hypotension.
- Discontinue trastuzumab for severe or life-threatening infusion reactions.
- Withhold trastuzumab for at least 4 weeks if
  - > 16% absolute decrease in LVEF from pretreatment values.
  - LVEF < institutional limits of normal and > 10% absolute decrease in LVEF from pretreatment value.

- Resume trastuzumab if within 4–8 weeks the LVEF returns to normal limits and absolute decrease from baseline is ≤ 15%.
- Permanently discontinue trastuzumab for persistent (> 8 weeks) LVEF decline or drug has been held on more than three occasions for cardiomyopathy.

Drug Preparation:

- Drug is available as a lyophilized sterile powder of 440 mg per vial for parenteral administration. Requires refrigeration at 2–8°C (36–46°F). DO NOT FREEZE.
- Reconstitute with 20 mL of bacteriostatic water for injection, USP, containing 1.1% benzyl alcohol, which is supplied with each vial. DO NOT SHAKE.
- Reconstituted solution contains 21 mg/mL. Further dilute desired dose in 250 mL of 0.9% sodium chloride injection, USP. DO NOT use dextrose (5%) solution.
- Vial is designed for multiple use, and is stable for 28 days following reconstitution at 2–8°C (36–46°F). If patient is hypersensitive to this bacteriostatic diluent, use 20 mL sterile water for injection without preservatives as a single solution (not multidose).

Drug Administration:

- Administered IV infusion; initial loading dose is administered over 90 minutes, and initial maintenance dose (week or dose 2) is administered over 30–60 minutes. Never give as IV push or bolus.
- Observe patient for 1 hour following completion of initial loading dose, and if well tolerated, observe patient for 30 minutes following completion of initial maintenance dose (week 2). If well tolerated, no further post-infusion observation is needed in subsequent weekly infusions.
- Subsequent maintenance doses are administered over 30 minutes if prior administration was well tolerated without fever, chills.
- Continue to administer over 90 minutes if fever, chills experienced in prior administrations.

Drug Interactions:

- Paclitaxel: 2 fold decrease in trastuzumab clearance in animals and a 1.5-fold increase in trastuzumab serum level in human clinical studies.
- Chemotherapy: increased neutropenia and febrile neutropenia.
- Doxorubicin, anthracyclines: additive cardiotoxicity; DO NOT GIVE CONCURRENTLY.

Lab Effects/Interference:

- Decreased LVEF; monitor baseline and throughout treatment.
- Decreased absolute neutrophil count when given with chemotherapy.

Special Considerations:

- Indications:
  - *Adjuvant breast cancer* (HER2 overexpressing node positive or high-risk node negative [ER/PR negative with one high risk feature]): (1) as part of a treatment regimen containing doxorubicin, cyclophosphamide, and either paclitaxel

or docetaxel; (2) with docetaxel and carboplatin; (3) as a single-agent after multimodality anthracycline based-therapy.
  - *Metastatic breast cancer* (HER2-overexpressing): (1) in combination with paclitaxel for first-line treatment; (2) as a single agent in patients who have received one or more chemotherapy regimens for metastatic disease.
- Phase III clinical trials studied co-administration together with doxorubicin/cyclophosphamide (AC) showed an increased risk of cardiomyopathy. DO NOT give trastuzumab concurrently with AC chemotherapy. Left ventricular function should be evaluated prior to and during treatment with trastuzumab therapy.
- Rarely, severe infusion reactions and pulmonary toxicity can occur within 24 hours of the drug dose. Interrupt treatment for dyspnea or significant hypotension. Discontinue drug if patient develops anaphylaxis, angioedema, pneumonitis, or ARDS.
- FISH (tests for HER2 gene amplification) appears more accurate in identifying HER2 overexpression; in some centers, patient tumors are tested with IHC (measures HER2 protein overexpression), and if 2+, sent for FISH testing. IHC 3+ demonstrates definite HER2 overexpression. Discordant lab values (false negatives or positives) occur more commonly in labs doing less than 100 tests per month (24%) compared with a lab doing 100 or more a month (3%) (Paik et al, 2002).
- Trastuzumab is very well tolerated; given that it is a humanized antibody, no premedication is recommended.
- Rarely, trastuzumab may cause hypersensitivity/allergic reactions, so emergency equipment should be available during infusions.
- Trastuzumab at a dose of 6–8 mg/kg q 3 weeks × 1 year in the adjuvant setting was shown to reduce the risk of breast cancer recurrence significantly. Interim analysis of the HERA study (2005) showed that the group receiving trastuzumab for 1–2 years after adjuvant chemotherapy in HER-2 positive women had an estimated 2-year survival of 86% compared to 77% for the observation group. $P < 0.01$. This translated to a 46% decrease in risk of recurrence. Cardiac toxicity was higher in the trastuzumab arm, with CHF occurring 3–4% more commonly in high risk patients in the trastuzumab arm, so cardiac function must be monitored (Piccart-Gebhart et al, 2005).
- Romond et al (2005) summarized the NSABP B-31 and NCCTG N0931 trials (Joint Analysis) showing that the addition of trastuzumab to paclitaxel (concurrent not sequential) following AC in the adjuvant setting, at 2 years, there was increased disease free and overall survival. Perez (2005) showed that after 4 years on study, 15% of the women treated with trastuzumab plus paclitaxel concurrently had recurrence, compared to 33% of women receiving paclitaxel alone. This translated into a 52% decrease in risk of recurrence. There was a 49% improvement in survival (Perez, 2005). While there was increased cardiotoxicity, it was within the 4% acceptable range (Tan-Chiu et al, 2005).
- In May 2008, the FDA approved the combination of docetaxel, carboplatin, and trastuzumab (TCH) as an adjuvant option. This regimen offers high efficacy with less risk of cardiotoxicity. In the Breast Canadian International Research Group (BCIRG) 006 trial, TCH reduced the risk of disease recurrence by 33% when

compared with AC followed by T alone but with the same risk of CHF (0.4%). When AC was followed by TC (Taxotere and Herceptin), the risk of recurrence was reduced by 39%, but the risk of CHF specifically was 2%, and that of cardiotoxicity 18%, compared with 9% in the THC group and 10% in the AC followed by T alone arm (Slamon et al, 2006). This regimen has a higher adjuvant therapy completion rate as it is only 12 months in duration as compared to AC followed by TC (15 months). Trastuzumab can be started at the same time as THC.

- Trastuzumab is being studied in combination with lapatinib to see whether the combination prevents brain metastases. O'Shaughnessy et al (2008) reported on a study of heavily pretreated women with HER2+ metastatic breast cancer who had progressed on an anthracycline, a taxane and trastuzumab who were then assigned to lapatinib or lapatinib plus trastuzumab arms of the study. Those receiving both lapatinib and trastuzumab had significantly longer PFS (12 weeks vs. 8 weeks, $p = 0.008$). Those receiving the combination also had longer median OS, which trended toward significance (51.6 vs. 39 wk). Adverse events were similar except for diarrhea and cardiac events (O'Shaughnessy et al, 2008).
- Also, in a large adjuvant breast cancer trial of 8000 patients, which is expected to conclude in 2011, trastuzumab will be compared head-to-head with lapatinib in patients with stage I or II breast cancer (ALTTO study).

Potential Toxicities/Side Effects and the Nursing Process

I. ALTERATION IN CIRCULATION related to CARDIOMYOPATHY

Defining Characteristics: Trastuzumab administration may result in ventricular dysfunction and congestive heart failure. The risk is significantly greater when given with doxorubicin (28% compared with 7% with AC alone), and thus, trastuzumab should NOT be given with doxorubicin and cyclophosphamide. It should begin after the completion of AC in the adjuvant setting. In addition, there is a theoretical slight increase when given together with paclitaxel, but clinical studies have shown a similar incidence of 2% when trastuzumab is given as monotherapy after adjuvant AC to that of AC followed by paclitaxel. Thus, the two drugs can be given concurrently. The 52-week incidence of trastuzumab-related cardiotoxicity when given to follow AC concurrent with paclitaxel for 12 weeks and then as a single agent is about 4%. If allowed to progress, failure may be severe, and the following have been reported: severe cardiac failure, death, and mural thrombosis leading to stroke. Thus, during adjuvant therapy, it is critical that cardiac function be monitored baseline and at least every 3 months. Rare events described following treatment with trastuzumab were vascular thrombosis, pericardial effusion, heart arrest, hypotension, syncope, hemorrhage, shock, and arrhythmia. Risk factors in the NSABP B-31 clinical trial were declining LVEF after completion of AC chemotherapy and increasing age.

Nursing Implications: Assess baseline cardiac function, including apical pulse, BP. Review history, and identify patients at risk who have CHF, hypertension, coronary artery disease. Patients should have baseline ECHO or gated blood pool scan to determine left ventricular ejection fraction (LVEF), and this should be monitored at least every 3 months during adjuvant trastuzumab therapy and at the conclusion of therapy. Repeat LVEF test every 4 weeks if trastuzumab is held for significant changes in LVEF. After completion of adjuvant therapy, assess LVEF every 6 months for at least 2 years. Assess for signs and symptoms at each visit: dyspnea, increased cough, paroxysmal nocturnal dyspnea, peripheral edema, S_3 gallop, and decrease in left ventricular function when tested. Teach patient to report cough, weight gain, edema of ankles, difficulty breathing, or need to use more pillows at night. If patient develops a significant decrease in LVEF, the drug should be held for at least 4 weeks and LVEF repeated every 4 weeks for either of the following: (1) ≥ 16% absolute decrease in LVEF from pretreatment values below ILLN and (2) ≥ 10% absolute decrease in LVEF from pretreatment values and below ILLN. Resume drug if within 4–8 weeks, the LVEF returns to normal limits, and the absolute decrease from baseline is 15% or less. Discontinue drug for a persistent (> 8 weeks) LVEF decline or for suspension of trastuzumab dosing on more than three occasions for cardiomyopathy.

II. POTENTIAL FOR INJURY related to HYPERSENSITIVITY

Defining Characteristics: Infusion-related reactions (e.g., fever and/or chills) were reported in about 40% of patients with their first treatment, and > 10% with subsequent infusions. Infusion reactions are characterized by a symptom complex of fever and chills, with or without nausea, vomiting, pain (may be at tumor site), headache, dizziness, dyspnea, hypotension, rash, and asthenia. Severe hypersensitivity reactions are rare but have been reported, including postmarketing serious and fatal infusion reactions. Bronchospasm, anaphylaxis, angioedema, hypoxia, and severe hypotension can occur during or immediately after the infusion but may have an initial improvement followed by rapid clinical deterioration. Severe deterioration may be delayed by hours to days after a serious infusion reaction.

Nursing Implications: Assess VS baseline and frequently during infusion, especially during initial loading and maintenance infusions. Observe patient for one hour following completion of loading dose, and 30 minutes after initial maintenance dose if loading dose was well tolerated. If not well tolerated, continue to monitor for 60 minutes until well tolerated. Notify physician if fever, chills develop and assess need for acetaminophen, and slowing of infusion. Although severe allergic reactions are uncommon, have emergency equipment available and nearby, and be prepared to provide emergency support if necessary. A drug must be stopped if dyspnea, severe bronchospasm, hypoxia, or severe hypotension occur. A reaction can occur within 24 hours of the drug dose, and thus, if the patient is symptomatic, consider admitting patient for observation. Discontinue drug for severe and life-threatening infusion reactions. If the patient is to receive the drug again after an infusion reaction during the prior administration, discuss with the physician, and ensure that the patient is premedicated with antihistamines and corticosteroids. Monitor the patient very carefully during the infusion, as despite the premedications, severe infusion reactions can still occur.

III. ALTERATION IN OXYGENATION, POTENTIAL, related to DYSPNEA, PULMONARY COMPLICATIONS

Defining Characteristics: After trastuzumab, patients have rarely developed serious and fatal pulmonary toxicity. Pulmonary events that have been described include dyspnea, interstitial pneumonitis, pulmonary infiltrates, pleural effusions, noncardiogenic pulmonary edema, pulmonary insufficiency, hypoxia, ARDS, and pulmonary fibrosis. These may be complications of infusion reactions.

Nursing Implications: Assess patient's baseline pulmonary status, including history of pulmonary disease, breath sounds, and respiratory rate. Patients at risk for developing pulmonary complications are (1) those with symptomatic intrinsic lung disease and (2) those patients with extensive tumor involvement of the lungs so that they are dyspneic at rest. Monitor patients closely during the infusion, and teach patient to report any changes in respiratory function or dyspnea right away. If dyspnea or other symptoms are severe, the patient should come to the emergency room right away for evaluation.

IV. ALTERATION IN COMFORT related to PAIN, ASTHENIA

Defining Characteristics: Generalized pain may affect 11% of patients, and asthenia 5%. Abdominal pain may specifically affect 3% of patients.

Nursing Implications: Teach patients to report alterations in comfort, especially pain and dyspnea. Distinguish new onset of symptoms versus those experienced prior to treatment due to malignancy. Discuss intensity of symptoms and need for pharmacologic and nonpharmacologic interventions. Monitor response to intervention between weekly treatments, and need for alternative strategies.

V. POTENTIAL FOR INFECTION related to EXACERBATION OF CHEMOTHERAPY-INDUCED NEUTROPENIA

Defining Characteristics: In patients with metastatic breast cancer, the incidences of grades 3 and 4 neutropenia, and febrile neutropenia were higher in patients receiving trastuzumab in combination with myelosuppressive chemotherapy.

Nursing Implications: For patients with metastatic breast cancer receiving chemotherapy and trastuzumab, monitor CBC, platelet count baseline and prior to each treatment. Assess for signs and symptoms of infection. Teach patient self-care measures to prevent or minimize the risk of infection. Teach patient self-assessment for signs and symptoms of infection and to call the provider immediately if they occur.

Drug: trastuzumab—MCC-DMI

Class: Antibody-drug conjugate.

Mechanism of Action: MAb trastuzumab is attached to a very toxic antimicrotubular poison DMI, via the linker molecule MMC, which provides a stable bond between the two agents. Trastuzumab goes directly to and binds to tumor-specific and/or overexpressed tumor cell specific antigens. The trastuzumab-linker-DMI is brought into the cell (internalized), and then the linker releases the DMI cellular poison. The resulting intracellular damage kills the cell and spares normal cells.

Trastuzumab in the conjugate drug has the same affinity to HER-2 as trastuzumab alone. The drug binds to HER-2 tightly, thus inhibiting cell signaling and cell proliferation. Trastuzumab alone is believed to act through three different mechanisms: (1) the antagonizing function of the growth-signaling properties of *HER*-2, (2) signaling immune cells to attack and kill malignant cells with this receptor (ADCC), and (3) synergistic and/or additive effects seen with many chemotherapeutic agents.

DMI is a mitotic tubulin inhibitor 20 times more potent than vincristine.

Metabolism: Trastuzumab alone has a mean half-life of 5.8 days when dosed weekly compared with a range of 1–32 days and a mean half-life is 16 days (range, 11–23 days) when given every 3 weeks. Steady state is reached between weeks 6 and 37. Metabolism of the conjugate molecule, including half-life and time to steady-state is currently being studied.

Dosage/Range:
- Per protocol, 1.2–2.9 mg/kg.
- MTD is 3.6 mg/kg when given every 3 weeks (ASCO, 2008 #1028).

Drug Preparation:
- Per protocol.

Drug Administration:
- Per protocol, one regimen was administered IV infusion every 3 weeks and another weekly (ASCO #1029).

Drug Interactions (Trastuzumab as a single agent):
- Paclitaxel: twofold decrease in trastuzumab clearance in animals and a 1.5-fold increase in trastuzumab serum level in human clinical studies.
- Chemotherapy: increased neutropenia and febrile neutropenia.

Lab Effects/Interference (Trastuzumab as a single agent):
- Decreased platelet count.
- Elevated hepatic transaminases.

Special Considerations:
- Conjugate drug shows activity in patients who have received extensive previous therapy with trastuzumab with tumor shrinkage.

- No cardiac toxicity.
- Infrequent and management toxicities; however, rarely, grade 4 thrombocytopenia occurred at dose greater than MTD.
- Being studied alone, with chemotherapy, other biologics.
- Most common toxicities were grade 1 thrombocytopenia, grade 1 fatigue, and less commonly, constipation, arthralgias, headache, muscular weakness, musculoskeletal chest pain, dyspnea, and pleural effusion.
- Uses ImmunoGen's maytansinoid TAP technology.

Potential Toxicities/Side Effects and the Nursing Process

I. ALTERATION IN COMFORT related to ARTHRALGIAS, MUSCULOSKELETAL CHEST PAIN, HEADACHE, FATIGUE, DYSPNEA

Defining Characteristics: Side effects seen in clinical trials included fatigue, arthralgias, headache, muscular weakness, musculoskeletal chest pain, which were mild and manageable.

Nursing Implications: Teach patients to report alterations in comfort, especially pain and dyspnea. Distinguish new onset of symptoms versus those experienced before treatment due to malignancy. Teach patient to manage arthralgias and musculoskeletal discomfort symptomatically as permitted on protocol, possibly improved with use of heat or cold. Teach patient to alternate rest and activity periods and to delegate heavy housekeeping and shopping chores to others to conserve energy. Discuss intensity of symptoms and need for pharmacologic and nonpharmacologic interventions. Monitor response to intervention and need for alternative strategies.

II. POTENTIAL FOR BLEEDING related to THROMBOCYTOPENIA

Defining Characteristics: Thrombocytopenia, when it occurs at doses < MTD, was grade 1.

Nursing Implications: Assess CBC, platelet count baseline and prior to each treatment. Assess for signs and symptoms of bleeding. Teach patient self-care measures to prevent or minimize the risk of bleeding, including avoidance of all OTC medications unless discussed with nurse or provider. Teach patient self-assessment for signs and symptoms of bleeding and to call the provider immediately if they occur.

III. POTENTIAL ALTERATION IN ELIMINATION related to CONSTIPATION

Defining Characteristics: DM1 is a microtubular poison that may cause constipation.

Nursing Implications: Assess bowel elimination pattern prior to each chemotherapy administration. Teach patient to include bulky and high-fiber foods in diet, increase fluids to 3 L/day, and exercise moderately to promote elimination. Suggest stool softeners if needed. Teach patient to use laxative if unable to move bowels at least once every 2 days. Instruct patient to report abdominal pain.

Drug: tretinoin (Vesanoid®, ATRA, All-Trans-Retinoic Acid)

Class: Retinoid.

Mechanism of Action: Induces maturation of acute promyelocytic leukemia (APL) cells, thus decreasing proliferation. In patients who achieve a complete response to this therapy, there is an initial maturation of primitive leukemic cells, and then cells in both the bone marrow and peripheral blood are normal, polyclonal blood cells. The exact mechanism is unknown.

Metabolism: This drug is well absorbed orally into the systemic circulation, with peak concentrations in 1–2 hours. Drug is > 95% protein-bound, primarily to albumin. Oxidative metabolism occurs via the cytochrome P450 enzyme system in the liver. Drug is excreted in the urine (63% in 72 hours) and feces (31% in 6 days).

Dosage/Range:
- 45 mg/m^2 per day.

Drug Preparation:
- None: oral.
- Available as 10–mg capsules.
- Protect from light.

Drug Administration:
- Drug is to be used for induction remission only.
- Administer in evenly divided doses until complete remission (CR) is achieved, then for an additional 30 days, or after 90 days of treatment, whichever comes first.

Drug Interactions:
- Drugs that either inhibit or induce the cytochrome P450 hepatic enzyme system potentially will interact with this drug, but there is no data to suggest that these drugs either increase or decrease tretinoin activity.
- Drugs that induce the enzyme system: rifampin, glucocorticoids, phenobarbital, pentobarbital; drugs that inhibit the enzyme system: ketoconazole, cimetidine, erythromycin, verapamil, diltiazem, cyclosporin.
- Antifibrinolytic agents.

Lab Effects/Interference:
- Increased cholesterol and triglyceride levels (60% of patients).
- Increased LFTs (50–60% of patients).

Special Considerations:

- Indicated for the induction remission of patients with APL (FAB-M3), characterized by the presence of the t(15:17) translocation and/or presence of the PML/RARα (alpha) gene.
- Absorption is enhanced when taken with food.
- Monitor CBC, platelets, coagulation studies, liver function tests, and triglyceride and cholesterol levels frequently during therapy.

Potential Toxicities/Side Effects and the Nursing Process

I. ALTERATION IN OXYGENATION, POTENTIAL, related to RETINOIC ACID-APL SYNDROME

Defining Characteristics: Syndrome occurs in approximately 25% of patients and varies in severity, but has resulted in death. Syndrome is characterized by fever, dyspnea, weight gain, pulmonary infiltrates on X-ray, and pleural and/or pericardial effusions. May also be accompanied by impaired myocardial contractility, hypotension, ± leukocytosis, and because of progressive hypoxemia and multisystem organ failure, some patients have died. Usually occurs during first month of treatment, but may follow initial drug dose.

Nursing Implications: Assess VS, pulmonary exam, and weight at each visit. Teach patient to do daily weights, and to report any SOB, fever, weight gain. If this occurs, notify physician and discuss obtaining CXR and focused exam. Discuss chest X-ray findings with physician. Be prepared to give high-dose steroids at the first sign of the syndrome, e.g., dexamethasone 10 mg IV q 12 h × 3 days or until symptom resolution (necessary in 60% of patients). Provide pulmonary and hemodynamic support as necessary. Discuss whether drug should be discontinued based on severity and patient's response to high-dose steroids.

II. ALTERATION IN COMFORT related to VITAMIN A TOXICITY

Defining Characteristics: Almost all patients experience some toxicity, but they do not usually have to discontinue the drug. Toxicity of high-dose vitamin A includes headache (86%) starting the first week of treatment, but fading after that; fever (83%); skin/mucous membrane dryness (77%); bone pain (77%); nausea/vomiting (57%); rash (54%); mucositis (26%); pruritus (20%); increased sweating (20%); visual disturbances (17%); ocular disorders (17%); skin changes (17%); alopecia (14%); changed visual acuity (6%); visual field defects (3%).

Nursing Implications: Teach patient about possible side effects of high-dose vitamin A as above and to report them if they occur. Teach patient symptom management. Assess severity of symptom(s) and discuss with physician symptom management of fever, headache unresponsive to acetaminophen, nausea/vomiting. If headache is severe in a child, have child evaluated for pseudotumor cerebri.

III. POTENTIAL FOR INJURY related to PSEUDOTUMOR CEREBRI

Defining Characteristics: Benign intracranial hypertension has occurred in children treated with retinoids. Early signs and symptoms are papilledema, headache, nausea and vomiting, and visual disturbances.

Nursing Implications: Teach patient/parents to report symptoms. Assess patient for symptomatology on regular basis. If headache is severe, discuss with physician analgesics and therapeutic lumbar puncture.

IV. POTENTIAL DISTURBANCE IN CIRCULATION

Defining Characteristics: The following disturbances may occur: arrhythmia (23%), flushing (23%), hypotension (14%), hypertension (11%), phlebitis (11%), cardiac failure (6%); 3% of patients studied developed cardiac arrest, myocardial infarction, enlarged heart, heart murmur, ischemia, stroke, and other serious disturbances.

Nursing Implications: Assess cardiac status baseline and presence of risk factors (e.g., hypertension). Assess VS at each visit and teach patient in a manner not to induce anxiety to report any symptoms such as chest pain, SOB, heart palpitations, or any changes that occur.

V. ALTERATION IN NUTRITION, LESS THAN BODY REQUIREMENTS, related to GI DYSFUNCTION

Defining Characteristics: Some problems are related to APL, and together with drug may emerge, such as GI bleeding/hemorrhage, which may occur in up to 34% of patients. Other GI problems include abdominal pain (31%), diarrhea (23%), constipation (17%), dyspepsia (14%), abdominal distention (11%), hepatosplenomegaly (9%), hepatitis (3%), and ulcer (3%).

Nursing Implications: Assess GI status and presence of GI dysfunction baseline. Teach patient to report any GI disturbances or changes in bowel status. If these occur, assess severity and need for symptom management, or discussion/intervention with physician. Monitor liver function studies frequently during therapy.

VI. SENSORY/PERCEPTUAL ALTERATIONS related to CHANGES IN EAR SENSATION/HEARING

Defining Characteristics: 23% of patients report earache or fullness in ears. Other ear problems that may occur are reversible hearing loss (5%) and irreversible hearing loss (1%).

Nursing Interventions: Teach patient that this may occur and to report it if it occurs. Assess severity and need for intervention.

VII. POTENTIAL FOR INJURY related to CNS, PERIPHERAL NERVOUS SYSTEM CHANGES, AND AFFECT CHANGES

Defining Characteristics: Changes that may occur include dizziness (20%), paresthesias (17%), anxiety (17%), insomnia (14%), depression (14%), confusion (11%), cerebral hemorrhage (9%), agitation (9%), and hallucinations (6%). Rarely, the following may occur: forgetfulness, gait disturbances, convulsions, coma, facial paralysis, tremor, leg weakness, somnolence, slow speech, aphasia, and other CNS changes.

Nursing Implications: Teach patient in a manner that does not cause anxiety to report any changes in affect, sensorium, or functional ability (e.g., to walk, speak). Assess severity of symptom(s) if they arise and potential for injury. If severe, modify patient's environment to minimize risk of injury and discuss medical intervention with physician.

VIII. ALTERED URINARY ELIMINATION, POTENTIAL, related to RENAL CHANGES

Defining Characteristics: Uncommonly, renal insufficiency may occur (11%), dysuria (9%), acute renal failure (3%), urinary frequency (3%), renal tubular necrosis (3%), and enlarged prostate (3%).

Nursing Implications: Assess baseline urinary elimination pattern. Teach patient to report any changes. Monitor BUN/creatinine periodically during therapy and discuss any abnormalities with physician.

Drug: liposomal tretinoin (Atragen®, All-Trans-Retinoic Acid Liposomal, AR-623. LipoATRA, Tretinoin Liposomal)

Class: Retinoid.

Mechanism of Action: Induces maturation of acute promyelocytic leukemia (APL) cells, thus decreasing proliferation. In patients who achieve a complete response to this therapy, there is an initial maturation of primitive leukemic cells, and then cells in both the bone marrow and peripheral blood are normal, polyclonal blood cells. The exact mechanism is unknown. Liposomal drug permits IV administration, with less toxicity, as it is believed the liposome overcomes resistance seen with continued oral therapy, possibly due to declining serum levels during oral administration since IV administration of liposome gives higher and more sustained plasma levels of drug (Estey et al, 1999).

Metabolism: IV administration of liposome gives higher and more sustained plasma levels of drug as compared to oral administration. Probably has oxidative metabolism via the cytochrome P450 enzyme system in the liver. Drug is probably excreted in the urine and feces.

Dosage/Range:
- Per research protocol.
- Newly diagnosed acute promyelocytic leukemia (APL) 90 mg/m^2 IV every other day for induction, followed by maintenance with the same dose 3 times a week × 9 months.
- AIDS-related Kaposi's sarcoma: 120 mg/m^2 three times a week × 4 weeks (Bernstein et al, 1998).

Drug Preparation:
- Per research protocol.

Drug Administration:
- IV, per research protocol.

Drug Interactions:
- Drugs that either inhibit or induce the cytochrome P450 hepatic enzyme system potentially will interact with this drug, but there is no data to suggest that these drugs either increase or decrease tretinoin activity.
- Drugs that induce the enzyme system: rifampin, glucocorticoids, phenobarbital, pentobarbital; drugs that inhibit the enzyme system: ketoconazole, cimetidine, erythromycin, verapamil, diltiazem, cyclosporin.

Lab Effects/Interference:
- Increased cholesterol and triglyceride levels.
- Elevated LFTs.
- Elevated renal function test.

Special Considerations:
- Has shown effectiveness in the induction remission of patients with APL (FAB-M3) characterized by the presence of the t(15:17) translocation and/or presence of the PML/RARα (alpha) gene. It should be considered in patients relapsing after oral tretinoin, refractory to oral tretinoin and chemotherapy, or unable to take oral tretinoin.
- In one clinical trial, for newly diagnosed patients with APL, time to hematologic complete remission (CR) was a median of 34 days (range, 22–64 days), but at this time only 10% had a molecular CR. However, after an additional three months of therapy, all patients with a hematologic CR achieved a molecular CR (Estey et al, 1999). Complete hematologic remission is defined as < 5% blasts and < 8% promyelocytes in bone marrow (with normal appearing myelocytes), ANC ≥ 1000/mm^3, and platelet count of ≥ 100,000/mm^3; molecular remission means the PML-RAR-alpha gene rearrangement has disappeared, as shown by PCR (polymerase chain reaction) at a sensitivity of 10 (–4).

- In newly diagnosed APL, high response rates were seen in patients with low white counts, e.g., < 10,000/mm^3, and were minimal in patients with high white counts (Estey et al, 1999).
- Drug appears to slow progression of lesions in AIDS-related Kaposi's sarcoma.
- Drug is being studied in cancer of the prostate, bladder (superficial), and non-Hodgkin's lymphoma.
- Toxicity profile is less than with oral tretinoin.
- Monitor CBC, platelets, coagulation studies, liver function tests, and triglyceride and cholesterol levels, renal function tests baseline, and frequently during therapy.
- Drug is contraindicated during pregnancy as drug is teratogenic, and women should not breast-feed while taking the drug; drug is contraindicated in patients hypersensitive to tretinoin or any of the liposomal components.
- Drug, as with oral version, can cause retinoic acid-acute promyelocytic leukemia syndrome (RA-APL): fever, dyspnea, joint pain.
- Drug should be used cautiously in patients with renal dysfunction; patients with prior sensitivity to acitretin, etretinate, isotretinoin, or other vitamin A derivatives; and patients with pretherapy leukocytosis, as the risk for developing RA-APL syndrome is increased.

Potential Toxicities/Side Effects and the Nursing Process

I. ALTERATION IN OXYGENATION, POTENTIAL, related to RETINOIC ACID-APL SYNDROME

Defining Characteristics: Syndrome occurs in approximately 25% of patients and varies in severity, but has resulted in death in studies of the oral drug. Syndrome is characterized by fever, dyspnea, weight gain, pulmonary infiltrates on X-ray, and pleural and/or pericardial effusions, and joint pain. May also be accompanied by impaired myocardial contractility, hypotension, ± leukocytosis, and because of progressive hypoxemia and multisystem organ failure, some patients have died in studies using the oral drug. Usually occurs during first month of treatment, but may follow initial drug dose. With liposomal drug, when dose was reduced and it was given with steroids, patients successfully continued/completed liposomal tretinoin treatment.

Nursing Implications: Assess VS, pulmonary exam, and weight at each visit. Teach patient to do daily weights, and to report any SOB, fever, weight gain. If this occurs, notify physician and discuss obtaining CXR and focused exam. Discuss chest X-ray findings with physician. Be prepared to give high-dose steroids at the first sign of the syndrome, e.g., dexamethasone 10 mg IV q 12 h × 3 days or until symptom resolution (necessary in 60% of patients). Provide pulmonary and hemodynamic support as necessary. Discuss whether drug should be discontinued based on severity and patient's response to high-dose steroids.

II. ALTERATION IN COMFORT related to VITAMIN A TOXICITY

Defining Characteristics: Toxicity is less with liposomal IV drug than when given orally. Almost all patients experience some toxicity, but they do not usually have to discontinue the drug. Toxicity of high-dose vitamin A includes headache starting the first week of treatment (87% incidence in one study), but fading after that; fever; skin/mucous membrane dryness; bone pain; nausea/vomiting; rash; mucositis; pruritus; increased sweating; visual disturbances (ocular disorders); skin changes; alopecia; changed visual acuity; visual field defects.

Nursing Implications: Teach patient about possible side effects of high-dose vitamin A as above and to report them if they occur. Teach patient symptom management. Assess severity of symptom(s) and discuss with physician symptom management of fever, headache unresponsive to acetaminophen, nausea/vomiting. Teach patient to avoid other administration of vitamin A preparations, e.g., beta carotene. If headache is severe in a child, have child evaluated for pseudotumor cerebri.

III. POTENTIAL FOR INJURY related to PSEUDOTUMOR CEREBRI

Defining Characteristics: Benign intracranial hypertension has occurred in children treated with retinoids. Early signs and symptoms are papilledema, headache, nausea and vomiting, and visual disturbances.

Nursing Implications: Teach patient/parents to report symptoms. Assess patient for symptomatology on regular basis. If headache is severe, discuss with physician analgesics and therapeutic lumbar puncture.

IV. POTENTIAL DISTURBANCE IN CIRCULATION

Defining Characteristics: Toxicity is less than in incidence of patients receiving oral tretinoin. The following disturbances may occur: arrhythmia, flushing, hypotension, hypertension, phlebitis, cardiac failure; one patient studied developed fatal acute heart failure myocardial infarction occurring day after starting therapy, with death the following day in a patient with a history of coronary artery disease and hypertension, and in whom ACE inhibitor was discontinued day prior to starting liposomal tretinoin. In oral studies, enlarged heart, heart murmur, ischemia, stroke, and other serious disturbances occurred.

Nursing Implications: Assess cardiac status baseline and presence of risk factors (e.g., hypertension). Assess VS at each visit and teach patient, in a manner not to induce anxiety, to report any symptoms such as chest pain, SOB, heart palpitations, or any changes that occur.

V. ALTERATION IN NUTRITION, LESS THAN BODY REQUIREMENTS, related to GI DYSFUNCTION

Defining Characteristics: Toxicity with liposomal tretinoin is less severe or frequent than with oral drug. Some problems are related to APL, and together with drug, may emerge, such as GI bleeding/hemorrhage, abdominal pain, diarrhea, constipation, dyspepsia, abdominal distention, hepatosplenomegaly, hepatitis, and ulcer.

Nursing Implications: Assess GI status and presence of GI dysfunction baseline. Teach patient to report any GI disturbances or changes in bowel status. If these occur, assess severity and need for symptom management, or discuss intervention with physician. Monitor liver function studies frequently during therapy.

VI. SENSORY/PERCEPTUAL ALTERATIONS related to CHANGES IN EAR SENSATION/HEARING

Defining Characteristics: Toxicity with liposomal tretinoin is less severe or frequent than with oral drug. Patients may report earache or fullness in ears, and hearing loss.

Nursing Interventions: Teach patient that this may occur and to report it if it occurs. Assess severity and need for intervention.

VII. POTENTIAL FOR INJURY related to CNS, PERIPHERAL NERVOUS SYSTEM CHANGES, AND AFFECT CHANGES

Defining Characteristics: Toxicity with liposomal tretinoin is less severe or frequent than with oral drug. Changes that may occur include dizziness, paresthesias, anxiety, insomnia, depression, confusion, cerebral hemorrhage, agitation, and hallucinations. Rarely, the following may occur: forgetfulness, gait disturbances, convulsions, coma, facial paralysis, tremor, leg weakness, somnolence, slow speech, aphasia, and other CNS changes.

Nursing Implications: Teach patient in a manner that does not cause anxiety to report any changes in affect, sensorium, or functional ability (e.g., to walk, speak). Assess severity of symptom(s) if they arise and potential for injury. If severe, modify patient's environment to minimize risk of injury and discuss medical intervention with physician.

VIII. ALTERED URINARY ELIMINATION, POTENTIAL, related to RENAL CHANGES

Defining Characteristics: Toxicity with liposomal tretinoin is less severe or frequent than with oral drug. Uncommonly, renal insufficiency may occur, dysuria, acute renal failure, urinary frequency, renal tubular necrosis, and enlarged prostate.

Nursing Implications: Assess baseline urinary elimination pattern. Teach patient to report any changes. Monitor BUN/creatinine periodically during therapy and discuss any abnormalities with physician.

Drug: vandetanib (D6474, Zactima) (investigational)

Class: Tyrosine kinase inhibitor.

Mechanism of Action: Vandetanib is a potent, selective inhibitor of multiple tyrosine kinases; it blocks vascular endothelial growth factor receptor (VEGFR-2), as well as the epidermal growth factor receptor (EGFR-1) tyrosine kinases. This blocks both the proliferation of cells (EGFR-1) and the primary endothelial cell receptor, preventing new blood vessel formation. It also blocks RET kinase, which may be important in certain tumors.

Metabolism: Unknown.

Dosage/Range:
- 100–300 mg/daily orally, in combination with docetaxel, pemetrexed, or alone, per protocol.

Drug Preparation:
- Oral.

Drug Interactions:
- Unknown.

Lab Effects/Interference:
- Unknown.

Special Considerations:
- Being studied in combination with pemetrexed (Alimta) in second-line treatment of patients with locally advanced or metastatic NSCLC.

Potential Toxicities/Side Effects and the Nursing Process

I. ALTERATION IN CIRCULATION, POTENTIAL, related to BLEEDING

Defining Characteristics: Unknown.

Nursing Implications: Teach patient bleeding may occur and to come to the emergency department and notify physician or nurse practitioner right away if bleeding (e.g., epistaxis) does not resolve in 15 minutes with local pressure and cooling. Ensure that major surgery is planned with adequate time for drug elimination from body and that it is not resumed until after adequate wound healing.

II. ALTERATION IN COMFORT related to RASH, FATIGUE, FLU-LIKE SYMPTOMS, HEADACHE

Defining Characteristics: Rash is usually mild to moderate. Rash and fatigue are common, with 5% of patients with advanced metastatic breast cancer reporting severe (grade 3) rash and fatigue.

Nursing Implications: Assess patient's baseline comfort, and teach that these symptoms may occur. Assess skin integrity baseline and during therapy. Teach symptom management strategies to minimize discomfort. Teach patient to notify nurse or physician if fatigue or rash is severe or does not resolve with local management. Interrupt or delay dose based on protocol.

III. ALTERATION IN NUTRITION, LESS THAN BODY REQUIREMENTS, related to DIARRHEA, NAUSEA, VOMITING, ANOREXIA, STOMATITIS, INCREASED LIVER FUNCTION TESTS

Defining Characteristics: In patients with metastatic breast cancer who were studied, diarrhea occurred commonly and was severe (grade 3) in 10% of patients.

Nursing Implications: Assess nutritional status, bowel elimination pattern, and appetite, including LFTs, at baseline and repeated periodically during treatment. Inform patient that these side effects may occur. Teach self-administration of antinausea and antidiarrheal medications (e.g., loperamide) according to protocol and to notify provider if symptoms persist so that dose can be interrupted per protocol. Teach patient dietary modification if nausea and vomiting or diarrhea occur (e.g., for diarrhea, bananas, rice, applesauce, and toast) and to increase oral fluids to prevent dehydration. Consult a dietitian to see the patient for dietary counseling for anorexia. Discuss any abnormalities with physician or nurse practitioner.

Drug: vatalanib (PTK787/ZK222584) (investigational)

Class: Angiogenesis inhibitor; protein tyrosine kinase inhibitor.

Mechanism of Action: Drug is a potent inhibitor of all known vascular endothelial growth factor (VEGF) tyrosine kinases (VEGFR-1, 2, 3) that are expressed on endothelial cells; also inhibits c-KIT and platelet-derived growth factor receptor (PDGFR).

Metabolism: Rapidly absorbed in 1–2 hours following oral ingestion; half-life of 4–5 hours.

Dosage/Range:

- Per protocol, e.g., 50–1500 mg/day; probably requires multiple dosing per day given half-life of q 4–5 hours.

Drug Preparation:
- Oral.

Drug Interactions:
- Unknown.

Lab Effects/Interference:
- Unknown.

Special Considerations:
- Drug is being studied in patients with colorectal cancer and glioblastoma multiforme.
- CONFIRM-1 (Colrectal Oral Novel Therapy for the Inhibition of Angiogenesis and Retarding of Metastases) trial: phase III trial comparing patients with advanced colorectal cancer receiving FOLFOX ± vetalinib. Although there appeared to be a significant difference favoring patients receiving the combination (17% reduction in risk of disease progression), this was not significant when reviewed by central reviewers. Survival data is being accrued. It is questioned that perhaps drug was not given frequently enough (daily instead of bid or more frequent) since the half-life of the drug is only 4–5 hours.
- CONFIRM 2: Phase III trial comparing patients with metastatic colorectal cancer who have progressed after 1st line irinotecan containing chemotherapy. Overall survival data did not show an advantage.
- Grade 3 thrombopenia and Grade 4 neutropenia higher in the patients receiving vatalinib and FOLFOX compared to patients receiving FOLFOX alone.

Potential Toxicities/Side Effects and the Nursing Process

I. ALTERATION IN HEMOSTASIS related to BLEEDING and THROMBOSIS

Defining Characteristics: In the CONFIRM trials, Grade 3 venous thrombosis occurred in 7% of patients compared to 4% in the FOLFOX alone arm, and Grade 4 pulmonary embolism occurred in 6% versus 1% in the FOLFOX only arm.

Nursing Implications: Assess baseline hematologic parameters and monitor during therapy. Teach patient to assess for and report right away signs/symptoms of thrombosis: new swelling, pain, skin warmth and/or change in color (e.g., erythema, mottling) on the legs or thighs; new onset pain in the abdomen; dyspnea or shortness of breath, rapid heartbeat, chest pain, or pressure that may signal a pulmonary embolism; and any changes in vision, new onset of severe headache, lightheadedness, or dizziness. Assess baseline mental status and neurological signs and monitor during therapy.

II. POTENTIAL ALTERATION IN CIRCULATION related to HYPERTENSION

Defining Characteristics: Grade 3 hypertension occurred in 21% of patients receiving the combination in the CONFIRM trial compared to 6% receiving FOLFOX alone.

Nursing Implications: Assess baseline BP prior to and during treatment, at least for the first treatment, then prior to each drug administration. If the patient has a history of hypertension, monitor BP more closely, although hypertension develops over time rather than during the drug infusion. Blood pressure should continue to be monitored after patient has stopped the drug. Teach patient drug administration, potential side-effects, and self care measures if prescribed antihypertensive medication, such as angiotensin-converting enzyme inhibitors, beta-blockers, diuretics, and calcium-channel blockers, consult protocol and expect that drug should be permanently discontinued if the patient develops hypertensive crisis (diastolic blood pressure > 120 mm Hg). Drug can be temporarily suspended in patients with severe hypertension until BP can be controlled with medical management per protocol.

III. POTENTIAL FOR ACTIVITY INTOLERANCE related to FATIGUE

Defining Characteristics: Fatigue occurs commonly in patients with advanced colorectal cancer treated with vatalinib and FOLFOX; dizziness was more common in the patients receiving the combination, and 7% of patients receiving the combination had grade 3 dizziness compared to 2% receiving FOLFOX alone.

Nursing Implications: Teach patient that fatigue and dizziness may occur and self-care measures. Teach patient to alternate rest and activity periods, to plan shopping and chores to minimize energy expenditure, and to explore whether family members can assist with necessary chores. Teach patient to slowly change position to minimize feeling dizzy, and to hold onto secure objects such as the wall and not a small table, when arising and moving from a sitting to a standing position. Teach patient to report increasing or severe dizziness.

Drug: volociximab (M200, investigational)

Class: Anti-$\alpha5\beta1$ integrin, chimeric MoAb. IgG4 chimeric monoclonal antibody against $\alpha5\beta1$ integrin, which is a protein found on activated endothelial cells and important in the migration of new blood vessels to the tumor.

Mechanism of Action: Binds to and blocks $\alpha5\beta1$ integrin, which is a protein found on activated endothelial cells and necessary for the endothelial cell to bind to fibronectin in the extracellular matrix around the blood vessel. This is important in the migration of sprouting new forming blood vessel to the tumor. Integrins act as grappling hooks that pull the newly forming endothelial tube to the tumor before blood starts to flow from the neighboring capillary to the tumor in the new vessel. Because the proliferating endothelial cell cannot bind via the integrin to fibronectin, it undergoes programmed cell death (apoptosis) and dies. This drug inhibits endothelial cell–cell interaction, the relationship of the endothelial cell to the surrounding extracellular matrix, and thus inhibits angiogenesis.

Metabolism: Unknown.

Dosage/Range:
- Per protocol, for example, 10-mg/kg IV infusion every 2 weeks (renal cell), 15 mg/kg (melanoma).

Drug Preparation:
- Per protocol.

Drug Administration:
- IV infusion per protocol; chimeric Mab so premedication per protocol; assess for hypersensitivity reactions.

Drug Interactions:
- Unknown.

Lab Effects/Interference:
- Unknown.

Special Considerations:
- Drug is being studied in patients with metastatic melanoma, or renal cell cancer, as well as other solid tumors.
- Most common side effects are fatigue (67%), nausea (35%), arthralgia (17.5%), vomiting (12.5%), hypertension (10%), and diarrhea.
- Subset of patients with malignant melanoma may respond (Barton, 2008).

Potential Toxicities/Side Effects and the Nursing Process

I. ALTERATION IN NUTRITION, LESS THAN BODY REQUIREMENTS, related to NAUSEA, DIARRHEA, VOMITING

Defining Characteristics: In clinical trials, most common side effects.

Nursing Implications: Assess weight, bowel elimination status, and baseline nutritional status, and monitor during therapy. Teach patient that symptoms can occur and ways to minimize this effect, such as self-administration of antinausea and antidiarrheal medications per protocol and to report symptoms that do not resolve with established plan. Teach patient to identify nutritionally dense (high calories and protein in the smallest amount) foods and to keep them handy in the refrigerator. Teach patient to eat small, frequent meals and to have a bedtime snack. Teach patient that goal is to drink a glass of fluid every hour while awake. Monitor closely patients, such as older persons, who are at risk for dehydration. Discuss any abnormalities with a physician.

II. ALTERATION IN COMFORT related to FATIGUE

Defining Characteristics: Fatigue is common in clinical trials.

Nursing Implications: Assess comfort and presence of discomfort, fatigue, baseline and at each visit. Teach patient that these side effects may occur and to report them. Teach patient local comfort measures as well as energy conservation, and discuss management plan with physician if ineffective.

Drug: vorinostat (Zolinza, suberoylanilide hydroxamic acid, SAHA)

Class: Histone deacetylase (HDAC) inhibitor.

Mechanism of Action: Histones are proteins that give structure and support to the DNA helix and DNA coils around the histones. Some tumors have excess HDAC, which causes the DNA to stay tightly packed. The DNA cannot be transcribed, and genes are not expressed and thus are silenced, like important tumor-suppressor genes. Vorinostat inhibits the enzymatic activity of histone deacetylases HDAC1, HDAC2, and HDAC3 (class I) and HDAC6 (class II). This results in increased histone acetylation and uncoiling of DNA so that the DNA is open; genes are expressed and can be transcribed for protein synthesis. These proteins are critical in normal cell-cycle regulation. The drug induces cell cycle arrest and apoptosis in some transformed cells; the mechanism of action of antineoplastic effect has not been fully characterized.

Metabolism: After oral ingestion, the drug becomes 71% protein bound. It is metabolized via glucuronidation and hydrolysis followed by β-oxidation, resulting in two inactive metabolites. Drug is eliminated primarily through metabolism, with < 1% of drug recoverable in the urine.

Dosage/Range:
- 400 mg orally once daily with food until disease progression or unacceptable toxicity.
- Dose reduce for thrombocytopenia, anemia.
- Dose reduction for intolerance: 300 mg orally once daily with food or daily for 5 consecutive days and repeated weekly.
- No information is available about drug tolerance in patients with renal or hepatic impairment.

Drug Preparation/Administration:
- Available in 100-mg gelatin capsules.
- Take with food; do not crush or open capsules.
- Monitor CBC, chemistry tests (electrolytes, glucose, serum creatinine, magnesium) every 2 weeks during first 2 months and then monthly thereafter; ECG with QTc measurement baseline and periodically during treatment.

Drug Interactions:
- Other HDACs (e.g., valproic acid): severe thrombocytopenia, GI bleeding; use together cautiously and monitor platelet count every 2 weeks during first 2 months.

Lab Effects/Interference:
- Decreased platelet and red blood cell count.
- Increased serum creatinine (46% of patients) and protein in urine (57% of patients).

Special Considerations:
- Indicated for the treatment of cutaneous manifestations of cutaneous T-cell lymphoma in patients who have progressive, persistent, or recurrent disease on or after two systemic therapies.
- Warnings:
  - Dose-related thrombocytopenia and anemia; requires dose modification.
  - Nausea, vomiting, diarrhea.
  - Hyperglycemia: monitor diabetic patients carefully.
  - QTc prolongation.
- Avoid pregnancy and breast-feeding while receiving the drug, as the drug is fetotoxic.
- Pulmonary embolism occurred in 4.7% of patients and squamous cell carcinoma in 3.5%.
- Most common side effects:
  - GI: diarrhea, nausea, anorexia, weight loss, vomiting, constipation.
  - Constitutional: fatigue, chills.
  - Hematologic: thrombocytopenia, anemia.
  - Taste disorders: dysgeusia, dry mouth.

Potential Toxicities/Side Effects and the Nursing Process

I. POTENTIAL FOR BLEEDING AND FATIGUE related to THROMBOCYTOPENIA AND ANEMIA

Defining Characteristics: Thrombocytopenia occurs in 25.6% (5.8% grade 3/4) of patients and anemia in 14% (gr 3/4, 2.3%).

Nursing Implications: Monitor CBC, platelet count baseline and periodically during therapy. Assess for signs and symptoms of bleeding, fatigue, and anemia. Teach patient to self-assess for signs and symptoms of bleeding and anemia and to call if they occur. Assess patient medication profile and any over-the-counter medications such as those containing aspirin or NSAIDs that would increase the risk of bleeding. Instruct patient to avoid these drugs and not to begin any over-the-counter medications without first discussing with nurse or physician. Teach patient to alternate rest and activity periods if feeling fatigued and to organize shopping and chores in a way to minimize energy expenditures.

II. ALTERATION IN NUTRITION, LESS THAN BODY REQUIREMENTS, related to NAUSEA, DIARRHEA, ANOREXIA, DEHYDRATION, VOMITING, DYSGEUSIA, HYPERGLYCEMIA

Defining Characteristics: In clinical trials these side effects occurred with the following frequency: diarrhea 52%, nausea 41%, dysgeusia 28%, anorexia 24%, dry mouth 16%, vomiting 15%, constipation 15%, and anorexia 14%.

Nursing Implications: Assess weight, bowel elimination status, baseline nutritional status, and glucose level, and monitor during therapy. Teach patient that symptoms can occur and ways to minimize this effect, such as self-administration of antinausea and antidiarrheal medications and to report symptoms that do not resolve with established plan. Teach patient to identify nutritionally dense (high calories and protein in the smallest amount) foods and to keep them handy in the refrigerator. Teach patient to eat small, frequent meals and to have a bedtime snack. Teach patient that goal is to take in at least 2 quarts of fluid a day and to try to drink a glass of fluid every hour while awake. Monitor patients at risk for dehydration closely such as elderly. Teach patient signs and symptoms of hyperglycemia (excessive thirst, frequent urination) and to report these. Discuss any abnormalities with a physician.

III. POTENTIAL ALTERATION IN CIRCULATION related to PULMONARY EMBOLISM, QTc PROLONGATION, PERIPHERAL EDEMA

Defining Characteristics: Pulmonary embolism occurred in 4.7% of patients, prolongation of the QTc interval occurred but has not been studied definitively, and peripheral edema occurred in 12% of patients.

Nursing Implications: Do baseline assessment of cardiac status, including the presence of peripheral edema, and ensure that baseline ECG with QTc interval has been done and that it is done periodically during treatment. Identify patients at risk for developing QTc prolongation, such as patients on antiarrhythmic agents and patients with hypomagnesemia or hypokalemia. Check electrolytes and magnesium every 2 weeks during first 2 months of therapy and then monthly after that. Replete magnesium and potassium as ordered, or teach patient about self-administration of medications. Teach patient to report new pain in the back of the leg, a red streak up the leg, or difficulty breathing right away and to come to the emergency department for evaluation.

Section 2
Symptom Management

Chapter 6
Pain

Pain in the patient with cancer may result from a variety of stimuli. A careful assessment is critical in order to identify the physical causes and psychosocial factors that modulate pain intensity and perception. Pain can be acute or chronic. Acute pain results from stimuli such as surgical procedures, pathological fractures, and obstruction of a hollow viscus, while chronic pain reflects the more common cancer pain resulting from tissue inflammation caused by tumor, but patients often have both acute and chronic components of pain. Acute pain lasts from minutes to months and ceases when the cause of pain is removed (e.g., pain caused by spinal cord compression is removed when the patient undergoes laminectomy or radiotherapy to relieve the compression). This type of pain is often associated with anxiety, and as well one sees symptoms of sympathetic nervous system arousal (increased heart rate, increased/decreased BP). In contrast, chronic pain lasts from months to years; the cause cannot be removed, and this type of pain is often associated with depression. The long duration of chronic pain dampens sympathetic response, so the patient does not manifest changes in heart rate or BP. Many patients with cancer pain have persistent pain that requires around-the-clock analgesia to prevent pain. In addition, patients can develop breakthrough pain, which may be precipitated by an anticipated event, such as movement, or it just may occur. It is estimated that 64–89% of patients with chronic cancer pain have breakthrough pain, with most episodes lasting 120 minutes or less, and a single patient having four to seven episodes a day (Zeppetella et al, 2000). Less commonly, pain can be intermittent, and this is characteristic of acute pain. Here analgesia is given intermittently.

Symptoms often accompanying unrelieved pain are sleeplessness, anorexia (loss of appetite), fatigue, irritability, and fear. Nurses play a critical role in advocating for effective cancer pain management and alleviation of other accompanying symptoms. Fortunately, there are a variety of available analgesic medications, including non-opioid and opioid, adjuvant agents such as antidepressants, as well as nonpharmacologic techniques such as relaxation exercises.

In addition, opioid agents are available in immediate-onset formulations for acute pain, and long-duration agents that allow superior control for chronic pain as long-acting preparations avoid the peaks and valleys of serum levels and relief associated with immediate preparations. While analgesics do not remove the source or stimulus for the pain, they decrease or modulate the impulse so that the pain impulse perceived by the patient is reduced or absent, thus decreasing the distress and discomfort perceived by the patient. *Non-opioid* medications are helpful for mild to moderate pain. Most non-opioid analgesics work peripherally to decrease prostaglandin synthesis (NSAIDs), but some agents may have a central action as well, possibly at the level of the hypothalamus (McEvoy, Litvak, and Welsh, 1992). Pain receptors appear to be sensitized to mechanical and chemical stimulation by prostaglandins, so interruption of prostaglandin synthesis diminishes the painful impulse. For example, bone destruction and pain from metastasis appear to be mediated by prostaglandins, so NSAIDs that inhibit prostaglandin synthesis are first-line analgesics (Foley 2000). In addition, the anti-inflammatory action of NSAIDs contributes to analgesia. Principal side effects of this class are alteration in hemostasis (aspirin inhibits platelet aggregation, while other salicylates may alter hepatic synthesis of blood coagulation factors); alteration in GI mucosal integrity (aspirin and other NSAIDs can erode GI mucosal surface, causing bleeding or ulceration); and altered renal elimination due to inhibition of renal prostaglandins responsible for renal blood flow and function.

COX-2 inhibitors came upon the healthcare scene in relation to the treatment of rheumatoid and osteoarthritis. Their role in the management of cancer-related bony pain is unclear, but the selective inhibition of prostaglandins responsible for inflammation is an achievement that will undoubtedly find a niche. In addition, these agents at slightly higher dosing may have anti-tumor effects as well as they decrease angiogenesis and increase apoptosis ability on the cellular level. NSAIDs achieve their anti-inflammatory effect by inhibiting the enzyme cyclooxygenase (COX), which is necessary for synthesis of prostaglandins and thromboxanes. There are two isoforms of the enzyme, COX-1, which appears to protect the gastric mucosa and is found in most tissues including platelets, and COX-2, which is found in brain and kidney tissue, as well as other body tissues at the site of inflammation. NSAIDs traditionally inhibit both COX-1 and COX-2 isoforms, resulting in a high risk of gastric ulceration and perforation. The risk of gastrointestinal bleeding is significantly less with the selective COX-2 inhibitors but still may occur. In addition, the selective COX-2 inhibitors do not affect bleeding time. The effect of the new COX-2 inhibitors on acute pain remains to be seen. In one study, 50 mg of rofecoxib was equally effective as 550 mg of naproxen sodium or 400 mg of ibuprofen. Two other selective COX-2 inhibitors are celecoxib (Celebrex®) and rofecoxib (Vioxx®). Of interest as the applications of these new agents are explored is their possible role in prevention or treatment of colon cancer. An American Cancer Society study (Thun et al, 1991) showed that the regular ingestion of aspirin diminished colon cancer mortality 40% in men and 42% in women over six years. In addition, it appears that prostaglandin E2 may have a role in colon cancer development, and it appears that a COX-2–derived prostanoid promotes survival of colonic adenomas (Lipsky, 1999). Currently, research is underway to better define the role of COX-2 inhibitors in the prevention and/or management of colon cancer.

Adjuvant analgesics play a vital role in cancer pain management. These drugs are indicated for purposes other than analgesia but can be combined with primary analgesics to increase analgesia and/or manage symptoms related to pain or the adverse effects of the opioids. There may be wide variations in patient responses. The major classes used as adjuvant drugs are antidepressant (Chapter 9), corticosteroid

(Chapter 1), anticonvulsant (Chapter 7), and specialty drugs for bony metastasis (Chapter 10).

The *antidepressants* enhance pain-modulating pathways that are mediated by serotonin and norepinephrine, and, interestingly, clomipramine and amitriptyline have been shown to increase morphine levels (Wilkie, 1995). Not only can these agents help reduce the depression associated with chronic pain, but they can also relieve sleep problems, and often offer significant benefit in the management of neuropathic pain. Most commonly, the tricyclic antidepressants are used, such as amitriptyline and desipramine. The drug selection should be individualized to the patient and the risk for developing side effects. The advent of serotonin-reuptake inhibitors (SSRI) brought great hope to oncology nurses. However, there have been conflicting reports of the efficacy of these SSRIs in managing chronic pain syndromes (Belcheva et al, 1995; Tokunaga et al, 1998). Of the non-tricyclic antidepressants, paroxetine (Paxil) has shown benefit in reducing the painful symptoms of peripheral neuropathy in diabetic patients (Sindrup et al, 1990) and itching in patients with advanced cancer (Zycliz, 1996). In dosing antidepressants, the starting dosage should be low (i.e., 10 mg amitriptyline for the elderly patient, or 25 mg for the young adult) and given at bedtime. The dose should be titrated up slowly to the usually effective range of 50–150 mg. It is important to allow one week between dose titrations to evaluate the benefit of a given dose. Side effects include sedation, orthostatic hypotension, constipation, dry mouth, dizziness and, less commonly, precipitation of acute angle-closure glaucoma, urinary retention, and arrhythmia.

Corticosteroids are useful in both acute and chronic pain management, such as that associated with metastatic bone pain, neuropathic pain, lymphedema, hepatic capsular distension, and brain metastasis. The dosing is individualized to the etiology of the pain and patient requirements, from low doses to high doses for patients with brain metastasis. It is important to identify patients at risk for peptic ulceration, and then to use corticosteroids cautiously if at all. In addition, patients need to be cautioned not to take concomitant aspirin.

Anticonvulsants may provide analgesia for lancinating, neuropathic pain. Drugs such as gabapentin, carbamazepine, phenytoin, clonazepam, and valproate are often used, and the dosing is the same as that used for seizure prevention. This year, pregabapentin was FDA approved (Lyrica) for treatment of pain resulting from diabetic peripheral neuropathy and postherpetic neuralgia.

Specialty drugs for the management of bony metastasis are bisphosphonate pamidronate disodium (Aredia) and zoledronate (Zometa), indicated for use in managing pain related to bony metastases. Pamidronate and zoledronate have been shown to inhibit osteoclast activity and reduce pain from bony metastasis. Treatment is given IV every four weeks. Radiopharmaceuticals such as Strontium-89 are taken up in bone mineral preferentially, in sites of metastasis. However, the subsequent development of acute leukemia has limited interest in radiopharmaceutical management of pain.

Opioid analgesics are the cornerstone of management of moderate to severe cancer pain. These drugs, opiate agonists, attach to specific opiate receptors in the limbic system, thalamus, hypothalamus, spinal cord, and organs such as intestines. This leads to altered pain perception at the spinal cord and higher CNS levels. Because of this action, side effects that may occur include suppressed cough reflex; alterations in consciousness and mood (drowsiness, sedation, euphoria, dysphoria, mental clouding); respiratory depression; nausea/vomiting; and constipation. Opiate agonists may cause physical dependence (causing physical signs and symptoms of withdrawal if drug is stopped abruptly after chronic usage) and addiction (psychological dependence). However, addiction is VERY RARE in cancer patients, occurring in less than 0.1% of patients. A recent study compared sustained-release oral morphine to transdermal fentanyl and oral methadone in cancer pain management (Mercadante et al, 2008). No differences in pain or symptom intensity were found or in adverse effects during titration or chronic treatment. Methadone was significantly less expensive.

Unfortunately, some patients with cancer pain suffer needlessly because healthcare providers (physicians) underprescribe and (nurses) undermedicate (Marks and Sacher, 1973). Chronic cancer pain requires the patient to self-administer opioids "around-the-clock" rather than "as needed (PRN)" to prevent moderate-to-severe pain. Tolerance is the ability to receive larger amounts of a drug without ill effect and to show decreased effect (i.e., pain relief) with continued use of the same drug dose. Tolerance occurs over time, depending on the drug and the route of administration. In addition, tolerance to the respiratory depressant effects of opiates develops over time with chronic usage for prevention of cancer pain. For instance, a patient with severe cancer pain who has been receiving escalating doses over a period of time may require very high doses to finally eliminate or reduce the pain to acceptable levels, as in the case of a patient with head and neck cancer who required 1200 mg/hour of morphine yet was still ambulatory and able to interact with family and friends. According to McCaffery (1982), pain is "whatever the patient says it is, occurring where the patient says it is." Use of quantifiable measurement tools is helpful to identify pain intensity (see Figure 6.1) and pain *relief* in response to intervention. The World Health Organization recommends a two-step approach to cancer pain management, beginning with non-opioids for slight-to-mild pain and adding an opioid as the pain intensity increases. Opioids have different potencies, and when a patient is changed from one opioid to another, it is imperative that equianalgesic dosages be used. Equianalgesic dose tables are based on comparative potencies to morphine (see Table 6.1). Opioids and non-opioids can be combined for additive analgesia. Opioid agonist-antagonists, such as pentazocine (e.g., Talwin), should be used with caution, if at all, since they may cause withdrawal syndrome. NSAIDs and opioid analgesics are available for oral, parenteral, and rectal administration. The United States Food and Drug Administration (FDA) approved ketorolac in 1996, and it is the only available *parenteral* NSAID. Also, transdermal patch delivery of fentanyl (20 times more potent than morphine) has been available for some time, and an immediate-release oral with mucosal absorption system is available (Actiq). A transdermal patch of hydromorphine was long awaited, but after FDA gave approval, it had to be withdrawn from the market because

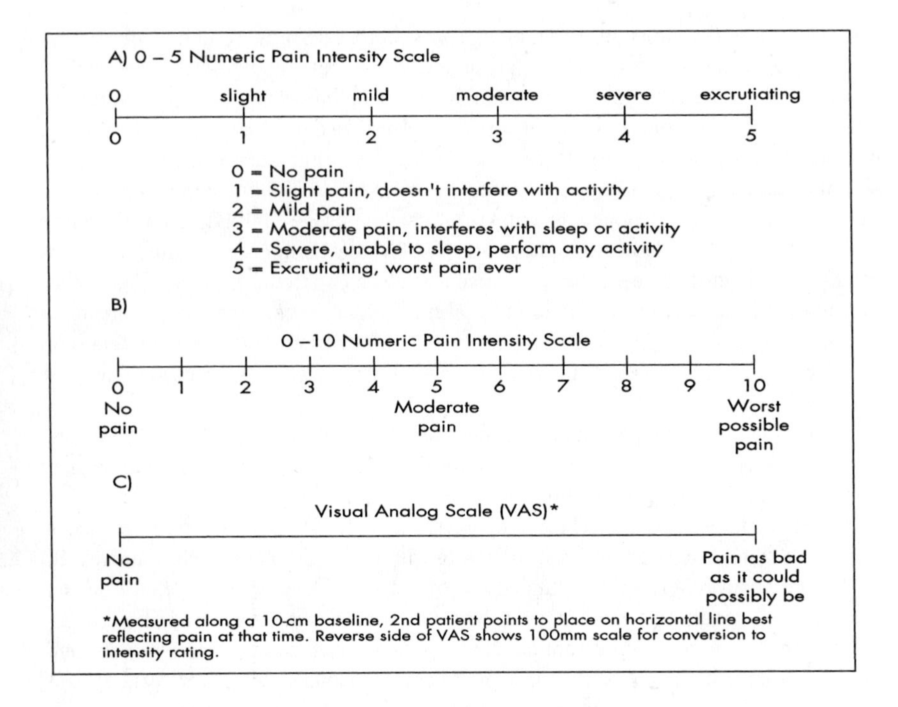

Figure 6.1 Examples of Measurement Tools of Pain Intensity

of improper use and morbidity. Other delivery approaches for fentanyl have led to the recent FDA approval of fentanyl buccal tablet (Fentora). Finally, awareness of the benefits of patient-controlled analgesia (PCA) has made this method of drug delivery for IV analgesics more widely available.

When trying to evaluate an opioid intervention, it is important to again recall that this is the century of genomics. It is now clear that there is considerable genetic polymorphism in the cytochrome P-450 family of enzymes (Bernard & Bruera, 2000), and that this can influence analgesic effect. For example, Payne (1998) states that 15% of Caucasians lack the enzyme CYPD211 that is required to metabolize codeine to morphine, so this group will require higher doses to achieve the same effect. As genotyping becomes more a part of designing a plan of care, it is important to remember this. In addition, as nurses have always done, when one opioid is ineffective, care planning with physician colleagues is to make sure that another opioid from a different class is tried.

Numerous practice guidelines are available, and most recently the National Comprehensive Cancer Network (NCCN) emphasizes the need for rapid titration of short-acting opioids to manage severe pain, before then determining the optimal analgesic regime to control the patient's pain (Grossman et al, 1999). The recommended

Table 6.1 Equianalgesic Dose Table

Drug			Recommended Starting Dose (Adults > 50 kg Body Weight)	
Opioid Agonist	**Approximate Equianalgesic Oral Dose**	**Approximate Equianalgesic Parenteral Dose**	**Oral**	**Parenteral**
Morphine	30 mg q 3–4 h (around-the-clock dosing)	10 mg q 3–4 h	30 mg q 3–4 h	10 mg q 3–4 h
	60 mg q 3–4 h (single dose or intermittent dosing)			
Codeine	130 mg q 3–4 h	75 mg q 3–4 h	60 mg q 3–4 h	60 mg q 2 h (IM, SQ)
Hydromorphone (Dilaudid)	7.5 mg q 3–4 h	1.5 mg q 3–4 h	6 mg q 3–4 h	1.5 mg q 3–4 h
Hydrocodone (in Lorcet, Lortab, Vicodin, others)	30 mg q 3–4 h	Not available	10 mg q 3–4 h	Not applicable
Levorphanol (Levo-Dromoran)	4 mg q 6–8 h	2 mg q 6–8 h	4 mg q 6–8 h	2 mg q 6–8 h
Meperidine (Demerol)	300 mg q 2–3 h	100 mg q 3 h	Not recommended	100 mg q 3 h
Methadone (Dolophine, others)	20 mg q 6–8 h	10 mg q 6–8 h	20 mg q 6–8 h	10 mg q 6–8 h
Oxycodone (Roxicodone, also in Percocet, Percodan, Tylox, others)	30 mg q 3–4 h	Not available	10 mg q 3–4 h	Not applicable
Oxymorphone (Numorphan)	Not available	1 mg q 3–4 h	Not available	1 mg q 3–4 h

Source: From AHCPR, Public Health Service, US Department of Health and Human Services. Rockville, MD AHCPR Publication No. 92-0032.

guidelines (version 1. 2008) are available on the Internet at http://www.nccn.org/professionals/physician_gls/PDF/pain.pdf.

New horizons are being explored, and new medications that act directly at the spinal cord level are being studied. Recently, research has identified alpha-adrenergic receptors for epinephrine at presynaptic and postjunctional sites in the dorsal horn of the spinal cord, located near the opioid receptors. Stimulation of these alpha-2 adrenergic receptors by agonists such as clonidine appears to block the transmission of the pain signal up the spinal cord to the brain, thus blocking pain perception, and this does not compete with opioids at opioid binding sites. One such agent that has been approved is clonidine hydrochloride (Duraclon), which is given along with opioids. Other agents being studied are *N*-methyl-D-aspartate (NMDA) antagonists (such as ketamine and dextromethorphan), which decrease pain due to inflammation and ischemia, and are effective in reducing neuropathic pain. NMDA receptors are found in the brain, spinal cord, and periphery, and are responsible for recognizing neuropathic pain. Unfortunately, side effects such as hallucinations and disassociation may be problematic.

Drugs intended to limit the development of tolerance are ongoing. Mu agonists (e.g., morphine) activate the mu-opioid receptor to inhibit the neuron from passing along incoming pain impulses, thus effecting analgesia. When morphine binds to the mu receptor, it increases the sensitization of the *N*-methyl-D-aspartate receptor, or NMDA receptor, and leads to an overactivation of protein-kinase C. This in turn leads to a desensitization of the mu-opioid receptor so that the effect of morphine is less, and tolerance may develop. By combining morphine with a NMDA antagonist, this stimulates the mu-opioid receptor and at the same time prevents activation of the protein-kinase C, thus preventing desensitization of the mu-opioid receptor, and theoretically increasing analgesia and preventing tolerance.

A second group that is being studied is the calcium-channel blockers, which may also offer analgesia. By antagonizing the voltage-sensitive calcium channels in the synaptic membranes of neurons, these *N*-type voltage-sensitive calcium channel (VSCC) antagonists have shown some success in relieving neuropathic pain. Intrathecal administration of selective neuronal channel is being studied and offers promise of relief of chronic intractable pain.

As a nurse negotiating with patients with cancer-related pain around goals, often patients choose a 2–3 on a scale of 0–10 as the goal because they would rather have some pain in exchange for not being too sleepy. One possible intervention that is being studied is the use of modafinil (Provigil) to help treat fatigue and help patients stay awake (NCI, accessed July 2002; Breitbart et al, 1998). This agent could also be useful to help patients try to achieve a goal of pain intensity of 0–1 and not be afraid of becoming too sleepy with a lower quality of life.

New entries to available analgesics included in this book include oxymorphone HCl, both in extended release and immediate release forms, for the treatment of moderate to severe pain in patients who require a long acting opioid for extended treatment. Although studies were based on patients with chronic back pain, this agent may find a niche in cancer care.

References

Algos Pharmaceutical Corporation. *Understanding NMDA-Enhanced Analgesia.* Neptune, NJ: Algos Pharmaceutical Corporation; 1999

Belcheva S, Petkov VD, Konstantinova E, et al. Effects on Nociception of the Calcium and 5-HT Antagonist Dotarizine and Other 5-HT Receptor Agonists and Antagonists. *Acta Physiol Pharmacol Bulg* 1995; 21 93–98

Bernard SA, Bruera E. Drug Interactions in Palliative Care. *J Clin Oncol* 2000; 18(8) 1780–1799

Breitbart W, Passik S, Payne D. Psychological and Psychiatric Interventions in Pain Control. Doyle D Hanks GW MacDonald N *Oxford Textbook of Palliative Medicine*, 2nd ed. New York: Oxford University Press; 1998; 437–454

Eliot L, Geiser R, Loewen G. Steady State Pharmacokinetic Comparison of a New Once-daily, Extended Release Morphine Formulation (Morphelan) and Oxy Contin Twice Daily. *J Oncol Pharm Pract* 2001; 7 1–8

Fan G-H, Zhao J, Wu Y-L, et al. *N*-methyl-D-aspartate Attenuates Opioid Receptor-Mediated G Protein Activation and This Process Involves Protein Kinase C. *Mol Pharmacol* 1998; 53 684–690

Ferrell BR, Rivera LM. Cancer Pain Education for Patients. *Semin Oncol Nurs* 1997; 13 42–48

Foley KM. The Treatment of Cancer Pain. *N Engl J Med* 1995; 313 84–95

Foley KM. Controlling Cancer Pain. *Hospital Practice* 2000; 35(4) 101–112

Grossman SA, Benedetti C, Payne R, Syrjala K, NCCN Practice Guidelines for Cancer Pain. *Oncology* 1999; 13(11A) 1–20

Jacox A, Carr DB, Payne R. Management of Cancer Pain. *Clinical Practice Guideline No 9 (AHCPR Pub No 94–0592).* Rockville, MD: Agency for Health Care Policy & Research USDHHS; 1994

Kaiko RF, Wallenstein SL, Rogers AG, et al. Opioids in the Elderly. *Med Clin North Am* 1982; 66 1079–1089

Lipsky PE. COX-2 Specific Inhibitors: Basic Science and Clinical Implications. *Am J Med* 1999; 106 (5B) 1–515 (proceeding of a symposium)

Lipsky PE. The Clinical Potential of Cyclooxygenase 2-Specific Inhibitors. *Am J Med* 1999; 106(5B) 515–575

Marks RM, Sacher EJ. Undertreatment of Medical Inpatients with Opioid Analgesics. *Ann Intern Med* 1973; 78 173–181

McCaffery M. *Nursing. Management of the Patient with Pain*, Philadelphia, PA: JB Lippincott Co.; 1982

Mercadante S, Porzio G, Ferrera P, et al. Sustained-Release Oral Morphine Versus Transdermal Fentanyl and Oral Methadone in Cancer Pain Management. *Eur J Pain* published online at DOI 10.1016/j.ejpain.2008.01.013. Accessed 24 June 2008

Miaskowski C. Innovations in Pharmacologic Therapies. *Semin Oncol Nurs* 1997; 13 30–35

National Cancer Institute. Fatigue PDQ: Intervention, Pschostimulants. July 2002; Available at http://www.nci.org. Accessed August 2002

Paice J. Pain, Yarbro CH, Frogge MH, Goodman M. *Cancer Symptom Management*, 3rd ed. Sudbury, MA: Jones and Bartlett Publishers; 2003

Payne R. Pharmacologic Management of Pain, Section IA3. Berger A Portenoy RK Weissman DE *Principles and Practice of Supportive Oncology*, Philadelphia, PA: Lippincott-Raven Publishers; 1998

Syndrup SH, Gram LF, Brosenk EO Jr. The Selective Serotonin Reuptake Inhibitor Paroxetine is Effective in the Treatment of Diabetic Neuropathy Symptoms. *Pain* 1990; 42 135–144

Thun MJ, Namboodri MM, Heath CW Jr. Aspirin Use and Reduced Risk of Fatal Colon Cancer. *N Engl J Med* 1991; 325 1593–1596

Tokunaga A, Saika M, Senba E. 5-HT2A Receptor Subtype is Involved in the Thermal Hyperalgesic Mechanism of Serotonin in the Periphery. *Pain* 1998; 76 349–355

Wilkie D. Neural Mechanisms of Pain: A Foundation for Cancer Pain Assessment and Management. *Maguire DB, Yarbro CH, Ferrell BR, Cancer Pain Management*, 2nd ed. Sudbury, MA: Jones and Bartlett Publishers; 1995; 61–87

Zeppetella G, O'Doherty CA, Collins S. Prevalence and Characteristics of Breakthrough Pain in Cancer Patients Admitted to a Hospice. *J Pain Symptom Manage* 2000; 20 87–92

Zycliz Z, Smits C, Krajnik M. Paroxetine for Pruritus in Advanced Cancer. *J Pain Symptom Management* 1996; 16 121–124

NON-OPIOID ANALGESICS

Drug: acetaminophen (Acephen, Actamin, Anacin-3, Apacet, Anesin, Dapa, Datril, Genapap, Genebs, Gentabs, Halenol, Liquiprin, Meda Cap, Panadol, Panex, Suppap, Tempra, Tenol, Ty Caps, Tylenol)

Class: Miscellaneous analgesic/antipyretic.

Mechanism of Action: Appears to inhibit prostaglandin synthesis centrally, thus preventing sensitization of pain receptors to chemical or mechanical stimulation. Mechanism is similar to salicylates but is not uricosuric. May have weak anti-inflammatory effects in nonrheumatoid conditions (e.g., after oral surgery). Reduces fever by direct effect on hypothalamus; heat is lost through vasodilation and increased peripheral blood flow. Analgesic and antipyretic action similar to aspirin.

Metabolism: Rapidly absorbed from GI tract; 25% serum protein-binding. Elimination half-life is 1–3 hours. Metabolized by the liver and excreted in the urine.

Dosage/Range:
- 325–650 mg every 4–6 hours PRN for pain, discomfort, not to exceed 4 g/24 hours. Some individuals may need increased single doses of 1 g.

Drug Preparation:
- Ensure seals on tamper-resistant package are intact when opening new package.

Drug Administration:
- Oral, rectal, elixir.

Drug Interactions:
- Hepatotoxicity of acetaminophen may be increased by chronic use of high doses of drugs using hepatic microsomal enzyme system: barbiturates, carbamazepine, rifampin, phenytoin, sulfinpyrazone.
- Alcohol: increased risk of hepatic damage with chronic, excessive use.
- Diflunisal: increased acetaminophen serum level; avoid concurrent use.
- Phenothiazines: possible severe hypothermia may occur when used concomitantly.

Lab Effects/Interference:
- None known.

Special Considerations:

- Elixirs contain alcohol (Tylenol, Valadol).
- Contraindicated in patients with known hypersensitivity; use cautiously, if at all, in patients with hepatic or renal dysfunction.
- Chronic ingestion of large doses of acetaminophen may slightly potentiate effects of coumarin and other anticoagulants.

Potential Toxicities/Side Effects and the Nursing Process

I. KNOWLEDGE DEFICIT related to SELF-ADMINISTRATION

Defining Characteristics: Fever curve or excessive fever can be masked by self-dosing with acetaminophen.

Nursing Implications: Instruct patient to report temperature over 38.3°C (101°F) or persistent or recurrent fever. Assess other over-the-counter (OTC) medicines the patient may be taking.

II. POTENTIAL INJURY related to HEPATOTOXICITY

Defining Characteristics: Excessive alcoholic intake and other drugs can increase risk for hepatotoxicity.

Nursing Implications: Assess total acetaminophen dosage/24 hours, taking into account OTC medications. Assess baseline LFTs, especially if the patient has primary hepatoma or liver metastasis. Teach patient to avoid excessive alcohol intake and/or excessive acetaminophen intake.

Drug: aspirin, acetylsalicylic acid (ASA, Aspergum, Bayer Aspirin, Easprin, Ecotrin, Empirin)

Class: Salicylate.

Mechanism of Action: Inhibits prostaglandin synthesis peripherally preventing sensitization of pain receptors by mechanical and chemical stimuli. Also, has anti-inflammatory effect, producing analgesic and antipyretic effects. Central action via hypothalamus unclear.

Metabolism: Rapidly and well absorbed from GI tract, and distributed throughout the body with high concentrations in liver and kidney. Drug is bound to serum proteins, especially albumin. Metabolized by liver and excreted in urine.

Dosage/Range:

- 325–650 mg PO or PR every 4 hours PRN for pain or fever (maximum 3.9 g/day).

Drug Preparation:

- Keep in closed container, away from heat, to prevent drug decomposition.
- Do not use if strong, vinegar-like odor is present. Do not crush enteric-coated aspirin.

Drug Administration:

- Oral or rectal suppositories. Give oral dose with 240 mL water or milk to decrease gastric irritation. Oral solution may be made from effervescent aspirin powders (e.g., Alka-Seltzer); Alka-Seltzer chewable aspirin tablets available.

Drug Interactions:

- Ammonium chloride, ascorbic acid, or methionine (urine acidifiers): Decrease ASA excretion, so increase risk of ASA toxicity.
- Antacids, urinary alkalizers: may increase ASA excretion, so may decrease the ASA effect. Alcohol increases the risk of GI ulceration, bleeding.
- Decreased effect of angiotensin-converting enzyme (ACE) inhibitors. When used together, the effect of anticoagulants may be enhanced (additive hypothrombinemic effect), leading to prolonged bleeding time. DO NOT USE TOGETHER.
- Beta-adrenergic blockers (e.g., propranolol): Possible decrease in antihypertensive effect.
- Corticosteroids: increase in aspirin excretion with decrease in aspirin effect.
- Methotrexate: increase in methotrexate serum levels with increased toxicity. DO NOT USE CONCURRENTLY.
- NSAIDs: decrease in NSAID serum concentration; may have increased incidence of GI side effects. Not recommended to be used together.
- Probenecid, sulfinpyrazone: aspirin (doses ≥ 3 g/day) antagonizes uricosuric drug effect.
- Spirolactone: aspirin may inhibit diuretic effect.
- Sulfonylureas, exogenous insulin: Aspirin may have hypoglycemic effect and may potentiate these drug actions. Monitor for hypoglycemia.
- Valproic acid: aspirin displaces drug and decreases its excretion, resulting in increased serum levels and possible valproic acid toxicity.

Lab Effects/Interference:

- Prolonged bleeding time, leukopenia, thrombocytopenia.

Special Considerations:

- Patients receiving myelosuppressive chemotherapy should be cautioned not to take aspirin due to increased risk of bleeding.
- Patients should be instructed to take drug with food or milk.
- Use cautiously in patients with asthma, rhinitis, or nasal polyps (can cause severe bronchospasm).
- Drug is contraindicated in patients with GI ulcer, GI bleeding, hypersensitivity to aspirin, increased bleeding tendencies.
- Use cautiously in patients with liver damage, hypoprothrombinemia, or with vitamin K deficiency.

Potential Toxicities/Side Effects and the Nursing Process

I. ALTERATION IN NUTRITION, LESS THAN BODY REQUIREMENTS, related to GI TOXICITY

Defining Characteristics: Nausea, dyspepsia (5–25% of patients), heartburn, epigastric discomfort, anorexia, and acute, reversible hepatotoxicity may occur. Risk increases with dose. May potentiate peptic ulcer disease.

Nursing Implications: Teach patient self-administration with 8 oz (240 mL) water or milk. If GI distress develops, discuss use of enteric-coated aspirin (e.g., Ecotrin). If patient receiving high doses of aspirin, monitor LFTs. Drug contraindicated in patients with peptic ulcer disease.

II. POTENTIAL FOR BLEEDING related to INHIBITION OF PLATELET AGGREGATION

Defining Characteristics: Aspirin may cause prolongation of bleeding time, leukopenia, thrombocytopenia, purpura, shortened erythrocyte survival time.

Nursing Implications: Teach patient to avoid aspirin and aspirin-containing drugs if receiving myelosuppressive chemotherapy. Review concurrent medications to identify risk for drug interactions. Monitor Hgb, HCT over time; teach patient signs/symptoms of anemia, and instruct to report them (headache, fatigue, chest pain, irritability). Monitor stool guaiacs.

III. INJURY related to MILD SALICYLISM

Defining Characteristics: Administration of large doses of salicylates may cause salicylism, characterized by dizziness, tinnitus, diminished hearing, nausea, vomiting, diarrhea, mental confusion, CNS depression, headache, sweating, and hyperventilation at serum salicylate concentration 150–300 μg/mL (use in cancer patients usually 100 μg/mL).

Nursing Implications: Teach patient to reduce dose, interrupt dose if signs/symptoms occur. Assess concurrent medications for possible drug interactions.

Drug: celecoxib (Celebrex®)

Class: Nonsteroidal anti-inflammatory drug.

Mechanism of Action: Drug has anti-inflammatory and antipyretic properties affected by inhibition of prostaglandin synthesis via selective inhibition of cyclooxygenase-2 (COX-2) pathway. It does not inhibit the cyclooxygenase-1 (COX-1) isoenzyme.

Metabolism: Following an oral dose, peak serum levels are reached at 3 hours, with a terminal half-life of 11 hours, and with multiple doses, steady-state is reached on or before 5 days. Drug is highly protein-bound (97%) and extensively distributed into tissue. Drug is metabolized in the liver via the cytochrome P450 2C9 system, with little unchanged drug recoverable in the urine or feces. Higher area under the curve (AUC) concentrations are found in the elderly (women > men), in African Americans, and in patients with moderate hepatic dysfunction.

Dosage/Range:

- Adults: 200 mg PO daily, or 100–200 mg PO.
- Patients with moderate hepatic dysfunction or weighing < 50 kg should get lowest dose.

Drug Preparation:

- Oral, available in 100-mg and 200-mg capsules.

Drug Administration:

- Administer orally in morning or evening, without regard to food.

Drug Interactions:

- Celecoxib inhibits cytochrome P450 2D6 system, so when given concurrently with drugs metabolized by this system, may result in increased doses of the second drug; also, celecoxib is metabolized primarily by P450 2C9 system, so if given concomitantly with drugs that inhibit this system, increased serum levels of celecoxib may result (e.g., fluconazole results in 2 × serum levels of celecoxib; use lowest dose possible of celecoxib, if at all).
- Angiotensin converting enzyme (ACE) inhibitors, e.g., lisinopril: may have decreased antihypertensive effect when used together.
- Furosemide, thiazide diuretics: reduced natriuretic effect due to inhibition of renal prostaglandin synthesis; assess diuretic effect and adjust dose as necessary.
- Lithium: use together cautiously, and monitor serum lithium levels if used together.
- Warfarin: monitor INR, PT closely, especially the first few days following initiation of celecoxib therapy or after changing the dose.
- Aspirin: low dose well tolerated, but higher doses may result in GI ulceration or other complications; use only together with low-dose aspirin.
- Methotrexate: no significant interaction.

Lab Effects/Interference:

- Increase in serum chloride, decrease in serum phosphate, and increased BUN; if there is GI bleeding, HCT and Hgb will be reduced. Also, rarely, borderline elevations of liver function tests (e.g., ALT, AST) may occur.

Special Considerations:

- Lowest doses should be used for individuals weighing < 50 kg or those with moderate hepatic impairment. DO NOT ADMINISTER to patients with severe hepatic impairment.

- DO NOT GIVE to pregnant women or nursing mothers unless benefits outweigh risk; DO NOT GIVE to women in last trimester of pregnancy.
- Celecoxib does not affect platelet aggregation or bleeding time. Studies showed significantly fewer GI ulcers in patients receiving celecoxib as compared to naproxen or ibuprofen.
- Indicated for the relief of signs and symptoms of osteoarthritis or rheumatoid arthritis in adults.
- Celecoxib is contraindicated in patients hypersensitive to celecoxib or allergic to sulfonamides, patients with severe hepatic disease, advanced renal disease, or patients who have or have had asthma, urticaria, or allergic-type reactions after taking aspirin or other NSAIDs, as anaphylaxis may occur.
- Use cautiously, if at all, in patients with preexisting asthma, preexisting kidney disease, fluid retention, cardiac failure, hypertension, prior history of ulcer disease or bleeding.

Potential Toxicities/Side Effects and the Nursing Process

I. ALTERATION IN NUTRITION, LESS THAN BODY REQUIREMENTS, related to GI SIDE EFFECTS

Defining Characteristics: Uncommon, but dyspepsia (8.8%), diarrhea (5.6%), abdominal pain (4.1%), nausea (3.4%), and flatulence (2.2%) have occurred. Rarely, the following may occur: diverticulitis, dysphagia, eructation, esophagitis, gastritis, gastroenteritis, gastroesophageal reflux, dry mouth, stomatitis, vomiting, tooth disorder, hemorrhoids, hiatal hernia, melena, vomiting, and tenesmus.

Nursing Implications: Assess history of GI symptoms and history of ulcer disease. Teach patient to take NSAID with meals or milk if possible. Teach patient potential side effects, to report them, and the importance of not taking aspirin. If symptoms are severe, discuss alternative NSAIDs with physician.

II. POTENTIAL FOR BLEEDING related to PEPTIC ULCERATION

Defining Characteristics: Although celecoxib causes fewer GI ulcers (< 0.1%), peptic ulceration and occult GI bleeding can occur and be life-threatening. Increased risk factors: most significant are presence or past history of peptic ulcer, and/or GI bleeding; other risk factors are: smoking, alcoholism, aspirin ingestion, oral corticosteroids, oral anticoagulants, longer duration of NSAID therapy, older age, poor general health status.

Nursing Implications: Assess risk, history of peptic ulcer disease or GI bleeding. Assess baseline Hgb, HCT and presence/absence of occult bleeding by guaiac of stools. Teach patient to report signs and symptoms of abdominal pain, black stools, blood per rectum, epistaxis, menorrhagia. If patient is at risk for bleeding, discuss use of misoprostol to protect GI mucosa with physician. Teach patient to avoid concurrent use of aspirin, other NSAIDs.

III. POTENTIAL SENSORY/PERCEPTUAL ALTERATIONS related to HEADACHE, DIZZINESS

Defining Characteristics: Headache (16%), insomnia (2.3%), dizziness (2%) may occur. Less commonly, migraine, neuralgia, neuropathy, paresthesia, vertigo, deafness, earache, tinnitus, taste perversion may occur.

Nursing Implications: Assess baseline neurologic and mental status. Teach patient to report changes in sensory/perceptual pattern. Teach patient symptom management of headache. If dizziness occurs, teach patient to change position slowly, and other safety measures. Discuss drug continuance with physician for significant symptoms.

IV. ALTERATION IN NUTRITION related to HEPATIC TOXICITY

Defining Characteristics: NSAIDs may cause elevations in LFTs, especially AST and ALK. Very rarely, severe hepatic reactions can occur: jaundice, fatal fulminant hepatitis, liver necrosis, hepatic failure, although this has not been reported with celecoxib.

Nursing Implications: Assess baseline LFTs and monitor periodically during long-term therapy. Teach patient to report the following symptoms immediately and to stop taking drug: nausea, fatigue, lethargy, itching, jaundice, tenderness in the RUQ, and flu-like symptoms, so that LFTs can be checked, as well as history and physical exam completed.

V. ALTERATION IN RENAL ELIMINATION related to INHIBITION OF RENAL PROSTAGLANDINS

Defining Characteristics: Long-term use of NSAIDs has rarely resulted in renal papillary necrosis. Rarely, acute renal failure (< 0.1%) may occur in patients with renal insufficiency or in patients with heart failure or liver dysfunction. The following have also been described: albuminuria, cystitis, dysuria, hematuria, urinary frequency, renal calculus, urinary incontinence, and urinary tract infection. Peripheral edema has also been described.

Nursing Implications: Assess baseline renal function. If patient has baseline renal insufficiency, use lowest dose possible initially and assess tolerance. Ensure that patient is well hydrated prior to beginning therapy with celecoxib. Teach patient to report any changes in urinary function, swelling of ankles, or weight gain. Monitor periodic serum BUN, creatinine during chronic therapy.

VI. POTENTIAL FOR INJURY related to ANAPHYLAXIS, ALLERGIC REACTION

Defining Characteristics: Although no patients developed anaphylactoid reactions while receiving celecoxib during clinical testing, there is a risk that this could occur, especially in patients with the "aspirin triad" (asthmatic patients who develop rhinitis with or without nasal polyps or who develop bronchospasm after taking aspirin or NSAIDs). Uncommonly, patients may develop rash, either erythematous or maculopapular (2.2%), dermatitis, photosensitivity reaction, pruritus, or urticaria.

Nursing Implications: Assess baseline allergies, including reaction to aspirin and/or NSAIDs. If patient has asthma and has had a reaction, the patient SHOULD NOT RECEIVE THIS DRUG. Assess baseline skin integrity and presence of lesions. Teach patient to stop drug and report rash immediately. Provide symptomatic relief for rash, pruritus.

Drug: choline magnesium trisalicylate (Trilisate)

Class: Choline and magnesium salicylate combination.

Mechanism of Action: Analgesic effect through peripheral and central pathways, decreasing pain perception. Prostaglandin inhibition probably involved in peripheral mechanism. Antipyretic effect via hypothalamic heat regulation center. Does not interfere with platelet aggregation.

Metabolism: Rapidly absorbed from GI tract. Metabolized by the liver and excreted in the urine.

Dosage/Range:
- Trilisate 750 mg bid or dose-increase to maximum 3200 mg/day.

Drug Preparation:
- Trilisate liquid 5 mL or Trilisate 500-mg tablet contains ASA equivalent of 650 mg.
- Trilisate 750-mg tablet contains 975 mg ASA.
- Trilisate 1000-mg tablet contains 1300 mg ASA.

Drug Administrations:
- Oral.

Drug Interactions:
- Antacids, urine alkalinizers: increase salicylate excretion and decrease drug effect. Do not administer with antacids.
- Ammonium chloride, ascorbic acid, methionine (urine acidifiers): decrease salicylate excretion, so increased risk of salicylate toxicity.

- Concomitant administration with alcohol, steroids, other NSAIDs may increase GI side effects.
- Corticosteroids: may increase salicylate excretion and decrease Trilisate effect.
- Warfarin: may have increased warfarin levels and increased PT; monitor patient closely, and reduce warfarin dosage as needed.

Lab Effects/Interference:

- Free T4 may be increased with a concurrent decrease in total plasma T4 (does not affect thyroid function).

Special Considerations:

- Drug does not interfere with platelet aggregation.
- Use cautiously in patients with chronic renal failure, gastritis.
- Contraindicated if known hypersensitivity to salicylates.
- Drug contains magnesium, so periodic evaluation of serum magnesium should be performed.

Potential Toxicities/Side Effects and the Nursing Process

I. ALTERATION IN NUTRITION, LESS THAN BODY REQUIREMENTS, related to GI TOXICITY

Defining Characteristics: Fewer GI side effects than aspirin. Nausea, dyspepsia (5–25% of patients), heartburn, epigastric discomfort, anorexia, and acute reversible hepatotoxicity may occur. Risk increases with dose. May potentiate peptic ulcer disease.

Nursing Implications: Teach patient self-administration with food, or 8 oz (240 mL) water or milk. If patient is receiving antacid, administer antacid two hours after meals and Trilisate before meals. Assess baseline liver and renal function and monitor if patient receiving high doses on ongoing basis. Guaiac stool to assess occult blood, as gastric ulceration may occur.

II. INJURY related to MILD SALICYLISM

Defining Characteristics: Administration of large doses of salicylates may cause salicylism, characterized by dizziness, tinnitus, diminished hearing, nausea, vomiting, diarrhea, mental confusion, CNS depression, headache, sweating, and hyperventilation at serum salicylate concentration 150–300 μg/mL (use in cancer patients usually 100 μg/mL).

Nursing Implications: Teach patient to reduce dose, interrupt dose if signs/symptoms occur. Assess concurrent medications for possible drug interactions.

III. POTENTIAL ALTERATION IN URINARY ELIMINATION related to RENAL PROSTAGLANDIN INHIBITION

Defining Characteristics: Rarely, elevated serum BUN and creatinine may occur.

Nursing Implications: Assess baseline serum BUN, creatinine, and monitor during therapy.

Drug: clonidine hydrochloride (Duraclon)

Class: Antiadrenergic agent.

Mechanism of Action: Acts centrally to stimulate alpha-2-adrenergic receptors in the CNS, thus inhibiting sympathetic vasomotor centers. When given epidurally, the drug is believed to mimic norepinephrine activity at presynaptic and postjunctional alpha-2-adrenoceptors in the dorsal horn of the spinal cord. Is administered together with opioids for severe cancer pain to maximize analgesia. Clonidine HCl shows best efficacy against neuropathic pain.

Metabolism: Drug is highly lipid-soluble and rapidly distributes into extravascular sites and into the CNS; enters the plasma via the epidural veins, leading to hypotensive effect. Drug is metabolized and excreted in the urine (72% of the administered dose in 96 hours, and 40–50% of that is unchanged drug).

Dosage/Range: *To be administered in combination with opioids via epidural route*:
- Initial: starting dose is 30 μg/hr.
- May be titrated up to 40 μg/hr or down, based on degree of pain relief and extent of side effects.

Drug Preparation:
- Preservative-free preparation.
- Given epidurally in combination with opioid via continuous epidural infusion device.

Drug Interactions:
- CNS depressants (e.g., alcohol, barbiturates): potentiation of CNS depression.
- Opioid analgesics: may potentiate hypotension due to clonidine.
- Tricyclic antidepressants: may antagonize hypotensive effect of clonidine.
- Beta-blockers: may exacerbate hypertensive symptoms of clonidine withdrawal.
- Epidural local anesthetics: clonidine may prolong pharmacologic effects of local anesthetic; both motor and sensory blockade.

Lab Effects/Interference:
- None known.

Special Considerations:

- Contraindicated in patients sensitive or allergic to clonidine HCl; epidural administration contraindicated if (1) injection site infection occurs, (2) patient is receiving anticoagulation, (3) patient has bleeding diathesis, (4) administered above the C4 dermatome, (5) patient has severe cardiac disease or is hemodynamically unstable, or (6) used in obstetrical or postoperative analgesia.
- Use cautiously in patients receiving digitalis, calcium-channel blockers, and beta-blockers, as there may be additive effects of bradycardia and AV block.
- Severe hypotension may occur during first 2 days of clonidine therapy, especially when drug is infused into the upper thoracic spinal segments—monitor vital signs frequently.
- Do not suddenly withdraw drug, as this may result in nervousness, agitation, headache, tremor, rapid increase in blood pressure; scrupulously maintain drug administration equipment to prevent accidental interruption of drug. Drug dose should be gradually decreased over 2–4 days. If patient is receiving a beta-blocker, the beta-blocker should be discontinued several days before the gradual discontinuation of epidural clonidine. Teach patient NOT to discontinue drug on own.

Potential Toxicities/Side Effects and the Nursing Process

I. ALTERED TISSUE PERFUSION related to HYPOTENSION

Defining Characteristics: Hypotension usually occurs within the first four days after beginning epidural clonidine but may also occur throughout treatment. Increased risk in patients receiving infusion into upper-thoracic spinal segments, in women, and in patients who have low body weight. Hypotension may be accentuated by concurrent opiate administration. Clonidine decreases sympathetic CNS outflow, decreasing peripheral resistance, decreasing renal vascular resistance, and decreasing heart rate and BP.

Nursing Implications: Monitor T, BP, HR frequently, especially during first few days of therapy. Notify physician of significant changes. Expect IV fluids to be given to correct hypotension, and if needed, IV ephedrine. Symptomatic bradycardia can be treated with atropine.

II. ALTERED TISSUE PERFUSION related to REBOUND HYPERTENSION

Defining Characteristics: Withdrawal symptoms can occur if drug is interrupted or stopped abruptly; characterized by nervousness, agitation, headache, tremor, rapid increase in BP. Increased risk in patients receiving high drug doses, patients receiving beta-blockers, or patients with a history of hypertension. Rarely, this may result in CVA, hypertensive encephalopathy, or death.

Nursing Implications: Scrupulously manage/maintain catheter and pump to prevent interruption in flow; teach patient catheter and pump care and use; instruct patient never to abruptly discontinue medicine; anticipate physician will discontinue beta-blockers prior to gradual taper of drug over 2–4 days when drug is being discontinued.

III. POTENTIAL FOR INFECTION related to IMPLANTED DEVICE

Defining Characteristics: Implanted epidural catheter may become infected, leading to epidural abscess or meningitis.

Nursing Implications: Scrupulously maintain catheter, using sterile technique; teach patient catheter care and management; monitor for signs/symptoms of infection and teach patient this assessment. If in the hospital, monitor for fever and pain and notify the physician immediately if either is found. Instruct patient to report fever, pain to the physician immediately if at home.

Drug: gabapentin (Neurontin)

Class: Anticonvulsant.

Mechanism of Action: Not clearly understood. Drug is structurally related to neurotransmitter GABA (gamma-amino-butyric acid), but drug does not bind to GABA receptor sites. It is unclear whether drug has activity at NMDA receptor sites. Drug has been shown to bind to receptor sites in neocortex and hippocampus.

Metabolism: Bioavailability of drug decreases as dose increases, and drug absorption unaffected by food. Drug half-life is 5–7 hours, and drug excreted unchanged in the urine. Plasma clearance may be reduced in elderly and is reduced in renal insufficiency.

Dosage/Range:
- Initial titration: 300 mg on day 1, 300 mg bid on day 2, and 300 mg tid on day 3.
- As needed, dose may be titrated up to 400 mg tid, in increments, to a maximum dose of 600 mg tid (1800 mg total dose per day).
- Dose-reduce in renal insufficiency:

Creatinine Clearance	Drug Dose
30–60 mL/min	300 mg bid
15–30 mL/min	300 mg/day
< 15 mL/min	300 mg every other day

Drug Preparation:
- Oral, take without regard to food intake.
- Take 1 hour before, or 2 hours after, antacid.
- Take initial dose at bedtime to enhance somnolence and minimize dizziness, fatigue and ataxia.
- Doses should not be separated by > 12 hours (must be tid, e.g., every 8 hours).
- If drug is discontinued or changed to another anticonvulsant, gradually discontinue drug over 1 week.

Drug Interactions:
- Antacids: decrease bioavailability of drug.
- Cimetidine: decreases renal excretion of drug with potential for excess toxicity; monitor patient closely and dose reduce if both drugs must be given concomitantly.

Lab Effects/Interference:
- Urinary protein test using Ames N-Multistix may be falsely positive.
- Drug may cause leukopenia, anemia, thrombocytopenia.

Special Considerations:
- Dose-reduce in patients with renal insufficiency, and consider dose reduction in the elderly.
- Drug helpful in the management of painful peripheral neuropathies.
- Drug may cause dizziness, fatigue, drowsiness, ataxia, so patient should be taught to avoid activities requiring mental acuity, such as driving, until after full effect of drug is known.

Potential Toxicities/Side Effects and the Nursing Process

I. SENSORY/PERCEPTUAL ALTERATIONS related to CNS CHANGES

Defining Characteristics: The most common side effects are somnolence, ataxia, dizziness, and fatigue. Less commonly, nystagmus, tremor, nervousness, dysarthria, amnesia, depression, abnormal thought processes, incoordination, headache, confusion, emotional lability, paresthesia, areflexia, anxiety, hostility, syncope, hypesthesia may occur. Seizures have been reported, as have suicidal tendencies. Other sensory side effects that rarely occur are diplopia, abnormal vision, dry eyes, photophobia, ptosis, and hearing loss.

Nursing Implications: Assess baseline neurological status and document. Instruct patient of general side effects that may occur, and to report them. Assess for suicidal ideation. If significant CNS changes occur, discuss dose reduction or change to an alternative drug with physician. Instruct patient not to drive a car or to do activities that require mental acuity until full effect of drug is known.

II. ALTERATION IN NUTRITION related to GI TOXICITY

Defining Characteristics: Nausea and vomiting may occur. Less commonly, dyspepsia, dry mouth, constipation, increased or decreased appetite, thirst, stomatitis, taste changes, increased salivation, fecal incontinence may occur.

Nursing Implications: Assess patient tolerance of GI side effects. Instruct patient to report side effects. If nausea and vomiting occur, discuss changing to another medication or adding antiemetic agent to regimen if relief of peripheral neuropathy is achieved.

III. ALTERATION IN SKIN INTEGRITY related to RASH

Defining Characteristics: Rash may occur, as may pruritus, acne, alopecia, hirsutism, herpes simplex, dry skin, and increased sweating.

Nursing Implications: Perform baseline skin assessment, and note any areas that are not intact. Teach patient to self-assess for rash, other changes, and to report them. If rash develops, instruct patient to notify provider immediately. If itch occurs, discuss symptomatic management.

IV. ALTERATION IN RESPIRATORY PATTERN related to RHINITIS, COUGH

Defining Characteristics: Rhinitis, pharyngitis, coughing, pneumonia, dyspnea may occur. Rarely, epistaxis and apnea have been reported.

Nursing Implications: Assess baseline respiratory pattern, and instruct patient to report any changes. Discuss any significant changes with physician, and discuss management versus change of drug.

V. ALTERATION IN URINARY ELIMINATION related to URINARY CHANGES

Defining Characteristics: Hematuria, dysuria, frequency, urinary incontinence, cystitis, urinary retention may occur.

Nursing Implications: Assess baseline urinary elimination pattern, and instruct patient of possible side effects and to report them. Discuss symptomatic management, or discuss drug change with physician if changes are significant.

VI. POTENTIAL FOR SEXUAL DYSFUNCTION related to VAGINAL CHANGES AND IMPOTENCE

Defining Characteristics: Vaginal hemorrhage, amenorrhea, dysmenorrhea, menorrhagia, inability to climax, abnormal ejaculation, and impotence have been reported.

Nursing Implications: Assess baseline sexuality, and instruct patient to report any changes. If changes occur, discuss impact and distress caused, and together with physician and patient, discuss drug alternatives.

VII. POTENTIAL ALTERATION IN OXYGENATION related to TACHYCARDIA, HYPOTENSION

Defining Characteristics: Rarely, hypertension, vasodilatation, hypotension, angina pectoris, peripheral vascular disease, palpitation, tachycardia, and appearance of a murmur may occur.

Nursing Implications: Assess baseline cardiovascular status, and instruct patient to notify provider if any changes occur. Instruct patient to report palpitations, fast heartbeat, dizziness, or chest pain immediately. If significant changes occur, discuss alternative drug therapy with physician.

Drug: ibuprofen (Advil, Genpril, Haltran, Ibuprin, Midol 200, Nuprin, Rufen)

Class: NSAID.

Mechanism of Action: Peripherally acting analgesic, anti-inflammatory, and antipyretic agent; anti-inflammatory action probably due to prostaglandin inhibition and/or release.

Metabolism: 80% of dose absorbed from GI tract, and absorption rate is slowed by administration with food. Peak serum concentrations with tablet occur in 2 hours; suspension in 1 hour. Highly protein bound (90–99%) and has a plasma half-life of 2–4 hours. Excreted in urine.

Dosage/Range:
- 200–800 mg every 4–8 hours PRN to maximum of 3200 mg/24 hours.

Drug Preparation:
- Tablets: 200 mg, 300 mg, 400 mg, 600 mg, 800 mg.
- Caplets: 200 mg.
- Oral suspension: 100 mg/5 mL.

Drug Administration:
- Oral.

Drug Interactions:
- Oral anticoagulants, thrombolytic agents: possible increase in PT with increased bleeding; use with caution and monitor patient closely.
- Other NSAIDs: possible increase in GI toxicity; do not administer concomitantly.
- Furosemide, thiazide diuretics: decreased diuretic effect when administered concomitantly.

Lab Effects/Interference:
- Slight decrease in Hgb not exceeding 1 g/dL without signs of bleeding; decrease in Hgb > 1 g/dL may be associated with signs of bleeding.

Special Considerations:
- Contraindicated in patients with known hypersensitivity, asthmatic patients with nasal polyps and other patients who develop bronchospasm or angioedema with aspirin or other NSAIDs, patients with peptic or duodenal ulcer.
- Use cautiously in patients with cardiac or renal dysfunction.

Potential Toxicities/Side Effects and the Nursing Process

I. ALTERATION IN NUTRITION, LESS THAN BODY REQUIREMENTS, related to GI SIDE EFFECTS

Defining Characteristics: Dyspepsia, heartburn, nausea, vomiting, anorexia, diarrhea, constipation, stomatitis, bloating, epigastric and abdominal pain may occur.

Nursing Implications: Assess history of GI symptoms and history of ulcer disease. Teach patient to take NSAID with meals or milk. Teach patient potential side effects, and instruct to report them. If symptoms are severe, discuss alternative NSAIDs with physician.

II. POTENTIAL FOR BLEEDING related to INHIBITION OF PLATELET AGGREGATION

Defining Characteristics: Drug can prolong bleeding time and inhibit platelet aggregation. Peptic ulceration and occult GI bleeding can occur and be life-threatening. Increased risk factors: smoking, alcoholism.

Nursing Implications: Assess risk, history of peptic ulcer disease or GI bleeding. Assess baseline Hgb, HCT, and presence/absence of occult bleeding by guaiac of stools. Instruct patient to report signs/symptoms of abdominal pain, black stools, blood per rectum, epistaxis, menorrhagia. If patient is at risk for bleeding, discuss with physician use of misoprostol to protect GI mucosa. Teach patient to avoid concurrent use of aspirin, other NSAIDs.

III. POTENTIAL SENSORY/PERCEPTUAL ALTERATIONS related to CNS CHANGES

Defining Characteristics: Dizziness, headache, nervousness, fatigue, drowsiness, malaise/light-headedness, anxiety, confusion, mental depression, and emotional lability may occur. Decreased hearing, visual acuity, changes in color vision, conjunctivitis, diplopia, and cataracts have been reported. In addition, though rare, aseptic meningitis has occurred.

Nursing Implications: Assess baseline neurologic and mental status. Instruct patient to report changes in sensory/perceptual pattern, especially VISUAL CHANGES. If visual changes occur, discuss with physician referral to ophthalmologist as soon as possible. Assess for rare occurrence of aseptic meningitis (fever, coma). Discuss drug continuance with physician for significant symptoms.

IV. ALTERATION IN NUTRITION, LESS THAN BODY REQUIREMENTS, related to HEPATIC TOXICITY

Defining Characteristics: Severe and sometimes fatal hepatotoxicity has occurred. Jaundice and hepatitis occur rarely. Borderline increase in LFTs occurs in 15% of patients, while values increase by three times in 1%.

Nursing Implications: Assess baseline LFTs and monitor periodically during long-term therapy. Instruct patient to report jaundice, abdominal pain. Discuss discontinuance of drug with physician for significant toxicity.

V. ALTERATION IN RENAL ELIMINATION related to INHIBITION OF RENAL PROSTAGLANDINS

Defining Characteristics: Acute renal failure may occur rarely within first few days of treatment in patients with preexisting renal dysfunction. Other signs/symptoms of renal dysfunction that may occur rarely are azotemia, cystitis, hematuria, increased serum BUN and creatinine, and decreased creatinine clearance. Peripheral edema has also been described.

Nursing Implications: Assess baseline renal function. Instruct patient to report any changes in urinary function. Monitor periodic serum BUN, creatinine during chronic therapy.

VI. ALTERATION IN SKIN INTEGRITY related to RASH

Defining Characteristics: Rash (urticaria, vesicles, or erythematous macular) may occur, as may Stevens-Johnson syndrome, flushes, alopecia, rectal itching, and acne.

Nursing Implications: Assess baseline skin integrity and presence of lesions. Teach patient to report abnormalities. Provide symptomatic relief for rashes, pruritus.

VII. POTENTIAL FOR FATIGUE AND INFECTION related to BONE MARROW INJURY

Defining Characteristics: Neutropenia, agranulocytosis, aplastic anemia, hemolytic anemia, and THROMBOCYTOPENIA may occur *rarely*.

Nursing Implications: Assess baseline CBC, WBC, differential, and platelet count. Discuss abnormalities with physician. Instruct patient to report severe fatigue, infection, bleeding. Monitor lab values periodically during treatment.

Drug: indomethacin (Indocin, Indocin SR, Indotech)

Class: NSAID, structurally related to sulindac.

Mechanism of Action: Actions similar to other NSAIDs: anti-inflammatory action, probably by inhibition of prostaglandin synthesis, as well as by inhibiting migration of leukocytes to infection site and stabilization of neutrophils so lysosomal enzymes can not be released; may also interfere with the production of autoantibodies (mediated by prostaglandins). Analgesic and antipyretic effects appear to result from inhibition of prostaglandin synthesis. Probably reduces tumor-associated fever by inhibition of synthesis of prostaglandin (PGE_1) in hypothalamus. However, drug has serious side effects, so should not be used routinely as an antipyretic.

Metabolism: Rapidly and completely absorbed from GI tract. When administered with food or antacid (aluminum and magnesium hydroxide), peak plasma drug concentrations may be slightly decreased or delayed. Drug is 99% bound to plasma proteins. Crosses BBB slightly, and placenta freely. Metabolized by liver, undergoes enterohepatic circulation, and is excreted in urine.

Dosage/Range:
- Capsules: 10 mg, 25 mg, 50 mg, 75 mg, given in 2–4 divided doses.
- Sustained release: 75 mg, given once or bid.
- Oral suspension: 25 mg/5 mL, given in 2–4 divided doses.
- Suppositories: 50 mg, given in 2–4 divided doses.

Drug Preparation:
- Drug is sensitive to light. Store capsules in well-closed containers at temperatures < 40°C (104°F).
- Oral suspension should be stored in tight, light-resistant containers at 30°C (86°F).
- Suppositories should be stored at temperatures < 30°C (86°F).

Drug Administration:
- Give with food or antacid to protect GI mucosa.
- Rectal suppository must remain in rectum for at least 1 hour for maximum absorption.
- Consider reduced dose in patients with renal dysfunction.
- Indocin suspension contains 1% alcohol.

Drug Interactions:

- Indomethacin can displace or be displaced by other protein-bound drugs: oral anticoagulants, hydantoins (e.g., phenytoin), salicylates, sulfonamides, sulfonylureas. Therefore, if taking any of these medications with indomethacin, the patient must be assessed for increased toxicity of each drug.
- Antihypertensive effect of hydralazine, captopril, furosemide, beta-adrenergic blockers, or thiazide diuretics may be decreased.
- NSAIDs: concurrent administration with salicylates does not improve drug effects but increases toxicity (GI, aplastic anemia) so should NOT be given concurrently. Diflunisal may decrease renal excretion of indomethacin and increase risk of GI hemorrhage; AVOID concurrent use.
- Triamterene: may precipitate renal failure. DO NOT USE CONCURRENTLY.
- Digoxin: serum levels may be increased and prolonged, so digoxin levels should be monitored closely.
- Methotrexate, especially HIGH DOSE: increased, prolonged serum methotrexate levels can be fatal; AVOID concurrent use.
- Potassium (K+) supplements, K+ sparing diuretics: indomethacin may increase serum K+ concentrations, especially in the elderly or patients with renal dysfunction. Use with caution and monitor K+ serum levels.
- Lithium: may increase plasma lithium levels; assess patient for lithium toxicity.
- Cyclosporine: possible increased nephrotoxicity; use with caution and monitor renal function.
- Probenecid: increased plasma level and therapeutic effects of indomethacin; decrease indomethacin dose.

Lab Effects/Interference:

- May prolong bleeding time.
- Rarely, hemolytic anemia, leukopenia, thrombocytopenia.

Special Considerations:

- Avoid use or use cautiously in the elderly or in patients with epilepsy, Parkinson's disease, renal dysfunction, mental illness.

Potential Toxicities/Side Effects and the Nursing Process

I. POTENTIAL SENSORY/PERCEPTUAL ALTERATIONS

Defining Characteristics: Dose-related headache occurs in 25–50% of patients (more severe in morning); may be associated with frontal throbbing, vomiting, tinnitus, ataxia, tremor, vertigo, and insomnia. Dizziness, depression, fatigue, and peripheral neuropathy may occur in 3–9% of patients; 1% of patients may have confusion, psychic disturbances, hallucinations, and nightmares. May accentuate epilepsy and Parkinson's disease symptomatology. Blurred vision, corneal and retinal damage, and hearing loss may occur with long-term use.

Nursing Implications: Assess baseline mental and neurologic status. Teach patient to report headache, changes in sensation or perception, and sleep problems. Discuss drug discontinuance with physician if neurologic side effects occur. Patients with visual disturbances or pain, or changes from baseline, should be seen by an ophthalmologist.

II. ALTERATION IN NUTRITION, LESS THAN BODY REQUIREMENTS, related to GI TOXICITY

Defining Characteristics: Nausea, with or without vomiting and indigestion, heartburn, and epigastric pain occur in ~ 10% of patients. Diarrhea, abdominal pain/distress, and constipation may occur in ~ 3%. Other effects occurring in ~ 1% are anorexia, distension, flatulence, gastroenteritis, rectal bleeding, stomatitis. Severe GI bleeding may occur in 1% of patients, as drug decreases platelet aggregation.

Nursing Implications: Teach patient potential side effects and to self-administer drug with food or antacid. Teach patient to avoid OTC aspirin-containing drugs, alcohol, or steroids, all of which can increase GI toxicity and risk for GI bleeding. Instruct patient to report any signs/symptoms of GI bleeding, abdominal pain immediately, and to stop taking the drug. Guaiac stool for occult blood periodically. If drug must be used, and risk of GI ulceration is high, discuss with physician use of misoprostol to protect the GI mucosa.

III. POTENTIAL FOR INFECTION, FATIGUE, BLEEDING related to BONE MARROW INJURY

Defining Characteristics: Although rare (1%), potential toxicities include hemolytic anemia, bone marrow depression (leukopenia, thrombocytopenia), aplastic anemia, thrombocytopenic purpura. Drug inhibits platelet aggregation but this will reverse to normal within 24 hours of drug discontinuance. May prolong bleeding time, especially in patients with underlying bleeding problems.

Nursing Implications: Assess all medicines the patient is taking and teach patient to avoid OTC aspirin-containing drugs. Teach patient to self-assess and instruct to report signs/symptoms of bleeding, fatigue, and infection.

IV. POTENTIAL FOR ALTERATION IN ELIMINATION PATTERN related to RENAL DYSFUNCTION

Defining Characteristics: Acute interstitial nephritis with hematuria, proteinuria, nephrotic syndrome may occur in 1% of patients. Patients with renal dysfunction may have worsening of renal function. Increased K+ levels may occur in the elderly or in patients with renal dysfunction. Risk increases with long-term therapy.

Nursing Implications: Assess baseline renal status. Discuss alternate drugs if renal dysfunction. Monitor serum K+, sodium (Na+), especially if receiving other drugs that affect serum K+ level (e.g., amphotericin, diuretics), or in the elderly.

V. POTENTIAL FOR ALTERATION IN CARDIAC OUTPUT related to CARDIAC EFFECTS

Defining Characteristics: CHF, tachycardia, chest pain, arrhythmias, palpitations, hypertension, and edema may occur in < 1% of patients.

Nursing Implications: Assess baseline cardiovascular status and monitor periodically while receiving the drug. Assess efficacy of antihypertensive medication due to possible drug interaction.

VI. POTENTIAL FOR INJURY related to DERMATOLOGIC AND SENSITIVITY REACTIONS

Defining Characteristics: Dermatologic effects occur in < 1% of patients and include pruritus, urticaria, rash, exfoliative dermatitis, and Stevens-Johnson syndrome. Allergic reactions occur in < 1%, characterized by asthma in aspirin-sensitive individuals, dyspnea, fever, acute anaphylaxis.

Nursing Implications: Assess baseline dermatologic, pulmonary status, and continue during drug use. Instruct patient to report any adverse reactions immediately.

Drug: ketorolac tromethamine (Toradol)

Class: NSAID.

Mechanism of Action: Inhibits prostaglandin synthesis peripherally to exert analgesic, anti-inflammatory, and antipyretic activity.

Metabolism: Drug completely absorbed following PO or IM administration of the drug, with peak serum levels in 44 minutes and 50 minutes, respectively. Drug is extensively bound to serum protein (99%). Terminal half-life is 2.4–9.2 hours. Excreted by the kidney.

Dosage/Range:

- Single dose: IM, 60 mg; IV, 30 mg.
- Multiple doses: IM/IV, 30 mg q 6 h (maximum daily dose is 120 mg).
- 50% dose reduction for patients aged ≥ 65 years, renal impaired, or weight < 50 kg.
- Oral: for continuation therapy.

- Patients < 65 years old: 20 mg × 1, then 10 mg q 4–6 h (max 40 mg/24 hours).
- Patients ≥ 65: 10 mg q 4–6 h (max 40 mg/24 hours).
- MAXIMUM USE OF KETOROLAC IS 5 DAYS.

Drug Preparation:
- Store at controlled room temperature of 15–30°C (59–86°F) and protect from light.

Drug Administration:
- PO, IM, or IV.

Drug Interactions:
- Other salicylates: displace ketorolac from protein binding. DO NOT USE together or dose-reduce ketorolac.
- Anticoagulants: possible increase in bleeding time; use with caution and monitor closely.
- Furosemide: decreased diuretic response; need to increase diuretic dose.
- Probenecid: causes prolonged, increased serum ketorolac levels; use cautiously, and reduce dose.
- Lithium, methotrexate: theoretically increased serum levels, so should be dose-reduced if given with ketorolac.

Lab Effects/Interference:
- None known.

Special Considerations:
- Drug indicated for the treatment of ACUTE, short-term pain, not chronic pain.
- Concurrent use with other NSAIDs NOT recommended due to risk of additive toxicity.
- Contraindicated in persons with hypersensitivity to ketorolac, or patients with asthma, nasal polyps, angioedema, and bronchospastic reaction to aspirin or other NSAIDs; also in patients with active peptic ulcer disease or GI bleeding, and patients with advanced renal insufficiency.

Potential Toxicities/Side Effects and the Nursing Process

I. ALTERATION IN NUTRITION, LESS THAN BODY REQUIREMENTS, related to GI SIDE EFFECTS

Defining Characteristics: Dyspepsia, heartburn, nausea, vomiting, anorexia, diarrhea, constipation, stomatitis, bloating, epigastric and abdominal pain may occur.

Nursing Implications: Assess history of GI symptoms and history of ulcer disease. Teach patient to take NSAID with meals or milk. Teach patient potential side effects and instruct to report them. If symptoms are severe, discuss alternative NSAIDs with physician.

II. POTENTIAL FOR BLEEDING related to INHIBITION OF PLATELET AGGREGATION

Defining Characteristics: Drug can prolong bleeding time and inhibit platelet aggregation. Peptic ulceration and occult GI bleeding can occur and be life-threatening. Increased risk factors: smoking, alcoholism.

Nursing Implications: Assess risk, history of peptic ulcer disease or GI bleeding. Assess baseline Hgb, HCT and presence/absence of occult bleeding by guaiac of stools. Instruct patient to report signs/symptoms of abdominal pain, black stools, blood per rectum, epistaxis, menorrhagia. If patient at risk for bleeding, discuss with physician use of misoprostol to protect GI mucosa. Teach patient to avoid concurrent use of aspirin, other NSAIDs.

III. POTENTIAL SENSORY/PERCEPTUAL ALTERATIONS related to CNS CHANGES

Defining Characteristics: Dizziness, headache, nervousness, fatigue, drowsiness, malaise/light-headed ness, anxiety, confusion, mental depression, and emotional lability may occur. Decreased hearing, visual acuity, changes in color vision, conjunctivitis, diplopia, and cataracts have been reported. In addition, though rare, aseptic meningitis has occurred.

Nursing Implications: Assess baseline neurologic and mental status. Instruct patient to report changes in sensory/perceptual pattern, especially VISUAL CHANGES. If visual changes occur, discuss with physician referral to ophthalmologist as soon as possible. Assess for rare occurrence of aseptic meningitis (fever, coma). Discuss drug continuance with physician for significant symptoms.

Equianalgesic Dosing:

Ketorolac	Meperidine		Morphine
IM			
30 or 90 mg	100 mg		12 mg
10 mg	50 mg		6 mg
Ketorolac	**Ibuprofen**	**Aspirin**	**Acetaminophen**
PO			
10 mg	400 mg	650 mg	600 mg

IV. ALTERATION IN NUTRITION, LESS THAN BODY REQUIREMENTS, related to HEPATIC TOXICITY

Defining Characteristics: Severe and sometimes fatal hepatotoxicity has occurred. Jaundice and hepatitis occur rarely. Borderline increase in LFTs occurs in 15% of patients, while values increase by three times in 1%.

Nursing Implications: Assess baseline LFTs and monitor periodically during long-term therapy. Instruct patient to report jaundice, abdominal pain. Discuss discontinuance of drug with physician for significant toxicity.

V. ALTERATION IN RENAL ELIMINATION related to INHIBITION OF RENAL PROSTAGLANDINS

Defining Characteristics: Acute renal failure may occur rarely within first few days of treatment in patients with preexisting renal dysfunction. Other signs/symptoms of renal dysfunction that may occur rarely are azotemia, cystitis, hematuria, increased serum BUN and creatinine, and decreased creatinine clearance. Peripheral edema has also been described.

Nursing Implications: Assess baseline renal function. Teach patient to report any changes in urinary function. Monitor periodic serum BUN, creatinine during chronic therapy.

VI. ALTERATION IN SKIN INTEGRITY related to RASH

Defining Characteristics: Rash (urticaria, vesicles, or erythematous macular) may occur, as may Stevens-Johnson syndrome, flushes, alopecia, rectal itching, and acne.

Nursing Implications: Assess baseline skin integrity and presence of lesions. Instruct patient to report abnormalities. Provide symptomatic relief for rashes, pruritus.

VII. POTENTIAL FOR FATIGUE AND INFECTION related to BONE MARROW INJURY

Defining Characteristics: Neutropenia, agranulocytosis, aplastic anemia, hemolytic anemia, and thrombocytopenia may occur rarely.

Nursing Implications: Assess baseline CBC, WBC, differential, and platelet count. Discuss abnormalities with physician. Instruct patient to report severe fatigue, infection, bleeding. Monitor lab values periodically during treatment.

Drug: pregabalin (Lyrica)

Class: Anti-convulsant, analgesic for peripheral neuropathy.

Mechanism of Action: Unknown, but believed to reduce the calcium-dependent release of several neurotransmitters, possibly by modulating the calcium channel function. In neuropathic pain, voltage-gated calcium channels let extra calcium into the neuron ending, which then binds to vesicles containing pain-causing chemicals (neurotransmitters). The vesicles then migrate to the neuronal membrane, and secrete them into the nerve endings. Pregabalin binds with the alpha$_2$-delta site (axillary subunit of the voltage-gated calcium channel) in CNS tissues (but not cardiac-related, voltage-gated calcium channels).

Metabolism: Well absorbed from GI tract with peak plasma levels in 1.5 hours; bioavailability is > .90% independent of dose. Drug does not bind to plasma proteins. Steady state is reached in 24–48 hours. Drug is not metabolized in the body, and 90% of intact drug is eliminated in the urine. Because of this, drug elimination rate is proportional to the creatinine clearance, so drug dose must be reduced in patients with renal compromise. Drug crosses blood–brain barrier in laboratory animals, so is presumed to do so in humans. The drug has an elimination half-life of 6 hours.

Dosage/Range:

- Diabetic peripheral neuropathy: Begin dosing at 50 mg PO tid, and increase to 100 mg PO tid over 1 week, with or without food, based on response and tolerability, in patients with creatinine clearance of > 60 mL/minute. Dose reduce for patients with creatinine clearance < 60 mL/minute.
- Postherpetic neuralgia: Begin dosing at 75 mg PO bid or 50 mg PO tid; may increase to 300 mg PO total dose over the course of 1 week based on response and tolerability, to 75–150 mg PO bid or 50–100 mg PO tid in patients with creatinine clearance of > 60 mL/minute. Dose reduce for patients with creatinine clearance < 60 mL/minute.
- Postherpetic neuralgia: Patients who do not experience adequate pain relief after 2–4 weeks of treatment, and who tolerate the drug well, can have their dose gradually increased to 300 mg PO bid or 200 mg PO tid.
- Epilepsy: Begin with a total daily dose of 150 mg PO total daily dose (either 75 mg PO bid or 50 mg PO tid) and gradually titrated up based on patient response and tolerability to a maximum daily dose of 600 mg PO/day (e.g., 150–600 mg PO as a total daily dose, given in equally divided doses either bid or tid).
- Patients with renal impairment: Dose should be reduced 50% if creatinine clearance is 30–60 mL/minute, another 50% if creatinine clearance is 15–30 mL/minute, and a further 50% if < 15 mL/minute (see package insert).
- If patient is being hemodialyzed, see package insert for supplementary doses.

Drug Preparation:

- Available 25-, 50-, 75-, 100-, 150-, 200-, 225-, 300-mg capsules.
- Oral; take with food or on an empty stomach.
- Teach patients to keep medication in a safe place, out of reach of children and pets.

Drug Interactions: None.

Lab Effects/Interference:
- ↑ Creatine kinase in 2% of patients.
- ↓ Platelets (20% below baseline in 3% of patients).
- ECG changes: PR interval prolongation by 3–6 msec.

Special Considerations:
- Drug is indicated for the management of neuropathic pain associated with diabetic peripheral neuropathy and post-herpetic neuralgia; also indicated as an adjunctive therapy for adult patients with partial onset seizures.
- As with any anti-elliptic drugs, the drug should be withdrawn gradually to minimize the potential of increased seizure frequency in patients with seizure disorders. If discontinued, the drug should be gradually reduced in dose over at least 1 week.
- Abrupt discontinuation of drug may result in insomnia, headache, nausea, and diarrhea (discontinue over a minimum of 1 week).
- Although uncommon, 2% of patients had creatine kinase > 3 times the ULN; patients should be taught to report immediately unexplained muscle pain or tenderness, especially if these muscle symptoms are associated with malaise or fever so that they can be further evaluated, and rhabdomyolysis or myopathy ruled out. Discontinue drug if myopathy is suspected or confirmed, or if patient develops markedly elevated creatine kinase.

Potential Toxicities/Side Effects and the Nursing Process

I. SENSORY/PERCEPTUAL ALTERATIONS related to CNS CHANGES

Defining Characteristics: The most common side effects are somnolence (22%), dizziness (29%), blurred vision (6%), abnormal thinking (concentration and attention). Somnolence and dizziness start right after the drug is initiated, increase in frequency as the dose is increased, and may persist throughout treatment. Less commonly, ataxia, vertigo, confusion, diplopia, euphoria, incoordination, and amnesia may occur. Increased sleepiness and dizziness if taking concomitant opioids for pain, alcohol, or anti-anxiety/sedatives.

Nursing Implications: Assess baseline neurological status and document. Instruct patient of general side effects that may occur, and to report them as well as any changes that may occur, such as reduced visual acuity. Assess for suicidal ideation. If significant CNS changes occur, discuss dose reduction or change to an alternative drug with physician. Instruct patient not to drive a car or to do activities that require mental acuity until full effect of drug is known. If blurred vision, dizziness, or weakness occurs, teach patient to report this immediately.

II. ALTERATION IN NUTRITION related to GI TOXICITY

Defining Characteristics: Gastroenteritis and increased appetite with weight gain (7% over baseline over 13 weeks) may occur. Weight gain of diabetic patients averaged 1.6 kg. Less commonly, cholecystitis, cholelithiasis, colitis, dysphagia, esophagitis, gastritis, GI hemorrhage, melena, mouth ulceration, pancreatitis, rectal hemorrhage, and tongue edema may occur. Rarely, aphthous stomatitis may occur.

Nursing Implications: Assess patient tolerance of GI side effects. Instruct patient to report side effects. Discuss symptomatic management depending upon symptoms. If patient is also taking rosiglitazone (Avandia) or pioglitazone (Actos), counsel about increased risk of weight gain.

III. ALTERATION IN SKIN INTEGRITY related to PRURITIS, EDEMA

Defining Characteristics: Pruritus is common; infrequently, patients may develop alopecia, dry skin, eczema, hirsutism, skin ulcer, urticaria, or vesiculobullous rash. Rarely, patients may develop exfoliative dermatitis. Edema, principally peripheral edema, occurs in 6% of patients, especially in diabetic patients taking thiazolidinedione antidiabetic agents (these drugs in and of themselves can cause fluid retention and weight gain).

Nursing Implications: Perform baseline skin assessment, and note any areas that are not intact, are swollen, or itch. Teach patient to self-assess for itch, swelling, other changes, and to report them. If rash develops, instruct patient to notify provider immediately. If itch occurs, discuss symptomatic management.

IV. ALTERATION IN COMFORT related to ARTHRALGIA, LEG CRAMPS, MYALGIA, EDEMA, PERIPHERAL EDEMA, ECCHYMOSIS, ABDOMINAL PAIN

Defining Characteristics: Although not common, arthralgias, leg cramps, myalgias, ecchymosis, and abdominal pain can occur.

Nursing Implications: Perform baseline comfort assessment, and teach patient to report these side effects if they occur. Develop a plan for symptomatic relief.

Drug: salsalate (Disalcid, Salsalate, Salflex)

Class: Salicylic acid derivative, NSAID.

Mechanism of Action: Hydrolyzed into two molecules of salicylic acid. Has central and peripheral action that decreases pain perception, probably through inhibition of prostaglandin synthesis. Anti-inflammatory action via prostaglandin inhibition.

Metabolism: Absorbed completely from small intestines and widely distributed into body tissues and fluids. Elimination half-life is 1 hour. Metabolized by liver and excreted in urine. Drug DOES NOT accumulate in plasma after multiple doses, unlike salicylates.

Dosage/Range:
- 500 mg q 4 h or 750 mg q 6 h, to maximum 3 g/24 hours.

Drug Preparation:
- Not significant.

Drug Administration:
- Oral: Administer with food or 8 oz (240 mL) of water or milk.

Drug Interactions:
- Antacids, urine alkalinizers: increase salicylate excretion and decrease drug effect. Do not administer with antacids.
- Ammonium chloride, ascorbic acid, methionine (urine acidifiers): decrease salicylate excretion, so increase risk of salicylate toxicity.
- Concomitant administration with alcohol, steroids, other NSAIDs may increase GI side effects.
- Corticosteroids may increase salicylate excretion and decrease drug effect.

Lab Effects/Interference:
- Competes with thyroid hormone for protein binding, so plasma T4 may be decreased but thyroid function is unaffected.

Special Considerations:
- Use cautiously if patient has history of GI bleeding, hepatic dysfunction, renal dysfunction, hypoprothrombinemia, vitamin K deficiency, bleeding hypersensitivity.
- Contraindicated if known Salsalate hypersensitivity.

Potential Toxicities/Side Effects and the Nursing Process

I. ALTERATION IN NUTRITION, LESS THAN BODY REQUIREMENTS, related to GI TOXICITY

Defining Characteristics: Fewer GI side effects than aspirin. Nausea, dyspepsia (5–25% of patients), heartburn, epigastric discomfort, anorexia, and acute reversible hepatotoxicity may occur. Risk increases with dose. May potentiate peptic ulcer disease.

Nursing Implications: Teach patient self-administration with food or 8 oz (240 mL) water or milk. If patient is receiving antacid, administer antacid two hours after meal and Salsalate before meal. Assess baseline liver and renal function, and monitor if patient is receiving high doses on ongoing basis.

II. INJURY related to MILD SALICYLISM

Defining Characteristics: Administration of large doses of salicylates may cause salicylism, characterized by dizziness, tinnitus, diminished hearing, nausea, vomiting, diarrhea, mental confusion, CNS depression, headache, sweating, and hyperventilation at serum salicylate concentration 150–300 μg/mL (use in cancer patients usually 100 μg/mL).

Nursing Implications: Teach patient to reduce dose, interrupt dose if signs/symptoms occur. Assess concurrent medications for possible drug interactions.

III. POTENTIAL FOR BLEEDING related to INHIBITION OF PLATELET AGGREGATION, OCCULT BLEEDING, BRUISING

Defining Characteristics: Salsalate may cause prolongation of bleeding time, leukopenia, thrombocytopenia, purpura, shortened erythrocyte survival time.

Nursing Implications: Teach patient to avoid aspirin and Salsalate-containing drugs if receiving myelosuppressive chemotherapy. Review concurrent medications to identify risk for drug interactions. Monitor Hgb, HCT over time; teach patient signs/symptoms of anemia, and instruct to report them (headache, fatigue, chest pain, irritability). Monitor stool guaiacs.

IV. POTENTIAL FOR INJURY related to ALLERGIC REACTION

Defining Characteristics: Rash; hypersensitivity characterized by asthma and anaphylaxis has occurred rarely.

Nursing Implications: Assess for reactions to prior salicylate-containing medications or salsalates. Teach patient to report rash, asthma-like symptoms. If these occur, discuss alternative non-opioid analgesics. Provide systemic support if anaphylaxis occurs.

Drug: ziconotide intrathecal infusion (Prialt)

Class: Selective blocker of neuronal N-type calcium channels in the nerves that normally conduct pain signals from the periphery to the spinal cord.

Mechanism of Action: Synthetic equivalent to a naturally occurring conopeptide found in a marine snail (*Conus magus*), which binds to N-type calcium channels on the primary afferent nerves (A-δ and C) of the dorsal horn of the spinal cord. Voltage sensitive calcium channels (VSCC) permit the cell to regulate the amount of calcium entering and leaving the cell; this directly influences membrane excitability, among other cellular processes. Ziconotide appears to block these channels so that pain messages from the periphery do not get passed through to the spinal cord and up the spinal cord where pain perception occurs.

Metabolism: Following 1 hour IT administration of 1–10 micrograms of drug, total and peak exposure were variable but dose proportional; as a continuous IT infusion, once a quantifiable serum level of drug is identified, the serum level remains constant at least up to 9 months. Drug is 50% bound to human plasma proteins, and CSF volume of distribution is the same as the total CSF volume of 140 mL. Terminal half-life in the CSF is 4.6 hours, and is cleared from the CSF at approximately the human CSF turnover rate of 0.3–0.4 mL/min. Drug passes across the blood–brain barrier into systemic circulation with a serum half-life of 1.3 hours. Drug is cleaved at multiple sites of the peptide; it is degraded via the ubiquitin-protease system in many organs (kidney, liver, lung) into component amino acids. < 1% of intact ziconotide is recovered in the urine.

Dosage/Range:

- Initial dose no more than 2.4 micrograms (mcg)/day (0.1 mcg/hr) and titrated to patient response.
- Increase dose by up to 2.4 mcg/day (0.1 mcg/hr) at intervals of no more than 2–3 times/week based on patient response, up to recommended MAXIMUM of 19.2 mcg/day (0.8 mcg/hr) by day 21.
- May use dose increases in increments of less than 2.4 mg/day less frequently than 2–3 times a week.
- With each dosage titration ensure that the pump infusion rate is adjusted correctly (either implanted microinfusion device or external microinfusion device and catheter).
- Available in 1, 2, 5 mL vials (100 micrograms/mL) for diluted use; and 20 mL vial (25 micrograms/mL) for undiluted use.
- Diluted ziconotide: use 0.9% sodium chloride injection USP (preservative free) using aseptic procedures to achieve pump manufacturer's recommended concentration.
- Once the appropriate dose has been established, the 100 micrograms/mL formulation may be used undiluted.
- Store unopened vials at 2°C–8°C (36°F–46°F) but do not freeze; Refrigerate (2°C–8°C) after preparation, protect from light, and use within 24 hours.
- **Initial (naïve) pump priming:** use 2 mL of undiluted 25-mcg/mL formulation to rinse the internal surfaces of the pump; repeat 2 × more for a total of 3 rinses.
- **Initial pump fill:** Use undiluted 25 mcg/mL ONLY to fill the naïve pump after priming; begin dosing NO HIGHER than 2.4 micrograms/day (0.1 micrograms/hr). Initial pump fill loses drug through adsorption on internal device surfaces and by dilution in the residual space in the device—this does not occur with subsequent pump filling. Refill the pump reservoir within 14 days of the initial fill to ensure accurate drug administration.

- **Pump Refills:** Fill the pump at least every 40 days if used diluted; if undiluted drug, fill the pump at least every 60 days. Use the Medtronic refill kit to empty the pump contents prior to refill with new drug. If an implanted pump must be surgically replaced while the patient is receiving the drug, the replacement pump should be primed, and the initial drug replaced in 14 days as above.

Drug Preparation:

Ziconotide IT infusion	Initial Fill (expiration)	Refill (expiration)
25 mcg/mL undiluted	14 days	60 days
100 mcg/mL undiluted	N/A	60 days
100 mcg/mL, diluted	N/A	60 days

Drug Preparation:

- Refer to manufacturer's pump manual for specific instructions. When using an external microinfusion device, and filling it the first time, use a concentration of 5 mcg/mL; dilute drug with 0.9% sodium chloride USP (preservative free); the flow rate for the external microinfusor usually starts at 0.02 mL/hr to deliver the initial dose rate of 2.4 mcg/day (0.1 mcg/hr).

Drug Administration:

- Continuous IT infusion via Medronic SynchroMed® EL (Medtronic Inc), SynchroMed® II Infusion System (Medtronic Inc), Simms Deltec Cadd Micro® (Ardus Medical, Inc.) External Microinfusion Device and Catheter pumps.
- Most patients continue to receive opioids.
- There is no known antidote for the drug; if overdosage, most patients recover within 24 hours after drug withdrawal; if inadvertent IV or epidural injection of drug, support blood pressure by recumbent positioning, and BP support as needed.

Drug Interactions:

- Additive effect when given with opioid medications as drug does not bind to opiate receptors.
- CNS depressant drugs: increased incidence of CNS adverse events (e.g., dizziness, confusion).

Lab Effects/Interference:

- Increased serum creatine kinase levels (40% of patients), which may be associated with muscle weakness; rare renal failure related to rhabdomyolysis and very high CK elevations.

Special Consideration:

- Severe psychiatric symptoms and neurological impairment may occur during ziconotide IT infusion; patients with a history of psychosis should NOT receive the drug; monitor patients frequently for signs/symptoms of cognitive impairment, hallucinations, or changes in mood or level of consciousness; interrupt or discontinue drug for severe psychiatric or neurological symptoms/signs.

- Drug can be interrupted or discontinued abruptly without risk of withdrawal syndrome.
- Drug is embryotoxic in animals.
- Use cautiously in elderly patients as incidence of confusion is higher; start at lower dose and titrate more slowly.
- Patients should be taught not to engage in hazardous activity, such as operation of heavy machinery.
- Patients should notify provider IMMEDIATELY for any of the following:
  - Change in mental status such as lethargy, confusion, disorientation, decreased alertness.
  - Change in mood or perception, such as hallucinations (e.g., unusual tactile sensations in oral cavity).
  - Symptoms of depression or suicidal ideation.
  - Nausea, vomiting, seizures, fever, headache, and/or stiff neck, as these may herald developing meningitis.

Potential Toxicities/Side Effects and the Nursing Process

I. SENSORY/PERCEPTUAL ALTERATIONS related to CNS CHANGES

Defining Characteristics: CNS depression and changes in mental status may occur, including psychiatric symptoms, cognitive impairment and decreased alertness/unresponsiveness. These are characterized by confusion (33%, with a higher incidence in the elderly), memory impairment (22%), speech disorder (14%), aphasia (12%), abnormal thinking (8%), and amnesia (1%). Psychiatric symptoms are more likely to occur in patients with pretreatment psychiatric disorders, and include hallucinations (12%), paranoid ideation (2%), hostility (2%), delirium (2%), psychosis (1%), and manic reactions (0.4%). Cognitive impairment may be gradual a few weeks after starting therapy. Once dose is interrupted or discontinued, symptoms usually resolve in 2 weeks. Patients may become depressed with suicidal ideation. Other sensory/perceptual alterations include: dizziness (47%), somnolence (22%), abnormal vision (22%), ataxia (16%), abnormal gait (15%), hypertonia (11%), nystagmus (8%), dysesthesia (7%), paresthesia (7%), and vertigo (7%).

Nursing Implications: Assess past medical history for psychiatric and neurological problems. Assess baseline gait, movement, mental, affective, and neurologic status. Assess medication profile to identify other contributions, i.e., CNS depressants, antiepileptics, neuroleptics, sedatives, diuretics. Teach patient and family that these side effects may occur, and instruct patient/family to report any changes. Teach patient/family to notify provider IMMEDIATELY for any of the following:

- Change in mental status such as lethargy, confusion, disorientation, decreased alertness.
- Change in mood or perception, such as hallucinations (e.g., unusual tactile sensations in oral cavity).
- Symptoms of depression or suicidal ideation.

Assess patient safety and measures to ensure safety. Discuss any significant changes with physician and need to interrupt/discontinue drug based on severity of symptoms.

OPIOID ANALGESICS

Drug: codeine (as Sulfate or Phosphate); may be combined with acetaminophen (Phenaphen with Codeine, Tylenol with Codeine, *nl Capital and Codeine, Codaphen [Odalan], or with aspirin (Empirin with Codeine, Soma Compound with Codeine, Fiorinal with Codeine)

Class: Opioid analgesic (opioid agonist).

Mechanism of Action: Resembles morphine but has milder action; binds to opiate receptors in CNS (limbic system, thalamus, striatum, hypothalamus, midbrain, spinal cord), altering pain perception at level of spinal cord and higher centers, as well as the emotional response to pain. Also suppresses cough reflex.

Metabolism: Well absorbed after oral or parenteral administration. Metabolized by liver; excreted in urine, and small amount in feces.

Dosage/Range:
- Mild pain: 30 mg q 4 h (range 15–60 mg), PO, subcutaneous, or IM.

Drug Preparation:
- Store tablets in tight, light-resistant containers at 15–30°C (59–86°F).
- Injection should be protected from light and stored at 15–40°C (59–104°F).
- At home, teach patient to store oral doses in a safe place away from children and pets.

Drug Administration:
- PO, subcutaneous, IM.

Drug Interactions:
- Injection is incompatible with solutions containing aminophylline, ammonium chloride, amobarbital sodium, chlorothiazide sodium, heparin sodium, methicillin sodium, nitrofurantoin, phenobarbital sodium, sodium bicarbonate.
- Alcohol, CNS depressants: additive effects.

Lab Effects/Interference:
- None known.

Special Considerations:
- Parenteral dose is 2/3 oral dose for equianalgesic effect.
- Onset of action after PO or subcutaneous dose is 15–30 minutes, with duration of analgesia 4–6 hours.
- Indicated for relief of mild-to-moderate pain unrelieved by nonopiate analgesia.
- Addition of acetaminophen or aspirin gives additive analgesia.

- Give smallest effective dose to prevent development of tolerance, physical dependency.
- Reduce dose in debilitated patients, or patients receiving other CNS depressants.
- Use with caution in patients with hepatic or renal dysfunction, hypothyroidism, Addison's disease, severe CNS depression, respiratory depression, head injury, elevated intracranial pressure.
- If required, naloxone HCl (Narcan) will reverse opiate toxicity (e.g., respiratory depression). However, it is important that acute withdrawal symptoms be prevented by giving only enough naloxone to reverse respiratory depression and that this be continued for opioid drug half-life.

Potential Toxicities/Side Effects and the Nursing Process

I. SENSORY/PERCEPTUAL ALTERATIONS related to CNS DEPRESSION

Defining Characteristics: Drowsiness, sedation, mood changes, euphoria, dysphoria, dizziness, mental clouding may occur. At high doses, may cause seizures. Miosis (papillary constriction) may occur.

Nursing Implications: Assess baseline neurologic status. Use cautiously, if at all, in patients with head injury, increased intracranial pressure, severe CNS depression, acute alcoholism, or who are elderly or debilitated. Assess other concurrent medications. Use with caution in patients receiving other opioids, tranquilizers, hypnotics, monoamine oxidase (MAO) inhibitors, since increasing CNS depressant effects can occur. Monitor neurologic status closely. Teach patient to avoid driving and operating machinery while taking the medicine, and to AVOID concurrent alcohol.

II. ALTERATION IN OXYGENATION related to RESPIRATORY DEPRESSION

Defining Characteristics: Opiate agonists directly depress respiratory center in brain stem, causing decreased sensitivity and responsiveness to increased pCO_2 (CO_2 tension in serum). Also may depress deep breathing and reflex to sigh. Tolerance to respiratory depressant effects occurs with chronic use.

Nursing Implications: Assess baseline pulmonary status, and monitor periodically during drug use. Use cautiously in patients with bronchial asthma, chronic obstructive pulmonary disease (COPD), respiratory depression, and monitor closely.

III. ALTERATION IN ELIMINATION related to CONSTIPATION, ILEUS

Defining Characteristics: Opium agonists bind to opiate receptors in bowel, slowing peristalsis, leading to constipation. Untreated constipation may result in bowel perforation.

Nursing Implications: Assess baseline elimination, fluid intake, diet, and exercise patterns. Teach patient about prevention of constipation: goal is to move bowels at least every two days by increasing fluid intake to 3 L/day, following a diet high in fiber (beans, vegetables, fruit), and taking moderate exercise. Assess need for bowel softeners, bulk-forming laxatives, and osmotic cathartics, and discuss prescription with physician. Teach patient self-administration of medications.

IV. ALTERATION IN NUTRITION, LESS THAN BODY REQUIREMENTS, related to GI TOXICITY

Defining Characteristics: Nausea, vomiting, dry mouth may occur. Gastric, biliary, and pancreatic secretions are decreased by opiate agonists; digestion is delayed. Biliary tract muscle tone is increased, and spasm of Oddi's sphincter may occur (morphine > meperidine > codeine).

Nursing Implications: Assess patient tolerance of GI side effects. Teach patient to report side effects. If nausea/vomiting occur, change to another opioid, or premedicate with antiemetic to prevent nausea/vomiting. Assess GI pain, biliary spasm, and consider alternative opioid.

V. ALTERATION IN CARDIAC OUTPUT related to HYPOTENSION, BRADYCARDIA

Defining Characteristics: Orthostatic hypotension, bradycardia due to cholinergic effect, and peripheral vasodilation may occur with rapid IV dosing. There may be histamine-related flushing, pruritus, diaphoresis with chronic drug usage; tolerance develops to this effect.

Nursing Implications: Assess baseline cardiovascular status. Teach patient to change position slowly and to hold onto stable, nearby structure for support as needed. Be careful when giving IV push opioids, and caution patient to remain in supine position for 15–20 minutes after injection. Monitor cardiovascular status after injection.

VI. ALTERATION IN URINE ELIMINATION related to URINARY RETENTION

Defining Characteristics: Increased smooth muscle tone in urinary tract and spasm may occur. Bladder tone is increased and may cause urgency. Vesical sphincter tone may be increased, leading to difficulty urinating. Increased risk of urinary retention in patients with prostatic hypertrophy or urethral stricture.

Nursing Implications: Assess baseline urinary elimination pattern. Teach patient to increase fluids to 3 L/day, and encourage voiding every 2–3 hours. Instruct patient to report problems with urination.

VII. KNOWLEDGE DEFICIT related to DRUG ADMINISTRATION, POTENTIAL FOR TOLERANCE, AND DEPENDENCY

Defining Characteristics: Psychological dependence (addiction) occurs rarely in patients taking opioid agonists for cancer pain (< 1%). Physical dependence (precipitation of withdrawal symptoms) occurs with chronic use of the drug for the relief of chronic cancer pain. In addition, tolerance, or less analgesic effect over time with the same drug dose, occurs and requires increased dosage of drug.

Nursing Implications: Assess baseline knowledge of opioid analgesics, and attitude about their use for cancer pain management. Teach patient about proper self-administration, possible side effects, and self-care measures. Suggest patient maintain diary of pain intensity, precipitating and alleviating factors, drug dose and time taken, and relief. Teach patient to self-administer opioid agonists for relief of chronic cancer pain around-the-clock, not PRN, to prevent pain. Explain use of prescribed short-acting opioid for rescue or to manage breakthrough pain. Discuss with physician dose increase or change in frequency of administration if tolerance develops. Teach patient that withdrawal symptoms may occur if chronic, around-the-clock dosing is interrupted. Withdrawal (abstinence) symptoms that may be seen are restlessness, lacrimation, rhinorrhea, yawning, perspiration, gooseflesh, restless sleep, mydriasis in first 24 hours. These are followed by twitching and leg spasm; severe aching of the back, abdomen, and legs; cramping in abdomen and legs; hot/cold flashes; insomnia; nausea/vomiting, diarrhea; severe sneezing; and increased heart rate, BP, and temperature (T), which peak at 36–72 hours. Withdrawal syndrome can be prevented by administration of at least 1/4 of previous opioid dose.

VIII. SEXUAL DYSFUNCTION related to IMPOTENCE, ↓ LIBIDO

Defining Characteristics: Opiate agonists may suppress gonadotropin, causing impotence and decreased libido.

Nursing Implications: Assess baseline sexual pattern. Discuss potential toxicity and impact on sexuality. Provide information, emotional support, and referral as needed.

Drug: fentanyl buccal tablet (Fentora)

Class: Opioid analgesic (opioid agonist).

Mechanism of Action: Fentanyl is a pure opioid agonist that binds to opioid μ-receptors located in the brain, spinal cord, and smooth muscle. Fentanyl in a buccal tablet is formulated using OraVescent technology so that when the tablet contacts saliva, the resulting reaction releases carbon dioxide, changes the local pH, allowing dissolution and passage of the fentanyl through the buccal membrane, the onset of analgesia at 15 minutes, with significant decrease in pain intensity at 30 minutes in 50% of patients, and duration of action of 60 minutes.

Metabolism: 48% of the drug is absorbed through the buccal mucosa, with an additional 17% absorbed via the GI tract (total 65% bioavailability). After buccal absorption, there is a steep rise in mean plasma fentanyl concentration, peaking at 46.8 minutes. Drug is highly lipophilic and highly protein bound (80–85%). Drug is taken up in tissues and eliminated primarily by biotransformation into inactive metabolites in the liver. It is metabolized in the liver primarily and to a lesser extent in the intestinal mucosa to norfentanyl by cytochrome P450 3A4 isoform. In population studies, patients with higher weight have a higher systemic exposure to the drug (men, Japanese subjects). Patients with renal and/or hepatic dysfunction who are receiving high doses of drug may have significantly decreased metabolic elimination of the drug. Four single 100-microgram tablets deliver 12–13% more drug than a single 400-microgram tablet. The dwell time (time tablet takes to disintegrate) does not affect early systemic exposure to fentanyl.

Dosage/Range:
- Starting dose is 100 micrograms; redose within a single breakthrough pain episode may occur 30 minutes after the start of administration of buccal fentanyl using the same dose strength.
- Prescription is written: place tablet above a rear molar between the upper cheek and gum; one tablet per breakthrough pain episode; may repeat once if pain is not relieved after 30 minutes.
- Titrate to adequate dose by patient diary and discussion with provider to achieve single tablet strength that provides relief; when doses above 100 micrograms needed, patient should place one 100 microgram tablet on buccal mucosa on each side of the mouth; if this is ineffective, increase dose by placing two 100-microgram tablets on each side of the mouth, for a total of four 100-microgram tablets.
- Titrating above 400 micrograms: increase dose in 200 microgram increments.
- When converting from oral transmucosal fentanyl (Actiq), a dose of buccal tablet is one half or less than the Actiq dose (e.g., Actiq 200 or 400 micrograms = Fentora 100 micrograms; Actiq 600 or 800 micrograms = Fentora 200 micrograms; Actiq 1200–1600 micrograms = Fentora 400 micrograms).
- The goal is to determine necessary dose in a single tablet.
- After an effective dose has been determined, when the patient requires more than four breakthrough pain episodes per day, increase the maintenance (around-the-clock) opioid by an equivalent amount.
- Increase the fentanyl buccal tablet dose when a patient requires more than one dose per breakthrough pain episode.

Preparation/Administration:
- Available in a carton of seven blister cards with four tablets in each card; blister pack is child resistant and encased in peelable foil.
- Available in 100-, 200-, 400-, 600-, and 800-microgram fentanyl base tablets.
- Open blister pack immediately before use: tear single blister unit from card, bend blister unit, and peel backing to expose the tablet (do not try to push through the backing).

- Remove tablet from blister unit, and place entire tablet in buccal cavity, usually above a rear molar, between the upper cheek and teeth; patient should NOT try to split the tablet and/or chew, suck, or swallow the tablet, as this results in lower plasma fentanyl levels.
- Leave the tablet against buccal mucosa until it has fully disintegrated (14–25 minutes).
- After 30 minutes, if tablet remnants remain, the patient can swallow them with a drink of water.
- Dispose of unused tablets from a prescription as soon as they are no longer needed (remove tablets from blister pack and flush down toilet).

Drug Interactions:
- CNS depressants (other opioids, sedatives, hypnotics, general anesthetics, phenothiazines, tranquilizers, skeletal muscle relaxants, sedating antihistamines), potent inhibitors of cytochrome P450 CYP3A4 isoform (erythromycin, ketoconazole, certain protease inhibitors), and alcohol: increased CNS depression, with risk of hypoventilation, hypotension, and profound sedation.
- Moderate CYP3A4 inhibitors (aprepitant, diltiazem, grapefruit juice, verapamil): may increase fentanyl plasma levels; use together cautiously.
- MAO inhibitors within 14 days: potentiation of opioid, do not give together.

Lab Effects/Interference:
- None known.

Special Considerations:
- Indicated for the management of breakthrough pain in patients with cancer who are already tolerant to opioid therapy for persistent cancer pain (taking at least 60 mg of oral morphine a day or 25 micrograms of fentanyl per hour or at least 30 mg of oxycodone daily or at least 8 mg of hydromorphone daily or an equianalgesic dose of another opioid, for at least 1 week or longer).
- Contraindicated in patients who are not opioid tolerant, have postoperative pain, who have received MAO inhibitors within 14 days, nursing mothers, as fentanyl is excreted in human milk causing potentially fatal respiratory depression, as well as physical dependence and withdrawal when no longer nursing.
- Use cautiously if at all in patients with hepatic and/or renal dysfunction, chronic pulmonary disease, head injuries with increased intracranial pressure, and bradyarrhythmias. If drug must be used in a pregnant woman, benefit must outweigh potential risk to the fetus.
- Teach patient drug must be kept out of reach of children and pets, as dose can be LETHAL to children and pets.
- Drug is an opioid and may cause physical dependence and withdrawal if stopped (along with maintenance opioid) abruptly.
- Application site reactions occur in about 10% of patients (range from paresthesia to irritation to ulceration and bleeding) but rarely cause drug discontinuation.

Potential Toxicities/Side Effects and the Nursing Process

I. POTENTIAL ALTERATION IN OXYGENATION related to HYPOVENTILATION

Defining Characteristics: Increased cough and/or dyspnea are rare, but the chief toxicity in naïve patients or if excessive dosing is respiratory depression. Drug may cause bradycardia; thus, use with caution in patients with bradyarrhythmias.

Nursing Implications: Assess baseline pulmonary status. Use with caution in patients with COPD, bradycardia, renal or hepatic dysfunction and in the older population. Teach patient to report any pulmonary difficulties immediately. Ensure that patient knows that if respiratory difficulty develops the drug must be removed from mouth and discarded immediately. Ensure that patient understands how to administer drug safely and to keep drug supply out of reach of children and pets.

II. SENSORY/PERCEPTUAL ALTERATIONS related to CNS CHANGES

Defining Characteristics: CNS depression and changes in mental status may occur, characterized by somnolence (9%) or dizziness (13%), confusion (7%), depression (8%), and insomnia (6%). Rarely, hypoesthesia, lethargy, balance problems, anxiety, disorientation, and hallucinations may occur.

Nursing Implications: Assess baseline gait, mental, affective, and neurologic status. Assess medication profile to identify other contributions (i.e., CNS depressants). Instruct patient to report any changes. Assess patient safety, and measures to ensure safety. Teach patient not to take alcohol, sleep aids, or tranquilizers, except as ordered by the oncology provider. Discuss any significant changes with provider.

III. ALTERATION IN COMFORT related to HEADACHE, PAIN, PERIPHERAL EDEMA

Defining Characteristics: Headache occurs in about 10% of patients, abdominal pain (9%), peripheral edema (12%), asthenia (11%), and fatigue (16%). Back pain (5%) and arthralgia (6%) were reported less commonly.

Nursing Implications: Assess baseline comfort. Assess baseline skin integrity, presence of peripheral edema, and weight. Teach patient to report symptoms and manage based on severity, including elevating legs if peripheral edema present. Assess impact on patient's quality of life. If severe, discuss alternative strategies with physician.

IV. ALTERATION IN NUTRITION, LESS THAN BODY REQUIREMENTS, related to NAUSEA/VOMITING

Defining Characteristics: Nausea occurred in 29% of patients, and vomiting occurred in 20% of patients. Dehydration occurred in 11% of patients, anorexia 8%, and hypokalemia 6%.

Nursing Implications: Assess baseline nutritional status, including electrolyte and fluid balance. Teach patient to take antiemetic agents as prescribed, to drink 8–10 ounces of fluid hourly while awake, and to eat small, frequent, calorie-dense foods. Teach patient to report nausea, vomiting, anorexia, and dehydration. Manage symptomatically. Assess severity and impact on quality of life. Discuss severe or unmanaged symptoms with physician.

V. ALTERATION IN ELIMINATION related to CONSTIPATION OR DIARRHEA

Defining Characteristics: Opium agonists bind to opiate receptors in bowel, slowing peristalsis, leading to constipation. Untreated constipation may result in bowel perforation. Constipation occurred in 12% of patients and diarrhea in 8% of patients.

Nursing Implications: Assess baseline elimination, fluid intake, diet, and exercise patterns. Instruct patient regarding prevention of constipation: goal is to move bowels at least every 2 days by increasing fluids to 3 L/day (drink 8- to 10-ounce glasses of fluid every hour while awake), following a diet high in fiber (beans, vegetables, fruit) and taking moderate exercise. Review bowel regimen, and assess need for additional bowel softeners, bulk-forming laxatives, and osmotic cathartics, and discuss prescription with physician. Teach patient self-administration of medications. However, all patients MUST be started on bowel regimen when receiving an opioid.

Drug: fentanyl citrate (Oral Transmucosal Fentanyl, Actiq)

Class: Opioid analgesic (opioid agonist).

Mechanism of Action: Fentanyl is a pure opioid agonist that binds to opioid μ-receptors located in the brain, spinal cord, and smooth muscle. The oral transmucosal preparation of the drug is a solid formulation of fentanyl citrate placed on a handle so the drug is sucked. Sucking, the drug dose coats the oral mucosa, through which 22% of the drug is rapidly absorbed, reportedly as fast as IV morphine. Onset of analgesia is approximately 5 minutes from onset of administration, with peak plasma fentanyl concentration at 90.8 minutes.

Metabolism: Initial rapid absorption of about 25% of total dose across buccal mucosa, into systemic circulation, and longer prolonged absorption of swallowed fentanyl (75% of dose) from GI tract. One-third of drug escapes first-pass elimination and enters the systemic circulation for a total of 50% of the total dose that is bioavailable. Following absorption, drug is rapidly distributed to brain, heart, lungs, kidneys, spleen. Plasma binding is 80–85%. The drug is primarily metabolized in the liver, and less than 7% of the dose is excreted in the urine. The terminal elimination half-life is approximately 219 minutes.

Dosage/Range:

Adult:

- Titrate to patient's individual needs: available in six strengths that are color coded: 200-, 400-, 600-, 800-, 1200-, and 1600-μg fentanyl base.
- Drug CANNOT be used in opioid-naïve patients, and is indicated for the management of chronic pain, especially breakthrough pain in patients who are ALREADY RECEIVING AND WHO ARE TOLERANT to opioid therapy (e.g., taking at least 60 mg of morphine/day, 50 μg/hr of transdermal fentanyl, or an equianalgesic dose of another opioid for a week or longer).
- Patient begins using 200 μg unit for breakthrough pain (BTP) and sucks the medicine for 15 minutes. If the pain is unrelieved, the patient waits an additional 15 minutes then administers a second 200-μg unit. If the pain is unrelieved, the patient waits another 15 minutes and administers a third 200-μg unit. Three units of any dosage is the maximum drug per BTP episode.
- If the patient required two units of 200-μg dosage, then the patient would give 400-μg dose for the next episode of BTP. If using two 200-μg units, the patient would wait 15 minutes between taking units.
- If the patient needed three units of 200-μg dose, the patient would take the 600-μg strength the next dose for BTP.
- The patient should notify the physician if drug is required more than four times per day, so that the long-acting opioid can be increased.

Drug Preparation:

- Drug is on a handle, sealed in a child-resistant foil pouch that requires scissors to open. The drug dose is color-coded.
- Open foil pack immediately before use. Patient should place drug dose unit in the mouth between cheek and lower gum. Patient should suck, NOT CHEW, the medication over 15 minutes.
- If the patient achieves adequate analgesia or develops excessive side effects, the drug should be removed from the mouth and discarded immediately. The remaining drug is very dangerous if a child or pet ingests it, so maximum precautions must be taken.
- To discard the remaining drug, twist drug off handle using tissue paper, and flush medicine down the toilet. Destroy any medication remaining on the handle by dissolving it under hot water.
- Keep medication away from patient's eyes, skin, or mucous membranes when not sucking the medication, and the patient should wash hands after discarding unused medication portion.
- At home, teach patient to store oral doses in a safe place away from children and pets.

Drug Interactions:

- CNS depressants (e.g., other opioids, alcohol, sedatives, hypnotics, general anesthetics, phenothiazines, tranquilizers, skeletal muscle relaxants, sedating antihistamines) may increase CNS depression (hypoventilation, hypotension, profound sedation, especially in opioid nontolerant patients).

Lab Effects/Interference:

- None known.

Special Considerations:

- CONTRAINDICATED in opioid-nontolerant patients, as life-threatening hypoventilation may occur; in children < 10 kg for management of acute postoperative pain; in patients with hypersensitivity to fentanyl; in patients with head injury and increased intracranial pressure (ICP); and in nursing mothers.
- Administer cautiously to patients with hepatic or renal dysfunction.
- Teach patient drug must be kept out of reach of children as dose can be LETHAL to children.
- Use cautiously in patients with chronic pulmonary disease (degree of hypoventilation), cardiac conduction disease (bradycardia), and the elderly.
- Respiratory depression may be associated with opioids, and patients should be monitored for this. This was not reported in the clinical trials with Actiq.
- Patients should be taught to call nurse or physician if taking four of the same strength units within 60 minutes without relief or if taking drug more than four times per day.
- Once effective dose determined, drug provides rapid relief of BTP.
- Some reported toxicities may be due to advanced malignancy rather than the drug.

Potential Toxicities/Side Effects and the Nursing Process

I. ALTERATION IN OXYGENATION related to HYPOVENTILATION

Defining Characteristics: Dyspnea (10%), increased cough and pharyngitis (3–10%).

Nursing Implications: Assess baseline pulmonary status. Use with caution in patients with COPD, bradycardia, renal or hepatic dysfunction, and in the elderly. Teach patient to report any pulmonary difficulties immediately. Ensure patient knows that if respiratory difficulty develops, the drug must be removed from mouth and discarded immediately; also, to suck and not chew drug. Ensure that patient understands how to handle drug safely to prevent additional absorption of unused drug.

II. SENSORY/PERCEPTUAL ALTERATIONS related to CNS CHANGES

Defining Characteristics: CNS depression and changes in mental status may occur, characterized by somnolence or dizziness (10%); abnormal gait, anxiety, confusion, depression, insomnia, hypesthesia, vasodilation, abnormal vision (3–10% incidence).

Nursing Implications: Assess baseline gait and mental, affective, and neurologic status. Assess medication profile to identify other contributions, i.e., CNS depressants. Instruct patient to report any changes. Assess patient safety, and measures to ensure safety. Discuss any significant changes with physician.

III. ALTERATION IN COMFORT related to HEADACHE, FEVER

Defining Characteristics: Headache, fever, asthenia are reported in ~ 10% of patients; less commonly, myalgia, pruritus, rash, sweating occur in 3–10% of patients.

Nursing Implications: Assess baseline comfort. Teach patient to report symptoms and manage based on severity. Assess impact on patient's quality of life. If severe, discuss alternative strategies with physician.

IV. ALTERATION IN NUTRITION, LESS THAN BODY REQUIREMENTS, related to NAUSEA/VOMITING

Defining Characteristics: Nausea and vomiting are reported in ~ 10% of patients; less commonly, anorexia, dehydration, edema, and dyspepsia occur in 3–10% of patients.

Nursing Implications: Assess baseline nutritional status. Teach patient to report nausea, vomiting, anorexia, dyspepsia. Manage symptomatically. Assess severity and impact on quality of life. Discuss severe or unmanaged symptoms with physician.

V. ALTERATION IN ELIMINATION related to CONSTIPATION OR DIARRHEA

Defining Characteristics: Opium agonists bind to opiate receptors in bowel, slowing peristalsis, leading to constipation. Untreated constipation may result in bowel perforation. Opiate receptors in bowel decrease peristalsis. Constipation and diarrhea were each reported in < 10% of patients.

Nursing Implications: Assess baseline elimination, fluid intake, diet, and exercise patterns. Instruct patient regarding prevention of constipation: goal is to move bowels at least every two days by increasing fluids to 3 L/day, following a diet high in fiber (beans, vegetables, fruit), and taking moderate exercise. Assess need for bowel softeners, bulk-forming laxatives, and osmotic cathartics, and discuss prescription with physician. Teach patient self-administration of medications. MUST be started on bowel regimen.

Drug: fentanyl transdermal system (Duragesic)

Class: Opioid analgesic (opioid agonist).

Mechanism of Action: Strong opioid analgesic; 20–30 times more potent than parenteral morphine when given transdermally to opioid-naïve patients. Drug interacts primarily with opioid μ-receptors, found in the brain, spinal cord, and other tissues, causing analgesia and sedation. Duragesic patches provide continuous-released fentanyl from a transdermal reservoir system at a constant amount per unit time. The drug moves from areas of higher concentration (patch) to areas of lower concentration (skin). Initially, the skin under the patch absorbs the fentanyl, and the drug is concentrated in the upper skin layers. The drug gradually enters the systemic circulation, leveling off 2–24 hours later, and remaining fairly constant for the 72-hour application period.

Metabolism: Primarily metabolized by the liver; 75% of IV dose excreted in urine, 9% in feces, and < 10% as unchanged drug. Peak levels occur 24–72 hours after a single application. Half-life is approximately 17 hours (after system removal, serum fentanyl concentrations fall to 50% in approximately 17 hours; range, 13–22 hours).

Dosage/Range:

- 25 μg/hour is initial dosage for non-opioid-tolerant patients. Doses for patients currently receiving opioid analgesics who are tolerant can be calculated from the following table:

Duragesic Dose Prescription Based on Daily Morphine Equivalence Dose

Oral 24-hour Morphine (mg/day)	IM 24-hour Morphine (mg/day)	DURAGESIC Dose (μg/hr)
45–134	8–22	25
135–224	23–37	50
225–314	38–52	75
315–404	53–67	100
405–494	68–82	125
495–584	83–97	150
585–674	98–112	175
675–764	113–127	200
765–854	128–142	225
855–944	143–157	250
945–1034	158–172	275
1035–1124	173–187	300

Drug Preparation:

- None.

Drug Administration:

- Apply to nonirritated and nonirradiated skin; clip hair (not shave) as needed. May cleanse with water only and dry completely if necessary. Apply patch immediately after removal from package. Press firmly into place with palm of hand for 10–20 seconds, making sure contact is complete, especially around edges. Patient wears for 72 hours, then changes patch. Some patients may need to reapply new patches every 48 hours. Short-acting opioids must be continued for 24 hours until serum fentanyl level achieved.

- Disposal: at home, patient must fold so adhesive side of system adheres to itself and then flush down toilet. In hospital, used patches must be returned to pharmacy for proper disposal.
- At home, teach patient to store oral doses in a safe place away from children and pets.

Drug Interactions:

- Potentiation of CNS depressant effects, when administered concurrently with other opioids, benzodiazepines, or other CNS depressants.

Lab Effects/Interference:

- None known.

Special Considerations:

- Indications: patients with chronic pain requiring opioid analgesia.
- Contraindicated in patients with known hypersensitivity to fentanyl or adhesives. Use with caution in the following patients: patients with COPD predisposed to hypoventilation; patients with head injuries, brain tumor (very sensitive to effects of CO_2 retention); patients with cardiac disease (may cause bradyarrhythmias); patients with hepatic dysfunction.
- Availability: Dosages: 25 μg/h, 50 μg/h, 75 μg/h, and 100 μg/h. Supplied in one carton containing five individually wrapped patches.

Potential Toxicities/Side Effects and the Nursing Process

I. ALTERATION IN OXYGENATION related to HYPOVENTILATION

Defining Characteristics: Dyspnea, hypoventilation, apnea (3–10% of patients); hemoptysis, pharyngitis, hiccups rare; stertorous breathing, asthma, respiratory dysfunction.

Nursing Implications: Assess baseline pulmonary status. Use with caution in patients with COPD, brain tumors, increased intracranial pressure (ICP), hepatic failure. NEVER exceed 25 μg/h if patient not tolerant to opioids. Must continue to observe patient for 17 hours after dose removed for signs/symptoms of toxicity—same is true if naloxone HCl (Narcan) required to reverse opioid. Theoretically, a temperature of 39°C (102°F) will increase serum fentanyl by 33% due to drug delivery and skin absorption. If patient develops fever, observe for signs/symptoms of overdosage. Elderly patients (> 60–65 years old) may have reduced ability to clear drug, so start at 25 μg/hr unless already tolerant of > 135 mg morphine sulfate/ 24 hours.

II. SENSORY/PERCEPTUAL ALTERATIONS related to CNS CHANGES

Defining Characteristics: CNS depression and changes in mental status may occur, characterized by somnolence, confusion, depression, asthenia (> 10%), dizziness, nervousness, hallucinations, anxiety, depression, euphoria (3–10%), tremors, abnormal coordination, speech disorder, abnormal thinking, dreams. Rare: aphasia, vertigo, stupor, hypotonia, hypertonia, hostility.

Nursing Implications: Assess baseline mental, neurologic status. Dose of other opioids and benzodiazepines should be 50%. Use cautiously in substance abusers.

III. ALTERATION IN CARDIAC OUTPUT related to ARRYTHMIA, ANGINA

Defining Characteristics: Arrhythmia, chest pain may occur; IV fentanyl has caused bradyarrhythmias.

Nursing Implications: Assess baseline cardiac status, and monitor during drug use. Instruct patient to report palpitations, chest pain.

IV. ALTERATION IN NUTRITION, LESS THAN BODY REQUIREMENTS, related to NAUSEA, VOMITING

Defining Characteristics: Nausea, vomiting, anorexia, dyspepsia, rare abdominal distension.

Nursing Implications: Assess baseline nutritional status. Instruct patient to report nausea, vomiting, anorexia, dyspepsia.

V. ALTERATION IN ELIMINATION related to CONSTIPATION, ILEUS

Defining Characteristics: Opium agonists bind to opiate receptors in bowel, slowing peristalsis, leading to constipation. Untreated constipation may result in bowel perforation. Opiate receptors in bowel decrease peristalsis.

Nursing Implications: Assess baseline elimination, fluid intake, diet, and exercise patterns. Instruct patient regarding prevention of constipation: goal is to move bowels at least every two days, by increasing fluids to 3 L/day, following a diet high in fiber (beans, vegetables, fruit), and taking moderate exercise. Assess need for bowel softeners, bulk-forming laxatives, and osmotic cathartics, and discuss prescription with physician. Teach patient self-administration of medications. MUST be started on bowel regimen.

VI. ALTERATION IN CARDIAC OUTPUT related to HYPOTENSION, BRADYCARDIA

Defining Characteristics: Orthostatic hypotension, bradycardia due to cholinergic effect, and peripheral vasodilation may occur with rapid IV dosing. There may be histamine-related flushing, pruritus, diaphoresis with chronic drug usage; tolerance develops to this effect.

Nursing Implications: Assess baseline cardiovascular status. Teach patient to change position slowly and to hold onto stable, nearby structure for support as needed. Be careful when giving IV push opioids, and caution patient to remain in supine position for 15–20 minutes after injection. Monitor cardiovascular status after injection.

VII. ALTERATION IN URINE ELIMINATION related to URINARY RETENTION

Defining Characteristics: Increased smooth muscle tone in urinary tract and spasm may occur. Bladder tone is increased, which may cause urgency. Vesical sphincter tone may be increased, leading to difficulty urinating. Increased risk of urinary retention in patients with prostatic hypertrophy or urethral stricture. Rare bladder pain, oliguria, urinary frequency.

Nursing Implications: Assess baseline urinary elimination pattern. Teach patient to increase fluids to 3 L/day, and encourage voiding every 2–3 hours. Instruct patient to report problems with urination.

VIII. ALTERATION IN SKIN INTEGRITY/COMFORT related to RASH, PRURITUS

Defining Characteristics: Sweating, pruritus, rash; erythema, papules, itching, edema, exfoliative dermatitis, pustules at application site; headache rare.

Nursing Implications: Teach patient proper drug application and to rotate sites.

Drug: hydromorphone (Dilaudid)

Class: Opioid analgesic (opioid agonist).

Mechanism of Action: Resembles morphine but has milder action; binds to opiate receptors in CNS (limbic system, thalamus, striatum, hypothalamus, midbrain, spinal cord), altering pain perception at level of spinal cord and higher centers as well as the emotional response to pain. Also suppresses cough reflex.

Metabolism: Well absorbed after oral, rectal, and parenteral administration. Onset of action is 15–30 minutes (more rapid than morphine), with a duration of action of 4–5 hours. Metabolized by liver and excreted in urine.

Dosage/Range:
- Use caution in patients who have not received opiates before and have not developed tolerance.
- Moderate pain: oral: 1–6 mg q 4–6 h; subcutaneous or IM: 2–4 mg q 4–6 h, 3 mg rectal suppository.
- Severe pain: oral: 4 mg or more q 4 h; subcutaneous or IM: 4 mg or more, then titrate based on patient response and tolerance.

Drug Preparation:
- Store tablets in tight, light-resistant containers at 15–30°C (59–86°F).
- Injection should be protected from light and stored at 15–40°C (59–104°F).

Drug Administration:
- PO, subcutaneous, IM. Use highly concentrated injectable solution for patients who are tolerant to opiate agonists.
- At home, teach patient to store oral doses in a safe place away from children and pets.

Drug Interactions:
- Alcohol, CNS depressants: Additive effects.

Lab Effects/Interference:
- None known.

Special Considerations:
- Parenteral dose is 1/5 oral dose for equianalgesic effect.
- Indicated for relief of moderate-to-severe pain.
- Additive benefit when combined with acetaminophen or aspirin.
- Give smallest effective dose to prevent development of tolerance, physical dependency.
- Reduce dose in debilitated patients or patients receiving other CNS depressants.
- Use with caution in patients with hepatic or renal dysfunction, hypothyroidism, Addison's disease, severe CNS depression, respiratory depression, head injury, elevated ICP.
- If required, naloxone HCl will reverse opiate toxicity (e.g., respiratory depression). However, it is important that acute withdrawal symptoms be prevented by giving only enough naloxone to reverse respiratory depression and that this be continued for opioid drug half-life.

Potential Toxicities/Side Effects and the Nursing Process

I. SENSORY/PERCEPTUAL ALTERATIONS related to CNS DEPRESSION

Defining Characteristics: Drowsiness, sedation, mood changes, euphoria, dysphoria, dizziness, mental clouding may occur. At high doses, may cause seizures. Miosis (papillary constriction) may occur.

Nursing Implications: Assess baseline neurologic status. Use cautiously, if at all, in patients with head injury, increased ICP, severe CNS depression, acute alcoholism, the elderly, and the debilitated. Assess other concurrent medications. Use with caution in patients receiving other opioids, tranquilizers, hypnotics, MAO inhibitors, since increasing CNS depressant effects can occur. Monitor neurologic status closely. Teach patient to avoid driving and operating machinery while taking the medicine, and to AVOID concurrent alcohol.

II. ALTERATION IN OXYGENATION related to RESPIRATORY DEPRESSION

Defining Characteristics: Opiate agonists directly depress respiratory center in brain stem, causing decreased sensitivity and responsiveness to increased pCO_2. Also may depress deep breathing and reflex to sigh. Tolerance to respiratory depressant effects occurs with chronic use.

Nursing Implications: Assess baseline pulmonary status, and monitor periodically during drug use. Use cautiously in patients with bronchial asthma, COPD, respiratory depression, and monitor closely.

III. ALTERATION IN ELIMINATION related to CONSTIPATION, ILEUS

Defining Characteristics: Opium agonists bind to opiate receptors in bowel, slowing peristalsis, leading to constipation. Untreated constipation may result in bowel perforation.

Nursing Implications: Assess baseline elimination, fluid intake, diet, and exercise patterns. Instruct patient about prevention of constipation: goal is to move bowels at least every two days by increasing fluids to 3 L/day, following a diet high in fiber (beans, vegetables, fruit), and taking moderate exercise. Assess need for bowel softeners, bulk-forming laxatives, and osmotic cathartics, and discuss prescription with physician. Teach patient self-administration of medications.

IV. ALTERATION IN NUTRITION related to GI TOXICITY

Defining Characteristics: Nausea, vomiting, and dry mouth may occur. Gastric, biliary, and pancreatic secretions are decreased by opiate agonists; digestion is delayed. Biliary tract muscle tone is increased, and spasm of Oddi's sphincter may occur (morphine > meperidine > codeine).

Nursing Implications: Assess patient tolerance of GI side effects. Teach patient to report side effects. If nausea/vomiting occur, change to another opioid, or premedicate with antiemetic to prevent nausea/vomiting. Assess GI pain, biliary spasm, and consider alternative opioid.

V. ALTERATION IN CARDIAC OUTPUT related to HYPOTENSION, BRADYCARDIA

Defining Characteristics: Orthostatic hypotension, bradycardia due to cholinergic effect, and peripheral vasodilation may occur with rapid IV dosing. There may be histamine-related flushing, pruritus, diaphoresis with chronic drug usage; tolerance develops to this effect.

Nursing Implications: Assess baseline cardiovascular status. Teach patient to change position slowly and to hold onto stable, nearby structure for support as needed. Be careful when giving IV push opioids, and caution patient to remain in supine position for 15–20 minutes after injection. Monitor cardiovascular status after injection.

VI. ALTERATION IN URINE ELIMINATION related to URINARY RETENTION

Defining Characteristics: Increased smooth muscle tone in urinary tract and spasm may occur. Bladder tone is increased, which may cause urgency. Vesical sphincter tone may be increased, leading to difficulty urinating. Increased risk of urinary retention in patients with prostatic hypertrophy or urethral stricture.

Nursing Implications: Assess baseline urinary elimination pattern. Teach patient to increase fluids to 3 L/day, and encourage voiding every 2–3 hours. Instruct patient to report problems with urination.

VII. KNOWLEDGE DEFICIT related to DRUG ADMINISTRATION, POTENTIAL FOR TOLERANCE, AND DEPENDENCY

Defining Characteristics: Psychological dependence (addiction) occurs rarely in patients taking opioid agonists for cancer pain (< 1%). Physical dependence (precipitation of withdrawal symptoms) occurs with chronic use of the drug for the relief of chronic cancer pain. In addition, tolerance, or less analgesic effect over time with the same drug dose, occurs and requires increased dosage of drug.

Nursing Implications: Assess baseline knowledge of opioid analgesics and attitude about their use for cancer pain management. Teach patient about proper self-administration, possible side effects, and self-care measures. Suggest patient maintain diary of pain intensity, precipitating and alleviating factors, drug dose and time taken, and relief. Teach patient to self-administer opioid agonists for relief of chronic cancer pain around-the-clock, not PRN, to prevent pain. Explain use of prescribed short-acting opioid for rescue or to manage BTP. Discuss with physician dose increase or change in frequency of administration if tolerance develops. Teach patient that withdrawal symptoms may occur if chronic, around-the-clock dosing is interrupted. Withdrawal (abstinence) symptoms that may be seen are restlessness, lacrimation, rhinorrhea, yawning, perspiration, gooseflesh, restless sleep, mydriasis in first 24 hours. These are followed by twitching and leg spasm; severe aching of the back, abdomen, and legs; cramping in abdomen and legs; hot/cold flashes; insomnia; nausea/vomiting, diarrhea; severe sneezing; and increased heart rate, BP, T, which peak at 36–72 hours. Withdrawal syndrome can be prevented by administration of at least 1/4 of previous opioid dose.

VIII. SEXUAL DYSFUNCTION related to IMPOTENCE, ↓ LIBIDO

Defining Characteristics: Opiate agonists may suppress gonadotropin, causing impotence and decreased libido.

Nursing Implications: Assess baseline sexual pattern. Discuss potential toxicity and impact on sexuality. Provide information, emotional support, and referral as needed.

Drug: levorphanol tartrate opioid (Levo-Dromoran)

Class: Opioid analgesic (opioid agonist).

Mechanism of Action: A synthetic opioid agonist, levorphanol resembles morphine but has milder action; binds to opiate receptors in CNS (limbic system, thalamus, striatum, hypothalamus, midbrain, spinal cord), altering pain perception at level of spinal cord and higher centers, as well as the emotional response to pain. Also suppresses cough reflex.

Metabolism: Well absorbed after oral (peak analgesia 60–90 minutes) or subcutaneous (peak analgesia 20 minutes) administration. Metabolized by liver and excreted in urine.

Dosage/Range:

For moderate to severe pain:

- PO: 2–3 mg PO q 6–8 h.
- Subcutaneous: 2–3 mg subcutaneous q 6–8 h.

Drug Preparation:

- Store tablets in tight, light-resistant containers at 15–30°C (59–86°F).
- Injectable preparation should be stored at 15–40°C (59–104°F).
- At home, teach patient to store oral doses in a safe place away from children and pets.

Drug Administration:

- PO, subcutaneous, IV.

Drug Interactions:

- Injection incompatible with solutions containing aminophylline, ammonium chloride, amobarbital sodium, chlorothiazide sodium, heparin sodium, methicillin sodium, nitrofurantoin, phenobarbital sodium, sodium bicarbonate.
- Alcohol, CNS depressants: additive effects.

Lab Effects/Interference:

- None known.

Special Considerations:

- Oral dose is twice parenteral dose.
- Produces less nausea, vomiting, constipation than morphine, but more sedation and smooth muscle stimulation.
- Additive benefit when combined with acetaminophen or aspirin.
- Give smallest effective dose to prevent development of tolerance, physical dependency.
- Reduce dose in debilitated patients, or patients receiving other CNS depressants.
- Use with caution in patients with hepatic or renal dysfunction, hypothyroidism, Addison's disease, severe CNS depression, respiratory depression, head injury, elevated ICP.
- If required, naloxone HCl will reverse opiate toxicity (e.g., respiratory depression). However, it is important that acute withdrawal symptoms be prevented by giving only enough naloxone to reverse respiratory depression and that this be continued for opioid drug half-life.

Potential Toxicities/Side Effects and the Nursing Process

I. SENSORY/PERCEPTUAL ALTERATIONS related to CNS DEPRESSION

Defining Characteristics: Drowsiness, sedation, mood changes, euphoria, dysphoria, dizziness, mental clouding may occur. At high doses, may cause seizures. Miosis (papillary constriction) may occur.

Nursing Implications: Assess baseline neurologic status. Use cautiously, if at all, in patients who are elderly, debilitated, have a head injury, increased ICP, severe CNS depression, acute alcoholism. Assess other concurrent medications. Use with caution in patients receiving other opioids, tranquilizers, hypnotics, MAO inhibitors, since increasing CNS depressant effects can occur. Monitor neurologic status closely. Instruct patient to avoid driving and operating machinery while taking the medicine, and to AVOID concurrent alcohol.

II. ALTERATION IN OXYGENATION related to RESPIRATORY DEPRESSION

Defining Characteristics: Opiate agonists directly depress respiratory center in brain stem, causing decreased sensitivity and responsiveness to increased pCO_2. Also may depress deep breathing and reflex to sigh. Tolerance to respiratory depressant effects occurs with chronic use.

Nursing Implications: Assess baseline pulmonary status, and monitor periodically during drug use. Use cautiously in patients with bronchial asthma, COPD, respiratory depression, and monitor closely.

III. ALTERATION IN ELIMINATION related to CONSTIPATION, ILEUS

Defining Characteristics: Opium agonists bind to opiate receptors in bowel, slowing peristalsis, leading to constipation. Untreated constipation may result in bowel perforation.

Nursing Implications: Assess baseline elimination, fluid intake, diet, and exercise patterns. Instruct patient regarding prevention of constipation: goal is to move bowels at least every two days by increasing fluids to 3 L/day, following a diet high in fiber (beans, vegetables, fruit), and taking moderate exercise. Assess need for bowel softeners, bulk-forming laxatives, and osmotic cathartics, and discuss prescription with physician. Teach patient self-administration of medications.

IV. ALTERATION IN NUTRITION, LESS THAN BODY REQUIREMENTS, related to GI TOXICITY

Defining Characteristics: Nausea, vomiting, dry mouth may occur. Gastric, biliary, and pancreatic secretions are decreased by opiate agonists; digestion is delayed. Biliary tract muscle tone is increased, and spasm of Oddi's sphincter may occur (morphine > meperidine > codeine).

Nursing Implications: Assess patient tolerance of GI side effects. Teach patient to report side effects. If nausea/vomiting occur, change to another opioid, or premedicate with antiemetic to prevent nausea/vomiting. Assess GI pain, biliary spasm, and consider alternative opioid.

V. ALTERATION IN CARDIAC OUTPUT related to HYPOTENSION, BRADYCARDIA

Defining Characteristics: Orthostatic hypotension, bradycardia due to cholinergic effect, and peripheral vasodilation may occur with rapid IV dosing. There may be histamine-related flushing, pruritus, and diaphoresis with chronic drug usage; tolerance develops to this effect.

Nursing Implications: Assess baseline cardiovascular status. Teach patient to change position slowly and to hold onto stable, nearby structure for support as needed. Be careful when giving IV push opioids, and caution patient to remain in supine position for 15–20 minutes after injection. Monitor cardiovascular status after injection.

VI. ALTERATION IN URINE ELIMINATION related to URINARY RETENTION

Defining Characteristics: Increased smooth muscle tone in urinary tract and spasm may occur. Bladder tone is increased, which may cause urgency. Vesical sphincter tone may be increased, leading to difficulty urinating. Increased risk of urinary retention in patients with prostatic hypertrophy or urethral stricture.

Nursing Implications: Assess baseline urinary elimination pattern. Teach patient to increase fluids to 3 L/day, and encourage voiding every 2–3 hours. Instruct patient to report problems with urination.

VII. KNOWLEDGE DEFICIT related to DRUG ADMINISTRATION, POTENTIAL FOR TOLERANCE, AND DEPENDENCY

Defining Characteristics: Psychological dependence (addiction) occurs rarely in patients taking opioid agonists for cancer pain (< 1%). Physical dependence (precipitation of withdrawal symptoms) occurs with chronic use of the drug for the relief of chronic cancer pain. In addition, tolerance, or less analgesic effect over time with the same drug dose, occurs and requires increased dosage of drug.

Nursing Implications: Assess baseline knowledge of opioid analgesics, and attitude about their use for cancer pain management. Teach patient about proper self-administration, possible side effects, and self-care measures. Suggest patient maintain diary of pain intensity, precipitating and alleviating factors, drug dose and time taken, and relief. Teach patient to self-administer opioid agonists for relief of chronic cancer pain around-the-clock, not PRN, to prevent pain. Explain use of prescribed short-acting opioid for rescue or to manage BTP. Discuss with physician dose increase or change in frequency of administration if tolerance develops. Teach patient that withdrawal symptoms may occur if chronic, around-the-clock dosing is interrupted. Withdrawal (abstinence) symptoms that may be seen are restlessness, lacrimation, rhinorrhea, yawning, perspiration, gooseflesh, restless sleep, mydriasis in first 24 hours. These are followed by twitching and leg spasm; severe aching of the back, abdomen, and legs; cramping in abdomen and legs; hot/cold flashes; insomnia; nausea/vomiting, diarrhea; severe sneezing; and increased heart rate, BP, and T, which peak at 36–72 hours. Withdrawal syndrome can be prevented by administration of at least 1/4 of previous opioid dose.

VIII. SEXUAL DYSFUNCTION related to IMPOTENCE, ↓ LIBIDO

Defining Characteristics: Opiate agonists may suppress gonadotropin, causing impotence and decreased libido.

Nursing Implications: Assess baseline sexual pattern. Discuss potential toxicity and impact on sexuality. Provide information, emotional support, and referral as needed.

Drug: meperidine hydrochloride (Demerol, Mepergan Fortis)

Class: Opioid analgesic (opioid agonist).

Mechanism of Action: A synthetic opioid agonist, meperidine resembles morphine but has milder action; binds to opiate receptors in CNS (limbic system, thalamus, striatum, hypothalamus, midbrain, spinal cord), altering pain perception at level of spinal cord and higher centers, as well as the emotional response to pain. Also suppresses cough reflex.

Metabolism: After oral administration, metabolized by liver (first pass) with 50–60% reaching systemic circulation; thus oral administration is < 50% as effective as IM dose. After IM dose, 80–85% of drug is absorbed. Peak analgesia is ~ 1 hour after oral administration, 40–60 minutes after subcutaneous, and 30–50 minutes after IM. Duration is 2–4 hours. Drug is 60–80% bound to plasma proteins. Metabolism is by the liver, into metabolites such as normeperidine, and excreted in the urine. Normeperidine has a longer half-life and accumulates in patients with decreased renal function. It is a potent CNS stimulant, producing seizures, agitation, irritability, nervousness, tremors, twitches, and myoclonus.

Dosage/Range:

For moderate to severe pain:

- PO: 50–150 mg q 3–4 h.
- IM: 50–150 mg q 3–4 h.
- Subcutaneous: 50–150 mg q 3–4 h.
- IV: 15–35 mg/hr by continuous IV infusion.

Drug Preparation:

- Store tablets in tight, light-resistant containers at 15–30°C (59–86°F).
- Injectable preparation should be stored at 15–40°C (59–104°F).

Drug Administration:

- PO, IM, subcutaneous, IV.
- At home, teach patient to store oral doses in a safe place away from children and pets.

Drug Interactions:

- May increase isoniazid side effects; use concurrently with caution.
- Enhanced toxicity with MAO inhibitors (coma, severe respiratory depression, hypotension), so drug is contraindicated for patients who have received MAO inhibitors in previous 14 days.
- Injection incompatible with solutions containing aminophylline, barbiturates, ephedrine sulfate, heparin sodium, hydrocortisone sodium succinate, methicillin sodium, methylprednisolone sodium succinate, morphine sulfate, tetracycline.
- Alcohol, CNS depressants: additive effects.

Lab Effects/Interference:

- None known.

Special Considerations:

- Drug has many side effects, unfavorable oral to parenteral ratio, so is not recommended in the treatment of cancer-related pain. Drug is NOT used to treat or prevent chronic cancer pain because of short duration of action, bioavailability, and severe risk of neurotoxicity related to metabolite normeperidine.
- Oral meperidine, 50 mg, is equivalent in analgesia (equianalgesic) to acetaminophen 650 mg or aspirin 650 mg.
- Sedative and euphoric effect greater than morphine (equianalgesic dose).
- Oral dose is three times parenteral dose for equianalgesic effect.
- Use with caution in patients with atrial flutter or other supraventricular tachycardias (drug can increase ventricular response rate via vagolytic action).
- Formulation may contain sodium metabisulfite, which may cause anaphylactic or other allergic reactions.
- Additive benefit when combined with acetaminophen or aspirin.
- Give smallest effective dose to prevent development of tolerance, physical dependency.

- Reduce dose in debilitated patients or patients receiving other CNS depressants.
- Use with caution in patients with hepatic or renal dysfunction, hypothyroidism, Addison's disease, severe CNS depression, respiratory depression, head injury, elevated ICP.
- If required, naloxone HCl will reverse opiate toxicity (e.g., respiratory depression). However, it is important that acute withdrawal symptoms be prevented by giving only enough naloxone to reverse respiratory depression and that this be continued for opioid drug half-life.

Potential Toxicities/Side Effects and the Nursing Process

I. SENSORY/PERCEPTUAL ALTERATIONS related to CNS DEPRESSION

Defining Characteristics: Drowsiness, sedation, mood changes, euphoria, dysphoria, dizziness, mental clouding may occur. At high doses, may cause seizures. Miosis (papillary constriction) may occur.

Nursing Implications: Assess baseline neurologic status. Use cautiously, if at all, in the elderly, the debilitated, and patients with head injury, increased ICP, severe CNS depression, acute alcoholism. Assess other concurrent medications. Use with caution in patients receiving other opioids, tranquilizers, hypnotics, MAO inhibitors, since increasing CNS depressant effects can occur. Monitor neurologic status closely. Instruct patient to avoid driving and operating machinery while taking the medicine, and to AVOID concurrent alcohol.

II. ALTERATION IN OXYGENATION related to RESPIRATORY DEPRESSION

Defining Characteristics: Opiate agonists directly depress respiratory center in brain stem, causing decreased sensitivity and responsiveness to increased pCO_2. Also may depress deep breathing and reflex to sigh. Tolerance to respiratory depressant effects occurs with chronic use.

Nursing Implications: Assess baseline pulmonary status, and periodically during drug use. Use cautiously in patients with bronchial asthma, COPD, respiratory depression, and monitor closely.

III. ALTERATION IN ELIMINATION related to CONSTIPATION, ILEUS

Defining Characteristics: Opium agonists bind to opiate receptors in bowel, slowing peristalsis, leading to constipation. Untreated constipation may result in bowel perforation.

Nursing Implications: Assess baseline elimination, fluid intake, diet, and exercise patterns. Instruct patient regarding prevention of constipation: goal is to move bowels at least every two days by increasing fluids to 3 L/day, following a diet high in fiber (beans, vegetables, fruit), and taking moderate exercise. Assess need for bowel softeners, bulk-forming laxatives, and osmotic cathartics, and discuss prescription with physician. Teach patient self-administration of medications.

IV. ALTERATION IN NUTRITION related to GI TOXICITY

Defining Characteristics: Nausea, vomiting, and dry mouth may occur. Gastric, biliary, and pancreatic secretions are decreased by opiate agonists; digestion is delayed. Biliary tract muscle tone is increased, and spasm of Oddi's sphincter may occur (morphine > meperidine > codeine).

Nursing Implications: Assess patient tolerance of GI side effects. Teach patient to report side effects. If nausea/vomiting occur, change to another opioid, or premedicate with antiemetic to prevent nausea/vomiting. Assess GI pain, biliary spasm, and consider alternative opioid.

V. ALTERATION IN CARDIAC OUTPUT related to HYPOTENSION, BRADYCARDIA

Defining Characteristics: Orthostatic hypotension, bradycardia due to cholinergic effect, and peripheral vasodilation may occur with rapid IV dosing. There may be histamine-related flushing, pruritus, diaphoresis with chronic drug usage; tolerance develops to this effect.

Nursing Implications: Assess baseline cardiovascular status. Teach patient to change position slowly and to hold onto stable, nearby structure for support as needed. Be careful when giving IV push opioids, and caution patient to remain in supine position for 15–20 minutes after injection. Monitor cardiovascular status after injection.

VI. ALTERATION IN URINE ELIMINATION related to URINARY RETENTION

Defining Characteristics: Increased smooth muscle tone in urinary tract and spasm may occur. Bladder tone is increased, which may cause urgency. Vesical sphincter tone may be increased, leading to difficulty urinating. Increased risk of urinary retention in patients with prostatic hypertrophy or urethral stricture.

Nursing Implications: Assess baseline urinary elimination pattern. Teach patient to increase fluids to 3 L/day, and encourage voiding every 2–3 hours. Instruct patient to report problems with urination.

VII. KNOWLEDGE DEFICIT related to DRUG ADMINISTRATION, POTENTIAL FOR TOLERANCE, AND DEPENDENCY

Defining Characteristics: Psychological dependence (addiction) occurs rarely in patients taking opioid agonists for cancer pain (< 1%). Physical dependence (precipitation of withdrawal symptoms) occurs with chronic use of the drug for the relief of chronic cancer pain. In addition, tolerance, or less analgesic effect over time with the same drug dose, occurs and requires increased dosage of drug.

Nursing Implications: Assess baseline knowledge of opioid analgesics and attitude about their use for cancer pain management. Teach patient about proper self-administration, possible side effects, and self-care measures. Suggest patient maintain diary of pain intensity, precipitating and alleviating factors, drug dose and time taken, and relief. Teach patient to self-administer opioid agonists for relief of chronic cancer pain around-the-clock, not PRN, to prevent pain. Explain use of prescribed short-acting opioid for rescue or to manage breakthrough pain. Discuss with physician dose increase or change in frequency of administration if tolerance develops. Teach patient that withdrawal symptoms may occur if chronic, around-the-clock dosing is interrupted. Withdrawal (abstinence) symptoms that may be seen are restlessness, lacrimation, rhinorrhea, yawning, perspiration, gooseflesh, restless sleep, mydriasis in first 24 hours. These are followed by twitching and leg spasm; severe aching of the back, abdomen, and legs; cramping in abdomen and legs; hot/cold flashes; insomnia; nausea/vomiting, diarrhea; severe sneezing; and increased heart rate, BP, T, which peak at 36–72 hours. Withdrawal syndrome can be prevented by administration of at least 1/4 of previous opioid dose.

VIII. SEXUAL DYSFUNCTION related to IMPOTENCE, ↓ LIBIDO

Defining Characteristics: Opiate agonists may suppress gonadotropin, causing impotence and decreased libido.

Nursing Implications: Assess baseline sexual pattern. Discuss potential toxicity and impact on sexuality. Provide information, emotional support, and referral as needed.

Drug: methadone (Dolophine, Methadose)

Class: Opioid analgesic (opioid agonist).

Mechanism of Action: A synthetic opioid agonist, methadone resembles morphine but has milder action; binds to opiate receptors in CNS (limbic system, thalamus, striatum, hypothalamus, midbrain, spinal cord), altering pain perception at level of spinal cord and higher centers, as well as the emotional response to pain. Also suppresses cough reflex.

Metabolism: Well absorbed from GI tract; onset and duration of single dose similar to morphine. With chronic administration (physical dependency) half-life is 22–48 hours. Highly tissue-bound; metabolized by liver, excreted by renal filtration, then is reabsorbed (pH dependent).

Dosage/Range:

For moderate to severe pain:

- PO: 5–20 mg q 6–8 h, or more for severe cancer pain.
- Subcutaneous, IM: 2.5–10 mg q 3–4 h.

Drug Preparation:

- Store tablets in tight, light-resistant containers at 15–30°C (59–86°F).
- Injection should be protected from light and stored at 15–40°C (59–104°F).
- At home, teach patient to store oral doses in a safe place away from children and pets.

Drug Administration:

- PO, IM, subcutaneous.

Drug Interactions:

- Injection incompatible with solutions containing aminophylline, ammonium chloride, amobarbital sodium, chlorothiazide sodium, heparin sodium, methicillin sodium, nitrofurantoin, phenobarbital sodium, sodium bicarbonate.
- Alcohol, CNS depressants: additive effects.

Lab Effects/Interference:

- None known.

Special Considerations:

- Oral dose is twice parenteral dose (equianalgesic effect).
- May produce similar or slightly greater respiratory depression than equivalent doses of morphine.
- Additive benefit when combined with acetaminophen or aspirin.
- Give smallest effective dose to prevent development of tolerance, physical dependency.
- Reduce dose in debilitated patients or patients receiving other CNS depressants.
- Use with caution in patients with hepatic or renal dysfunction, hypothyroidism, Addison's disease, severe CNS depression, respiratory depression, head injury, elevated ICP.
- If required, naloxone HCl will reverse opiate toxicity (e.g., respiratory depression). However, it is important that acute withdrawal symptoms be prevented by giving

only enough naloxone to reverse respiratory depression and that this be continued for opioid drug half-life.

Potential Toxicities/Side Effects and the Nursing Process

I. SENSORY/PERCEPTUAL ALTERATIONS related to CNS DEPRESSION

Defining Characteristics: Drowsiness, sedation, mood changes, euphoria, dysphoria, dizziness, mental clouding may occur. At high doses, may cause seizures. Miosis (papillary constriction) may occur.

Nursing Implications: Assess baseline neurologic status. Use cautiously, if at all, in the elderly, the debilitated, and patients with head injury, increased ICP, severe CNS depression, acute alcoholism. Assess other concurrent medications. Use with caution in patients receiving other opioids, tranquilizers, hypnotics, MAO inhibitors, since increasing CNS depressant effects can occur. Monitor neurologic status closely. Instruct patient to avoid driving and operating machinery while taking the medicine, and to AVOID concurrent alcohol.

II. ALTERATION IN OXYGENATION related to RESPIRATORY DEPRESSION

Defining Characteristics: Opiate agonists directly depress respiratory center in brain stem, causing decreased sensitivity and responsiveness to increased pCO_2. Also may depress deep breathing and reflex to sigh. Tolerance to respiratory depressant effects occurs with chronic use.

Nursing Implications: Assess baseline pulmonary status, and periodically during drug use. Use cautiously in patients with bronchial asthma, COPD, respiratory depression, and monitor closely.

III. ALTERATION IN ELIMINATION related to CONSTIPATION, ILEUS

Defining Characteristics: Opium agonists bind to opiate receptors in bowel, slowing peristalsis, leading to constipation. Untreated constipation may result in bowel perforation.

Nursing Implications: Assess baseline elimination, fluid intake, diet, and exercise patterns. Instruct patient regarding prevention of constipation: goal is to move bowels at least every two days by increasing fluids to 3 L/day, following a diet high in fiber (beans, vegetables, fruit), and taking moderate exercise. Assess need for bowel softeners, bulk-forming laxatives, and osmotic cathartics, and discuss prescription with physician. Teach patient self-administration of medications.

IV. ALTERATION IN NUTRITION, LESS THAN BODY REQUIREMENTS, related to GI TOXICITY

Defining Characteristics: Nausea, vomiting, and dry mouth may occur. Gastric, biliary, and pancreatic secretions are decreased by opiate agonists; digestion is delayed. Biliary tract muscle tone is increased, and spasm of Oddi's sphincter may occur (morphine > meperidine > codeine).

Nursing Implications: Assess patient tolerance of GI side effects. Instruct patient to report side effects. If nausea/vomiting occur, change to another opioid, or premedicate with antiemetic to prevent nausea/vomiting. Assess GI pain, biliary spasm, and consider alternative opioid.

V. ALTERATION IN CARDIAC OUTPUT related to HYPOTENSION, BRADYCARDIA

Defining Characteristics: Orthostatic hypotension, bradycardia due to cholinergic effect, and peripheral vasodilation may occur with rapid IV dosing. There may be histamine-related flushing, pruritus, diaphoresis with chronic drug usage; tolerance develops to this effect.

Nursing Implications: Assess baseline cardiovascular status. Teach patient to change position slowly and to hold onto stable, nearby structure for support as needed. Be careful when giving IV push opioids, and caution patient to remain in supine position for 15–20 minutes after injection. Monitor cardiovascular status after injection.

VI. ALTERATION IN URINE ELIMINATION related to URINARY RETENTION

Defining Characteristics: Increased smooth muscle tone in urinary tract and spasm may occur. Bladder tone is increased, which may cause urgency. Vesical sphincter tone may be increased leading to difficulty urinating. Increased risk of urinary retention in patients with prostatic hypertrophy or urethral stricture.

Nursing Implications: Assess baseline urinary elimination pattern. Teach patient to increase fluids to 3 L/day, and encourage voiding every 2–3 hours. Instruct patient to report problems with urination.

VII. KNOWLEDGE DEFICIT related to DRUG ADMINISTRATION, POTENTIAL FOR TOLERANCE, AND DEPENDENCY

Defining Characteristics: Psychological dependence (addiction) occurs rarely in patients taking opioid agonists for cancer pain (< 1%). Physical dependence (precipitation of withdrawal symptoms) occurs with chronic use of the drug for the relief of chronic cancer pain. In addition, tolerance, or less analgesic effect over time with the same drug dose, occurs and requires increased dosage of drug.

Nursing Implications: Assess baseline knowledge of opioid analgesics, and attitude about their use for cancer pain management. Teach patient about proper self-administration, possible side effects, and self-care measures. Suggest patient maintain diary of pain intensity, precipitating and alleviating factors, drug dose and time taken, and relief. Teach patient to self-administer opioid agonists for relief of chronic cancer pain around-the-clock, not PRN, to prevent pain. Explain use of prescribed short-acting opioid for rescue or to manage BTP. Discuss with physician dose increase or change in frequency of administration if tolerance develops. Teach patient that withdrawal symptoms may occur if chronic, around the-clock dosing is interrupted. Withdrawal (abstinence) symptoms that may be seen are restlessness, lacrimation, rhinorrhea, yawning, perspiration, gooseflesh, restless sleep, mydriasis in first 24 hours. These are followed by twitching and leg spasm; severe aching of the back, abdomen, and legs; cramping in abdomen and legs; hot/cold flashes; insomnia; nausea/vomiting, diarrhea; severe sneezing; and increased heart rate, BP, T, which peak at 36–72 hours. Withdrawal syndrome can be prevented by administration of at least 1/4 of previous opioid dose.

VIII. SEXUAL DYSFUNCTION related to IMPOTENCE, ↓ LIBIDO

Defining Characteristics: Opiate agonists may suppress gonadotropin, causing impotence and decreased libido.

Nursing Implications: Assess baseline sexual pattern. Discuss potential toxicity and impact on sexuality. Provide information, emotional support, and referral as needed.

Drug: morphine (Astramorph, Avinza, Duramorph, Infumorph, Kadian Morphine Sulfate Sustained Release, MS Contin, MSIR, Morphelan, Oramorph, Roxanol)

Class: Opioid analgesic (opioid agonist).

Mechanism of Action: Binds to opiate receptors in CNS (limbic system, thalamus, striatum, hypothalamus, midbrain, spinal cord). This opioid agonist alters pain perception at level of spinal cord and higher centers, as well as the emotional response to pain. Also suppresses cough reflex.

Metabolism: Variable absorption from GI tract; increased absorption when taken with food. Peak analgesia 60 minutes (oral), 20–60 minutes (rectal), 50–90 minutes (subcutaneous), 30–60 minutes (IM), 20 minutes (IV). Duration is 4–7 hours. Maximum respiratory depression is 30 minutes (IM), 7 minutes (IV), 90 minutes (subcutaneous). Drug is slowly absorbed into systemic circulation after intrathecal (IT) administration. Peak CSF concentrations occur 60–90 minutes after epidural dose. Metabolized by liver and excreted in urine and, to a small degree, feces.

Dosage/Range:

For moderate to severe pain:

- Oral: 10–60 mg PO q 3–4 h titrated to pain; 10–240 mg sustained release q 8–12 h, titrated to pain.
- Rectal: 10–60 mg q 4 h.
- Subcutaneous, IM: 4–15 mg q 3–4 h.
- IV: 1–100 mg/h, and higher, titrated to need in physically dependent patients.
- Intrathecal: dose is 1/10 the epidural dose.
- Epidural: 5 mg q 24 h.
- At home, teach patient to store oral doses in a safe place away from children and pets.

Drug Preparation:

- Store tablets in tight, light-resistant containers at 15–30°C (59–86°F).
- Injection should be protected from light, and stored at 15–40°C (59–104°F).

Drug Administration:

- Begin morphine therapy using immediate-release oral preparations and increase dose to control pain; once optimal dose identified, convert to sustained-release formulation by dividing 24-hour total morphine dose by 2, giving two (q 12 h) doses.
- Intrathecal or epidural: use preservative-free morphine only, e.g., Astramorph PF, Duramorph PF, Infumorph; consult individual policies/procedures for administration.

Drug Interactions:

- Injection incompatible with solutions containing aminophylline, ammonium chloride, amobarbital sodium, chlorothiazide sodium, heparin sodium, methicillin sodium, nitrofurantoin, phenobarbital sodium, sodium bicarbonate.
- Alcohol, CNS depressants: additive effects.

Lab Effects/Interference:

- None known.

Special Considerations:

- Oral to parenteral dose is 3–6 to 1 (equianalgesic dose).
- Highly concentrated formulations are available and are for use in continuous infusion pumps.

- Do not crush sustained-release formulations (e.g., MS Contin, Oramorph).
- When epidural or intrathecal route is used, refer to institutional policy/procedure for administration and patient monitoring.
- Additive benefit when combined with acetaminophen or aspirin.
- Give smallest effective dose to prevent development of tolerance, physical dependency.
- Reduce dose in debilitated patients, or patients receiving other CNS depressants.
- Use with caution in patients with hepatic or renal dysfunction, hypothyroidism, Addison's disease, severe CNS depression, respiratory depression, head injury, elevated intracranial pressure.
- If required, naloxone HCl will reverse opiate toxicity (e.g., respiratory depression). However, it is important that acute withdrawal symptoms be prevented by giving only enough naloxone to reverse respiratory depression and that this be continued for opioid drug half-life.
- Kadian as well as Avinza are sustained-release morphine formulated for once-a-day dosing; available in 20-, 50-, and 100-mg tablets (Kadian) and 30-, 60-, 90-, and 120 mg capsules (Avinza).

Potential Toxicities/Side Effects and the Nursing Process

I. SENSORY/PERCEPTUAL ALTERATIONS related to CNS DEPRESSION

Defining Characteristics: Drowsiness, sedation, mood changes, euphoria, dysphoria, dizziness, mental clouding may occur. At high doses, may cause seizures. Miosis (papillary constriction) may occur.

Nursing Implications: Assess baseline neurologic status. Use cautiously, if at all, in the elderly, the debilitated, and patients with head injury, increased intracranial pressure, severe CNS depression, acute alcoholism. Assess other concurrent medications. Use with caution in patients receiving other opioids, tranquilizers, hypnotics, MAO inhibitors, since increasing CNS depressant effects can occur. Monitor neurologic status closely. Instruct patient to avoid driving and operating machinery while taking the medicine, and to AVOID concurrent alcohol.

II. ALTERATION IN OXYGENATION related to RESPIRATORY DEPRESSION

Defining Characteristics: Opiate agonists directly depress respiratory center in brain stem, causing decreased sensitivity and responsiveness to increased pCO_2. Also may depress deep breathing and reflex to sigh. Tolerance to respiratory depressant effects occurs with chronic use.

Nursing Implications: Assess baseline pulmonary status, and periodically during drug use. Use cautiously in patients with bronchial asthma, COPD, respiratory depression, and monitor closely.

III. ALTERATION IN ELIMINATION related to CONSTIPATION, ILEUS

Defining Characteristics: Opium agonists bind to opiate receptors in bowel, slowing peristalsis, leading to constipation. Untreated constipation may result in bowel perforation.

Nursing Implications: Assess baseline elimination, fluid intake, diet, and exercise patterns. Instruct patient regarding prevention of constipation: goal is to move bowels at least every two days by increasing fluids to 3 L/day, following a diet high in fiber (beans, vegetables, fruit), and taking moderate exercise. Assess need for bowel softeners, bulk-forming laxatives, and osmotic cathartics, and discuss prescription with physician. Teach patient self-administration of medications.

IV. ALTERATION IN NUTRITION, LESS THAN BODY REQUIREMENTS, related to GI TOXICITY

Defining Characteristics: Nausea, vomiting, and dry mouth may occur. Gastric, biliary, and pancreatic secretions are decreased by opiate agonists; digestion is delayed. Biliary tract muscle tone is increased, and spasm of Oddi's sphincter may occur (morphine > meperidine > codeine).

Nursing Implications: Assess patient tolerance of GI side effects. Teach patient to report side effects. If nausea/vomiting occur, change to another opioid, or premedicate with antiemetic to prevent nausea/vomiting. Assess GI pain, biliary spasm, and consider alternative opioid.

V. ALTERATION IN CARDIAC OUTPUT related to HYPOTENSION, BRADYCARDIA

Defining Characteristics: Orthostatic hypotension, bradycardia due to cholinergic effect, and peripheral vasodilation may occur with rapid IV dosing. There may be histamine-related flushing, pruritus, diaphoresis with chronic drug usage; tolerance develops to this effect.

Nursing Implications: Assess baseline cardiovascular status. Teach patient to change position slowly and to hold onto stable, nearby structure for support as needed. Be careful when giving IV push opioids, and caution patient to remain in supine position for 15–20 minutes after injection. Monitor cardiovascular status after injection.

VI. ALTERATION IN URINE ELIMINATION related to URINARY RETENTION

Defining Characteristics: Increased smooth muscle tone in urinary tract and spasm may occur. Bladder tone is increased, which may cause urgency. Vesical sphincter tone may be increased, leading to difficulty urinating. Increased risk of urinary retention in patients with prostatic hypertrophy or urethral stricture.

Nursing Implications: Assess baseline urinary elimination pattern. Teach patient to increase fluids to 3 L/day, and encourage voiding every 2–3 hours. Instruct patient to report problems with urination.

VII. KNOWLEDGE DEFICIT related to DRUG ADMINISTRATION, POTENTIAL FOR TOLERANCE, AND DEPENDENCY

Defining Characteristics: Psychological dependence (addiction) occurs rarely in patients taking opioid agonists for cancer pain (< 1%). Physical dependence (precipitation of withdrawal symptoms) occurs with chronic use of the drug for the relief of chronic cancer pain. In addition, tolerance, or less analgesic effect over time with the same drug dose, occurs and requires increased dosage of drug.

Nursing Implications: Assess baseline knowledge of opioid analgesics, and attitude about their use for cancer pain management. Teach patient about proper self-administration, possible side effects, and self-care measures. Suggest patient maintain diary of pain intensity, precipitating and alleviating factors, drug dose and time taken, and relief. Teach patient to self-administer opioid agonists for relief of chronic cancer pain around-the-clock, not PRN, to prevent pain. Explain use of prescribed short-acting opioid for rescue or to manage breakthrough pain. Discuss with physician dose increase or change in frequency of administration if tolerance develops. Teach patient that withdrawal symptoms may occur if chronic, around-the-clock dosing is interrupted. Withdrawal (abstinence) symptoms that may be seen are restlessness, lacrimation, rhinorrhea, yawning, perspiration, gooseflesh, restless sleep, mydriasis in first 24 hours. These are followed by twitching and leg spasm; severe aching of the back, abdomen, and legs; cramping in abdomen and legs; hot/cold flashes; insomnia; nausea/vomiting, diarrhea; severe sneezing; and increased heart rate, BP, T, which peak at 36–72 hours. Withdrawal syndrome can be prevented by administration of at least 1/4 of previous opioid dose.

VIII. SEXUAL DYSFUNCTION related to IMPOTENCE, ↓ LIBIDO

Defining Characteristics: Opiate agonists may suppress gonadotropin, causing impotence and decreased libido.

Nursing Implications: Assess baseline sexual pattern. Discuss potential toxicity and impact on sexuality. Provide information, emotional support, and referral as needed.

Drug: oxycodone (Percodan, Endodan, Roxiprin)

Class: Opioid analgesic (opioid agonist).

Mechanism of Action: A synthetic opioid agonist, oxycodone resembles morphine but has milder action; binds to opiate receptors in CNS (limbic system, thalamus, striatum, hypothalamus, midbrain, spinal cord), altering pain perception at level of spinal cord and higher centers, as well as the emotional response to pain. Also suppresses cough reflex.

Metabolism: Onset of analgesia in 10–15 minutes, peaks 30–60 minutes, duration 3–6 hours. Metabolized by liver and kidney; excreted in urine.

Dosage/Range:
For moderate to moderately severe pain:
- 5 mg q 6 h (Roxicodone).
- 5 mg q 6 h, combined with acetaminophen: 300 mg (e.g., Oxycet, Percocet, Roxicet caplets), OR 500 mg (e.g., Roxicet caplets, Tylox); OR combined with aspirin: 325 mg (e.g., Percodan, Codoxy, Roxiprin); OR combined with ibuprofen 5 mg/400 mg (e.g., Combunox).
- Oral solution: 5 mg/5 mL (Roxicodone); 20 mg/mL (Roxicodone, Intensol).
- Oxycontin 10-mg, 20-mg, 40-mg (sustained-release) tablets q 12 h.

Drug Preparation:
- Store tablets in tight, light-resistant containers at 15–30°C (59–86°F) and protect from light.
- At home, teach patient to store oral doses in a safe place away from children and pets.

Drug Administration:
- Oral.

Drug Interactions:
- Alcohol, CNS depressants: additive CNS depressant effects.
- Anticoagulants, chemotherapy: aspirin-oxycodone combination may increase bleeding risk; AVOID concurrent use.

Lab Effects/Interference:
- None known.

Special Considerations:
- Adverse effects are milder than morphine.
- Preparations may contain sodium metabisulfite and may cause allergic reactions, including anaphylaxis and severe asthma-like reactions.

- Additive benefit when combined with acetaminophen or aspirin.
- Give smallest effective dose to prevent development of tolerance, physical dependency.
- Reduce dose in debilitated patients or patients receiving other CNS depressants.
- Use with caution in patients with hepatic or renal dysfunction, hypothyroidism, Addison's disease, severe CNS depression, respiratory depression, head injury, elevated ICP.
- If required, naloxone HCl will reverse opiate toxicity (e.g., respiratory depression). However, it is important that acute withdrawal symptoms be prevented by giving only enough naloxone to reverse respiratory depression and that this be continued for opioid drug half-life.
- Oxycontin is a sustained-release oxycodone preparation that is taken q 12 h; available in 10-mg, 20-mg, and 40-mg tablets.

Potential Toxicities/Side Effects and the Nursing Process

I. SENSORY/PERCEPTUAL ALTERATIONS related to CNS DEPRESSION

Defining Characteristics: Drowsiness, sedation, mood changes, euphoria, dysphoria, dizziness, mental clouding may occur. At high doses, may cause seizures. Miosis (papillary constriction) may occur.

Nursing Implications: Assess baseline neurologic status. Use cautiously, if at all, in the elderly, the debilitated, and patients with head injury, increased ICP, severe CNS depression, acute alcoholism. Assess other concurrent medications. Use with caution in patients receiving other opioids, tranquilizers, hypnotics, MAO inhibitors, since increasing CNS depressant effects can occur. Monitor neurologic status closely. Instruct patient to avoid driving and operating machinery while taking the medicine, and to AVOID concurrent alcohol.

II. ALTERATION IN OXYGENATION related to RESPIRATORY DEPRESSION

Defining Characteristics: Opiate agonists directly depress respiratory center in brain stem, causing decreased sensitivity and responsiveness to increased pCO_2. Also may depress deep breathing and reflex to sigh. Tolerance to respiratory depressant effects occurs with chronic use.

Nursing Implications: Assess baseline pulmonary status, and periodically during drug use. Use cautiously in patients with bronchial asthma, COPD, respiratory depression, and monitor closely.

III. ALTERATION IN ELIMINATION related to CONSTIPATION, ILEUS

Defining Characteristics: Opium agonists bind to opiate receptors in bowel, slowing peristalsis, leading to constipation. Untreated constipation may result in bowel perforation.

Nursing Implications: Assess baseline elimination, fluid intake, diet, and exercise patterns. Instruct patient regarding prevention of constipation: goal is to move bowels at least every two days by increasing fluids to 3 L/day, following a diet high in fiber (beans, vegetables, fruit), and taking moderate exercise. Assess need for bowel softeners, bulk-forming laxatives, and osmotic cathartics, and discuss preparation with physician. Teach patient self-administration of medications.

IV. ALTERATION IN NUTRITION, LESS THAN BODY REQUIREMENTS, related to GI TOXICITY

Defining Characteristics: Nausea, vomiting, dry mouth may occur. Gastric, biliary, and pancreatic secretions are decreased by opiate agonists; digestion is delayed. Biliary tract muscle tone is increased, and spasm of Oddi's sphincter may occur (morphine > meperidine > codeine).

Nursing Implications: Assess patient tolerance of GI side effects. Teach patient to report side effects. If nausea/vomiting occur, change to another opioid, or premedicate with antiemetic to prevent nausea/vomiting. Assess GI pain, biliary spasm, and consider alternative opioid.

V. ALTERATION IN CARDIAC OUTPUT related to HYPOTENSION, BRADYCARDIA

Defining Characteristics: Orthostatic hypotension, bradycardia due to cholinergic effect, and peripheral vasodilation may occur with rapid IV dosing. There may be histamine-related flushing, pruritus, diaphoresis with chronic drug usage; tolerance develops to this effect.

Nursing Implications: Assess baseline cardiovascular status. Teach patient to change position slowly and to hold onto stable, nearby structure for support as needed. Be careful when giving IV push opioids, and caution patient to remain in supine position for 15–20 minutes after injection. Monitor cardiovascular status after injection.

VI. ALTERATION IN URINE ELIMINATION related to URINARY RETENTION

Defining Characteristics: Increased smooth muscle tone in urinary tract and spasm may occur. Bladder tone is increased, which may cause urgency. Vesical sphincter tone may be increased, leading to difficulty urinating. Increased risk of urinary retention in patients with prostatic hypertrophy or urethral stricture.

Nursing Implications: Assess baseline urinary elimination pattern. Teach patient to increase fluids to 3 L/day, and encourage voiding every 2–3 hours. Instruct patient to report problems with urination.

VII. KNOWLEDGE DEFICIT related to DRUG ADMINISTRATION, POTENTIAL FOR TOLERANCE, AND DEPENDENCY

Defining Characteristics: Psychological dependence (addiction) occurs rarely in patients taking opioid agonists for cancer pain (< 1%). Physical dependence (precipitation of withdrawal symptoms) occurs with chronic use of the drug for the relief of chronic cancer pain. In addition, tolerance, or less analgesic effect over time with the same drug dose, occurs and requires increased dosage of drug.

Nursing Implications: Assess baseline knowledge of opioid analgesics, and attitude about their use for cancer pain management. Teach patient about proper self-administration, possible side effects, and self-care measures. Suggest patient maintain diary of pain intensity, precipitating and alleviating factors, drug dose and time taken, and relief. Teach patient to self-administer opioid agonists for relief of chronic cancer pain around-the-clock, not PRN, to prevent pain. Explain use of prescribed short-acting opioid for rescue or to manage breakthrough pain. Discuss with physician dose increase or change in frequency of administration if tolerance develops. Teach patient that withdrawal symptoms may occur if chronic, around-the-clock dosing is interrupted. Withdrawal (abstinence) symptoms that may be seen are restlessness, lacrimation, rhinorrhea, yawning, perspiration, gooseflesh, restless sleep, mydriasis in first 24 hours. These are followed by twitching and leg spasm; severe aching of the back, abdomen, and legs; cramping in abdomen and legs; hot/cold flashes; insomnia; nausea/vomiting, diarrhea; severe sneezing; and increased heart rate, BP, T, which peak at 36–72 hours. Withdrawal syndrome can be prevented by administration of at least 1/4 of previous opioid dose.

VIII. SEXUAL DYSFUNCTION related to IMPOTENCE, ↓ LIBIDO

Defining Characteristics: Opiate agonists may suppress gonadotropin, causing impotence and decreased libido.

Nursing Implications: Assess baseline sexual pattern. Discuss potential toxicity and impact on sexuality. Provide information, emotional support, and referral as needed.

Drug: oxymorphone hydrochloride (Opana)

Class: Opioid analgesic (opioid agonist).

Mechanism of Action: A semi-synthetic opioid agonist, oxymorphone HCl resembles morphine but has milder action; binds to opiate receptors in CNS (limbic system, thalamus, striatum, hypothalamus, midbrain, spinal cord), altering pain perception at level of spinal cord and higher centers, as well as the emotional response to pain. Also suppresses cough reflex.

Metabolism: Absolute oral bioavailability is about 10%, and steady state serum levels occurred after 3 days of multiple doses. Food increases absorption by 38%, so it should not be taken with food. Drug is not bound to plasma proteins to any degree (10–12%), and is highly metabolized by the liver by reduction or conjugation with glucuronide into active and inactive metabolites. In studies of drug in extended formulation, bioavailability is higher in patients with hepatic or renal impairment, and plasma levels in the elderly were 40% higher than younger controls. Drug and metabolites are excreted in the urine and feces.

Dosage/Range:

For moderate to severe acute pain:

- Usual initial dose in opioid-naïve patients is 10–20 mg PO q 4–6 hr PRN depending on initial pain intensity; alternatively, a dose of 5 mg may be used initially.
- If patient is receiving parenteral oxymorphone, given the 10% bioavailability, multiply the total parenteral dose of oxymorphone by 10, and administer in 4 or 6 equally divided doses.
- Beginning dose for elderly patient should be 5 mg PO q 4–6 hr PRN.
- Administer cautiously and in reduced doses in patients with creatinine clearance rates < 50 mL/min.
- Drug is contraindicated in patients with moderate and severe hepatic dysfunction; use cautiously and start at the lowest dose in patients with mild hepatic dysfunction, and titrate dose up.
- If patient is receiving CNS depressants (sedatives, hypnotics, general anesthetics, phenothiazines, tranquilizers, or alcohol) concurrently, start at ⅓ to ½ of the usual dose.
- If opioids are discontinued, drug should be gradually tapered to prevent withdrawal.

Drug Preparation:

- Drug available in 5- and 10-mg tablets.
- At home, teach patient to store oral doses in a safe place away from children and pets.

Drug Administration:
- Oral, on an empty stomach (at least 1 hour before or 2 hours after food ingestion).

Drug Interactions:
- Alcohol, CNS depressants: Additive CNS depressant effects (hypotension, respiratory depression, profound sedation).
- Mixed agonist/antagonist analgesics (pentazocine, nalbuphine, butorphanol, buprenorphine) should not be given concurrently, as they may reduce the analgesic effect of oxymorphone and/or precipitate withdrawal.

Lab Effects/Interference:
- None known.

Special Considerations:
- Indicated for the relief of moderate to severe acute pain.
- Additive benefit when combined with acetaminophen or aspirin.
- Give smallest effective dose to prevent development of tolerance, physical dependency.
- Reduce dose in debilitated patients or patients receiving other CNS depressants.
- If required, naloxone HCl will reverse opiate toxicity (e.g., respiratory depression). However, it is important that acute withdrawal symptoms are prevented by giving only enough naloxone to reverse respiratory depression, and that this be continued for opioid drug half-life.
- Opioids cause peripheral vasodilation, which may cause hypotension; in addition, many cause the release of histamine, which can further intensify the hypotension. Oxymorphone has a lower likelihood of causing histamine release than other opioids.

Potential Toxicities/Side Effects and the Nursing Process

I. SENSORY/PERCEPTUAL ALTERATIONS related to CNS DEPRESSION

Defining Characteristics: Adverse effects were < 10%: Drowsiness, sedation, mood changes, euphoria, dysphoria, dizziness, confusion.

Nursing Implications: Assess baseline neurologic status. Use cautiously in the elderly, and start with lowest dose and titrate up. Use cautiously, if at all, in patients who are debilitated, and patients with head injury, increased ICP, severe CNS depression, or acute alcoholism. Assess other concurrent medications. Use with caution in patients receiving other opioids, tranquilizers, hypnotics, MAO inhibitors, since increasing CNS depressant effects can occur. Monitor neurologic status closely. Instruct patient to avoid driving and operating machinery while taking the medicine, and to AVOID concurrent alcohol.

II. ALTERATION IN OXYGENATION related to RESPIRATORY DEPRESSION

Defining Characteristics: Opiate agonists directly depress respiratory center in brain stem, causing decreased sensitivity and responsiveness to increased pCO_2. May also depress deep breathing and reflex to sigh. Tolerance to respiratory depressant effects occurs with chronic use.

Nursing Implications: Assess baseline pulmonary status, and periodically during drug use. Use cautiously in patients with bronchial asthma, COPD, respiratory depression, and monitor closely.

III. ALTERATION IN ELIMINATION related to CONSTIPATION, ILEUS

Defining Characteristics: Opium agonists bind to opiate receptors in bowel, slowing peristalsis, leading to constipation. Untreated constipation may result in bowel perforation. Incidence of constipation in clinical trials was 4%.

Nursing Implications: Assess baseline elimination, fluid intake, diet, and exercise patterns. Instruct patient regarding prevention of constipation: goal is to move bowels at least every two days by increasing fluids to 3 L/day, following a diet high in fiber (beans, vegetables, fruit), and taking moderate exercise. Assess need for bowel softeners, bulk-forming laxatives, and osmotic cathartics, and discuss preparation with physician. Teach patient self-administration of medications.

IV. ALTERATION IN NUTRITION, LESS THAN BODY REQUIREMENTS, related to GI TOXICITY

Defining Characteristics: Nausea, vomiting, dry mouth may occur. Gastric, biliary, and pancreatic secretions are decreased by opiate agonists; digestion is delayed. Biliary tract muscle tone is increased, and spasm of Oddi's sphincter may occur (morphine > meperidine > codeine).

Nursing Implications: Assess patient tolerance of GI side effects. Teach patient to report side effects. If nausea/vomiting occur, change to another opioid, or premedicate with antiemetic to prevent nausea/vomiting. Assess GI pain, biliary spasm, and consider alternative opioid.

V. ALTERATION IN URINE ELIMINATION related to URINARY RETENTION

Defining Characteristics: Rarely, increased smooth muscle tone in urinary tract and spasm may occur. Bladder tone is increased, which may cause urgency. Vesical sphincter tone may be increased, leading to difficulty urinating. Increased risk of urinary retention in patients with prostatic hypertrophy or urethral stricture.

Nursing Implications: Assess baseline urinary elimination pattern. Teach patient to increase fluids to 3 L/day, and encourage voiding every 2–3 hours. Instruct patient to report problems with urination.

VI. KNOWLEDGE DEFICIT related to DRUG ADMINISTRATION, POTENTIAL FOR TOLERANCE, AND DEPENDENCY

Defining Characteristics: Psychological dependence (addiction) occurs rarely in patients taking opioid agonists for cancer pain (< 1%). Physical dependence (precipitation of withdrawal symptoms) occurs with chronic use of the drug for the relief of chronic cancer pain. In addition, tolerance, or less analgesic effect over time with the same drug dose, occurs and requires increased dosage of drug.

Nursing Implications: Assess baseline knowledge of opioid analgesics, and attitude about their use for cancer pain management. Teach patient about proper self-administration, possible side effects, and self-care measures. Suggest patient maintain diary of pain intensity, precipitating and alleviating factors, drug dose and time taken, and relief. Teach patient to self-administer opioid agonists for relief of chronic cancer pain around-the-clock, not PRN, to prevent pain. Explain use of prescribed short-acting opioid for rescue or to manage breakthrough pain. Discuss with physician dose increase or change in frequency of administration if tolerance develops. Teach patient that withdrawal symptoms may occur if chronic, around-the-clock dosing is interrupted. Withdrawal (abstinence) symptoms that may be seen in the first 24 hours are restlessness, lacrimation, rhinorrhea, yawning, perspiration, gooseflesh, restless sleep, mydriasis. These are followed by twitching and leg spasms; severe aching of the back, abdomen, and legs; cramping in abdomen and legs; hot/cold flashes; insomnia; nausea/vomiting, diarrhea; severe sneezing; and increased heart rate, BP, T, which peak at 36–72 hours. Withdrawal syndrome can be prevented by administration of at least ¼ of previous opioid dose.

Drug: oxymorphone hydrochloride extended release (Opana ER)

Class: Opioid analgesic (opioid agonist).

Mechanism of Action: A semi-synthetic opioid agonist, oxymorphone HCl resembles morphine but has milder action; binds to opiate receptors in CNS (limbic system, thalamus, striatum, hypothalamus, midbrain, spinal cord), altering pain perception at level of spinal cord and higher centers, as well as the emotional response to pain. Also suppresses cough reflex.

Metabolism: Absolute oral bioavailability is about 10%, and steady state serum levels occurred after 3 days of multiple doses. Food increases absorption by 38% so it should not be taken with food. Drug is not bound to plasma proteins to any degree (10–12%), and is highly metabolized by the liver by reduction or conjugation with glucuronide into active and inactive metabolites. In studies of drug in extended formulation, bioavailability is higher in patients with hepatic or renal impairment, and plasma levels in the elderly were 40% higher than younger controls. Drug and metabolites are excreted in the urine and feces.

Dosage/Range:

For moderate to severe:

- Usual initial dose in opioid-naïve patients is 5 mg every 12 hours; thereafter, the dose should be individually titrated in increments of 5–10 mg q 12 hours every 3–7 days to an effective dose that provides adequate analgesia and minimal side effect.
- To convert a patient from oxymorphone immediate release (Opana), give half the total daily dose of Opana as Opana ER every 12 hours.
- If patient is receiving parenteral oxymorphone, given the 10% bioavailability, multiply the total parenteral dose of oxymorphone by 10 and administer in 2 equally divided doses.
- Beginning dose for elderly patient should be 5 mg PO q 4–6 hr PRN.
- Administer cautiously and in reduced doses in patients with creatinine clearance rates < 50 mL/min.
- Drug is contraindicated in patients with moderate and severe hepatic dysfunction; use cautiously and start at the lowest dose in patients with mild hepatic dysfunction, and titrate dose up.
- If patient is receiving CNS depressants (sedatives, hypnotics, general anesthetics, phenothiazines, tranquilizers, or alcohol) concurrently, start at ⅓ to ½ of the usual dose.
- If opioids are discontinued, drug should be gradually tapered to prevent withdrawal.
- If converting from other opioids to oxymorphone, use the following equianalgesic table (Opana ER package insert, June 2006); generally, start oxymorphone ER by giving half of the calculated total daily dose in 2 divided doses, every 12 hours; gradually titrate dose until pain is adequately controlled.

Opioid	Approximate equivalent dose (oral)	Oral conversion ration
Oxymorphone	10 mg	1
Hydrocodone	20 mg	0.5
Oxycodone	20 mg	0.5
Methadone	20 mg	0.5
Morphine	30 mg	0.333

Drug Preparation:
- Drug available in 5-, 10-, 20-, and 40-mg tablets.
- At home, teach patient to store oral doses in a safe place away from children and pets.

Drug Administration:
- Oral on an empty stomach (at least 1 hour before or 2 hours after food ingestion); drug must be swallowed whole and is not to be broken, chewed, dissolved, or crushed, as this would lead to a rapid release and absorption of a potentially fatal dose of oxymorphone.

Drug Interactions:
- Alcohol, CNS depressants: Additive CNS depressant effects (hypotension, respiratory depression, profound sedation); alcohol must NOT be used concurrently as it may result in a potentially fatal overdose of oxymorphone.
- Mixed agonist/antagonist analgesics (pentazocine, nalbuphine, butorphanol, buprenorphine) should not be given concurrently, as they may reduce the analgesic effect of oxymorphone and/or precipitate withdrawal.
- Anticholinergic medications: If used concurrently, may increase risk of urinary retention, and/or severe constipation, which may lead to paralytic ileus.
- Cimetidine: Reported increase in CNS side effects (confusion, disorientation, respiratory depression, apnea, seizures).

Lab Effects/Interference:
- None known.

Special Considerations:
- Indicated for the relief of moderate to severe pain when a continuous, around-the-clock opioid analgesic is needed for an extended period of time.
- Drug is contraindicated in patients who (1) have acute pain and need a PRN analgesic, as this drug is intended only for extended analgesia, (2) are in immediate post-operative period (12–24 hours after surgery), (3) have hypersensitivity to morphine analogues, such as codeine, (4) have post-op pain that is mild and not expected to persist, (5) have other contraindications to opioids (e.g., acute/severe bronchial asthmas, hypercarbia, paralytic ileus), (6) have moderate or severe hepatic impairment.
- Additive benefit when combined with acetaminophen or aspirin.
- Opioids cause peripheral vasodilation, which may cause hypotension; in addition, may cause the release of histamine, which can further intensify the hypotension. Oxymorphone has a lower likelihood of causing histamine release than other opioids.
- Give smallest effective dose to prevent development of tolerance, physical dependency.
- Reduce dose in debilitated patients or patients receiving other CNS depressants.

- If required, naloxone HCl will reverse opiate toxicity (e.g., respiratory depression). However, it is important that acute withdrawal symptoms are prevented by giving only enough naloxone to reverse respiratory depression, and that this be continued for opioid drug half-life.

Potential Toxicities/Side Effects and the Nursing Process

I. SENSORY/PERCEPTUAL ALTERATIONS related to CNS DEPRESSION

Defining Characteristics: Adverse effects were < 10% drowsiness, sedation, mood changes, euphoria, dysphoria, dizziness, confusion.

Nursing Implications: Assess baseline neurologic status. Use cautiously in the elderly, and start with lowest dose and titrate up. Use cautiously, if at all, in patients who are debilitated, and patients with head injury, increased ICP, severe CNS depression, or acute alcoholism. Assess other concurrent medications. Use with caution in patients receiving other opioids, tranquilizers, hypnotics, MAO inhibitors, since increasing CNS depressant effects can occur. Monitor neurologic status closely. Instruct patient to avoid driving and operating machinery while taking the medicine, and to AVOID concurrent alcohol.

II. ALTERATION IN OXYGENATION related to RESPIRATORY DEPRESSION

Defining Characteristics: Opiate agonists directly depress respiratory center in brain stem, causing decreased sensitivity and responsiveness to increased pCO_2. May also depress deep breathing and reflex to sigh. Tolerance to respiratory depressant effects occurs with chronic use.

Nursing Implications: Assess baseline pulmonary status, and periodically during drug use. Use cautiously in patients with bronchial asthma, COPD, respiratory depression, and monitor closely.

III. ALTERATION IN ELIMINATION related to CONSTIPATION, ILEUS

Defining Characteristics: Opium agonists bind to opiate receptors in bowel, slowing peristalsis, leading to constipation. Untreated constipation may result in bowel perforation. Incidence of constipation in clinical trials was 4%.

Nursing Implications: Assess baseline elimination, fluid intake, diet, and exercise patterns. Instruct patient regarding prevention of constipation: goal is to move bowels at least every two days by increasing fluids to 3 L/day, following a diet high in fiber (beans, vegetables, fruit), and taking moderate exercise. Assess need for bowel softeners, bulk-forming laxatives, and osmotic cathartics, and discuss preparation with physician. Teach patient self-administration of medications.

IV. ALTERATION IN NUTRITION, LESS THAN BODY REQUIREMENTS, related to GI TOXICITY

Defining Characteristics: Nausea, vomiting, and dry mouth may occur. Gastric, biliary, and pancreatic secretions are decreased by opiate agonists; digestion is delayed. Biliary tract muscle tone is increased, and spasm of Oddi's sphincter may occur (morphine > meperidine > codeine).

Nursing Implications: Assess patient tolerance of GI side effects. Teach patient to report side effects. If nausea/vomiting occur, change to another opioid, or premedicate with antiemetic to prevent nausea/vomiting. Assess GI pain, biliary spasm, and consider alternative opioid.

V. ALTERATION IN URINE ELIMINATION related to URINARY RETENTION

Defining Characteristics: Rarely, increased smooth muscle tone in urinary tract and spasm may occur. Bladder tone is increased, which may cause urgency. Vesical sphincter tone may be increased, leading to difficulty urinating. Increased risk of urinary retention in patients with prostatic hypertrophy or urethral stricture.

Nursing Implications: Assess baseline urinary elimination pattern. Teach patient to increase fluids to 3 L/day, and encourage voiding every 2–3 hours. Instruct patient to report problems with urination.

VI. KNOWLEDGE DEFICIT related to DRUG ADMINISTRATION, POTENTIAL FOR TOLERANCE, AND DEPENDENCY

Defining Characteristics: Psychological dependence (addiction) occurs rarely in patients taking opioid agonists for cancer pain (< 1%). Physical dependence (precipitation of withdrawal symptoms) occurs with chronic use of the drug for the relief of chronic cancer pain. In addition, tolerance, or less analgesic effect over time with the same drug dose, occurs and requires increased dosage of the drug.

Nursing Implications: Assess baseline knowledge of opioid analgesics, and attitude about their use for cancer pain management. Teach patient about proper self-administration, possible side effects, and self-care measures. Suggest patient maintain diary of pain intensity, precipitating and alleviating factors, drug dose and time taken, and relief. Teach patient to self-administer opioid agonists for relief of chronic cancer pain around-the-clock, not PRN, to prevent pain. Explain use of prescribed short-acting opioid for rescue or to manage breakthrough pain. Discuss with physician dose increase or change in frequency of administration if tolerance develops. Teach patient that withdrawal symptoms may occur if chronic, around-the-clock dosing is interrupted. Withdrawal (abstinence) symptoms that may be seen in the first 24 hours are restlessness, lacrimation, rhinorrhea, yawning, perspiration, gooseflesh, restless sleep, mydriasis. These are followed by twitching and leg spasms; severe aching of the back, abdomen, and legs; cramping in abdomen and legs; hot/cold flashes; insomnia; nausea/vomiting, diarrhea; severe sneezing; and increased heart rate, BP, T, which peak at 36–72 hours. Withdrawal syndrome can be prevented by administration of at least 1/4 of previous opioid dose.

ADJUVANT AGENTS

Drug: modafinil (Provigil)

Class: Wakeful promoting agent, symptom management.

Mechanism of Action: Promotes wakefulness without generalized CNS stimulation by an unknown mechanism. Drug acts in selected brain areas thought to regulate normal wakefulness in the hypothalamus: increased neuronal activity in tuberomammillary nucleus (wake-promoting center), which then projects into cerebral cortex; decreases activity in the ventrolateral preoptic area (sleep promoting); does not affect suprachiasmatic nucleus (regulated circadian rhythm). Action is different from amphetamines.

Metabolism: Rapidly absorbed from the GI system with peak plasma concentrations in 2–4 hours. Taking with food delays absorption by 1 hour, but does not affect bioavailability. About 60% protein bound (albumin), but at steady state does not displace protein binding of warfarin. Metabolized in the liver, with renal excretion of metabolites. Drug clearance may be reduced in the elderly. Drug is a reversible inhibitor of drug metabolizing enzyme CYP2C19. Elimination half-life 15 hours.

Dosage/Range:

- 200 mg PO daily as a single dose in the morning.
- 50% dose reduction in patients with severe liver impairment.
- Consider dose reduction in elderly patients with renal impairment and/or hepatic impairment.

Drug Preparation:

- Oral, available in 100-mg and 200-mg tablets.

Drug Administration:

- Oral, in the morning, with a glass of water.

Drug Interactions:

- Potentially, due to reversible inhibition of CYP2C19 enzyme system:
— Diazepam, phenytoin, propranolol: drug may increase serum levels of these drugs; monitor closely for toxicity and dose reduce if needed.
— Patients with CYP2C19 deficiency: increased serum levels of tricyclic antidepressants, SSRIs; monitor closely for toxicity and dose reduce if needed.
— Patients taking drug chronically may have increased induction of metabolism enzyme CYP3A4, resulting in theoretical decreased serum levels of steroidal contraceptives, cyclosporine, theophylline; monitor closely and dose increase as necessary.
— Methylphenidate: delays absorption of modafinil by 1 hour when given together.
— Use in pregnancy or breast-feeding women only if risk outweighs benefit as drug potentially teratogenic.

Lab Effects/Interference:

- Unknown.

Special Considerations:

- Anecdotal success in reducing in non-anemia cancer or HIV-related fatigue (Breitbart).
- Contraindicated in people with a sensitivity to modafinil.
- Contraindicated in patients with history of left ventricular hypertrophy or ischemic EKG changes, chest pain, arrhythmia, or mitral valve prolapse.
- Use with caution in patients who have had a recent MI or unstable angina.
- Use cautiously in patients with a history of psychosis.
- Women using steroidal contraceptives should use alternative or concomitant methods of contraception while taking the drug and for one month following discontinuation of the drug.
- Drug may produce psychoactive and euphoric effects, alterations in mood, perception, thinking, and feelings typical of other CNS stimulants. Drug binds to dopamine reuptake site and causes an increase in extracellular dopamine but no increase in dopamine release. Drug is reinforcing.
- Incidence of insomnia was 3% (placebo 1%).
- Drug is indicated in the treatment of narcolepsy, and does not cause a withdrawal when drug is stopped.

Potential Toxicities/Side Effects (dose and schedule dependent) and the Nursing Process

I. ALTERATION IN COMFORT related to HEADACHE, NAUSEA, DEPRESSION, NERVOUSNESS, RHINITIS

Defining Characteristics: In controlled clinical trials, headache occurred 10% more frequently than placebo, nausea occurred 9% more than placebo, depression 1% more than placebo, rhinitis 11% (placebo 8%), and nervousness 2% more than placebo.

The few patients who discontinued the drug did so due to headache (1%), nausea (1%), depression (1%), and nervousness (1%).

Nursing Implications: Teach patient that these effects are rare but may occur. Teach symptom management strategies and if these do not work, to notify provider. If this occurs, discuss drug discontinuance versus more aggressive symptom management if drug is effective in reducing fatigue.

II. ALTERATION IN NUTRITION, POTENTIAL, related to NAUSEA, DRY MOUTH, DIARRHEA, ANOREXIA, THIRST

Defining Characteristics: Although rare, these symptoms may occur: nausea occurs in 13% (placebo 4%), diarrhea 8% (placebo 4%), dry mouth 5% (placebo 1%), anorexia 5% (placebo 1%), and thirst 1%.

Nursing Implications: Perform baseline patient nutritional assessment, history of nausea and vomiting, bowel elimination pattern, oral assessment, and usual appetite. Teach patient these are rare, but to report these side effects so that they can be evaluated. Teach patient self-care measures, including dietary modification, local comfort measures as well as pharmacologic management as determined by the nurse/physician team. Teach patient to report symptoms that persist and do not respond to the planned therapy.

Chapter 7
Nausea and Vomiting

Nausea and/or vomiting can occur commonly during the course of the cancer experience, related to disease, such as liver metastases, or to treatment, such as with chemotherapy or radiation to the abdomen. In addition, if acute nausea and vomiting were not prevented following cancer chemotherapy, delayed nausea and vomiting often followed. This problem continues. Nausea is often underreported and under-assessed (Wickham, 2003). A replication of the Coates et al (1983) study by de Boer-Dennert et al (1997) showed that patients rated nausea as more distressing than vomiting since much has been done to prevent and control chemotherapy-induced nausea and vomiting (CINV). Complete control of CINV has improved greatly with the advent of serotonin 5-hydroxytryptamine type 3 (5-HT_3) receptor antagonists used in combination with dexamethasone, bringing complete control to about 70% for patients receiving high-dose cisplatin. This new century of genomics has led to the understanding that the effectiveness of many drugs, and in particular, 5-HT_3 receptor antagonists, is influenced by the recipient's genotype. This is because the liver's microenzyme system, Cytochrome P450, and subtypes are determined by an individual's genotype. If the genotype is an ultrarapid metabolizer, the drug is rapidly cleared and eliminated from the body with decreased effect and undertreatment, while slow or poor metabolizers slowly clear the drug from the body with the risk of overtreatment. A study by Kaiser et al (2002) evaluated whether patients who vomited after receiving their first cycle of emetogenic chemotherapy with 5-HT_3 receptor antagonist protection by either ondansetron or tropisetron were either ultrarapid or slow metabolizers of the P450 subsystem CYP 2D6. They found that 30% had nausea and vomiting. The ultrarapid metabolizers had a higher incidence of nausea and vomiting, which was more marked for tropisetron- than ondansetron-receiving patients, and the poor metabolizers had higher serum concentrations and were protected. As we look to the future, not only do we see patients having genotypic evaluation of their tumors for an individualized prescription of anti-cancer treatment, but it will also include individual prescription of antiemetic dose based on genotype.

CHEMOTHERAPY INDUCED NAUSEA AND VOMITING

CINV appears mediated by multiple pathways. Nausea usually precedes vomiting, and is controlled by cerebral and autonomic input, with common accompanying signs and symptoms of tachycardia, pallor, and diaphoresis. Vomiting involves the ejection of stomach contents and is a critical protection mechanism that helps the body excrete poisons. Most commonly, receptors in the gut enterochromaffin cells are stimulated and release serotonin. Serotonin binds to 5-HT_3 receptors which stimulate the vagus nerve. This leads to stimulation of the chemotherapy trigger zone (CTZ) in the area postrema on the floor of the 4th ventricle, leading to activation of the vomiting center (VC) in the medulla, or to stimulation of the vomiting center directly. The 5-HT_3 receptor antagonists, such as dolasetron, granisetron, and ondansetron, block the emetic impulses from reaching the CTZ and VC. In addition, other neuroreceptors in the CTZ can transmit impulses to the VC, such as dopamine, endorphin, and Substance P. Other neuroreceptors that are found in the VC and vestibular center and that appear to have a role in emesis are acetylcholine, corticosteroid, histamine, cannabinoid, opiate, and neurokinin-1 (NK_1). Dopamine antagonists include phenothiazines and butyrophenones, and Substance P/Neurokinin-1 receptor antagonist antiemetics include aprepitant and its IV formulation fosaprepitant, which has been newly FDA approved, as well as the investigational agent casopitant. Emotional and cognitive factors can influence the occurrence and severity of CINV through a descending pathway from the cerebral cortex to the vomiting center, such as with anticipatory nausea and vomiting. Here a conditioned response is set up based on 3–4 past episodes of severe nausea and/or vomiting. The benzodiazepine lorazepam has been effective in preventing or lessening this effect through the drug's amnesiac qualities.

Dexamethasone has long been known to reduce the incidence of CINV, through a probable anti-inflammatory effect, leading to a closing of spaces in the gut wall that would permit leakage of emetogens into the bloodstream (Wickham, 2003). However, the exact mechanism is unknown.

Delayed nausea and vomiting are difficult to control, but appears to be influenced by slowed gastric emptying. Thus, delayed antiemetic regimes usually include metoclopramide to speed gastric emptying, along with dexamethasone, and a phenothiazine or serotonin antagonist. Recently, it became clear that Substance P and its receptor Neurokinin-1 (NK_1), in the gut and brainstem, were important mediators in delayed CINV. The NK_1 receptors are located near the vomiting center, the "final common pathway" for emesis, so it is expected the NK_1 receptor antagonists will have broader application (Wickham, 2003). Although great strides have been made in the prevention and control of CINV, even with maximal pharmacologic blockade of known pathways, 100% protection is not obtained, so it is clear other pathways await discovery. See Figure 7.1 for a review of pathophysiology of CINV. See Table 7.1 for the emetogenicity of cancer chemotherapy agents, and Table 7.2 for a schematic for antiemetic drugs and doses for CINV.

CINV can occur *acutely*, during the first 24 hours following chemotherapy administration, *delayed*, occurring after the first 24 hours, or in anticipation (*anticipatory*).

Factors that influence the occurrence and severity of CINV include sex (female has higher risk than male), age (younger have higher risk than older), drug dose and emetogenic potential, combination of drugs versus single agent, history of alcohol

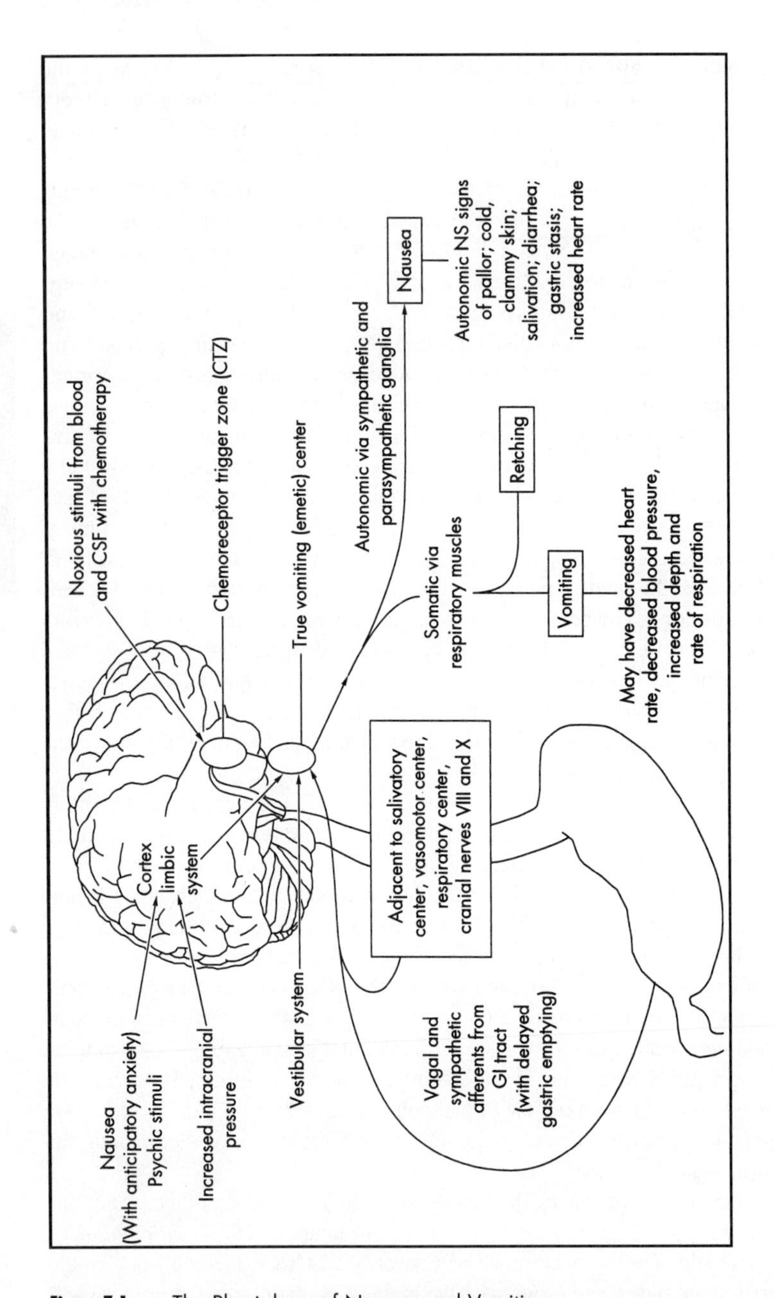

Figure 7.1 The Physiology of Nausea and Vomiting.
Source: Reproduced from Burke MM, Wilkes GM, Ingwersen K et al (1996) *Chemotherapy and the Nursing Process*, Sudbury, MA, Jones and Bartlett Publishers. *Drawing adapted from original by Gail Wilkes.*

Table 7.1 Emetogenic Risk by Antineoplastic Agent

High Risk > 90%	Moderate Risk 30–90%	Low Risk 10–30%	Minimal Risk < 10%
Altretamine Carmustine > 250 mg/m^2	Aldesleukin > 12–15 million units/m^2 Amifostine > 300 mg/m^2 Arsenic trioxide Azacitidine Busulfan > 4 mg/d Carboplatin Carmustine ≤ 250 mg/m^2	Amifostine < 300 mg/m^2	Alemtuzumab Alpha interferon Asparaginase Bevacizumab Bleomycin Bortezomib Melphalan Busulfan < 4 mg/d
Cisplatin ≥ 50 mg/m^2	Cisplatin < 50 mg/m^2	Asparaginase Bexarotene Capecitabine Cytarabine 100–200 mg/m^2	Capecitabine Cetuximab Chlorambucil (PO) Cladribine Decitabine Denileukin diftitox Dasatinib Dexrazoxane Erlotinib
Cyclophosphamide > 1500 mg/m^2	Cyclophosphamide ≤ 1500 mg/m^2	Docetaxel	Etoposide IV
Dacarbazine > 500 mg/m^2	Cyclophosphamide PO	Doxorubicin < 20 mg/m^2 Doxorubicin (liposomal)	Fludarabine Gefitinib Gemtuzumab ozogamicin Hydroxyurea (PO) Lapatinib Lenalidomide Melphalan PO
Dactinomycin	Cytarabine > 1 g/m^2 Daunorubicin	Etoposide PO Fludarabine (PO)	Methotrexate ≤ 50 mg/m^2 Nelarabine Panitumumab Pentostatin
Lomustine > 60 mg/m^2	Doxorubicin	5-Fluorouracil	Rituximab Sorafinib Sunitinib Temsirolimus
Mechlorethamine Melphalan HD IV	Epirubicin Etoposide (PO)	Gemcitabine	Thalidomide Thioguanine (PO)

(continued)

Table 7.1 *(Continued)*

High Risk > 90%	Moderate Risk 30–90%	Low Risk 10–30%	Minimal Risk < 10%
Pentostatin Procarbazine	Hexamethylmelamine	Methotrexate > 50 mg/m^2 < 250 mg/m^2	Trastuzumab Valrubicin
Streptozocin	Idarubicin	Mitomycin C	Vinblastine Vincristine
AC regimen (Doxorubicin or epirubicin plus cyclophosphamide)	Ifosfamide Imatinib (PO)	Mitoxantrone < 12 mg/m^2	Vinorelbine IV
	Irinotecan Lomustine	Paclitaxel Paclitaxel-albumin bound	
	Melphalan > 50 mg/m^2 Methotrexate 250–1000 mg/m^2	Pemetrexed	
	Mitoxantrone > 12 mg/m^2	Thiotepa	
	Oxaliplatin > 75 mg/m^2	Topotecan Vorinostat	
	Temozolomide (PO) Vinorelbine (PO)		

Source: From Wickham R (2003) Nausea and Vomiting, Chapter 11. In Yarbro CH, Goodman M, and Frogge MH *Cancer Symptom Management*, 3rd ed. Sudbury, MA, Jones and Bartlett Publishers; Consensus Report of the Multinational Association of Supportive Care in Cancer (MASCC), June 2004; National Comprehensive Cancer Network. *Clinical Practice Guideline Antiemesis*, version 3. 2008; http://www.nccn.org. Accessed June 9, 2008.

intake (increased alcohol intake confers protection), and past experience with nausea and vomiting, such as air sickness, which increase risk.

Delayed nausea and vomiting are influenced by the effectiveness of control/prevention of the acute phase of CINV (Roila, 2000; Koeller et al, 2002), as well as the half-life of the antineoplastic agent. For example, the metabolites of cisplatin continue to be excreted for 3–5 days after drug administration, so protection must be provided for that period of time; and for cyclophosphamide, the half-life is at least 12 hours, so only half the drug is excreted by that time, and full antiemetic protection must continue for at least 24 hours to prevent delayed nausea and vomiting. Common delayed regimens begin on days 2–4 for highly emetogenic regimens (aprepitant 80 mg PO

Table 7.2 Antiemetic Agents Used in CINV

Antiemetic Agent	IV Doses *nl (Acute)	Oral Doses (Acute)	Oral (Delayed)
Serotonin Receptor Antagonists			
• Dolasetron	100 mg or 1.8 mg/kg IV	100 mg (acute)	100 mg qd delayed
• Granisetron	0.01 mg/kg or 1 mg IV	1–2 mg oral (acute)	1 mg bid delayed
• Ondansetron	0.15 mg/kg or 8mg IV	24 mg oral (acute)	8 mg bid delayed
Corticosteroids			
• Dexamethasone	20 mg	20 mg	8 mg bid days 2–4 highly emetogenic 4–8 mg bid days 2–3 moderately emetogenic
Substance P/NK_1 Receptor Antagonist			
• Aprepitant		125 mg PO day 1 with dexamethasone 12 mg PO with serotonin receptor antagonist	80 mg day 2, 3 with dexamethasone 8 mg PO
• Fosaprepitant		115 mg IV day 1 with dexamethasone 12 mg PO with serotonin receptor antagonist	80 mg day 2, 3 with dexamethasone 8 mg PO
Dopamine Receptor Antagonists			
• Metoclopramide			20–40 mg bid-qid
• Prochlorperazine			15–30mg LA spansules bid PRN
Benzodiazepines			
• Lorazepam	0.5–1 mg	1–2 mg	

Source: Modified from Wickham R (2003) Nausea and Vomiting, Chapter 11. In Yarbro CH, Goodman M, and Frogge MH *Cancer Symptom Management*, 3rd ed. Sudbury, MA, Jones and Bartlett Publishers.

daily × 2 plus dexamethasone 8 mg PO daily × 3; or a serotonin antagonist such as granisetron 1 mg PO bid or ondansetron 8 mg PO twice daily, plus dexamethasone 8 mg PO daily × 3; or metoclopramide 30–40 mg PO twice daily plus dexamethasone 8 mg PO twice daily × 3 days. For moderately emetogenic regimens, delayed emesis regimens are given on days 2–3 and include a serotonin antagonist or dexamethasone or metoclopramide alone or in combination (Grunberg and Siebel, 2007).

Insofar as CINV involves multiple pathways, multiple antiemetics to block these pathways are needed, especially for aggressive antiemesis. Antiemetics must be administered to prevent nausea and vomiting, so the drug(s) should be administered prior to chemotherapy administration in order to block stimulation of the pathways. Oral antiemetics should be administered 30–40 minutes before treatment; rectal (PR) preparations 60 minutes before; intramuscular (IM) injections 20–30 minutes before; and intravenous bolus (IVB) 10–30 minutes prior to chemotherapy (Barton-Burke et al, 2001).

In order to better identify treatment approaches for CINV, American Society for Clinical Oncology (ASCO) published "Recommendations for the Use of Antiemetics: Evidence-Based Clinical Practice Guidelines" and stated that "at equivalent doses, serotonin receptor antagonists have equivalent safety and efficacy and can be used interchangeably based on convenience, availability, and cost" (Gralla et al, 1999). They listed four agents in this class, three of which are commercially available in the United States: dolasetron, granisetron, and ondansetron. Finally, key members of the Supportive Care in Cancer organization have developed consensus guidelines for the study and prescription of antiemetic care (Koeller et al, 2002).

In addition, the National Community Network (NCCN, 2008) has developed supportive care guidelines for antiemesis, which identify the following principles of emesis control in patients with cancer:

- The goal is the prevention of nausea/vomiting.
- Patients receiving moderately to highly emetogenic chemotherapy should receive antiemetic protection for at least 4 days.
- Oral and IV antiemetics have equivalent efficacy.
- Use the lowest fully efficacious dose before chemotherapy or radiation therapy.
- Choose antiemetic(s) based on emetogenicity of the therapy, prior experience with antiemetics, patient factors, and antiemetic(s) potential side effect(s).
- Ensure that other potential causes of emesis in patients with cancer are not overlooked:
  - Partial or complete bowel obstruction.
  - Vestibular dysfunction.
  - Brain metastases.
  - Electrolyte imbalance (hypercalcemia, hyperglycemia, hyponatremia).
  - Uremia.
  - Concomitant drug treatment, including opiates.
  - Gastroparesis (tumor, chemotherapy such as vincristine).
  - Psychophysiologic causes (anxiety, anticipatory nausea/vomiting).

Aprepitant (Emend) is the first substance P/Neurokinin-1 receptor antagonist indicated for the prevention of acute and delayed nausea and vomiting related to highly emetogenic chemotherapy, in combination with other antiemetic agents. First identified in 1931 and reaching notoriety in 1950 when linked with pain transmission, substance P has continued to be prominent in the symptom management field. Substance P is a member of the tachykinin family of peptides and, together with NK_1 receptors, is found in high concentrations in the chemotherapy trigger zone (CTZ, in the medulla oblongata) and the dorsal horn of the spinal cord (posterior column of gray matter), as well as the gut. Substance P is released from peripheral sensory as well as central sensory nerve endings and plays a key role in transmitting noxious sensory information to the brain. Substance P initiates its activity by binding to the neurokinin-1 (NK_1) receptor, a site distinctly different from the serotonin-mediated $5HT_3$ site (Hesketh, 2001).

In an effort to design a serotonin-antagonist with a long half-life, and activity against delayed chemotherapy-induced nausea and vomiting, palonosetron (Aloxi) was created. Recently approved for the prevention of chemotherapy-induced nausea and vomiting, palonosetron is the only serotonin-antagonist with an indication for delayed nausea and vomiting. Given these advances, complete protection from chemotherapy-induced nausea and vomiting should be the standard (Hesketh, 2008); however, there continues to be a minority of patients who have significant nausea and vomiting.

The NCCN (2008) recommends the following algorithm for emesis prevention:

- *Highly emetogenic chemotherapy*:
  - Start aprepitant 125 mg PO day 1; 80 mg PO daily on days 2 and 3 (fosaprepitant dimeglumine 115 mg IV over 15 minutes may be substituted for aprepitant 125 mg 30 minutes prior to chemotherapy on day 1 only of the regimen).
  - Dexamethasone 12 mg PO or IV day 1; 8 mg PO or IV daily on days 2–4.
  - Serotonin receptor antagonist day 1 (ondansetron 16–24 mg PO or 8–12 mg [maximum 32 mg] IV; granisetron 2 mg PO or 1 mg IV; or dolasetron 100 mg PO or IV; or palonosetron 0.25 mg IV).
  - Lorazepam 0.5–2 mg PO or IV or SL either every 4 or every 6 hours on days 1–4, as needed.
- *Moderately emetogenic chemotherapy*:
  - Day 1: as day 1 in highly emetogenic.
  - Days 2–4: aprepitant as above, dexamethasone as above or 4 mg PO or IV bid, serotonin receptor antagonist (ondansetron 8 mg PO bid or 16 mg PO daily, granisetron 1–2 mg PO daily or 1 mg PO bid or 1 mg IV daily; or dolasetron 100 mg PO daily or 1 mg PO bid or 1.8 mg/kg IV; lorazepam as in highly emetogenic.
- *Low emetogenic chemotherapy*:
  - Start antiemesis before chemotherapy.
  - Repeat daily for fractionated doses of chemotherapy.

        - Dexamethasone 12 mg PO or IV daily OR
        - Prochlorperazine 10 mg PO or IV every 4 or 6 hours or metoclopramide 20–40 mg PO either every 4 or 6 hours or 1–2 mg/kg IV either every 3 or every 4 hours plus/minus diphenhydramine 24–50 mg PO or IV either every 4 or 6 hours.
        - Lorazepam 0.5–2 mg PO or IV either every 4 or 6 hours.
- *Minimal emetogenic chemotherapy*:
    - No routine prophylaxis.
    - If nausea or emesis within 24 hours, consider using drugs in low emetogenicity category.
- *Rescue or breakthrough emesis management*:
    - Add an additional agent from different drug class, such as prochlorperazine (25 mg supp PR every 12 hr or 10 mg PO or IV every 4 or 6 hours) OR
    - Metoclopramide 10–40 mg PO or IV either every 4 or 6 hours with or without diphenhydramine 25–50 mg PO or IV every 4 or 6 hours OR
    - Lorazepam 0.5–2.0 mg PO every 4 or 6 hours OR
    - Different serotonin receptor antagonist (such as ondansetron 16 mg PO or 8 mg IV daily) OR granisetron 1–2 mg PO daily or 1 mg PO bid or 0.01 mg/kg (maximum 1 mg IV) OR dolasetron 100 mg PO daily or 1.8 mg/kg IV or 100 mg IV OR
    - Haloperidol 1–2 mg PO every 4–6 hours PRN OR
    - Dronabinol 5–10 mg PO every 3 or 6 hours, OR
    - Nabilone 1–2 mg PO bid OR
    - Dexamethasone 12 mg PO or IV daily if not previously given OR
    - Olanzapine 2.5–5 mg PO bid OR
    - Promethazine 12.5–25 mg PO or IV every 4 hours.
    - Multiple concurrent agents may be necessary, in alternating schedules or routes.
    - Dopamine antagonists (e.g., metoclopramide), haloperidol, corticosteroids, and lorazepam may be required.
    - If the patient has dyspepsia, consider antacid therapy (H_2 blocker or proton pump inhibitor).
    - Consider around-the-clock NOT PRN dosing.
    - Ensure adequate hydration or fluid repletion, along with correction of any electrolyte imbalance.
    - FOR THE NEXT CYCLE, change the regimen (both day 1 and postchemotherapy regimen).
    - Monitor for dystonic reactions when phenothiazines are used, and administer diphenhydramine as needed to resolve reaction.
- *Prevention of Anticipatory Emesis*
    - Use optimal antiemetic therapy during every cycle of treatment.
    - Behavioral therapy: relaxation/systematic desensitization; hypnosis/guided imagery; music therapy; acupuncture/acupressure.
    - Alprazolam 0.5 mg PO tid beginning on the night before treatment OR
    - Lorazepam 0.5–2.0 mg PO on the night before and morning of treatment.

RADIATION INDUCED NAUSEA AND VOMITING

Radiation therapy to the gastrointestinal tract usually causes nausea and vomiting. Highest risk (90%) is when Total Body Irradiation (TBI) or external beam radiation is administered to the upper or total abdomen or upper hemithorax, with emesis occurring within 10–15 minutes with TBI or hemithorax treatment, and within 1–2 hours when external beam therapy is administered to the upper abdomen (Wickham, 2003). Antiemesis is effective using serotonin-antagonists with or without dexamethasone, which should be administered at a time before RT when the drug can be absorbed (NCCN Antiemesis Guidelines, 2008). NCCN (2008) recommends to protect against upper abdomen RT, that ondansetron 8 mg PO bid with or without dexamethasone 4 mg PO daily prior to RT. Recommended prophylaxis for TBI is ondansetron 8 mg PO bid-tid or granisetron 2 mg PO daily or 3 mg IV daily with or without dexamethasone 2 mg PO tid. For breakthrough nausea and vomiting from RT to other sites, pretreat with ondansetron 8 mg PO bid/tid. Antiemesis for patients receiving combined chemotherapy and RT, refer to recommended antiemetics for the chemotherapy agent.

DISEASE INDUCED NAUSEA AND VOMITING

Site of advanced disease is a strong predictor of the risk for nausea and vomiting. Metastases to the liver are often associated with difficult to control nausea and vomiting. Pressure from ascites or obstruction of a hollow viscus, as with advanced ovarian cancer, can also lead to intractable nausea and vomiting. A factor here, along with advanced pancreatic cancer, may be delayed gastric emptying, or gastric outlet syndrome. Increased intracranial pressure (ICP) from a malignant brain tumor often causes nausea and vomiting. Other conditions related to disease that cause nausea and vomiting include hypercalcemia, hyperglycemia, electrolyte imbalance, and severe constipation. Strategies to relieve nausea and vomiting in these circumstances vary with the cause, and range from aggressive antiemesis to correction of delayed gastric emptying (metoclopramide) or the obstruction (stent if possible, or if not, release of gastric contents via a gastrostomy tube), to correction of electrolyte abnormalities

Currently, antiemetics are available as oral, intravenous, or rectal suppositories. Fortunately, a new and less invasive formulation is being studied: transdermal delivery of antiemetic agents. Transdermal granisetron is being reviewed by the FDA. This delivery modality will increase the benefit to many more patients with cancer.

In summary then, nausea and/or vomiting can arise from treatment or complications of disease. There are a variety of agents useful for blocking a number of neurotransmitter pathways to prevent or control nausea and vomiting in cancer. Specifically, it is known that chemotherapy stimulates nausea and vomiting via multiple pathways and often, therefore, multiple drugs are necessary for the prevention of nausea and vomiting associated with aggressive chemotherapy.

References

Barnhart ER. *Physicians' Desk Reference*. Oradell, NJ, Medical Economics Data 1998

Barton-Burke M, Wilkes G, Berg D, et al. *Cancer Chemotherapy: A Nursing Process Approach*, 3rd ed. Sudbury, MA, Jones and Bartlett Publishers; 2001

Barton-Burke M, Wilkes G, Ingwersen K. *Chemotherapy Care Plans: Designs for Nursing Care*. Sudbury, MA, Jones and Bartlett Publishers 1997

Coates A, Abraham S, Kaye SB, et al. On the Receiving End–Patient Perception of the Side-Effects of Cancer Chemotherapy. *Eur J Cancer Clin Oncol* 1983; 19 203–208

Cotanch PM, Stum S. Progressive Muscle Relaxation as Antiemetic Therapy for Cancer Patients. *Oncol Nurs Forum* 1987; 14(1) 33–37

de Boer-Dennert M, de Wit R, Schmitz PIM, et al. Patient Perceptions of the Side-effects of Chemotherapy: The Influence of 5HT3 Antagonists. *Br J Cancer* 1997; 76 1055–1061

Gralla RJ, Osoba D, Kris MG, et al. ASCO Special Article: Recommendations for the Use of Antiemetics: Evidence-Based Clinical Practice Guidelines. *J Clin Oncol* 1999; 17(9) 2971–2994

Grunberg SM, Siebel M. Management of Nausea and Vomiting. In Pazdur R, Coia LR, Hoskins WJ, Wagman LD (eds). *Cancer Management: A Multidisciplinary Approach*, 10th ed. Lawrence, KS, CMP Healthcare Media LLC; 2007

Grunberg SM, Gabrial NY, Clark G. Phase III Trial of Transdermal Granisetron Patch (Sancuso) Compared With Oral Granisetron in the Management of Chemotherapy-Induced Nausea and Vomiting (CINV). Multinational Association of Supportive Care (MASCC) 20th Annual Symposium, abstract #18, 2007

Grunberg SM, Aziz Z, Shaharyar A, et al. Phase III Results of a Novel Neurokinin-1 (NK-1) Receptor Antagonist, Casopitant: Single Oral and 3-Day Oral Dosing Regimens for Chemotherapy-induced Nausea and Vomiting (CINV) in Patients (Pts) Receiving Moderately Emetogenic Chemotherapy (MEC). *J Clin Oncol* 26: 2008 (May 20 suppl: abstract #9540)

Herrstedt J, Grunberg SM, Rolski J, et al. Phase III Results for the Novel Neurokinin-1 (NK-1) Receptor Antagonist, Casopitant: Single Oral Dosing Regimen for Chemotherapy-induced Nausea and Vomiting (CINV) in Patients (Pts) Receiving Highly Emetogenic Chemotherapy (HEC). *J Clin Oncol* 26: 2008 (May 20 suppl: Abstract #9549)

Hesketh PJ. Chemotherapy-induced nausea and vomiting. *N Engl J Med* 2008; 358 2482–2494

Hesketh PJ. Potential Role of the NK1 Receptor Antagonists in Chemotherapy-induced Nausea and Vomiting. *Supportive Care in Cancer* 2001; 9 350–354

Hesketh PJ, Beck TM, Uhlenhopp M, et al. Adjusting the Dose of Intravenous Ondansetron plus Dexamethasone to the Emetogenic Potential of the Chemotherapy Regimen. *J Clin Oncol* 1995; 13(8) 2117–2122

Hesketh PJ, Kris MG, Grunberg SM, et al. Proposal for Classifying the Acute Emetogenicity of Cancer Chemotherapy. *J Clin Oncol* 1997; 15(1) 103–109

Kaiser R, Sezer O, Papies A, et al. Patient-tailored Antiemetic Treatment with 5-hydroxytryptamine Type 3 Receptor Antagonists According to Cytochrome P-450 Genotypes. *J Clin Oncol* 2002; 20(12) 2805–2811

Koeller JM, Aapro MS, Gralla RJ, et al. Antiemetic Guidelines: Creating a More Practical Treatment Approach. *Supportive Care in Cancer* 2002; 10 519–522

National Comprehensive Cancer Network. *Clinical Practice Guideline Antiemesis*, version 3.2008; http://www.nccn.org. Accessed June 9, 2008.

Roila F, Ballatori E, Ruggeri B, Dexamethasone Alone or in Combination with Ondansetron for the Prevention of Delayed Nausea and Vomiting Induced by Chemotherapy. *New Engl J Med* 2000; 342(21) 1554–1559

Sylvester RK, Etzell R, Levitt R, et al. Comparison of 16-mg vs 32-mg Ondansetron and Dexamethasone in Patients Receiving Cisplatin. *Proc Am Soc Clin Oncol* 1996; 15 547 (abstract 1781)

Van Belles, Cocquyt V, DeSmet M. Comparison of a Neurokinin-1 Antagonist L-758, 298 to Ondansetron in the Prevention of Cisplatin-induced Emesis. *Proc American Society of Clinical Oncologists* 1998; 17 51a (abstract 198)

Wickham R. Nausea and Vomiting, chapter 11. Yarbro CH, Frogge MH, Goodman M. Cancer Symptom Management, 3rd ed. Sudbury, MA: Jones and Bartlett Publishers 2003

Drug: aprepitant (Emend® oral formulation)

Class: Substance P/Neurokinin-1 Receptor Antagonist. For IV preparation, see Fosaprepitant dimeglumine.

Mechanism of Action: Selective Substance P/Neurokinin-1 (NK_1) receptor antagonist (high affinity). Drug has no affinity for $5HT_3$, dopamine, or corticosteroid receptors. Drug crosses the blood–brain barrier to saturate brain NK_1 receptors. Drug increases the activity of serotonin receptor antagonists and corticosteroids in preventing acute nausea and vomiting, and inhibits both acute and delayed nausea and vomiting related to cisplatin chemotherapy.

Metabolism: Drug is well absorbed after oral administration with 60–65% bioavailability. Drug is 95% bound to plasma proteins and crosses the placenta and blood–brain barrier. Aprepitant undergoes extensive metabolism in the liver by the P450 hepatic microenzyme system, specifically CYP3A4, and minor metabolism by CYP1A2 and CYP2C19. Seven inactive metabolites have been found in the plasma. The drug is excreted in the urine (57%) and the feces (45%). The terminal half-life of the drug is 9–13 hours.

Dosage/Range:

- Day 1, 125 mg PO 1 hour before chemotherapy, together with a serotonin (HT3) receptor antagonist and dexamethasone (dose reduced to 12 mg day 1, 8 mg days 2 & 3); days 2 and 3, 80 mg PO each morning.

Drug Preparation:

- Oral drug supplied as (1) 80 mg capsules in bottle of 30 capsules or in unit dose packs of 5 capsules, (2) 125 mg tablets in bottle of 30 capsules or in unit dose packs of 5 capsules, and (3) trifold pack containing 1–125 mg capsule, and 2–80 mg capsules. Capsules should be stored at room temperature.
- Day 1, give 125 mg capsule PO 1 hour before chemotherapy, and then the 80 mg capsule in the morning on days 2 and 3. Give with or without food.

Drug Interactions:

- Drugs that inhibit the CYP3A4 isoenzyme system can increase the serum level of aprepitant: ketoconazole, itraconazole, nefazodone, clarithromycin, ritonavir,

nelfinavir; diltiazem (2-fold increase in aprepitant plasma concentration), so coadminister cautiously and monitor for aprepitant toxicity or dose reduce aprepitant.
- Drugs that strongly induce CYP3A4 isoenzyme system can lower aprepitant serum levels: rifampin, carbamazepine, phenytoin; assess for efficacy of aprepitant and need for drug dose increase.
- Drug is a moderate inhibitor of P450 hepatic isoenzyme system CYP3A4, so the plasma concentrations of the following drugs can theoretically be increased if coadministered:
  - Chemotherapy agents are docetaxel, paclitaxel, etoposide, irinotecan, ifosfamide, imatinib, vinorelbine, vinblastine, and vincristine.
  - dexamethasone (dose-reduce dexamethasone by 50%).
  - methylprednisolone (dose-reduce 25% if IV, 50% if PO).
  - benzodiazepines: midazolam, lorazepam, alprazolam, triazolam.
- Drug is an inducer of CYP2C9, and the plasma concentrations of the following drugs can theoretically be decreased if coadministered:
  - Warfarin (34% decrease with 14% decrease in INR; closely monitor INR 7–10 days after 3-day antiemetic regime, and modify warfarin dose as needed).
  - Phenytoin, tolbutamide, oral contraceptives.

Lab Effects/Interference:
- Decreased INR if patient taking warfarin.

Special Considerations:
- Contraindications: do not give concomitantly with pimozide, terfenadine, astemizole, or cisapride; do not give if hypersensitive to aprepitant or any of its components; use cautiously if at all during pregnancy or breast-feeding; no studies have been done in patients with severe liver failure.
- Indications: in combination, with other antiemetic agents, for the prevention of acute and delayed nausea and vomiting associated with initial and repeat courses of highly emetogenic chemotherapy, including high-dose cisplatin.
- Significant drug interactions (see above).
- Drug is well tolerated with few side effects.

Potential Toxicities/Side Effects and the Nursing Process

I. ALTERATION IN NUTRITION, LESS THAN BODY REQUIREMENTS related to CONSTIPATION, DIARRHEA, NAUSEA, ANOREXIA, HICCUPS

Defining Characteristics: Gastrointestinal side effects may occur but are infrequent with the following incidences: constipation (10.3%), diarrhea (10.3%), nausea (12.7%), vomiting (7.5%), hiccups (10.8%), and anorexia (10.1%).

Nursing Implications: Teach patient that these side effects may occur, and to report them if unrelieved by symptom-management measures. Teach patient self-care measures to manage and prevent symptoms.

II. ALTERATION IN COMFORT related to ASTHENIA/FATIGUE, ABDOMINAL PAIN, HEADACHE

Defining Characteristics: Asthenia/fatigue occurred in 17.8% of patients; abdominal pain 4.6%; headache 8.5%.

Nursing Implications: Teach patient that these side effects may occur and measures to minimize their occurrence. Teach energy-conserving measures, management of abdominal pain and headache. Teach patient to report signs and symptoms that worsen or are unrelieved.

Drug: Casopitant mesylate [Rezonic (US), Zunrisa (UK), investigational]

Class: Neurokinin-1 (NK_1) receptor antagonist.

Mechanism of Action: Chemotherapy-induced nausea and vomiting (CINV) is mediated by a number of pathways, including the NK_1 receptor pathway. The NK_1 receptor is found in the area postrema, which houses the Chemoreceptor Trigger Zone (CTZ), and the nucleus tractus solitarii in the brain stem. Vagal afferent fibers innervate both the area postrema and nucleus tractus solitarii and can be stimulated by endogenous tachykinin neuropeptide substance P. Casopitant mesylate competitively binds to the NK_1 receptor so that it cannot bind with substance P in the neurons of the vagal afferent fibers. This is believed to reduce CINV. Drug has both antiemetic and antidepressant qualities.

Metabolism: Unknown. Crosses blood–brain barrier.

Dosage/Range: Per protocol, for example, single oral dose of 150 mg PO or 3 day regimen of day 1 90 mg IV, together with ondansetron, and 50 mg PO days 2 and 3.

Drug Preparation: Oral and IV formulation per protocol.

Drug Administration: Administered together with ondansetron and dexamethasone per protocol.

Drug Interactions: Unknown but probably similar to aprepitant.

Lab Effects/Interference: Unknown but probably similar to aprepitant.

Special Considerations:
- Phase III clinical trials show 73 (3-day regimen)–86% (single oral dose) complete response rates in patients receiving highly and moderately emetogenic chemotherapy (Herrstedt et al, 2008; Grunberg et al, 2008).
- Neutropenia, anemia, alopecia, fatigue and constipation were the primary adverse effects.

Potential Toxicities/Side Effects and the Nursing Process

I. ALTERATION IN NUTRITION, LESS THAN BODY REQUIREMENTS, related to CONSTIPATION

Defining Characteristics: Constipation may occur.

Nursing Implications: Teach patient that these side effects may occur and to report them if unrelieved by symptom-management measures. Teach patient self-care measures to manage and prevent symptoms.

II. POTENTIAL FOR INFECTION AND FATIGUE related to BONE MARROW DEPRESSION

Defining Characteristics: Incidence of neutropenia, leukopenia, and anemia were higher (1–4%) in two studies in the patients receiving casopitant than in the arm receiving ondansetron and decadron alone.

Nursing Implications: Assess CBC, WBC, differential, and platelet count before each cycle of drug administration, as well as for signs/symptoms of infection or bleeding. Teach patient signs/symptoms of infection and bleeding, and instruct to report them immediately. Teach self-care measures to minimize risk of infection and bleeding, including avoidance of OTC aspirin-containing medications. Assess energy and activity tolerance and discuss strategies to conserve energy and reduce expenditure such as shopping tips and alternating rest and activity.

Drug: dexamethasone (Decadron)

Class: Glucocorticoid steroid.

Mechanism of Action: May inhibit prostaglandin release by stabilizing lysosomal membranes, thereby interrupting hypothalamic prostaglandin release and subsequent stimulation of nausea and vomiting. Causes demargination of marginated WBCs, with leukocytosis. Decreases inflammation by suppression of migration of polymorphonuclear leukocytes.

Metabolism: Half-life is 3–4 hours; oral dose peaks in 1–2 hours, with duration of two days; IM peaks in 8 hours, with duration of six days.

Dosage/Range:

Adult (as antiemetic):

- Oral: 4 mg q 4 h × four doses beginning 1–8 hours before chemotherapy.
- IV: 10–20 mg prior to chemotherapy, then q 4–6 h.

Drug Preparation:

- Oral: administer with food or milk.
- IV: may be given with H_2-antagonist (e.g., ranitidine) to prevent gastric irritation.

Drug Interactions:

- Indomethacin, aspirin: increased GI irritation and bleeding; avoid concurrent administration.
- Barbiturates, phenytoin, rifampin: decreased dexamethasone effect; increase dose as needed.

Lab Effects/Interference:

- Increased WBC may occur due to demargination.
- Increased serum glucose level.
- May cause decreased K.

Special Considerations:

- Contraindicated in patients with psychosis, hypersensitivity, idiopathic thrombocytopenia, acute glomerulonephritis, amebiasis, fungal infections, and nonasthmatic bronchial disease.
- Indicated in the management of inflammation, allergies, neoplasms, cerebral edema, and in combination antiemetic therapy.
- If patient received dexamethasone chronically, drug must be tapered to prevent withdrawal (i.e., signs/symptoms of adrenal insufficiency, rebound weakness, arthralgia, fever, dizziness, orthostatic hypotension, dyspnea, hypoglycemia).

Potential Toxicities/Side Effects and the Nursing Process

I. ALTERATION IN NUTRITION, LESS THAN BODY REQUIREMENTS, related to GI TOXICITY

Defining Characteristics: Increased appetite, abdominal distension, pancreatitis, GI hemorrhage; diarrhea may occur.

Nursing Implications: Assess baseline nutritional status and monitor throughout therapy. Discuss symptomatic management of diarrhea, abdominal distension, and increased appetite with patient. Assess stool for occult blood and notify physician if positive. Monitor Hgb and HCT values.

II. ALTERATIONS IN SENSORY/PERCEPTUAL PATTERNS related to CHANGES IN MOOD, VASODILATION, CATARACTS

Defining Characteristics: Euphoria, insomnia, depression, flushing, sweating, headache, mood changes, and cataracts may occur.

Nursing Implications: Assess baseline mental status and monitor during therapy. Discuss symptomatic management or drug discontinuance, based on severity, with physician.

III. ALTERATION IN CARDIAC OUTPUT related to CHF

Defining Characteristics: Congestive heart failure (CHF), hypertension, fluid retention, and edema may occur.

Nursing Implications: Assess baseline vital signs (VS), and monitor during therapy. Discuss hypertension with physician, monitor daily weights, and assess for edema.

IV. ALTERATION IN CARBOHYDRATE METABOLISM related to CARBOHYDRATE INTOLERANCE

Defining Characteristics: May cause hyperglycemia, hypokalemia, and carbohydrate intolerance.

Nursing Implications: Assess baseline blood glucose, K, and monitor during therapy. Teach patient signs/symptoms of hyperglycemia (polyuria, polydipsia), especially if receiving drug for extended period.

Drug: diphenhydramine hydrochloride (Benadryl)

Class: Antihistamine.

Mechanism of Action: Inhibits histamine, and has slight, if any, antiemetic activity by blocking the CTZ and decreasing vestibular stimulation. Acts on blood vessels, GI, respiratory systems by competing with histamine for H_1-receptor site; decreases allergic response by blocking histamine.

Metabolism: Biologically transformed in the liver; half-life is 2.4–9.3 hours; 80–85% protein-bound; excreted by the kidney. Metabolized in the liver, crosses placenta, and is excreted in breast milk.

Dosage/Range:

Adult:
- Oral: 25–50 mg q 4 h.
- IM: 25–50 mg q 4 h.
- IV: 50 mg prior to chemotherapy or 25 mg q 4 h × 4 doses, beginning prior to antiemetic.

Drug Preparation:
- Available forms include 25-, 50-mg capsules; elixir 12.5 mg/mL; syrup 12.5 mg/mL; injection available as 10 mg/mL and 50 mg/mL.
- Administer IM deep in large muscle mass.

Drug Interactions:
- CNS depressants: increased sedation; monitor patient closely.

Lab Effects/Interference:
- None known.

Special Considerations:
- Useful in treatment or prevention of extrapyramidal side effects (EPS) related to antiemetics (dopamine antagonists).
- Contraindicated in patients with prior hypersensitivity to H_1-receptor antagonist, acute asthma attack, or lower respiratory tract disease.

Potential Toxicities/Side Effects and the Nursing Process

I. ALTERATIONS IN SENSORY/PERCEPTUAL PATTERNS related to CNS CHANGES

Defining Characteristics: Sedation/drowsiness, dizziness, confusion (especially in the elderly), hyperexcitability, blurred vision/diplopia, tinnitus, dry mouth/nose/throat may all occur.

Nursing Implications: Assess patient's level of consciousness and risk for increased sedation (i.e., elderly, concomitant CNS depressant drugs). Monitor neurologic VS closely if sedated. Instruct patient to avoid alcohol ingestion, operation of equipment, or driving a car while drowsy. Teach strategies to protect safety.

II. ALTERED URINARY ELIMINATION related to URINARY RETENTION, DYSURIA

Defining Characteristics: Urinary retention, dysuria, frequency may occur.

Nursing Implications: Assess baseline urinary elimination pattern. Teach patient potential side effects and instruct to report them. Use drug cautiously in men with prostatic hypertrophy; if side effect occurs, instruct patient not to take drug and discuss with physician.

III. ALTERATION IN COMFORT related to RASH

Defining Characteristics: Rash, urticaria, photosensitivity, hypotension, palpitations may occur.

Nursing Implications: Assess baseline drug allergy history. Instruct patient to report rash, itching, and to avoid sunlight while taking the drug. Assess VS and monitor patient closely for hypotension, especially if patient is elderly or sedated, or taking other sedating drugs.

IV. POTENTIAL FOR INJURY related to BONE MARROW DEPRESSION

Defining Characteristics: Thrombocytopenia, agranulocytosis, hemolytic anemia may occur rarely.

Nursing Implications: Assess baseline CBC, platelet count. Discuss abnormalities with physician.

Drug: dolasetron mesylate (Anzemet)

Class: Serotonin antagonist.

Mechanism of Action: Together with the active metabolite hydrodolasetron, drug is a selective serotonin 5-HT_3 receptor antagonist, blocking transmission of impulses via the vagus nerve peripherally and centrally in the chemotherapy receptor trigger zone (CTZ). Blocks chemotherapy-induced nausea and vomiting produced by the release of serotonin from the enterochromaffin cells of the small intestines, which otherwise would stimulate the 5-HT_3 receptors on the vagus efferents that begin the vomiting reflex.

Metabolism: IV: Parent drug is rapidly eliminated from the plasma and completely metabolized into the major metabolite hydrodolasetron, as is the oral drug. Hydrodolasetron is metabolized by the cytochrome P-450 enzyme system in the liver, with an approximate half-life of 7.3 hours. Oral and orally administered IV solution are bioequivalent, and apparent absolute bioavailability of oral dolasetron is 75%, determined by the active metabolite; 66% of drug is excreted in the urine unchanged, and 33% in the feces. Metabolite is 77% protein-bound.

Dosage/Range: For the prevention of cancer chemotherapy-induced nausea and vomiting:
Adult:
- IV: 1.8 mg/kg IV, 30 minutes prior to chemotherapy, diluted in 50 mL and infused over a period of up to 15 min, or 100-mg IV fixed dose for most adults given IV over 30 sec.
- Oral: 100 mg given within 1 hour prior to chemotherapy.

Pedi (2–16 years of age):
- IV: the recommended intravenous dosage is 1.8 mg/kg given as a single dose approximately 30 minutes before chemotherapy, up to a maximum of 100 mg. Safety and effectiveness in pediatric patients under 2 years of age have not been established.
- Oral: Anzemet injection mixed in apple or apple-grape juice may be used for oral dosing of pediatric patients. When Anzemet injection is administered orally, the

recommended dosage in pediatric patients 2–16 years of age is 1.8 mg/kg, up to a maximum 100-mg dose given within 1 hour before chemotherapy. For the prevention or treatment of postoperative nausea and/or vomiting:

Adult:

- IV: 12.5 mg given as a single dose 15 minutes before the cessation of anesthesia for prevention, or as soon as nausea or vomiting presents (treatment).
- Oral: 100 mg given within 2 hours before surgery.

Pedi (2–16 years of age):

- IV: 0.35 mg/kg, with a maximum dose of 12.5 mg, given as a single dose 15 minutes prior to the cessation of anesthesia (prevention), or as soon as nausea or vomiting presents (treatment).
- Oral: Anzemet injection mixed in apple or apple-grape juice may be used for oral dosing of pediatric patients. When Anzemet injection is administered orally, the recommended dose is 1.2 mg/kg, up to a maximum 100-mg dose given within 2 hours before surgery.
- Safety and efficacy have not been established for children less than 2 years of age.
- Diluted product can be up to 2 hours at room temperature before use. The recommended dose of Anzemet should not be exceeded.

Drug Preparation:

- Injectable drug available in 100-mg/5-mL single-use vials, and 12.5-mg/0.625 mL single-use vials.
- Tablets available in 50-mg and 100-mg doses, each in a 5-count bottle or blister pack, or in a 10-count unit dose.
- IV dose given IVP over 30 sec or further diluted in 50 mL of 0.9% NS, 5% D_5W, D_5 1/2 NS, D_5LR, LR, or 10% mannitol injection and infused over a period of up to 15 minutes. Diluted drug stable 24 hours at room temperature, or 48 hours refrigerated.
- Oral: administer within 1 hour before chemotherapy or within 2 hours prior to surgery.

Drug Interactions:

- Anzemet injection has been safely coadministered with other drugs used in chemotherapy and surgery. As with other agents that prolong ECG intervals, caution should be exercised in patients taking other drugs that prolong ECG intervals, particularly QT_c. See Special Considerations section.
- Increased hydrodolasetron serum levels (24%) when given with cimetidine (nonselective inhibitor of cytochrome P-450 enzyme system).
- Decreased hydrodolasetron serum levels (28%) when combined with rifampin (potent inducer of P-450 enzyme system).

Lab Effects/Interference:

- Transient increased liver transaminases (AST, ALT) in $< 1\%$ of patients; rare increase in bili, GGT, alk phos.

Special Considerations:

- Administer with caution in patients who have or may develop cardiac conduction defects, especially prolongation of QT interval (e.g., patients with hypokalemia, hypomagnesemia, receiving diuretics, congenital QT syndrome, receiving antiarrhythmic drugs or other drugs causing QT segment prolongation, and with high cumulative doses of anthracycline chemotherapy). Prolongation of PR, QRS, and QT_c intervals was observed in some patients. These changes are mild, transient, asymptomatic, and do not require medical treatment. Of note, other 5-HT_3 antagonists were also associated with similar electrocardiographic changes.
- Rare anaphylaxis, facial edema, urticaria.
- No dosage modifications necessary in elderly or patients with hepatic or renal impairment.
- IV preparation indicated for highly emetogenic chemotherapy, including high-dose cisplatin; oral dose indicated for prevention of chemotherapy-induced nausea and vomiting due to moderately emetogenic chemotherapy.

Potential Toxicities/Side Effects and Nursing Process

I. ALTERATION IN COMFORT related to HEADACHE

Defining Characteristics: Headache (24%), fever (4%), fatigue (4%), and, rarely, arthralgia, myalgia occur.

Nursing Implications: Assess baseline comfort. Teach patient to report any unusual occurrence. Provide symptomatic management.

II. ALTERATION IN NUTRITION, LESS THAN BODY REQUIREMENTS, related to CONSTIPATION, DYSPEPSIA

Defining Characteristics: Constipation, dyspepsia, anorexia, and, rarely, pancreatitis may occur. In less than 1% of patients, there is an increase in LFTs.

Nursing Implications: Assess baseline weight, nutritional pattern. Instruct patient to report alterations, and manage symptomatically. Discuss alterations in LFTs and/or abdominal pain suggestive of pancreatitis with physician.

III. POTENTIAL ALTERATIONS IN SENSORY/PERCEPTUAL PATTERNS related to VERTIGO, PARESTHESIA

Defining Characteristics: Rarely, flushing, vertigo, paresthesia, agitation, sleep disorder, depersonalization may occur, as may ataxia, twitching, confusion, anxiety, abnormal dreams.

Nursing Implications: Teach patient to report any changes, and assess patient safety. Discuss any significant alterations with physician and consider alternative antiemetics.

Drug: dronabinol (Marinol)

Class: Cannabinoid.

Mechanism of Action: Active ingredient is δ-9-tetrahydrocannabinol (THC). Probably depresses CNS and may disrupt higher cortical input, inhibit prostaglandin synthesis, or bind to opiate receptors in the brain to indirectly block the VC.

Metabolism: Metabolized by the liver.

Adult:

- Oral: 5 mg/m^2–7.5 mg/m^2 1–3 hours prior to chemotherapy, then 2–4 hours post-chemotherapy for 4–6 doses per day.

Drug Preparation:

- If ineffective at above dose and no toxicity, may be increased by 2.5 mg/m^2 to a maximum of 15 mg/m^2/day.

Drug Interactions:

- CNS depressants: increased sedation; avoid concurrent use.

Lab Effects/Interference:

- None known.

Special Considerations:

- More effective than placebo and in some instances may be better than prochlorperazine.
- Indicated in the management of chemotherapy-induced nausea and vomiting refractory to usual antiemetics.
- Can produce physical and psychological dependency.
- May increase appetite.
- May produce dry mouth.

Potential Toxicities/Side Effects and the Nursing Process

I. ALTERATIONS IN SENSORY/PERCEPTUAL PATTERNS related to CNS CHANGES

Defining Characteristics: Mood changes, disorientation, drowsiness, muddled thinking, dizziness, and brief impairment of perception, coordination, and sensory functions may occur. Increased toxicity in elderly (up to 35%).

Nursing Implications: Explain to patient these changes may occur to decrease anxiety, fear. Assess baseline mental status, and monitor during therapy. Assess patient safety and implement measures to ensure this. Avoid use in the elderly.

II. ALTERATION IN CARDIAC OUTPUT related to TACHYCARDIA

Defining Characteristics: Tachycardia, orthostatic hypotension may occur.

Nursing Implications: Assess baseline VS, and monitor during therapy. If hypotension occurs, notify physician and anticipate increasing rate of IV fluids to increase BP.

Drug: droperidol (Inapsine)

Class: Butyrophenone.

Mechanism of Action: Neuroleptic compound that produces a state of quiescence with reduced motor activity, reduced anxiety, and indifference to surroundings. Dopamine antagonist that suppresses CTZ and VC; more potent than phenothiazines. Decreases stimulation of the VC along vestibular pathway.

Metabolism: When given IM/IV, has onset of action in 3–10 minutes, peak 30 minutes, duration 3–6 hours; metabolized in liver, excreted in urine as metabolites; crosses placenta.

Dosage/Range:

Adults:

- IM/IV: 0.5–2.5 mg q 4–6 h or drip, but reports suggest large loading dose, then intermittent IVB or continuous infusion for 6–10 hours.

Drug Preparation:

- IM: 2.5 mg/mL.
- IV: 2.5 mg/mL initial reconstitution then further dilute in at least 25 mL 0.9% sodium chloride or 5% dextrose.

Drug Interactions:

- Epinephrine: reversal of vasopressor effects; avoid concurrent use.
- CNS depressants: increased sedation; monitor patient closely.

Lab Effects/Interference:

- None known.

Special Considerations:

- Contraindicated in patients with hypersensitivity or who are pregnant.
- Indicated for premedication prior to surgery; induction and maintenance of general anesthesia; also useful as an antiemetic prior to chemotherapy for some patients.

Potential Toxicities/Side Effects and the Nursing Process

I. ALTERATIONS IN SENSORY/PERCEPTUAL PATTERNS related to SEDATION, RESTLESSNESS

Defining Characteristics: Sedation, restlessness, and EPS may occur, although are less severe than with phenothiazines. Tardive dyskinesia may occur in older patients.

Nursing Implications: Assess baseline level of consciousness and monitor during therapy. Assess for signs/symptoms of EPS (dystonia, tongue protrusion, trismus, opisthotonus), and administer diphenhydramine as ordered.

II. ALTERATION IN OXYGENATION/PERFUSION related to RESPIRATORY DEPRESSION

Defining Characteristics: Can induce respiratory depression when used with narcotic analgesics; rarely, laryngospasm or bronchospasm may occur.

Nursing Implications: Assess baseline pulmonary status and monitor during therapy. Identify risk factors (concomitant narcotics, CNS depressants), notify physician, and hold drug if respiratory depression occurs or is suspected. Be prepared to institute respiratory support if necessary, and to reverse opiate.

III. ALTERATION IN CARDIAC OUTPUT related to TACHYCARDIA

Defining Characteristics: Tachycardia and hypotension may occur.

Nursing Implications: Assess baseline VS, and monitor during therapy. If hypotension occurs, notify physician and anticipate increasing rate of IV fluids to increase BP. Epinephrine should not be used since drug reverses vasopressor effect; rather, metaraminol or norepinephrine should be used.

IV. ALTERATION IN COMFORT related to CHILLS, FACIAL SWEATING

Defining Characteristics: Rarely, chills, facial sweating, and shivering occur.

Nursing Implications: Assess baseline comfort. Teach patient to report any unusual occurrence. Provide symptomatic management.

Drug: fosaprepitant dimeglumine (Emend® for injection)

Class: Substance P/Neurokinin-1 receptor antagonist. For oral formulation, see aprepitant.

Mechanism of Action: Drug is a prodrug of aprepitant. Selective Substance P/Neurokinin-1 (NK_1) receptor antagonist (high affinity). Drug has no affinity for $5HT_3$, dopamine, or corticosteroid receptors. Drug crosses the blood–brain barrier to saturate brain NK_1 receptors. Drug increases the activity of serotonin receptor antagonists and corticosteroids in preventing acute nausea and vomiting and inhibits both acute and delayed nausea and vomiting related to cisplatin chemotherapy.

Metabolism: Drug is rapidly converted to aprepitant after IV administration, and the prodrug is neglig1e 30 minutes following administration. The mean aprepitant serum concentrations at 24 hours postdose were similar between a 125-mg oral dose and a 115-mg IV fosaprepitant dose. Aprepitant is 95% bound to plasma proteins and crosses the placenta and blood–brain barrier. Aprepitant undergoes extensive metabolism in the liver by the P450 hepatic microenzyme system, specifically CYP3A4, and minor metabolism by CYP1A2 and CYP2C19. Seven inactive metabolites have been found in the plasma. The drug is excreted in the urine (57%) and the feces (45%). The terminal half-life of the drug is 9–13 hours. The C_{max} is 16% higher for females than males, and the half-life of aprepitant is lower in females than males; however, this is not believed to be clinically important. No dosage adjustment necessary for patients with renal insufficiency or requiring dialysis or patients with mild to moderate hepatic insufficiency.

Dosage/Range:

- Day 1, 115 mg IV over 15 minutes before chemotherapy, together with a serotonin (HT_3) receptor antagonist and dexamethasone (dose reduced to 12 mg day 1, 8 mg days 2 and 3); days 2 and 3, aprepitant 80 mg PO each morning.

Drug Preparation:

- IV formulation supplied as single dose of 115-mg lyophilized white to white off solid in 10-mL glass vial. Vial should be stored at 2–8°C (36–46°F). Aseptically add 5-mL 0.9% sodium chloride for injection into the vial; gently swirl the contents until dissolved (do not shake or jet the diluent into the vial). Aseptically withdraw entire contents, and add to previously prepared 110-ml bag of 0.9% sodium chloride infusion bag. This results in a final concentration of 1 mg/mL.
- Oral drug supplied as (1) 80-mg capsules in bottle of 30 capsules or in unit dose packs of 5 capsules, (2) 125-mg tablets in bottle of 30 capsules or in unit dose packs of 5 capsules, and (3) trifold pack containing 1- to 125-mg capsule and 2- to 80-mg capsules. Capsules should be stored at room temperature.

- Day 1, give 125-mg capsule PO 1 hour before chemotherapy and then the 80-mg capsule in the morning on days 2 and 3. Give with or without food.

Drug Interactions:
- Drugs that inhibit the CYP3A4 isoenzyme system can increase the serum level of aprepitant: ketoconazole, itraconazole, nefazodone, clarithromycin, ritonavir, nelfinavir; diltiazem (twofold increase in aprepitant plasma concentration), and thus, coadminister cautiously and monitor for aprepitant toxicity or dose reduce aprepitant.
- Drugs that strongly induce CYP3A4 isoenzyme system can lower aprepitant serum levels: rifampin, carbamazepine, phenytoin; assess for efficacy of aprepitant and need for drug dose increase.
- Drug is a moderate inhibitor of P450 hepatic isoenzyme system CYP3A4, and thus, the plasma concentrations of the following drugs can theoretically be increased if coadministered:
  - Chemotherapy agents are docetaxel, paclitaxel, etoposide, irinotecan, ifosfamide, imatinib, vinorelbine, vinblastine, and vincristine.
  - Dexamethasone (dose-reduce dexamethasone by 50%).
  - Methylprednisolone (dose reduce 25% if IV, 50% if PO).
  - Pimozide, terfenadine, astemizole: do not use together.
  - Benzodiazepines: midazolam, lorazepam, alprazolam, triazolam.
- Drug is an inducer of CYP2C9, and the plasma concentrations of the following drugs can theoretically be decreased if co-administered:
  - Warfarin (34% decrease with 14% decrease in INR; closely monitor during 2 weeks following antiemetic treatment, especially as the INR 7–10 days after 3-day antiemetic regime may be significantly lowered, and modify warfarin dose as needed).
  - Phenytoin, tolbutamide serum levels can be decreased.
  - Oral contraceptives can become ineffective.

Lab Effects/Interference:
- Decreased INR if patient taking warfarin.

Special Considerations:
- Contraindications: do not give concomitantly with pimozide, terfenadine, astemizole, or cisapride. Do not give if hypersensitive to aprepitant or any of its components. Use cautiously if at all during pregnancy or breast-feeding; no studies have been done in patients with severe liver failure.
- Indications: in combination, with other antiemetic agents, for the prevention of acute and delayed nausea and vomiting associated with initial and repeat courses of highly emetogenic chemotherapy, including high-dose cisplatin.
- Significant drug interactions (discussed previously here).
- Drug is well tolerated with few side effects.

Potential Toxicities/Side Effects and the Nursing Process

I. ALTERATION IN NUTRITION, LESS THAN BODY REQUIREMENTS, related to CONSTIPATION, DIARRHEA, NAUSEA, ANOREXIA, HICCUPS

Defining Characteristics: Gastrointestinal side effects may occur but are infrequent with the following incidences: constipation (10.3%), diarrhea (10.3%), nausea (12.7%), vomiting (7.5%), hiccups (10.8%), and anorexia (10.1%).

Nursing Implications: Teach patient that these side effects may occur and to report them if unrelieved by symptom management measures. Teach patient self-care measures to manage and prevent symptoms.

II. ALTERATION IN COMFORT related to ASTHENIA/FATIGUE, ABDOMINAL PAIN, HEADACHE

Defining Characteristics: Asthenia/fatigue occurred in 17.8% of patients; abdominal pain 4.6%; headache 8.5%.

Nursing Implications: Teach patient that these side effects may occur and measures to minimize their occurrence. Teach energy-conserving measures and management of abdominal pain and headache. Teach patient to report signs and symptoms that worsen or are unrelieved.

Drug: granisetron hydrochloride (Kytril)

Class: Serotonin antagonist.

Mechanism of Action: Binds to vagal afferents (serotonin receptors) adjacent to the enterochromaffin cells in the GI mucosa, thus preventing the stimulation of afferent fibers that would otherwise stimulate the VC and CTZ. In addition, granisetron inhibits a positive feedback loop located on the enterochromaffin cells that normally responds to high levels of serotonin released from chemotherapy injury to the gut mucosa by releasing a surge of additional serotonin. Thus, granisetron blocks two pathways of serotonin release to prevent chemotherapy-induced nausea and vomiting.

Metabolism: Rapidly and extensively metabolized by the liver using the P-450 cytochrome enzymes; 12% of unchanged drug is eliminated in the urine at 48 hours. The half-life of IV granisetron in cancer patients is 9 hours.

Dosage/Range:
- IV: 10 μg/kg IV over 5 minutes, beginning within 30 minutes prior to chemotherapy.
- Oral: 1 mg bid (q 12 h).

Drug Preparation:
- Dilute in 20–50 mL 0.9% sodium chloride or 5% dextrose.

Drug Administration:
- IV infusion over 5 minutes.
- Drug can also be given IV push over 5 minutes.

Drug Interactions:
- None known, but, because the drug is metabolized by the P-450 cytochrome enzymes, drugs that induce or inhibit this may theoretically change the drug serum levels and half-life.

Lab Effects/Interference:
- Rarely, increased AST, ALT.

Special Considerations:
- Useful in the management of high-dose cisplatin, in combination with dexamethasone, either with oral tablets or IV preparation.
- Preliminary study data showed little difference in efficacy between oral dosing of 1 mg bid versus a single dose of 2 mg.
- Both IV and tablet formulation are indicated for the prevention of nausea and vomiting associated with initial and repeat courses of emetogenic chemotherapy, including cisplatin.

Potential Toxicities/Side Effects and the Nursing Process

I. ALTERATION IN COMFORT related to HEADACHE, ASTHENIA, SOMNOLENCE

Defining Characteristics: Side effects are uncommon but may include headache, asthenia, and somnolence.

Nursing Implications: Teach patient that side effects may occur. Headache is usually relieved by OTC analgesics such as acetaminophen.

II. ALTERATION IN ELIMINATION related to CONSTIPATION OR DIARRHEA

Defining Characteristics: A small percentage of patients may experience constipation or diarrhea.

Nursing Implications: Assess baseline elimination pattern. Instruct patient to report alterations. Identify patients at risk, such as those receiving narcotic analgesics for cancer pain, who may develop constipation. Assist patient in modifying bowel regimen.

Drug: granisetron hydrochloride transdermal (Sancuso, investigational)

Class: Serotonin antagonist.

Mechanism of Action: Drug, in a transdermal patch, is delivered via the transdermal route. Granisetron binds to vagal afferents (serotonin receptors) adjacent to the enterochromaffin cells in the GI mucosa, thus preventing the stimulation of afferent fibers that would otherwise stimulate the VC and CTZ. In addition, granisetron inhibits a positive feedback loop located on the enterochromaffin cells that normally responds to high levels of serotonin released from chemotherapy injury to the gut mucosa by releasing a surge of additional serotonin. Thus, granisetron blocks two pathways of serotonin release to prevent chemotherapy-induced nausea and vomiting.

Metabolism: Drug contains 34 mg of drug and delivers drug over 5 days. Once absorbed, drug is rapidly and extensively metabolized by the liver using the P-450 cytochrome enzymes; 12% of unchanged drug is eliminated in the urine at 48 hours. The half-life of IV granisetron in cancer patients is 9 hours.

Dosage/Range:
- 34.3-mg transdermal patch providing antiemesis for 7 days.

Drug Preparation: None

Drug Administration:
- Remove plastic backing and apply to clean, dry skin.
- Apply 24–48 hr before chemotherapy.

Drug Interactions:
- None known, but because the drug is metabolized by the P-450 cytochrome enzymes, drugs that induce or inhibit this may theoretically change the drug serum levels and half-life.

Lab Effects/Interference:
- Rarely, increased AST, ALT.

Special Considerations:
- In a noninferiority trial, transdermal formulation was as good as oral granisetron in the management of patients with cancer receiving first cycle of multiday (3–5 day), moderate or highly emetogenic chemotherapy (Grundberg et al, 2007). This phase III trial was a randomized, double-blind, multinational (nine countries) trial that enrolled 641 patients. Complete protection was achieved in 60.2% of patients receiving the transdermal granisetron and 64.9% of those receiving oral granisetron. Ninety percent of the patients in the transdermal granisetron arm had ≥ 75% patch adherence. Side effects were identical (constipation and headache were most common), and there was no significant irritation at the patch site.

Potential Toxicities/Side Effects and the Nursing Process

I. ALTERATION IN COMFORT related to HEADACHE, ASTHENIA, SOMNOLENCE

Defining Characteristics: Side effects are uncommon but may include headache, asthenia, and somnolence.

Nursing Implications: Teach patient that side effects may occur. Headache is usually relieved by OTC analgesics such as acetaminophen.

II. ALTERATION IN ELIMINATION related to CONSTIPATION OR DIARRHEA

Defining Characteristics: A small percentage of patients may experience constipation or diarrhea.

Nursing Implications: Assess baseline elimination pattern. Instruct patient to report alterations. Identify patients at risk, such as those receiving narcotic analgesics for cancer pain, who may develop constipation. Assist patient in modifying bowel regimen.

Drug: haloperidol (Haldol)

Class: Butyrophenone.

Mechanism of Action: Tranquilizer that depresses cerebral cortex, hypothalamus, limbic system (controls activity and aggression); appears to block dopamine receptors in CTZ, giving antiemetic activity.

Metabolism: Metabolized by the liver, excreted in the urine, bile, and crosses placenta. Enters breast milk. Half-life is 21 hours.

Dosage/Range:

Adult:

- Oral: 3–5 mg q 2 h × 3–4 doses, beginning 30 minutes before chemotherapy.
- IM: 0.5–2 mg (dose reduce in older patients).

Drug Preparation:

- Available as 0.5-, 1-, 2-, 5-, 10-, 20-mg tablets; injection: 5 mg/mL.

Drug Interactions:

- Epinephrine: reversal of vasopressor effects; avoid concurrent use.
- CNS depressants: increased sedation; monitor patient closely.

Lab Effects/Interference:
- Rarely, increased alk phos, bili, serum transaminases (AST, ALT).
- Rarely, decreased PT (if patient on warfarin).
- Rarely, decreased serum cholesterol.

Special Considerations:
- Indicated for the management of psychotic disorders, short-term treatment of hyperactive children showing excessive motor activity, schizophrenia; may be used in the management of nausea and vomiting.
- Contraindicated in severe toxic CNS depression or comatose states; individuals with hypersensitivity; patients with Parkinson's disease, blood dyscrasias, brain damage, bone marrow depression, and alcohol or barbiturate withdrawal states.
- Shown to be equivalent to THC and superior to phenothiazines when tested as an antiemetic.

Potential Toxicities/Side Effects and the Nursing Process

I. ALTERATIONS IN SENSORY/PERCEPTUAL PATTERNS related to TARDIVE DYSKINESIA

Defining Characteristics: With chronic use, tardive dyskinesia syndrome occurs, characterized by involuntary, dyskinetic movements; sedation, EPS may occur when used as an antiemetic.

Nursing Implications: Assess baseline level of consciousness and monitor during therapy. Assess for signs/symptoms of EPS (dystonia, tongue protrusion, trismus, opisthotonus), and administer diphenhydramine as ordered.

II. ALTERATION IN OXYGENATION related to LARYNGOSPASM

Defining Characteristics: Laryngospasm and respiratory depression occur rarely.

Nursing Implications: Assess baseline pulmonary status, and monitor during therapy. Identify risk factors (concomitant narcotics, CNS depressants). Notify physician, and hold drug if respiratory depression occurs or is suspected. Be prepared to institute respiratory support if necessary and to reverse opiate.

III. ALTERATION IN CARDIAC OUTPUT/PERFUSION related to ORTHOSTATIC HYPOTENSION

Defining Characteristics: Orthostatic hypotension may occur and may precipitate angina; also, tachycardia, EKG changes, and rare cardiac arrest may occur.

Nursing Implications: Assess VS baseline, and monitor during therapy. If hypotension occurs, notify physician and anticipate increasing rate of IV fluids to increase BP. Epinephrine should NOT be used because the drug reverses vasopressor effect; rather, metaraminol or norepinephrine should be used.

Drug: metoclopramide hydrochloride (Reglan)

Class: Substituted benzamide.

Mechanism of Action: Procainamide derivative without cardiac effects. Acts both centrally and peripherally. Acts peripherally to enhance the action of acetylcholine at muscarinic synapses and in the CNS to antagonize dopamine. Is primarily a dopamine antagonist blocking the CTZ; also stimulates upper GI tract motility, thus increasing gastric emptying, and opposes retrograde peristalsis of retching.

Metabolism: Metabolized by the liver, excreted in the urine, with a half-life of 4 hours.

Dosage/Range:

Adult:

- Oral: 10 mg qid (gastroparesis).
- IV: 2 mg/kg q 2 h × 3–5 doses OR 3 mg/kg q 2 h × 2 doses, beginning 30 minutes prior to chemotherapy. Dose-reduce if renal insufficiency.

Drug Preparation:

- IV: further dilute in 50 mL 0.9% sodium chloride or 5% dextrose and administer over 15 minutes.

Drug Interactions:

- Digoxin: may decrease absorption; monitor digoxin effectiveness and modify dose as needed.
- Aspirin, acetaminophen, tetracycline, ethanol, levodopa, diazepam: may increase absorption; monitor for drug toxicity.
- CNS depressants: increased depressant effects; monitor patient closely.

Lab Effects/Interference:

- None known.

Special Considerations:

- Indicated as an antiemetic to prevent nausea and vomiting from chemotherapy, delayed gastric emptying, gastroesophageal reflux.
- There is an increased incidence of dystonic reactions in men under 35 years old. Consider diphenhydramine q 4 h or lorazepam and decadron to minimize dystonic reactions.
- Efficacy as an antiemetic: 60% complete protection against high-dose cisplatin, and increased to 66% with the addition of steroids and lorazepam.

- Contraindicated in patients with prior hypersensitivity to this drug, procaine, or procainamide; patients with seizure disorder, pheochromocytoma, GI obstruction.
- Use cautiously in patients with breast cancer, as may increase prolactin levels, and in patients with renal insufficiency.

Potential Toxicities/Side Effects and the Nursing Process

I. ALTERATIONS IN SENSORY/PERCEPTUAL PATTERNS related to SEDATION, EPS

Defining Characteristics: Sedation, akathisia (restlessness), adverse dystonic or extrapyramidal effects may occur; increased risk in patients < 30 years old.

Nursing Implications: Assess baseline neurologic status, and monitor during therapy. Protect patient safety, and keep all necessary patient equipment at the bedside, e.g., commode. Assess for extrapyramidal side effects, and administer diphenhydramine as ordered. In addition, lorazepam administered as part of combination antiemetics helps to decrease akathisia.

II. POTENTIAL FOR ALTERED BOWEL ELIMINATION related to DIARRHEA

Defining Characteristics: Increase in both esophageal sphincter pressure and gastric emptying, leading to diarrhea with high doses. Action antagonized by narcotics.

Nursing Implications: Assess baseline bowel elimination status. Teach patient to report diarrhea, and administer kaolin/pectin as ordered, or other antidiarrheals. Arrange for commode at the bedside if bathroom far from bed. Also, diarrhea may be prevented by administration of dexamethasone as part of antiemetic regimen.

III. ALTERATION IN COMFORT related to DRY/MOUTH, RASH

Defining Characteristics: Dry mouth, rash, urticaria, hypotension may occur.

Nursing Implications: Assess baseline comfort. Teach patient to report rash, urticaria, and treat symptomatically. Monitor VS, and slow infusion rate if hypotensive, as well as replace IV fluids per physician's order.

Drug: nabilone (Cesamet)

Class: Cannabinoid antiemetic.

Mechanism of Action: Drug acts as an omnineuromodulator, interacting with the cannabinoid receptors CB1 and CB2, which are involved in regulating nausea and vomiting. CB1 and CB2 receptors are found throughout the human body.

Metabolism: After oral administration, drug and its carbinol metabolite achieve peak plasma levels in 2 hours, but this amount represents only 10–20% of total drug. Plasma half-life of nabilone is about 2 hours, while that of the total radio-carbon dose was 35 hours. Drug is primarily metabolized by direct enzymatic oxidation, and excreted via the biliary system. Drug and its metabolites are excreted primarily in the feces (65%), with 20% excreted in the urine.

Dosage/Range:
- 1–2 mg PO BID, beginning 1–3 hours before planned chemotherapy; beginning with the lower dose is recommended, with dose increase as needed. Some patients have benefited from a beginning dose the night before chemotherapy.
- Give drug during the entire course of each cycle of chemotherapy, and if needed, for 48 hours after the last dose of each cycle of chemotherapy.
- The maximum daily dose is 6 mg given orally in divided doses 3 times a day.

Drug Preparation:
- None, oral capsule.

Drug Interactions:
- Additive CNS depressant effects with alcohol, sedatives, hypnotics, or other psychotomimetic substances. DO NOT give concomitantly.
- Diazepam: Significantly impaired psychomotor function; DO NOT give concurrently.

Lab Effects/Interference:
- Leukopenia.

Special Considerations:
- Indicated for the management of nausea and vomiting related to chemotherapy in patients who have been refractory to other anti-nausea agents.
- Use cautiously, if at all, in patients with severe liver dysfunction, and in those with a history of non-psychotic emotional disorders. Use cautiously in patients with a substance abuse history.
- Drug should NOT be taken with alcohol, sedatives, hypnotics, or other psychotomimetic substances.
- Drug should not be used during pregnancy, in nursing mothers, or in pediatric patients, as safety has not been established.
- Adverse psychiatric reactions can persist for 48–72 hours after drug is taken.
- Use cautiously in elderly patients with hypertension or heart disease, as drug elevates supine and standing heart rates, and causes postural hypotension.
- Common side effects are unsteadiness, dizziness, difficulty concentrating, drowsiness, mouth dryness, and/or headache.

Potential Toxicities/Side Effects and the Nursing Process

I. ALTERATIONS IN SENSORY/PERCEPTUAL PATTERNS related to SEDATION, EPS

Defining Characteristics: Frequency of symptoms was drowsiness (66%), psychological high (39%), depression (14%), ataxia (13%), blurred vision (13%), sensation disturbance (12%), euphoria (4%), and hallucinations (2%). Rarely, syncope, nightmares, distortion in the perception of time, confusion, disassociation, dysphoria, psychotic reactions, and seizures occurred in < 1% of patients. Anxiety, insomnia, and emotional lability may all occur. Increased toxicity in the elderly.

Nursing Implications: Explain to patient these changes may occur, and strategies to decrease anxiety, fear. Assess baseline mental status, and monitor during therapy. Assess patient's comfort and ability to cope with side effects that occur. Assess patient safety and implement measures to ensure this. Teach patient to avoid driving a car and operating machinery until effect of drug is known and safety assured. Develop safety plan for home care, and involve family or significant caregiver in plan. Avoid use of drug in the elderly. Teach patient to notify physician or NP immediately if patient experiences changes in mood (depression, anxiety), confusion, difficulty breathing, fainting, irregular heartbeats, tremors, hallucinations, and increased blood pressure as they may indicate an overdose.

If psychotic episodes occur, manage patient conservatively if possible. If moderate episode or anxiety reaction, provide verbal support and comforting. If severe, discuss need for antipsychotic drugs, although this has not been studied. Monitor patient closely for additive CNS depressant effects if antipsychotic therapy is used. Protect patient's airway, and support ventilation and perfusion. Consider administration of activated charcoal to decrease GI absorption of drug and to hasten drug elimination.

II. ALTERATION IN CARDIAC OUTPUT related to TACHYCARDIA, ORTHOSTATIC HYPOTENSION

Defining Characteristics: Tachycardia, syncope, orthostatic hypotension may rarely occur.

Nursing Implications: Assess baseline VS, and monitor during therapy. Teach patient to change position from lying to sitting gradually and from sitting to standing so that dizziness is minimized. If hypotension occurs, notify physician and anticipate increasing IV fluids to increase BP during chemotherapy administration.

Drug: ondansetron hydrochloride (zofran)

Class: Serotonin antagonist.

Mechanism of Action: Selective 5-HT_3 (serotonin) receptor antagonist and may block 5-HT_3 receptors found peripherally on the vagus nerve terminals and centrally in the CTZ, thus preventing chemotherapy-induced vomiting.

Metabolism: Extensively metabolized, with only 5% of parent compound found in urine.

Dosage/Range:

Adults:

- IV: 0.15 mg/kg q 4 h × 3 doses OR as a single 32-mg dose, beginning 30 minutes prior to chemotherapy.
- Highly emetogenic chemo: 24 mg PO 30 minutes before chemotherapy.
- Moderately emetogenic chemotherapy.
- Oral: 8 mg PO bid, beginning 30 minutes before chemotherapy, and continuing for 1–2 days after chemotherapy.

Drug Preparation:

- IV available as 2 mg/mL or 32 mg/50 mL; mix in 50 mL 5% dextrose or 0.9% sodium chloride and infuse over 15 minutes.
- Note: single-dose ondansetron (> 22 mg) needs to be given over at least 30 minutes to minimize risk of headache/hypotension.
- Tablets available as either regular tablet or ODT (oral disintegrating tablet), which is freeze-dried and dissolves instantly on the tongue, available in 4-mg and 8-mg strengths.
- Available as an oral solution, 4 mg/5 mL.

Drug Interactions:

- None significant.

Lab Effects/Interference:

- Rarely, increased LFTs.

Special Considerations:

- Contraindicated in patients hypersensitive to the drug.
- Does not affect the dopamine system, so does not cause EPS.
- Approved for use to prevent nausea/vomiting related to chemotherapy, radiation therapy to the abdomen or total body, and following surgery (postoperative).

Potential Toxicities/Side Effects and the Nursing Process

I. ALTERATION IN ELIMINATION related to DIARRHEA or CONSTIPATION

Defining Characteristics: Patients may experience diarrhea (22%) or constipation (11%).

Nursing Implications: Assess baseline elimination status. Teach patient to report alterations, and treat symptomatically.

II. ALTERATION IN COMFORT related to HEADACHE

Defining Characteristics: Headache may occur (16%).

Nursing Implications: Assess comfort level. Teach patient to report headache. Administer acetaminophen as ordered.

III. ALTERATION IN NUTRITION, LESS THAN BODY REQUIREMENTS, related to ↑ LFTs

Defining Characteristics: Transient increases in LFTs may occur (5%).

Nursing Implications: Assess LFTs baseline, and monitor during therapy.

Drug: palonosetron (Aloxi)

Class: Serotonin subtype 3 (5-HT_3) receptor antagonist antiemetic.

Mechanism of Action: Selective serotonin antagonist with strong binding affinity to receptor.

Metabolism: Drug is excreted via renal and metabolic pathways.

Dosage/Range:
- CINV:
  - Single 0.25 mg IV over 30 seconds 30 minutes before the start of chemotherapy.
  - Give once every 7 days OR
  - 0.5 mg capsule PO given 60 minutes prior to the start of moderately emetogenic chemotherapy, with or without food.
- Adult postoperative nausea and vomiting: a single 0.075-mg dose given IV over 10 seconds immediately before the induction of anesthesia.

Drug Preparation:
- Draw up in a syringe to administer IVP over 30 seconds; flush line with Normal Saline prior to and after drug administration.
- Oral capsule: 0.5 mg available in a bottle containing 5 capsules. Store at 25°C (77° F) and protect from light.

Drug Interactions:
- None known.

Lab Effects/Interference:
- Rare prolongation of QTc interval on ECG (> 500 msec, changes > 60 msec from baseline).

Special Considerations:

- Drug is indicated for:
  - Prevention of nausea and vomiting related to moderately emetogenic chemotherapy, both acute and delayed, associated with initial and repeat courses.
  - Prevention of acute nausea and vomiting related to highly emetogenic chemotherapy, associated with initial and repeat courses.
  - Prevention of postoperative nausea and vomiting (PONV) for up to 24 hours after surgery.
- Palonosetron has greater potency, higher binding affinity to the 5-HT_3 receptor, and has a longer half-life (40 hours) than any of the 1st generation serotonin antagonists.
- Rarely, patients hypersensitive to other HT_3 receptor antagonists may be hypersensitive to palonestron.
- Most common side effects are:
  - CINV (occurring in > 5%): headache, constipation.
  - PONV (occurring in > 2%) : QT prolongation, bradycardia, headache, constipation.

Potential Toxicities/Side Effects and the Nursing Process

I. ALTERATION IN COMFORT related to HEADACHE

Defining Characteristics: Headache occurs in 3.7% (capsule) 0–9% (IV) of patients.

Nursing Implications: Teach patients that this may occur, and to take acetaminophen to relieve headache if it occurs.

II. ALTERATION IN BOWEL ELIMINATION related to CONSTIPATION

Defining Characteristics: Constipation occurs in about 0.6% (capsule) to 5% (injection) of patients.

Nursing Implications: Assess baseline bowel elimination status. Teach patients that constipation may occur, and to use usual strategies to prevent constipation. If constipation occurs, teach patient to use bowel softeners, laxatives as needed, and to increase oral fluids, fiber, and exercise to promote peristalsis.

III. ALTERATION IN OXYGENATION related to RARE CARDIAC EVENTS

Defining Characteristics: Cardiovascular events are rare and occur in 1% of patients. These include nonsustained tachycardia, bradycardia, hypotension or hypertension, sinus arrhythmia, supraventricular extrasystoles, sinus tachycardia, and QT prolongation. The relationship to palonestron was not clear in all instances. In nonclinical studies, palonosetron has the ability to block ion channels involved in ventricular depolarization and repolarization and to prolong action potential duration.

Nursing Implications: Assess baseline cardiac status, and monitor closely during therapy. Teach patient to notify the provider if any abnormalities occur, such as rapid or slow heartbeat.

Drug: perphenazine

Class: Phenothiazine.

Mechanism of Action: Antipsychotic agent. Blocks dopamine receptors in CTZ; also decreases vagal stimulation of VC by peripheral afferents.

Metabolism: Metabolized by the liver, excreted in the urine, crosses placenta, enters breast milk.

Dosage/Range:

Adult:

- Oral: 4 mg q 4–6 h.
- IM/IV: 5 mg IVB q 4–6 h OR 5 mg IVB then infusion at 1 mg/hour for 10 hours.
- Maximum: 30 mg in 24 hours (inpatient), or 15 mg in 24 hours (outpatient).

Drug Preparation:

- Further dilute IV drug in 50 mL 0.9% sodium chloride, and infuse over 20 minutes.

Drug Interactions:

- Antacids: decreased perphenazine absorption; take 2 hours before or after antacid.
- Antidepressants: increased Parkinsonian symptoms; avoid concomitant use or use cautiously.
- Barbiturates: increased CNS depressant effect; use together cautiously, if at all.

Lab Effects/Interference:

- Rarely, increased LFTs.

Special Considerations:

- Effective in management of nausea and vomiting related to moderately emetogenic drugs.
- Contraindicated in patients hypersensitive to the drug, or who have blood dyscrasias, coma.
- Increased incidence of dystonic reactions in men less than 35 years old. Consider diphenhydramine or lorazepam and decadron q 4 h to minimize risk of dystonia.
- Indicated in the treatment of psychotic disorders, schizophrenia, alcoholism, intractable hiccups; and is used to prevent chemotherapy-induced nausea and vomiting.

Potential Toxicities/Side Effects and the Nursing Process

I. ALTERATIONS IN SENSORY PERCEPTUAL PATTERNS related to SEDATION, EPS

Defining Characteristics: Sedation, blurred vision, and EPS reactions may occur, especially dystonia; also, seizure threshold may be lowered.

Nursing Implications: Assess baseline mental status. Instruct patient to report signs/symptoms of EPS, and assess for them during treatment (tongue protrusion, trismus, akathisia or restlessness, tremor, insomnia, dizziness). Administer diphenhydramine as ordered to reverse reaction. Diphenhydramine should be ordered prior to drug to prevent EPS.

II. ALTERATION IN NUTRITION related to CONSTIPATION, ↑APPETITE, CHOLESTATIC JAUNDICE

Defining Characteristics: Dry mouth, constipation, increased appetite and weight gain, cholestatic jaundice may occur.

Nursing Implications: Assess baseline nutritional patterns, moistness of mucous membranes, and elimination pattern. Assess baseline liver function, and monitor during therapy.

III. ALTERATION IN SKIN INTEGRITY related to RASH

Defining Characteristics: Mild photosensitivity, rash, urticaria, and, rarely, exfoliative dermatitis may occur.

Nursing Implications: Assess baseline skin integrity. Instruct patient to report any changes.

Drug: prochlorperazine (Compazine)

Class: Phenothiazine.

Mechanism of Action: Blocks dopamine receptors in CTZ; also decreases vagal stimulation of VC by peripheral afferents.

Metabolism: Metabolized by liver, excreted in kidney, crosses placenta, excreted in breast milk. Onset of action for oral is 30–40 minutes, duration 3–4 hours; extended-release 30–40 minutes with duration 10–13 hours; PR onset 60 minutes, duration 3–4 hours; and IM onset 10–20 minutes, duration 12 hours.

Dosage/Range:

Adult:

- Oral: 5–25 mg q 4–6 h; slow-release: 10–75 mg q 12 h.
- IM/IV: 5–40 mg q 3–4 h; dilute in 50 mL 5% dextrose or 0.9% sodium chloride and administer IV over 20–30 minutes.
- PR: 25 mg q 4–6 h.

Drug Preparation:

- Store in tight, light-resistant containers. Administer IM injection deep into large muscle mass.

Drug Interactions:

- Antacids: decreased prochlorperazine absorption; take 2 hours before or after antacid.
- Antidepressants: increased Parkinsonian symptoms; avoid concomitant use or use cautiously.
- Barbiturates: decreased prochlorperazine effect; may need to increase dose of prochlorperazine.

Lab Effects/Interference:

- Rarely, may cause increased LFTs.

Special Considerations:

- Indicated in the management of chemotherapy-induced nausea and vomiting.
- Increased risk of dystonic reactions in men under 35 years old. Consider diphenhydramine or lorazepam and decadron q 4 h to minimize risk of dystonia.
- Dose-reduce in the elderly.
- Use cautiously in combination with CNS depressants.
- Contraindicated in patients with hypersensitivity to phenothiazines or with coma, seizure, encephalopathy.

Potential Toxicities/Side Effects and the Nursing Process

I. ALTERATIONS IN SENSORY PERCEPTUAL PATTERN related to SEDATION, EPS

Defining Characteristics: Sedation, blurred vision, EPS reactions may occur, especially dystonia; also, seizure threshold may be lowered.

Nursing Implications: Assess baseline mental status. Teach patient to report signs/symptoms of EPS and assess for them during treatment (tongue protrusion, trismus, akathisia or restlessness, tremor, insomnia, dizziness). Administer diphenhydramine as ordered to reverse reaction. Diphenhydramine may be ordered prior to drug to prevent EPS.

II. ALTERATION IN NUTRITION related to CONSTIPATION, ↑APPETITE, CHOLESTATIC JAUNDICE

Defining Characteristics: Dry mouth, constipation, increased appetite and weight gain, cholestatic jaundice may occur.

Nursing Implications: Assess baseline nutritional patterns, moistness of mucous membranes, and elimination pattern. Assess baseline liver function, and monitor during therapy.

III. ALTERATION IN SKIN INTEGRITY related to RASH

Defining Characteristics: Mild photosensitivity, rash, urticaria, and, rarely, exfoliative dermatitis may occur.

Nursing Implications: Assess baseline skin integrity. Teach patient to report any changes.

IV. ALTERATION IN CARDIAC OUTPUT related to ORTHOSTATIC HYPOTENSION

Defining Characteristics: Orthostatic hypotension, tachycardia, and EKG changes may occur.

Nursing Implications: Assess baseline VS prior to and during IV infusions, especially with high doses. Discuss with physician and anticipate increasing IV fluid rate if hypotensive.

Drug: promethazine hydrochloride (Anergan, Phenameth, Phenergan)

Class: Antihistamine; phenothiazine derivative with sedative, antihistamine, and mild antiemetic properties.

Mechanism of Action: Drug is anticholinergic and has CNS depressant effects; specific CNS mechanism is unknown.

Dosage/Range:

Adult:

- Antiemetic: Oral/IM/IV: 12.5–25 mg q 4 h PRN.

Drug Preparation:

- Drug must not be given subcutaneously or intra-arterially.
- IV: administer a dilute solution < 25 mg/mL, at < 25 mg/min.
- IM: administer deep IM in large muscle mass.

Drug Preparation:
- CNS depressants: increased sedation; avoid concurrent use.
- Epinephrine: may reverse vasopressor effects and further decrease BP; avoid concurrent use.
- Phenothiazines: increased toxicity; avoid concurrent use.

Special Considerations:
- Contraindicated in patients with increased intraocular pressure, prostatic hypertrophy, epilepsy, coma, CNS depression, intestinal obstruction.
- Use cautiously in the elderly and patients with asthma, hypertension, and seizure disorder.

Potential Toxicities/Side Effects and the Nursing Process

I. ALTERATIONS IN SENSORY/PERCEPTUAL PATTERNS related to CONFUSION, RESTLESSNESS

Defining Characteristics: Increased risk in the elderly for confusion, sedation, drowsiness, restlessness, tremors; blurred vision may also occur.

Nursing Implications: Assess baseline level of consciousness, and monitor during therapy. Assess for signs/symptoms of EPS (dystonia, tongue protrusion, trismus, opisthotonus), and administer diphenhydramine as ordered.

II. ALTERATION IN CARDIAC OUTPUT related to HYPOTENSION

Defining Characteristics: Hypotension may occur, especially with high or IV dosing.

Nursing Implications: Assess baseline VS, and monitor during IV administration. Administer drug slowly, and notify physician if hypotension occurs. Anticipate increasing IV fluids.

III. ALTERATION IN NUTRITION, LESS THAN BODY REQUIREMENTS, related to GI SIDE EFFECTS

Defining Characteristics: Dry mouth, nausea, vomiting, and constipation may occur.

Nursing Implications: Assess baseline nutritional status. Instruct patient to report GI side effects. Discuss alternative antiemetic if these occur. Assess elimination status; teach patient importance of diet high in bulk and fiber, increased fluids, and exercise to prevent constipation.

IV. ALTERATION IN URINARY ELIMINATION related to URINARY RETENTION

Defining Characteristics: Urinary retention may occur.

Nursing Implications: Instruct patient to report this symptom; discuss alternative drug with physician for control of emesis.

Drug: scopolamine

Class: Antimuscarinic; used as an antiemetic.

Mechanism of Action: Appears to prevent nausea/vomiting associated with motion sickness by blocking cholinergic impulses, thus preventing stimulation of the VC.

Dosage/Range:

Adult:

- Patch: transdermal patch 1.5 mg q 72 h.

Drug Preparation:

- Apply 4 hours prior to time protection is needed.
- Apply to clean and dry hairless area behind ear; remove clear plastic cover, exposing adhesive layer; apply directly to skin behind ear and press firmly; wash hands.

Drug Interactions:

- None significant.

Lab Effects/Interference:

- None known.

Special Considerations:

- Use cautiously in patients with glaucoma, urinary bladder-neck obstruction.
- Wash hands after handling patch to prevent exposure to scopolamine.
- If patch falls off, wash area, then reapply new patch in another location.

Potential Toxicities/Side Effects and the Nursing Process

I. ALTERATION IN MUCOUS MEMBRANE INTEGRITY related to DRY MOUTH

Defining Characteristics: Dry mouth occurs in 67% of patients.

Nursing Implications: Teach patient this may occur. Suggest patient suck ice chips, sugar-free candy, or practice usual oral hygiene regimen more frequently.

II. ALTERATIONS IN SENSORY/PERCEPTUAL PATTERNS related to DROWSINESS, BLURRED VISION

Defining Characteristics: Drowsiness, blurred vision, mydriasis may occur; rarely, disorientation, restlessness, confusion may occur.

Nursing Implications: Assess baseline mental status. Instruct patient to report changes in vision or feeling state. Assess patient safety needs, and provide safe environment.

Drug: thiethylperazine (Torecan)

Class: Phenothiazine derivative; antiemetic.

Mechanism of Action: Blocks stimulation of CTZ and VC.

Metabolism: Metabolized by liver, excreted by kidneys, crosses placenta, and may be excreted in breast milk.

Dosage/Range:
Adult:
- Oral/PR/IM: 10 mg daily-tid.

Drug Preparation:
- IM: give deep IM into large muscle mass.
- Do not give IV (causes hypotension).

Drug Interactions:
- Barbiturates: may decrease antiemetic effect; increase dose as needed.
- Antacids: may decrease absorption of thiethylperazine; administer 2 hours before or after antacid.
- Epinephrine: may reverse vasopressor effect of epinephrine; avoid concurrent use.

Lab Effects/Interference:
- Rarely, increased LFTs.

Special Considerations:
- Contraindicated in patients with severe CNS depression, coma, prior sensitivity reaction.
- Contraindicated in patients allergic to dye tartrazine (FD&C Yellow No. 5) as it may cause bronchial asthma.
- Torecan injection contains sodium metabisulfite; contraindicated in patients allergic to sulfites.
- Increased risk of dystonic reactions in men under 35 years old. Consider diphenhydramine or lorazepam and decadron every 4 hours to minimize dystonia.

Potential Toxicities/Side Effects and the Nursing Process

I. ALTERATIONS IN SENSORY/PERCEPTUAL PATTERNS related to DROWSINESS, EPS

Defining Characteristics: Drowsiness may occur after IM injection. Rarely, extrapyramidal side effects may occur (i.e., dystonia, torticollis, akathisia, gait disturbances), as may blur vision and tinnitus.

Nursing Implications: Assess baseline level of consciousness, and monitor during therapy. Assess for signs/symptoms of EPS (dystonia, tongue protrusion, trismus, opisthotonus), and administer diphenhydramine as ordered.

II. ALTERATION IN CARDIAC OUTPUT related to HYPOTENSION

Defining Characteristics: Hypotension may occur after IM dosing; rarely, tachycardia, EKG changes occur.

Nursing Implications: Assess baseline VS, and monitor during IV administration. Administer drug slowly, and notify physician if hypotension occurs. Anticipate increasing IV fluids.

Chapter 8
Anorexia and Cachexia

Anorexia and weight loss may be presenting symptoms of cancer, or symptoms of advanced disease. No other symptoms may cause more powerful distress to a patient than being confronted with weight loss and inability to eat due to anorexia. Consequences of severe anorexia include nutritional depletion and further weight loss, which result in decreased functional status, diminished treatment responses to chemotherapy, and apparent decreased quality of life. Primary cachexia, or wasting syndrome, occurs in at least two-thirds of patients with advanced cancer or human immunodeficiency virus (HIV) disease. The associated extreme weakness and fatigue lead to incapacity, dependency, social isolation, and again, apparent diminished quality of life.

In addition, anorexia and cachexia can be terrifying and frustrating to family members. The patient's spouse may be used to nurturing the patient and preparing meals, and feel rejected and frightened by a loved one's inability to eat. This may symbolize personal failure on the part of the spouse, as well as failure of current treatment to reverse the disease process and a poor prognosis.

Metabolically, cachexia appears to result from chronic, systemic inflammation with the release of acute-phase proteins and orchestration by cytokines such as tumor necrosis factor, IL-1 and IL-6 (Laviano et al, 2002). Morley et al (2006) suggest that other potential mediators of cachexia are testosterone, insulin-like growth factor I deficiency, excess myostatin, and excess glucocorticoids. This leads to the preferential breakdown of skeletal muscle protein and body fat, resulting in the profound wasting syndrome characterized by anorexia, early satiety, weight loss, decreased function, and death (Inui, 2002). Secondary cachexia is simple starvation from decreased food intake or defective nutrient absorption, and results from situations such as nausea, vomiting, and anorexia due to chemotherapy. As expected, patients responding to chemotherapy will show a weight gain.

Pharmacologic agents used to stimulate appetite are varied in mechanism of action, efficacy, and strength of evidence. Corticosteroids have been tried for many years, with usual effect within 1–3 weeks (Ottery et al, 1998; Loprinzi et al, 1999). However, side effects, such as insomnia, muscle catabolism, hyperglycemia, have limited their usefulness. When compared with megestrol acetate 800 mg/day, dexamethasone (0.75 mg four times daily) patients had similar responses but different toxicities: megestrol acetate caused thromboembolism, whereas dexamethasone caused myopathy, peptic ulcers, and problems related to Cushingoid side effects

(Loprinzi et al, 1999). Of the studies of pharmacologic agents in the treatment of anorexia and cachexia in cancer, megestrol acetate has shown statistical improvement in nonfluid weight gain (Ottery, 1998). Mantovani et al (1998) suggest that megestrol acetate, in fact, downregulates cytokine production, resulting in increased appetite and anabolism. There appears to be a dose-response effect, and Loprinzi et al (1992) showed optimal weight gain at a dose of 800 mg/day. Patients showed increased appetite, increased food intake, weight gain, and less nausea and vomiting. The incidence of thrombophlebitis was 6%. Loprinzi et al also demonstrated that the weight gain resulting from megestrol acetate is increased fat and lean body mass, not water gain (i.e., edema, ascites).

Thalidomide, an agent originally developed as a nonbarbiturate sedative but which was never marketed as such due to its teratogenicity, has been shown to increase weight gain and lean body mass in HIV-infected individuals with cachexia (Ottery, 1998). Metoclopramide, at low doses for stimulation of GI motility, has been shown to decrease early satiety and postprandial fullness, and may be helpful for some patients (Kris et al, 1985). Cannabinoid derivatives, such as δ-9-tetrahydrocannabinol (THC) and dronabinol, appear to stimulate appetite and possible weight gain in some patients (Beal et al, 1997; Klausner et al, 1996; Kaplan et al, 1998; Jatoi, 2006). Eicosapentaenoic (EPA) acid (fish oil, thought to stabilize acute phase proteins) in a nutritional supplement was compared with megestrol acetate or a combination of both; megestrol acetate was found more effective in stimulating appetite (Jatoi et al, 2004). Studies continue to explore whether other agents, such as melatonin (regulation of circadian rhythm), can be of benefit (Cunningham, 2003).

The ONS Putting Evidence into Practice (PEP) cards for "Anorexia" recommend for practice based on strong evidence from rigorously conducted studies corticosteroids (reserved for those with anorexia with advanced disease or who may have disease regression, where a short-term benefit is needed) and progestins. In addition, they point out that dietary counseling is likely to be effective, as individual dietary counseling has been shown to improve nutritional intake and body weight. They point out that effectiveness is not established for cyproheptadine, eicosapentaenoic acid (EPA), erythropoietin, ghrelin, metoclopramide, oral branched chain amino acids, pentoxifylline, and thalidomide. Effectiveness is unlikely with cannabinoids, hydrazine sulfate, and melatonin (Adams et al, 2008).

It is exciting to think that perhaps nutritional stimulation might improve the patient's ability to tolerate aggressive therapy or in some way improve efficacy of the treatment; however, a randomized, double-blind, controlled trial compared megestrol acetate or placebo together with chemotherapy and radiation therapy for newly diagnosed patients with extensive SCLC. Unfortunately, there was no difference in patient response (efficacy), quality of life, or overall survival between the two groups (Loprinzi and Jatoi, 2007). In an earlier study (1999) with chemotherapy only, patients receiving megestrol acetate had more thromboembolic events and edema, inferior response to chemotherapy and survival (Rowland et al, 1996).

References

Adams L, Cunningham R, Caruso RA, Norling M, Shepard N. *Anorexia: What Interventions Are Effective in Managing Anorexia in People With Cancer*. Pittsburgh PA: Oncology Nursing Society, 2008.

Beal JE. Long-term Efficacy and Safety of Dronabinol for Acquired Immunodeficiency Syndrome-associated Anorexia. *J Pain Symptom Manage.* 1997; 14(1) 7–14

Brown JK. A Systematic Review of the Evidence on Symptom Management of Cancer-related Anorexia and Cachexia. *Oncol Nurs Forum* 2002; 29 517–530

Bruera E, Macmillan K, Kuehn N, et al. A Controlled Trial of Megestrol Acetate on Appetite, Caloric Intake, Nutritional Status, and Other Symptoms in Patients with Advanced Cancer. *Cancer* 1990; 66 1279–1282

Chlebowski RT, Bulcavage L, Grosvenor M, et al. Hydrazine Sulfate Influence on Nutritional Status and Survival in NSCLC. *J Clin Oncol* 1990; 8 9–15

Cunningham RS. The Anorexia-Cachexia Syndrome, chapter 9. Yarbro CH, Frogge MH, Goodman M, (eds). Cancer Symptom Management, 3rd ed. Sudbury, MA: Jones and Bartlett Publishers 2003; 137–155

Dreizen S, McCredie KB, Keating MJ, et al. Nutritional Deficiencies in Patients Receiving Cancer Chemotherapy. *Postgrad Med J* 1990; 87 163–170

Enck RE. Anorexia and Cachexia: An Update. *Am J Hospice Palliative Care* 1990; 7(5) 13–15

Inui A. Cancer Anorexia-Cachexia Syndrome: Current issues in Research and Management. *CACancer J Clin* 2002; 52 72–91

Jatoi A. Pharmacologic Therapy for the Cancer Anorexia/Weight Loss Syndrome: A Data Driven, Practical Approach. *J Support Oncol* 2006; 4(10) 499–502

Jatoi A, Rowland K, Loprinzi CL, et al. An Eicosapentaenoic Acid Supplement Versus Megestrol Acetate Versus Both for Patients with Cancer-Associated Wasting: A North Central Cancer Treatment Group and National Cancer Institute of Canada Collaborative Effort. *J Clin Oncol* 2004; 22 2469–2476

Kaplan G, Schambelan M, Gottleib C, et al. Thalidomide Reverses Cachexia in HIV-Wasting Syndrome. 5th International Conference on Retroviruses and Opportunistic Infections, Abstract 476. February 1–5, 1998, *Chicago, IL* 1998

Klausner JD, Makonkawkeyoon S, Akarasewi P, et al. The Effect of Thalidomide on the Pathogenesis of Human Immunodeficiency Virus Type 1 and M. tuberculosis Infection. *J Acquir Immune Defic Syndr and Hum Retrovirology* 1996; 11 247–257

Kornblith AB, Hollis D, Phillips CA, et al. Effect of Megestrol Acetate upon Quality of Life in Advanced Breast Cancer Patients in a Dose Response Trial. *Proc American Society of Clinical Oncologists* 1992; 11 377

Kris MG, Yeh SDJ, Gralla RJ, et al. Symptomatic Gastroparesis in Cancer Patients: Possible Cause of Anorexia That Can Be Improved with Oral Metoclopramide. *Proc American Society of Clinical Oncologists* 1985; 4 267

Laviano A, Russo M, Freda F, et al. Neurochemical Mechanisms for Cancer Cachexia. *Nutrition* 2002; 18 100–105

Loprinzi C, Jatoi A. Anorexia and cachexia. In Pazdur R, Coia LR, Hoskins WJ, Wagman LD (eds). *Cancer Management: A Multidisciplinary Approach*, 10th ed. Lawrence, KS: CMP Healthcare Media LLC; 2007

Loprinzi CL, Ellison NM, Schard OJ, et al. Controlled Trial of Megestrol Acetate for the Treatment of Cancer Anorexia and Cachexia. *J Natl Cancer Inst* 1990; 82 1127–1132

Loprinzi CL, Jensen M, Burnham N, et al. Body Composition Changes in Cancer Patients Who Gain Weight from Megestrol Acetate. *Proc American Society of Clinical Oncologists* 1992; 11 378

Loprinzi CL, Kugler JW, Sloan JA, et al. Randomized Comparison of Megestrol Acetate versus Dexamethasone versus Fluoxymesterone for the Treatment of Cancer Anorexia/Cachexia. *J Clin Oncol* 1999; 17 3299–3306
Loprinzi CL, Mailliard J, Schaid D, et al. Dose/Response Evaluation of Megestrol Acetate for the Treatment of Cancer Anorexia/Cachexia: A Mayo Clinic and North Central Cancer Treatment Group Trial. *Proc American Society of Clinical Oncologists* 1992; 11 378
Mantovani G, Maccio A, Paola L, et al. Cytokine Activity in Cancer-related Anorexia/Cachexia: Role of Megestrol Acetate and Medroxyprogesterone Acetate. *Semin Oncol* 1998; 25 (suppl) 45–52
Morley JE, Thomas DR, Wilson MMG. Cachexia: Pathophysiology and Relevance. *Am J Clin Nutr* 2006; 83 735–743
Ottery FD, Walsh D, Strawford A. Pharmacologic Management of Anorexia/Cachexia. *Semin Oncol* 1998; 25 (suppl) 35–44
Rowland KM, Loprinzi CL, Shaw EG, et al. Randomized Double Blind Placebo Controlled Trial of Cisplatin and Etoposide Plus Megestrol Acetate/Placebo in Extensive-Stage Small Cell Lung Cancer: A North Central Cancer Treatment Group Study. *J Clin Oncol* 1996; 14 135–141

Drug: dronabinol (Marinol)

Class: Cannabinoid.

Mechanism of Action: Stimulates appetite in acquired immunodeficiency syndrome (AIDS) patients, leading to trends toward improved body weight and mood.

Metabolism: 90–95% absorption after oral dose, but because of first-pass effect of the liver and high lipid solubility, only about 20% of the dose reaches the systemic circulation. Large area of distribution so that drug continues to be excreted for a long period of time. The appetite stimulation effect may persist for 24 hours from a single dose.

Dosage/Range:

- 2.5 mg bid before lunch and supper, or if patient is intolerant, a single 2.5-mg dose may be taken at bedtime.

Drug Preparation:

- Available in 2.5-, 5-, or 10-mg gel capsules that harden under refrigeration.

Drug Administration:

- Oral.

Drug Interactions:

- Amphetamines, cocaine: additive hypertension, tachycardia.
- Atropine, scopolamine: tachycardia, drowsiness.
- Amitriptyline, tricyclic antidepressants: additive tachycardia, hypertension.
- Barbiturates, CNS depressants, buspirone: drowsiness and additive CNS depression.
- Theophylline: increased metabolism.

Lab Effects/Interference:
- None known.

Special Considerations:
- Drug has antiemetic qualities.

Potential Toxicities/Side Effects and the Nursing Process

I. ALTERATIONS IN SENSORY/PERCEPTUAL PATTERNS related to CNS CHANGES

Defining Characteristics: Drug can cause changes in mood, cognition, memory, and perception. In addition, nervousness, anxiety, confusion, dizziness, depersonalization, euphoria, paranoid reaction, somnolence, and thinking abnormalities can occur. Drug has abuse potential.

Nursing Implications: Assess appropriateness of drug for patient, as this would not be the drug of choice for a substance abuser, either one who is actively using or who has withdrawn and is abstaining because of abuse potential. Teach patient of possible side effects, and self-care strategies to avoid heightened fear or anxiety.

II. POTENTIAL FOR ALTERATION IN OXYGENATION related to SYMPATHOMIMETIC EFFECTS

Defining Characteristics: Tachycardia and conjunctival injection may occur. Drug interactions may cause hypertension.

Nursing Implications: Review patient medication profile to identify any possible drug interactions. Monitor appetite stimulation effects, and weigh these against any sympathomimetic changes.

Drug: megestrol acetate (Megace)

Class: Synthetic progestin.

Mechanism of Action: Alters malignant cell environment in hormonally sensitive tumors, discouraging tumor cell proliferation; appears to stimulate appetite and weight gain in cancer cachexia directly or indirectly through antagonism of TNF. Designated as orphan drug by FDA for management of anorexia, cachexia, or weight loss > 10% of baseline. Approved for AIDS-related cachexia.

Metabolism: Well absorbed from GI tract. Metabolized in liver and excreted by kidneys.

Dosage/Range:
- Optimal dose for management of cachexia is 800 mg/day in a single dose.
- Available in Megace ES formulation (concentrated suspension) delivering 625 mg (125 mg/mL), which has been shown equivalent to the 800 mg of Megace oral suspension (40 mg/mL) (in volunteers under fed conditions).

Drug Preparation:
- Store in tight container at temperature < 40°C (104°F).
- Oral administration.

Drug Administration
- 5 mL of Megace ES (625 mg) or 20 mL Megase OS (800 mg).

Drug Interactions:
- None.

Lab Effects/Interference:
- May increase glucose, lactic dehydrogenase (LDH).
- Rare leukopenia.

Special Considerations:
- Drug is expensive.
- One-third of patients with metastatic cancer gain weight.
- Weight gain appears to be from increased fat stores rather than water gain (Loprinzi et al 1992).

Potential Toxicities/Side Effects and the Nursing Process

I. ALTERATIONS IN PERFUSION related to DEEP VEIN THROMBOSIS

Defining Characteristics: Rarely, 6% of patients may experience deep vein thrombosis (DVT) or pulmonary emboli.

Nursing Implications: Assess baseline peripheral vascular status and monitor during therapy. Teach patient to report pain in calf, erythema, shortness of breath, chest pain immediately.

II. ALTERATION IN NUTRITION related to HYPERGLYCEMIA

Defining characteristics: Hyperglycemia is uncommon but may be significant if it occurs.

Nursing Implications: Assess baseline FBS, and monitor during therapy. Teach patient signs and symptoms of hyperglycemia and to report them (polydipsia, polyuria, polyphagia).

III. ALTERATION IN COMFORT related to CARPAL TUNNEL SYNDROME, NAUSEA AND VOMITING, TUMOR FLARE

Defining Characteristics: Carpal tunnel syndrome, nausea, vomiting, tumor flare may occur rarely.

Nursing Implications: Instruct patient to report any signs/symptoms. Discuss with patient, physician symptomatic measures.

IV. ANXIETY related to ABNORMAL UTERINE BLEEDING

Defining Characteristics: Breakthrough vaginal bleeding, discharge often occur in females, and can cause anxiety.

Nursing Implications: Teach female patient that this is an expected side effect. Encourage patient to verbalize feelings, provide patient with emotional support and information about cause and management.

Drug: thalidomide (Thalomid)

Class: Inhibitor of TNF-α; nonbarbiturate sedative.

Mechanism of Action: Selective inhibitor of TNF-α. TNF-α is implicated as a principal mediator in the complex syndrome of HIV or cancer cachexia. TNF-α has been shown to cause effects similar to many of those seen in cancer cachexia: weight loss, anorexia, fever, metabolic abnormalities such as hyperlipidemia, insulin resistance, muscle wasting.

Metabolism: Well absorbed after oral administration. Mean peak serum level reached at 4–5 hours. Elimination half-life is 4–12 hours, with drug found in the plasma after 24 hours. NOT metabolized using P-450 hepatic enzyme system, and has low renal excretion.

Dosage/Range:
Adult:
- 100 mg/day at bedtime (range 50–200 mg/day).
- If needed, increase by 100 mg/day at intervals of 1–2 weeks.

Drug Preparation:
- Oral, give at bedtime.
- Available for investigational or compassionate use in 50-mg capsules.

Drug Interactions:
- Barbiturates, alcohol, chlorpromazine, reserpine: increased sedation.

Lab Effects/Interference:
- May slightly increase HIV viral load.
- Rare neutropenia, especially in HIV-infected patients.

Special Considerations:
- Studies in HIV wasting have showed a mean gain of 6.5% in body weight in 3 weeks vs 0.9% in controls (Klausner et al, 1996), and other studies have shown that weight gain is lean body mass (Kaplan et al, 1998).
- ABSOLUTE CONTRAINDICATION IS PREGNANCY. Pregnancy test must be routinely negative prior to beginning therapy in women of child-bearing age. Contraception is mandatory for men and women.
- Women taking hormonal contraception, as well as any of the following—barbiturates, glucocorticoids, phenytoin, carbamazepine—have decreased efficacy of the hormonal contraception and must use barrier contraception as well.
- Drug is being studied in higher doses as an anticancer agent in tumors that are TNF-α dependent (e.g., Kaposi's sarcoma) as well as in other tumors (metastatic breast cancer, prostate cancer); also being studied in graft-versus-host disease.
- Patient must be enrolled in a government-monitored registry, and prescriptions can be written or dispensed by precertified doctors and pharmacists, respectively. Only a 28-day supply will be given, and women must have a negative pregnancy test before next prescription is written.

Potential Toxicities/Side Effects and the Nursing Process

I. ALTERATION IN SEXUALITY/REPRODUCTION related to POTENTIAL TERATOGENICITY

Defining Characteristics: Drug is teratogenic and a single dose can cause birth defects. Unclear if drug is excreted in semen.

Nursing Implications: Assess reproductive status, sexual activity, and birth control measures used for both men and women. Instruct male patients to use barrier contraception, and women to use both barrier and hormonal contraception. Women of childbearing age must have a negative pregnancy test baseline to begin the drug, and pregnancy test should be repeated every two weeks for two months then every month. Instruct patient to continue contraception one month after drug is discontinued. Physicians, patients, and pharmacists must participate in drug manufacturer (Celgene, Warren, NJ) STEPS program (System for Thalidomid Education and Prescription Safety).

II. ALTERATION IN SENSORY/PERCEPTUAL PATTERNS related to PERIPHERAL NEUROPATHY

Defining Characteristics: Peripheral neuropathy occurs in about 25% of patients (range, 10–50%). If drug is discontinued at the first sign of neuropathy, symptoms are reversible. Neuropathy is a distal axonal degeneration affecting long and large-diameter motor and sensory axons in hands and feet. Initially, there is numbness of toes/feet, described often as a "tightness around the feet." There may be decreased sensitivity to light touch, pinprick (sensory loss) in hands and feet, muscle cramps, symmetrical sensorimotor neuropathy, painful paresthesias in hands and feet, distal hypoesthesia, proximal weakness in lower limbs, slight postural tremor, leg cramps, absent ankle jerks. IF treatment is continued, there are permanent paresthesias of feet and hands, which progresses proximally. Increased risk of occurrence with increased age (> 70 years old) and high total doses > 14 g (40–50 g).

Nursing Implications: Assess baseline neurologic status, especially presence of peripheral neuropathy. Teach patient to stop drug and report immediately dysesthesias, numbness, and/or muscle cramps. Perform assessment for peripheral neuropathy at every visit.

III. ALTERATION IN SENSORY/PERCEPTUAL PATTERNS related to DROWSINESS

Defining Characteristics: Drug has nonbarbiturate sedative qualities, and drowsiness is the most frequent side effect. Tolerance to daytime drowsiness occurs over several weeks of use. Drowsiness and dizziness are more frequent at doses of 20–400 mg/day than at lower doses. HIV-infected patient studies reported drowsiness, dizziness, and mood changes 33–100% of the time.

Nursing Implications: Assess baseline alertness, sleep patterns. Assess other drugs taken, especially those with sedating qualities, and alcohol ingestion. Instruct patient to avoid alcohol and to take drug at bedtime. Assess degree of drowsiness and dizziness and safety of patient. If significant, teach measures to ensure safety. Tell patient that tolerance develops over 2–3 weeks.

IV. ALTERATION IN SKIN INTEGRITY, POTENTIAL, related to RASH

Defining Characteristics: Pruritic, erythematous macular rash may appear over trunk and back 2–13 days after initiation of therapy. Increased incidence in patients with HIV infection with low CD4 counts. Drug rechallenge often results in immediate reaction of rash, tachycardia, and fever. Rash resolves with drug discontinuation.

Nursing Implications: Teach patient to self-assess for rash, and instruct to discontinue drug and report rash to nurse or physician immediately. If necessary, manage symptomatic itching with antihistamines.

V. ALTERATION IN ELIMINATION related to CONSTIPATION

Defining Characteristics: Mild constipation occurs in 3–30% of patients.

Nursing Implications: Instruct patient to prevent constipation by using stool softeners, mild laxatives if needed (e.g., milk of magnesia), and to use bulk (e.g., psyllium). In addition, teach dietary interventions (e.g., increased fiber, fluids of 3 qt/day), and mild exercise. Instruct patient to report constipation unresponsive to these interventions.

VI. POTENTIAL FOR INFECTION related to NEUTROPENIA

Defining Characteristics: Rare (< 1%) in most patients, but increased incidence of 2–20% in HIV-infected patients. Average onset 6–7 weeks after initiation of treatment (range, 3–12 weeks).

Nursing Implications: Determine baseline WBC and absolute neutrophil count (ANC). Do not initiate therapy if ANC $< 750/mm^3$. If on treatment, ANC $< 750/ mm^3$, consider drug discontinuance, but definitely drug should be discontinued if ANC $< 500/mm^3$. Drug may be reinstituted after neutrophil recovery (e.g., G-CSF). WBC and ANC should be monitored closely in HIV-infected patients (e.g., every other week for three months), and then at least every month. In non-HIV-infected patients, monitor baseline and monthly.

Chapter 9
Anxiety and Depression

Anxiety and depression in response to uncertainty and hopelessness are frequently associated with the cancer experience. Studies have shown that anxiety increases with the cancer diagnosis and remains elevated to some degree throughout treatment, regardless of modality or setting (Clark, 1990). Nursing efforts are aimed at anxiety-reducing strategies such as helping the patient explore the anxiety and find anxiety-reducing activities (e.g., relaxation exercises, verbalization of feelings). Nurses can also refer patients for specialized support if necessary, and, as appropriate, teach patients and their families about prescribed anxiolytic medications. Depression is an often expected response to the cancer experience, to an actual or perceived loss of health, role, and life. The reported incidence of depression in hospitalized cancer patients is 25–42% (Trask, 2004). It also may be associated with chronic cancer pain and can clearly adversely affect quality of life. Prominent features may be perceived loss of self-esteem, worthlessness, hopelessness, guilt, and sadness. There is a continuum of depression, ranging from everyday sadness to severe, debilitating depression with physical and/or psychological symptoms that constitute a major depressive disorder (Valentine, 2007). Most commonly in practice, nurses assess patient symptoms of changes in appetite, sleeplessness, lethargy, and social withdrawal. Nurses use caring and compassion to help patients who are depressed acknowledge and explore their feelings. Through patient teaching and supportive counseling, short-term realistic and achievable goals can often be negotiated by patient and nurse. Now, nurses are helping patients to make the "mountain" more "manageable."

Patients cope individually with the multiple threats that cancer brings. Patients with depression may have a variety of symptoms that fall within one or more categories of functioning, and the ASCO (2007) has developed an excellent patient educational brochure that is helpful for oncology patients (PLWC, 2007). These symptoms may include

- Mood symptoms: feelings of sadness, helplessness, hopelessness; irritability; feelings of guilt or worthlessness
- Cognitive symptoms: decreased ability to concentrate, decreased memory, suicidal thoughts
- Physical symptoms: fatigue or low energy, poor appetite, inability to experience pleasure
- Behavioral symptoms: social withdrawal, crying spells, loss of interest in activities or hobbies, decreased sex drive

Of course, pharmacotherapy is also very important. It is generally accepted that depression results from a deficiency in key neurotransmitters, resulting in either an overexpression or underexpression of neurotransmitters that control the release or breakdown of the neurotransmitters (Barsevick and Much, 2003).

The tricyclic antidepressant (TCA) medications have long been the cornerstone of managing cancer-related depression, partially because of their ability to improve sleeplessness and to enhance analgesia. These drugs include amitriptyline (Elavil). However, these drugs also have undesirable side effects, such as dry mouth, constipation, and blurred vision related to their anticholinergic, α-adrenergic–blocking, and antihistamine properties (Valentine, 2007). Serotonin antagonist reuptake inhibitors (SARIs) raise serotonin levels and include trazodone (Desyrel). Common side effects include dry mouth, dizziness, sedation, orthostasis, and rarely priapism in men. Monamine oxidase inhibitors (MAOIs) are not used often because of the many drug interactions that can occur. These drugs are phenelzine (Nardil) and tranylcypromine (Parnate) and prevent the breakdown of neurotransmitters, thus increasing their levels. Side effects include insomnia and orthostasis.

Newer antidepressant medications are more commonly used and have found a firm niche in oncology care. The selective serotonin reuptake inhibitors (SSRIs) are quite effective for many patients and have few side effects, together with a short half-life. In addition, they differ from the TCAs in that they are generally less lethal if a patient accidentally overdoses (except citalopram hydrobromide). They also do not posses anticholinergic or α-adrenergic–blocking properties and thus are safer in medically complex patients (Valentine, 2007). These agents block serotonin reuptake, and thus, more serotonin is available as a neurotransmitter and include fluoxetine (Prozac), sertraline (Zoloft), citalopram (Celexa), escitalopram (Lexapro), and paroxetine (Paxil). Common side effects are nausea, insomnia, headache, and sexual problems. More recently, serotonin-norepinephrine reuptake inhibitors (SNRIs) have been developed that increase the levels of norepinephrine as well as serotonin to act as neurotransmitters. Drugs in this category are venlafaxine (Effexor), duloxetine (Cymbalta), and mirtazapine (Remeron), and common side effects are nausea, dry mouth, headache, and sedation. This year, a new SNRI, desvenlafaxine (Pristiq), was FDA approved for the treatment of depression. Because this drug is a synthetic form of the active metabolite of venlafaxine, it is being studied as a nonhormonal treatment for menopausal symptoms.

Because of an increased risk of suicidality (suicidal thinking and behavior) in young adults 18–24 years old during the initial treatment (first 1–2 months), the FDA has required that all antidepressant drugs indicate this risk as a black box warning (FDA, 2007).

Massie and Popkin (1998) suggest principles to guide antidepressant therapy in patients with cancer: start with a lower dose, slowly increase the dose as the therapeutic dose may be lower than that in non-cancer patients, and monitor very carefully for side effects as there may be overlapping toxicity in organ systems (with chemotherapy, the malignancy).

In addition, it is important to do a thorough assessment of herbs used in the management of anxiety and depression, as these may be interacting with anti-cancer drug therapy. For example, St. John's wort induces the metabolism of SN-38 via the cytochrome P450 CYP3A4 subsystem, lowering serum levels by up 42% with an effect lasting up to 3 weeks (Mathijssen et al, 2002). Table 9.1 depicts anti-anxiety and antidepressant agents commonly prescribed.

Table 9.1 Agents Commonly Used in the Management of Anxiety and Depression in Patients with Cancer

Drug	Dose Range (oral)	Half-Life or Onset of Therapeutic Effect	Common Side Effects	Comments
Anti-anxiety				
Alprazolam (Xanax)	0.25–1.0 mg PO every 6–24 hours	10–15 hours half-life	Sedation, confusion, motor incoordination, somnolence	Short half-life; rapid onset; tolerance may develop rapidly
Clonazepam (Klonopin)	0.5–2.0 PO every 6–24 hours	Peak serum level 1–2 hours; half-life 18–60 hours, median 30–40 hours	Drowsiness, dizziness, motor incoordination, orthostasis, ↓ mental alertness	Increased CNS depressant effects when combined with CNS depressants
Diazepam (Valium, Valrelease)	2–10 mg every 6–24 hours PO, IM, IV	20–70 hours half-life	Drowsiness, fatigue, lethargy, weakness, rash, vivid dreams, feeling "hung over"	Long half-life, so accumulation of active metabolites; fast absorption; difficult to use in older patients
Lorazepam (Ativan)	0.5–2.0 mg PO, IM, IV every 4–12 hours	10–20 hr half-life	Drowsiness, fatigue, lethargy, weakness, rash, vivid dreams	Short half-life with intermediate absorption; continuous IV infusion in severe cases
Oxazepam (Serax)	30–120 mg/day (usual max dose 60 mg/day)	5–15 hours	Drowsiness, fatigue, lethargy, weakness, rash, vivid dreams	Short half-life

(continued)

Table 9.1 *(Continued)*

Drug	Dose Range (oral)	Half-Life or Onset of Therapeutic Effect	Common Side Effects	Comments
Antidepressants SSRIs				
Paroxetine (Paxil)	20 mg to start PO (morning) to 50 mg every day	Onset 3–10 days	Nausea, dry mouth, rash, headache, drowsiness, loss of libido, postural hypotension, mild nausea, anxiety; sedation	Caution in elderly, patients with renal or hepatic dysfunction, suicidal ideation; Dose ↑ if needed after 2–3 weeks; if renal or hepatic dysfunction, begin with one-half to one-fourth of the normal starting dose to start
Sertraline (Zoloft)	50 PO to start (morning), up to 200 mg every day	Onset 7 days	Same as paroxetine, except, no sedation, sexual dysfunction	Same
Fluoxetine (Prozac)		Onset 2–4 weeks	Same as paroxetine; sexual dysfunction	Same
Escitalopram (Lexapro)	10 mg PO daily; if ↑ to 20 mg daily, do so after at least 1 week	half-life of 27–32 hours; steady-state plasma levels in 1 week	Same as paroxetine, no sedation	Same
Citalopram Hydrobromide (Celexa)	20 mg PO to start (morning); 40 mg PO daily after at least 1 week	Terminal half-life of 25 hours; steady state in 1 week	Same as paroxetine, except may be fatal if over-dosed	Same

(continued)

Table 9.1 *(Continued)*

Drug	Dose Range (oral)	Half-Life or Onset of Therapeutic Effect	Common Side Effects	Comments
TCAs				
Amitriptyline (Elavil)	25–250 mg	Onset 4–6 weeks	Anticholinergic (urinary retention, dry mouth, thirst, blurred vision, sedation) and antihistaminic (sedation); tachycardia, orthostatic hypotension, arrhythmia; withdrawal reaction	Caution in patients with suicidal ideation, cardiac/renal or hepatic dysfunction; don't stop drug abruptly; do baseline EKG and assess toxicity
Desipramine (Norpramin)	25–150 mg	4–6 weeks	Same as amitriptyline	Same as amitriptyline; serum level correlates with therapeutic effect
Doxepin (Sinequan)	50–150 mg	4–6 weeks	Same as amitriptyline	Same as amitriptyline
Imipramine (Tofranil)	25–150 mg	4–6 weeks	Same as amitriptyline	Same as amitriptyline; serum level correlates with therapeutic effect
Nortriptyline (Pamelor)	50–150 mg	4–6 weeks	Same as amitriptyline	Same as amitriptyline; serum level correlates with therapeutic effect
Trazodone (Dyseril)	50–250 mg	1–4 weeks	Same as amitriptyline	Same as amitriptyline

(continued)

Table 9.1 *(Continued)*

Drug	Dose Range (oral)	Half-Life or Onset of Therapeutic Effect	Common Side Effects	Comments
SNRI				
Venlafaxine HCl (Effexor)	75–225 mg/day	1–4 weeks	Emotional lability, vertigo, trismus, nausea	Use cautiously in elderly, patients with cardiac/renal or hepatic dysfunction; also helpful with hot flashes
Nefazodone HCl (Serzone)	200–600 mg/day	1–4 weeks	Dizziness, drowsiness, dry mouth, headache	Use cautiously in elderly, patients with cardiac/renal or hepatic dysfunction
Duloxetine (Cymbalta)	40 mg daily to start, ↑ to 60 mg PO daily	Half-life of 12 hours, steady-state achieved in 3 days	Nausea, dry mouth, constipation, diarrhea, insomnia, decreased appetite, somnolence	Contraindicated if narrow angle glaucoma; indicated in patients with peripheral neuropathic pain
Mirtazapine (Remeron)	15 mg PO daily to start; ↑ to 45 mg PO daily after 2–4 weeks if needed	Elimination half-life of 20–40 hours; steady state in 3–4 days	↑ appetite, weight gain, peripheral edema; CNS effects, drowsiness, orthostasis	Use cautiously and monitor closely hepatic or renal insufficiency, epilepsy, organic brain syndrome, heart disease, BPH, acute narrow angle glaucoma, DM; rare BMD
Desvenlafaxine (Pristiq)	50 mg recommended dose; may slowly ↑ dose to 400 mg in clinical trials	Elimination half-life 11 hrs; time to steady state 4–5 days	Nausea, headache, dry mouth, sweating, dizziness, insomnia	Dose reduction for severe renal impairment; Use cautiously in older persons or in patients with cardiac/renal or hepatic dysfunction

(continued)

Table 9.1 *(Continued)*

Drug	Dose Range (oral)	Half-Life or Onset of Therapeutic Effect	Common Side Effects	Comments
Atypical (unknown MOA)				
Bupropion hydrochloride (Wellbutrin)	100 mg PO twice daily for at last 3 days, may ↑ to 100 mg three times daily; after 4 weeks may ↑ to 150 mg three times daily if needed	Half-life of 14 hours	Weight loss, restlessness, agitation, insomnia, dizziness, tachycardia, changes in BP, dry mouth, anorexia, nausea, vomiting, urinary retention	Drug increases activity, so useful if psychomotor slowing; rare sexual dysfunction; may cause seizures; contraindicated if history of seizures, bulimia, anorexia nervosa

BPH: benign prostatic hypertrophy, DM: diabetes mellitus, BMD: bone marrow depression.
Source: Modified from Barsevick AM and Much JK (2003) Depression, Chapter 34 in *Cancer Symptom Management*, 3rd ed., Yarbro CH, Frogge MH, Goodman M (eds). Sudbury, MA, Jones and Bartlett Publishers, pp. 668–692; Goebel BH (2003) Anxiety, Chapter 33 in *Cancer Symptom Management*, 3rd ed., Yarbro CH, Frogge MH, Goodman M (eds). Sudbury, MA, Jones and Bartlett Publishers, pp. 651–668

References

American Society of Clinical Oncology. Depression, in Mental Health and Cancer, *People Living with Cancer (PLWC)*. http://www.plwc.org/portal/site/PLWC/menuitem.034b98abc65a8f566343cc10ee37a01d/?vgnextoid=a2c7ea97a56d9010VgnVCM100000f2730ad1RCRD. Accessed 2 July 2007

Barsevick AM, Much JK. Depression, chapter 34. Yarbro CH Frogge MH Goodman M *Cancer Symptom Management*, 3rd ed. Sudbury, MA: Jones and Bartlett Publishers 2003; 668–692

Buclin T, Mazzocato C, Berney A, et al. Psychopharmacology in Supportive Care of Cancer: A Review for the Clinician. *Support Care Cancer* 2001; 9 213–222

Clark J. Psychosocial Dimensions: The Patient. Groenwald S, Frogge MH, Goodman M, Yarbro CH. *Cancer Nursing Principles and Practice*, 2nd ed. Sudbury, MA: Jones and Bartlett Publishers 1990

Federal Drug Administration. FDA Proposes New Warnings About Suicidal Thinking, Behavior in Young Adults Who Take Antidepressant Medications. http://www.fda.gov/bbs/topics/NEWS/2007/NEW01624.html. Accessed 2 July 2007

Gerchufsky M. The Art and Science of Prescribing Psychiatric Medications. *ADVANCE for Nurse Practitioners* 1997; 4(3) 33–36

Goebel BH. Anxiety, chapter 33. Yarbro CH, Frogge MH, Goodman M. *Cancer Symptom Management*, 3rd ed. Sudbury, MA: Jones and Bartlett Publishers 2003; 651–668

Massie MJ, Popkin MK. Depressive disorders, chapter 10. Holland JC *Psycho-Oncology*. New York NY: Oxford University Press 1998; 518–540

Mathijssen RH, Verweij J, de Bruijn P, et al. Effects of St. John's Wort on Irinotecan Metabolism. *J Natl Cancer Inst* 2002; 94(16) 1247–9
Trask PC. Assessment of Depression in Cancer Patients. *J Natl Cancer Inst* 2004; 32 80–92
Valentine A. Depression, Anxiety, and Delirium. In Pazdur R, Coia LR, Hoskins WJ, Wagman LD (eds). *Cancer Management: A Multidisciplinary Approach*. Lawrence, KS: CMP Media LLC; 2007

Drug: alprazolam (Xanax)

Class: Benzodiazepine (anxiolytic).

Mechanism of Action: Binds to benzodiazepine receptors in the CNS (limbic and cortical areas, cerebellum, brain stem, and spinal cord), resulting in the following effects: anxiolytic, ataxia, anticonvulsant, muscle relaxation. Appears to potentiate the effects of γ-aminobutyric acid (GABA).

Metabolism: Well absorbed from GI tract. Widely distributed in body tissues and fluids, including CSF. Crosses placenta and is excreted in breast milk. Highly bound to plasma proteins. Metabolized in liver and excreted in urine. Short elimination time; half-life of 12–15 hours. May produce psychological and physical dependence. Indicated for management of anxiety, the short-term relief of anxiety associated with depression, and panic disorder.

Dosage/Range:
Adult:
- Anxiety: 0.25–0.5 mg PO tid (may gradually increase dose q 3–4 days over time to maximum 4 mg/day in divided doses).
- Elderly/debilitated: 0.25 mg PO bid.
- Discontinue drug by decreasing dose by 0.25–0.5 mg q 3–7 days.
- Drug should be used for short-term use only (< 4 months).
- Panic: optimal dosage not determined; titrate dose and increase slowly.

Drug Preparation:
- Store in tight, light-resistant containers at 15–30°C (59–86°F).

Drug Administration:
- Orally, in divided doses.
- May take with food if stomach upset occurs.

Drug Interactions:
- CNS depressants (alcohol, anticonvulsants, phenothiazines, opiates): additive CNS depression; avoid concurrent use or use cautiously and monitor carefully.
- Oral contraceptives, isoniazid, ketoconazole, or cimetidine: decrease plasma clearance of alprazolam so may increase effect (e.g., sedation); monitor patient closely.
- Tricyclic antidepressants: increased serum levels of antidepressant possible; use together cautiously.
- Digoxin: may decrease renal excretion of digoxin; monitor for overdosage; may need to decrease digoxin.

Lab Effects/Interference:
- No consistent pattern of interaction between benzodiazepines and laboratory tests.

Special Considerations:
- Wide margin of safety between therapeutic and toxic doses.
- May impair ability to perform activities requiring mental alertness (e.g., driving a car, operating machinery).
- May produce psychological and physical dependence.
- Administer cautiously in patients with liver or renal impairment.
- Use cautiously in patients with chronic pulmonary disease or sleep apnea.
- Contraindicated in patients with depressive neuroses, psychotic reactions (without prominent anxiety), acute alcoholic intoxication (with depressed VS), known hypersensitivity to the drug, or acute angle-closure glaucoma.
- May cause fetal damage so should not be used during pregnancy or if the mother is breast-feeding.
- Withdrawal symptoms (including seizure, delirium) can occur with rapid drug discontinuance in patients taking high or chronic doses.
- If manic episodes or hyperactivity occur soon after drug started, drug should be discontinued.
- Drug should not be used to manage "everyday stress."

Potential Toxicities/Side Effects and the Nursing Process

I. ALTERATIONS IN SENSORY/PERCEPTUAL PATTERNS related to CNS DEPRESSION

Defining Characteristics: CNS depressant effects include drowsiness, fatigue, lethargy, confusion, weakness, headache, which may occur initially and resolve with continued therapy or dose reduction. Vivid dreams, suicidal ideation, and bizarre behavior also may occur. Patient risk factors: elderly, debilitated, liver dysfunction, low serum albumin.

Nursing Implications: Assess baseline neurologic status and risk factors, and monitor during treatment. Instruct patient to report signs/symptoms and discuss drug modification with physician. Evaluate patient satisfaction with drug efficacy. If patient expresses suicidal ideation (more common in panic disorders), refer patient for psychiatric evaluation and drug modification. Instruct patient to avoid alcohol while taking drug. Teach patient prescribed schedule for discontinuing drug when used chronically: assess for signs/symptoms of withdrawal (increased anxiety, rebound insomnia; may also include agitation, dysphoria, nausea/vomiting, irritability, muscle cramps, hallucinations, seizures).

II. ALTERATION IN NUTRITION, LESS THAN BODY REQUIREMENTS, related to GI SIDE EFFECTS

Defining Characteristics: Nausea, vomiting, weight increase or decrease, dry mouth, constipation may occur; also, elevated serum LFTs.

Nursing Implications: Assess baseline nutrition and elimination patterns and LFTs, and monitor during therapy. Discuss abnormalities and drug modification with physician. Teach patient to self-administer prescribed antiemetics as appropriate.

III. POTENTIAL FOR INJURY related to DECREASE IN MENTAL ALERTNESS, PHYSICAL COORDINATION

Defining Characteristics: Drug may cause drowsiness, dizziness, and impair physical coordination, mental alertness.

Nursing Implications: Assess other medications that may increase risk (e.g., opiates, phenothiazines) and response to drug. Instruct patient to avoid potentially hazardous activities, including driving a car, operating machinery.

IV. ALTERATIONS IN CARDIAC OUTPUT related to RHYTHM DISTURBANCES, VASODILATION

Defining Characteristics: Drug may cause bradycardia, tachycardia, hyper- or hypotension, palpitations, edema.

Nursing Implications: Assess baseline VS, and monitor during therapy. Discuss abnormalities with physician. Instruct patient to report dizziness on standing or other changes.

V. ALTERATIONS IN SKIN INTEGRITY related to RASH

Defining Characteristics: Urticaria, pruritus, rash (morbilliform, urticarial, or maculopapular) may occur.

Nursing Implications: Assess baseline skin integrity, and instruct patient to report changes. Teach symptomatic skin management, and discuss drug discontinuance with physician if severe.

Drug: amitriptyline hydrochloride (Elavil)

Class: Tricyclic antidepressant.

Mechanism of Action: Blocks reuptake of neurotransmitters at neuronal membrane, thus increasing available serotonin, norepinephrine in CNS, and potentiating their effects. Appears to have analgesic effect separate from antidepressant action. May increase bioavailability of morphine. Indicated in the treatment of depressive (affective) mood disorders. Also used as an adjuvant analgesic in cancer pain management.

Metabolism: Well absorbed from GI tract. Distributed to lungs, heart, brain, liver; highly bound to plasma, proteins. Plasma half-life of 10–50 hours. Metabolized in liver, excreted in urine and, to a lesser degree, in bile and feces.

Dosage/Range:

Adult:

- Oral: 25–100 mg PO hs divided or single dose; may increase to 200–300 mg/day (300 mg maximum).
- Cancer pain: 25 mg/day hs; may increase by 25 mg of 1–2 days to 75–150 mg, when desired relief level is reached; may start at 10 mg in elderly.
- Elderly: 30 mg/day in divided doses.
- Intramuscular (IM): 20–30 mg qid or as single dose at bedtime.

Drug Preparation:

- Oral: store in well-closed containers at 15–30°C (59–86°F); store Elavil 10-mg capsules away from light. Administer as a single bedtime dose.
- IM: administer IM in large muscle mass; change to oral as soon as possible.

Drug Interactions:

- Monamine oxidase inhibitors (MAOIs): increased excitation, hyperpyrexia, seizures; use together cautiously (especially if high dose is used).
- CNS depressants (alcohol, sedatives, hypnotics): increase CNS depression; use together cautiously.
- Sympathomimetic (epinephrine, amphetamines): increased hypertension; AVOID concurrent use.
- Cimetidine methylphenidate: increased amitriptyline levels, increased toxicity; use cautiously and monitor for increased toxicity.
- Warfarin: may increase PT; monitor closely and decrease dose of warfarin as needed.

Lab Effects/Interference:

- None known; bone marrow depression uncommon.

Special Considerations:

- Antidepressant effect may take two weeks or longer.
- Adjuvant analgesic useful in cancer pain management.
- May also decrease depression associated with chronic cancer pain and promote improved sleep.
- Contraindicated in patients with myocardial infarction, seizure disorder, or benign prostatic hypertrophy.
- Use cautiously in patients with urine retention, narrow-angle glaucoma, hyperthyroidism, hepatic dysfunction, or suicidal ideation.
- Drug should be gradually discontinued rather than abruptly withdrawn to prevent anxiety, malaise, dizziness, nausea/vomiting.
- May be helpful in treating hiccups.
- Increased anticholinergic side effects in older persons.

- Teach all patients/families: call provider right away if thoughts of suicide or dying; attempts to commit suicide; new or worse depression; new or worse anxiety; feeling very agitated or restless; panic attacks; trouble sleeping (insomnia); new or worse irritability; aggressive, angry, or violent behavior; acting on dangerous impulses; extreme increase in activity or talking (mania); any unusual changes in behavior or mood.

Potential Toxicities/Side Effects and the Nursing Process

I. ALTERATIONS IN SENSORY/PERCEPTUAL PATTERNS related to DROWSINESS, FATIGUE, EPS

Defining Characteristics: Drowsiness, dizziness, weakness, lethargy, and fatigue are common; confusion, disorientation, hallucinations may occur in the elderly. Extrapyramidal symptoms may occur (fine tremor, rigidity, dystonia, dysarthria, dysphagia), as may peripheral neuropathy and blurred vision.

Nursing Implications: Assess baseline gait, neurologic and mental status, and monitor during therapy. Instruct patient to report signs/symptoms; discuss benefit/risk ratio with physician. Assess for signs/symptoms of suicidal ideation; if they occur, refer for psychiatric evaluation. Inform patient that drowsiness, dizziness will resolve after 1–2 weeks; instruct to avoid hazardous activities while drowsy (e.g., driving a car, operating machinery).

II. ALTERATION IN CARDIAC OUTPUT related to POSTURAL HYPOTENSION, TACHYCARDIA

Defining Characteristics: Postural hypotension, EKG changes, tachycardia, hypertension may occur.

Nursing Implications: Assess baseline orthostatic BP, heart rate, and monitor during therapy. Instruct patient to report abnormalities, including postural dizziness, palpitations. Drug should be stopped several days before surgery to prevent hypertensive crisis, especially if high dose.

III. ALTERATION IN NUTRITION, LESS THAN BODY REQUIREMENTS, related to GI SIDE EFFECTS

Defining Characteristics: Dry mouth, anorexia, nausea, vomiting, diarrhea, abdominal cramping may occur; also, elevated LFTs.

Nursing Implications: Assess baseline nutrition and elimination patterns and LFTs, and monitor during therapy. Discuss abnormalities with physician, and discuss drug modification. Teach patient to self-administer prescribed antiemetics as appropriate. LFTs should be repeated, and if still elevated, the drug should be discontinued. Teach patient to take full dose at bedtime. Suggest patient use sugar-free hard candy, frequent ice chips, or artificial saliva for dry mouth.

IV. ALTERATION IN URINARY ELIMINATION related to URINARY RETENTION

Defining Characteristics: Urinary retention may occur. Increased risk if patient has history of urinary retention.

Nursing Implications: Assess baseline urinary elimination pattern and risk. Assess for urinary retention, and instruct patient to report signs/symptoms. Discuss alternative drug with physician if this occurs.

V. ALTERATIONS IN SKIN INTEGRITY related to ALLERGY

Defining Characteristics: Urticaria, erythema, rash, and photosensitivity may occur.

Nursing Implications: Assess baseline drug allergy history and skin integrity. Instruct patient to report skin changes. If angioedema of face, tongue develops, discuss drug discontinuance with physician. Instruct patient to avoid sunlight or to use sunblock protection.

Drug: bupropion hydrochloride (Wellbutrin)

Class: Aminoketone antidepressant.

Mechanism of Action: Unknown. Does block reuptake of serotonin, norepinephrine, and dopamine weakly; does not inhibit MAO; has CNS stimulant effects.

Metabolism: Peak plasma level 2 hours after oral administration, and it appears that only a small percentage of the dose reaches the systemic circulation. Half-life about 14 hours (8–24 hours average). Four major metabolites, with significantly longer elimination half-lives. Primarily excreted in the urine (87%) and to a lesser extent in the feces (10%).

Dosage/Range:

Adult:

- Initial dose: 100 mg bid for at least 3 days.
- Based on response, may increase to usual dose of 100 mg tid (300 mg total dose/day).
- If after 4 weeks of treatment there is no clinical response, may increase to a maximum of 450 mg/day (150 mg tid).

Drug Preparation:

- Available in 75-mg and 100-mg tablets.
- Protect tablets from light and moisture.
- Ensure at least 4 hours between doses (optimally, give in morning and evening).

Drug Interactions:

- Because of extensive drug metabolism by liver, when given with other drugs that have hepatic metabolism may have decreased effect of that drug (e.g., carbamazepine, cimetidine, phenobarbital, phenytoin).
- MAOIs may increase drug toxicity.
- Use cautiously in patients receiving L-dopa, starting with small initial dose, and slowly increasing dose.
- Use cautiously in patients receiving other seizure-threshold-lowering drugs, starting with small initial dose, and slowly and gradually increasing dose.
- Bupropion, (Zyban; smoking cessation aid): DO NOT USE TOGETHER, as will increase risk of seizures.

Lab Effects/Interference:

- Rarely, anemia and pancytopenia.

Special Considerations:

- Contraindicated in patients with seizure disorder, present/past history of bulimia, or anorexia nervosa.
- Contraindicated in patients receiving MAOI; if MAOI is discontinued, wait at least 14 days before starting bupropion HCl.
- Risk of seizures for patients receiving drug at a dose of 450 mg is 0.4% and appears related to dose and predisposing factors, such as prior seizure, head trauma, CNS tumor, and concomitant medications that lower seizure threshold (e.g., antipsychotics, other antidepressants, abrupt cessation of a benzodiazepine medication, use or abrupt cessation of alcohol).
- Avoid alcohol when taking drug.
- Can precipitate manic episodes in patients with bipolar manic depression or can activate latent psychoses.
- Use cautiously, if at all, in individuals who are underweight, as drug may cause weight loss of at least 2.25 kg (5 lb) (28% of patients), and most patients do not gain weight (only 9% of patients gain weight).
- Drug contains same ingredient found in bupropion, which is used in smoking cessation. DO NOT USE TOGETHER.
- Use cautiously in patients with a recent history of myocardial infarction or unstable heart disease.
- Teach all patients/families: call provider right away if thoughts of suicide or dying; attempts to commit suicide; new or worse depression; new or worse anxiety; feeling very agitated or restless; panic attacks; trouble sleeping (insomnia); new or worse irritability; aggressive, angry, or violent behavior; acting on dangerous impulses; extreme increase in activity or talking (mania); any unusual changes in behavior or mood.

Potential Toxicities/Side Effects and the Nursing Process

I. ALTERATIONS IN SENSORY/PERCEPTUAL PATTERNS related to RESTLESSNESS, AGITATION, INSOMNIA

Defining Characteristics: Many patients experience increased restlessness, agitation, anxiety, and insomnia, especially after initiation of therapy. This may be severe enough to require treatment with sedative/hypnotic or drug discontinuation. Restlessness, agitation, hostility, decreased concentration, ataxia, incoordination, confusion, paranoia, anxiety, manic episodes in bipolar manic depressives, migraine, insomnia, euphoria, and psychoses may occur. Akathisia, dyskinesia, dystonia, muscle spasms, bradykinesia, and sensory disturbances may occur.

Nursing Implications: Assess baseline gait, neurologic and mental status, and monitor during therapy. Teach patient to report signs/symptoms; discuss benefit/risk ratio with physician. Assess for signs/symptoms of suicidal ideation; if they occur, refer for psychiatric evaluation. Inform patient that drowsiness, dizziness will resolve after 1–2 weeks; instruct to avoid hazardous activities while drowsy (e.g., driving a car, operating machinery). Instruct patient to avoid alcohol ingestion, as this may precipitate seizures.

II. ALTERATION IN CARDIAC OUTPUT related to CHANGES IN BP, HR

Defining Characteristics: Dizziness, tachycardia, hypertension or hypotension, palpitations, edema, syncope, and cardiac arrhythmias may occur.

Nursing Implications: Assess baseline orthostatic BP, heart rate, presence of peripheral edema, and monitor during therapy. Patient should have a baseline EKG. Instruct patient to report abnormalities including postural dizziness, palpitations. Discuss any significant changes with physician, and discuss interventions. If the patient has had a recent myocardial infarction, expect that dose of drug may be reduced.

III. ALTERATION IN NUTRITION, LESS THAN BODY REQUIREMENTS, related to GI SIDE EFFECTS

Defining Characteristics: Dry mouth, anorexia, nausea, vomiting, diarrhea, constipation, weight loss of up to 2.25 kg (5 lb), dyspepsia, weight gain and increased appetite, increased salivation, taste changes, stomatitis may occur rarely.

Nursing Implications: Assess baseline nutrition and elimination patterns, weight, and monitor during therapy. Discuss abnormalities with physician, and discuss drug modification. Teach patient to self-administer prescribed antiemetics as appropriate. Suggest patient use sugar-free hard candy, frequent ice chips, or artificial saliva for dry mouth.

IV. ALTERATION IN URINARY ELIMINATION related to URINARY RETENTION

Defining Characteristics: Urinary retention, frequency, and nocturia may occur. Increased risk in patients with history of urinary retention.

Nursing Implications: Assess baseline urinary elimination pattern and risk. Assess for urinary retention, and instruct patient to report signs/symptoms. Discuss alternative drug with physician if this occurs.

V. ALTERATIONS IN SKIN INTEGRITY related to ALLERGY

Defining Characteristics: Urticaria, erythema, rash, pruritus may occur.

Nursing Implications: Assess baseline drug allergy history and skin integrity. Instruct patient to report skin changes. If angioedema of face or tongue develops, tell patient to stop drug and discuss drug discontinuance with physician.

VI. POTENTIAL SEXUAL DYSFUNCTION related to IMPOTENCE, IRREGULAR MENSES

Defining Characteristics: Impotence in men and irregular menses in women may occur.

Nursing Considerations: Assess baseline sexual functioning. Inform patient that alterations may occur, and instruct to report them. If severe, discuss dysfunction with physician, and whether another antidepressant would provide equal benefit with less dysfunction.

Drug: buspirone hydrochloride (BuSpar)

Class: Antianxiety agent.

Mechanism of Action: Unclear; drug is considered a midbrain modulator and affects many neurotransmitters (serotonin, dopamine, and cholinergic and noradrenergic systems).

Metabolism: Rapid and complete GI absorption. Food may delay absorption but does not affect total serum drug level. Distributed to body tissues and fluids, especially brain. Metabolized in liver and excreted in urine.

Dosage/Range:

Adult:

- Oral: 10–15 mg in 2–3 divided doses.
- May be increased in 5-mg increments every 2–4 days to achieve goal (maximum 60 mg/day).
- Maintenance: usual is 5–10 mg tid.

Drug Preparation:
- Store tablets in tight, light-resistant containers at < 30°C (86°F).
- Administer with food.

Drug Interactions:
- MAOIs: increased BP; AVOID CONCURRENT USE.
- Haloperidol: increased haloperidol serum levels; AVOID CONCURRENT USE or reduce haloperidol dose.
- Alcohol: may increase fatigue, drowsiness, dizziness; AVOID CONCURRENT USE.
- Other CNS depressants (analgesics, sedatives): may increase fatigue, drowsiness, dizziness; AVOID CONCURRENT USE.

Lab Effects/Interference:
- None known.

Special Considerations:
- Selective anxiolytic; causes little sedation or psychomotor dysfunction.
- Anxiolytic effect comparable to oral diazepam.
- Onset slower, so patients should be told to expect full anxiolytic effect in 3–4 weeks.
- Use with caution if renal insufficiency; dose-reduce in anuric patients.

Potential Toxicities/Side Effects and the Nursing Process

I. ALTERATIONS IN SENSORY/PERCEPTUAL PATTERNS related to DIZZINESS, DROWSINESS

Defining Characteristics: Far less sedation than with other anxiolytics. May cause dizziness, drowsiness, headache in 10% of patients; fatigue, nightmares, weakness, paresthesia occur less frequently.

Nursing Implications: Assess baseline neurologic status, and monitor during therapy. Instruct patient to report signs/symptoms, and discuss drug modification with physician. Instruct patient to avoid alcohol while taking drug.

II. ALTERATION IN NUTRITION, LESS THAN BODY REQUIREMENTS, related to GI SIDE EFFECTS

Defining Characteristics: Nausea occurs in 8% of patients; less common is dry mouth, vomiting, diarrhea, or constipation.

Nursing Implications: Assess baseline nutrition and elimination patterns, and monitor during therapy. Instruct patient to report signs/symptoms.

Drug: citalopram hydrobromide (Celexa®)

Class: Antidepressant.

Mechanism of Action: Selective serotonin reuptake inhibitor (SSRI) with unique structure unlike other antidepressants (racemic bicyclic phthalane derivative). Drug inhibits the reuptake of neurotransmitter serotonin in the CNS, thus potentiating serotonin activity in the CNS and relieving depressive symptoms.

Metabolism: Steady-state plasma level reached in one week. Bioavailability is 80% following single daily dose, unaffected by food intake, and peak plasma level is reached in 4 hours. Metabolism is primarily hepatic, with a terminal half-life of 25 hours. Renal excretion accounts for 20% of drug excretion. In the elderly, drug is more slowly cleared, with increases in area under the curve (AUC) by 23% and half-life by 30%. Patients with hepatic dysfunction have reduced drug clearance (37%), with half-life of drug extended to 8 hours.

Dosage/Range:

Adult:

- 20 mg daily, increased 40 mg daily after at least 1 week.
- Patients with hepatic dysfunction or elderly: 20 mg daily.
- If changing to or from monamine oxidase inhibitor therapy, wait at least 14 days between drugs.

Drug Preparation:

- Oral: available in 20-mg (pink) and 40-mg (white) oval, scored tablets.

Drug Administration:

- Administer orally in morning or evening, without regard to food.

Drug Interactions:

- Monamine oxidase inhibitors: potential for serious, sometimes fatal interactions (hyperthermia, rigidity, myoclonus, autonomic instability, mental status changes, including coma). DO NOT USE TOGETHER, and if changing to/from citalopram HBr, drugs MUST be separated by at least 14 days.
- Alcohol: possible potentiation of depression of cognitive and motor function; DO NOT USE TOGETHER.
- Cimetidine: increases AUC of citalopram HBr by 43%. Use together with caution, if at all; assess for toxicity and reduce dose as needed if must use together.
- Lithium: use together cautiously, and monitor serum lithium levels if used together.
- Warfarin: monitor INR, PT closely.
- Carbamazepine, ketoconazole, itraconazole, fluconazole, erythromycin: possible increase in clearance of citalopram HBr, monitor drug effectiveness and increase dose as needed.

- Metoprolol: may increase metoprolol levels; monitor BP and HR.
- Tricyclic antidepressants, e.g., imipramine: possible increases in plasma tricyclic antidepressant level; use together cautiously, if at all.

Lab Effects/Interference:
- Infrequently, increased liver function tests, alk phos, and abnormal glucose tolerance test.
- Rarely, bilirubinemia, hypokalemia, and hypoglycemia.

Special Considerations:
- At high doses in animals, drug is teratogenic, and, in some tests, mutagenic and carcinogenic (> 20 times the human maximum dose). DO NOT give to pregnant women or nursing mothers.
- Most responses occur within 1–4 weeks of therapy, but if no benefit has yet occurred, patients should be taught to continue taking medicine as prescribed.
- Use cautiously in patients with a seizure disorder, and monitor closely during therapy.
- Teach all patients/families: call provider right away if thoughts of suicide or dying; attempts to commit suicide; new or worse depression; new or worse anxiety; feeling very agitated or restless; panic attacks; trouble sleeping (insomnia); new or worse irritability; aggressive, angry, or violent behavior; acting on dangerous impulses; extreme increase in activity or talking (mania); any unusual changes in behavior or mood.

Potential Toxicities/Side Effects and the Nursing Process

I. ALTERATION IN NUTRITION related to GI SIDE EFFECTS

Defining Characteristics: Nausea (21%) and dry mouth (20%) are common. Less common are diarrhea (8%), dyspepsia (5%), vomiting (4%), and abdominal pain (3%). Infrequent are gastritis, stomatitis, eructation, dysphagia, teeth grinding, change in weight, and gingivitis. The following were rare: colitis, cholecystitis, gastroesophageal reflux, diverticulitis, and hiccups.

Nursing Implications: Assess baseline nutrition and elimination patterns, and monitor during therapy. Discuss abnormalities with physician, and discuss drug modification. Teach patient to self-administer prescribed antiemetics as appropriate. Suggest patient use sugar-free hard candy, frequent ice chips, or artificial saliva for dry mouth.

II. ALTERATION IN CARDIAC OUTPUT, POTENTIAL, related to CHANGES IN BLOOD PRESSURE

Defining Characteristics: Tachycardia, postural hypotension, and hypotension are common. The following are infrequent: hypertension, bradycardia, peripheral edema, angina, arrhythmias, flushing, and cardiac failure. Rarely, transient ischemic attacks, phlebitis, changes in cardiac conduction (atrial fibrillation, bundle branch block), and cardiac arrest.

Nursing Implications: Assess baseline orthostatic BP, heart rate, and monitor during therapy. Teach patient to report abnormalities, including postural dizziness, palpitations. Discuss significant changes with physician. If patient has orthostatic hypotension, teach patient to change position slowly and to hold on to support.

III. SENSORY/PERCEPTUAL ALTERATIONS related to CHANGES IN MENTAL STATUS

Defining Characteristics: The following may occur: somnolence (18%), insomnia (15%), agitation (3%), impaired concentration, amnesia, apathy, confusion, taste perversion, abnormal ocular accommodation, and possibly worsening depression and suicide attempt. Infrequently, increased libido, aggressive reaction, depersonalization, hallucination, euphoria, paranoia, emotional lability, and panic reaction may occur.

Nursing Implications: Assess baseline gait, neurologic, affective, and mental status, and monitor during therapy. Teach patient to report signs and symptoms; discuss benefit/risk ratio with physician. Assess for signs and symptoms of suicidal ideation; if they occur, refer for psychiatric evaluation. Teach patient that drowsiness may occur, and teach to avoid hazardous activities while drowsy (e.g., driving a car, operating machinery).

IV. POTENTIAL FOR INJURY related to DRUG OVERDOSE

Defining Characteristics: Although rare, drug overdoses have resulted in fatalities (total drug 3920 mg and 2800 mg in two cases resulting from this drug only) while other total doses of 6000 mg have not resulted in death. Symptoms resulting from overdose include: dizziness, sweating, nausea, vomiting, tremor, somnolence, sinus tachycardia, amnesia, confusion, coma, convulsions, hyperventilation, cyanosis, rhabdomyolysis, and EKG changes (QT interval prolongation, nodal rhythm, and ventricular arrhythmias).

Nursing Implications: Teach patient self-administration schedule and to keep drug in tightly closed container out of reach of children and pets. Teach patient not to double doses if a dose is missed. Give prescriptions in smallest number of pills possible (e.g., one month's worth at a time). In the event of an overdosage, teach patient to come to nearest emergency department where focus is on maintaining a patent airway and oxygenation, gastric evacuation by lavage and use of activated charcoal, and close monitoring of cardiac and overall status. Because of large area of drug distribution, dialysis is unlikely to be beneficial.

V. ALTERATIONS IN SKIN INTEGRITY related to RASH, SKIN CHANGES

Defining Characteristics: Rash and pruritus may occur. Less commonly, photosensitivity, urticaria, eczema, acne, dermatitis, alopecia, and dry skin may occur. Rarely, angioedema, epidermal necrolysis, erythema multiforme have been reported.

Nursing Implications: Assess baseline skin integrity. Teach patient to report skin changes. If angioedema of face, tongue develops, discuss drug discontinuance with physician. Assess impact of changes on patient and discuss strategies to minimize distress and preserve skin integrity and comfort.

VI. SEXUAL DYSFUNCTION, POTENTIAL, related to ↓ LIBIDO, IMPOTENCE, ANORGASMIA

Defining Characteristics: While difficult to separate from sexual dysfunction related to depression, the following have been reported in men: decreased ejaculation disorder (6.1%), libido (3.8%), and impotence (2.8%), and in women: decreased libido (1.3%) and anorgasmia (1.1%). Dysmenorrhea and amenorrhea may occur in female patients.

Nursing Implications: Assess baseline sexual functioning. Teach patient that alterations may occur and to report them. If severe, discuss dysfunction with physician and whether an antidepressant other than an SSRI would provide equal benefit with less dysfunction.

VII. ALTERATION IN URINE ELIMINATION related to CHANGES IN PATTERNS

Defining Characteristics: Polyuria is common. Less commonly, the following may occur: urinary frequency, incontinence, retention, and dysuria. Rarely, hematuria, liguria, pyelonephritis, renal calculus, and renal pain have been reported.

Nursing Implications: Assess baseline urinary elimination pattern and risk for alterations. Assess for changes in urinary elimination and teach patient to report signs and symptoms. Discuss alternative drug with physician if severe or bothersome symptoms occur.

Drug: clonazepam (Klonopin)

Class: Benzodiazepine.

Mechanism of Action: Appears to enhance the activity of γ-aminobutyric acid (GABA), which inhibits neurotransmitter activity in the CNS. Drug is able to suppress absence seizures (petit mal) and decrease the frequency, amplitude, and duration of minor motor seizures. Unclear mechanism in relieving panic episodes.

Metabolism: Completely absorbed after oral administration, with peak plasma levels of 1–2 hours. Drug half-life is 18–60 hours (typically 30–40 hours), and therapeutic serum level is 20–80 ng/mL; 80% protein-bound, metabolized by the liver via the P-450 cytochrome enzyme system, and inactive metabolites are excreted in the urine.

Dosage/Range:

Adult (panic attacks):
- Initial: 0.25 mg bid.
- May increase as needed to target dose of 1 mg/day after at least 3 days on the previous dose. Some individuals may require doses of up to 4 mg/day in divided doses, and dose is titrated up to that dose in increments of 0.125–0.25 mg bid every 3 days until panic disorder is controlled or as limited by side effects.
- Withdrawal of treatment must be gradual, with a decrease of 0.125 mg bid every 3 days until drug is completely withdrawn.

Adult (seizure disorders):
- Initial dose: 1.5 mg/day in 3 divided doses.
- Dosage may be increased in increments of 0.5–1 mg every 3 days until seizures are controlled or as limited by side effects.
- Maximum recommended daily dose is 20 mg/day.

Drug Preparation:
- Oral.
- Available in 0.5-, 1-, and 2-mg tablets.
- Discontinuance of drug when used for panic attacks: gradually discontinue, by 0.125 mg bid every 3 days, until drug is completely withdrawn.

Drug Interactions:
- CNS depressants (narcotics, barbiturates, hypnotics, anxiolytics, phenothiazines): potentiation of CNS depressive effects; use together cautiously, if at all, and monitor patient closely.
- Alcohol: potentiates CNS depressant effects; DO NOT use together.
- Phenobarbital: increases hepatic metabolism of clonazepam so that decreased serum levels lead to decreased clonazepam effect; assess patient for drug efficacy and need for increased drug dose.
- Phenytoin: increased hepatic metabolism of clonazepam so that decreased serum levels lead to decreased clonazepam effect; assess patient for drug efficacy and need for increased drug dose.
- Valproic acid: increased risk of absence seizure activity.

Lab Effects/Interference:
- Rarely, anemia, leukopenia, thrombocytopenia, eosinophilia.
- Transient elevation of liver function studies (serum transaminases and alk phos).

Special Considerations:
- Contraindicated during pregnancy, for breast-feeding mothers, and patients with severe liver dysfunction or acute narrow-angle glaucoma.
- May cause psychological and physical dependency.

I. ALTERATIONS IN SENSORY/PERCEPTUAL PATTERNS related to CNS DEPRESSION

Defining Characteristics: CNS depressant effects include drowsiness (37%), and, less commonly, dizziness (8%); abnormal coordination (6%); ataxia (5%); dysarthria (2%); depression (7%); memory disturbance (4%); nervousness (3%); decreased intellectual ability (2%); emotional lability; confusion; paresthesia; feeling of drunkenness; paresis; tremor; head fullness; hyperactivity, or hypoactivity. Rarely, suicidal ideation.

Nursing Implications: Assess baseline gait, neurologic status, affects, and monitor during treatment. Instruct patient to report signs/symptoms, and discuss drug modification with physician. Evaluate patient satisfaction with drug efficacy. Instruct patient to avoid alcohol while taking drug. Instruct patient prescribed schedule for discontinuing drug when used chronically: assess for signs/symptoms of withdrawal. Assess patient risk for suicide, and if at risk, refer to psychiatry for supportive counseling.

II. ALTERATION IN NUTRITION, LESS THAN BODY REQUIREMENTS, related to GI SIDE EFFECTS

Defining Characteristics: Constipation (1%), decreased appetite (1%), and less commonly, abdominal pain, flatulence, increased salivation, dyspepsia, decreased appetite; also elevated serum transaminases and alk phos.

Nursing Implications: Assess baseline nutrition and elimination patterns and serum transaminases, alk phos, and monitor during therapy. Assess degree of discomfort and interference with nutrition. Discuss significant abnormalities with physician and discuss drug modification.

III. INJURY related to DECREASE IN MENTAL ALERTNESS, PHYSICAL COORDINATION

Defining Characteristics: Drug may cause drowsiness, dizziness, and impair physical coordination, mental alertness.

Nursing Implications: Assess other medications that may increase risk (e.g., opiates, phenothiazines) and response to drug. Instruct patient to avoid potentially hazardous activities, including driving a car, operating machinery. Instruct patient to avoid alcohol.

IV. ALTERATIONS IN CARDIAC OUTPUT related to POSTURAL HYPOTENSION

Defining Characteristics: Drug may cause postural hypotension, palpitations, chest pain, edema.

Nursing Implications: Assess baseline VS, and monitor during therapy. Discuss abnormalities with physician. Instruct patient to report dizziness on standing or other changes, and to change position slowly and hold on to support if this occurs.

V. ALTERATIONS IN SKIN INTEGRITY related to SKIN DISORDERS

Defining Characteristics: Acne flare, xeroderma, contact dermatitis, pruritus, skin disorders may occur.

Nursing Implications: Assess baseline skin integrity, and instruct patient to report changes. Teach symptomatic skin management, and discuss drug discontinuance with physician if severe.

VI. SEXUAL DYSFUNCTION related to CHANGES IN LIBIDO, MENSTRUAL IRREGULARITIES

Defining Characteristics: Loss or increase in libido, menstrual irregularities in women; decreased ejaculation in men.

Nursing Implications: Assess baseline sexual functioning. Inform patient that alterations may occur, and instruct to report them. If severe, discuss dysfunction with physician, and whether another antidepressant would provide equal benefit with less dysfunction.

VII. ALTERATION IN ELIMINATION, URINARY, related to DYSURIA, BLADDER DYSFUNCTION

Defining Characteristics: Dysuria, polyuria, cystitis, urinary incontinence, bladder dysfunction, urinary retention, urine discoloration, and urinary bleeding may occur uncommonly.

Nursing Implications: Assess baseline urinary elimination pattern. Instruct patient to report any changes. Discuss impact on patient, and severity, and discuss significant problems with physician.

Drug: desipramine hydrochloride (Norpramin, Pertofrane)

Class: Tricyclic antidepressant.

Mechanism of Action: Blocks reuptake of neurotransmitters at neuronal membrane, thus increasing available serotonin, norepinephrine in CNS, and potentiating their effects. Appears to have analgesic effect separate from antidepressant action. May increase bioavailability of morphine. Indicated in the treatment of depressive (affective) mood disorders. Also used as an adjuvant analgesic in cancer pain management.

Metabolism: Well absorbed from GI tract. Highly protein-bound. Plasma half-life of 7–60 hours. Metabolized in liver, and primarily excreted in urine.

Dosage/Range:

Adult:

- Oral: 75–150 mg hs, or in divided doses.
- May be gradually increased to 300 mg/day if needed.
- Elderly: 25–50 mg/day, maximum 150 mg/day.

Drug Preparation:

- Store in tight containers at < 40°C (104°F).
- Administer as a single bedtime dose.

Drug Interactions:

- MAOIs: increased excitation, hyperpyrexia, seizures; use together cautiously (especially if high dose used).
- Sympathomimetic (epinephrine, amphetamines): increased hypertension; AVOID concurrent use.
- Cimetidine methylphenidate: increased amitriptyline levels, increased toxicity; use cautiously and monitor for increased toxicity.
- Warfarin: may increase PT; monitor closely and decrease dose of warfarin as needed.
- Barbiturates: may decrease desipramine serum level; monitor for decreased antidepressant effect; may need increased dose.
- Alcohol: may antagonize antidepressant effects; AVOID CONCURRENT USE.

Lab Effects/Interference:

- Rarely, altered liver function studies.
- Rarely, increased or decreased serum glucose levels.
- Rarely, increased pancreatic enzymes.
- Rarely, bone marrow depression with agranulocytosis, eosinophilia, purpura, thrombocytopenia.

Special Considerations:

- Antidepressant effect may take two weeks or longer.
- Adjuvant analgesic useful in cancer pain management.
- May also decrease depression associated with chronic cancer pain and promote improved sleep.
- Contraindicated in patients with myocardial infarction, seizure disorder, or benign prostatic hypertrophy.
- Use cautiously in patients with urine retention, narrow-angle glaucoma, hyperthyroidism, hepatic dysfunction, or suicidal ideation.
- Drug should be gradually discontinued rather than abruptly withdrawn to prevent anxiety, malaise, dizziness, nausea/vomiting.

- May be helpful in treating hiccups.
- Increased anticholinergic side effects in elderly.
- Teach all patients/families: call provider right away if thoughts of suicide or dying; attempts to commit suicide; new or worse depression; new or worse anxiety; feeling very agitated or restless; panic attacks; trouble sleeping (insomnia); new or worse irritability; aggressive, angry, or violent behavior; acting on dangerous impulses; extreme increase in activity or talking (mania); any unusual changes in behavior or mood.

Potential Toxicities/Side Effects and the Nursing Process

I. ALTERATIONS IN SENSORY/PERCEPTUAL PATTERNS related to DROWSINESS, EPS

Defining Characteristics: Drowsiness, dizziness, weakness, lethargy, fatigue are common; confusion, disorientation, hallucinations may occur in the elderly. Extrapyramidal symptoms may occur (fine tremor, rigidity, dystonia, dysarthria, dysphagia), as may peripheral neuropathy and blurred vision. Less sedation than amitriptyline.

Nursing Implications: Assess baseline gait, neurologic and mental status, and monitor during therapy. Instruct patient to report signs/symptoms; discuss benefit/risk ratio with physician. Assess for signs/symptoms of suicidal ideation; if they occur, refer for psychiatric evaluation. Inform patient that drowsiness, dizziness will resolve after 1–2 weeks; instruct to avoid hazardous activities while drowsy (e.g., driving a car, operating machinery).

II. ALTERATION IN CARDIAC OUTPUT related to POSTURAL HYPOTENSION, TACHYCARDIA

Defining Characteristics: Postural hypotension, EKG changes, tachycardia, hypertension may occur. Less severe than with other tricyclics.

Nursing Implications: Assess baseline orthostatic BP, heart rate, and monitor during therapy. Instruct patient to report abnormalities, including postural dizziness, palpitations. Drug should be stopped several days before surgery to prevent hypertensive crisis, especially if high dose is used.

III. ALTERATION IN NUTRITION, LESS THAN BODY REQUIREMENTS, related to GI SIDE EFFECTS

Defining Characteristics: Dry mouth, anorexia, nausea, vomiting, diarrhea, abdominal cramping may occur; also, elevated LFTs.

Nursing Implications: Assess baseline nutrition and elimination patterns and LFTs, and monitor during therapy. Discuss abnormalities with physician, and discuss drug modification. Teach patient to self-administer prescribed antiemetics as appropriate. LFTs should be repeated, and if still elevated, the drug should be discontinued. Instruct patient to take full dose at bedtime. Suggest patient use sugar-free hard candy, frequent ice chips, or artificial saliva for dry mouth.

IV. ALTERATION IN URINARY ELIMINATION related to URINARY RETENTION

Defining Characteristics: Urinary retention may occur. Increased risk in patients with history of urinary retention.

Nursing Implications: Assess baseline urinary elimination pattern and risk. Assess for urinary retention, and instruct patient to report signs/symptoms. Discuss alternative drug with physician if this occurs.

V. ALTERATIONS IN SKIN INTEGRITY related to ALLERGY

Defining Characteristics: Urticaria, erythema, rash, and photosensitivity may occur.

Nursing Implications: Assess baseline drug allergy history and skin integrity. Instruct patient to report skin changes. If angioedema of face or tongue develops, discuss drug discontinuance with physician. Instruct patient to avoid sunlight or to use sunblock protection.

Drug: desvenlafaxine succinate (Pristiq)

Class: Serotonin-norepinephrine reuptake inhibitor (SNRI) antidepressant.

Mechanism of Action: Drug is synthetic active metabolite of venlafaxine. It appears to potentiate neurotransmitter activity by inhibiting neuronal serotonin and norepinephrine reuptake.

Metabolism: Drug is well absorbed after oral administration (80% bioavailability, with mean time to peak plasma level of 7.5 hours after the dose). With once-daily dosing, steady state is reached in 4–5 days. The terminal half-life is 11 hours. Drug is 30% protein bound. Metabolized primarily by conjugation (UGT isoforms) and to a minor extent through oxidation (CYP3A4); 45% of the drug is excreted unchanged in the urine 72 hours after oral administration. Elimination half-lives significantly prolonged in severe renal dysfunction or end-stage renal disease (ESRD), and thus, dose should be adjusted in this population.

Dosage/Range:

- Adult (indicated for the treatment of depression): Extended release tablet 50 mg daily, with or without meals.
- In clinical studies, doses 50–400 mg daily were used. There is no evidence a dose higher than 50 mg daily offers increased benefit.
- Patients with hepatic dysfunction: do not escalate dose above 100 mg/day.
- Patients with renal impairment:
  - Mild (CrCl 50–80 mL/min): no dose adjustment.
  - Moderate (CrCl 30–50 mL/min) dysfunction: 50 mg PO daily but do not escalate dose.
  - Severe renal dysfunction (CrCl M 30 mL/min) or ESRD, 50 mg PO every other day; do not escalate dose. Do not give supplemental doses after hemodialysis.
- In older patients, ensure renal function when considering dose.

Drug Preparation/Administration:

- XL capsule available in 50- and 100-mg strengths.
- Administer PO daily with or without food at about the same time each day; tablets must be swallowed whole (DO NOT dissolve, crush, divide, or chew).
- Drug can cause HTN: monitor BP and correct HTN before initiating treatment, and monitor BP during therapy.
- When changing from an MAOI to venlafaxine HCl, wait at least 14 days after MAOI is stopped; when stopping desvenlafaxine and beginning an MAOI, wait at least 7 days.
- If drug is discontinued, taper with gradual dose reduction if possible (e.g., decrease frequency).

Drug Interactions:

- MAOIs: tremor, myoclonus, diaphoresis, nausea, vomiting, flushing, dizziness, hyperthermia resembling neuroleptic malignant syndrome, and may be fatal. DO NOT USE TOGETHER. See Administration section.
- Central nervous system (CNS) active agents: concomitant use has not been studied; use cautiously and monitor closely if required.
- Serotonergic drugs: use cautiously together if at all, and monitor closely.
- Drugs interfering with hemostasis (aspirin, NSAIDs, warfarin): serotonin important in hemostasis, and when reuptake blocked, risk of upper GI bleeding increased.
  - Aspirin, NSAIDs: increased risk of bleeding; do not use together concomitantly if possible.
  - Warfarin: altered anticoagulant effects, including increased bleeding; monitor INR and signs/symptoms bleeding closely, especially when drug started or stopped.
- Ethanol: no increased impairment, but because of CNS-active drug interaction, patients should be instructed not to drink alcohol.
- Venlafaxine: desvenlafaxine is the active metabolite in venlafaxine, and thus, the patient will overdose; do not coadminister.

- Inhibitors of CYP3A4 (e.g., ketoconazole increases area under the curve of desvenlafaxine by 43%): may increase serum level of desvenlafaxine, and thus, do not coadminister if possible.
- Drugs metabolized by CYP2D6: concomitant administration with desvenlafaxine may increase concentration of that drug.

Lab Effects/Interference:

- Elevated cholesterol, low-density lipids (LDL), and triglycerides: monitor baseline and throughout therapy.
- Hyponatremia.
- Rare abnormal LFTs, increased prolactin serum level.

Special Considerations:

- Drug is indicated for the treatment of patients with major depressive disorder.
- Avoid drug use during pregnancy and in nursing mothers. Drug exposure to fetus in third trimester resulted in neonates developing complications requiring prolonged hospitalization with respiratory support and tube feedings.
- Contraindicated in patients hypersensitive to desvenlafaxine succinate, venlafaxine HCl, or any excipients of drug; patients receiving MAO inhibitors (see Administration).
- Warnings:
  - Mydriasis may occur, and thus, patients with angle-closure and narrow angle glaucoma are at risk: monitor patients with raised intraocular pressure (or at risk of developing it) closely.
  - Drug can activate mania/hypomania states. Use cautiously in patients with bipolar disorder; screen patients initially for bipolar disorder, as drug is not approved for treatment of related depression. The risk of mania is 0.1%. Use cautiously in patients with a history of or family history of mania or hypomania about the risk of activation of mania/hypomania.
  - Use cautiously in patients with cardiovascular, cerebrovascular disease, or lipid metabolism diseases.
  - Rarely seizures can occur: use cautiously in patients with a history of seizures.
  - Rarely interstitial lung disease and eosinophilic pneumonia can occur; if patients develop progressive dyspnea, cough, or chest discomfort, stop drug and fully evaluate patient's pulmonary status.
- Monitor for clinical worsening and suicide risk.
- Drug was studied for short-term (8 week) treatment; monitor continued need of drug past that time.
- Rarely, serotonin syndrome may occur with desvenlafaxine (Pristiq), especially when used together with SSRIs, SNRIs, 5-hydroxytryptamine receptor agonists (triptans), and with drugs that reduce serotonin metabolism (including MAOIs), characterized by mental status changes (agitation, hallucinations, coma), autonomic instability (labile BP, hyperthermia), neuromuscular abnormalities (hyperreflexia, incoordination), with or without gastrointestinal symptoms (nausea, vomiting, diarrhea). Caution patient not to take other anti-depressants or tryptophan supplements (serotonin precursors) while taking this drug.

- Teach all patients/families: call provider right away if thoughts of suicide or dying; attempts to commit suicide; new or worse depression; new or worse anxiety; feeling very agitated or restless; panic attacks; trouble sleeping (insomnia); new or worse irritability; aggressive, angry, or violent behavior; acting on dangerous impulses; extreme increase in activity or talking (mania); any unusual changes in behavior or mood.

Potential Toxicities/Side Effects and the Nursing Process

I. ALTERATION IN OXYGENATION, POTENTIAL, related to CHANGES IN BP, TACHYCARDIA, HYPERLIPIDEMIA

Defining Characteristics: At all doses, some patients experienced sustained hypertension defined as a treatment emergent diastolic BP of ≥ 90 mm Hg and ≥ 10 mm Hg above baseline for three consecutive visits. This occurred at all doses with the following incidence: placebo 0.5%, 50 mg/da: 1.3%, 100 mg/da: 0.7%, 200 mg/da 1.1%, and 400 mg/da 2.3%. Orthostatic hypotension also occurred. Rarely, small increases in heart rate occurred in patients during clinical studies (incidence 1–2%). Patients with a history of MI, unstable heart disease, uncontrolled HTN were excluded from studies. Dose-related increases in LDL, total serum cholesterol, and triglycerides were seen during clinical studies, affecting 3–10% of patients depending on dose.

Nursing Implications: Assess baseline weight, cardiac status and BP at each visit. If BP elevated, reassess × 3, and if patient has three successive episodes as defined previously here, discuss dose reduction or change to another antidepressant with physician. Teach patient to change position slowly as risk of orthostatic hypotension. Instruct patient to report any headache, edema, palpitations, chest pain, or any changes in condition. Discuss any symptoms with the physician depending on severity. Monitor baseline cholesterol, LDL, and triglycerides, and monitor during therapy.

II. ALTERATIONS IN SENSORY/PERCEPTUAL PATTERNS related to DIZZINESS, INSOMNIA, SOMNOLENCE, ANXIETY

Defining Characteristics: Infrequently, dizziness, fatigue, or somnolence can occur. Insomnia occurs in 9–15% of patients depending on dose. Anxiety occurs in 3–5% of patients. Rarely, blurred vision, mydriasis (2% incidence at 50 mg dose and 6% at 400 mg dose), tinnitus, taste perversion, irritability, manic or hypomanic reaction, seizure, depersonalization, syncope, extrapyramidal disorder, and abnormal dreams may occur.

Nursing Implications: Assess baseline neurologic status, affective state, and risk factors, and monitor during treatment. Instruct patient to avoid alcohol while taking drug. Assess effect on older persons and/or patients with hepatic or renal dysfunction. Assess for symptoms at each visit, and instruct patient to report changes. If symptoms occur, discuss strategies to ensure patient safety and comfort.

III. ALTERATION IN NUTRITION, LESS THAN BODY REQUIREMENTS, related to GI SIDE EFFECTS, HYPONATREMIA

Defining Characteristics: Nausea (22–41% of patients), vomiting (3–9% compared with 3% placebo), dry mouth (11–25%), diarrhea (11%), constipation (9–14%), and decreased appetite (5–10%). Hyponatremia is rare and appears related to syndrome of inappropriate anti-diuretic hormone (SIADH). Rarely, cases of serum sodium < 110 mmol/L have occurred. Patients at risk are older persons who are volume depleted or on diuretic therapy.

Nursing Implications: Assess baseline nutrition and gastrointestinal functional status, and instruct the patient to report any GI disturbances or changes. Discuss measures to reduce nausea and/or stimulate appetite. Assess baseline serum sodium and risk factors for developing hyponatremia (SIADH), and monitor closely during therapy. Teach patients at risk signs and symptoms (headache, difficulty concentrating, memory impairment, confusion, weakness and unsteadiness; severe signs and symptoms are hallucination, syncope, seizure, coma) and to call their provider (mild) or to come to the emergency room or clinic right away (severe) if they occur.

IV. SEXUAL DYSFUNCTION, POTENTIAL, related to EJACULATORY DISTURBANCES

Defining Characteristics: Anorgasmia occurred in 0% at the 50-mg dose, 3% at the 100-mg dose, 5% at 200-mg dose, and 8% at 400-mg dose; decreased libido in 3–6% of patients, abnormal orgasm in 1–3%, and delayed ejaculation in 1–7% of patients; and ejaculation disfunction in 3–11% of patients depending on the dose. Women rarely experienced anorgasmia (1–3%).

Nursing Implications: Assess baseline sexual functioning. Inform patient that alterations may occur, and instruct to report them. If severe, discuss dysfunction with physician and whether another antidepressant would provide equal benefit with less dysfunction.

V. ALTERATION IN COMFORT related to HYPERHIDROSIS, HEADACHE

Defining Characteristics: Hyperhidrosis (excessive sweating) occurs in 10% at a 50-mg dose, 18% at 200-mg dose, and 21% at a 400-mg dose. Headache may occur uncommonly.

Nursing Implications: Assess baseline comfort level. Instruct patient to report any changes in comfort, and discuss strategies to reduce discomfort. If hyperhidrosis is severe, teach patient to change clothes frequently to see if this increases comfort.

Drug: diazepam (Valium)

Class: Benzodiazepine (anxiolytic).

Mechanism of Action: Binds to benzodiazepine receptors in the CNS (limbic and cortical areas, cerebellum, brain stem, and spinal cord), resulting in the following effects: anxiolytic, ataxia, anticonvulsant, muscle relaxation. Appears to potentiate the effects of GABA.

Metabolism: Well absorbed from GI tract. Widely distributed in body tissues and fluids, including CSF. Crosses placenta and is excreted in breast milk. Highly bound to plasma proteins. Metabolized in liver and excreted in urine. Half-life of 20–80 hours. May produce psychological and physical dependence. Indicated for management of anxiety, the relief of reflex spasm or spasticity, and as an anticonvulsant for termination of status epilepticus.

Dosage/Range:

Adult:

- Oral: 2–10 mg tid–qid or 15–30 mg/day extended-release preparation.
- Intravenous (IV) (tension): 5–10 mg IV, maximum 30 mg/8 h.
- IV (seizures): 5–10 mg IV, maximum 30 mg; may repeat in 2–4 hours if needed.
- IV (status epilepticus): 5–20 mg slow IV push (IVP) (2–5 mg/min), q 5–10 min, maximum 60 mg.
- IV (elderly, debilitated): 2–5 mg slow IVP.

Drug Preparation:

- Oral: protect tablets from light and store at 15–30°C (59–86°F).
- IV: do not administer with other drugs; drug may absorb to sides of plastic syringe or to plastic IV bag and tubing if added to IV infusion bag; consult hospital pharmacist for IV infusion protocol; administer IVP slowly 2–5 mg/min; have emergency equipment available.

Drug Interactions:

- CNS depressants (alcohol, anticonvulsants, phenothiazines, opiates): additive CNS depression; avoid concurrent use or use cautiously and monitor carefully.
- Oral contraceptives, isoniazid, ketoconazole, or cimetidine: decrease plasma clearance of diazepam so may increase effect (e.g., sedation); monitor patient closely.
- Tricyclic antidepressants: increased serum levels of antidepressant possible; use together cautiously.
- Digoxin: may decrease renal excretion of digoxin; monitor for overdosage; may need to decrease digoxin.
- Levodopa: may decrease levodopa effect; monitor patient response; may have to increase levodopa dose.

Lab Effects/Interference:

- Rarely, altered liver function studies.
- Rarely, neutropenia.

Special Considerations:

- Wide margin of safety between therapeutic and toxic doses.
- May impair ability to perform activities requiring mental alertness (e.g., driving a car, operating machinery).
- May produce psychological and physical dependence.
- Administer cautiously in patients with liver or renal impairment.
- Use cautiously in patients with chronic pulmonary disease or sleep apnea.
- Contraindicated in patients with depressive neuroses, psychotic reactions (without prominent anxiety), acute alcoholic intoxication (with depressed VS), known hypersensitivity to the drug, or acute angle-closure glaucoma.
- May cause fetal damage, so should not be used during pregnancy or if the mother is breast-feeding.
- Withdrawal symptoms (including seizure, delirium) can occur with rapid drug discontinuance in patients taking high or chronic doses.

Potential Toxicities/Side Effects and the Nursing Process

I. ALTERATIONS IN SENSORY/PERCEPTUAL PATTERNS relating to CNS DEPRESSION

Defining Characteristics: CNS depressant effects include drowsiness, fatigue, lethargy, confusion, weakness, headache, which may occur initially and resolve with continued therapy or dose reduction. Vivid dreams, visual disturbances, slurred speech, "hangover," and bizarre behavior may also occur. Patient risk factors: elderly, debilitated, liver dysfunction, low serum albumin.

Nursing Implications: Assess baseline neurologic status and risk factors, and monitor during treatment. Instruct patient to report signs/symptoms and discuss drug modification with physician. Evaluate patient satisfaction with drug efficacy. Instruct patient to avoid alcohol while taking drug. Teach patient prescribed schedule for discontinuing drug when used chronically: assess for signs/symptoms of withdrawal (increased anxiety, rebound insomnia; may also include agitation, dysphoria, nausea/vomiting, irritability, muscle cramps, hallucinations, seizures).

II. ALTERATION IN NUTRITION, LESS THAN BODY REQUIREMENTS, related to GI SIDE EFFECTS

Defining Characteristics: Nausea, vomiting, abdominal discomfort may occur; also, elevated LFTs.

Nursing Implications: Assess baseline nutrition and elimination patterns and LFTs, and monitor during therapy. Discuss abnormalities with physician and discuss drug modification. Teach patient to self-administer prescribed antiemetics as appropriate.

III. INJURY related to DECREASE IN MENTAL ALERTNESS, PHYSICAL COORDINATION

Defining Characteristics: Drug may cause drowsiness, dizziness, and impair physical coordination, mental alertness.

Nursing Implications: Assess other medications that may increase risk (e.g., opiates, phenothiazines) and response to drug. Instruct patient to avoid potentially hazardous activities, including driving a car, operating machinery.

IV. ALTERATIONS IN PERFUSION related to CARDIOPULMONARY COMPROMISE

Defining Characteristics: Drug may cause transient hypotension, bradycardia, cardiovascular collapse, respiratory depression.

Nursing Implications: Assess baseline VS; have resuscitation equipment nearby. Monitor q 5–15 min and before IV dose of drug. Discuss abnormalities with physician.

V. ALTERATIONS IN SKIN INTEGRITY related to RASH

Defining Characteristics: Urticaria, rash may occur; also phlebitis, pain at injection site.

Nursing Implications: Assess baseline skin integrity, and instruct patient to report changes. Teach symptomatic skin management, and discuss drug discontinuance with physician if severe. Assess IV site for evidence of pain, phlebitis, and change site; apply heat as needed.

Drug: doxepin hydrochloride (Sinequan)

Class: Antidepressant of the dibenzoxepine tricyclic class.

Mechanism of Action: Appears to exert adrenergic effect at the synapses, preventing deactivation of norepinephrine by reuptake into the nerve terminals.

Metabolism: Metabolized in the liver by the P-450 enzyme system, into active metabolite. Effective serum level of doxepin and metabolite is 100–200 mg/mL. Takes 2–8 days to reach steady-state.

Dosage/Range:

Adult:

- Initial dose of 75 mg/day is recommended; in elderly, dose should start at 25–50 mg/day.
- Dose may be titrated up or down based on response. Usual dose is 75 mg/day to 150 mg/day.

- Patients with mild symptoms may require only 25 mg/day to 50 mg/day.
- Patients with severe symptoms may require gradual titration up to 300 mg/day.

Drug Preparation:
- Oral, taken in a single dose (maximum 150-mg dose) or in divided doses. Single dose given at bedtime enhances sleep.
- Available in 10-, 25-, 50-, 75-, 100-, and 150-mg capsules.
- If changing a patient from MAOI to doxepin HCl, wait at least 14 days before the careful initiation of doxepin.

Drug Interactions:
- Alcohol: do not use concomitantly, as increases drug toxicity.
- MAOI: severe reaction, including death may occur; DO NOT USE TOGETHER.
- Cimetidine: increased serum levels of drug and anticholinergic side effects (severe dry mouth, urinary retention, blurred vision); avoid concurrent use.
- Tolazamide: may cause severe hypoglycemia; monitor patient's serum glucose carefully.

Lab Effects/Interference:
- Rarely, eosinophilia, bone marrow depression (e.g., agranulocytosis, leukopenia, thrombocytopenia, purpura).
- Increased or decreased blood glucose levels.

Special Considerations:
- Contraindicated in patients with glaucoma or urinary retention.
- Antianxiety effect appears before the antidepressant effect, which takes 2–3 weeks.
- Most sedating of antidepressants, so useful in enhancing sleep, and single dose (up to 150 mg) should be taken at bedtime.
- Recommended for the treatment of depression accompanied by anxiety and insomnia, depression associated with organic illness or alcohol, psychotic depressive disorders with associated anxiety.
- Teach all patients/families: call provider right away if thoughts of suicide or dying; attempts to commit suicide; new or worse depression; new or worse anxiety; feeling very agitated or restless; panic attacks; trouble sleeping (insomnia); new or worse irritability; aggressive, angry, or violent behavior; acting on dangerous impulses; extreme increase in activity or talking (mania); any unusual changes in behavior or mood.

Potential Toxicities/Side Effects and the Nursing Process

I. ALTERATIONS IN SENSORY/PERCEPTUAL related to DROWSINESS, EPS

Defining Characteristics: Drowsiness, which may disappear as therapy continues. Rarely, dizziness, confusion, disorientation, hallucinations, numbness, paresthesia, ataxia, extrapyramidal symptoms, seizures, blurred vision, tardive dyskinesia, tremor may occur.

Nursing Implications: Assess baseline gait, neurologic, affective and mental status, and monitor during therapy. Instruct patient to report signs/symptoms; discuss benefit/risk ratio with physician and measures to reduce extrapyramidal side effects if they occur. Assess for signs/symptoms of suicidal ideation; if they occur, refer for psychiatric evaluation. Inform patient that drowsiness will decrease after 1–2 weeks, and instruct to avoid hazardous activities while drowsy (e.g., driving a car, operating machinery). Instruct patient to avoid alcohol while taking drug.

II. ALTERATION IN CARDIAC OUTPUT related to BLOOD PRESSURE CHANGES

Defining Characteristics: Hypotension or hypertension, tachycardia may occur.

Nursing Implications: Assess baseline orthostatic BP, heart rate, and monitor during therapy. Instruct patient to report abnormalities, including postural dizziness, palpitations.

III. ALTERATION IN NUTRITION, LESS THAN BODY REQUIREMENTS, related to GI SIDE EFFECTS

Defining Characteristics: Dry mouth, anorexia, nausea, vomiting, diarrhea, indigestion, taste changes, aphthous stomatitis may occur rarely.

Nursing Implications: Assess baseline nutrition and elimination patterns. Discuss abnormalities with physician, and discuss drug modification. Teach patient to self-administer prescribed antiemetics as appropriate. Instruct patient to take full dose at bedtime (if 150 mg or less). Suggest patient use sugar-free hard candy, frequent ice chips, or artificial saliva for dry mouth.

IV. ALTERATION IN URINARY ELIMINATION related to URINARY RETENTION

Defining Characteristics: Urinary retention may occur. Increased risk in patients with history of urinary retention.

Nursing Implications: Assess baseline urinary elimination pattern and risk. Assess for urinary retention, and instruct patient to report signs/symptoms. Discuss alternative drug with physician if this occurs.

V. ALTERATIONS IN SKIN INTEGRITY related to ALLERGY

Defining Characteristics: Urticaria, erythema, rash, and photosensitivity may occur.

Nursing Implications: Assess baseline drug allergy history and skin integrity. Instruct patient to report skin changes. If severe changes occur, discuss drug discontinuance with physician. Instruct patient to avoid sunlight or to use sunblock protection.

VI. SEXUAL DYSFUNCTION related to CHANGES IN LIBIDO

Defining Characteristics: Increased or decreased libido, testicular swelling, gynecomastia in males; enlargement of breasts and galactorrhea in women.

Nursing Implications: Assess baseline sexual functioning. Inform patient that alterations may occur, and instruct to report them. If severe, discuss dysfunction with physician and whether another antidepressant would provide equal benefit with less dysfunction.

Drug: duloxetine hydrochloride (Cymbalta)

Class: Antidepressant.

Mechanism of Action: Selective serotonin and norepinephrine uptake inhibitor (SSNRI), resulting in potentiation of serotonergic and noradrenergic activity in the CNS, and antidepressant, central pain inhibition, and anxiolytic qualities.

Metabolism: After oral ingestion, drug undergoes extensive metabolism, but metabolites do not appear to contribute to the drug effect. The drug is highly protein bound. Elimination half-life is about 12 hours, achieving steady-state plasma levels in 3 days of dosing. When taken with food, the time to reach peak concentration increases from 6 to 10 hours and reduces absorption by about 10%. When the drug is taken in the evening, there is a 3-hour delay in absorption and a 33% increase in drug clearance compared with taking the drug in the morning. The drug is metabolized by the CYP1A2 and CYP2D6 P450 hepatic enzymes. Metabolites are excreted in the urine primarily (70%) with 20% excreted in the feces. Drug area under the curve is about 25% higher, and the half-life of the drug about 4 hours longer in older women. Smoking reduces the bioavailability by 33%, but the manufacturer does not recommend dose modification in smokers. Drug is not recommended for patients with severe renal impairment (urinary creatinine clearance < 30 mL/min), including patients on dialysis or patients with hepatic insufficiency.

Dosage/Range:

Adult: Depression

- 20 mg orally twice daily to 60 mg/day (given either once a day or as 30 mg twice daily) without regard to meals.

Adult: Diabetic Peripheral Neuropathy

- 60 mg orally once daily without regard to meals (start with a lower dose if renal impairment and gradually increase dose).

Adult: Generalized Anxiety Disorder

- 60 mg orally once daily without regard to meals.

Drug Preparation/Administration:

- Oral, available as delayed release capsules in 20-, 30-, and 60-mg strengths.

- When discontinuing fluoxetine, the drug should be gradually reduced in dose (tapered), as otherwise, discontinuation symptoms such as dizziness, nausea, headache, paresthesia, vomiting, irritability, nightmares, insomnia, diarrhea, anxiety, hyperhidrosis, and vertigo may occur.
- Allow at least 14 days between stopping an MAOI and beginning fluoxetine; when stopping fluoxetine to begin an MAOI, wait at least 5 days after stopping duloxetine before beginning the MAOI.

Drug Interactions:
- CYP1A2 inhibitors (cimetidine, ciprofloxacin, levofloxacin, enoxacin): increased serum levels and terminal half-life of duloxetine; avoid concurrent administration.
- CYP2D6 inhibitors (paroxetine, quinidine): increased duloxetine serum levels by 60%; avoid concurrent use.
- Drugs metabolized by CYP1A2: no effect on the other drugs.
- Drugs metabolized by CYP2D6 (tricyclic antidepressants (TCA), phenothiazines, type 1C antiarrhythmics such as propafenone and flecainide): increased serum levels of these drugs; use together cautiously if at all and monitor TCA serum levels; do not give concurrently with thioridazine as increased risk of ventricular arrhythmias and sudden death.
- Alcohol: DO NOT USE CONCOMITANTLY, as this may increase the risk of hepatic injury in heavy alcohol imbibers.
- CNS acting drugs: use together cautiously if at all.
- Serotonergic drugs (triptans, linezolid, lithium, tramadol, St. John's wort): increased risk for serotonin syndrome (mental status changes such as agitation, hallucinations, coma); autonomic instability such as tachycardia, labile BP, hyperthermia; neuromuscular aberrations such as hyperreflexia, incoordination; and/or GI symptoms such as nausea, vomiting, diarrhea. DO NOT use concurrently.
- Drugs that affect gastric acidity: drug requires a pH of 5.5 to dissolve the enteric coating. No effect with magnesium or aluminum containing antacids but caution advised in patients with slow gastric emptying (diabetics). It is not known whether concurrent administration with proton-pump inhibitors affects drug absorption.
- MAOIs: when drug is given concomitantly or within a short time period, severe, potentially life-threatening interactions may occur, including symptoms resembling neuroleptic malignant syndrome. DO NOT GIVE TOGETHER, AND END SEPARATELY, as stated in the administration section.

Lab Effects/Interference:
- Increased liver transaminases.
- Rare anemia, leucopenia, thrombocytopenia.
- Rare hypercholesteremia, hyperlipidemia, hypoglycemia, dyslipidemia, hypertriglyceridemia.
- Rare increased serum creatinine.

Special Considerations:

- FDA approved for the treatment of major depressive disorder, the management of neuropathic pain associated with diabetic peripheral neuropathy, and the treatment of generalized anxiety disorder (associated with at least three symptoms such as restlessness, easy fatigability, difficulty concentrating, irritability, muscle tension, and/or sleep disturbance).
- Contraindicated in patients who are (1) taking MAOIs, (2) have uncontrolled narrow-angle glaucoma, (3) have end-stage renal disease or severe renal impairment (urinary creatinine clearance < 30 mL/min), (4) have hepatic insufficiency, and (5) nursing mothers.
- Women who are pregnant in the third trimester: neonates exposed to SSRIs, SNRIs developed complications requiring prolonged hospitalization; must consider risk versus benefit, and consider tapering drug during third trimester.
- Increased risk of suicidality (thinking and behavior) in young adults aged 18–24 years, as well as children and adolescents, especially during the first 2 months of treatment; monitor closely for signs/symptoms of suicidality (emergency of agitation, irritability, unusual changes in behavior, emergence of suicidality).
- Teach all patients/families: call provider right away if thoughts of suicide or dying; attempts to commit suicide; new or worse depression; new or worse anxiety; feeling very agitated or restless; panic attacks; trouble sleeping (insomnia); new or worse irritability; aggressive, angry, or violent behavior; acting on dangerous impulses; extreme increase in activity or talking (mania); any unusual changes in behavior or mood.

Potential Toxicities/Side Effects and the Nursing Process

I. ALTERATIONS IN SENSORY/PERCEPTUAL PATTERNS related to CNS EFFECTS

Defining Characteristics: Blurred vision, vertigo, lethargy, dizziness, somnolence, tremor, paresthesia/hypoesthesia, hot flushes, agitation, anxiety, nervousness, nightmare/abnormal dreams, sleep disorder may occur in at least 1 of 100 patients. Patients aged 18–24 years are at risk for suicide or others at risk for suicide may commit suicide during initial period of treatment.

Nursing Implications: Assess baseline neurologic status and risk factors, and monitor during treatment. Instruct patient to report signs/symptoms, and discuss drug modification with physician. Evaluate patient satisfaction with drug efficacy. Instruct patient to avoid alcohol while taking drug. Assess suicide risk, and if at high risk, monitor closely and provide supportive counseling and referral to a psychiatrist. The patient should receive only a small number of pills to prevent overdose.

II. ALTERATION IN NUTRITION, LESS THAN BODY REQUIREMENTS, related to GI SIDE EFFECTS

Defining Characteristics: Nausea and less commonly vomiting, diarrhea, constipation, dry mouth, dyspepsia, anorexia, abdominal discomfort, flatulence, taste changes, and gastroenteritis may occur.

Nursing Implications: Assess baseline nutrition and elimination patterns. Discuss abnormalities with physician and discuss drug modification. Teach patient to self-administer prescribed antiemetics as appropriate. If patient is losing weight, instruct patient to report this and involve nutritionist in care.

III. SEXUAL DYSFUNCTION, POTENTIAL, related to IMPOTENCE

Defining Characteristics: Sexual dysfunction and anorgasmia and erectile dysfunction in men can occur uncommonly.

Nursing Implications: Assess baseline sexual functioning. Inform patient that alterations may rarely occur and that they should be reported. If severe, discuss dysfunction with a physician and whether another antidepressant would provide equal benefit with less dysfunction.

Drug: escitalalopram oxalate (Lexapro)

Class: Antidepressant.

Mechanism of Action: Selective inhibitor of neuronal reuptake of serotonin (SSRI) in the CNS, resulting in potentiation of serotonin activity in the CNS; has minimal effect on reuptake of norepinephrine or dopamine.

Metabolism: After oral administration, 80% of the drug is absorbed, with peak plasma levels in 5 hours and steady-state plasma concentrations in about 1 week. Drug is 56% bound to plasma proteins. The terminal half-life of the drug is 27–32 hours. Drug undergoes hepatic biotransformation, with CYP3A4 and CYP 2C19 liver microsomes primarily involved in drug metabolism. Bioavailability of tablet is the same as the oral solution.

Dosage/Range:

- Recommended dose is 10 mg/day orally (20 mg daily has not shown improved benefit); however, if dose is increased to 20 mg daily, wait at least 1 week before increasing the dose.

Drug Preparation/Administration:
- Available in 5-, 10-, and 20-mg tablets, as well as 5-mg/5-mL oral solution.
- May be given in morning or evening and with or without food.
- When discontinuing drug, the dose should be gradually tapered rather than abruptly stopped.

Drug Interactions:
- CYP1A2 inhibitors (cimetidine): increased serum levels of escitalalopram oxalate by 43%; avoid concurrent administration.
- Drugs metabolized by CYP2D6 (tricyclic antidepressants (TCA), phenothiazines, metoprolol): possible, increased serum levels of these drugs; use together cautiously and monitor TCA serum levels.
- Alcohol: DO NOT USE CONCOMITANTLY, as this may increase the risk of hepatic injury in heavy alcohol imbibers.
- CNS acting drugs: use together cautiously if at all.
- Serotonergic drugs (triptans, linezolid, lithium, tramadol, St. John's wort): increased risk for serotonin syndrome (mental status changes such as agitation, hallucinations, coma); autonomic instability such as tachycardia, labile BP, hyperthermia; neuromuscular aberrations such as hyperreflexia, incoordination; and/or GI symptoms such as nausea, vomiting, diarrhea. DO NOT use concurrently.
- Drugs that interfere with hemostasis (NSAIDs, aspirin, warfarin): increased risk of upper-GI bleeding; use cautiously if at all, and monitor closely.
- MAOIs: when drug is given concomitantly or within a short time period, severe, potentially life-threatening interactions may occur, including symptoms resembling neuroleptic malignant syndrome. DO NOT GIVE TOGETHER AND END SEPARATELY, as stated in the administration section.
- Lithium: enhanced serotonergic effects, monitor patient closely; monitor lithium levels.
- Pimozide: increased QTc by 10 msec; avoid concurrent use.
- Sumatriptan: weakness, hyperreflexia, and incoordination; avoid concurrent use.

Lab Effects/Interference: None known.

Special Considerations:
- FDA approved for the treatment of major depressive disorder, the management of neuropathic pain associated with diabetic peripheral neuropathy, and the treatment of generalized anxiety disorder (associated with at least three symptoms, such as restlessness, easy fatigability, difficulty concentrating, irritability, muscle tension, and/or sleep disturbance).
- Contraindicated in patients who are (1) taking MAOIs, (2) have uncontrolled narrow-angle glaucoma, (3) have end-stage renal disease or severe renal impairment (urinary creatinine clearance < 30 mL/min), (4) have hepatic insufficiency, and (5) nursing mothers.
- Women who are pregnant in the third trimester: neonates exposed to SSRIs, SNRIs developed complications requiring prolonged hospitalization; must consider risk versus benefit and consider tapering drug during third trimester.

- Increased risk of suicidality (thinking and behavior) in young adults aged 18–24, as well as children and adolescents, especially during the first 2 months of treatment; monitor closely for signs/symptoms of suicidality (emergency of agitation, irritability, unusual changes in behavior, emergence of suicidality).
- Teach all patients/families: call provider right away if thoughts of suicide or dying; attempts to commit suicide; new or worse depression; new or worse anxiety; feeling very agitated or restless; panic attacks; trouble sleeping (insomnia); new or worse irritability; aggressive, angry, or violent behavior; acting on dangerous impulses; extreme increase in activity or talking (mania); any unusual changes in behavior or mood.

Potential Toxicities/Side Effects and the Nursing Process

I. ALTERATIONS IN SENSORY/PERCEPTUAL PATTERNS related to CNS EFFECTS

Defining Characteristics: Somnolence (13%), insomnia (12%), abnormal dreaming (3%), lethargy (3%), and dizziness (2%) may occur. Patients aged 18–24 years are at risk for suicide, or others at risk for suicide may commit suicide during initial period of treatment.

Nursing Implications: Assess baseline neurologic status, sleep patterns, and risk factors, and monitor during treatment. Instruct patient to report signs/symptoms, and discuss drug modification with physician. Evaluate patient satisfaction with drug efficacy. Instruct patient to avoid alcohol while taking drug. Assess suicide risk, and if at high risk, monitor closely and provide supportive counseling and referral to a psychiatrist. The patient should receive only a small number of pills to prevent overdose.

II. ALTERATION IN NUTRITION, LESS THAN BODY REQUIREMENTS, related to GI SIDE EFFECTS

Defining Characteristics: Nausea (18%), dry mouth (9%), diarrhea (8%), constipation (5%), indigestion (3%), vomiting (3%), and rarely abdominal discomfort and flatulence may occur. Weight changes were no different from placebo group.

Nursing Implications: Assess baseline nutrition and elimination patterns. Discuss abnormalities with physician, and discuss drug modification. Teach patient to self-administer prescribed antiemetics as appropriate. If patient is losing weight, instruct patient to report this and involve nutritionist in care.

III. SEXUAL DYSFUNCTION, POTENTIAL, related to IMPOTENCE

Defining Characteristics: Sexual dysfunction, including ejaculation disorder (primarily ejaculatory delay), decreased libido, and impotence in men and decreased libido and anorgasmia in women can occur uncommonly. SSRIs have a rare incidence of priapism.

Nursing Implications: Assess baseline sexual functioning. Inform patient that alterations may rarely occur and should be reported. If severe, discuss dysfunction with physician and whether another antidepressant would provide equal benefit with less dysfunction.

Drug: fluoxetine hydrochloride (Prozac)

Class: Antidepressant.

Mechanism of Action: Inhibits CNS neuronal uptake of serotonin.

Metabolism: Well absorbed after oral administration, and peak serum levels occur in 6–8 hours. Peak plasma concentrations are 15–55 mg/mL. Time to steady-state in serum level is 2–4 weeks; 94.5% protein-bound. Drug is extensively metabolized in the liver to norfluoxetine and other metabolites using P-450 enzyme pathway; inactive metabolites are excreted in the urine. Elimination half-life is 1–3 days when administered acutely, and 4–6 days with chronic administration.

Dosage/Range:

Adult (for depression):

- 20 mg/day initially.
- After several weeks of therapy, if no response, may increase dose gradually to a maximum dose of 80 mg/day.
- Patients with hepatic dysfunction, elderly, or patients with concurrent diseases: start at lower dose or give less frequently.
- Weekly 90 mg tablets: begin 7 days after last 20-mg daily dose.

Drug Preparation:

- Give orally with or without food in the morning; with higher doses, e.g., 80 mg/day, may give two doses, one in the morning and one at noon.
- Available in pulvules of 10 mg and 20 mg; liquid/oral solution available as 20 mg/5 mL; weekly 90-mg tablets.
- Allow at least 14 days between stopping an MAOI and beginning fluoxetine; when stopping fluoxetine to begin an MAOI, wait at least five weeks before beginning the MAOI.

Drug Interactions:

- Alcohol: DO NOT USE CONCOMITANTLY, as increases impaired judgment, thinking, and motor skills.
- Tricyclic antidepressants (TCA): decreased metabolism and increased serum levels of TCA; monitor for increased toxicity and dose-reduce TCA as necessary when drug is given concomitantly with fluoxetine.

- MAOIs: when drug is given concomitantly or within a short time period, severe, potentially life-threatening interactions may occur, including symptoms resembling neuroleptic malignant syndrome. DO NOT GIVE TOGETHER, AND END SEPARATELY, as stated in Administration section.
- Buspirone: reduced effects of buspirone; assess need to increase dose.
- Carbamazepine: increased serum levels of carbamazepine, with potential increased toxicity; monitor closely and dose-reduce as necessary.
- Cyproheptadine: decreased fluoxetine serum levels, so that effect was reduced or reversed; avoid concomitant administration if possible.
- Dextromethorphan: increased risk of hallucinations.
- Diazepam: increased diazepam half-life with increased circulating serum levels, leading to increased toxicity (e.g., excessive sedation or impaired psychomotor skills); dose-reduce diazepam or avoid concurrent administration.
- Digoxin: displaces fluoxetine from plasma protein binding, leading to increased fluoxetine serum levels and effect; monitor for toxicity and dose reduce as necessary.
- Lithium: increased lithium serum levels leading to possible increased neurotoxicity; monitor patient closely, and reduce lithium dose as needed.
- Phenytoin: increased phenytoin serum levels; monitor effect and serum levels, and modify dose accordingly.
- Thioridazine: DO NOT administer together. Discontinue fluoxetine at least 5 weeks before starting thioridazine.
- Tryptophan: increased risk of CNS toxicity (e.g., headache, sweating, dizziness, agitation, aggressiveness) and peripheral toxicity (e.g., nausea, vomiting); use together cautiously if at all; avoid if possible.
- Warfarin: displaces fluoxetine from plasma protein binding sites, leading to increased fluoxetine serum levels, and effect; monitor for toxicity and dose reduce as necessary.
- Teach all patients/families: call provider right away if thoughts of suicide or dying; attempts to commit suicide; new or worse depression; new or worse anxiety; feeling very agitated or restless; panic attacks; trouble sleeping (insomnia); new or worse irritability; aggressive, angry, or violent behavior; acting on dangerous impulses; extreme increase in activity or talking (mania); any unusual changes in behavior or mood.

Lab Effects/Interference:

- None known.

Special Considerations:

- Weekly dosing is for patients whose depression is stable on daily dosing. Diarrhea and cognitive changes are more common with weekly dosing.
- May take up to four weeks of therapy before benefit is seen.
- Possibility of suicide attempt may exist in depression and persist until depression managed by drug; monitor high-risk patients closely and give smallest prescription of tablets possible to ensure frequent follow-up and reduce the risk of overdosage.

- Has slight-to-no anticholinergic, sedative, or orthostatic hypotensive side effects.
- Avoid use in women who are pregnant or breast-feeding.
- Drug is also indicated for treatment of obsessive-compulsive disorder and bulimia disorder.

Potential Toxicities/Side Effects and the Nursing Process

I. ALTERATIONS IN SKIN INTEGRITY related to RASH

Defining Characteristics: Urticaria, rash may occur (7%). In initial trials, in one-third of patients developing rash, rash was associated with fever, leukocytosis, arthralgias, edema, carpal tunnel syndrome, respiratory distress, lymphadenopathy, proteinuria, and/or mildly elevated liver transaminase levels that required drug discontinuation, which largely resolved symptoms.

Nursing Implications: Assess baseline skin integrity, and instruct patient to report rash immediately. Discuss drug discontinuance with physician if severe or associated with other symptoms as above. Teach symptomatic skin management.

II. ALTERATIONS IN SENSORY/PERCEPTUAL PATTERNS related to CNS EFFECTS

Defining Characteristics: CNS effects include headache and, less commonly, activation of mania or hypomania, insomnia, anxiety, decreased ability to concentrate, tremor, sensory disturbances, abnormal dreams, nervousness, dizziness, fatigue, sedation, lightheadedness, blurred vision. Rarely, seizures may occur. Patients at risk for suicide may commit suicide during initial period of treatment.

Nursing Implications: Assess baseline neurologic status and risk factors, and monitor during treatment. Instruct patient to report signs/symptoms, and discuss drug modification with physician. Evaluate patient satisfaction with drug efficacy. Instruct patient to avoid alcohol while taking drug. Assess suicide risk, and if at high risk, monitor closely, provide supportive counseling, and prescribe only small numbers of pills to prevent overdosage. May take up to four weeks for therapeutic effect to be seen.

III. ALTERATION IN NUTRITION, LESS THAN BODY REQUIREMENTS, related to GI SIDE EFFECTS

Defining Characteristics: Nausea and, less commonly, vomiting, diarrhea, constipation, dry mouth, dyspepsia, anorexia, abdominal discomfort, flatulence, taste changes, gastroenteritis, and increased hunger may occur. Significant weight loss can occur in underweight, depressed patients.

Nursing Implications: Assess baseline nutrition and elimination patterns. Discuss abnormalities with physician and discuss drug modification. Teach patient to self-administer prescribed antiemetics as appropriate. If patient is losing weight, instruct patient to report this immediately, and discuss benefit of continuation of drug with physician.

IV. INJURY related to DECREASE IN MENTAL ALERTNESS, PHYSICAL COORDINATION

Defining Characteristics: Drug may cause drowsiness, dizziness, and impair physical coordination, mental alertness.

Nursing Implications: Assess other medications that may increase risk (e.g., opiates, phenothiazines) and response to drug. Instruct patient to avoid potentially hazardous activities, including driving a car, operating machinery.

V. SEXUAL DYSFUNCTION, POTENTIAL, related to IMPOTENCE

Defining Characteristics: Sexual dysfunction, impotence, anorgasmia may occur.

Nursing Implications: Assess baseline sexual functioning. Inform patient that alterations may occur, and instruct to report them. If severe, discuss dysfunction with physician, and whether another antidepressant would provide equal benefit with less dysfunction.

VI. ALTERATION IN OXYGENATION, POTENTIAL, related to ALTERED BREATHING PATTERNS

Defining Characteristics: Bronchitis, upper respiratory infections, pharyngitis, cough, dyspnea, rhinitis, nasal congestion, and sinusitis may occur infrequently.

Nursing Implications: Assess baseline respiratory status, and instruct patient to report any changes. Discuss serious changes with physician, and interventions necessary.

VII. ALTERATION IN COMFORT, POTENTIAL, related to PAIN

Defining Characteristics: Pain in muscles, joints, or back may occur; flu-like symptoms are infrequent, as are asthenia, chest pain, and limb pain.

Nursing Implications: Assess baseline comfort level; instruct patient to report any changes. Discuss symptom management strategies, unless severe, and then discuss benefit of changing to another antidepressant medicine.

Drug: imipramine pamoate (Tofranil-PM)

Class: Tricyclic antidepressant.

Mechanism of Action: Blocks reuptake of neurotransmitters at neuronal membrane, thus increasing available serotonin, norepinephrine in CNS, and potentiating their effects. Appears to have analgesic effect separate from antidepressant action. May increase bioavailability of morphine. Indicated in the treatment of depressive (affective) mood disorders. Also used as an adjuvant analgesic in cancer pain management.

Metabolism: Completely absorbed from GI tract; highly protein bound. Plasma half-life is 8–16 hours. Metabolized in liver; excreted in urine and, to lesser degree, in bile and feces.

Dosage/Range:

Adult:

- Oral: 75–100 mg/day (may increase on patient response, to maximum 300 mg; reduce dose in elderly, 30–40 mg/day, to maximum 100 mg).
- IM: used only when oral route can not be used.

Drug Preparation:

- Oral: store in well-closed containers at 15–30°C (59–86°F). Administer as a single bedtime dose.
- IM: administer IM in large muscle mass; change to oral as soon as possible.

Drug Interactions:

- MAOIs: increased excitation, hyperpyrexia, seizures; use together cautiously (especially if high dose is used).
- CNS depressants (alcohol, sedatives, hypnotics): increase CNS depression; use together cautiously.
- Sympathomimetic (epinephrine, amphetamines): increased hypertension; AVOID concurrent use.
- Cimetidine methylphenidate: increased imipramine levels, increased toxicity; use cautiously and monitor for increased toxicity.
- Warfarin: may increase PT; monitor closely and decrease dose of warfarin as needed.
- Barbiturates: may decrease imipramine level; monitor patient response; may need to increase dose.

Lab Effects/Interference:

- Increased metanephrine (Pisano test).
- Decreased urinary 5-HIAA.

Special Considerations:

- Antidepressant effect may take two weeks or longer.
- Adjuvant analgesic useful in cancer pain management.
- May also decrease depression associated with chronic cancer pain and promote improved sleep.

- Contraindicated in patients with myocardial infarction, seizure disorder, or benign prostatic hypertrophy.
- Use cautiously in patients with urine retention, narrow-angle glaucoma, hyperthyroidism, hepatic dysfunction, or suicidal ideation.
- Drug should be gradually discontinued rather than abruptly withdrawn to prevent anxiety, malaise, dizziness, nausea/vomiting.
- May be helpful in treating hiccups.
- Increased anticholinergic side effects in elderly.
- Some preparations may contain sodium bisulfite, which can cause allergic reactions, including anaphylaxis, in hypersensitive individuals. Check ingredients. Assess allergy history.
- Teach all patients/families: call provider right away if thoughts of suicide or dying; attempts to commit suicide; new or worse depression; new or worse anxiety; feeling very agitated or restless; panic attacks; trouble sleeping (insomnia); new or worse irritability; aggressive, angry, or violent behavior; acting on dangerous impulses; extreme increase in activity or talking (mania); any unusual changes in behavior or mood.

Potential Toxicities/Side Effects and the Nursing Process

I. ALTERATIONS IN SENSORY/PERCEPTUAL PATTERNS related to DROWSINESS, CNS EFFECT

Defining Characteristics: Drowsiness, dizziness, weakness, lethargy, fatigue are common; confusion, disorientation, hallucinations may occur in the elderly. Extrapyramidal symptoms may occur (fine tremor, rigidity, dystonia, dysarthria, dysphagia), as may peripheral neuropathy and blurred vision.

Nursing Implications: Assess baseline gait, neurologic and mental status, and monitor during therapy. Instruct patient to report signs/symptoms; discuss benefit/risk ratio with physician. Assess for signs/symptoms of suicidal ideation; if they occur, refer for psychiatric evaluation. Inform patient that drowsiness, dizziness will resolve after 1–2 weeks; instruct to avoid hazardous activities while drowsy (e.g., driving a car, operating machinery).

II. ALTERATION IN CARDIAC OUTPUT related to POSTURAL HYPOTENSION, TACHYCARDIA

Defining Characteristics: Postural hypotension, EKG changes, tachycardia, hypertension may occur.

Nursing Implications: Assess baseline orthostatic BP, heart rate, and monitor during therapy. Instruct patient to report abnormalities, including postural dizziness, palpitations. Drug should be stopped several days before surgery to prevent hypertensive crisis (especially if high dose is used).

III. ALTERATION IN NUTRITION related to GI SIDE EFFECTS

Defining Characteristics: Dry mouth, anorexia, nausea, vomiting, diarrhea, and abdominal cramping may occur; also, elevated LFTs.

Nursing Implications: Assess baseline nutrition and elimination patterns and LFTs, and monitor during therapy. Discuss abnormalities with physician, and discuss drug modification. Teach patient to self-administer prescribed antiemetics as appropriate. LFTs should be repeated, and if still elevated, the drug should be discontinued. Instruct patient to take full dose at bedtime. Suggest patient use sugar-free hard candy, frequent ice chips, or artificial saliva for dry mouth.

IV. ALTERATION IN URINARY ELIMINATION related to URINARY RETENTION

Defining Characteristics: Urinary retention may occur. Increased risk in patients with history of urinary retention.

Nursing Implications: Assess baseline urinary elimination pattern and risk. Assess for urinary retention, and instruct patient to report signs/symptoms. Discuss alternative drug with physician if this occurs.

V. ALTERATIONS IN SKIN INTEGRITY related to ALLERGY

Defining Characteristics: Urticaria, erythema, rash, photosensitivity may occur.

Nursing Implications: Assess baseline drug allergy history and skin integrity. Instruct patient to report skin changes. If angioedema of face, tongue develops, discuss drug discontinuance with physician. Instruct patient to avoid sunlight or to use sunblock protection.

Drug: lorazepam (Ativan)

Class: Benzodiazepine (anxiolytic).

Mechanism of Action: Binds to benzodiazepine receptors in the CNS (limbic and cortical areas, cerebellum, brain stem, and spinal cord), resulting in the following effects: anxiolytic, ataxia, anticonvulsant, muscle relaxation. Appears to potentiate the effects of GABA.

Metabolism: Well absorbed from GI tract. Widely distributed in body tissues and fluids, including CSF. Crosses placenta and is excreted in breast milk. Highly bound to plasma proteins. Metabolized in liver and excreted in urine. Short half-life of 10–20 hours. May produce psychological and physical dependence. Indicated for management of anxiety and short-term relief of anxiety associated with depression.

Dosage/Range:

Adult:

- Oral: 1–6 mg/day in divided doses (maximum 10 mg/day).
- IM: 0.044 mg/kg or 2 mg, whichever is smaller (initial dose).
- IV: 0.044 mg/kg (up to 2 mg) given 15–20 minutes prior to surgery; 1.4 mg/m^2 given 30 minutes prior to chemotherapy; or 0.05 mg/kg (maximum 4 mg) if perioperative amnesia is desired.
- Use maximum dose (2 mg) in patients > 50 years old.

Drug Preparation:

- Oral: may administer with food to decrease stomach upset; has been given sublingually for more rapid onset (investigational).
- IM and IV: store drug in refrigerator until use.
- IM: administer undiluted, deep IM in large muscle mass (e.g., gluteus maximus).
- IV: dilute in equal volume of 0.9% sodium chloride or 5% dextrose for IVP administration (administer slowly; not > than 2 mg/min) OR dilute in 50 mL 0.9% sodium chloride or 5% dextrose immediately prior to administering IVB over 15 minutes.

Drug Interactions:

- CNS depressants (alcohol, anticonvulsants, phenothiazines, opiates): additive CNS depression; avoid concurrent use or use cautiously and monitor carefully.
- Oral contraceptives, isoniazid, ketoconazole: decrease plasma clearance of lorazepam so may increase effect (e.g., sedation); monitor patient closely.
- Tricyclic antidepressants: increased serum levels of antidepressant possible; use together cautiously.
- Digoxin: may decrease renal excretion of digoxin; monitor for overdosage; may need to decrease digoxin.

Lab Effects/Interference:

- Rarely, leukopenia, elevated LDH.
- Less frequently, elevated liver function studies.

Special Considerations:

- Wide margin of safety between therapeutic and toxic doses.
- May impair ability to perform activities requiring mental alertness (e.g., driving a car, operating machinery).
- May produce psychological and physical dependence.
- Administer cautiously in patients with liver or renal impairment.
- Use cautiously in patients with chronic pulmonary disease or sleep apnea.

- Contraindicated in patients with depressive neuroses, psychotic reactions (without prominent anxiety), acute alcoholic intoxication (with depressed VS), known hypersensitivity to the drug, or acute angle-closure glaucoma.
- May cause fetal damage, so should not be used during pregnancy or if the mother is breast-feeding.
- Withdrawal symptoms (including seizure, delirium) can occur with rapid drug discontinuance in patients taking high or chronic doses.
- If manic episodes or hyperactivity occur soon after drug started, drug should be discontinued.
- Drug should not be used to manage "everyday stress."
- Causes anterograde amnesia.

Potential Toxicities/Side Effects and the Nursing Process

I. ALTERATIONS IN SENSORY/PERCEPTUAL PATTERNS related to CNS DEPRESSION

Defining Characteristics: CNS depressant effects include drowsiness, fatigue, lethargy, confusion, weakness, headache, which may occur initially and resolve with continued therapy or dose reduction. Vivid dreams, suicidal ideation, and bizarre behavior may also occur. Patient risk factors: elderly, debilitated, liver dysfunction, low serum albumin.

Nursing Implications: Assess baseline neurologic status and risk factors, and monitor during treatment. Instruct patient to report signs/symptoms and discuss drug modification with physician. Evaluate patient satisfaction with drug efficacy. If patient expresses suicidal ideation (more common in panic disorders), refer patient for psychiatric evaluation and drug modification. Instruct patient to avoid alcohol while taking drug. Teach patient prescribed schedule for discontinuing drug when used chronically; assess for signs/symptoms of withdrawal (increased anxiety, rebound insomnia; may also include agitation, dysphoria, nausea/vomiting, irritability, muscle cramps, hallucinations, seizures).

II. ALTERATION IN NUTRITION, LESS THAN BODY REQUIREMENTS, related to GI SIDE EFFECTS

Defining Characteristics: Nausea, vomiting, weight increase or decrease, dry mouth, constipation may occur; also elevated serum LFTs.

Nursing Implications: Assess baseline nutrition and elimination patterns and LFTs, and monitor during therapy. Discuss abnormalities with physician and discuss drug modification. Teach patient to self-administer prescribed antiemetics as appropriate.

III. INJURY related to DECREASE IN MENTAL ALERTNESS, PHYSICAL COORDINATION

Defining Characteristics: Drug may cause drowsiness, dizziness, and impair physical coordination, mental alertness. Sedation, amnesia may last hours, impaired thinking and coordination 24–48 hours, and longer in the elderly.

Nursing Implications: Assess other medications that may increase risk (e.g., opiates, phenothiazines) and response to drug. Instruct patient to avoid potentially hazardous activities, including driving a car, operating machinery. For 8 hours following IV injection, assess level of consciousness and instruct patient to call nurse for assistance in ambulating if needed. Instruct patient to avoid alcohol for 24–48 hours after drug injection.

IV. ALTERATIONS IN CARDIAC OUTPUT related to CHANGES IN BP, HR

Defining Characteristics: Drug may cause bradycardia, tachycardia, hypertension or hypotension, palpitations, edema.

Nursing Implications: Assess baseline VS, and monitor during therapy. Discuss abnormalities with physician. Instruct patient to report dizziness upon standing or other changes.

V. ALTERATIONS IN SKIN INTEGRITY related to RASH

Defining Characteristics: Urticaria, pruritus, rash (morbilliform, urticarial, or maculopapular) may occur.

Nursing Implications: Assess baseline skin integrity, and instruct patient to report changes. Teach symptomatic skin management, and discuss drug discontinuance with physician if severe.

Drug: mirtazapine (Remeron)

Class: Antidepressant.

Mechanism of Action: Centrally active presynaptic a2-antagonist, which increases central noradrenergic and serotonergic neurotransmission (via 5-HT_1 receptors). Drug also blocks 5-HT_2 and 5-HT_3 receptors that contribute to antidepressant action. Thus, drug increases brain levels of both serotonin and norepinephrine. Antagonizes histamine H_1 causing some sedation but has limited anticholinergic or cardiovascular effects.

Metabolism: Active ingredient mirtazapine is rapidly absorbed from the GI tract with > 50% bioavailability. Peak plasma level is reached in about 2 hours, with approximately 85% of drug protein bound. Mean elimination half-life is 20–40 hours with rare variation (up to 65 hours vs shorter in young men). Steady state reached in 3–4 days. Drug extensively metabolized (demethylation, oxidation, conjugation) and eliminated via urine and feces in a few days. Renal or hepatic insufficiency can delay drug clearance.

Dosage/Range:

Adults:

- 15 mg PO daily to start, increasing in 2–4 weeks to a maximum of 45 mg daily if no response.
- If no response at maximal dose in 2–4 weeks, stop drug.
- Monitor elderly patients during dose titration. Use lowest dose, and monitor patients with renal or hepatic insufficiency closely due to reduced drug clearance.
- Response should be seen in 2–4 weeks of treatment at optimal dose.
- Once a response is obtained, drug is usually continued until the patient is symptom free for 4–6 months, and then the drug is gradually discontinued.

Drug Preparation:

- Tablets available in 15-, 30-, and 45-mg strengths, as well as in SolTab Orally Disintegrating Tablets (ODT), which dissolve on the tongue within 30 seconds.
- Administer tablets in a single daily dose at bedtime or in 2 divided doses (morning and evening).
- Administer SolTab ODT with or without water, to be chewed or allowed to disintegrate on the tongue.
- Store drug in the dark at 2–30° C.

Drug Interactions:

- Alcohol: AVOID concurrent use as potentiation of CNS depressant effects.
- Monamine Oxidase Inhibitors (MAOI): AVOID concurrent use; DO NOT start mirtazapine until at least 2 weeks after the cessation of MAOI, and do not start a MAOI until at least 2 weeks after cessation of mirtazapine.
- Benzodiazepines: Potentiate CNS depressant effects of drug. Use together cautiously, if at all.

Lab Effects/Interference:

- Transient increase in hepatic transaminases (SGOT/AST and SGPT/ALT).

Special Considerations:

- Rarely, granulocytopenia or agranulocytosis may occur, usually after 4–6 weeks of treatment.
- Possibility of suicide attempt may exist in depression and persist until depression is managed by drug. Monitor high-risk patients closely and give smallest prescription of tablets to ensure frequent follow-up and reduce the risk of overdosage.
- Avoid use in women who are pregnant or breast-feeding.

- Discontinue the drug if jaundice develops.
- Abrupt termination of drug after long-term therapy can result in nausea, headache, and malaise.
- Patients requiring close monitoring for toxicity: include those with epilepsy or organic brain syndrome; hepatic or renal insufficiency; heart disease, including conduction disturbances, and angina pectoris, or history of myocardial infarction; hypotension; prostatic hypertrophy or other voiding (micturition) disturbances; acute narrow angle glaucoma; and diabetes mellitus.
- Teach all patients/families: call provider right away if thoughts of suicide or dying; attempts to commit suicide; new or worse depression; new or worse anxiety; feeling very agitated or restless; panic attacks; trouble sleeping (insomnia); new or worse irritability; aggressive, angry, or violent behavior; acting on dangerous impulses; extreme increase in activity or talking (mania); any unusual changes in behavior or mood.

Potential Toxicities/Side Effects and the Nursing Process

I. ALTERATION IN NUTRITION, MORE THAN BODY REQUIREMENTS, related to INCREASED APPETITE, WEIGHT GAIN, EDEMA

Defining Characteristics: Increased appetite and weight gain are common. Peripheral edema may occur, resulting in increased weight. Drug may be chosen for its appetite stimulation in patients with advanced cancer who are depressed and losing weight.

Nursing Implications: Assess baseline nutrition pattern and weight, and monitor during therapy. Assess baseline fluid status and presence of edema, and monitor during therapy. Teach patient that these side effects may occur and to report them, especially edema. If patient develops significant edema, assess cardiopulmonary status (heart rate, orthostatic blood pressure, respiratory rate at rest and with activity, oxygen saturation). Discuss significant edema with physician.

II. ALTERATIONS IN SENSORY/PERCEPTUAL PATTERNS related to CNS EFFECTS

Defining Characteristics: CNS effects include drowsiness and sedation, especially during the first few weeks of treatment. Rarely, seizure, tremor, or myoclonus may occur. Worsening of psychotic symptoms may occur in patients with schizophrenia or other psychotic disturbances, and paranoid thoughts may become intensified. Mania may become activated in patients with manic depressive psychosis. Patients at risk for suicide may attempt/commit suicide during initial period of treatment.

Nursing Implications: Assess baseline neurologic status and risk factors, and monitor during treatment. Instruct patient to report signs/symptoms, and discuss drug modification with physician. Evaluate patient satisfaction with drug efficacy. Teach patient to avoid alcohol while taking drug, and to avoid benzodiazepines unless physician feels benefits outweigh risks. Assess suicide risk, and if at high risk, monitor closely, provide supportive counseling, and prescribe only a small number of pills to prevent overdosage. May take up to 4 weeks for therapeutic effect to be seen.

III. POTENTIAL FOR INJURY related to DECREASE IN MENTAL ALERTNESS, PHYSICAL COORDINATION, ORTHOSTATIC HYPOTENSION

Defining Characteristics: Drug may cause drowsiness, decreased mental alertness, and orthostatic hypotension.

Nursing Implications: Assess other medications patient is taking that may increase the risk (e.g., opiates, phenothiazines) and response to drug. Instruct patient to avoid potentially hazardous activities, such as driving a car or other vehicle, and operating machinery. Assess baseline orthostatic blood pressure and heart rate, and monitor during therapy. Teach patient that orthostatic hypotension may occur, and to report symptoms such as dizziness when changing position. Teach patient self-care measures to minimize risk of injury, such as changing position slowly over the course of 5 minutes, going from lying to sitting, and then from sitting to standing positions, holding on to walls or fixed railings when walking, and removing scatter rugs from walkways.

IV. POTENTIAL FOR INFECTION, BLEEDING, AND FATIGUE related to RARE BONE MARROW DEPRESSION

Defining Characteristics: Rare granulocytopenia or agranulocytosis may occur, usually after 4–6 weeks of treatment. If it occurs, it is usually reversible following drug discontinuance.

Nursing Implications: Teach patient that this rare side effect may occur. Instruct patient to stop the drug and to report signs and symptoms of infection, such as fever, sore throat, productive cough, or dysuria right away. If the patient develops any signs and symptoms of infection, the drug should be stopped and a complete blood count with differential checked. Assess baseline CBC/differential, and periodically during therapy, especially at 4–6 weeks after drug initiated.

V. POTENTIAL ALTERATION IN SKIN INTEGRITY related to EXANTHEMA

Defining Characteristics: Rarely, skin rash resembling chicken pox, measles, or rubella may develop.

Nursing Implications: Assess baseline skin integrity, and instruct patient to report rash immediately. Discuss drug cessation or discontinuance with physician. Teach patient symptomatic skin management.

Drug: nefazodone HCl (Serzone)

Class: Antidepressant, synthetically derived phenylpiperazine.

Mechanism of Action: Appears to inhibit neuronal uptake of serotonin and norepinephrine. Drug occupies central serotonin (5-HT_2) receptors and acts as an antagonist. In addition, it antagonizes α-adrenergic receptors that may explain the associated postural hypotension.

Metabolism: Rapidly and completely absorbed after oral administration, but extensively metabolized by the liver using the P-450 cytochrome enzyme system. Food delays absorption and decreases bioavailability by 20%. Peak plasma concentrations occur at 1 hour, and half-life of the drug is 2–4 hours. Drug is extensively protein-bound (> 99%). Time to steady-state is 4–5 days. Only 1% of drug is excreted unchanged in the urine.

Dosage/Range:

Adult:

- Initial: 200 mg/day, administered in two divided doses.
- If no or slight response, increase dose by 100–200 mg/day in two divided doses after at least one week at the previous dose; usual dose requirements are 300–600 mg/day in two divided doses.
- Elderly (especially women) or debilitated patients: begin at 50% of dose or 100 mg/day in two divided doses, and titrate up to therapeutic dose very slowly and gradually.

Drug Preparation/Administration:

- Oral, total dose given in two divided, bid doses on an empty stomach.
- Available in 100-, 150-, 200-, and 250-mg tablets.
- If changing from an MAOI to nefazodone HCl, allow at least 14 days after discontinuance of the MAOI before starting nefazodone; if changing from nefazodone to an MAOI, allow at least 7 days after stopping nefazodone before starting the MAOI.

Drug Interactions:

- Terfenadine, astemizole, cisapride: are metabolized by the P-450 hepatic enzyme system; nefazodone can inhibit their metabolism, resulting in QT elongation and potential cardiac arrest; DO NOT GIVE CONCOMITANTLY WITH NEFAZODONE.
- MAOIs: may cause symptoms resembling neuroleptic malignant syndrome, including death. DO NOT USE CONCURRENTLY. See administration guidelines above when changing from/to MAOIs.

- Alprazolam: increased serum levels of alprazolam; monitor effect and toxicity, and determine need for dose reduction.
- Digoxin: increased plasma levels of digoxin; assess effect and toxicity, and need for dose reduction of digoxin.
- Propranolol: decreased plasma levels of propranolol; assess effect and need for increased dosage.
- Triazolam: increased plasma levels of triazolam; assess effect, toxicity, and need for dosage reduction.

Lab Effects/Interference:
- Rarely, increased AST, ALT, LDH.
- Rarely, decreased HCT, anemia, leukopenia.
- Rarely, hypercholesterolemia, hypoglycemia.

Special Considerations:
- Contraindications: coadministration with terfenadine, astemizole, cisapride, or MAOIs.
- Drug produces slight anticholinergic effects, moderate sedation, and slight orthostatic hypotension.
- May take several weeks until therapeutic effect is known.
- Use with caution in patients recovering from myocardial infarction, who have unstable heart disease and are taking digoxin, and patients with a history of mania.
- Monitor patients at risk for suicide carefully, as attempts may be made during initial period before significant antidepressant effects of the drug are seen.
- Avoid use during pregnancy or in nursing mothers.
- Teach all patients/families: call provider right away if thoughts of suicide or dying; attempts to commit suicide; new or worse depression; new or worse anxiety; feeling very agitated or restless; panic attacks; trouble sleeping (insomnia); new or worse irritability; aggressive, angry, or violent behavior; acting on dangerous impulses; extreme increase in activity or talking (mania); any unusual changes in behavior or mood.

Potential Toxicities/Side Effects and the Nursing Process

I. ALTERATIONS IN SENSORY/PERCEPTUAL PATTERNS related to DROWSINESS, DIZZINESS

Defining Characteristics: Dizziness (17% incidence), drowsiness (25%), insomnia (17%), lightheadedness (10%), activation of mania or hypomania, agitation, blurred vision (9%), confusion (7%), decreased concentration (3%), memory impairment (4%), paresthesia (4%), ataxia (2%), incoordination (2%), psychomotor retardation (2%), tremor (1%), hypertonia (1%), vertigo, twitching, hallucinations, abnormal dreams (3%), and paranoia may occur. Neuroleptic malignant syndrome is rare (e.g., hyperthermia, seizures).

Nursing Implications: Assess baseline gait, neurologic and mental status, and monitor during therapy. Instruct patient to report signs/symptoms; depending upon severity and dysfunction, discuss benefit/risk ratio with physician. Assess for signs/symptoms of suicidal ideation; if they occur, refer for psychiatric evaluation. Inform patient that drowsiness, dizziness will resolve after 1–2 weeks; instruct to avoid hazardous activities while drowsy (e.g., driving a car, operating machinery).

II. ALTERATION IN CARDIAC OUTPUT related to POSTURAL HYPOTENSION, TACHYCARDIA

Defining Characteristics: Infrequent postural hypotension (4% incidence), hypotension (2%), tachycardia, hypertension, syncope, ventricular ectopic beats, angina pectoris, and CVA may occur rarely.

Nursing Implications: Assess baseline orthostatic BP, heart rate, and monitor during therapy. Instruct patient to report abnormalities, including postural dizziness, palpitations. If patient has orthostatic hypotension, teach patient to change position slowly and to hold on to supportive structure. If symptoms are significant, discuss changing to another antidepressant with physician.

III. ALTERATION IN NUTRITION, LESS THAN BODY REQUIREMENTS, related to GI SIDE EFFECTS

Defining Characteristics: Dry mouth (25% incidence), nausea (22%), vomiting (rare), diarrhea (5%), constipation (14%), dyspepsia (9%), and rarely eructation, gastritis, stomatitis, peptic ulceration, rectal hemorrhage have been reported.

Nursing Implications: Assess baseline nutrition and elimination patterns and LFTs, and monitor during therapy. Discuss abnormalities with physician, and discuss drug modification. Teach patient to self-administer prescribed antiemetics, and other symptom management interventions as ordered. Suggest patient use sugar-free hard candy, frequent ice chips, or artificial saliva for dry mouth.

IV. ALTERATION IN URINARY ELIMINATION related to URINARY FREQUENCY

Defining Characteristics: Infrequently, (2% incidence) urinary frequency, urinary retention, and urinary tract infections may occur.

Nursing Implications: Assess baseline urinary elimination pattern and risk. Assess for urinary frequency, retention, and infection, and instruct patient to report signs/symptoms. Discuss alternative drug with physician if this occurs.

V. ALTERATION IN COMFORT related to HEADACHE

Defining Characteristics: Headache (36% incidence), asthenia (11%), arthralgia (1%) may occur.

Nursing Implications: Assess baseline comfort. Instruct patient to report unrelieved symptoms, and consider symptom-management strategies. Discuss severe discomfort that is unrelieved with physician and consider alternative antidepressant therapy.

Drug: nortriptyline hydrochloride (Aventyl, Pamelor)

Class: Tricyclic antidepressant.

Mechanism of Action: Blocks reuptake of neurotransmitters at neuronal membrane, thus increasing available serotonin, norepinephrine in CNS, and potentiating their effects. May increase bioavailability of morphine. Indicated in the treatment of depressive (affective) mood disorders. Also used as an adjuvant analgesic in cancer pain management.

Metabolism: Distributed to lungs, heart, brain, liver; highly bound to plasma, proteins. Plasma half-life is 16–90 hours. Metabolized in liver, excreted in urine, and, to a lesser degree, in bile and feces.

Dosage/Range:

Adult:

- Oral: 75–100 mg/day (maximum 100 mg or serum levels should be monitored; therapeutic dose: 50–150 mg/mL).
- Elderly: 30–50 mg/day.

Drug Preparation:

- Store oral solution in tight, light-resistant containers; store tablets in tight containers; keep at temperature of 15–30°C (59–86°F).
- Administer in single bedtime dose.

Drug Interactions:

- MAOIs: increased excitation, hyperpyrexia, seizures; use together cautiously (especially if high dose is used).
- CNS depressants (alcohol, sedatives, hypnotics): increase CNS depression; use together cautiously.
- Sympathomimetic (epinephrine, amphetamines): increased hypertension; AVOID concurrent use.
- Cimetidine methylphenidate: increased nortriptyline levels, increased toxicity; use cautiously and monitor for increased toxicity.
- Warfarin: may increase PT; monitor closely and decrease dose of warfarin as needed.
- Barbiturates: may decrease nortriptyline levels; monitor patient response; may need to increase dose.

Lab Effects/Interference:
- Rarely, bone marrow depression (agranulocytosis, eosinophilia, purpura, thrombocytopenia).
- Rarely, increased or decreased serum glucose levels.

Special Considerations:
- Antidepressant effect may take two weeks or longer.
- Adjuvant analgesic useful in cancer pain management.
- May also decrease depression associated with chronic cancer pain and promote improved sleep.
- Contraindicated in patients with myocardial infarction, seizure disorder, or benign prostatic hypertrophy.
- Use cautiously in patients with urine retention, narrow-angle glaucoma, hyperthyroidism, hepatic dysfunction, or suicidal ideation.
- Drug should be gradually discontinued rather than abruptly withdrawn to prevent anxiety, malaise, dizziness, nausea/vomiting.
- May be helpful in treating hiccups.
- Increased anticholinergic side effects in elderly.
- Some preparations may contain sodium bisulfite, which can cause allergic reactions, including anaphylaxis, in hypersensitive individuals. Check ingredients and assess allergy history.
- Teach all patients/families: call provider right away if thoughts of suicide or dying; attempts to commit suicide; new or worse depression; new or worse anxiety; feeling very agitated or restless; panic attacks; trouble sleeping (insomnia); new or worse irritability; aggressive, angry, or violent behavior; acting on dangerous impulses; extreme increase in activity or talking (mania); any unusual changes in behavior or mood.

Potential Toxicities/Side Effects and the Nursing Process

I. ALTERATIONS IN SENSORY/PERCEPTUAL PATTERNS related to DROWSINESS, DIZZINESS

Defining Characteristics: Drowsiness, dizziness, weakness, lethargy, fatigue are common; confusion, disorientation, hallucinations may occur in the elderly. Extrapyramidal symptoms may occur (fine tremor, rigidity, dystonia, dysarthria, dysphagia), as may peripheral neuropathy and blurred vision.

Nursing Implications: Assess baseline gait, neurologic and mental status, and monitor during therapy. Instruct patient to report signs/symptoms; discuss benefit/risk ratio with physician. Assess for signs/symptoms of suicidal ideation; if they occur, refer for psychiatric evaluation. Inform patient that drowsiness, dizziness will resolve after 1–2 weeks; instruct to avoid hazardous activities while drowsy (e.g., driving a car, operating machinery).

II. ALTERATION IN CARDIAC OUTPUT related to POSTURAL HYPOTENSION, TACHYCARDIA

Defining Characteristics: Low incidence of postural hypotension; EKG changes, tachycardia, and hypertension may occur.

Nursing Implications: Assess baseline orthostatic BP, heart rate, and monitor during therapy. Instruct patient to report abnormalities, including postural dizziness, palpitations. Drug should be stopped several days before surgery to prevent hypertensive crisis (especially if high dose is used).

III. ALTERATION IN NUTRITION, LESS THAN BODY REQUIREMENTS, related to GI SIDE EFFECTS

Defining Characteristics: Dry mouth, anorexia, nausea, vomiting, diarrhea, abdominal cramping may occur; also, elevated LFTs.

Nursing Implications: Assess baseline nutrition and elimination patterns and LFTs, and monitor during therapy. Discuss abnormalities with physician, and discuss drug modification. Teach patient to self-administer prescribed antiemetics as appropriate. LFTs should be repeated, and if still elevated, the drug should be discontinued. Instruct patient to take full dose at bedtime. Suggest patient use sugar-free hard candy, frequent ice chips, or artificial saliva for dry mouth.

IV. ALTERATION IN URINARY ELIMINATION related to URINARY FREQUENCY

Defining Characteristics: Urinary retention may occur. Increased risk if history of urinary retention.

Nursing Implications: Assess baseline urinary elimination pattern and risk. Assess for urinary retention, and instruct patient to report signs/symptoms. Discuss alternative drug with physician if this occurs.

V. ALTERATIONS IN SKIN INTEGRITY related to ALLERGY

Defining Characteristics: Urticaria, erythema, rash, photosensitivity may occur.

Nursing Implications: Assess baseline drug allergy history and skin integrity. Instruct patient to report skin changes. If angioedema of face, tongue develops, discuss drug discontinuance with physician. Instruct patient to avoid sunlight or to use sunblock protection.

Drug: oxazepam (Serax)

Class: Benzodiazepine (anxiolytic).

Mechanism of Action: Binds to benzodiazepine receptors in the CNS (limbic and cortical areas, cerebellum, brain stem, and spinal cord), resulting in the following effects: anxiolytic, ataxia, anticonvulsant, muscle relaxation. Appears to potentiate the effects of GABA.

Metabolism: Well absorbed from GI tract. Widely distributed in body tissues and fluids, including CSF. Crosses placenta and is excreted in breast milk. Highly bound to plasma proteins. Metabolized in liver and excreted in urine. Short half-life of 5–20 hours. May produce psychological and physical dependence. Indicated for management of anxiety, the short-term relief of anxiety associated with depression, and alcohol withdrawal.

Dosage/Range:

Adult:

- Oral: 10–30 mg tid–qid.
- Elderly: 10 mg tid OR 15 mg tid–qid.

Drug Preparation:

- Store tablets in tight container at < 40°C (104°F).

Drug Interactions:

- CNS depressants (alcohol, anticonvulsants, phenothiazines, opiates): additive CNS depression; avoid concurrent use or use cautiously and monitor carefully.
- Oral contraceptives, isoniazid, ketoconazole, or cimetidine: decrease plasma clearance of oxazepam, so may increase effect (e.g., sedation); monitor patient closely.
- Tricyclic antidepressants: increased serum levels of antidepressant possible; use together cautiously.
- Digoxin: may decrease renal excretion of digoxin; monitor for overdosage; may need to decrease digoxin.

Lab Effects/Interference:

- Rarely, leukopenia.
- Rarely, altered liver function studies.

Special Considerations:

- Wide margin of safety between therapeutic and toxic doses.
- May impair ability to perform activities requiring mental alertness (e.g., driving a car, operating machinery).
- May produce psychological and physical dependence.
- Administer cautiously in patients with liver or renal impairment.
- Use cautiously in patients with chronic pulmonary disease or sleep apnea.

- Contraindicated in patients with depressive neuroses, psychotic reactions (without prominent anxiety), acute alcoholic intoxication (with depressed VS), known hypersensitivity to the drug, or acute angle-closure glaucoma.
- May cause fetal damage, so should not be used during pregnancy or if the mother is breast-feeding.
- Withdrawal symptoms (including seizure, delirium) can occur with rapid drug discontinuance in patients taking high or chronic doses.
- If manic episodes or hyperactivity occur soon after drug started, drug should be discontinued.
- Drug should not be used to manage "everyday stress."
- Serax 15-mg tablet contains dye tartrazine, which may cause allergic reactions in sensitive individuals, especially if sensitive to aspirin.

Potential Toxicities/Side Effects and the Nursing Process

I. ALTERATIONS IN SENSORY/PERCEPTUAL PATTERNS related to CNS DEPRESSION

Defining Characteristics: CNS depressant effects include drowsiness, fatigue, lethargy, weakness. Cumulative effects are less, as there is a short plasma half-life. Risk factors: elderly, debilitated, liver dysfunction, low serum albumin.

Nursing Implications: Assess baseline neurologic status and risk factors, and monitor during treatment. Instruct patient to report signs/symptoms. Instruct patient to avoid alcohol while taking drug. Teach patient prescribed schedule for discontinuing drug when drug is used chronically.

II. ALTERATION IN NUTRITION, LESS THAN BODY REQUIREMENTS, related to GI SIDE EFFECTS

Defining Characteristics: Nausea, vomiting, weight increase or decrease, dry mouth, constipation may occur; also, elevated LFTs.

Nursing Implications: Assess baseline nutrition and elimination patterns and LFTs, and monitor during therapy. Discuss abnormalities with physician and discuss drug modification. Teach patient to self-administer prescribed antiemetics as appropriate.

III. INJURY related to DECREASE IN MENTAL ALERTNESS, PHYSICAL COORDINATION

Defining Characteristics: Drug may cause drowsiness, dizziness, and impair physical coordination, mental alertness.

Nursing Implications: Assess other medications that may increase risk (e.g., opiates, phenothiazines) and response to drug. Instruct patient to avoid potentially hazardous activities, including driving a car, operating machinery.

IV. ALTERATIONS IN CARDIAC OUTPUT related to TRANSIENT HYPOTENSION

Defining Characteristics: Transient hypotension may occur.

Nursing Implications: Assess baseline VS, and monitor during therapy. Discuss abnormalities with physician. Instruct patient to report dizziness on standing or other changes.

V. ALTERATIONS IN SKIN INTEGRITY related to RASH

Defining Characteristics: Urticaria, pruritus, rash (morbilliform, urticarial, or maculopapular) may occur.

Nursing Implications: Assess baseline skin integrity, and instruct patient to report changes. Teach symptomatic skin management, and discuss drug discontinuance with physician if severe.

Drug: paroxetine hydrochloride (Paxil)

Class: Antidepressant with mechanism of action different from selective serotonin reuptake inhibitors, tricyclic, or tetracyclic antidepressants.

Mechanism of Action: Appears to potentiate serotonergic activity of the CNS by potent and selective inhibition of serotonin reuptake by the neurons.

Metabolism: Completely absorbed after oral administration and metabolized to some degree by the P-450 hepatic enzyme system. Distributed throughout the body, including the CNS, and is extensively protein-bound (95%). Increased serum levels occur in patients with hepatic or renal dysfunction (twofold), and in elderly patients. Time to peak plasma levels 5.2 hours, and time to reach steady-state is 10–24 days. Largely excreted in the urine (64%) over a 10-day period, and approximately 36% is excreted in the feces.

Dosage/Range:

Adult (depression):

- Initial: 20 mg/day PO in the morning. Initial response may be delayed; if no response, may increase dose in 10 mg/day increments after an interval of at least one week, to a maximum of 50 mg/day.

- Patients who are elderly, or who have severe hepatic or renal dysfunction: initial dose of 10 mg/day, with increased dose adjustments made after at least one week, in 10 mg/day increments up to a maximum of 40 mg/day.

Drug Preparation:
- Oral, available in 10-, 20-, 30-, and 40-mg tablets.
- Administer as a single daily dose, usually in the morning.
- Allow at least 14 days when changing from an MAOI to paroxetine, or when changing from paroxetine to an MAOI.

Drug Interactions:
- Tryptophan: when administered concomitantly, headache, nausea, sweating, and dizziness may occur; avoid concomitant administration.
- MAOIs: reactions including death have occurred (hyperthermia, rigidity, myoclonus, autonomic instability, mental status changes including delirium/coma); allow at least 14 days between changing to or from paroxetine to an MAOI.
- Warfarin: increased bleeding despite a normal PT; give together cautiously if at all.
- Sumatriptan: may cause hyperreflexia, weakness; incoordination may occur; monitor patient closely.
- Drugs inhibiting the P-450 cytochrome hepatic metabolic pathway (e.g., cimetidine): paroxetine serum levels may be increased by up to 50%; assess response and toxicity carefully and need to decrease paroxetine dosage.
- Drugs inducing the P-450 cytochrome hepatic metabolic pathway (e.g., phenobarbital, phenytoin): paroxetine serum levels may be reduced by up to 25–50%; assess response and need to increase paroxetine dosage.
- Drugs metabolized by the P-450 cytochrome hepatic metabolic pathway (other antidepressant medications, phenothiazines, type 1C antiarrhythmics): paroxetine may inhibit the metabolism of these drugs, resulting in increased toxicity.
- Tricyclic antidepressants should be given together with caution, and the dose of the tricyclic antidepressant may need to be reduced.
- Drugs that are highly bound to plasma proteins: paroxetine may displace the other drug from serum proteins, thus increasing the serum level of the other drug, resulting in toxicity. Give together cautiously and monitor/reduce drug as needed.
- Alcohol: avoid concurrent administration.
- Lithium, digoxin: use together cautiously; digoxin levels may be reduced.
- Procyclidine: increased anticholinergic effects possible; decrease dose of procyclidine if necessary to co-administer.
- Theophylline: may elevate serum theophylline levels; monitor and adjust dose accordingly.

Lab Effects/Interference:
- None known.

Special Considerations:
- Drug excreted in breast milk; drug should be administered cautiously, if at all, in breast-feeding mothers.

- Drug is teratogenic, so women of childbearing age should use contraception if sexually active.
- Drug indicated for the treatment of depression, panic disorder, obsessive/compulsive disorder.
- Teach all patients/families: call provider right away if thoughts of suicide or dying; attempts to commit suicide; new or worse depression; new or worse anxiety; feeling very agitated or restless; panic attacks; trouble sleeping (insomnia); new or worse irritability; aggressive, angry, or violent behavior; acting on dangerous impulses; extreme increase in activity or talking (mania); any unusual changes in behavior or mood.

Potential Toxicities/Side Effects and the Nursing Process

I. ALTERATIONS IN SENSORY/PERCEPTUAL PATTERNS related to DIZZINESS, SOMNOLENCE

Defining Characteristics: Somnolence, dizziness, insomnia, tremor, nervousness, and asthenia occur in more than 5% of patients. Less common are headache, agitation, seizures, anxiety, activation of mania or hypomania, paresthesia, confusion, impaired concentration, emotional lability, depression.

Nursing Implications: Assess baseline neurologic status, affective state, and risk factors, and monitor during treatment. Instruct patient to avoid alcohol while taking drug. Assess effect on elderly and/or patients with hepatic or renal dysfunction. Inform patient that daytime drowsiness may occur, and instruct to use caution if driving or operating heavy machinery. Assess for symptoms at each visit, and instruct patient to report changes. If symptoms occur, discuss strategies to ensure patient safety and comfort.

II. ALTERATION IN NUTRITION, LESS THAN BODY REQUIREMENTS, related to GI SIDE EFFECTS

Defining Characteristics: Nausea and decreased appetite may occur.

Nursing Implications: Assess baseline nutrition status, and instruct patient to report any nausea or loss of appetite. Discuss measures to reduce nausea and/or stimulate appetite.

III. ALTERATION IN COMFORT related to SWEATING

Defining Characteristics: Sweating may occur.

Nursing Implications: Inform patient that this may occur, and assess impact on patient and need for intervention.

IV. SEXUAL DYSFUNCTION, POTENTIAL, related to EJACULATORY DISTURBANCES

Defining Characteristics: Incidence of ejaculatory disturbances is 13%; other disorders may occur (10%), including erectile difficulties, delayed ejaculation/orgasm, impotence, and other sexual dysfunction.

Nursing Implications: Assess baseline sexual functioning. Inform patient that alterations may occur, and instruct to report them. If severe, discuss dysfunction with physician, and whether another antidepressant would provide equal benefit with less dysfunction.

Drug: sertraline hydrochloride (Zoloft)

Class: Antidepressant.

Mechanism of Action: Inhibits CNS neuronal uptake of serotonin.

Metabolism: Undergoes extensive first-pass metabolism by the liver and is excreted in the urine (45% by 9 days) and the feces (40–45%). Time to peak plasma levels is 4.5–8.4 hours, and peak plasma levels are 20–55 mg/mL. Food reduces time to reach peak serum levels. Highly protein bound (98%). Time to steady-state plasma levels is 7 days but is increased to 2–3 weeks in the elderly.

Dosage/Range:

Adult:
- Initial: 50 mg/day.
- If no response after a period of 1–2 weeks, may titrate gradually up to a maximum dose of 200 mg/day.

Drug Preparation/Administration:
- Oral, once daily in morning or evening.
- Available in 25-, 50-, and 100-mg tablets.
- When changing from an MAOI to sertraline HCl, wait at least 14 days after stopping the MAOI before initiating sertraline; when changing from sertraline HCl to an MAOI, wait at least 14 days after stopping sertraline before beginning the MAOI.

Drug Interactions:
- MAOIs: severe reactions, similar to neuroleptic malignant syndrome, including death may occur; DO NOT ADMINISTER CONCURRENTLY; see Administration section.
- Alcohol: DO NOT give concurrently.
- Benzodiazepines: decreased metabolism of benzodiazepine drugs, which are metabolized by the P-450 enzyme system in the liver, resulting in increased serum levels and toxicity; monitor for toxicity and adjust dose accordingly.

- Tolbutamide: decreased clearance with increased serum levels; monitor blood-sugar levels closely.
- Warfarin: increased PT and delayed normalization of same; monitor PT values closely.
- CNS active drugs: monitor effects closely and modify drug doses accordingly (e.g., lithium).

Lab Effects/Interference:

- Increased AST or ALT, total cholesterol, triglycerides.
- Decreased serum uric acid.

Special Considerations:

- Teach all patients/families: call provider right away if thoughts of suicide or dying; attempts to commit suicide; new or worse depression; new or worse anxiety; feeling very agitated or restless; panic attacks; trouble sleeping (insomnia); new or worse irritability; aggressive, angry, or violent behavior; acting on dangerous impulses; extreme increase in activity or talking (mania); any unusual changes in behavior or mood.

Potential Toxicities/Side Effects and the Nursing Process

I. ALTERATIONS IN SENSORY/PERCEPTUAL PATTERNS related to HEADACHE, INSOMNIA

Defining Characteristics: Commonly, headache, insomnia. Less commonly, drowsiness, dizziness, agitation, nervousness, anxiety, tremor, fatigue, impaired concentration, paresthesia, yawning, hypoesthesia, twitching, confusion, abnormal coordination (ataxia), abnormal gait, hyperesthesia, hyperkinesia, abnormal dreams, amnesia, apathy, hallucinations. Suicidal ideation or attempt is uncommon, but patients at risk may attempt suicide during initial treatment before therapeutic effects of drug are felt.

Nursing Implications: Assess baseline gait, neurologic, affective, and mental status, and monitor during therapy. Instruct patient to report signs/symptoms; discuss benefit/risk ratio with physician. Assess for signs/symptoms of suicidal ideation; if they occur, refer for psychiatric evaluation. Inform patient that drowsiness may occur, and instruct to avoid hazardous activities while drowsy (e.g., driving a car, operating machinery).

II. ALTERATION IN CARDIAC OUTPUT, POTENTIAL, related to CHANGES IN BP

Defining Characteristics: Rarely, palpitations, edema, hypertension or hypotension, peripheral ischemia, postural hypotension, tachycardia, and syncope may occur.

Nursing Implications: Assess baseline orthostatic BP, heart rate, and monitor during therapy. Instruct patient to report abnormalities, including postural dizziness, palpitations.

Discuss significant changes with physician. If patient has orthostatic hypotension, teach patient to change position slowly and to hold on to support.

III. ALTERATION IN NUTRITION, LESS THAN BODY REQUIREMENTS, related to GI SIDE EFFECTS

Defining Characteristics: Nausea and diarrhea are common. Less common are dry mouth, constipation, dyspepsia, increased or decreased appetite, vomiting, increased salivation, abdominal pain, gastroenteritis, dysphagia, eructation, taste changes; also, elevated LFTs.

Nursing Implications: Assess baseline nutrition and elimination patterns and LFTs, and monitor during therapy. Discuss abnormalities with physician, and discuss drug modification. Teach patient to self-administer prescribed antiemetics as appropriate. Suggest patient use sugar-free hard candy, frequent ice chips, or artificial saliva for dry mouth.

IV. ALTERATION IN URINARY ELIMINATION related to URINARY FREQUENCY

Defining Characteristics: Urinary frequency, dysuria, urinary incontinence, nocturia, polyuria may occur.

Nursing Implications: Assess baseline urinary elimination pattern and risk. Assess for changes in urinary elimination, and instruct patient to report signs/symptoms. Discuss alternative drug with physician if this occurs.

V. ALTERATIONS IN SKIN INTEGRITY related to RASH

Defining Characteristics: Maculopapular rash, acne, facial edema, pruritus, excessive sweating, alopecia, and dry skin may occur rarely.

Nursing Implications: Assess baseline skin integrity. Instruct patient to report skin changes. If angioedema of face, tongue develops, discuss drug discontinuance with physician. Assess impact of changes on patient and discuss strategies to minimize distress.

VI. SEXUAL DYSFUNCTION, POTENTIAL, related to MENSTRUAL IRREGULARITY, ↓ LIBIDO

Defining Characteristics: Menstrual disorders, dysmenorrhea, intermenstrual bleeding, sexual dysfunction, decreased libido may occur.

Nursing Implications: Assess baseline sexual functioning. Inform patient that alterations may occur, and instruct to report them. If severe, discuss dysfunction with physician, and whether another antidepressant would provide equal benefit with less dysfunction.

Drug: trazodone hydrochloride (Desyrel, Trialodine)

Class: Antidepressant.

Mechanism of Action: Appears to selectively inhibit the uptake of serotonin by brain synaptosomes and potentiates the behavioral changes induced by the serotonin precursor, 5-hydroxytryptophan.

Metabolism: Well absorbed after oral administration, with peak plasma levels occurring at 1 hour when taken on an empty stomach and at 2 hours when taken with food. Metabolized by the liver and excreted in the urine and feces. Time to steady-state is 3–7 days. Elimination half-life initially is 3–6 hours, followed by slower phase with a half-life of 5–9 hours.

Dosage/Range:

Adult:

- Initial dose of 150 mg in divided doses.
- Increase dose by 50 mg/day q 3–4 days (maximum outpatient dosage is 300 mg/day, and inpatient is 600 mg/day in divided doses).

Maintenance:

- Lowest possible dose; once therapeutic effect reached, may be able to gradually reduce dose.

Elderly:

- 75 mg/day in divided doses; increase dose as needed and tolerated, every 3–4 days.

Drug Preparation:

- Oral administration, shortly after a meal or light snack, in divided doses.
- If drowsiness, may take majority of dose at bedtime.

Drug Interactions:

- Alcohol, CNS depressants: increased CNS depression; DO NOT GIVE TOGETHER.
- Antihypertensives: additive hypotension; evaluate and modify dose of antihypertensive as needed.
- Barbiturates: increased CNS depression; avoid concomitant use.
- Clonidine: reduced effect of clonidine; assess need for increased clonidine dosage.
- Digoxin: trazodone may increase serum digoxin levels; assess effects, and need to decrease digoxin dosage.
- MAOIs: initiate combined therapy cautiously and monitor patient for toxicity.
- Phenytoin: serum phenytoin levels may be increased; monitor levels and therapeutic effect and need for reduced phenytoin dosage.

Lab Effects/Interference:
- Occasional decreased WBC and neutrophil count.

Special Considerations:
- 75% of patients will respond within 2 weeks of therapy, and the remainder within 2–4 weeks.
- Drug causes moderate sedative effects and orthostatic hypotension, with slight anticholinergic effects.
- Contraindicated in patients during recovery from myocardial infarction, or patients receiving electroshock therapy.
- Elderly may be more vulnerable to sedative and hypotensive effects of drug.
- Teach all patients/families: call provider right away if thoughts of suicide or dying; attempts to commit suicide; new or worse depression; new or worse anxiety; feeling very agitated or restless; panic attacks; trouble sleeping (insomnia); new or worse irritability; aggressive, angry, or violent behavior; acting on dangerous impulses; extreme increase in activity or talking (mania); any unusual changes in behavior or mood.

Potential Toxicities/Side Effects and the Nursing Process

I. SEXUAL DYSFUNCTION related to PRIAPISM

Defining Characteristics: Priapism (prolonged or inappropriate penile erection) may occur, and has required surgical intervention in some cases, and in others there was permanent dysfunction.

Nursing Implications: Teach male patients that this may occur. If it does, patient should immediately discontinue the drug and call physician. Make certain the patient understands the instructions and knows how to contact the physician. If priapism has persisted for 24 hours or more, a urologist should be consulted.

II. ALTERATIONS IN SENSORY/PERCEPTUAL PATTERNS related to CNS DEPRESSION

Defining Characteristics: CNS depressant effects include drowsiness, fatigue, nightmares, confusion, anger, excitement, decreased ability to concentrate, disorientation, insomnia, nervousness, impaired memory, dizziness, lightheadedness; rarely, hallucinations, impaired speech, hypomania, incoordination, tremors, paresthesias may occur.

Nursing Implications: Assess baseline gait, neurologic status, affective state, and risk factors, and monitor during treatment. Instruct patient to report worsening depression, and assess for any suicidal ideation. Instruct patient to avoid alcohol while taking drug. Assess effect on elderly and/or debilitated patients (cognition, motor function, other sensitivities). Assess effect of drug side effects on patient, and weigh against benefit. Inform patient that daytime drowsiness may occur, and instruct to use caution if driving or operating heavy machinery. If sleep problems, have patient take majority of dose at bedtime to enhance sleep.

III. ALTERATION IN NUTRITION, LESS THAN BODY REQUIREMENTS, related to GI SIDE EFFECTS

Defining Characteristics: Diarrhea, nausea, vomiting, flatulence may occur rarely.

Nursing Implications: Assess baseline nutrition status, and instruct the patient to report any nausea or vomiting. If required, discuss with physician antiemetic to manage symptoms. If severe, discuss alternative antidepressant medications.

IV. INJURY related to DECREASE IN MENTAL ALERTNESS, PHYSICAL COORDINATION

Defining Characteristics: Drug may cause drowsiness, dizziness, blurred vision, and impair physical coordination, mental alertness.

Nursing Implications: Assess baseline mental alertness, and teach patient to assess tolerance of medication before driving a car or operating heavy machinery. Assess medication profile to identify other medications that may increase risk (e.g., opiates, phenothiazines) and response to drug.

V. ALTERATION IN OXYGENATION, POTENTIAL, related to CHANGES IN BP, SYNCOPE

Defining Characteristics: Rarely, hypotension or hypertension, syncope, palpitations, tachycardia, shortness of breath, and chest pain may occur.

Nursing Implications: Assess baseline cardiovascular status, and vital signs, and monitor during therapy at each visit. Instruct patient to report any palpitations, chest pain, or any changes in condition. Discuss significant symptoms with the physician. If patient is hypotensive and receiving antihypertensive medication, discuss with physician discontinuing or dose-reducing the antihypertensive medication. Prior to elective surgery, because interaction with anesthesia is unknown, temporarily discontinue drug.

Drug: venlafaxine hydrochloride (Effexor)

Class: Serotonin-norepinephrine reuptake inhibitor (SNRI) antidepressant.

Mechanism of Action: Appears to potentiate neurotransmitter activity by inhibiting neuronal serotonin and norepinephrine reuptake.

Metabolism: Well absorbed after oral administration, and eliminated via the kidneys; time to reach steady-state is 3–4 days. Drug and metabolite half-lives are 5 ± 2 and 11 ± 2 hours. Increased drug serum levels in patients with renal or hepatic dysfunction.

Dosage/Range:

Adult (indicated for the treatment of depression and generalized anxiety disorder):

- Initial (extended-release capsule): 75 mg once a day, at the same time each day; if indicated, can start dose at 37.5 mg once daily for 4–7 days, increasing to 75-mg capsule strength; if no response after adequate trial at 75 mg per day, may increase dose in 75-mg increments after at least a 4-day trial at the previous dose, up to a maximum of 225 mg per day in a single dose.
- Initial (immediate-release tablets): 75 mg/day in two or three divided doses.
- If little or no response, dose may be increased in dose increments of up to 75 mg/day after at least 4 days at the previous dose, to 150 mg/day, and up to a maximum of 225 mg/day for moderately depressed patients. Severely depressed patients may need up to 350–375 mg/day in three divided doses.
- Patients with hepatic dysfunction: daily dose should be reduced at least 50%.
- Patients with renal impairment: Mild to moderate dysfunction: reduce daily dose by 25%; patients receiving hemodialysis: 50% dose reduction; dose is given after dialysis.

Drug Preparation/Administration:

- Effexor XR tablets available in a 225-mg dose (uses Osmodex controlled-release technology).
- XL capsule available in 37.5-mg, 75-mg, and 150-mg strengths.
- Immediate-release tablets available as 25-, 37.5-, 50-, 75-, and 100-mg tablets.
- Drug should be administered orally with food in a single dose in morning or at night (same time every day) for extended-release capsule, or in two to three divided doses for tablets.
- When changing from an MAOI to venlafaxine HCl, wait at least 14 days after MAOI is stopped; when stopping venlafaxine HCl and beginning an MAOI, wait at least 7 days.
- When discontinuing drug after > 1 week of therapy, taper dose. If more than 6 weeks of therapy, taper over 2 weeks.

Drug Interactions:

- MAOIs: tremor, myoclonus, diaphoresis, nausea, vomiting, flushing, dizziness, hyperthermia resembling neuroleptic malignant syndrome, and may be fatal. DO NOT USE TOGETHER. See Administration section.
- Cimetidine: may increase venlafaxine HCl serum levels that are significant in patients with existing hypertension, hepatic dysfunction, or who are elderly; use with caution in these patients and monitor closely.
- Haloperidol: may increase haloperidol serum levels; monitor patient when drugs are administered concomitantly.

Lab Effects/Interference:

- Infrequent increased alk phos, creatinine, transaminases AST, ALT.

- Infrequent hyperglycemia with glycosuria, hyperlipemia, bilirubinemia, hyperuricemia, hypercholesterolemia, hypoglycemia, hypokalemia, hyperkalemia, hyperphosphatemia, hyponatremia, hypophosphatemia, hypoproteinemia, uremia, albuminuria.

Special Considerations:
- Avoid drug use during pregnancy and in nursing mothers.
- Dose-reduce in patients with hepatic or renal dysfunction.
- Use caution in patients with mania.
- Use for more than 4–6 weeks has not been evaluated.
- Contraindicated in patients receiving MAOIs.
- Studies have shown equal efficacy to fluoxetine (Costa, 1998; Silverstone and Ravindran, 1999).
- Serious adverse reactions have occurred in patients changing from MAOIs to venlafaxine HCl or from venlafaxine to an MAOI. It is imperative to wait 14 days changing from MAOIs to venlafaxine HCl or 7 days after stopping venlafaxine before starting an MAOI.
- Teach all patients/families: call provider right away if thoughts of suicide or dying; attempts to commit suicide; new or worse depression; new or worse anxiety; feeling very agitated or restless; panic attacks; trouble sleeping (insomnia); new or worse irritability; aggressive, angry, or violent behavior; acting on dangerous impulses; extreme increase in activity or talking (mania); any unusual changes in behavior or mood.

Potential Toxicities/Side Effects and the Nursing Process

I. ALTERATION IN OXYGENATION, POTENTIAL, related to CHANGES IN BP

Defining Characteristics: Rarely, hypertension, vasodilation, tachycardia, postural hypotension, angina, extrasystoles, syncope, thrombophlebitis, peripheral edema occur. Migraine headaches are frequent.

Nursing Implications: Assess baseline weight, presence of peripheral edema, cardiac status and vital signs, and monitor during therapy at each visit. Instruct patient to report any edema, palpitations, chest pain, or any changes in condition. Discuss any symptoms with the physician depending on severity.

II. ALTERATIONS IN SENSORY/PERCEPTUAL PATTERNS related to EMOTIONAL LABILITY, VERTIGO

Defining Characteristics: Emotional lability, trismus, vertigo occur frequently; infrequently, apathy, ataxia, circumoral paresthesia, CNS stimulation, euphoria, hallucinations, hostility, blurred vision, abnormal accommodation, photophobia, tinnitus, taste perversion, manic reaction, psychosis, sleep disturbance, abnormal dreams, and stupor may occur.

Nursing Implications: Assess baseline neurologic status, affective state, and risk factors, and monitor during treatment. Instruct patient to avoid alcohol while taking drug. Assess effect on elderly and/or patients with hepatic or renal dysfunction. Assess for symptoms at each visit, and instruct patient to report changes. If symptoms occur, discuss strategies to ensure patient safety and comfort.

III. ALTERATION IN NUTRITION, LESS THAN BODY REQUIREMENTS, related to GI SIDE EFFECTS

Defining Characteristics: Nausea (37% of patients), anorexia (11%), constipation (15%) may occur. Less commonly, dry mouth, diarrhea, dyspepsia, flatulence, dysphagia, melena, gastroenteritis, and eructation may occur.

Nursing Implications: Assess baseline nutrition and gastrointestinal functional status, and instruct the patient to report any GI disturbances or changes. Discuss measures to reduce nausea and/or stimulate appetite.

IV. SEXUAL DYSFUNCTION, POTENTIAL, related to EJACULATORY DISTURBANCES

Defining Characteristics: Incidence of ejaculatory disturbances is 12%, and other disorders may occur (1–6%), including erectile difficulties, delayed ejaculation/orgasm, impotence, and other sexual dysfunction. Rarely, women with uterine fibroids may develop enlargement, uterine hemorrhage, or vaginal hemorrhage; in addition, women may develop vaginitis and metrorrhagia and, rarely, amenorrhea.

Nursing Implications: Assess baseline sexual functioning. Inform patient that alterations may occur, and instruct to report them. If severe, discuss dysfunction with physician, and whether another antidepressant would provide equal benefit with less dysfunction.

V. ALTERATION IN COMFORT related to PAIN

Defining Characteristics: Malaise, neck pain, hangover-like effect, arthritis, bone pain may occur infrequently.

Nursing Implications: Assess baseline comfort level. Instruct patient to report any changes in comfort, and discuss strategies to reduce discomfort.

VI. ALTERATION IN OXYGENATION, POTENTIAL, related to altered BREATHING PATTERNS

Defining Characteristics: Bronchitis, dyspnea may occur frequently; infrequently, asthma, chest congestion, hyperventilation, laryngitis may occur.

Nursing Implications: Assess baseline respiratory status, and instruct patient to report any changes. Discuss serious changes with physician, and interventions necessary.

VII. ALTERATION IN SKIN INTEGRITY, POTENTIAL, related to RASH

Defining Characteristics: Infrequently, acne, alopecia, brittle nails, contact dermatitis, dry skin, maculopapular rash, urticaria, and herpes simplex and zoster may occur.

Nursing Implications: Assess baseline skin integrity, and instruct patient to report any changes. Discuss serious changes with the physician, and need for changing to another antidepressant depending on severity.

VIII. POTENTIAL FOR INJURY related to EFFECTS ON BLOOD CELL ELEMENTS

Defining Characteristics: Frequently, ecchymosis may occur; less commonly, anemia, leucocytosis, leukopenia, lymphadenopathy, lymphocytosis, thrombocytopenia, thrombocythemia may occur.

Nursing Implications: Assess baseline CBC and presence of bruising on skin. Instruct patient to report any bleeding, bruising, infection, or any changes in condition. Check CBC as indicated and discuss any changes with physician.

IX. ALTERATION IN URINARY ELIMINATION related to DYSURIA

Defining Characteristics: Frequently, dysuria, hematuria, metrorrhagia, impaired urination, or vaginitis may occur. Infrequently, albuminuria, kidney calculus, cystitis, nocturia, bladder pain, kidney pain, polyuria, prostatitis, pyelonephritis, pyuria, incontinence, urinary urgency may occur.

Nursing Implications: Assess baseline urinary status. Instruct patient to report any changes, and discuss interventions with physician.

Drug: zolpidem tartrate (Ambien)

Class: Benzodiazepine-like hypnotic.

Mechanism of Action: Despite a chemical structure unlike the benzodiazepines, it selectively binds to one of the GABA complexes that the benzodiazepines non-selectively bind to, producing deep sleep (stages 3 and 4) without muscle relaxant or anticonvulsant properties.

Metabolism: Well absorbed from GI tract, with 70% of drug reaching the systemic circulation. Absorption and distribution affected by food intake. Widely distributed in body tissues and fluids, including CSF. Crosses placenta and is excreted in breast milk. Highly bound to plasma proteins. Metabolized in liver and excreted in urine, bile, and feces. Onset of action in 7–27 minutes, with a peak of 0.5–2.3 hours, and duration of 6–8 hours. Elimination half-life is 1.7–2.5 hours.

Dosage/Range:

Adult (for insomnia):
- Oral: 10–20 mg PO at hs.
- Elderly or debilitated individuals: 5 mg PO.

Drug Preparation:
- Store tablets in tight container at < 40°C (104°F).
- Administer on an empty stomach immediately before bedtime.

Drug Interactions:
- CNS depressants (e.g., alcohol, phenothiazines): additive CNS depression; avoid concurrent use or use cautiously and monitor carefully.

Lab Effects/Interference:
- None.

Special Considerations:
- Indicated for the short-term treatment of insomnia, generally 7–10 days of use.
- Contraindications: nursing mothers.
- Administer cautiously in patients with liver or renal dysfunction, pregnancy, pulmonary compromise, or who are depressed.
- May cause increased depression in patients who are already depressed.

Potential Toxicities/Side Effects and the Nursing Process

I. ALTERATIONS IN SENSORY/PERCEPTUAL PATTERNS related to CNS DEPRESSION

Defining Characteristics: CNS depressant effects include drowsiness, fatigue, lethargy, drugged feeling, depression, anxiety, irritability.

Nursing Implications: Assess baseline neurologic status, affective state, and risk factors, and monitor during treatment. Instruct patient to report worsening depression, and assess for any suicidal ideation. Instruct patient to avoid alcohol while taking drug. Assess effect on elderly and/or debilitated patients (cognition, motor function, other sensitivities). Assess effect of drug side effects on patient, and weigh against benefit. Inform patient that daytime drowsiness may occur, and instruct to use caution if driving or operating heavy machinery.

II. ALTERATION IN NUTRITION, LESS THAN BODY REQUIREMENTS, related to GI SIDE EFFECTS

Defining Characteristics: Nausea, vomiting, dyspepsia may occur.

Nursing Implications: Assess baseline nutrition status, and instruct the patient to report any nausea or vomiting.

III. INJURY related to DECREASE IN MENTAL ALERTNESS, PHYSICAL COORDINATION

Defining Characteristics: Drug may cause drowsiness, dizziness, diplopia, and impair physical coordination, mental alertness. At doses > 10 mg, patients may experience anterograde amnesia or memory impairment.

Nursing Implications: Assess other medications that may increase risk (e.g., opiates, phenothiazines) and response to drug. Instruct patient to avoid potentially hazardous activities, including driving a car, operating machinery.

Section 3
Complications

Chapter 10
Hypercalcemia

Hypercalcemia is a metabolic complication of malignant disease and is evidenced by a serum calcium of > 10.5 mg/dL. Potentially fatal, hypercalcemia occurs in 10–20% of patients with cancer, principally in patients with breast cancer, multiple myeloma, squamous cell cancers of head and neck and esophagus, prostate cancer, and adult T-cell lymphoma. Hypercalcemia is compounded by problems of advanced disease, such as immobility and dehydration. Hypercalcemia of malignancy is either humoral or related to tumor invasion of bone. In humoral hypercalcemia, osteoclasts are activated and break down bone (resorption) as a result of tumor-released factors such as parathyroid hormone-related protein. This type may occur in patients with squamous-cell malignancies of the lung, head, and neck or with genitourinary cancers such as renal cell or ovarian cancer. This group of patients in most cases does not have bony involvement by tumor. In contrast, patients with bony metastases in which a tumor has invaded the bone have tumors that release local substances that cause the bone to undergo resorption by osteoclasts (bone is broken down) with the release of calcium. Malignancies commonly associated with this type of hypercalcemia are breast cancer and multiple myeloma.

In reviewing normal calcium homeostasis, calcium is found primarily in bone. As such, 99% of the body's calcium is in the form of insoluble crystals, giving the human skeleton strength and durability. The remaining 1% is distributed between the body's intracellular and extracellular fluids: 45% is ionized in the serum, 45% is bound by protein, and 10% is found in insoluble complexes.

The ionized fraction of calcium is necessary for excitation of nerves, voluntary skeletal muscle, cardiac muscle, and involuntary muscles in the gut. If the body has too much ionized calcium, there is decreased excitability of these tissues. For instance, symptoms of early hypercalcemia (calcium of 10–12 mg/dL) are fatigue, lethargy, constipation, anorexia, nausea and vomiting, and polyuria. Later symptoms, when the calcium is > 12 mg/dL, are altered mental status, coma, decreased deep tendon reflexes, increased cardiac contractility, and oliguric renal failure. In contrast, if there is too little ionized calcium in the body, there is increased excitability of nerves and muscle. The body attempts to regain more calcium to raise the level of ionized calcium by "raiding" the bone matrix.

Because 45% of the calcium outside of bone is bound to albumin, it is important to correct the value of ionized calcium in the serum if the albumin is low (normally bound calcium is now free in the serum, and the serum level may actually be higher than the laboratory value). The formula to determine ionized serum calcium, corrected for low serum albumin is:

$$\text{Corrected serum calcium} = \text{measured total serum calcium (mg/dL)} + [4.0\text{-serum albumin (g/dL)}] \times 0.8$$

For example, a patient has a serum calcium of 10.0 mg/dL but has a serum albumin of 2.2 (normal is 3.5–5.5 g/dL). The corrected serum calcium is 10.0 mg/dL + (4.0 – 2.2 = 1.8 g/dL) × 0.8 = 10.0 + 1.44 = 11.44. Thus, a serum calcium level that appears normal may be abnormal (high) in the presence of a low serum albumin level.

The human skeleton undergoes constant remodeling, where there is an exquisite balance between bone formation and bone resorption (breakdown). Bone formation is mediated by osteoblasts and bone resorption by osteoclasts. Calcium balance is maintained by a number of factors. First, parathyroid hormone (PTH) released by the parathyroid gland increases serum calcium levels by stimulating bone resorption, increasing renal absorption of calcium, and stimulating the production of $1{,}25(OH)_2D_3$, which increases the intestinal absorption of calcium. In contrast, calcitonin balances these effects by reducing serum calcium: it inhibits bone resorption (breakdown) and decreases renal absorption of calcium. Normally, intestinal absorption of calcium is balanced by an approximately equal loss of calcium through urinary excretion. In most individuals before midlife, bone formation balances bone resorption.

There are many potential causes of hypercalcemia of malignancy. These include:

- Secretion of parathyroid-related protein by tumor.
- Secretion of other bone-resorbing substances by tumor (i.e., cytokines, transforming growth factor [TGF-α], IL-1, tumor necrosis factor [TNF]).
- Conversion of 25-hydroxyvitamin D_3 to 1,25-dihydroxyvitamin D_3 by tumor.
- Local effects of osteolytic bony metastasis.

Therapeutic efforts to lower serum calcium in hypercalcemia of malignancy are based on rehydration to restore glomerular filtration and excretion of calcium (normally up to 600 mg/day), and drugs that promote calcium excretion or inhibit osteoclastic bone resorption. Today, bisphosphonate agents have been shown to decrease the development of osteoclastic bone lesions from breast and prostate cancer metastases and multiple myeloma. For patients with advanced disease, general management principles are based on palliation of symptoms. Diet restriction of calcium is not necessary, as calcium absorbed from the gut is often less than normal and patients are malnourished. Patients with T-cell lymphoma, who have increased 1,25-dihydroxyvitamin D_3, are an exception to this rule. These patients have high levels of 1,25-dihydroxyvitamin D_3 and should avoid intake of dairy products. It is important for patients to bear weight if possible, since immobility increases osteoclastic activity and decreases osteoblastic activity. Since calcium is a potent diuretic, patients are often dehydrated with the loss of sodium and water. Further, as the serum calcium increases, the distal renal tubules become less able to retain sodium, and there is further sodium loss from the kidneys. Patients are usually rehydrated with 3–4 liters per day of 0.9% sodium chloride over 48 hours to restore fluid volume. Loop diuretics are administered, such as furosemide (Lasix), which increase calcium excretion. Thiazide diuretics are avoided, since they increase tubular reabsorption of calcium. This usually provides symptomatic improvement, but it is important to monitor the patient closely for possible fluid overload on the one hand, or intravascular dehydration with electrolyte imbalance on the other.

A number of drugs inhibit osteoclastic bone activity. The bisphosphonates have potent hypocalcemic activity, binding tightly to the calcified bone matrix. Some of the drugs inhibit lymphokine- and prostaglandin-mediated bone resorption, and the drugs vary in their inhibition of bone mineralization. Pamidronate (Aredia) and zoledronic acid (Zometa) inhibit bone resorption at low doses without decreasing mineralization and normalizing serum calcium in 80–90% of patients within 48–96 hours (Fitton and McTavish, 1991). Pamidronate and zolendronic acid are effective in reducing pain from bony metastases and decrease the incidence of bone metastasis in patients with multiple myeloma or breast cancer. Zolendronic acid was shown to reduce skeletal events in patients with prostate cancer (Berenson et al, 2001). More recently, studies have determined that bone resorption markers such as N-telopeptide of type I collagen (NTX) correlate with the extent of bone metastases and reflect the extent of bony metastases in patients (Lipton et al, 2007). Furthermore, studies have suggested that the normalization of NTX as a result of bisphosphonate therapy results in decreased progression of bony metastases and lower incidence of fractures (Brown et al, 2005). Lipton et al (2007) demonstrated in a retrospective subset analysis of a phase III randomized controlled trial patients with breast cancer that early normalization of elevated baseline NTX through zolendronic acid therapy was associated with higher event-free survival (e.g., fewer fractures) and higher overall survival. Similarly, Hirsch et al (2008) found statistically significant correlations between zolendronic acid and increased survival compared to placebo in patients with high baseline NTX levels. Well, what about prevention of bony metastases and improved survival in the adjuvant breast cancer setting? In a very exciting presentation, Ghant (2008) reported that in a randomized, open-label phase III trial of patients with early premenopausal breast cancer there was improved outcome when zoledronic acid was added to endocrine therapy (either tamoxifen or anastrozole) [Austrian Breast and Colorectal Cancer Study Group, ABCSG-12]. Adjuvant zolendronic acid was included in the study both to counter the significant bone loss associated with ovarian suppression (goserelin) and to see whether the antitumor effects seen in the metastatic setting would be seen in the adjuvant setting as well as measured by time to disease recurrence and overall survival. At a median follow-up of 60 months, patients receiving zolendronic acid had improved disease free survival ($p = 0.011$), as evidenced by less contralateral breast cancer, distant metastases, and local regional recurrence, as well as longer relapse-free survival ($p = 0.014$) and a trend toward improved overall survival ($p = 0.101$)

There were no reported renal toxicity or confirmed osteonecrosis of the jaw during the study.

Etidronate (Didronel) inhibits osteoclastic resorption, but with long-term use, the drug inhibits bone mineralization, causing osteomalacia and pathologic fractures. A class effect of the drugs is potential renal insufficiency (zolendronic acid > pamidronate) and also rarely osteonecrosis of the jaw. Patients should have a serum creatinine assessed before each treatment, as well as serial urinalyses for protein. In addition, patients should have a baseline oral exam by a dentist or oral surgeon, and patients at highest risk for osteonecrosis of the jaw (e.g., poor dental health) should be seen regularly.

As more is understood about the process of bone resorption and metastases, new agents are being explored. One such agent is denosumab, a human monoclonal antibody that blocks the receptor activator of nuclear factor-κB ligand (RANKL) (Lipton et al, 2007). Denosumab is being studied in postmenopausal osteoporosis, aromatase inhibitor-induced osteoporosis, bone metastases from breast and prostate cancers, bone metastases from multiple myeloma, and the prevention of bone metastases from prostate cancer. Osteoclast differentiation, activation, and survival are regulated by three molecules: receptor activator of nuclear factor κB (RANK), the cytokine, RANKL, and osteoprotegerin, a soluble decoy receptor of RANKL, which can turn off RANKL to stop bone loss (Body et al, 2006). RANKL binds to RANK on pre and mature osteoclasts and regulates their differentiation, function, and survival (Body et al, 2006). The seed and soil hypothesis suggests that breast or prostate cancer cells are the "seeds," which secrete substances that create a microenvironment in the skeleton (bone) where various cytokines and growth factors make a very rich "soil" that attracts circulating tumor cells and fosters tumor growth in the bone. RANKL appears to regulate cancer cell migration and bone metastases in cells that express the receptor RANK, such as breast cancer cells (Jones et al, 2006). RANK is also expressed by prostate cancer where again RANKL has been found to act directly on RANK expressing prostate tumor cells, guiding tumor cell migration to bone, and expression of tumor metastases genes that further stimulate tumor growth (Armstrong et al, 2008).

Other hypocalcemic agents include the following, but are less often used. Oral phosphates inhibit bone resorption and stimulate bone formation, as well as precipitate calcium. However, the side effect of diarrhea limits their usefulness. Glucocorticoids have an unpredictable effect, and their value is limited by side effects of high drug doses. However, they are often used in steroid-responsive malignancies such as multiple myeloma and lymphoma. Calcitonin inhibits bone resorption and promotes urinary calcium excretion with a rapid, but brief, response (2–3 days). Plicamycin (Mithramycin) inhibits osteoclastic bone resorption by killing the osteoclasts. It is potent, lowering calcium in 24–72 hours, but rebound hypercalcemia often occurs within one week. The high toxicity of the drug prevents wide usage.

After symptomatic hypercalcemia is resolved, the malignant disease is treated if appropriate to prevent recurrence (e.g., with chemotherapy or radiotherapy to lytic bone lesions). Nursing implications revolve around management of the patient receiving aggressive hydration and hypocalcemic medications. Patient education is prominent, as patients and their families are taught about the disease, as well as self-assessment of signs and symptoms of hypercalcemia, fluid balance, activity, and oral care. For patients receiving bisphosphonates for the prevention of bony metastases, nursing priorities include assessment of renal function before each treatment, oral assessment and patient education about potential, albeit rare, osteonecrosis of the jaw, and teaching patients about self-administration of calcium and vitamin D supplements to prevent osteoporosis.

References

Armstrong AP, Miller RE, Jones JC, Zhang J, Keller ET, Dougall WC. RANKL Acts Directly on RANK-Expressing Prostate Tumor Cells and Mediates Migration and expression of Tumor Metastasis Genes. *Prostate* 2008; 68(1) 92–104

Berenson JR, Rosen LS, Howell A. Zoledronic Acid Reduces Skeletal-related Events in Patients with Osteolytic Metastases. A Double-blind, Randomized Dose-response Study. *Cancer* 2001; 91 144–154

Blum RH, Novetsky D, Shasha D, Fleishman S. The Multidisciplinary Approach to Bone Metastases. *Oncology* 2003; 17 845–857

Body JJ, Facon T, Coleman RE et al. A Study of the Biological Receptor Activator of Nuclear Factor κB-Ligand Inhibitor, Denosumab, in Patients With Multiple Myeloma or Bone Metastases From Breast Cancer. *Clin Cancer Res* 2006; 12 1221–1228

Bone HG, Bolognese MA, Yuen CK, Kendler DL, Wang H, Liu Y, San Martin J. Effects of Denosumab on Bone Mineral Density and Bone Turnover in Postmenopausal Women. *J Clin Endocrinology and Metabolism* 2008; 93(6) 2149–2157

Ghant M, Mlineritsch B, Schippinger W, et al. Adjuvant Ovarian Suppression Combined With Tamoxifen or Anastrozole, Alone or in Combination With Zoledronic Acid, in Premenopausal Women With Hormone-Responsive, Stage I and II Breast Cancer: First Efficacy Results From ABCSG-12. *J Clin Oncol* 26; 2008 (May 20 suppl: abstract LBA4)

Hirsch V, Major PP, Lipton A, et al. Zoledronic Acid and Survival in Patients With Metastatic Bone Disease From Lung Cancer and Elevated Markers of Osteoclast Activity. *Thorac Oncol* 2008; 3(3) 228–236

Jones DH, Nakashima T, Sanchez OH, et al. Regulation of Cancer Cell Migration and Bone Metastasis by RANKL. *Nature* 2006; 440(7084) 692–696

Lipton A, Cook RJ, Major P, Smith MR, Coleman RE. Zoledronic Acid and Survival in Breast Cancer Patients With Bone Metastases and Elevated Markers of Osteoclast Activity. *The Oncologist* 2007; 12 1035–1043

Lipton A, Steger GG, Figueroa J, et al. Randomized Active Controlled Phase II Study of Denosumab Efficacy and Safety in Patients With Breast Cancer Related Bone Metastases. *J Clin Oncol* 2007; 25(28) 4431–4437

Major P, Lortholary A, Hon J. Zoledronic Acid Is Superior to Pamidronate in the Treatment of Hypercalcemia of Malignancy: A Pooled Analysis of Two Randomized, Controlled Clinical Trials. *J Clin Oncol* 2001; 19 558–567

Reich CD. Advances in the Treatment of Bone Metastases. *Clin J Oncol Nurs* 2003; 7 641–646

Viale PH, Sanchez, Yamamoto D. Bisphosphonates: Expanded Roles in the Treatment of Patients with Cancer. *Clin J Oncol Nurs* 2003; 7 393–401

Drug: calcitonin-salmon (Calcimar, Miacalcin)

Class: Thyroid hormone.

Mechanism of Action: Inhibits bone absorption (breakdown) by inhibiting bone osteoclasts and blocking osteolysis. Decreases high serum calcium concentrations in hypercalcemia of malignancy, beginning 2 hours after dose and lasting 6–8 hours. Promotes renal excretion of calcium, phosphate; also, acts on GI tract to decrease volume, acidity of gastric fluid, and enzyme content in pancreatic fluid.

Metabolism: Rapidly converted to smaller fragments by kidneys; excreted in urine.

Dosage/Range:

Adult (hypercalcemia):

- Subcutaneous (SQ) or intramuscular (IM): 4 international units/kg q 12 h × 2 days; if no effect, increase dose to 8 international units/kg q 12 h × 2 days, then to 8 international units q 6 h (maximum).

Drug Preparation:

- Refrigerate for 2–6 hours (36–43°F, 2–6°C).
- Reconstitute according to manufacturer's recommendations.
- If allergy suspected, perform skin test first: withdraw 0.05 mL of the 200 international units/mL solution in tuberculin syringe, then fill syringe with 1 mL 0.9% sodium chloride. After mixing, discard 0.9 mL; inject 0.1 mL intradermally on forearm and inspect for urticaria or wheal at 15 minutes.

Drug Interactions:

- None.

Lab Effects/Interference:

- Decreased alk phos.
- Decreased 24-hour urinary excretion of hydroxyproline.
- Casts in urine (indicate kidney damage).
- Decreased Ca++.

Special Considerations:

- Calcitonin-salmon consists of a foreign protein, so allergic reactions may occur. Perform skin test first if sensitivity is suspected. Do not use drug if wheal forms.
- It is unknown whether drug crosses placenta or is excreted in breast milk; use cautiously in pregnancy or breast-feeding.
- Patient should receive adequate saline hydration to keep urinary output at ~2 L/day throughout treatment.
- 80% of patients have reduction in calcium in 24 hours.
- Antibodies to drug may develop with long-term use.
- Rapid onset of action and mild side effects.
- Short duration of response.

Potential Toxicities/Side Effects and the Nursing Process

I. INJURY related to HYPERSENSITIVITY

Defining Characteristics: Rare hypersensitivity may occur.

Nursing Implications: Perform skin testing as ordered when sensitivity suspected; if positive, suggest use of human calcitonin or other hypocalcemic agent. Assess for signs/symptoms of hypersensitivity (generalized itching, agitation, dizziness, nausea, sense of impending doom, urticaria, angioedema, respiratory distress, hypotension). If this develops, stop drug immediately, notify physician, maintain IV access, and be prepared to administer epinephrine, hydrocortisone, diphenhydramine.

II. ALTERATION IN NUTRITION, LESS THAN BODY REQUIREMENTS, related to GI SIDE EFFECTS

Defining Characteristics: Transient nausea/vomiting is mild and tolerance develops; anorexia, diarrhea, epigastric discomfort, and abdominal pain may occur as well.

Nursing Implications: Assess baseline nutrition and elimination patterns. Since nausea/vomiting may occur within 30 minutes after injection, administer at bedtime to decrease distress.

III. ALTERATION IN COMFORT related to DRUG EFFECTS

Defining Characteristics: Flushing of face, hands, and feet may occur soon after injection, as well as tingling of palms and soles. Rarely, rash (maculopapular), erythema, urticaria, headache, chills have developed. Inflammation may occur at IM or subcutaneous injection site.

Nursing Implications: Assess comfort level. Administer drug at bedtime if possible. If symptoms are uncomfortable, consider symptomatic relief measures (e.g., heat, cold). Reassure patient that flushing lasts ~1 hour and is transient. Assess rash if severe; discuss with physician drug discontinuance.

IV. ALTERATIONS IN ELECTROLYTES related to HYPOCALCEMIA, HYPERCALCEMIA

Defining Characteristics: Rarely, if drug is very effective, hypocalcemia may occur; conversely, if drug is ineffective, hypercalcemia may occur.

Nursing Implications: Monitor serum Ca+ closely. Assess for signs/symptoms of hypocalcemia (muscle twitching, spasm tetany, seizures) and hypercalcemia (bone pain, nausea, vomiting, polyuria, polydipsia, constipation, bradycardia, lethargy, muscle weakness, psychosis). Notify physician, recheck serum calcium immediately, and institute corrective measures as ordered.

Drug: cinacalcet HCl (Sensipar)

Class: Hypocalcemic agent

Mechanism of Action: The calcium-sensing receptor on the surface of the chief cell of the parathyroid gland regulates PTH secretion. PTH is responsible for telling the bones to break down bone (osteoclastic) and release calcium into the blood when it is needed. Cinacalcet HCl directly decreases PTH levels by increasing the sensitivity of calcium-sensing receptors to activation by extracellular calcium. As PTH levels decrease, the level of calcium in the blood decreases.

Metabolism: Oral drug is well absorbed, and maximum plasma levels are achieved in 2–6 hours. Drug AUC levels are increased 82% when ingested with a high fat meal. Drug is metabolized by CYP3A4, CYP2D6, and CYP1A2 enzymes of the P450 microenzyme system. Drug is excreted in the urine (80%) primarily, and to a lesser degree in the feces (15%). Drug is poorly excreted in patients with moderate-to-severe hepatic impairment, with a half-life prolonged 33% and 70% respectively. Drug is highly protein bound so hemodialysis does not treat over dosage.

Dosage/Range:

- 30 mg PO bid, titrated every 2–4 weeks through sequential doses of 30 mg PO bid, then 60 mg PO bid, then 90 mg PO bid, and 90 mg tid or quid as necessary to normalize serum calcium levels.
- Monitor patients with moderate or severe hepatic impairment closely.
- Do not administer if serum calcium is < 8.4 mg/dL.
- Monitor calcium levels frequently during dose titration.

Drug Preparation:

- Drug available in 30, 60, and 90 mg tablets.
- Administer with food or shortly after a meal.

Drug Interactions:

- Drug is a potent inhibitor of CYP2D6: Dosage adjustment may be needed for flecainide, vinblastine, thioridazine, tricyclic antidepressants.
- Ketoconazole: increased AUC by 2.3 times of cinacalcet HCl.
- Amitriptyline: increased amitriptyline and nortriptyline by 20% in CYP2D6 extensive metabolizers.
- Warfarin: no effect.

Lab Effects/Interference:

- Hypocalcemia
- Hyperphosphatemia

Special Considerations:

- Drug is indicated for treatment of hypercalcemia in patients with parathyroid carcinoma.
- Patients should be monitored for signs and symptoms of hypocalcemia.
- Drug should not be used by pregnant or breast-feeding mothers, unless benefit outweighs risk.

Potential Toxicities/Side Effects and the Nursing Process

I. POTENTIAL FOR INJURY related to HYPOCALCEMIA

Defining Characteristics: Drug lowers serum calcium. Signs and symptoms of hypocalcemia are paresthesia, myalgias, cramping, tetany, and seizures.

Nursing Implications: Assess baseline serum calcium, phosphate, magnesium levels, as well as PTH level. Develop a plan for titration with the patient, and frequency of laboratory monitoring. Teach patient symptoms of hypocalcemia, and to report them right away if they occur. Serum calcium should be assessed within 1 week after initiation or dose adjustment. Once dose has been established, serum calcium should be assessed q month. If serum calcium > 7.5 mg/dL but < 8.4 mg/dL, or if symptoms of hypocalcemia occur, discuss with physician the addition of calcium-containing phosphate binders and/or vitamin D sterols to raise the serum calcium. If the serum calcium falls to < 7.5 mg/dL or if symptoms of hypocalcemia persist, stop drug until serum calcium level reaches 8.0 mg/dL and/or symptoms resolve. Resume dose per physician, at next lowest dose of drug.

II. ALTERATION IN NUTRITION, LESS THAN BODY REQUIREMENTS, related to GI SIDE EFFECTS

Defining Characteristics: Nausea (31%), vomiting (27%) are most common adverse effects, but diarrhea may also occur (21%).

Nursing Implications: Assess baseline nutritional and elimination status, and monitor during treatment. Ensure adequate hydration and urinary output of 2 L/day. Teach patient to administer oral antiemetics prior to taking drug, and as needed between drug doses. Assess food preferences, and suggest small, frequent feedings. Teach patient to report symptoms that worsen or do not resolve with supportive care.

III. ALTERATION IN COMFORT related to MYALGIA AND DIZZINESS

Defining Characteristics: Myalgia affects about 15% of patients and dizziness 10% of patients.

Nursing Implications: Assess baseline hydration, comfort status, and teach patient that these side effects may occur. Teach patient to change position slowly if dizziness occurs, and to notify nurse or physician if dizziness worsens or does not resolve. Teach patient symptom management strategies such as local application of heat for myalgias, and to notify provider if myalgias worsen.

Drug: denosumab (AMG-162, investigational)

Class: Receptor activator of nuclear factor-κB ligand (RANKL) inhibitor.

Mechanism of Action: Human monoclonal antibody directed against RANKL, thus inhibiting or turning off osteoclast function and bone resorption. It mimics the effect of the RANK modulator osteoprotegerin.

Metabolism: Unknown.

Dosage/Range: Per protocol, such as 60 mg SQ every 6 months (postmenopausal osteoporosis) to 120 mg SQ either every 4 weeks (bone metastases).

Drug Preparation: Per protocol.

Drug Interactions: Unknown.

Lab Effects/Interference: Unknown.

Special Considerations:
- Efficacy and side effect profile similar to IV bisphosphonates (Lipton et al, 2007).
- Most common side effects were nausea and fatigue compared with fever, arthralgia, and asthenia in the bisphosphonate group.
- In a randomized controlled trial of denosumab compared with placebo in postmenopausal women with low bone mineral density (BMD), denosumab significantly increased BMD in the lumbar spine, hip, radius, and total body (Bone et al, 2008).
- RANKL and RANK function in other body processes, and thus, it is unclear what long term effects of antagonism of this cytokine are.

Potential Toxicities/Side Effects and the Nursing Process

I. ALTERATIONS IN NUTRITION, LESS THAN BODY REQUIREMENTS, related to GI SIDE EFFECTS

Defining Characteristics: Diarrhea, nausea, vomiting, constipation may occur in > 10% of patients.

Nursing Implications: Assess baseline nutritional and elimination status, and monitor during treatment. Instruct patient to report nausea and vomiting, and discuss appropriate antiemetic with physician or nurse practitioner. Discuss bowel elimination plan with patient, foods that minimize diarrhea or constipation, and use of over-the-counter medications to correct bowel elimination problems.

Drug: etidronate disodium (Didronel)

Class: Bisphosphonate; hypocalcemic agent.

Mechanism of Action: Inhibits osteoclastic bone resorption (bone breakdown), thereby decreasing calcium release, and serum calcium levels. Indicated in the management of hypercalcemia of malignancy.

Metabolism: Oral absorption is variable and decreased by food. Following IV injection, drug is distributed into bone, then excreted unchanged in the urine.

Dosage/Range:
Adult (hypercalcemia of malignancy):
- IV (induction): 7.5* mg/kg/day × 3 days (may increase to 7 days; if hypercalcemia recurs, wait at least 7 days before treatment using same induction regimen).
- Oral (maintenance): 20 mg/kg/day beginning on day after last IV dose, for up to 90 days if effective.

Drug Preparation:
- Oral: give as single oral dose (may be advised if GI distress); give at least 2 hours before or after a meal.
- IV: dilute drug in at least 250 mL 0.9% sodium chloride and infuse over at least 2 hours.

Drug Interactions:
- Nephrotoxic drugs: additive nephrotoxicity; AVOID concurrent use.

Lab Effects/Interference:
- Decreased P, decreased Mg.
- Abnormal renal function tests.
- Decreased Ca.

Special Considerations:
- Saline hydration should be maintained during treatment to keep urinary output at 2 L/day.
- Use with caution.
- It is unknown whether drug crosses placenta or is excreted in breast milk; use with caution, if at all, in pregnant or breast-feeding women.

---

*Dose reduction necessary in patients with renal insufficiency.

- 60–70% response rate when given with hydration and diuresis, and one-half of this when based on corrected calcium value.

Potential Toxicities/Side Effects and the Nursing Process

I. ALTERATIONS IN NUTRITION, LESS THAN BODY REQUIREMENTS, related to GI SIDE EFFECTS

Defining Characteristics: Diarrhea, nausea, vomiting, abdominal discomfort, and guaiac-positive stools may occur rarely.

Nursing Implications: Assess baseline nutritional and elimination status and monitor during treatment. Instruct patient to report nausea and vomiting, and consider dividing dose (if oral) or slowing infusion rate > 2 hours. Guaiac stools and notify physician if positive.

II. ALTERATION IN URINE ELIMINATION related to NEPHROTOXICITY

Defining Characteristics: Drug is nephrotoxic and may cause rises in serum BUN and creatinine. Increased risk when concurrent nephrotoxic drugs administered.

Nursing Implications: Assess baseline hydration status and total body fluid balance to ensure adequate urinary output (> 2 L/day). Assess baseline serum BUN and creatinine, and monitor throughout treatment. Dose reduction necessitated by renal insufficiency.

III. ALTERATIONS IN ELECTROLYTES related to HYPOCALCEMIA, HYPERCALCEMIA

Defining Characteristics: Rarely, if drug is very effective, hypocalcemia may occur; conversely, if drug is ineffective, hypercalcemia may occur. Increased sodium phosphate levels may occur during oral therapy but are less frequent with IV dosing (serum phosphate levels are inversely proportional to serum calcium).

Nursing Implications: Monitor serum calcium closely. Assess for signs/symptoms of hypocalcemia (muscle twitching, spasm tetany, seizures) and hypercalcemia (bone pain, nausea, vomiting, polyuria, polydipsia, constipation, bradycardia, lethargy, muscle weakness, psychosis). Notify physician, recheck serum calcium immediately, and institute corrective measures as ordered.

Drug: furosemide (Lasix)

Class: Loop diuretic.

Mechanism of Action: Inhibits renal reabsorption of sodium and chloride in proximal loop of Henle. Useful in management of edema, hypertension related to CHF or renal disease, and with 0.9% sodium chloride IV hydration/diuresis to increase renal excretion of calcium in patients with hypercalcemia of malignancy.

Metabolism: Variable GI absorption of oral drug. Diuretic effect of oral dose occurs within 30–60 minutes, lasting 6–8 hours; with IV dose, occurs within 5 minutes, maximal 20–60 minutes, and lasts 2 hours. Highly protein-bound. Slight hepatic metabolism and is excreted in urine.

Dosage/Range:
- Edema: 20–80 mg PO in morning; if no response, dose-increase in 20–40 mg increments q 6–8 h.
- Hypertension: 10–20 mg PO bid, increasing to 40 mg bid based on BP response.
- Hypercalcemia: 80–100 mg IV q 1–2 h.

Drug Preparation:
- Oral: store in tight, light-resistant containers.
- IV: slow IVP over 1–2 minutes (use multidose vial or draw up drug from ampule through filtered needles).

Drug Interactions:
- Ascorbic acid, tetracycline, epinephrine form a precipitate; DO NOT give together with IV.
- Diuretics: enhanced diuretic effect; dose-reduce furosemide.
- Digoxin: toxicity enhanced by furosemide-induced hypokalemia; keep potassium level 4.5–5.0 mEq/dL.
- Drugs causing potassium loss (corticosteroids, amphotericin B): enhanced hypokalemia; monitor potassium level closely.
- Antidiabetic agents: decreases effect of insulin or oral hypoglycemics; monitor blood glucose and adjust antidiabetic drug as needed.
- Indocin: may decrease diuretic effect; monitor patient response and increase furosemide dose as needed.
- Aminoglycosides: increased ototoxicity; use cautiously.
- High doses of salicylates: increase salicylate toxicity at lower doses; monitor carefully and decrease salicylate dose.

Lab Effects/Interference:
- Decreased potassium, decreased chloride, decreased sodium, increased uric acid.
- Rarely, anemia, thrombocytopenia, neutropenia, leukopenia.

Special Considerations:

- Contraindicated in anuric patients and patients hypersensitive to the drug.
- May produce profound diuresis and electrolyte depletion.
- Should not be used by pregnant women, and breast-feeding should be interrupted during drug therapy.
- Use with caution in patients with liver cirrhosis.

Potential Toxicities/Side Effects and the Nursing Process

I. ALTERATIONS IN FLUID AND ELECTROLYTE BALANCE related to HYDRATION/DIURESIS

Defining Characteristics: Aggressive hydration with 0.9% sodium chloride and IV furosemide is used to promote calcium excretion. Hypokalemia, hypochloremia, hyperuricemia, hypomagnesemia may occur.

Nursing Implications: Assess baseline electrolyte (K+, Mg++, Cl–, Ca++), renal BUN, creatinine, and fluid balance, and monitor during therapy. Strictly monitor intake/output (I/O), assess daily weights, and maintain total body fluid balance (I = O). Administer prescribed replacement electrolytes. Assess for signs/symptoms of hypokalemia. Assess orthostatic BP, heart rate, and monitor during therapy.

II. ALTERATION IN SENSORY/PERCEPTUAL PATTERNS related to OTOTOXICITY, CNS EFFECTS

Defining Characteristics: Tinnitus and reversible or permanent hearing impairment may occur, often related to high doses of drug given IVP (high serum drug concentrations). Headache, vertigo, paresthesias can occur.

Nursing Implications: Assess baseline hearing (ability to hear spoken voice) and neurologic status. Teach patient to report tinnitus, decreased hearing, and any other symptoms. Discuss administration of high doses as IV infusion (4 mg/min).

III. ALTERATIONS IN SKIN INTEGRITY related to RASH, SENSITIVITY

Defining Characteristics: Purpura, photosensitivity, rash, urticaria, pruritus, exfoliative dermatitis, and erythema multiforme may occur. Anaphylaxis has occurred in patients allergic to sulfonamides.

Nursing Implications: Assess drug allergies, especially to furosemide and sulfonamides. Assess baseline skin integrity, and instruct patient to report changes. Discuss drug discontinuance if severe reaction occurs.

Drug: gallium nitrate (Ganite)

Class: Hypocalcemic agent.

Mechanism of Action: Inhibits calcium release from bone by inhibiting bone resorption and turnover. Indicated for the treatment of hypercalcemia of malignancy refractory to hydration.

Metabolism: Excreted by kidneys.

Dosage/Range:

Adult:

- IV: Severe hypercalcemia: 200 mg/m^2 as continuous 24-hour infusion × 5 days (or when serum calcium normalizes if before 5 days). Moderate hypercalcemia: 100 mg/m^2 as continuous 24-hour infusion × 5 days (or less if patient achieves normal serum calcium).

Drug Preparation:

- Dilute daily dose in 1 L 0.9% sodium chloride or 5% dextrose injection, and infuse over 24 hours (42 mL/hour) via infusion pump.

Drug Interactions:

- Nephrotoxic drugs (amphotericin B, aminoglycosides, and cisplatin): additive nephrotoxicity; avoid concurrent use.

Lab Effects/Interference:

- Increased BUN, creatinine.
- Decreased calcium; transient decrease in phosphorus, decrease in bicarbonate.
- Rarely, anemia, leukopenia.

Special Considerations:

- Contraindicated in patients with severe renal dysfunction (serum creatinine > 2.5 mg/dL).
- Unknown if drug crosses placenta or is excreted in breast milk; use cautiously in pregnancy, and suggest mother interrupt breast-feeding while taking drug.
- 92% patient response (reduction in serum calcium corrected for albumin), lasting for 7.5 days.
- Saline hydration to maintain urinary output of 2 L/day should be maintained during treatment.

Potential Toxicities/Side Effects and the Nursing Process

I. ALTERATION IN URINE ELIMINATION related to NEPHROTOXICITY

Defining Characteristics: Increased serum BUN, creatinine in 13% of patients. Decreased risk if concurrent administration of other nephrotoxic drugs.

Nursing Implications: Assess baseline hydration status and total body fluid balance to ensure adequate urinary output (> 2 L/day). Assess baseline serum BUN and creatinine, and monitor throughout treatment. Dose reduction necessitated by renal insufficiency. Drug should NOT be given if serum creatinine > 2.5 mg/dL.

II. ALTERATIONS IN ELECTROLYTES related to HYPOCALCEMIA, HYPERCALCEMIA

Defining Characteristics: Rarely, if drug is very effective, hypocalcemia may occur; conversely, if drug is ineffective, hypercalcemia may occur. Transient hypophosphatemia occurs in up to 79% of hypercalcemic patients after treatment with drug. Also, decreased serum bicarbonate occurs in 40–50% of patients.

Nursing Implications: Monitor serum calcium closely. Assess for signs/symptoms of hypocalcemia (muscle twitching, spasm tetany, seizures) and hypercalcemia (bone pain, nausea, vomiting, polyuria, polydipsia, constipation, bradycardia, lethargy, muscle weakness, psychosis). Notify physician, recheck serum calcium immediately, and institute corrective measures as ordered. Monitor serum phosphate levels, and administer replacement oral phosphates as ordered.

III. ALTERATIONS IN NUTRITION, LESS THAN BODY REQUIREMENTS, related to GI SIDE EFFECTS

Defining Characteristics: Diarrhea, nausea, vomiting, constipation may occur.

Nursing Implications: Assess baseline nutritional and elimination status, and monitor during treatment. Instruct patient to report nausea and vomiting. Administer ordered antiemetics. Ensure adequate hydration with urinary output > 2 L/day.

Drug: pamidronate disodium (Aredia)

Class: Bisphosphonate; hypocalcemic agent.

Mechanism of Action: Probably inhibits osteoclast activity in bone (bone breakdown) and may also block dissolution of minerals (hydroxyapatite) in bone, thus preventing calcium release from bone. Does not inhibit bone formation or bone mineralization. Indicated for the treatment of hypercalcemia of malignancy, in conjunction with adequate hydration, as well as prevention of osteolytic lesions in breast cancer and multiple myeloma.

Metabolism: Excreted by kidneys.

Adult (hypercalcemia of malignancy):

- IV (moderate hypercalcemia, 12–13.5 mg/dL corrected): 60–90 mg as continuous infusion over 2–24 hours.
- IV (severe hypercalcemia > 13.5 mg/dL): 90 mg as continuous infusion over 2–24 hours.
- If retreatment required, wait a minimum of 7 days between treatments.

Osteolytic bone metastases of breast cancer:

- 90 mg in 250 mL of IV fluid via 2-hour infusion every 3–4 weeks.

Osteolytic lesions of multiple myeloma:

- 90 mg in 500 mL IV fluid via a 2- to 4-hour infusion every month.

Drug Preparation/Administration:

- Reconstitute by adding 10 mL sterile water for injection to 30-mg vial. Further dilute in 1 L 0.9% sodium chloride or 5% dextrose injection as per manufacturer's directions.
- Infuse over 2–24 hours via infusion pump or rate controller.
- When drug is given to prevent lytic lesions in the bone, patients should take an oral calcium supplement of 500 mg and a multiple vitamin containing 400 IU of vitamin D daily.

Drug Interactions:

- None.

Lab Effects/Interference:

- Decreased calcium.
- Decreased K+, decreased Mg, decreased P (phosphate).
- Increased serum creatinine, urinary excretion of protein (proteinuria).

Special Considerations:

- Use cautiously when combined with renally toxic drugs such as aminoglycoside antibiotics or loop diuretics. Use cautiously in patients who have aspirin-sensitive asthma.
- The drug may rarely cause osteonecrosis of the jaw, often in conjunction with a dental procedure, such as tooth extraction. Patients should have an oral examination and preventative dentistry completed before starting bisphosphonate therapy and periodically during treatment if high risk or symptoms arise. Patients should avoid dental work being done while receiving bisphosphonate therapy.

- Drug may rarely cause renal insufficiency: assess serum creatinine at baseline and before each treatment, and perform periodic urinalyses for protein. Hold the drug for increased serum creatinine or proteinuria.
- Saline hydration to maintain urinary output of 2 L/day should be maintained during treatment for hypercalcemia.
- Clinical studies show 64% of patients have corrected serum calcium levels by 24 hours after beginning therapy, and after 7 days 100% of the 90-mg group had normal corrected levels. For some (33–53%), normal or partially corrected calciums in 60-mg and 90-mg groups persisted × 14 days.
- Has been shown to reduce bony metastasis in patients with multiple myeloma and to reduce pain.
- Patients with preexisting anemia, leukopenia, or thrombocytopenia should be monitored closely for 2 weeks after pamidronate disodium treatment.

Potential Toxicities/Side Effects and the Nursing Process

I. ALTERATIONS IN NUTRITION, LESS THAN BODY REQUIREMENTS, related to GI SIDE EFFECTS

Defining Characteristics: Nausea, vomiting, abdominal discomfort, constipation, and anorexia may occur rarely.

Nursing Implications: Assess baseline nutritional and elimination status and monitor during treatment. Ensure adequate hydration and urinary output of 2 L/day. Administer ordered antiemetics. Administer oral phosphates as cathartics if ordered. Assess food differences and offer small, frequent feedings.

II. ALTERATION IN ELECTROLYTES related to HYPOCALCEMIA, HYPERCALCEMIA

Defining Characteristics: Rarely, if drug is very effective, hypocalcemia may occur; conversely, if drug is ineffective, hypercalcemia may occur. Hypokalemia, hypomagnesemia, hypophosphatemia may occur. Women with breast cancer taking the drug to prevent lytic lesions are at risk for developing osteoporosis.

Nursing Implications: Monitor serum calcium closely. Assess for signs/symptoms of hypocalcemia (muscle twitching, spasm tetany, seizures) and hypercalcemia (bone pain, nausea, vomiting, polyuria, polydipsia, constipation, bradycardia, lethargy, muscle weakness, psychosis). Notify physician, recheck serum calcium immediately, and institute corrective measures as ordered. Monitor serum potassium, magnesium, phosphate levels and notify physician of abnormalities. Women receiving drug to prevent lytic lesions should receive calcium and vitamin D supplements and should be encouraged to exercise. If a smoker, she should be encouraged to stop smoking to reduce the risk of osteoporosis.

III. ALTERATIONS IN COMFORT related to LOCAL VEIN IRRITATION

Defining Characteristics: Transient fever (1°C or 3°F elevation) may occur 24–48 hours after drug administration (27% of patients), local reactions (pain, irritation, phlebitis) are common with 90-mg dose.

Nursing Implications: Assess baseline temperature, and monitor during and after infusion. Administer antipyretics as ordered. Assess IV site and restart new IV as needed for 90-mg dose in large vein where drug can be rapidly diluted. Apply warm packs as needed to site.

IV. ALTERATIONS IN FLUID BALANCE related to AGGRESSIVE HYDRATION

Defining Characteristics: Patients receive aggressive saline hydration to ensure urinary output of 2 L/day. Hypertension may occur. Patients with history of heart disease or renal insufficiency are at risk for fluid overload.

Nursing Implications: Assess baseline hydration status, total body fluid balance; monitor q 4 h. Discuss with physician need for diuretics once hydrated to keep body fluid balance equal (I = O). Monitor vital signs q 4 h during hydration, and notify physician of changes.

Drug: zoledronic acid (Zometa)

Class: Third-generation bisphosphonate.

Mechanism of Action: Inhibits bone resorption. Inhibits tumor-related osteoclast activity in bone (bone breakdown), promotes apoptosis of osteoclasts, and blocks dissolution of minerals (hydroxyapatite) in bone, thus preventing calcium release from bone, as well as osteoclastic resorption of cartilage. It also inhibits osteoclast activity and the release of calcium from the bones that is caused by tumor-related stimulatory factors. It does not inhibit bone formation or bone mineralization. Drug is very rapidly taken up in the bone, but very slowly released. Drug appears to inhibit endothelial cell proliferation and to inhibit the beta fibroblast growth factor (βFGF)-mediated angiogenesis. The drug is 100–850 times more potent than pamidronate.

Metabolism: Drug is primarily eliminated intact via the kidney. Long terminal half-life in plasma of 167 hours. Rapid injection results in 30% increase in serum drug concentration and renal damage.

Dosage/Range: Hypercalcemia of malignancy (corrected calcium ≥ 12 mg/dL): 4 mg (maximum) IV over at least 15 minutes; if retreatment required, wait at least 7 days before administering again and monitor renal function closely.

Multiple myeloma and metastatic bone lesions from solid tumors with urinary creatinine clearance of at least 60 mL/min is 4 mg IV over at least 15 minutes every 3–4 weeks. If urinary creatinine clearance is ≤ 60 mL/min

- 50–60 mL/min: dose is 3.5 mg
- 40–49 mL/min: dose is 3.3 mg
- 30–39 mL/min: dose is 3.0 mg

Drug Preparation:

- Drug is available in 4-mg vials. Reconstitute drug by adding 5-mL sterile water for injection, USP so that 4 mg = 5 mL. If the patient is receiving a reduced dose, withdraw the appropriate volume.
- Further dilute in 100 ml 5% dextrose injection, USP or 0.9% sodium chloride injection, USP. DO NOT use any other IV solution such as Lactated Ringer's Solution.
- If not used immediately, it may be refrigerated at 2–8°C (36–46°F) for up to 24 hours but must complete administration within 24 hours of the initial dilution.

Drug Administration:

- Administer as a single IV dose over *at least* 15 minutes. Use a separate line from all other drugs.
- Assure that patient has been adequately rehydrated prior to drug administration, and the BUN and creatinine are WNL.
- Patients who require retreatment and who have had altered renal status after receiving the drug (manufacturer's recommendations):
  - Normal serum creatinine before receiving drug, but have an increase of 0.5 mg/dL within 2 weeks of their next dose: hold drug until serum creatinine is at least within 10% of their baseline value.
  - Abnormal serum creatinine before receiving drug, but have an increase of 1.0 mg/dL within 2 weeks of next dose; drug should be held until serum creatinine is at least within 10% of their baseline value.
- When drug is given to prevent lytic lesions in the bone, patients should take an oral calcium supplement of 500 mg and a multiple vitamin containing 400 IU of vitamin D daily.

Drug Interactions:

- Incompatible with calcium-containing fluids, such as Lactated Ringer's.
- Use cautiously together with aminoglycoside antibiotics, as there may be an additive effect resulting in hypocalcemia for prolonged periods as well as renal toxicity.

- Use cautiously together with loop diuretics, as the risk of hypocalcemia and nephrotoxicity may be increased.

Lab Effects/Interference:
- Hypocalcemia.
- Hypophosphatemia.
- Hypomagnesemia.
- Increased BUN and serum creatinine.

Special Considerations:
- Indicated for the treatment of (1) hypercalcemia of malignancy; (2) patients with multiple myeloma and patients with documented bone metastases from solid tumors, in conjunction with standard antineoplastic therapy; (3) patients with prostate cancer who have progressed after treatment with at least one hormonal therapy.
- Contraindicated in patients with bone metastases and severe renal impairment (serum creatinine ≥ 4.5 mg/dL), pregnant women, or nursing mothers.
- Use cautiously when combined with renally toxic drugs such as aminoglycoside antibiotics or loop diuretics. Use drug cautiously in patients who have aspirin-sensitive asthma, as well as in older patients.
- Monitor serum creatinine before each dose, and serum electrolytes, magnesium, phosphate, and hematocrit/hemoglobin baseline and regularly during treatment.
- Drug may rarely cause osteonecrosis of the jaw, often in conjunction with a dental procedure, such as tooth extraction. Patients should have an oral examination and preventative dentistry completed before starting bisphosphonate therapy and periodically during treatment if high risk or symptoms arise. Patients should avoid dental work being done while receiving bisphosphonate therapy.
- Serum creatinine must be monitored prior to each treatment, and abnormal values discussed with physician, as risk must be weighed against benefit. Risk factors for deteriorating renal function, possibly renal failure are (1) impaired renal function and (2) multiple cycles of bisphosphonate therapy.
- Teach patients to use effective birth control measures.
- As compared with pamidronate in the management of hypercalcemia of malignancy, Zometa had a 45.3% response rate by day 4 and an 82.6% response rate by day 7, as compared with a 33.3% response rate and a 63.6% response rate, respectively, when pamidronate was given. Time to relapse was 30 days with Zometa, and 17 days with pamidronate.

Potential Toxicities/Skin Effects and the Nursing Process

I. ALTERATION IN COMFORT, related to FEVER, NAUSEA AND VOMITING, INSOMNIA, AND FLU-LIKE SYMPTOMS

Defining Characteristics: Fever occurred in 44% of patients during clinical trials. Flu-like symptoms of chills, bone pain, and/or arthralgias and myalgias may occur less commonly. Nausea occurred in 29% of patients, and vomiting 14%. Insomnia affects 15%. The symptom frequency was similar to the pamidronate and placebo groups.

Nursing Implications: Assess baseline comfort and temperature. Teach patient that these side effects may occur and to report them. Administer or teach patient self-administration of acetaminophen or over-the-counter NSAIDs as appropriate to manage fever, arthralgias myalgias, if they occur. Teach patient to report if symptoms do not resolve. Administer antiemetics as ordered to minimize nausea and vomiting.

II. ALTERATION IN BOWEL ELIMINATION PATTERN related to CONSTIPATION, DIARRHEA, ABDOMINAL PAIN, AND ANOREXIA

Defining Characteristics: Diarrhea affected 24% (versus 18% placebo) of patients in clinical trials, while 31% developed constipation (compared to 38% in placebo). 14% of patients developed abdominal pain (versus 11% in placebo), and 22% anorexia (compared to 23% in placebo).

Nursing Implications: Assess baseline bowel elimination status, and teach patient to report alterations. Teach patient to use diet modifications depending upon changes, and over-the-counter antidiarrheals or laxatives as necessary. Teach patient to report persistent diarrhea or constipation (lasting more than 24 hours), presence of blood, abdominal cramping, or pain.

III. ALTERATION IN ACTIVITY TOLERANCE related to ANEMIA, FATIGUE

Defining Characteristics: Anemia occurred in 33% of patients (compared to 23% in placebo arm) during clinical trials.

Nursing Implications: Assess baseline hemoglobin and hematocrit. Teach patient to report fatigue, and discuss strategies to conserve energy, such as alternating rest and activity. Discuss with physician transfusion if symptoms are severe.

IV. ALTERATION IN FLUID AND ELECTROLYTE BALANCE related to CHANGES IN RENAL EXCRETION

Defining Characteristics: Drug will cause renal dysfunction with rise in serum creatinine if drug is given rapidly or in less than 15 minutes. Hypophosphatemia occurred in 13% of patients during clinical trials, hypokalemia in 12%, and hypomagnesemia in 10%.

Nursing Implications: Assess baseline renal function and electrolytes prior to initial therapy, post therapy, and prior to any additional therapy as needed. Hold drug if renal abnormalities do not correct, as indicated in administration section.

V. POTENTIAL FOR INJURY related to OSTEOPOROSIS

Defining Characteristics: Women with breast cancer and men with prostate cancer are at risk for osteoporosis from various cancer treatments, including hormonal manipulation.

Nursing Implications: Teach patients to take calcium and vitamin D supplements (or multivitamin) while receiving bisphosphonates and be encouraged to exercise regularly. If a smoker, encourage the patient to stop smoking to reduce the risk of osteoporosis.

Chapter 11
Infection

Patients with cancer are susceptible to infections related to their treatments. Chemotherapy, radiation therapy, and even the malignancy itself result in immunosuppression. The risk for infection results from damage to bone marrow stem cells. Additionally, patients receiving newer treatments, such as hematopoietic stem cell transplant, and those receiving high-dose corticosteroids, purine analogues, and alemtuzumab are populations of cancer patients who are at risk for life-threatening infection.

Leukocytes, or white blood cells (WBCs), are composed of five different cell types; they are further divided into cells that contain granules in the cytoplasm (granulocytes) and those that do not. Granulocytes include the neutrophils, basophils, and eosinophils. Neutrophils fight against invading microorganisms by migrating to the site of infection. See Figure 11.1 for maturation of the formed blood cell elements.

The risk of infection is related to the degree and duration of neutropenia, as shown in Table 11.1. The frequency and severity of infection are inversely proportional to the neutrophil count; therefore, the rate of decline and the length of time the patient is neutropenic result in a greater risk of infection. Infection and fever in a neutropenic patient represent a medical emergency, and, if untreated, can result in sepsis and death. The absolute neutrophil count (ANC), the number of neutrophils in the body, determines the risk for infection. This calculation is shown in Table 11.2.

Recently, the National Comprehensive Cancer Network (NCCN) v.1.2008 has expanded the thinking about fever and neutropenia and has presented a comprehensive evidenced-based guideline to prevent as well as treat cancer-related infections. The NCCN (v.1.2008) guidelines delineate the prevention, diagnosis, and treatment for major common and opportunistic infections. In Table 11.3, the NCCN (v.1.2008) Guideline for Risk of Infection and Antimicrobial Prophylaxis highlights the risk of infections in cancer patients and suggests the fever and neutropenia risk along with the recommended antimicrobial prophylaxis.

Gram-negative bacilli are responsible for the high incidence of life-threatening infections (*Escherichia coli*, *Klebsiella* spp., *Proteus* spp., and *Pseudomonas aeruginosa*); however, gram-positive organisms such as *Staphylococcus epidermidis* and streptococci have become more prominent, probably because of a decrease in gram-negative sepsis resulting from prompt empiric antimicrobial therapy against gram-negative organisms, as well as the wide use of central venous access lines that become infected by gram-positive organisms.

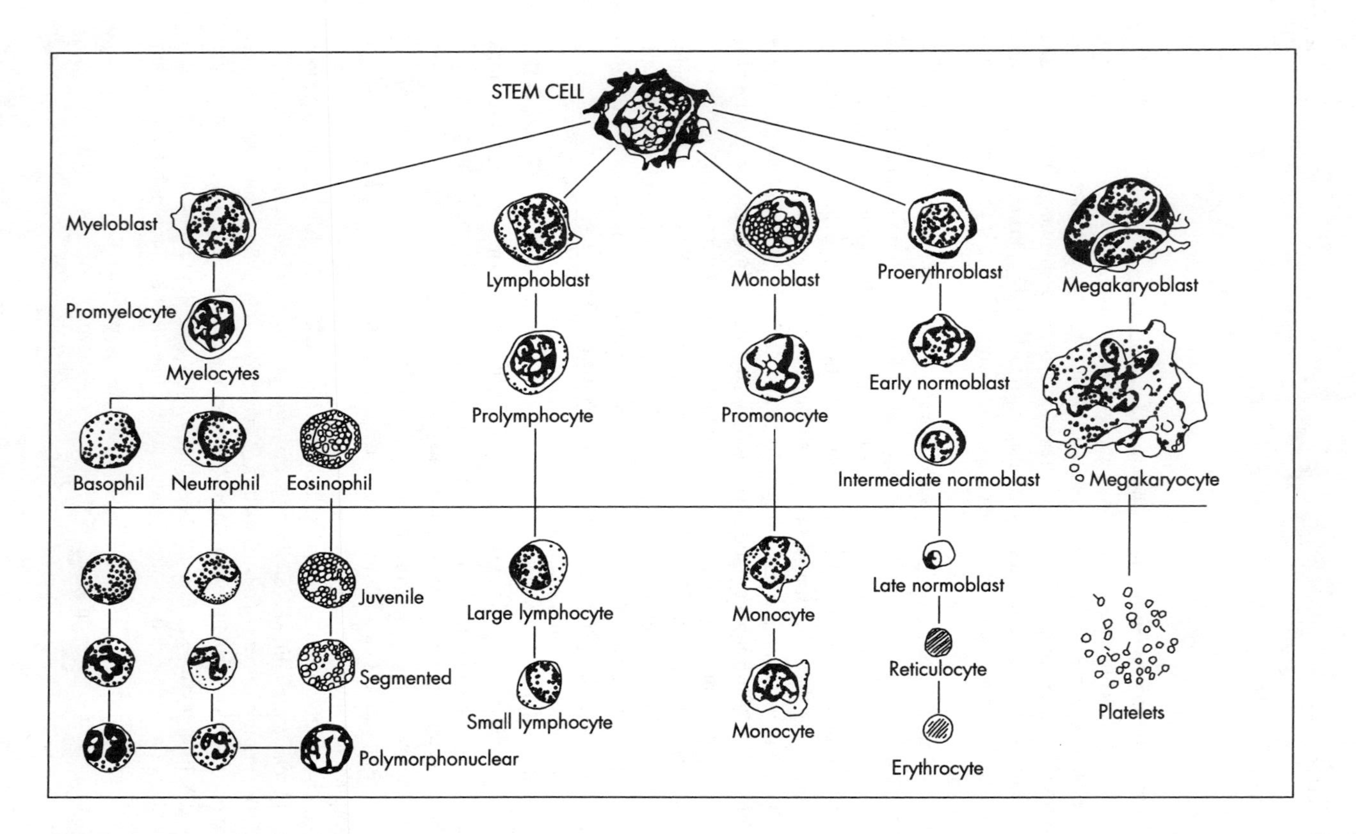

Figure 11.1 The development of formed blood cell elements

Table 11.1 Relative Risk of Infection

Risk	Number/Neutrophils
No significant risk	> 1500–2000/mm^3
Minimal risk	1000–1500/mm^3
Moderate risk	500–1000/mm^3
Severe risk	< 500/mm^3

Table 11.2 Calculation of Absolute Neutrophil Count (ANC)

Patient Example	Normal Values
1. Lab results: total white blood count (WBC) = 4000/mm^3	5000–10,000/mm^3
neutrophils = 40	50–70%
lymphocytes = 50	20–40%
monocytes = 6	2–6%
eosinophils = 1	0.5–1%
bands = 2	
2. Total WBC × % (neutrophils + bands)	2500–7000/mm^3
4000 × % (40 + 2) =	
4000 × 42/100 =	
4000 × 0.42 = 1680/mm^3	

Disease-related immunosuppression is related to defects in the cell-mediated immunity (thymus-dependent lymphocytes), such as with certain lymphomas. This leads to an increased risk for bacterial infections (*Mycobacterium, Nocardia asteroides, Legionella, Salmonella*), as well as infections caused by fungi (*Cryptococcus, Histoplasma, Candida, Aspergillus*), parasites (*Pneumocystis carinii* pneumonia, *Toxoplasma gondii*), and viruses (varicella zoster, cytomegalovirus). Other malignancies may have defects in the humoral immune system (B lymphocytes), as in multiple myeloma and chronic lymphocytic leukemia (CLL). Patients with these malignancies are at risk for infection from bacteria (*Streptococcus pneumoniae, Haemophilus influenzae, Neisseria meningitidis, Klebsiella pneumoniae,* and *Staphylococcus aureus*) and certain enteroviruses.

Another antibiotic-related concern is the emergence of antibiotic resistance, such as vancomycin-resistant enterococci (VRE) and methicillin-resistant *Staphylococcus aureus* (MRSA). Since 1989, US hospitals report a rapid increase in the incidence of infection and colonization with vancomycin-resistant enterococci (VRE). This increase poses important problems, including (a) the lack of available antimicrobial therapy for VRE infections, since most VRE infections are also resistant to drugs previously used

Table 11.3 Infection Risk

Overall Infection Risk in Cancer Patients	Disease/Therapy Examples	Fever and Neutropenia Risk Category	Antimicrobial Prophylaxis
LOW	• Standard chemotherapy for most solid tumors • Anticipated neutropenia less than 7 days	LOW	• Bacterial—none • Fungal—none • Viral—none unless prior HSV episode
INTERMEDIATE	• Autologous HSCT • Lymphoma • Multiple myeloma • CLL • Purine analogue therapy (i.e., fludarabine, 2-CdA) • Anticipated neutropenia 7 to 10 days	Usually HIGH, but some experts suggest modifications depending on patient status	• Bacterial—consider fluoroquinolone prophylaxis • Fungal—consider fluconazole during neutropenia and for anticipated mucositis • Viral—during neutropenia and at least 30 days after HSCT

HIGH	• Allogenic HSCT
	• Acute leukemia
	  • Induction
	  • Consolidation
	• Alemtuzumab therapy
	• GVHD treated with high dose steroids
	• Anticipated neutropenia greater than 10 days
		Usually HIGH, but significant variability exists related to duration of neutropenia, immunosuppressive agents, and status of underlying malignancy	• Bacterial—consider fluoroquinolone prophylaxis
			• Fungal— NCCN Guidelines suggests specific antifungals for specific conditions
			• Viral—during neutropenia and at least 30 days after HSCT

2-CdA = chlorodeoxyadenosine (cladribine), CLL = chronic lymphocytic leukemia, GVHD = graft versus host disease, HSCT = hematopoietic stem cell transplant, HSV = herpes simplex virus.

Source: Reprinted with permission NCCN.v1.2008.

to treat these infections (e.g., aminoglycosides and ampicillin), and (b) the possibility that the vancomycin-resistant genes present in VRE can be transferred to other gram-positive microorganisms (e.g., *Staphylococcus aureus*).

The increased risk for VRE infection and colonization is associated with previous vancomycin and/or multiantimicrobial therapy, severe underlying disease or immunosuppression, and intra-abdominal surgery. Because enterococci are found in the normal gastrointestinal and female genital tracts, most enterococcal infections are attributed to endogenous sources within the patient. Whenever possible, empiric antimicrobial therapy should be modified based on culture and sensitivity results so that the most specific therapy is administered.

Antimicrobial medications are intended to kill or to inhibit the growth of the organism without harming the patient. Antimicrobial agents may be bacteriostatic (inhibit growth of organisms) or bactericidal (kill microorganisms). Drug activity varies, so that at low concentrations a drug may be bacteriostatic, but bactericidal at higher concentrations. Usually antimicrobial drugs target some difference between the microorganism and the host. Overall, antibiotics are prescribed based on patient factors—the condition of the renal and hepatic systems, as well as drug allergies, the spectrum of antibiotic activity, and the site of infection.

This section focuses on antimicrobial medications used to treat infections in patients with cancer: antibacterial, antiviral, and antifungal. These drugs target specific cellular mechanisms of the infectious agent. For example, sulfonamide antibiotics inhibit para-aminobenzoic acid, an essential requirement for nucleic acid synthesis in many bacteria but not in humans. Penicillins and the cephalosporins contain a β-lactam ring that disrupts the synthesis of peptidoglycan. Peptidoglycan gives shape and strength to the bacterial cell wall. Table 11.4 provides an overview of one of the oldest (penicillins/cephalosporins) as well as the newest groups of antibacterials (streptogramins/oxazolidinones).

Within the past few years, the FDA approved daptomycin and telithromycin. These new antibiotics have largely been developed by making minor modifications to an existing class of drugs. Daptomycin is the first drug in a new structural class, the cyclic lipopeptides. Its mode of action is to rapidly kill gram-positive bacteria by disrupting multiple aspects of bacterial membrane function. Telithromycin, a first-in-class antibiotic group called the ketolides, is structurally related to the macrolide antibiotics and specifically designed to offer optimal spectrum activity for the first-line treatment of upper and lower respiratory tract infections. The latest antibiotic group, the glycylcyclines, is structurally similar to the tetracyclines and tigecycline is the first agent in this class to be FDA-approved for the treatment of MRSA.

Another class of antimicrobial agents, the echinocandins or glucan synthesis inhibitors, has recently been added to the options available for treating opportunistic fungal infections. Caspofungin, the first-in-class, inhibits the synthesis of a key component of the fungal cell wall. Caspofungin demonstrates fungicidal activity against *Candida* species; it is indicated for the treatment of invasive *Aspergillus* in patients who are refractory to, or intolerant of, other therapies. Ideal candidates for this drug

Table 11.4 Comparison of Antibiotic Categories

Antibacterial Category	Examples	Mechanism of Action, Including Differences Among or Between Categories or Unique Characteristics
Penicillins		Penicillins are derived from the fungus *Penicillium* and contain a β-lactam ring.
Natural penicillins	• penicillin V • penicillin G	The first group comprises natural penicillins, which are active against many aerobic gram-positive cocci (*S. aureus, Streptococcus*), Gram-negative aerobic cocci (*N. meningitidis,* some *H. influenzae*), and some spirochetes. However, they are resistant to *Pseudomonas*, most *Enterobacter*, and to bacteria that produce the enzyme penicillinase, which inactivates the penicillin molecule.
Penicillinase-resistant penicillins	• cloxacillin • dicloxacillin • nafcillin • oxacillin	The second group contains the penicillinase-resistant penicillins. These are semisynthetic drugs that can withstand the action of the enzyme penicillinase and continue to exert their antibiotic action. They are primarily used to treat *S. aureus* and *S. epidermidis* strains that secrete penicillinase; they also have some activity against gram-negative bacteria and spirochetes.

(continued)

Table 11.4 *(Continued)*

Antibacterial Category	Examples	Mechanism of Action, Including Differences Among or Between Categories or Unique Characteristics
Aminopenicillins	• amoxicillin • ampicillin • bacampicillin	The third group includes the aminopenicillins; this group has heightened activity against gram-negative bacteria as compared to the first two groups. These drugs are resistant to penicillinase-producing bacteria.
Extended-spectrum penicillins	• carbenicillin • mezlocillin • piperacillin • ticarcillin	The fourth group is composed of the extended-spectrum penicillins; drugs in this group have enhanced activity against gram-negative bacilli, both aerobic and nonaerobic.
Cephalosporins		The cephalosporins are derived from cephalosporin C (produced by a fungus) and have broad bactericidal activity. They contain a β-lactam ring and may also be referred to as β-lactam antibiotics. Bacterial resistance can develop, and a major mechanism is the development by the bacteria of an enzyme, β-lactamase, which inactivates the cephalosporin antibiotic by destroying the β-lactam ring.
First generation	• cefadroxil • cephalothin • cefazolin • cephalexin • cephapirin • cephradine	First-generation cephalosporins are active against gram-positive cocci (*Staphylococcus* and *Streptococcus*) and have only limited activity against gram-negative bacteria (e.g., *E. coli*); they have no activity against enterococci.

(continued)

Table 11.4 *(Continued)*

Antibacterial Category	Examples	Mechanism of Action, Including Differences Among or Between Categories or Unique Characteristics
Second generation	• cefaclor • cefamandole • cefmetazole • cefonicid • ceforanide • cefotetan • cefoxitin • cefprozil • cefuroxime • cefuroxime axetil	Second-generation cephalosporins are active against the same organisms as the first-generation drugs but are slightly more active against gram-negative bacteria. In addition, they are active against *H. influenzae*.
Third generation	• cefdinir • cefixime • cefoperazone • cefotaxime • cefpodoxime • ceftazidime • ceftibuten • ceftizoxime • ceftriaxone • loracarbef	Third-generation cephalosporins are less active against gram-positive organisms but have broader activity against gram-negative organisms than either first- or second-generation drugs.
Fourth generation	• cefepime	Fourth-generation cephalosporins are projected to have many attributes including: • Extended spectrum of activity for gram-negative and gram-positive organisms (different from third-generation cephalosporins) • Minimal β-lactamase activity due to rapid periplasmic penetration and high penicillin-binding protein (PBP) access • Spectrum of activity to include gram-negative organisms with multiple drug resistance patterns (*Enterobacter* and *Klebsiella*)

(continued)

Table 11.4 *(Continued)*

Antibacterial Category	Examples	Mechanism of Action, Including Differences Among or Between Categories or Unique Characteristics
Streptogramins	• quinupristin/dalfopristin	This new class of antibiotics, the streptogramin group, is a separate family of antimicrobials. Synercid is an intravenous combination of two semisynthetic, water-soluble derivatives of naturally occurring pristinamycin. The two distinct compounds are quinupristin and dalfopristin, derived from pristinamycin I and pristinamycin II. These two compounds work synergistically to kill susceptible bacteria through a two-pronged attack on protein synthesis in bacterial cells. Each component of the drug binds irreversibly to different sites on the bacterial cell's ribosomal subunit to form a stable quinupristin-ribosome-dalfopristin complex, which disables the cell's ability to make cellular protein. Without the ability to manufacture new proteins, the bacterial cell dies.
Oxazolidinones	• linezolid	Inhibits initiation of protein synthesis by binding to a site on bacterial 23S ribosomal RNA of the 50S subunit. This mechanism of inhibiting protein synthesis is not shared by other antibacterials. Cross-resistance is unlikely.

(continued)

Table 11.4 *(Continued)*

Antibacterial Category	Examples	Mechanism of Action, Including Differences Among or Between Categories or Unique Characteristics
Macrolides	• azithromycin • clarithromycin • erythromycin	Binds to 50S ribosomal subunit resulting in inhibition of protein synthesis. In some cases the drug metabolite is twice as active as the parent compound.
Lipopeptides	• daptomycin	Derived from the fermentation of *Streptomyces roseosporus*. The mechanism of action is not fully understood. Binds to bacterial membranes and causes a rapid depolarization of membrane potential. This loss of membrane potential leads to inhibition of protein, DNA, and RNA synthesis resulting in bacterial cell death.
Ketolide	• telithromycin	Similar to that of macrolides and is related to the 50S-ribosomal subunit binding with inhibition of bacterial protein synthesis. Telithromycin appears to have greater affinity for the ribosomal binding site than macrolides. It concentrates in phagocytes where it exhibits activity against intracellular respiratory pathogens.

are patients with amphotericin B–induced nephrotoxicity. Caspofungin appears to be well tolerated. Micafungin inhibits the synthesis of 1,3-β-D-glucan, an essential component of fungal cell walls. It is indicated for the treatment of patients with esophageal candidiasis and as prophylaxis for *Candida* infections in patients undergoing hematopoietic stem cell transplantation.

The latest echinocandin, anidulafungin, was FDA-approved for the treatment of candidemia and esophageal candidiasis. All three echinocandins are well tolerated and have some use in febrile neutropenia. There have been anecdotal reports of the use of these agents to treat less common fungal infections and limited use as a component of antifungal therapy. Their benefits are few, if any drug interactions and the ability to be used in patients with impaired renal and hepatic function. The echinocandins are an important addition to the antifungal armentarium in the treatment of fungal infections in immunocompromised patients.

Posaconazole is a new broad-spectrum triazole that is used for the treatment and prevention of invasive fungal infections. It is a lipophilic antifungal triazole that is similar to other members in this class, effective against Candida species, Cryptococcus neoformans, Aspergillus species, Fusarium species, zygomycetes, and endemic fungi. The compound is available as an oral suspension and appears to be well-tolerated, even in long-term courses.

On the horizon are some agents that are newly discovered and that are now in development as anti-infective agents. Platensimycin is a previously unknown class of antibiotics produced by *Streptomyces platensis*. Platensimycin demonstrates strong, broad-spectrum gram-positive antibacterial activity by selectively inhibiting cellular lipid biosynthesis in animal models. It remains to be seen whether this new class of antibiotic will be effective against microorganisms in humans.

Finally polyketides are a large family of structurally diverse, natural products with a broad range of biological activities, including antibiotic and pharmacologic properties. Many important antibiotics such as tetracyclines, erythromycin, Adriamycin, monensin, rifamycin and avermectins are polyketides. Work has begun on a general strategy for biosynthesis of polyketides through the cloning of various gene clusters. Currently these bioengineered anti-infectives are being developed in the laboratory; someday we may see these genetically modified agents in the clinical setting.

COMPLICATIONS

References

American Thoracic Society. Guidelines for the management of adults with hospital-acquired, ventilatory-associated and health care-associated pneumonia. *Am J Respiratory Critical Care* 2005; 171 388–416

Ampicillin sodium/sulbactam sodium. Available at http://hcunviweb05/mdxcgi/quiklocn.exe?CTL=E:/Mdx/mdxcgi/MEGAT.SYS&SET=1C573 June 2005

Courtney R, Pai S, Laughlin M, Lim J, Batra V. Pharmacokinetics, Safety, and Tolerability of Oral Posaconazole administered in Single and Multiple Doses in healthy Adults. *Antimicrobial Agents and Chemotherapy* 2003; 47(9) 2788–2795

Cubicin. Product Information. Cubist Pharmaceutical Inc. September 2003

Declomycin. Product Information. Lederle Pharmaceutical Division, American Cynamid Co. Pearl River, NY: 2003

Declomycin. Available at http://www.rxmed.com/b.main/b2.pharmaceutical/b2.1monographs/CPS-%20 Monographs. Accessed June 2004

Drugs.com. Drug Information Online. Daptomycin. Available at http://www.drugs.com/MTM/daptomycin.html. Accessed June 2004

Freifeld AG, Segal BH, Baden LR, et al. NCCN Prevention and Treatment of Cancer-related Infections, v.2. 2007. http://www.canceradvocacy.org/. Accessed June 15, 2007

Gemifloxacin mesylate [package insert]. http://hcunviweb05/mdxcgi/quiklocn.exe?CTL=E:/Mdx/mdxcgi/MEGAT.SYS&SET=1C573. June 2005

Goh KP, Management of hyponatremia. *AM Fam Physician* 2004; 69(10) 2387–2394

Ketek. Product Information. Aventis Pharmaceutical Inc. March 2004

Medline. Drug Information: Daptomycin. Available at http://www.nlm.nih.gov/medline. Accessed June 2004

Meropenem [package insert]. http://hcunviweb05/mdxcgi/quiklocn.exe?CTL=E:/Mdx/mdxcgi/MEGAT.SYS&SET=1C573. June 2005

Mycamine [Package Insert]. Osaka Japan: Fujisawa Pharmaceutical Company LTD; 2005

Raad II, Graybill JR, Bustamante AB, et al. Safety of Long-Term Oral Posaconazole Use in the Treatment of refractory Invasive Fungal Infections. *Clinical Infectious Diseases* 2006; 42(15 June) 1726–1734

Rifaximin [package insert]. http://hcunviweb05/mdxcgi/quiklocn.exe?CTL=E:/Mdx/mdxcgi/MEGAT.SYS&SET=1C573. June 2005

Segal BH, Baden LR, Brown, AE, et al. NCCN Prevention and Treatment of Cancer-Related Infections, v.1.2008. http://www.canceradvocacy.org/. Accessed June 1, 2008

Telithromycin. Thompson Center Watch. Clinical Trials Listing Service. Drugs approved by the FDA. Available at http://www.mcromedex.com/products/updates/drugdex_updates/de/tilithromycinfull.html. Accessed June 2004.

Telithromycin. Available at http://www.centerwatch.com/patient/drugs/dru853.html. Accessed June 2004

Torres HA, Hachem RY, Chemaly RF, et al. Posaconazole: a broad spectrum triazole antifungal. *Lancet Infect Dis* 2005; 5(12) 775–785

Tygacil [package insert]. Philadelphia, PA: Wyeth Pharmaceuticals, Inc.; 2005

United States Pharmacopoeia Drug Information for Health Care Professionals. Rockville, MD: 18th ed.

The United States Pharmacopoeia Convention, Inc.; 1998

Vasquez JA, Sobel JD. Anidulafungin: A Novel Echinocandin. *Clinical Infectious Diseases* 2006; 43 215–222

VHA Pharmacy Benefits Management Strategic Healthcare Group and Medical Advisor Panel. Daptomycin

Warner-Lambert Co. Omnicef Package Insert. Morris Plains, NJ: Parke-Davis; 1998

Wujik D. Infection. Groenwald SL, Frogge MH, Goodman M, Yarbro CH. *Cancer Symptom Management*. Sudbury, MA: Jones and Bartlett; 1996; 289–308

ANTIBIOTICS

Drug: amikacin sulfate (Amikin)

Class: Aminoglycoside antibacterial antibiotic.

Mechanism of Action: Synthetic antibiotic derived from kanamycin; bactericidal, most probably by inhibition of protein synthesis. Active against aerobic microorganisms: many sensitive gram-negative organisms (including *Acinetobacter*, *Citrobacter*, *Enterobacter*, *E. coli*, *Klebsiella*, *Proteus*, *Pseudomonas*, *Salmonella*, *Serratia*, and

Shigella), and some sensitive gram-positive organisms (*S. aureus* and *S. epidermidis*). Over time, bacterial resistance may develop, either naturally or acquired.

Metabolism: Well absorbed following parenteral administration, but variability in absorption after IM injection (peak serum level 0.5–2 hours, duration 8–12 hours). Widely distributed into body fluids. Minimally protein-bound. Readily crosses placenta and into breast milk. Drug excreted unchanged in the urine.

Dosage/Range:

- 15 mg/kg/day given in 8-hour or 12-hour doses IV or IM.
- Desired peak serum concentration is 15–30 μg/mL, and trough serum concentration is 5–10 μg/mL. DOSE-REDUCE IF RENAL IMPAIRMENT.

Drug Preparation:

- Store injectable at < 40°C (104°F).
- Potency not affected by pale yellow color that may develop.
- Stable for 24 hours at concentrations of 0.25 and 5 mg/mL in 0.9% sodium chloride, 5% dextrose.

Drug Administration:

- IV: in 100–200 mL IV fluid (e.g., 0.9% sodium chloride or 5% dextrose injection), infused over 30–60 minutes.

Drug Interactions:

- Increased risk of toxicity with other ototoxic drugs: acyclovir, other aminoglycosides, amphotericin B, bacitracin, cephalosporins, colistin, cisplatin, ethacrynic acid, furosemide, vancomycin.
- Potentiation of neuromuscular blockade when given concurrently with general anesthetics (succinylcholine, tubocurarine)—use cautiously; observe for signs/symptoms of respiratory depression.
- Synergism with extended-spectrum penicillins, but must be administered separately.

Lab Effects/Interference:

- Serum ALT, serum alk phos, serum AST, serum bili, and serum LDH values all may be increased.
- BUN and serum creatinine values may be increased.
- Serum Ca+, serum Mg+, serum K+, and serum Na+ concentrations may be decreased.

Special Considerations:

- Used as first-line treatment in short-term treatment of serious gram-negative infections (e.g., septicemia, respiratory tract infections).
- Use against gram-positive organisms only as second-line treatment.
- Use in pregnancy only if infection is life-threatening and no safer drug exists; drug crosses placenta and may cause fetal toxicity.

Potential Toxicities/Side Effects and the Nursing Process

I. ALTERATIONS IN SENSORY/PERCEPTUAL PATTERNS related to OTOTOXICITY

Defining Characteristics: Damage to eighth cranial nerve (auditory) may result in dizziness, nystagmus, vertigo, ataxia (vestibular damage) and less commonly, tinnitus, roaring sound in ears, and impaired hearing (auditory damage). Hearing loss usually begins with high-frequency loss, followed by clinical hearing loss, then permanent hearing loss if damage continues. Increased risk in elderly or renally impaired patients.

Nursing Implications: Assess baseline hearing (ability to hear spoken voice) and continue during therapy. Teach patient potential side effects, and instruct patient to report any hearing/perceptual problems (e.g., tinnitus, vertigo, decreased hearing). Discuss drug discontinuance and audiogram with physician to confirm hearing dysfunction if symptoms arise. Assess for increased risk if given concurrently with other ototoxic medications (e.g., cisplatin, furosemide).

II. ALTERATION IN URINARY ELIMINATION related to NEPHROTOXICITY

Defining Characteristics: Renal damage characterized by tubular necrosis with increased serum BUN, creatinine; decreased urine creatinine clearance and specific gravity; proteinuria and casts in urine. Azotemia usually not associated with oliguria. Rarely, electrolyte wasting with hypomagnesemia, hypocalcemia, and hypokalemia may occur. Renal dysfunction usually reversible after drug discontinuance. Increased risk in elderly and in patients with preexisting renal dysfunction. Risk is low in well-hydrated patients with normal renal function when normal doses given.

Nursing Implications: Assess baseline renal function and electrolytes, and monitor periodically during therapy. Discuss any abnormalities with physician, as drug should be dose-reduced or discontinued if renal dysfunction develops. Assess baseline total body fluid balance, weight, and monitor periodically during antibiotic therapy. Monitor hydration status to keep patient well hydrated. Assess drug peak and trough levels as ordered so that drug dosage is correctly titrated. Increased risk of toxicity if peak serum concentration > 30–35 μg/mL. Draw blood for peak drug concentration 30 minutes after end of 30-minute infusion or at the end of a 60-minute infusion; draw trough immediately before next dose.

III. ALTERATIONS IN SENSORY/PERCEPTUAL PATTERNS related to CNS EFFECTS, NEUROMUSCULAR BLOCKADE

Defining Characteristics: Headache, tremor, lethargy may occur. Peripheral neuropathy or encephalopathy (numbness, skin tingling, muscle twitching) may occur rarely.

Neuromuscular blockade is dose related, self-limiting, and uncommon: risk is greater with topical application or when drug is administered to patient with neuromuscular disease (myasthenia gravis) or hypocalcemia.

Nursing Implications: Assess baseline neurologic status. Assess coexisting risk factors, neuroblockade medications. Teach patient about side effects, and instruct to report headache, tremor, and lethargy. Observe for respiratory depression. If signs/symptoms arise, discuss drug discontinuance with physician.

IV. POTENTIAL FOR INJURY related to HYPERSENSITIVITY

Defining Characteristics: Rash, urticaria, pruritus, fever, and eosinophilia have occurred rarely. CROSS-SENSITIVITY between AMINOGLYCOSIDES exists!

Nursing Implications: Assess for drug allergies to any aminoglycoside—amikacin, gentamicin, kanamycin, neomycin, netilmicin, streptomycin, tobramycin—prior to drug administration. Instruct patient to report any allergic reactions. Assess for signs/ symptoms of allergic reaction after drug dose.

V. ALTERATION IN NUTRITION, LESS THAN BODY REQUIREMENTS, related to GI SIDE EFFECTS

Defining Characteristics: Nausea, vomiting, anorexia have occurred rarely. Also, transient hepatomegaly with elevated LFTs—AST, ALT, LDH, alk phos—has occurred.

Nursing Implications: Assess baseline nutritional status, preexisting nausea/vomiting, anorexia. Assess baseline LFTs and monitor periodically during treatment. Instruct patient to report side effects. Provide symptomatic interventions if side effects occur; discuss with physician use of alternative drug(s).

VI. POTENTIAL FOR FATIGUE, INFECTION, AND BLEEDING related to BONE MARROW INJURY

Defining Characteristics: Anemia, leukopenia, granulocytopenia, and thrombocytopenia may occur. Also, patients receiving antibiotics are at risk for overgrowth of nonsusceptible microorganisms, such as fungi (superinfection). Rare.

Nursing Implications: Assess baseline CBC, differential, and monitor periodically during treatment. Instruct patient to report signs/symptoms of fatigue, infection, or bleeding immediately. Assess for signs/symptoms of superinfection. Discuss any adverse effects with physician.

Drug: amoxicillin (Amoxil, Polymox, Trimox, Wymox; amoxicillin plus potassium clavulanate is Augmentin)

Class: Penicillin (aminopenicillin antibiotic); β-lactam.

Mechanism of Action: Semisynthetic antibiotic prepared from fungus *Penicillium*. Contains β-lactam ring and is bactericidal by inhibiting cell wall synthesis. Aminopen icillins have increased activity against gram-negative bacilli (*H. influenzae*, *E. coli*), as well as some activity against gram-positive bacilli (*Streptococci* and *Staphylococci*). Used for treatment of infections of upper and lower respiratory tract, genitourinary (GU) tract, and skin by sensitive organisms.

Metabolism: Well absorbed from GI tract; rate of absorption slowed by food but total amount of drug absorbed remains unchanged. Widely distributed in body tissues and fluids. Crosses placenta and is found in breast milk. Excreted in urine and bile.

Dosage/Range:

Adult:

- 125–500 mg PO q 8 h 48–72 hours after infection eradicated; for uncomplicated urinary tract infection, may use single dose of 3 gm PO.
- Drug dose should be reduced if severe renal failure occurs.
- Augmentin dose: mild to moderate infection: 500 mg PO 2 × /day; severe infection: 875 mg PO 2 × /day.

Drug Preparation:

- Store capsules in tight container at 15–30°C (59–86°F).
- Administer on empty stomach.

Drug Interactions:

- Aminoglycosides: synergism.
- Aminoglycosides (e.g., gentamicin): incompatible when mixed together; administer at separate sites at different times. Also, penicillinase-resistant penicillins can inactivate aminoglycoside serum samples from patients receiving both drugs.
- Rifampin: possible antagonism, only at high doses of penicillin.
- Probenecid: increased serum level of penicillin; may be coadministered to exert this effect.
- Allopurinol: increased incidence of rash; avoid concurrent administration if possible.
- Clavulanic acid (β-lactamase inhibitor): synergistic bactericidal effect. Amoxicillin plus potassium clavulanate = Augmentin.

Lab Effects/Interference:

Major clinical significance:

- Urine glucose: high urinary concentrations of a penicillin may produce false-positive or falsely elevated test results with copper-reduction tests (Benedict's, Clinitest, or Fehling's); glucose enzymatic tests (Clinistix or Testape) are not affected.

Clinical significance:

- Coombs' tests: false-positive result may occur during therapy with any penicillin.
- ALT, alk phos, AST, serum bili, and serum LDH values may be increased.
- Estradiol, total conjugated estriol, estriol-glucuronide, or conjugated estrone concentrations may be transiently decreased in pregnant women following administration of amoxicillin.
- WBC: leukopenia or neutropenia is associated with the use of all penicillins; the effect is more likely to occur with prolonged and severe hepatic function impairment.

Special Considerations:

- Contraindicated in patients with prior hypersensitivity to penicillins. Use with caution in patients sensitive to other β-lactams (e.g., cephalosporins) since partial cross-allergenicity exists.
- Obtain ordered specimen and send for culture and sensitivity prior to first antibiotic dose.
- Consider alternative antibiotic therapy if eosinophilia, drug fever or rash, arthralgia, hematuria, or unexplained rise in BUN and serum creatinine occur.
- Monitor electrolytes and renal, hepatic, and hematologic laboratory parameters during extended treatment periods.
- Use with caution in pregnancy or with nursing women.
- Amoxicillin rash may occur that is distinct from drug-allergic rash; increased risk if concurrent use of allopurinol.
- Less diarrhea as a GI side effect than ampicillin.
- May cause false-positive with Clinitest glucose testing.

Potential Toxicities/Side Effects and the Nursing Process

I. POTENTIAL FOR INJURY related to HYPERSENSITIVITY REACTION

Defining Characteristics: Urticaria, pruritus, rash (maculopapular or erythematous), fever and chills, eosinophilia, myalgia, edema, erythema, angioedema, Stevens-Johnson syndrome, and exfoliative skin reactions occur in 5% of patients. Increased risk in individuals allergic to cephalosporin antibiotics. A nonimmunologic rash may occur 3–14 days after drug started, characterized as a generalized erythematous/ maculopapular rash, and worse over pressure areas of elbows and knees. Rash usually subsides in 6–14 days, even if drug is continued. If drug is stopped, resolves in 1–7 days.

Nursing Implications: Assess allergy to cephalosporin antibiotics and penicillin: if patient states "yes," determine actual response, e.g., "swollen lips = angioedema." If angioedema, patient SHOULD NOT receive drug. Discuss other patient responses with physician to determine whether drug should be given. Assess baseline skin condition, including integrity and allergy history to drugs. Instruct patient to report rash, itching, other skin changes. Teach patient skin care and symptomatic measures as appropriate. If skin rash develops, discuss drug discontinuance with physician. If rash progresses, drug should be discontinued, as fatal Stevens-Johnson syndrome may develop. Be prepared to treat severe acute hypersensitivity reactions with airway management, oxygen, epinephrine, corticosteroids, and antihistamines as ordered.

II. ALTERATION IN NUTRITION, LESS THAN BODY REQUIREMENTS, related to GI SIDE EFFECTS

Defining Characteristics: Nausea, vomiting, diarrhea, and anorexia may occur; rarely, pseudomembranous colitis caused by *Clostridium difficile* resistant to the antibiotic occurs. Rarely, transient increases in LFTs—AST, ALT, alk phos, bili—may occur.

Nursing Implications: Assess baseline nutritional status. Instruct patient to report GI disturbances. Administer and instruct patient to self-administer antiemetics as needed and as ordered. Teach patient importance of nutritious diet, and suggest small, frequent, high-calorie, high-protein meals as appropriate. Assess baseline LFTs and monitor periodically during treatment. Discuss abnormalities and drug interruption with physician.

III. FUNGAL SUPERINFECTION related to OVERGROWTH of ENDOGENOUS MICROORGANISMS

Defining Characteristics: Vaginal candidiasis, vaginitis may occur as endogenous bacteria are eliminated, and normal fungal population expands.

Nursing Implications: Teach female patient to report vaginal itching or discharge. Discuss appropriate antifungal treatment with physician. Teach perineal hygiene and symptomatic management.

IV. ALTERATIONS IN PROTECTIVE MECHANISMS (RARE) related to TRANSIENT LEUKOPENIA

Defining Characteristics: Rarely, transient leukopenia, lymphocytosis, anemia, eosinophilia may occur. Prolonged PT, prolonged activated partial thromboplastin time (APTT), and hypoprothrombinemia have occurred rarely, especially in elderly or debilitated patients, or in individuals with vitamin K deficiency.

Nursing Implications: Assess baseline laboratory parameters, and monitor periodically during treatment. Assess patient for response to antibiotics. Discuss abnormalities with physician.

V. KNOWLEDGE DEFICIT related to SELF-ADMINISTRATION OF MEDICATION

Defining Characteristics: Increased compliance when patient is instructed in self-care activities.

Nursing Implications: Assess knowledge regarding infection and planned treatment. Teach drug action, potential side effects, and when and how to take drug (take medication as directed, 1 hour before or 2 hours after food). Instruct patient to report any possible drug side effects that occur.

Drug: ampicillin sodium/sulbactam sodium (UNASYN)

Class: Penicillin (aminopenicillin antibiotic).

Mechanism of Action: Semisynthetic antibiotic prepared from fungus *Penicillium*. Contains β-lactam ring and is bactericidal by inhibiting cell wall synthesis. Aminopenicillins have increased activity against gram-negative bacilli (*H. influenzae, E. coli*), as well as some activity against gram-positive bacilli (*Streptococci* and *Staphylococci*). Although sulbactam alone possesses little useful antibacterial activity, whole organism studies have shown that sulbactam restores ampicillin activity against beta-lactamase producing strains of bacteria. Used for treatment of infections of the skin, intra-abdominal infections, and gynecologic infections by sensitive organisms. In combination with sulbactam there is irreversible inhibition of beta lactamases, thus making ampicillin effective against beta lactamase bacteria that would otherwise be resistant to it.

Metabolism: Well absorbed from GI tract, but rate and amount of drug absorbed is decreased with food. Widely distributed in body tissues and fluids. Crosses placenta and is found in breast milk. Excreted in urine and bile.

Dosage/Range:

Adult:

- Dose modification necessary if renal impairment occurs. See manufacturer's package insert.
- UNASYN: 1.5–3 grams ampicillin and 0.5–1 gram sulbactam IV/IM every 6 hours (dose not to exceed 4 g sulbactam a day).

Drug Preparation:

- IV dilute with Normal Saline only, give over 10–30 minutes.
- IM: reconstitute per manufacturer's directions and use within 1 hour after reconstitution.

Drug Interaction:

- Aminoglycosides: synergism.
- Aminoglycosides (e.g., gentamicin): incompatible when mixed together; administer at separate sites at different times. Also, penicillinase-resistant

penicillins can inactivate aminoglycoside serum samples from patients receiving both drugs.
- Rifampin: possible antagonism, only at high doses of ampicillin.
- Probenecid: decreases renal tubular secretion of ampicillin and sulbactam.
- Oral contraceptives: may decrease efficacy of contraceptive and increase incidence of breakthrough bleeding. Suggest additional use of barrier contraception.
- Sulbactam: broadens antibacterial coverage of ampicillin against resistant beta lactamase-producing microorganisms.
- Concurrent administration of allopurinol and ampicillin increases the incidence of rashes.

Lab Effects/Interference:
- Urine glucose: high urinary concentrations of a penicillin may produce false-positive or falsely elevated test results with copper-reduction tests (Benedict's Clinitest, or Fehling's); glucose enzymatic tests (Clinistix or Testape) are not affected.
- Estradiol, total conjugated estriol, estriol-glucuronide or conjugated estrone concentrations may be transiently decreased in pregnant women following administration of ampicillin.
- Increased AST (SGOT), ALT (SGPT), alkaline phosphatase, and LDH.
- Decreased serum albumin and total protein.
- WBC: leukopenia or neutropenia is associated with the use of all penicillins; the effect is more likely to occur with prolonged and severe hepatic function impairment.
- BUN and serum creatinine: increased concentrations have been associated with ampicillin.

Special Considerations:
- Contraindicated in patients with prior hypersensitivity to penicillins. Use with caution in patients sensitive to other β-lactams (e.g., cephalosporins) since partial cross-allergenicity exists.
- Obtain ordered specimen and send for culture and sensitivity prior to first antibiotic dose.
- Consider alternative antibiotic therapy if eosinophilia, drug fever or rash, arthralgia, hematuria, or unexplained rise in BUN and serum creatinine occur.
- Monitor electrolytes and renal, hepatic, and hematologic laboratory parameters during extended treatment periods.
- Use with caution in pregnancy or with nursing women.
- Renal dysfunction: Unasyn dose must be reduced.

Potential Toxicities/Side Effects and the Nursing Process

I. POTENTIAL FOR INJURY related to HYPERSENSITIVITY REACTION and LOCAL REACTIONS (pain at injection site & thrombophlebitis)

Defining Characteristics: Urticaria, pruritus, rash (maculopapular or erythematous), fever and chills, eosinophilia, myalgia, edema, erythema, angioedema,

Stevens-Johnson syndrome, and exfoliative skin reactions occur in 5% of patients. Increased risk in individuals allergic to cephalosporin antibiotics.

Nursing Implications: Assess allergy to cephalosporin antibiotics and penicillin: if patient states "yes," determine actual response, e.g., "swollen lips = angioedema." If angioedema, patient SHOULD NOT receive drug. Discuss other patient responses with physician to determine whether drug should be given. Assess baseline skin condition, including integrity and allergy history to drugs. Instruct patient to report rash, itching, other skin changes. Teach patient skin care and symptomatic measures as appropriate. If skin rash develops, discuss drug discontinuance with physician. If rash progresses, drug should be discontinued, as fatal Stevens-Johnson syndrome may develop. Be prepared to treat severe acute hypersensitivity reactions with airway management, oxygen, epinephrine, corticosteroids, and antihistamines as ordered.

II. ALTERATION IN NUTRITION, LESS THAN BODY REQUIREMENTS, related to GI SIDE EFFECTS

Defining Characteristics: Nausea, vomiting, diarrhea may occur; rarely, pseudomembranous colitis caused by *C. difficile* resistant to the antibiotic occurs. Rarely, transient increases in LFTs—AST, ALT, alk phos, bili—may occur.

Nursing Implications: Assess baseline nutritional status. Instruct patient to report GI disturbances. Administer and teach patient to self-administer antiemetics as needed and as ordered. Teach patient importance of nutritious diet, and suggest small, frequent, high-calorie, high-protein meals as appropriate. Assess baseline LFTs, and monitor periodically during treatment. Discuss abnormalities and drug interruption with physician.

III. FUNGAL SUPERINFECTION related to REDISTRIBUTION OF ENDOGENOUS MICROORGANISMS

Defining Characteristics: Vaginal candidiasis, vaginitis may occur as endogenous bacteria are eliminated, and normal fungal population expands.

Nursing Implications: Instruct female patient to report vaginal itching or discharge. Discuss appropriate antifungal treatment with physician. Teach perineal hygiene and symptomatic management.

IV. KNOWLEDGE DEFICIT related to SELF-ADMINISTRATION OF MEDICATION

Defining Characteristics: Increased compliance when patient is instructed in self-care activities.

Nursing Implications: Assess knowledge regarding infection and planned treatment. Teach about drug action, potential side effects, and when and how to take drug. (Take medication as directed, 1 hour before or 2 hours after food.) Instruct patient to report any possible drug side effects.

Drug: azithromycin (Zithromax)

Class: Antibacterial (macrolide).

Mechanism of Action: Azithromycin binds to the 50S ribosomal subunit of the 70S ribosome of susceptible organisms, thereby inhibiting RNA-dependent protein synthesis. Bactericidal for *S. pyogenes*, *S. pneumoniae*, and *H. influenzae*. It is bacteriostatic for staphylococci and most aerobic gram-negative species.

Metabolism: Rapidly and widely distributed throughout the body; concentrates intracellularly, resulting in tissue concentrations 10 to 100 times those in plasma and serum. Rapidly absorbed with decreased absorption when given with food. Azithromycin is highly concentrated in phagocytes and fibroblasts. Over 50% of the dose is eliminated through biliary excretion as unchanged drug; approximately 4.5% of the dose is excreted unchanged in the urine within 72 hours.

Dosage/Range:
- Oral: loading dose of 500 mg as a single dose on day 1, then 250 mg once a day on days 2–5.
- No adjustment in dose is required in patients with mild renal function impairment. No data available for patients with more severe renal function impairment.
- IV: if indicated, 500 mg may be given daily × 1–2 days, then followed by oral therapy 250 mg to complete course.

Drug Preparation
- Reconstitute 500-mg vial with 4.8 mL sterile water for concentration of 100 mg/mL.
- Further dilute with 250 or 500 mL of compatible IV solution.

Drug Administrations:
- Oral: give at least 1 hour before and 2 hours after meals. Give at least 1 hour before and 2 hours after aluminum- and magnesium-containing antacids.
- IV: infuse 500 mg/500 mL over 3 hours and 500 mg/250 mL over 1 hour.

Drug Interactions:
- Concurrent use with antacids has decreased the peak serum concentration by approximately 24%.

Lab Effects/Interference:
- Serum SGPT, serum SGOT values may be increased.
- Creatinine clearance ≥ 40 mL per minute is desired.

Special Considerations:

- Do not use when there is a known hypersensitivity to erythromycins or other macrolides.
- Use with caution in patients with severe, impaired hepatic function.

Potential Toxicities/Side Effects and the Nursing Process

I. POTENTIAL FOR INJURY related to HYPERSENSITIVITY

Defining Characteristics: Rarely, serious allergic reactions such as anaphylaxis and angioedema have been known to occur. Fever, joint pain, skin rash, urticaria, pruritus, difficulty breathing, swelling of face, mouth, neck, hands, and feet have occurred rarely.

Nursing Implications: Assess for drug allergies to erythromycin or macrolide antibiotic prior to drug administration. Teach patient to report any allergic reactions. Assess for signs/symptoms of allergic reaction after drug dose.

II. ALTERATION IN NUTRITION related to GI SIDE EFFECTS

Defining Characteristics: Abdominal pain, diarrhea, nausea, and vomiting have occurred rarely.

Nursing Implications: Assess baseline nutritional status, preexisting nausea/vomiting, anorexia. Assess baseline LFTs and monitor periodically during treatment. Teach patient to report side effects. Provide symptomatic interventions if side effects occur; discuss with physician use of alternative drug(s).

III. ALTERATION IN URINARY ELIMINATION related to ACUTE INTERSTITIAL NEPHRITIS

Defining Characteristics: Risk is low, but patient may manifest symptoms of acute interstitial nephritis—fever, joint pain, skin rash.

Nursing Implications: Assess baseline renal function and electrolytes, and monitor periodically during therapy. Monitor hydration status to keep patient well hydrated.

IV. SENSORY/PERCEPTUAL ALTERATIONS related to CNS EFFECTS OF DIZZINESS AND HEADACHE

Defining Characteristics: Dizziness and headache may occur.

Nursing Implications: Assess baseline neurological status. Teach patient about side effects and to report dizziness or headache. If signs/symptoms arise, discuss drug discontinuance with physician.

Drug: aztreonam (Azactam)

Class: Antibacterial (systemic).

Mechanism of Action: Bactericidal by inhibition of cell wall synthesis, which results in cell wall disintegration, lysis, and cell death. Narrow-spectrum of activity against aerobic, gram-negative microorganisms (*Enterobacteriaceae* and *P. aeruginosa*). Used to treat gram-negative infections of urinary and lower respiratory tract, septicemia, and gynecologic and intra-abdominal infections.

Metabolism: Poorly absorbed from GI tract. Widely distributed in body tissue and fluids, including CSF and peritoneal fluid. Crosses placenta and is excreted in breast milk. Partially metabolized, and excreted primarily in urine.

Dosage/Range:
- Given IV or IM (IV preferred for doses > 1 g, and for serious infections).
- Adults: 500 mg–2 g IV/IM q 6–12 h (maximum 8 g/day).
- Dose modification needed for renal dysfunction (creatinine clearance < 30 mL/min); may need to modify dosage in hepatic impairment.

Drug Preparation:
- IV: reconstitute by adding 10 mL sterile water for injection or compatible IV fluid. Further dilute by adding to a volume of IV fluid (50 mL for each gram of drug) so final concentration is < 20 mg/mL. Administer over 20–60 minutes. Flush line with plain IV fluid before and after drug infusion to prevent incompatibilities.
- IM: reconstitute drug with 3 mL for each gram of drug using sterile or bacteriostatic water for injection, or 0.9% sodium chloride. Do not mix with local anesthetics. Administer deep IM in large muscle mass (e.g., gluteus maximus).

Drug Interactions:
- Probenecid: increased serum concentrations of antibiotic; monitor and decrease dose if needed.
- Aminoglycosides, penicillins: may have synergistic antibacterial effect against some organisms.
- Nephrotoxic drugs (aminoglycosides, colistin, vancomycin): may increase risk of renal dysfunction; avoid if possible.
- Magnesium, calcium: incompatible in IV fluid.
- Oral anticoagulants, ASPIRIN: may increase risk of bleeding.
- Alcohol: disulfiram-like reaction (flushing, throbbing headache, dyspnea, nausea, vomiting, diaphoresis, chest pain, palpitation, hyperventilation, tachycardia, hypertension, syncope, weakness, blurred vision) when alcohol is ingested within 48–72 hours of aztreonam; does not occur if alcohol is ingested prior to first antibiotic dose. If no alcohol prior to first dose, avoid alcohol for 72 hours after last dose.

Lab Effects/Interference:
- Coombs' (antiglobulin) tests may become positive during therapy.

- Serum ALT, serum alk phos, serum AST, and serum LDH values may be transiently increased during therapy.
- Serum creatinine concentrations may be transiently increased during therapy.
- PTT and PT may be prolonged during therapy.

Special Considerations:

- Obtain and send specimen for culture and sensitivity prior to first drug dose.
- May cause false-positive Clinitest glucose result.
- Use with caution in patients with renal or hepatic dysfunction.
- Drug crosses placenta and is excreted in breast milk. Use with caution if patient is pregnant; weigh potential risks and benefits carefully if lactating; suggest interruption of breast-feeding during antibiotic therapy.
- Use cautiously if prior immediate hypersensitivity reaction to penicillins or cephalosporins; little risk of cross-allergenicity, but monitor patient closely.
- Comparable anti-infective effectiveness to aminoglycosides against gram-negative organisms without ototoxicity or nephrotoxicity.

Potential Toxicities/Side Effects and the Nursing Process

I. ALTERATIONS IN SKIN INTEGRITY related to ALLERGY HYPERSENSITIVITY REACTION

Defining Characteristics: 1–2% incidence of rash that is mild, transient, pruritic, and/or erythematous. Less than 1% of patients develop purpura, erythema multiforme, urticaria, or exfoliative dermatitis. Less than 1% incidence occurs of immediate hypersensitivity reaction characterized by angioedema, bronchospasm, severe shock. Little cross-allergenicity with penicillins, cephalosporins (less than 1%).

Nursing Implications: Assess baseline skin integrity and presence of drug allergies; if anaphylactic reaction to penicillins or cephalosporins, monitor patient closely during drug infusions. Instruct patient to report immediately signs/symptoms of rash, pruritus, shortness of breath, and adverse sensation. Teach patient skin care and symptomatic measures as appropriate. If skin rash develops, discuss drug discontinuance with physician. If rash progresses, especially in HIV-infected patients, drug should be discontinued, as fatal Stevens-Johnson syndrome may develop. Be prepared to treat severe acute hypersensitivity reactions with airway management, oxygen, epinephrine, corticosteroids, antihistamines as ordered.

II. ALTERATION IN NUTRITION, LESS THAN BODY REQUIREMENTS, related to GI SIDE EFFECTS

Defining Characteristics: Nausea, vomiting, diarrhea, anorexia may occur; rarely, pseudomembranous colitis caused by *C. difficile* resistant to the antibiotic occurs.

Rarely, transient increases in LFTs—AST, ALT, alk phos—may occur. May develop taste alteration and halitosis.

Nursing Implications: Assess baseline nutritional status. Instruct patient to report GI disturbances. Administer and teach patient to self-administer antiemetics as needed and as ordered. Teach patient importance of nutritious diet, and suggest small, frequent, high-calorie, high-protein meals as appropriate. Assess baseline LFTs, and monitor periodically during treatment. Discuss abnormalities and drug interruption with physician. Encourage oral hygiene after meals and at bedtime.

III. FUNGAL SUPERINFECTION related to REDISTRIBUTION OF ENDOGENOUS MICROORGANISMS

Defining Characteristics: Vaginal candidiasis, vaginitis may occur as endogenous bacteria are eliminated, and normal fungal population expands.

Nursing Implications: Instruct female patient to report vaginal itching or discharge. Discuss appropriate antifungal treatment with physician. Teach perineal hygiene and symptomatic management.

IV. ALTERATIONS IN PROTECTIVE MECHANISMS (RARE) related to PANCYTOPENIA

Defining Characteristics: Pancytopenia, neutropenia, thrombocytopenia, anemia, leukocytosis, thrombocytosis may occur rarely. Eosinophilia occurs in 11% of patients. May have slight prolongation of bleeding time with high doses (e.g., 2-gm IV q 6 h).

Nursing Implications: Assess baseline laboratory parameters, and monitor periodically during treatment. Assess patient for response to antibiotics. Discuss abnormalities with physician. Assess for signs/symptoms of bleeding. If taking anticoagulants, assess for increased PT, signs/symptoms of bleeding.

V. ALTERATIONS IN SENSORY/PERCEPTUAL PATTERNS related to DIZZINESS, SOMNOLENCE

Defining Characteristics: Dizziness, headache, somnolence, seizures occur rarely.

Nursing Implications: Assess baseline neurologic function and comfort, and monitor during treatment. Instruct patient to report any changes. Discuss any abnormalities with physician.

VI. ALTERATIONS IN COMFORT related to LOCAL INJECTION IRRITATION

Defining Characteristics: 2–3% incidence of phlebitis and thrombophlebitis when administering IV; 3% incidence of pain and swelling at injection site when given IM.

Nursing Implications: Rotate IM injection sites, and administer drug deep IM in large muscle mass (e.g., gluteus maximus). Use IM injection when IV administration is not possible. Change IV sites q 48 h, and assess for signs/symptoms of phlebitis prior to each administration. Administer drug slowly. Apply warm packs to increase comfort.

VII. ALTERATIONS IN CARDIAC OUTPUT related to CARDIOVASCULAR CHANGES

Defining Characteristics: Rare, ~1% incidence of hypotension, transient EKG changes (e.g., premature ventricular contractions), bradycardia, flushing, and chest pain.

Nursing Implications: Assess baseline heart rate and BP; monitor during therapy, at least with initial dose.

Drug: carbenicillin indanyl sodium (Geocillin, Geopen)

Class: Extended-spectrum penicillin antibacterial.

Mechanism of Action: Semisynthetic penicillin prepared from fungus *Penicillium*. Contains β-lactam ring and is bactericidal by inhibiting cell wall synthesis. Active against gram-positive and gram-negative organisms, but most active against *Pseudomonas* and *Proteus,* except those that have developed resistance to carbenicillin.

Metabolism: After oral administration, rapidly converted to carbenicillin by hydrolysis. Widely distributed in body tissues and fluids. Crosses placenta and is excreted in breast milk. Excreted via urine and bile.

Dosage/Range:

Adult:

- 1 tablet (382 mg).
- Urinary tract infections:
  - *Escherichia coli*, *Proteus* species, *Enterobacter*: 1–2 tabs QID (QID = 4 times a day).
  - *Pseudomonas*, *Enterococcus*: 2 tabs QID.

- Prostatitis due to *Escherichia coli*, *Proteus mirabilis*, *Enterobacter*, *Enterococcus*: 2 tabs QID.

Drug Preparation:
- Oral, none.

Drug Interactions:
- Probenecid: increased serum level of penicillin; may be coadministered to exert this effect.

Lab Effects/Interference:
Major clinical significance:
- Urine glucose: high urinary concentrations of a penicillin may produce false positive or falsely elevated test results with copper sulfate tests (Benedict's, Clinitest, or Fehling's); glucose enzymatic tests (Clinistix or Testape) are not affected.
- PTT and PT: an increase has been associated with intravenous carbenicillin.

Clinical significance:
- Coombs' (direct antiglobulin) tests: false-positive result may occur during therapy with any penicillin.
- ALT, alk phos, AST, and serum LDH values may be decreased.
- WBC: leukopenia or neutropenia is associated with the use of all penicillins; the effect is more likely to occur with prolonged therapy and severe hepatic function impairment.

Special Considerations:
- Contraindicated in patients with prior hypersensitivity to penicillins. Use with caution in patients sensitive to other β-lactams (e.g., cephalosporins) since partial cross-allergenicity exists.
- Obtain ordered specimen and send for culture and sensitivity prior to first antibiotic dose.
- Consider alternative antibiotic therapy if eosinophilia, drug fever or rash, arthralgia, hematuria, or unexplained rise in BUN and serum creatinine occur.
- Use with caution in pregnancy or with nursing women.

Potential Toxicities/Side Effects and the Nursing Process

I. POTENTIAL FOR INJURY related to HYPERSENSITIVITY REACTION

Defining Characteristics: Urticaria, pruritus, rash (maculopapular or erythematous), fever and chills, eosinophilia, myalgia, edema, erythema, angioedema, Stevens-Johnson syndrome, and exfoliative skin reactions occur in 5% of patients. Increased risk in individuals allergic to cephalosporin antibiotics.

Nursing Implications: Assess allergy to cephalosporin antibiotics and penicillin: if patient states "yes," determine actual response, e.g., "swollen lips = angioedema."

If angioedema, patient SHOULD NOT receive drug. Discuss other patient responses with physician to determine whether drug should be given. Assess baseline skin condition, including integrity and allergy history to drugs. Instruct patient to report rash, itching, other skin changes. Teach patient skin care and symptomatic measures as appropriate. If skin rash develops, discuss drug discontinuance with physician. If rash progresses, drug should be discontinued, as fatal Stevens-Johnson syndrome may develop.

II. ALTERATION IN NUTRITION, LESS THAN BODY REQUIREMENTS, related to GI SIDE EFFECTS

Defining Characteristics: Nausea, vomiting, diarrhea may occur; rarely, "furry" tongue, abdominal cramps, transient increases in LFTs—AST, ALT, alk phos, bili—may occur.

Nursing Implications: Assess baseline nutritional status. Instruct patient to report GI disturbances. Administer and teach patient to self-administer antiemetics as needed and as ordered. Teach patient importance of nutritious diet, and suggest small, frequent, high-calorie, high-protein meals as appropriate. Assess baseline LFTs and monitor periodically during treatment. Discuss abnormalities and drug interruption with physician.

III. FUNGAL SUPERINFECTION related to REDISTRIBUTION OF ENDOGENOUS MICROORGANISMS

Defining Characteristics: Vaginal candidiasis, vaginitis may occur as endogenous bacteria are eliminated, and normal fungal population expands.

Nursing Implications: Instruct female patient to report vaginal itching or discharge. Discuss appropriate antifungal treatment with physician. Teach perineal hygiene and symptomatic management.

IV. ALTERATIONS IN PROTECTIVE MECHANISMS (RARE) related to LEUKOPENIA

Defining Characteristics: Rarely, transient leukopenia, lymphocytosis, anemia, eosinophilia may occur. Prolonged PT, prolonged APTT, and hypoprothrombinemia have occurred rarely, especially in elderly or debilitated patients, or in individuals with vitamin K deficiency.

Nursing Implications: Assess baseline laboratory parameters, and monitor periodically during treatment. Assess patient for response to antibiotics. Discuss abnormalities with physician. Assess for signs/symptoms of bleeding.

Drug: cefaclor (Ceclor)

Class: Second-generation cephalosporin antibiotic.

Mechanism of Action: Semisynthetic derivative of cephalosporin C (produced by fungus); contains β-lactam ring and is related to penicillins and cephamycins (e.g., cefoxitin). Bactericidal through inhibition of cell wall synthesis, with resulting cell wall instability and cell lysis. Active against organisms causing lower respiratory tract infections (*H. influenzae, Klebsiella, Proteus, S. aureus, Streptococcus pneumoniae*); urinary tract infections (*Enterobacter, E. coli*); skin and soft tissue infections (*S. aureus, E. coli*); septicemia; and biliary infections. (Active against *H. influenzae, S. pneumoniae, Streptococcus pyogenes, E. coli, Proteus mirabilis, Klebsiella,* and staphylococci.)

Metabolism: Well absorbed from GI tract; delayed GI absorption if taken with food, but total amount of drug absorption is the same. Widely distributed in body tissues, fluids except CSF; readily crosses placenta and is excreted in breast milk. Unchanged drug rapidly excreted by the kidneys.

Dosage/Range:
- Oral: 250–500 mg q 8 h (maximum total 4 gm/day).

Drug Preparation:
- Store in tight container at 15–30°C (59–86°F).

Drug Interactions:
- Probenecid: increased serum concentrations of cefaclor, but does not usually require dose reduction of antibiotic.

Lab Effects/Interference:
Major clinical significance:
- Coombs' (antiglobulin) tests: a positive reaction frequently appears in patients who receive large doses of cephalosporins; hemolysis rarely occurs, but it has been reported; test may be positive in neonates whose mothers received cephalosporins before delivery.
- Urine glucose: cefaclor may produce false-positive or falsely elevated test results with copper sulfate tests (Benedicts, Clinitest, or Fehling's); glucose enzymatic tests (Clonistix or Testape) are not affected.
- PT: may be prolonged; cephalosporins may inhibit vitamin K synthesis by suppressing gut flora.

Clinical significance:
- Serum ALT, serum alk phos, serum AST, serum bili, or serum LDH values may be increased.
- BUN and serum creatinine concentrations may be increased.
- CBC or platelet count: transient leukopenia, neutropenia, agranulocytosis, thrombocytopenia, eosinophilia, lymphocytosis, and thrombocytosis have been seen on rare occasions.

Special Considerations:

- Use cautiously if renal impairment is present.
- Contraindicated if hypersensitive to other cephalosporins, or if has had angioedema response to penicillin.
- Urine glucose testing with Clinitest may result in false-positive.

Potential Toxicities/Side Effects and the Nursing Process

I. POTENTIAL FOR INJURY related to HYPERSENSITIVITY REACTION

Defining Characteristics: Urticaria, pruritus, rash (maculopapular or erythematous), fever and chills, eosinophilia, myalgia, edema, erythema, angioedema, Stevens-Johnson syndrome, and exfoliative skin reactions occur in 5% of patients. Increased risk in individuals allergic to penicillin.

Nursing Implications: Assess allergy to cephalosporin antibiotics and penicillin: if patient states "yes," determine actual response, e.g., "swollen lips = angioedema." If angioedema, patient SHOULD NOT receive drug. Discuss other patient responses with physician to determine whether drug should be given. Assess baseline skin condition, including integrity and allergy history to drugs. Instruct patient to report rash, itching, and other skin changes. Teach patient skin care and symptomatic measures as appropriate. If skin rash develops, discuss drug discontinuance with physician. If rash progresses, drug should be discontinued, as fatal Stevens-Johnson syndrome may develop. Be prepared to treat severe acute hypersensitivity reactions with airway management, oxygen, epinephrine, corticosteroids, antihistamines as ordered.

II. ALTERATION IN NUTRITION, LESS THAN BODY REQUIREMENTS, related to GI SIDE EFFECTS

Defining Characteristics: Nausea, vomiting, diarrhea, and anorexia may occur; rarely, pseudomembranous colitis caused by *C. difficile* resistant to the antibiotic occurs. May cause transient increases in LFTs.

Nursing Implications: Assess baseline nutritional status. Instruct patient to report GI disturbances. Administer and teach patient to self-administer antiemetics as needed and as ordered. Teach patient importance of nutritious diet, and suggest small, frequent, high-calorie, high-protein meals as appropriate. Assess baseline LFTs and monitor periodically during treatment. Discuss abnormalities and drug interruption with physician.

III. FUNGAL SUPERINFECTION related to REDISTRIBUTION OF ENDOGENOUS MICROORGANISMS

Defining Characteristics: Vaginal candidiasis, vaginitis may occur as endogenous bacteria are eliminated, and normal fungal population expands.

Nursing Implications: Instruct female patient to report vaginal itching or discharge. Discuss appropriate antifungal treatment with physician. Teach perineal hygiene and symptomatic management.

IV. ALTERATIONS IN PROTECTIVE MECHANISMS (RARE) related to CHANGES IN BLOOD CELL ELEMENTS, CLOTTING FACTOR

Defining Characteristics: Rarely, transient leukopenia, lymphocytosis, anemia, eosinophilia may occur. Prolonged PT, prolonged APTT, and hypoprothrombinemia have occurred rarely, especially in elderly or debilitated patients, or in individuals with vitamin K deficiency.

Nursing Implications: Assess baseline laboratory parameters, and monitor periodically during treatment. Assess patient for response to antibiotics. Discuss abnormalities with physician.

V. ALTERATIONS IN SENSORY/PERCEPTUAL PATTERNS related to DIZZINESS, SOMNOLENCE

Defining Characteristics: Dizziness, headache, somnolence occur rarely.

Nursing Implications: Assess baseline neurologic function and comfort, and monitor during treatment. Instruct patient to report any changes. Discuss any abnormalities with physician.

VI. KNOWLEDGE DEFICIT related to SELF-ADMINISTRATION OF MEDICATION

Defining Characteristics: Increased compliance when patient is instructed in self-care activities.

Nursing Implications: Assess knowledge regarding infection and planned treatment. Teach about drug action, potential side effects, and when and how to take drug. Instruct patient to report any possible side effects that occur.

Drug: cefadroxil (Duracef)

Class: First-generation cephalosporin antibacterial.

Mechanism of Action: Semisynthetic derivative of cephalosporin C, contains β-lactam ring, and is related to penicillins and cephamycins. Bactericidal through inhibition of cell wall synthesis by binding to one or more of the penicillin-binding proteins (PBPs) that in turn inhibit the final transpeptidation step of peptidoglycan synthesis in bacterial cell walls, thus inhibiting cell wall biosynthesis. Bacteria eventually lyse due to ongoing activity of cell wall autolytic enzymes (autolysins and murein hydrolases) while cell wall assembly is arrested.

Metabolism: Well absorbed from GI tract; delayed GI absorption if taken with food, but total amount of drug absorption is the same. Widely distributed in body tissues, fluids except cerebrospinal fluid; readily crosses placenta and is excreted in breast milk. Unchanged drug rapidly excreted by the kidneys.

Dosage/Range:
- Adults: 1–2 g/day every 12 hours.
- Dose: reduce if creatinine clearance is reduced per manufacturer's recommendations.

Drug Preparation:
- Store suspension in refrigerator, discard after 14 days.
- Oral administration.

Drug Interactions:
- Furosemide and aminoglycosides increase nephrotic potential and increase toxicity.
- Probenecid may decrease cephalosporin elimination and increase effect.

Lab Effects/Interference:
- Serum SGPT, serum alk phos, serum SGOT, serum bilirubin, or serum LDH—values may be increased.
- BUN and serum creatinine—concentrations may be increased.

Special Considerations:
- Use with caution in patients with renal dysfunction—dose reduction required if severe impairment exists.
- Contraindicated in patients hypersensitive to other cephalosporin antibiotics.
- Use cautiously if sensitive to penicillin; contraindicated if angioedema reaction to penicillin.
- Obtain ordered specimen and send for culture and sensitivity prior to first drug dose.

COMPLICATIONS

Potential Toxicities/Side Effects and the Nursing Process

I. POTENTIAL FOR INJURY related to HYPERSENSITIVITY REACTION

Defining Characteristics: Urticaria, pruritus, rash (maculopapular or erythematous), fever and chills, eosinophilia, myalgia, edema, erythema, angioedema. Increased risk in individuals allergic to penicillin.

Nursing Implications: Assess allergy to cephalosporin antibiotics and penicillin: if patient states "yes," determine actual response, e.g., "swollen lips = angioedema."

If angioedema, patient SHOULD NOT receive drug. Discuss other patient responses with physician to determine whether drug should be given. Assess baseline skin condition, including integrity and allergy history to drugs. Teach patient to report rash, itching, other skin changes. Teach patient skin care and symptomatic measures as appropriate. If skin rash develops, discuss drug discontinuance with physician.

II. ALTERATION IN NUTRITION, LESS THAN BODY REQUIREMENTS, related to GI SIDE EFFECTS

Defining Characteristics: Nausea and vomiting, diarrhea, and anorexia may occur. Rarely, transient increases in LFTs—AST (SGOT), ALT (SGPT), ALKPHOS, BR—may occur.

Nursing Implications: Assess baseline nutritional status. Teach patient to report GI disturbances. Administer and teach patient to self-administer medication as needed and as ordered. Teach patient importance of nutritious diet, and suggest small, frequent, high-calorie, high-protein meals as appropriate. Assess baseline LFTs and monitor periodically during treatment. Discuss abnormalities and drug interruption with physician.

III. FUNGAL SUPERINFECTION related to REDISTRIBUTION OF ENDOGENOUS MICROORGANISMS

Defining Characteristics: Vaginal moniliasis, vaginitis may occur as endogenous bacteria are eliminated and normal fungal population expands.

Nursing Implications: Teach female patient to report vaginal itching or discharge. Discuss appropriate antifungal treatment with physician. Teach perineal hygiene and symptomatic management.

Drug: cefamandole nafate (Mandol)

Class: Second-generation cephalosporin antibacterial.

Mechanism of Action: Semisynthetic derivative of cephalosporin C (produced by fungus); contains β-lactam ring and is related to penicillins and cephamycins (e.g., cefoxitin). Bactericidal through inhibition of cell wall synthesis, with resulting cell wall instability and cell lysis. Active against organisms causing lower respiratory tract infections (*H. influenzae, Klebsiella, Proteus, S. aureus, S. pneumoniae*); urinary tract infections (*Enterobacter, E. coli*); skin and soft tissue infections (*S. aureus, E. coli*); septicemia; and biliary infections.

Metabolism: Not absorbed from GI tract, so must be given IV or IM. Rapidly hydrolyzed to active metabolite. Widely distributed to body tissues and fluids except CSF; 65–75% bound to serum proteins. Readily crosses placenta and is excreted in breast milk. Rapidly excreted by kidneys in urine.

Dosage/Range:

Adult:

- 500 mg–1 g q 4–8 h; severe infections: 1–2 g q 4–6 h.
- Dose modification if renal impairment, based on creatinine clearance: refer to manufacturer's package insert.

Drug Preparation:

- Store powder for injection at T < 40°C (104°F). Reconstituted solution stable for 24 hours at room temperature, or 96 hours refrigerated.
- IV or deep IM injection. IV: reconstitute with 10 mL sterile water for injection, 5% dextrose or 0.9% sodium chloride injection, then further dilute in 100-mL piggyback set and infuse over 30 minutes. IM: reconstitute 1-g vial with 3 mL sterile or bacteriostatic water for injection, 0.9% sodium chloride. Administer deep IM into large muscle mass (e.g., gluteus maximus).

Drug Interactions:

- Probenecid: increased serum concentrations of antibiotic; monitor and decrease dose if needed.
- Aminoglycosides, penicillins: may have synergistic antibacterial effect against some organisms.
- Nephrotoxic drugs (aminoglycosides, colistin, vancomycin): may increase risk of renal dysfunction; avoid if possible.
- Magnesium, calcium: incompatible in IV fluid.
- Oral anticoagulants, ASPIRIN: may increase risk of bleeding.
- Alcohol: disulfiram-like reaction (flushing, throbbing headache, dyspnea, nausea, vomiting, diaphoresis, chest pain, palpitations, hyperventilation, tachycardia, hypertension, syncope, weakness, blurred vision) when alcohol ingested within 48–72 hours of cefamandole; does not occur if alcohol ingested prior to first antibiotic dose. If no alcohol prior to first dose, avoid alcohol for 72 hours after last dose.

Lab Effects/Interference:

Major clinical significance:

- Coombs' (antiglobulin) tests: a positive reaction frequently appears in patients who receive large doses of cephalosporins; hemolysis rarely occurs, but it has been reported; test may be positive in neonates whose mothers received cephalosporins before delivery.
- Urine glucose: cefamandole may produce false-positive or falsely elevated test results with copper sulfate tests (Benedicts, Clinitest, or Fehling's); glucose enzymatic tests (Clonistix or Testape) are not affected.

- PT: may be prolonged; cephalosporins may inhibit vitamin K synthesis by suppressing gut flora; also, cephalosporins with the NMTT side chain (cefamandole) have been associated with an increased incidence of hypoprothrombinemia; patients who are critically ill, malnourished, or have liver function impairment may be at the highest risk of bleeding.

Clinical significance:

- Urine protein may produce false-positive tests for proteinuria with acid and denaturization-precipation tests.
- Serum ALT, serum alk phos, serum AST, serum bili, or serum LDH values may be increased.
- BUN and serum creatinine concentrations may be increased.
- CBC or platelet count: transient leukopenia, neutropenia, agranulocytosis, thrombocytopenia, eosinophilia, lymphocytosis, and thrombocytosis have been seen on rare occasions.

Special Considerations:

- Use with caution in patients with renal dysfunction—dose reduction required if severe impairment exists.
- Use cautiously if history of colitis exists.
- Contraindicated in patients hypersensitive to other cephalosporin antibiotics.
- Use cautiously if sensitive to penicillin; contraindicated if angioedema reaction to penicillin.
- Obtain ordered specimen and send for culture and sensitivity prior to first drug dose.
- May cause false-positive direct Coombs' test.
- May cause false-positive Clinitest glucose result.

Potential Toxicities/Side Effects and the Nursing Process

I. POTENTIAL FOR INJURY related to HYPERSENSITIVITY REACTION

Defining Characteristics: Urticaria, pruritus, rash (maculopapular or erythematous), fever and chills, eosinophilia, myalgia, edema, erythema, angioedema, Stevens-Johnson syndrome, and exfoliative skin reactions occur in 5% of patients. Increased risk in individuals allergic to penicillin.

Nursing Implications: Assess allergy to cephalosporin antibiotics and penicillin: if patient states "yes," determine actual response, e.g., "swollen lips = angioedema." If angioedema, patient SHOULD NOT receive drug. Discuss other patient responses with physician to determine whether drug should be given. Assess baseline skin condition, including integrity and allergy history to drugs. Instruct patient to report rash, itching, other skin changes. Teach patient skin care and symptomatic measures as appropriate. If skin rash develops, discuss drug discontinuance with physician.

If rash progresses, drug should be discontinued, as fatal Stevens-Johnson syndrome may develop. Be prepared to treat severe acute hypersensitivity reactions with airway management, oxygen, epinephrine, corticosteroids, antihistamines as ordered.

II. ALTERATION IN NUTRITION, LESS THAN BODY REQUIREMENTS, related to GI SIDE EFFECTS

Defining Characteristics: Nausea, vomiting, diarrhea, anorexia may occur; rarely, pseudomembranous colitis caused by *C. difficile* resistant to the antibiotic occurs. Rarely, transient increases in LFTs—AST, ALT, alk phos, bili—may occur.

Nursing Implications: Assess baseline nutritional status. Instruct patient to report GI disturbances. Administer and teach patient to self-administer antiemetics as needed and as ordered. Teach patient importance of nutritious diet, and suggest small, frequent, high-calorie, high-protein meals as appropriate. Assess baseline LFTs, and monitor periodically during treatment. Discuss abnormalities and drug interruption with physician.

III. FUNGAL SUPERINFECTION related to REDISTRIBUTION OF ENDOGENOUS MICROORGANISMS

Defining Characteristics: Vaginal candidiasis, vaginitis may occur as endogenous bacteria are eliminated and normal fungal population expands.

Nursing Implications: Teach female patient to report vaginal itching or discharge. Discuss appropriate antifungal treatment with physician. Teach perineal hygiene and symptomatic management.

IV. ALTERATIONS IN PROTECTIVE MECHANISMS (RARE) related to TRANSIENT LEUKOPENIA

Defining Characteristics: Rarely, transient leukopenia, lymphocytosis, anemia, eosinophilia may occur. Prolonged PT, prolonged APTT, and hypoprothrombinemia have occurred rarely, especially in elderly or debilitated patients, or in individuals with vitamin K deficiency.

Nursing Implications: Assess baseline laboratory parameters, and monitor periodically during treatment. Assess patient for response to antibiotics. Discuss abnormalities with physician. Assess for signs/symptoms of bleeding. If they occur, especially in elderly or debilitated patients, discuss vitamin K administration with physician. Instruct patient to avoid aspirin. If taking oral anticoagulants, assess for increased PT, signs/symptoms of bleeding.

V. ALTERATIONS IN SENSORY/PERCEPTUAL PATTERNS related to DIZZINESS, HEADACHE, SOMNOLENCE

Defining Characteristics: Dizziness, headache, somnolence occur rarely.

Nursing Implications: Assess baseline neurologic function and comfort, and monitor during treatment. Instruct patient to report any changes. Discuss any abnormalities with physician.

VI. ALTERATIONS IN COMFORT related to LOCAL INJECTION IRRITATION

Defining Characteristics: Pain, induration, sterile abscesses may form in IM injection sites; phlebitis may develop in IV sites.

Nursing Implications: Rotate IM injection sites, and administer drug deep IM in large muscle mass (e.g., gluteus maximus). Use IM injection when IV administration is not possible. Change IV sites q 48 h, and assess for signs/symptoms of phlebitis prior to each administration. Administer drug slowly. Apply warm packs to increase comfort.

Drug: cefazolin sodium (Ancef)

Class: First-generation cephalosporin antibacterial.

Mechanism of Action: Semisynthetic derivative of cephalosporin C (produced by fungus); contains β-lactam ring and is related to penicillins and cephamycins (e.g., cefoxitin). Bactericidal through inhibition of cell wall synthesis, with resulting cell wall instability and cell lysis. Active against many gram-positive aerobic cocci (*S. aureus*, groups A and B streptococci); some susceptible gram-negative organisms (*E. coli, H. influenzae, Klebsiella, Proteus*); and gram-negative organisms causing intra-abdominal and biliary infections.

Metabolism: Not absorbed from GI tract, so must be given IV or IM. Widely distributed to body tissues and fluids, including bile; 74–86% bound to serum proteins. Excreted unchanged in urine. Crosses placenta and is excreted in breast milk.

Dosage/Range:
- IV is same as IM.
- Adults: 250 mg–1.5 g q 6–8 h (maximum 12 g/day in life-threatening infections).
- May give loading dose of 500 mg.
- Dose-reduce if serum creatinine = 1.5 mg/dL according to manufacturer's package insert.

Drug Preparation:

- Store powder at < 40°C (104°F) and protect from light. Is available as frozen solution that should be stored at T < −20°C (−4°F).
- Reconstitute powder with sterile water for injection, bacteriostatic water for injection, or 0.9% sodium chloride; solution stable for 24 hours at room temperature or 96 hours at 5°C (41°F).
- Further dilute in 50–100 mL 0.9% sodium chloride or 5% dextrose for IV administration.
- For IM administration, reconstitute with 2–2.5 mL sterile or bacteriostatic water for injection or 0.9% sodium chloride injection. Administer deep IM in large muscle mass (e.g., gluteus maximus).

Drug Interactions:

- Probenecid: increased serum concentrations of antibiotic; monitor and decrease dose if needed.
- Aminoglycosides, penicillins: may have synergistic antibacterial effect against some organisms.
- Nephrotoxic drugs (aminoglycosides, colistin, vancomycin): may increase risk of renal dysfunction; avoid if possible.

Lab Effects/Interference:

Major clinical significance:

- Coombs' (antiglobulin) tests: a positive reaction frequently appears in patients who receive large doses of cephalosporins; hemolysis rarely occurs, but it has been reported; test may be positive in neonates whose mothers received cephalosporins before delivery.
- Urine glucose: cefazolin may produce false-positive or falsely elevated test results with copper sulfate tests (Benedicts, Clinitest, or Fehling's); glucose enzymatic tests (Clonistix or Testape) are not affected.
- PT may be prolonged; cephalosporins may inhibit vitamin K synthesis by suppressing gut flora.

Clinical significance:

- Serum ALT, serum alk phos, serum AST, serum bili, or serum LDH values may be increased.
- BUN and serum creatinine concentrations may be increased.
- CBC or platelet count: transient leukopenia, neutropenia, agranulocytosis, thrombocytopenia, eosinophilia, lymphocytosis, and thrombocytosis have been seen on rare occasions.

Special Considerations:

- Used in treatment of serious infections of respiratory tract, urinary tract, skin and soft tissues, and biliary tree.
- Use with caution in patients with renal dysfunction—dose reduction required if severe impairment exists.
- Use cautiously if history of colitis exists.

- Contraindicated in patients hypersensitive to other cephalosporin antibiotics.
- Use cautiously if sensitive to penicillin; contraindicated if angioedema reaction to penicillin.
- Obtain ordered specimen and send for culture and sensitivity prior to first drug dose.
- May cause false-positive direct Coombs' test.
- May cause false-positive Clinitest glucose result.

Potential Toxicities/Side Effects and the Nursing Process

I. POTENTIAL FOR INJURY related to HYPERSENSITIVITY REACTION

Defining Characteristics: Urticaria, pruritus, rash (maculopapular or erythematous), fever and chills, eosinophilia, myalgia, edema, erythema, angioedema, Stevens-Johnson syndrome, and exfoliative skin reactions occur in 5% of patients. Increased risk in individuals allergic to penicillin.

Nursing Implications: Assess allergy to cephalosporin antibiotics and penicillin: if patient states "yes," determine actual response, e.g., "swollen lips = angioedema." If angioedema, patient SHOULD NOT receive drug. Discuss other patient responses with physician to determine whether drug should be given. Assess baseline skin condition, including integrity and allergy history to drugs. Instruct patient to report rash, itching, other skin changes. Teach patient skin care and symptomatic measures as appropriate. If skin rash develops, discuss drug discontinuance with physician. If rash progresses, drug should be discontinued, as fatal Stevens-Johnson syndrome may develop. Be prepared to treat severe acute hypersensitivity reactions with airway management, oxygen, epinephrine, corticosteroids, antihistamines as ordered.

II. ALTERATION IN NUTRITION, LESS THAN BODY REQUIREMENTS, related to GI SIDE EFFECTS

Defining Characteristics: Nausea, vomiting, diarrhea, anorexia may occur; rarely, pseudomembranous colitis caused by *C. difficile* resistant to the antibiotic occurs. Rarely, transient increases in LFTs—AST, ALT, alk phos, bili—may occur.

Nursing Implications: Assess baseline nutritional status. Instruct patient to report GI disturbances. Administer and teach patient to self-administer antiemetics as needed and as ordered. Teach patient importance of nutritious diet, and suggest small, frequent, high-calorie, high-protein meals as appropriate. Assess baseline LFTs, and monitor periodically during treatment. Discuss abnormalities and drug interruption with physician.

III. FUNGAL SUPERINFECTION related to REDISTRIBUTION OF ENDOGENOUS MICROORGANISMS

Defining Characteristics: Vaginal candidiasis, vaginitis may occur as endogenous bacteria are eliminated and normal fungal population expands.

Nursing Implications: Teach female patient to report vaginal itching or discharge. Discuss appropriate antifungal treatment with physician. Teach perineal hygiene and symptomatic management.

IV. ALTERATIONS IN PROTECTIVE MECHANISMS (RARE) related to CHANGES IN FORMED BLOOD CELL ELEMENTS

Defining Characteristics: Rarely, transient leukopenia, lymphocytosis, anemia, eosinophilia may occur. Prolonged PT, prolonged APTT, and hypoprothrombinemia have occurred rarely, especially in elderly or debilitated patients, or in individuals with vitamin K deficiency.

Nursing Implications: Assess baseline laboratory parameters, and monitor periodically during treatment. Assess patient for response to antibiotics. Discuss abnormalities with physician. Assess for signs/symptoms of bleeding. If they occur, especially in elderly or debilitated patients, discuss vitamin K administration with physician. Instruct patient to avoid aspirin. If taking oral anticoagulants, assess for increased PT, signs/symptoms of bleeding.

V. ALTERATIONS IN SENSORY/PERCEPTUAL PATTERNS related to DIZZINESS, SOMNOLENCE

Defining Characteristics: Dizziness, headache, somnolence occur rarely.

Nursing Implications: Assess baseline neurologic function and comfort, and monitor during treatment. Teach patient to report any changes. Discuss any abnormalities with physician.

VI. ALTERATIONS IN COMFORT related to LOCAL INJECTION IRRITATION

Defining Characteristics: Pain, induration, sterile abscesses may form in IM injection sites; phlebitis may develop in IV sites.

Nursing Implications: Rotate IM injection sites, and administer drug deep IM in large muscle mass (e.g., gluteus maximus). Use IM injection when IV administration is not possible. Change IV sites q 48 h, and assess for signs/symptoms of phlebitis prior to each administration. Administer drug slowly. Apply warm packs to increase comfort.

Drug: cefdinir (Omnicef)

Class: Cephalosporin broad-spectrum antibiotic.

Mechanism of Action: Inhibits cell wall synthesis, thus destroying microorganisms. Stable in presence of some β-lactamase enzymes, so active against many microorganisms that are resistant to the penicillins and other cephalosporin antibiotics.

Metabolism: Well absorbed from the GI tract following oral dosing, with maximal plasma concentration in 2–4 hours. Drug largely unmetabolized and eliminated by the kidneys. Mean plasma half-life is 1.7 hours. Dose must be adjusted in patients with severe renal dysfunction or who receive hemodialysis.

Dosage/Range:

Adults with:

- Community-acquired pneumonia: 300 mg PO q 12 h × 10 days.
- Acute exacerbation of chronic bronchitis: 300 mg PO q 12 h or 600 mg PO q 24 h × 10 days.
- Acute maxillary sinusitis: 300 mg PO q 12 h or 600 mg PO q 24 h × 10 days.
- Pharyngitis/tonsillitis: 300 mg PO q 12 h × 5–10 days or 600 mg PO q 24 h × 10 days.
- Uncomplicated skin/skin structures: 300 mg PO q 12 h × 10 days.
- Patients with renal insufficiency (creatinine clearance < 30 mL/min) is 300 mg PO q 24 h.
- Patients on hemodialysis: 300 mg PO every other day with 300 mg given at the end of each dialysis.

Drug Preparation:

- Oral, available as 300-mg tablets or oral suspension that, when reconstituted as directed, results in 125 mg/5 mL in 60- or 100-mL bottles.

Drug Administrations:

- Take orally without regard to meals or food intake.

Drug Interactions:

- Antacids containing magnesium or aluminum decrease absorption of cefdinir; take cefdinir at least 2 hours before or after the antacid.
- Iron or iron supplements decrease absorption by up to 80%; separate drugs by at least 2 hours.
- Probenecid inhibits the renal excretion of cefdinir, increasing peak plasma levels by 54% and prolonging half-life by 50%; decrease cefdinir dose if must use together.

Lab Effects/Interference:

- False-positive reaction for ketones in testing using nitroprusside.
- False-positive test for glucose in the urine using Clinitest, Benedict's solution, or Fehling's solution (suggest using Clinistix or Testape).
- False-positive Coombs' test (rare).
- Increased gamma glutamyltransferase (1%); rarely other liver function tests.

Special Considerations: Indicated for the treatment of adults with mild-to-moderate infections:

- Community-acquired pneumonia caused by *Haemophilus influenzae* (including β-lactamase–producing strains), penicillin-susceptible strains of *Streptococcus pneumoniae, Moraxella catarrhalis* (including β-lactamase–producing strains).
- Acute exacerbation of chronic bronchitis cased by *Haemophilus influenzae*, (including β-lactamase–producing strains), penicillin-susceptible strains of *Streptococcus pneumoniae, Moraxella catarrhalis* (including β-lactamase–producing strains).
- Acute maxillary sinusitis caused by *Haemophilus influenzae* (including β-lactamase–producing strains), penicillin-susceptible strains of *Streptococcus pneumoniae, Moraxella catarrhalis* (including β-lactamase–producing strains).
- Pharyngitis/tonsillitis caused by *Streptococcus pyogenes*.
- Uncomplicated skin and skin structure infections caused by *Staphylococcus aureus* (including β-lactamase–producing strains) and *Streptococcus pyogenes*.
- Contraindicated in patients with an allergy to the cephalosporin class of antibiotics as well as penicillin (cross-sensitivity in 10% of patients).
- Use cautiously, if at all, in patients with a history of colitis.
- Use in pregnancy only when benefits outweigh risks.
- If patient has severe renal dysfunction as evidenced by creatinine clearance < 30 mL/min, the dose should be reduced to 300 mg q day.
- Diabetic patients should know that the oral suspension has 2.86 g of sucrose per teaspoon.

Potential Toxicities/Side Effects and the Nursing Process

I. ALTERATION IN NUTRITION related to GI SIDE EFFECTS

Defining Characteristics: Diarrhea occurs in approximately 16% of patients, and nausea in 3%. Less common are abdominal discomfort (1%), vomiting < 1%, anorexia (< 1%). The following rarely occur: dyspepsia, flatulence, constipation, abnormal stools (red-colored in patients taking iron). As with all antibiotics, pseudomembranous colitis may occur, ranging in severity from mild to life-threatening. Treatment with antibiotics changes the intestinal microflora, so *Clostridiaum difficile* bacteria may overgrow. Once diagnosis is made, mild diarrhea may stop with cessation of drug; if moderate to severe, it will require, in addition, hydration, electrolyte replacement, nutritional support, and antibacterial coverage against *C. difficile*.

Nursing Implications: Assess baseline nutritional and elimination status. Teach patient to report GI disturbances. Teach patient to report diarrhea immediately, consider whether this is pseudomembranous colitis, and send stool specimen for *C. difficile*; if positive, discuss drug discontinuance with physician. Administer and teach patient to self-administer antiemetics, antidiarrheals as needed and as ordered. Teach patient importance of nutritious diet, and suggest small, frequent, high-calorie, high-protein meals as appropriate. Assess baseline LFTs and monitor periodically during treatment. Discuss abnormalities and drug interruption with physician.

II. SENSORY/PERCEPTUAL ALTERATIONS related to CNS EFFECTS

Defining Characteristics: Headaches occur in 2% of patients, and less common (< 1%) are dizziness, asthenia, insomnia, somnolence.

Nursing Implications: Assess baseline neurological function and comfort, and monitor during treatment. Teach patient to report any changes. Teach patient how to manage symptoms. If unrelieved or persistent, discuss any abnormalities with physician.

III. ALTERATION IN SKIN INTEGRITY related to ALLERGY/HYPERSENSITIVITY

Defining Characteristics: Uncommonly (< 1%) rash and pruritus may occur; other manifestations include eosinophilia, urticaria, flushing, fever, chills, photosensitivity, angioedema. Rarely, Stevens-Johnson reaction, toxic epidermal necrolysis, and exfoliative dermatitis have occurred. Anaphylactic reactions have occurred rarely.

Nursing Implications: Assess baseline skin condition, including integrity and drug allergy history. Teach patient to report rash, itching, other skin changes. Teach patient skin care and symptomatic measures as appropriate. If skin rash develops, discuss drug discontinuance with physician. If rash progresses, drug should be discontinued, as fatal Stevens-Johnson syndrome may develop. Be prepared to treat severe acute hypersensitivity reactions with airway management, oxygen, epinephrine, corticosteroids, antihistamines as ordered.

IV. FUNGAL SUPERINFECTION related to REDISTRIBUTION OF ENDOGENOUS MICROORGANISMS

Defining Characteristics: Vaginal moniliasis, vaginitis may occur as endogenous bacteria are eliminated and normal fungal population expands.

Nursing Implications: Teach female patient to report vaginal itching or discharge. Discuss appropriate antifungal treatment with physician. Teach perineal hygiene and symptomatic management.

Drug: cefditoren pivoxil (Spectracef)

Class: Cephalosporin antibacterial.

Mechanism of Action: Semisynthetic derivative of cephalosporin C, contains β-lactam ring, and is related to penicillins and cephamycins. Bactericidal through inhibition of cell wall synthesis, with resulting cell wall instability and cell lysis.

Metabolism: Well absorbed from GI tract.

Dosage/Range:
- Oral (adult 12 years and older): 200–400 mg q 12 hours.
- Dose modification if renal impairment, based on creatinine clearance—refer to manufacturer's recommendations.
- Dose modification if hepatic impairment, based on LFTs—refer to manufacturer's recommendations.

Drug Preparation:
- Take with food.

Drug Interactions:
- Probenecid: increased serum concentrations of antibiotic; monitor and decrease dose if needed.
- Histamine H_2 antagonists: Famotidine decreases oral absorption; concomitant use should be avoided.
- Nephrotoxic drugs: may increase risk of renal dysfunction; avoid if possible.
- Magnesium- and aluminum-containing antacids decrease oral absorption; concomitant use should be avoided.

Lab Effects/Interference:
- Serum ALT (SGPT), serum alk phos, serum AST (SGOT), and serum bilirubin—values may be increased.
- BUN and serum creatinine—concentrations may be increased.

Special Considerations:
- Use cautiously if renal impairment is present.
- Contraindicated if hypersensitive to other cephalosporins, or if has had angioedema response to penicillin.

Potential Toxicities/Side Effects and the Nursing Process

I. POTENTIAL FOR INJURY related to HYPERSENSITIVITY REACTION

Defining Characteristics: Urticaria, pruritus, rash (maculopapular or erythematous), fever and chills, eosinophilia, myalgia, edema, erythema, angioedema. Increased risk in individuals allergic to penicillin.

Nursing Implications: Assess allergy to cephalosporin antibiotics and penicillin: if patient states "yes," determine actual response, e.g., "swollen lips = angioedema." If angioedema, patient SHOULD NOT receive drug. Discuss other patient responses with physician to determine whether drug should be given. Assess baseline skin condition, including integrity and allergy history to drugs. Teach patient to report rash, itching, other skin changes. Teach patient skin care and symptomatic measures as appropriate. If skin rash develops, discuss drug discontinuance with physician.

II. ALTERATION IN NUTRITION, LESS THAN BODY REQUIREMENTS, related to GI SIDE EFFECTS

Defining Characteristics: Nausea, vomiting, diarrhea, and anorexia may occur.

Nursing Implications: Assess baseline nutritional status. Teach patient to report GI disturbances. Administer and teach patient to self-administer antiemetics as needed and as ordered. Teach patient importance of nutritious diet, and suggest small, frequent, high-calorie, high-protein meals as appropriate. Discuss abnormalities and drug interruption with physician.

III. FUNGAL SUPERINFECTION related to REDISTRIBUTION OF ENDOGENOUS MICROORGANISMS

Defining Characteristics: Vaginal moniliasis, vaginitis may occur as endogenous bacteria are eliminated and normal fungal population expands.

Nursing Implications: Teach female patient to report vaginal itching or discharge. Discuss appropriate antifungal treatment with physician. Teach perineal hygiene and symptomatic management.

Drug: cefepime (Maxipime)

Class: Fourth-generation cephalosporin antibacterial.

Mechanism of Action: Exerts bactericidal action by inhibiting cell wall synthesis. Highly resistant to hydrolysis by β-lactamases, and exhibits rapid penetration into gram-negative bacterial cells. Active against gram-negative and gram-positive organisms. Spectrum of activity includes gram-negative organisms with multiple drug resistance patterns (*Enterobacter* and *Klebsiella*.) Drug is used for treatment of infections in lower respiratory tract, skin, abdomen, and urinary tract.

Metabolism: Given intramuscularly and parenterally. Widely distributed into body tissues and fluids. Serum protein binding is less than 19% and is independent of its concentration in the serum. Excreted in urine. The average elimination half-life is approximately 2 hours.

Dosage/Range:
Adult:
- IV and IM are similar.
- Mild–mod UTI: 0.5–1 g IV or IM q 12 h × 7–10 days.
- Severe UTI, Klebsiella pneumonia: 2 g IV q 12 h × 10 days.
- Mod–severe pneumonia: 1–2 g IV q 12 h × 10 days.
- Febrile neutropenia: 2 g IV q 8 h × 7 days or neutrophil recovery.

Drug Preparation:
- IV or IM: add diluent recommended by manufacturer into vial.

Drug Interactions:
- Solutions of cefepime should not be added to solutions of metronidazole, vancomycin hydrochloride, gentamicin sulfate, tobramycin sulfate, or netilmicin sulfate and aminophylline because of potential side effects. If necessary, administer each drug separately.

Lab Effects/Interference:
Major clinical significance:
- Coombs' (antiglobulin) tests: a positive reaction has appeared in clinical trials without evidence of hemolysis.
- PT or PTT: may be prolonged; cephalosporins may inhibit vitamin K synthesis by suppressing gut flora.

Clinical significance:
- Serum SGPT, serum alk phos, serum SGOT, serum bilirubin, or serum LDH: values may be increased.
- BUN and serum creatinine: concentrations may be increased.
- CBC or platelet count: transient leukopenia, neutropenia, agranulocytosis, thrombocytopenia, eosinophilia, lymphocytosis, and thrombocytosis have been seen on rare occasions.

Special Considerations:
- Contraindicated in patients hypersensitive to other cephalosporin antibiotics.
- Use cautiously if sensitive to penicillin; contraindicated if angioedema reaction to penicillin.
- Obtain specimen and send for culture and sensitivity prior to first drug dose.
- May cause false-positive Clinitest glucose result.

Potential Toxicities/Side Effects and the Nursing Process

I. POTENTIAL FOR INJURY related to HYPERSENSITIVITY REACTION

Defining Characteristics: Urticaria, pruritus, rash (maculopapular or erythematous), fever and chills, eosinophilia, myalgia, edema, erythema, angioedema, Stevens-Johnson syndrome, and exfoliative skin reactions occur in 5% of patients. Increased risk in individuals allergic to penicillin.

Nursing Implications: Assess allergy to cephalosporin antibiotics and penicillin: if patient states "yes," determine actual response, e.g., "swollen lips = angioedema." If angioedema, patient SHOULD NOT receive drug. Discuss other patient responses with physician to determine whether drug should be given. Assess baseline skin condition, including integrity and allergy history to drugs. Teach patient to report rash, itching, other skin changes. Teach patient skin care and symptomatic measures as appropriate. If skin rash develops, discuss drug discontinuance with physician. If rash progresses, drug should be discontinued, as fatal Stevens-Johnson syndrome may develop. Be prepared to treat severe acute hypersensitivity reactions with airway management, oxygen, epinephrine, corticosteroids, antihistamines as ordered.

II. ALTERATION IN NUTRITION, LESS THAN BODY REQUIREMENTS, related to GI SIDE EFFECTS

Defining Characteristics: Nausea, vomiting, diarrhea, constipation, abdominal pain, and dyspepsia may occur; rarely, pseudomembranous colitis caused by *C. difficile* resistant to the antibiotic occurs. Rarely, transient increases in LFTs—AST (SGOT), ALT (SGPT), alk phos, BR—may occur.

Nursing Implications: Assess baseline nutritional status. Teach patient to report GI disturbances. Administer and teach patient to self-administer antiemetics, antidiarrheals as needed and as ordered. Teach patient importance of nutritious diet, and suggest small, frequent, high-calorie, high-protein meals as appropriate. Assess baseline LFTs and monitor periodically during treatment. Discuss abnormalities and drug interruption with physician.

III. FUNGAL SUPERINFECTION related to REDISTRIBUTION OF ENDOGENOUS MICROORGANISMS

Defining Characteristics: Vaginal moniliasis, vaginitis may occur as endogenous bacteria are eliminated and normal fungal population expands.

Nursing Implications: Teach female patient to report vaginal itching or discharge. Discuss appropriate antifungal treatment with physician. Teach perineal hygiene and symptomatic management.

IV. ALTERATIONS IN PROTECTIVE MECHANISMS (RARE) related to CHANGES IN FORMED BLOOD CELL ELEMENTS

Defining Characteristics: Rarely, transient leukopenia, lymphocytosis, anemia, eosinophilia may occur. Prolonged PT, prolonged APTT, and hypoprothrombinemia have occurred rarely, especially in elderly or debilitated patients, or in individuals with vitamin K deficiency.

Nursing Implications: Assess baseline laboratory parameters and monitor periodically during treatment. Assess patient for response to antibiotics. Discuss abnormalities with physician. Assess for signs and symptoms of bleeding. If they occur, especially in elderly or debilitated patients, discuss vitamin K administration with physician. Teach patient to avoid aspirin. If taking oral anticoagulants, assess for increased PT, signs and symptoms of bleeding.

V. SENSORY/PERCEPTUAL ALTERATIONS related to DIZZINESS, SOMNOLENCE

Defining Characteristics: Dizziness, headache, somnolence occur rarely.

Nursing Implications: Assess baseline neurological function and comfort, and monitor during treatment. Teach patient to report any changes. Discuss any abnormalities with physician.

Drug: cefixime (Suprax)

Class: Third-generation cephalosporin antibacterial.

Mechanism of Action: Semisynthetic derivative of cephalosporin C (produced by fungus); contains β-lactam ring and is related to penicillins and cephamycins (e.g., cefoxitin). Bactericidal through inhibition of cell wall synthesis, with resulting cell wall instability and cell lysis. Active against sensitive gram-negative bacteria (e.g., urinary tract infections caused by *E. coli, Proteus, H. influenzae*), as well as *S. pneumoniae* and *H. influenzae* related to acute bronchitis and acute exacerbations of chronic bronchitis.

Metabolism: 30–50% absorbed from GI tract; rate of absorption slowed by food but does not affect total dose absorbed; 65–70% protein-bound. Eliminated unchanged in urine, and to a lesser degree in bile and feces.

Dosage/Range:
- Adult: 400 mg/day PO (single, or two divided doses q 12 h).
- Duration: 5–10 days for uncomplicated urinary tract infection or upper respiratory infection; 10–14 days for lower respiratory tract infections.
- Dose-reduce if creatinine clearance < 60 mL/min per manufacturer's package insert.

Drug Preparation:
- Store tablets in tight container at 15–30°C (59–86°F).
- Oral administration.

Drug Interactions:
- Probenecid: increased serum concentrations of antibiotic; monitor and decrease dose if needed.

Lab Effects/Interference:
Major clinical significance:
- Coombs' (antiglobulin) tests: a positive reaction frequently appears in patients who receive large doses of cephalosporins; hemolysis rarely occurs, but it has been reported; test may be positive in neonates whose mothers received cephalosporins before delivery.
- PT: may be prolonged; cephalosporins may inhibit vitamin K synthesis by suppressing gut flora.

Clinical significance:
- Serum ALT, serum alk phos, serum AST, serum bili, or serum LDH values may be increased.
- BUN and serum creatinine concentrations may be increased.
- CBC or platelet count: transient leukopenia, neutropenia, agranulocytosis, thrombocytopenia, eosinophilia, lymphocytosis, and thrombocytosis have been seen on rare occasions.

Special Considerations:
- Use with caution in patients with renal dysfunction; dose reduction required if severe impairment exists.
- Use cautiously if history of colitis exists.
- Contraindicated in patients hypersensitive to other cephalosporin antibiotics.
- Use cautiously if sensitive to penicillin; contraindicated if angioedema reaction to penicillin.
- Obtain ordered specimen and send for culture and sensitivity prior to first drug dose.
- May cause false-positive direct Coombs' test.
- May cause false-positive Clinitest glucose result.

Potential Toxicities/Side Effects and the Nursing Process

I. POTENTIAL FOR INJURY related to HYPERSENSITIVITY REACTION

Defining Characteristics: Urticaria, pruritus, rash (maculopapular or erythematous), fever and chills, eosinophilia, myalgia, edema, erythema, angioedema, Stevens-Johnson syndrome, and exfoliative skin reactions occur in 5% of patients. Increased risk in individuals allergic to penicillin.

Nursing Implications: Assess allergy to cephalosporin antibiotics and penicillin: if patient states "yes," determine actual response, e.g., "swollen lips = angioedema."

If angioedema, patient SHOULD NOT receive drug. Discuss other patient responses with physician to determine whether drug should be given. Assess baseline skin condition, including integrity and allergy history to drugs. Instruct patient to report rash, itching, other skin changes. Teach patient skin care and symptomatic measures as appropriate. If skin rash develops, discuss drug discontinuance with physician. If rash progresses, drug should be discontinued, as fatal Stevens-Johnson syndrome may develop. Be prepared to treat severe acute hypersensitivity reactions with airway management, oxygen, epinephrine, corticosteroids, antihistamines as ordered.

II. ALTERATION IN NUTRITION, LESS THAN BODY REQUIREMENTS, related to GI SIDE EFFECTS

Defining Characteristics: Nausea, vomiting, diarrhea, anorexia may occur; rarely, pseudomembranous colitis caused by *C. difficile* resistant to the antibiotic occurs. Rarely, transient increases in LFTs—AST, ALT, alk phos, bili—may occur.

Nursing Implications: Assess baseline nutritional status. Instruct patient to report GI disturbances. Administer and teach patient to self-administer antiemetics as needed and as ordered. Teach patient importance of nutritious diet, and suggest small, frequent, high-calorie, high-protein meals as appropriate. Assess baseline LFTs and monitor periodically during treatment. Discuss abnormalities and drug interruption with physician.

III. FUNGAL SUPERINFECTION related to REDISTRIBUTION OF ENDOGENOUS MICROORGANISMS

Defining Characteristics: Vaginal candidiasis, vaginitis may occur as endogenous bacteria are eliminated, and normal fungal population expands.

Nursing Implications: Teach female patient to report vaginal itching or discharge. Discuss appropriate antifungal treatment with physician. Teach perineal hygiene and symptomatic management.

IV. ALTERATIONS IN PROTECTIVE MECHANISMS (RARE) related to TRANSIENT LEUKOPENIA

Defining Characteristics: Rarely, transient leukopenia, lymphocytosis, anemia, eosinophilia may occur. Prolonged PT, prolonged APTT, and hypoprothrombinemia have occurred rarely, especially in elderly or debilitated patients, or in individuals with vitamin K deficiency.

Nursing Implications: Assess baseline laboratory parameters, and monitor periodically during treatment. Assess patient for response to antibiotics. Discuss abnormalities with physician. Assess for signs/symptoms of bleeding. If they occur, especially in elderly or debilitated patients, discuss vitamin K administration with physician. Instruct patient to avoid aspirin. If taking oral anticoagulants, assess for increased PT, signs/symptoms of bleeding.

V. ALTERATIONS IN SENSORY/PERCEPTUAL PATTERNS related to DIZZINESS, SOMNOLENCE

Defining Characteristics: Dizziness, headache, somnolence occur rarely.

Nursing Implications: Assess baseline neurologic function and comfort, and monitor during treatment. Instruct patient to report any changes. Discuss any abnormalities with physician.

Drug: cefoperazone sodium (Cefobid)

Class: Third-generation cephalosporin antibacterial.

Mechanism of Action: Semisynthetic derivative of cephalosporin C, contains β-lactam ring, and is related to penicillins and cephamycins. Bactericidal through inhibition of cell wall synthesis, with resulting cell wall instability and cell lysis.

Metabolism: Not absorbed from GI tract so must be given IV or IM. Widely distributed in body fluids, including bile and cerebrospinal fluid at high doses, and body tissues. Metabolized by liver and excreted by kidneys into urine.

Dosage/Range:
- IV route when possible, but IV and IM doses are the same.
- Adults: 2–12 gm q 6–12 hours IM/IV; MAX 16 gm/day.
- Pediatrics: 100–150 mg/kg/day q 8–12 hours IV; MAX 6 gm/day.

Drug Preparation:
- Store vial containing powder at < 30°C (86°F).
- IV: Reconstitute with sterile water for injection, and further dilute in 50–100 mL of 0.9% sodium chloride or 5% dextrose injection and infuse over 15–30 minutes at maximum concentration of 50 mg/ml.
- IM: Reconstitute by adding sterile or bacteriostatic water for injection. Depending on dose, divide dose and give in separate IM sites; may need to administer large doses to avoid discomfort. Administer IM injections deeply into large muscle (e.g., gluteus maximus).

Drug Interactions:

- Probenecid: increased serum concentrations of antibiotic; monitor and decrease dose if needed.
- Aminoglycosides, penicillins: may have synergistic antibacterial effect against some organisms.
- Nephrotoxic drugs (aminoglycosides, colistin, vancomycin): may increase risk of renal dysfunction; avoid if possible.
- Heparin and warfarin-cephalosporins may inhibit vitamin K synthesis by suppressing gut flora.
- Typhoid vaccine.

Lab Effects/Interference:

- PT: may be prolonged; cephalosporins may inhibit vitamin K synthesis by suppressing gut flora.
- Serum SGPT, serum alk phos, serum SGOT, serum bilirubin, or serum LDH: values may be increased.
- BUN and serum creatinine: concentrations may be increased.

Special Considerations:

- Use with caution in patients with renal dysfunction; dose reduction required if severe impairment exists.
- Contraindicated in patients hypersensitive to other cephalosporin antibiotics.
- Use cautiously if sensitive to penicillin; contraindicated if angioedema reaction to penicillin.
- Obtain ordered specimen and send for culture and sensitivity prior to first drug dose.

Potential Toxicities/Side Effects and the Nursing Process

I. POTENTIAL FOR INJURY related to HYPERSENSITIVITY REACTION

Defining Characteristics: Urticaria, pruritus, rash (maculopapular or erythematous), fever and chills, eosinophilia, myalgia, edema, erythema, and angioedema. Increased risk in individuals allergic to penicillin.

Nursing Implications: Assess allergy to cephalosporin antibiotics and penicillin: if patient states "yes," determine actual response, e.g., "swollen lips = angioedema." If angioedema, patient SHOULD NOT receive drug. Discuss other patient responses with physician to determine whether drug should be given. Assess baseline skin condition, including integrity and allergy history to drugs. Teach patient to report rash, itching, or other skin changes. Teach patient skin care and symptomatic measures as appropriate. If skin rash develops, discuss drug discontinuance with physician.

II. ALTERATION IN NUTRITION, LESS THAN BODY REQUIREMENTS, related to GI SIDE EFFECTS

Defining Characteristics: Diarrhea or anorexia may occur.

Nursing Implications: Assess baseline nutritional status. Teach patient to report GI disturbances. Administer and teach patient to self-administer antidiarrheal agent as needed and as ordered.

III. FUNGAL SUPERINFECTION related to REDISTRIBUTION OF ENDOGENOUS MICROORGANISMS

Defining Characteristics: Vaginal moniliasis, vaginitis may occur as endogenous bacteria are eliminated and normal fungal population expands.

Nursing Implications: Teach female patient to report vaginal itching or discharge. Discuss appropriate antifungal treatment with physician. Teach perineal hygiene and symptomatic management.

IV. ALTERATIONS IN PROTECTIVE MECHANISMS (RARE)

Defining Characteristics: Prolonged PT, prolonged APTT, and hypoprothrombinemia have occurred rarely, especially in elderly or debilitated patients, or in individuals with vitamin K deficiency.

Nursing Implications: Assess baseline laboratory parameters, and monitor periodically during treatment. Assess patient for response to antibiotics. Discuss abnormalities with physician. Assess for signs/symptoms of bleeding. If they occur, especially in elderly or debilitated patients, discuss vitamin K administration with physician. Teach patient to avoid aspirin. If taking oral anticoagulants, assess for increased PT, signs/symptoms of bleeding.

V. ALTERATIONS IN COMFORT related to LOCAL INJECTION IRRITATION

Defining Characteristics: Pain, induration, and sterile abscesses may form in IM injection sites; phlebitis may develop in IV sites.

Nursing Implications: Rotate IM injection sites, and administer drug deep IM in large muscle mass (e.g., gluteus maximus). Use IM injection when IV administration is not possible. Change IV sites q 48 hours, and assess for signs/symptoms of phlebitis prior to each administration. Administer drug slowly. Apply warm packs to increase comfort.

Drug: cefotaxime sodium (Claforan)

Class: Third-generation cephalosporin antibacterial.

Mechanism of Action: Semisynthetic derivative of cephalosporin C (produced by fungus); contains β-lactam ring and is related to penicillins and cephamycins (e.g., cefoxitin). Bactericidal through inhibition of cell wall synthesis, with resulting cell wall instability and cell lysis. Active against gram-negative cocci (*Enterobacter*, some strains of *Pseudomonas, E. coli, Klebsiella, Serratia*), as well as gram-positive *S. aureus* and *Staphylococcus epidermidis*, and *S. pneumoniae*. Used to treat serious lower respiratory tract, urinary tract, gynecologic, CNS, blood, and skin infections caused by sensitive bacteria.

Metabolism: Not absorbed from GI tract, so must be given IV or IM. Widely distributed in body fluids, including bile and CSF at high doses, and body tissues. Crosses placenta and is excreted in breast milk. Metabolized by liver and excreted by kidneys into urine.

Dosage/Range:
- IV route when possible, but IV and IM doses are the same.
- Adults: 1–2 g q 6–8 h (severe, 2 g q 4 h) × 48–72 hours after infection eradicated.

Drug Preparation:
- Store vial containing powder at < 30°C (86°F).
- Frozen injection should be stored at < −20°C (−4°F).
- IV: reconstitute with 10 mL sterile water for injection, and further dilute in 50–100 mL of 0.9% sodium chloride or 5% dextrose injection and infuse over 20–30 minutes.
- IM: reconstitute by adding 2–5 mL sterile or bacteriostatic water for injection. Depending on dose, divide dose and give in separate IM sites; may need to administer large doses (2 g) IV to avoid discomfort. Administer IM injections deeply into large muscle (e.g., gluteus maximus).

Drug Interactions:
- Probenecid: increased serum concentrations of antibiotic; monitor and decrease dose if needed.
- Aminoglycosides, penicillins: may have synergistic antibacterial effect against some organisms.
- Nephrotoxic drugs (aminoglycosides, colistin, vancomycin): may increase risk of renal dysfunction; avoid if possible.

Lab Effects/Interference:

Major clinical significance:
- Coombs' (antiglobulin) tests: a positive reaction frequently appears in patients who receive large doses of cephalosporins; hemolysis rarely occurs, but it has been

reported, test may be positive in neonates whose mothers received cephalosporins before delivery.
- PT: may be prolonged; cephalosporins may inhibit vitamin K synthesis by suppressing gut flora.

Clinical significance:
- Serum ALT, serum alk phos, serum AST, serum bili, or serum LDH values may be increased.
- BUN and serum creatinine concentrations may be increased.
- CBC or platelet count: transient leukopenia, neutropenia, agranulocytosis, thrombocytopenia, eosinophilia, lymphocytosis, and thrombocytosis have been seen on rare occasions.

Special Considerations:
- Use with caution in patients with renal dysfunction; dose reduction required if severe impairment exists.
- Use cautiously if history of colitis exists.
- Contraindicated in patients hypersensitive to other cephalosporin antibiotics.
- Use cautiously if sensitive to penicillin; contraindicated if angioedema reaction to penicillin.
- Obtain ordered specimen and send for culture and sensitivity prior to first drug dose.
- May cause false-positive direct Coombs' test.

Potential Toxicities/Side Effects and the Nursing Process

I. POTENTIAL FOR INJURY related to HYPERSENSITIVITY REACTION

Defining Characteristics: Urticaria, pruritus, rash (maculopapular or erythematous), fever and chills, eosinophilia, myalgia, edema, erythema, angioedema, Stevens-Johnson syndrome, and exfoliative skin reactions occur in 5% of patients. Increased risk in individuals allergic to penicillin.

Nursing Implications: Assess allergy to cephalosporin antibiotics and penicillin: if patient states "yes," determine actual response, e.g., "swollen lips = angioedema." If angioedema, patient SHOULD NOT receive drug. Discuss other patient responses with physician to determine whether drug should be given. Assess baseline skin condition, including integrity and allergy history to drugs. Instruct patient to report rash, itching, other skin changes. Teach patient skin care and symptomatic measures as appropriate. If skin rash develops, discuss drug discontinuance with physician. If rash progresses, drug should be discontinued, as fatal Stevens-Johnson syndrome may develop. Be prepared to treat severe acute hypersensitivity reactions with airway management, oxygen, epinephrine, corticosteroids, antihistamines as ordered.

II. ALTERATION IN NUTRITION, LESS THAN BODY REQUIREMENTS, related to GI SIDE EFFECTS

Defining Characteristics: Nausea, vomiting, diarrhea, anorexia may occur; rarely, pseudomembranous colitis caused by *C. difficile* resistant to the antibiotic occurs. Rarely, transient increases in LFTs—AST, ALT, alk phos, bili—may occur.

Nursing Implications: Assess baseline nutritional status. Instruct patient to report GI disturbances. Administer and teach patient to self-administer antiemetics as needed and as ordered. Teach patient importance of nutritious diet, and suggest small, frequent, high-calorie, high-protein meals as appropriate. Assess baseline LFTs, and monitor periodically during treatment. Discuss abnormalities and drug interruption with physician.

III. FUNGAL SUPERINFECTION related to REDISTRIBUTION OF ENDOGENOUS MICROORGANISMS

Defining Characteristics: Vaginal candidiasis, vaginitis may occur as endogenous bacteria are eliminated and normal fungal population expands.

Nursing Implications: Instruct female patient to report vaginal itching or discharge. Discuss appropriate antifungal treatment with physician. Teach perineal hygiene and symptomatic management.

IV. ALTERATIONS IN PROTECTIVE MECHANISMS (RARE) related to TRANSIENT LEUKOPENIA

Defining Characteristics: Rarely, transient leukopenia, lymphocytosis, anemia, eosinophilia may occur. Prolonged PT, prolonged APTT, and hypoprothrombinemia have occurred rarely, especially in elderly or debilitated patients, or in individuals with vitamin K deficiency.

Nursing Implications: Assess baseline laboratory parameters, and monitor periodically during treatment. Assess patient for response to antibiotics. Discuss abnormalities with physician. Assess for signs/symptoms of bleeding. If they occur, especially in elderly or debilitated patients, discuss vitamin K administration with physician. Instruct patient to avoid aspirin. If taking oral anticoagulants, assess for increased PT, signs/symptoms of bleeding.

V. ALTERATIONS IN SENSORY/PERCEPTUAL PATTERNS related to DIZZINESS, SOMNOLENCE

Defining Characteristics: Dizziness, headache, somnolence occur rarely.

Nursing Implications: Assess baseline neurologic function and comfort, and monitor during treatment. Instruct patient to report any changes. Discuss any abnormalities with physician.

VI. ALTERATIONS IN COMFORT related to LOCAL INJECTION IRRITATION

Defining Characteristics: Pain, induration, and sterile abscesses may form in IM injection sites; phlebitis may develop in IV sites.

Nursing Implications: Rotate IM injection sites, and administer drug deep IM in large muscle mass (e.g., gluteus maximus). Use IM injection when IV administration is not possible. Change IV sites q 48 h, and assess for signs/symptoms of phlebitis prior to each administration. Administer drug slowly. Apply warm packs to increase comfort.

Drug: cefotetan (Cefotan)

Class: Second-generation cephalosporin antibiotic.

Mechanism of Action: Semisynthetic derivative of cephalosporin C; contains β-lactam ring, and is related to penicillins and cephamycins. Bactericidal through inhibition of cell wall synthesis by binding to one or more of the penicillin-binding proteins (PBPs) that in turn inhibit the final transpeptidation step of peptidoglycan synthesis in bacterial cell walls, thus inhibiting cell wall biosynthesis. Bacteria eventually lyse due to ongoing activity of cell wall autolytic enzymes (autolysins and murein hydrolases) while cell wall assembly is arrested.

Metabolism: Widely distributed in body tissues, fluids except cerebrospinal fluid; readily crosses placenta and is excreted in breast milk. Unchanged drug rapidly excreted by the kidneys.

Dosage/Range:
- Oral (adult): 1–6 g/day in divided doses every 12 hours, usual dose: 1–2 g every 12 hours for 5–10 days; 1–2 g may be given every 24 hours for urinary tract infection.
- Oral (child): 20–40 mg/kg/dose q 12 hours.

Drug Preparation:
- Refrigerate suspension.

Drug Interactions:
- Probenecid: increased serum concentrations of cefotetan but does not usually require dose reduction of antibiotic.

- Aminoglycosides and furosemide can increase nephrotoxicity.
- Disulfiram-like reaction has been reported when taken within 72 hours of ethanol consumption.

Lab Effects/Interference:
- Serum ALT (SGPT), serum alk phos, serum AST (SGOT), and serum bilirubin—values may be increased.
- BUN and serum creatinine—concentrations may be increased.

Special Considerations:
- Use cautiously if renal impairment is present.
- Contraindicated if hypersensitive to other cephalosporins, or if has had angioedema response to penicillin.

Potential Toxicities/Side Effects and the Nursing Process

I. POTENTIAL FOR INJURY related to HYPERSENSITIVITY REACTION

Defining Characteristics: Urticaria, pruritus, rash (maculopapular or erythematous), fever and chills, eosinophilia, myalgia, edema, erythema, angioedema. Increased risk in individuals allergic to penicillin.

Nursing Implications: Assess allergy to cephalosporin antibiotics and penicillin: if patient states "yes," determine actual response, e.g., "swollen lips = angioedema." If angioedema, patient SHOULD NOT receive drug. Discuss other patient responses with physician to determine whether drug should be given. Assess baseline skin condition, including integrity and allergy history to drugs. Teach patient to report rash, itching, and other skin changes. Teach patient skin care and symptomatic measures as appropriate. If skin rash develops, discuss drug discontinuance with physician.

II. ALTERATION IN NUTRITION, LESS THAN BODY REQUIREMENTS, related to GI SIDE EFFECTS

Defining Characteristics: Nausea, vomiting, diarrhea, and anorexia may occur. May cause transient increases in LFTs.

Nursing Implications: Assess baseline nutritional status. Teach patient to report GI disturbances. Administer and teach patient to self-administer antiemetics as needed and as ordered. Teach patient importance of nutritious diet, and suggest small, frequent, high-calorie, high-protein meals as appropriate. Assess baseline LFTs and monitor periodically during treatment. Discuss abnormalities and drug interruption with physician.

III. FUNGAL SUPERINFECTION related to REDISTRIBUTION OF ENDOGENOUS MICROORGANISMS

Defining Characteristics: Vaginal moniliasis, vaginitis may occur as endogenous bacteria are eliminated, and normal fungal population expands.

Nursing Implications: Teach female patient to report vaginal itching or discharge. Discuss appropriate antifungal treatment with physician. Teach perineal hygiene and symptomatic management.

IV. KNOWLEDGE DEFICIT related to SELF-ADMINISTRATION OF MEDICATION

Defining Characteristics: Increased compliance when patient is instructed in self-care activities.

Nursing Implications: Assess knowledge regarding infection and planned treatment. Teach about drug action, potential side effects, and when and how to take drug. Teach patient to report any possible side effects that occur.

Drug: cefoxitin sodium (Mefoxin)

Class: Considered second-generation cephalosporin based on activity spectrum; technically, a cephamycin antibacterial.

Mechanism of Action: β-lactam antibiotic that inhibits bacterial cell wall synthesis, leading to cell lysis. Active against sensitive gram-negative bacteria causing lower respiratory infections (*H. influenzae, E. coli, Klebsiella*); GU infections (*E. coli, Klebsiella, Proteus*); septicemia; pelvic infections (*E. coli, Neisseria gonorrheae*); or skin infections (*E. coli, Klebsiella*). Also, some gram-positive infections, including lower respiratory tract infections (*S. aureus, S. pneumoniae*, streptococci).

Metabolism: Not absorbed from GI tract, so must be administered IV or IM.

Dosage/Range:
- IV route preferred; IV and IM dosages the same.
- Adult: 1–2 g q 6–8 h (maximum 12 g/day in divided doses).
- Dose—reduce for renal compromise (based on manufacturer's package insert).

Drug Preparation:
- Store sterile powder at < 30°C (86°F); frozen injection should be stored at < −20°C (−4°F).
- IV: reconstitute drug by adding 10 mL sterile water for injection. Further dilute in 50–100 mL 0.9% sodium chloride or 5% dextrose injection and infuse over 30–60 minutes.

- IM: reconstitute drug by adding 2 mL sterile water for injection or 0.5% or 1% lidocaine HCl injection without epinephrine to 1 g of cefoxitin. Administer IM deeply into large muscle mass (e.g., gluteus maximus). Using proper technique, ensure that injection is not into blood vessel. (Make certain patient is NOT ALLERGIC to lidocaine.)

Drug Interactions:

- Probenecid: increased serum concentrations of antibiotic; monitor and decrease dose if needed.
- Aminoglycosides, penicillins: may have synergistic antibacterial effect against some organisms.
- Nephrotoxic drugs (aminoglycosides, colistin, vancomycin): may increase risk of renal dysfunction; avoid if possible.
- Magnesium, calcium: incompatible in IV fluid.
- Oral anticoagulants, ASPIRIN: may increase risk of bleeding.
- Alcohol: disulfiram-like reaction (flushing, throbbing headache, dyspnea, nausea, vomiting, diaphoresis, chest pain, palpitation, hyperventilation, tachycardia, hypertension, syncope, weakness, blurred vision) when alcohol ingested within 48–72 hours of cefoxitin; does not occur if alcohol ingested prior to first antibiotic dose. If no alcohol prior to first dose, avoid alcohol for 72 hours after last dose.

Lab Effects/Interference:

Major clinical significance:

- Coombs' (antiglobulin) tests: a positive reaction frequently appears in patients who receive large doses of cephalosporins; hemolysis rarely occurs, but it has been reported; test may be positive in neonates whose mothers received cephalosporins before delivery.
- Urine glucose: some cephalosporins (cefoxitin) may produce false-positive or falsely elevated test results with copper sulfate tests (Benedict's, Fehling's, or Clinitest); glucose enzymatic tests (Clinistix and Testape) are not affected.
- PT: may be prolonged; cephalosporins may inhibit vitamin K synthesis by suppressing gut flora.

Clinical significance:

- Serum and urine creatinine may falsely elevate test values when the Jaffe reaction is used; serum samples should not be obtained within 2 hours of administration.
- Serum ALT, serum alk phos, serum AST, serum bili, or serum LDH values may be increased.
- BUN and serum creatinine concentrations may be increased.
- CBC or platelet count: transient leukopenia, neutropenia, agranulocytosis, thrombocytopenia, eosinophilia, lymphocytosis, and thrombocytosis have been seen on rare occasions.

Special Considerations:

- Use with caution in patients with renal dysfunction; dose reduction required if severe impairment exists.
- Use cautiously if history of colitis exists.
- Contraindicated in patients hypersensitive to other cephalosporin antibiotics.
- Use cautiously if sensitive to penicillin; contraindicated if angioedema reaction to penicillin.
- Obtain ordered specimen and send for culture and sensitivity prior to first drug dose.
- May cause false-positive direct Coombs' test.
- May cause false-positive Clinitest glucose result.

Potential Toxicities/Side Effects and the Nursing Process

I. POTENTIAL FOR INJURY related to HYPERSENSITIVITY REACTION

Defining Characteristics: Urticaria, pruritus, rash (maculopapular or erythematous), fever and chills, eosinophilia, myalgia, edema, erythema, angioedema, Stevens-Johnson syndrome, and exfoliative skin reactions occur in 5% of patients. Increased risk in individuals allergic to penicillin.

Nursing Implications: Assess allergy to cephalosporin antibiotics and penicillin: if patient states "yes," determine actual response, e.g., "swollen lips = angioedema." If angioedema, patient SHOULD NOT receive drug. Discuss other patient responses with physician to determine whether drug should be given. Assess baseline skin condition, including integrity and allergy history to drugs. Instruct patient to report rash, itching, and other skin changes. Teach patient skin care and symptomatic measures as appropriate. If skin rash develops, discuss drug discontinuance with physician. If rash progresses, drug should be discontinued, as fatal Stevens-Johnson syndrome may develop. Be prepared to treat severe acute hypersensitivity reactions with airway management, oxygen, epinephrine, corticosteroids, antihistamines as ordered.

II. ALTERATION IN NUTRITION, LESS THAN BODY REQUIREMENTS, related to GI SIDE EFFECTS

Defining Characteristic: Nausea, vomiting, diarrhea, anorexia may occur; rarely, pseudomembranous colitis caused by *C. difficile* resistant to the antibiotic occurs. Rarely, transient increases in LFTs—AST, ALT, alk phos, bili—may occur.

Nursing Implications: Assess baseline nutritional status. Instruct patient to report GI disturbances. Administer and teach patient to self-administer antiemetics as needed and as ordered. Teach patient importance of nutritious diet, and suggest small, frequent, high-calorie, high-protein meals as appropriate. Assess baseline LFTs and monitor periodically during treatment. Discuss abnormalities and drug interruption with physician.

III. FUNGAL SUPERINFECTION related to REDISTRIBUTION OF ENDOGENOUS MICROORGANISMS

Defining Characteristics: Vaginal candidiasis, vaginitis may occur as endogenous bacteria are eliminated and normal fungal population expands.

Nursing Implications: Instruct female patient to report vaginal itching or discharge. Discuss appropriate antifungal treatment with physician. Teach perineal hygiene and symptomatic management.

IV. ALTERATIONS IN PROTECTIVF MECHANISMS (RARE) related to TRANSIENT LEUKOPENIA

Defining Characteristics: Rarely, transient leukopenia, lymphocytosis, anemia, eosinophilia may occur. Prolonged PT, prolonged APTT, and hypoprothrombinemia have occurred rarely, especially in elderly or debilitated patients, or in individuals with vitamin K deficiency.

Nursing Implications: Assess baseline laboratory parameters, and monitor periodically during treatment. Assess patient for response to antibiotics. Discuss abnormalities with physician. Assess for signs/symptoms of bleeding. If they occur, especially in elderly or debilitated patients, discuss vitamin K administration with physician. Instruct patient to avoid aspirin. If taking oral anticoagulants, assess for increased PT, signs/symptoms of bleeding.

V. ALTERATIONS IN SENSORY/PERCEPTUAL PATTERNS related to DIZZINESS, SOMNOLENCE

Defining Characteristics: Dizziness, headache, somnolence occur rarely.

Nursing Implications: Assess baseline neurologic function and comfort, and monitor during treatment. Instruct patient to report any changes. Discuss any abnormalities with physician.

VI. ALTERATIONS IN COMFORT related to LOCAL INJECTION IRRITATION

Defining Characteristics: Pain, induration, sterile abscesses may form in IM injection sites; phlebitis may develop in IV sites.

Nursing Implications: Rotate IM injection sites, and administer drug deep IM in large muscle mass (e.g., gluteus maximus). Use IM injection when IV administration is not possible. Change IV sites q 48 h, and assess for signs/symptoms of phlebitis prior to each administration. Administer drug slowly. Apply warm packs to increase comfort.

Drug: cefpodoxime proxetil (Vantin)

Class: Cephalosporin antibacterial.

Mechanism of Action: Semisynthetic derivative of cephalosporin C; contains β-lactam ring and is related to penicillins and cephamycins. Bactericidal through inhibition of cell wall synthesis, with resulting cell wall instability and cell lysis.

Metabolism: Well absorbed from GI tract.

Dosage/Range:
- Oral (adult 13 years and older): 100–400 mg q 12 hours.
- Oral (gonorrhea indication): 200-mg single dose.
- Oral (child 6 months–12 years): 10 mg/kg/daily (divided daily-BID), (MAX 400 mg/day).
- Dose modification if renal impairment, based on creatinine clearance: refer to manufacturer's recommendations.

Drug Preparation:
- Take with food.

Drug Interactions:
- Probenecid: increased serum concentrations of antibiotic; monitor and decrease dose if needed.
- Aminoglycosides, penicillins: may have synergistic antibacterial effect against some organisms.
- Nephrotoxic drugs: may increase risk of renal dysfunction; avoid if possible.
- Magnesium and aluminum.

Lab Effects/Interference:
- Serum ALT (SGPT), serum alk phos, serum AST (SGOT), and serum bilirubin: values may be increased.
- BUN and serum creatinine: concentrations may be increased.

Special Considerations:
- Use cautiously if renal impairment is present.
- Contraindicated if hypersensitive to other cephalosporins, or if has had angioedema response to penicillin.

Potential Toxicities/Side Effects and the Nursing Process

I. POTENTIAL FOR INJURY related to HYPERSENSITIVITY REACTION

Defining Characteristics: Urticaria, pruritus, rash (maculopapular or erythematous), fever and chills, eosinophilia, myalgia, edema, erythema, angioedema. Increased risk in individuals allergic to penicillin.

Nursing Implications: Assess allergy to cephalosporin antibiotics and penicillin: if patient states "yes," determine actual response, e.g., "swollen lips = angioedema." If angioedema, patient SHOULD NOT receive drug. Discuss other patient responses with physician to determine whether drug should be given. Assess baseline skin condition, including integrity and allergy history to drugs. Teach patient to report rash, itching, other skin changes. Teach patient skin care and symptomatic measures as appropriate. If skin rash develops, discuss drug discontinuance with physician.

II. ALTERATION IN NUTRITION, LESS THAN BODY REQUIREMENTS, related to GI SIDE EFFECTS

Defining Characteristics: Nausea, vomiting, diarrhea, and anorexia may occur.

Nursing Implications: Assess baseline nutritional status. Teach patient to report GI disturbances. Administer and teach patient to self-administer antiemetics as needed and as ordered. Teach patient importance of nutritious diet, and suggest small, frequent, high-calorie, high-protein meals as appropriate. Discuss abnormalities and drug interruption with physician.

III. FUNGAL SUPERINFECTION related to REDISTRIBUTION OF ENDOGENOUS MICROORGANISMS

Defining Characteristics: Vaginal moniliasis, vaginitis may occur as endogenous bacteria are eliminated and normal fungal population expands.

Nursing Implications: Teach female patient to report vaginal itching or discharge. Discuss appropriate antifungal treatment with physician. Teach perineal hygiene and symptomatic management.

Drug: cefprozil (Cefzil)

Class: Second-generation cephalosporin antibiotic.

Mechanism of Action: Semisynthetic derivative of cephalosporin C; contains β-lactam ring, and is related to penicillins and cephamycins. Bactericidal through inhibition of cell wall synthesis, with resulting cell wall instability and cell lysis.

Metabolism: Well absorbed from GI tract; delayed GI absorption if taken with food, but total amount of drug absorption is the same. Widely distributed in body tissues and fluids, except cerebrospinal fluid; readily crosses placenta and is excreted in breast milk. Unchanged drug rapidly excreted by the kidneys.

Dosage/Range:
- Oral (adult 13 years and older): 250–500 mg q 12–24 hours.
- Oral (child 7 months–12 years): 7.5–15 mg/kg q 12 hours (MAX 1 gm/day).

Drug Preparation:
- Refrigerate suspension.
- Discard after 14 days.

Drug Interactions:
- Probenecid: increased serum concentrations of cefprozil but does not usually require dose reduction of antibiotic.
- Aminoglycosides, penicillins: may have synergistic antibacterial effect against some organisms.
- Typhoid vaccine.

Lab Effects/Interference:
- Serum ALT (SGPT), serum alk phos, serum AST (SGOT), and serum bilirubin: values may be increased.
- BUN and serum creatinine: concentrations may be increased.

Special Considerations:
- Use cautiously if renal impairment is present.
- Contraindicated if hypersensitive to other cephalosporins, or if has had angioedema response to penicillin.

Potential Toxicities/Side Effects and the Nursing Process

I. POTENTIAL FOR INJURY related to HYPERSENSITIVITY REACTION

Defining Characteristics: Urticaria, pruritus, rash (maculopapular or erythematous), fever and chills, eosinophilia, myalgia, edema, erythema, angioedema. Increased risk in individuals allergic to penicillin.

Nursing Implications: Assess allergy to cephalosporin antibiotics and penicillin: if patient states "yes," determine actual response, e.g., "swollen lips = angioedema." If angioedema, patient SHOULD NOT receive drug. Discuss other patient responses with physician to determine whether drug should be given. Assess baseline skin condition, including integrity and allergy history to drugs. Teach patient to report rash, itching, and other skin changes. Teach patient skin care and symptomatic measures as appropriate. If skin rash develops, discuss drug discontinuance with physician.

II. ALTERATION IN NUTRITION, LESS THAN BODY REQUIREMENTS, related to GI SIDE EFFECTS

Defining Characteristics: Nausea, vomiting, diarrhea, and anorexia may occur. May cause transient increases in LFTs.

Nursing Implications: Assess baseline nutritional status. Teach patient to report GI disturbances. Administer and teach patient to self-administer antiemetics as needed and as ordered. Teach patient importance of nutritious diet, and suggest small, frequent, high-calorie, high-protein meals as appropriate. Assess baseline LFTs and monitor periodically during treatment. Discuss abnormalities and drug interruption with physician.

III. FUNGAL SUPERINFECTION related to REDISTRIBUTION OF ENDOGENOUS MICROORGANISMS

Defining Characteristics: Vaginal moniliasis, vaginitis may occur as endogenous bacteria are eliminated and normal fungal population expands.

Nursing Implications: Teach female patient to report vaginal itching or discharge. Discuss appropriate antifungal treatment with physician. Teach perineal hygiene and symptomatic management.

IV. KNOWLEDGE DEFICIT related to SELF-ADMINISTRATION OF MEDICATION

Defining Characteristics: Increased compliance when patient is instructed in self-care activities.

Nursing Implications: Assess knowledge regarding infection and planned treatment. Teach about drug action, potential side effects, and when and how to take drug. Teach patient to report any possible side effects that occur.

Drug: ceftazidime (Fortaz, Tazicef, Tazidime)

Class: Third-generation cephalosporin antibacterial.

Mechanism of Action: Semisynthetic derivative of cephalosporin C (produced by fungus); contains β-lactam ring and is related to penicillins and cephamycins (e.g., cefoxitin). Bactericidal through inhibition of cell wall synthesis, with resulting cell wall instability and cell lysis. Active against sensitive microorganisms causing lower respiratory tract, urinary tract, skin, bone and joint, gynecologic, intra-abdominal infections. These include primarily gram-negative bacteria (*Enterobacter, E. coli, Klebsiella, Proteus, Serratia,* and *Pseudomonas*) and, to a lesser degree, some gram-positive bacteria (*S. aureus, S. epidermidis*, streptococci).

Metabolism: Not absorbed from GI tract so must be administered parenterally. Small degree of protein binding (5–24%). Widely distributed in body fluids (including CSF and bile) and body tissues. Crosses placenta and is excreted unchanged in urine.

Dosage/Range:
- IV and IM doses are the same.
- Adult: maximum 6 g/d.
- Uncomplicated pneumonia, skin/structure infections: 0.5–1 g IV q 8 h.
- Bone, joint infection: 2 g q 12 h.
- Severe GYN, abdominal infections or febrile neutropenia: 2 g IV q 8 h.
- Lung infection by pseudomonas in patients with cystic fibrosis: 30–50 mg/kg q 8 h.
- Dose should be reduced in renal insufficiency according to manufacturer's package insert.

Drug Preparation:
- Store sterile powder vials at 15–30°C (59–86°F) and protect from light; frozen injection containers should be stored at < −20°C (−4°F).
- IV: reconstitute according to manufacturer's package insert, as some preparations contain sodium carbonate. Further dilute in 100 mL of 0.9% sodium chloride or 5% dextrose and infuse over 30–60 minutes.
- IM: reconstitute according to manufacturer's package insert, which may suggest the addition of 0.5–1% lidocaine HCl to decrease discomfort. Make certain patient is NOT ALLERGIC to lidocaine. Administer deep IM in large muscle mass (e.g., gluteus maximus).

Drug Interactions:
- Probenecid: increased serum concentrations of antibiotic; monitor and decrease dose if needed.
- Aminoglycosides, penicillins: may have synergistic antibacterial effect against some organisms.
- Nephrotoxic drugs (aminoglycosides, colistin, vancomycin): may increase risk of renal dysfunction; avoid if possible.
- Sodium bicarbonate: incompatible; DO NOT administer concurrently through same IV site.

Lab Effects/Interference:

Major clinical significance:
- Coombs' (antiglobulin) tests: a positive reaction frequently appears in patients who receive large doses of cephalosporins; hemolysis rarely occurs, but it has been reported; test may be positive in neonates whose mothers received cephalosporins before delivery.

- PT: may be prolonged; cephalosporins may inhibit vitamin K synthesis by suppressing gut flora.

Clinical significance:

- Serum ALT, serum alk phos, serum AST, serum bili, or serum LDH values may be increased.
- BUN and serum creatinine concentrations may be increased.
- CBC or platelet count: transient leukopenia, neutropenia, agranulocytosis, thrombocytopenia, eosinophilia, lymphocytosis, and thrombocytosis have been seen on rare occasions.

Special Considerations:

- Empiric use in management of febrile neutropenic patient appears to be as effective as combination antibiotic regimens; vancomycin may need to be added to ceftazidime to better cover gram-positive bacteria (e.g., *S. epidermidis*).
- Has excellent coverage against *P. aeruginosa*.
- Use with caution in patients with renal dysfunction; dose reduction required if severe impairment exists.
- Use cautiously if history of colitis exists.
- Contraindicated in patients hypersensitive to other cephalosporin antibiotics.
- Use cautiously if sensitive to penicillin; contraindicated if angioedema reaction to penicillin.
- Obtain specimen and send for culture and sensitivity prior to first drug dose.
- May cause false-positive direct Coombs' test.
- May cause false-positive Clinitest glucose result.

Potential Toxicities/Side Effects and the Nursing Process

I. POTENTIAL FOR INJURY related to HYPERSENSITIVITY REACTION

Defining Characteristics: Urticaria, pruritus, rash (maculopapular or erythematous), fever and chills, eosinophilia, myalgia, edema, erythema, angioedema, Stevens-Johnson syndrome, and exfoliative skin reactions occur in 5% of patients. Increased risk in individuals allergic to penicillin.

Nursing Implications: Assess allergy to cephalosporin antibiotics and penicillin: if patient states "yes," determine actual response, e.g., "swollen lips = angioedema." If angioedema, patient SHOULD NOT receive drug. Discuss other patient responses with physician to determine whether drug should be given. Assess baseline skin condition, including integrity and allergy history to drugs. Instruct patient to report rash, itching, other skin changes. Teach patient skin care and symptomatic measures as appropriate. If skin rash develops, discuss drug discontinuance with physician. If rash progresses, drug should be discontinued, as fatal Stevens-Johnson syndrome may develop. Be prepared to treat severe acute hypersensitivity reactions with airway management, oxygen, epinephrine, corticosteroids, antihistamines as ordered.

II. ALTERATION IN NUTRITION, LESS THAN BODY REQUIREMENTS, related to GI SIDE EFFECTS

Defining Characteristics: Nausea, vomiting, diarrhea, anorexia may occur; rarely, pseudomembranous colitis caused by *C. difficile* resistant to the antibiotic occurs. Rarely, transient increases in LFTs—AST, ALT, alk phos, bili—may occur.

Nursing Implications: Assess baseline nutritional status. Instruct patient to report GI disturbances. Administer and teach patient to self-administer antiemetics as needed and as ordered. Teach patient importance of nutritious diet, and suggest small, frequent, high-calorie, high-protein meals as appropriate. Assess baseline LFTs, and monitor periodically during treatment. Discuss abnormalities and drug interruption with physician.

III. FUNGAL SUPERINFECTION related to REDISTRIBUTION OF ENDOGENOUS MICROORGANISMS

Defining Characteristics: Vaginal candidiasis, vaginitis may occur as endogenous bacteria are eliminated, and normal fungal population expands.

Nursing Implications: Instruct female patient to report vaginal itching or discharge. Discuss appropriate antifungal treatment with physician. Teach perineal hygiene and symptomatic management.

IV. ALTERATIONS IN PROTECTIVE MECHANISMS (RARE) related to TRANSIENT LEUKOPENIA

Defining Characteristics: Rarely, transient leukopenia, lymphocytosis, anemia, eosinophilia may occur. Prolonged PT, prolonged APTT, and hypoprothrombinemia have occurred rarely, especially in elderly or debilitated patients, or in individuals with vitamin K deficiency.

Nursing Implications: Assess baseline laboratory parameters, and monitor periodically during treatment. Assess patient for response to antibiotics. Discuss abnormalities with physician.

V. ALTERATIONS IN SENSORY/PERCEPTUAL PATTERNS related to DIZZINESS, SOMNOLENCE

Defining Characteristics: Dizziness, headache, somnolence occur rarely.

Nursing Implications: Assess baseline neurologic function and comfort, and monitor during treatment. Instruct patient to report any changes. Discuss any abnormalities with physician.

VI. ALTERATIONS IN COMFORT related to LOCAL INJECTION IRRITATION

Defining Characteristics: Pain, induration, sterile abscesses may form in IM injection sites; phlebitis may develop in IV sites.

Nursing Implications: Rotate IM injection sites, and administer drug deep IM in large muscle mass (e.g., gluteus maximus). Use IM injection when IV administration is not possible. Change IV sites q 48 h, and assess for signs/symptoms of phlebitis prior to each administration. Administer drug slowly. Apply warm packs to increase comfort.

Drug: ceftibuten (Cedax)

Class: Third-generation cephalosporin antibacterial.

Mechanism of Action: Semisynthetic derivative of cephalosporin C, contains β-lactam ring, and is related to penicillins and cephamycins. Bactericidal through inhibition of cell wall synthesis, with resulting cell wall instability and cell lysis.

Metabolism: Well absorbed from GI tract; delayed GI absorption if taken with food, but total amount of drug absorption is the same. Widely distributed in body tissues and fluids, except cerebrospinal fluid; readily crosses placenta and is excreted in breast milk. Unchanged drug rapidly excreted by the kidneys.

Dosage/Range:
- Adults: 400 mg orally daily × 10 days.
- Dose reduce if creatinine clearance is reduced per manufacturer's recommendations.

Drug Preparation:
- Store suspension in refrigerator; discard after 14 days.
- Oral administration.

Drug Interactions:
- Aminoglycosides, penicillins: may have synergistic antibacterial effect against some organisms.
- Typhoid vaccine.

Lab Effects/Interference:
- Serum SGPT, serum alk phos, serum SGOT, serum bilirubin, or serum LDH: values may be increased.
- BUN and serum creatinine: concentrations may be increased.

Special Considerations:
- Use with caution in patients with renal dysfunction; dose reduction required if severe impairment exists.
- Contraindicated in patients hypersensitive to other cephalosporin antibiotics.

- Use cautiously if sensitive to penicillin; contraindicated if angioedema reaction to penicillin.
- Obtain ordered specimen and send for culture and sensitivity prior to first drug dose.

Potential Toxicities/Side Effects and the Nursing Process

I. POTENTIAL FOR INJURY related to HYPERSENSITIVITY REACTION

Defining Characteristics: Urticaria, pruritus, rash (maculopapular or erythematous), fever and chills, eosinophilia, myalgia, edema, erythema, angioedema. Increased risk in individuals allergic to penicillin.

Nursing Implications: Assess allergy to cephalosporin antibiotics and penicillin: if patient states "yes," determine actual response, e.g., "swollen lips = angioedema." If angioedema, patient SHOULD NOT receive drug. Discuss other patient responses with physician to determine whether drug should be given. Assess baseline skin condition, including integrity and allergy history to drugs. Teach patient to report rash, itching, other skin changes. Teach patient skin care and symptomatic measures as appropriate. If skin rash develops, discuss drug discontinuance with physician.

II. ALTERATION IN NUTRITION, LESS THAN BODY REQUIREMENTS, related to GI SIDE EFFECTS

Defining Characteristics: Nausea, vomiting, diarrhea, and anorexia may occur. Rarely, transient increases in LFTs—AST (SGOT), ALT (SGPT), alk phos, bili—may occur.

Nursing Implications: Assess baseline nutritional status. Teach patient to report GI disturbances. Administer and teach patient to self-administer medication as needed and as ordered. Teach patient importance of nutritious diet, and suggest small, frequent, high-calorie, high-protein meals as appropriate. Assess baseline LFTs and monitor periodically during treatment. Discuss abnormalities and drug interruption with physician.

III. FUNGAL SUPERINFECTION related to REDISTRIBUTION OF ENDOGENOUS MICROORGANISMS

Defining Characteristics: Vaginal moniliasis, vaginitis may occur as endogenous bacteria are eliminated and normal fungal population expands.

Nursing Implications: Teach female patient to report vaginal itching or discharge. Discuss appropriate antifungal treatment with physician. Teach perineal hygiene and symptomatic management.

Drug: ceftriaxone sodium (Rocephin)

Class: Third-generation cephalosporin antibacterial.

Mechanism of Action: Semisynthetic derivative of cephalosporin C (produced by fungus); contains β-lactam ring and is related to penicillins and cephamycins (e.g., cefoxitin). Bactericidal through inhibition of cell wall synthesis, with resulting cell wall instability and cell lysis. Active primarily against gram-negative cocci (*H. influenzae, Enterobacter, E. coli, Klebsiella, Proteus, Pseudomonas*) and, to a lesser degree, gram-positive cocci (*S. aureus* and streptococci). Drug is used for treatment of infections in lower respiratory tract, skin, bone and joint, abdomen, urinary tract, and pelvis (gonorrhea), as well as for treatment of meningitis and sepsis.

Metabolism: Not absorbed from GI tract and must be given parenterally. Widely distributed into body tissues and fluids, including bile and CSF. Crosses placenta and excreted in breast milk. Protein binding depends on drug concentration, and varies from 58–96%. Excreted in urine and feces to a lesser extent. Has a long half-life.

Dosage/Range:
- IV and IM doses same.
- 1–2 g/day, or in equally divided doses q 12 h.
- CNS infections may require maximum recommended of 4 g/day in divided doses.

Drug Preparation:
- Store vial of sterile drug powder at ≤ 25°C (77°F) and protect from light. Frozen injection containers should be stored at ≤ −20°C (−4°F).
- IV: Add diluent recommended by manufacturer into vial, then further dilute in 100 mL 0.9% sodium chloride or 5% dextrose. Infuse over 30–60 minutes.
- IM: Add 0.9–7.2 mL of sterile or bacteriostatic water for injection, or 1% lidocaine HCl without epinephrine to appropriate vial, resulting in 250 mg/mL. Administer deep IM into large muscle mass (e.g., gluteus maximus). Make certain patient is NOT ALLERGIC to lidocaine.

Drug Interactions:
- Probenecid: increased serum concentrations of antibiotic; monitor and decrease dose if needed.
- Aminoglycosides, penicillins: may have synergistic antibacterial effect against some organisms.
- Nephrotoxic drugs (aminoglycosides, colistin, vancomycin): may increase risk of renal dysfunction; avoid if possible.

Lab Effects/Interference:

Major clinical significance:
- Coombs' (antiglobulin) tests: a positive reaction frequently appears in patients who receive large doses of cephalosporins; hemolysis rarely occurs, but it has been reported; test may be positive in neonates whose mothers received cephalosporins before delivery.

- PT: may be prolonged; cephalosporins may inhibit vitamin K synthesis by suppressing gut flora.

Clinical significance:

- Serum ALT, serum alk phos, serum AST, serum bili, or serum LDH values may be increased.
- BUN and serum creatinine concentrations may be increased.
- CBC or platelet count: transient leukopenia, neutropenia, agranulocytosis, thrombocytopenia, eosinophilia, lymphocytosis, and thrombocytosis have been seen on rare occasions.

Special Considerations:

- Use cautiously if history of colitis exists.
- Contraindicated in patients hypersensitive to other cephalosporin antibiotics.
- Use cautiously if sensitive to penicillin; contraindicated if angioedema reaction to penicillin.
- Obtain specimen and send for culture and sensitivity prior to first drug dose.
- May cause false-positive direct Coombs' test.
- May cause false-positive Clinitest glucose result.

Potential Toxicities/Side Effects and the Nursing Process

I. POTENTIAL FOR INJURY related to HYPERSENSITIVITY REACTION

Defining Characteristics: Urticaria, pruritus, rash (maculopapular or erythematous), fever and chills, eosinophilia, myalgia, edema, erythema, angioedema, Stevens-Johnson syndrome, and exfoliative skin reactions occur in 5% of patients. Increased risk in individuals allergic to penicillin.

Nursing Implications: Assess allergy to cephalosporin antibiotics and penicillin: if patient states "yes," determine actual response, e.g., "swollen lips = angioedema." If angioedema, patient SHOULD NOT receive drug. Discuss other patient responses with physician to determine whether drug should be given. Assess baseline skin condition, including integrity and allergy history to drugs. Instruct patient to report rash, itching, other skin changes. Teach patient skin care and symptomatic measures as appropriate. If skin rash develops, discuss drug discontinuance with physician. If rash progresses, drug should be discontinued, as fatal Stevens-Johnson syndrome may develop. Be prepared to treat severe acute hypersensitivity reactions with airway management, oxygen, epinephrine, corticosteroids, antihistamines as ordered.

II. ALTERATION IN NUTRITION, LESS THAN BODY REQUIREMENTS, related to GI SIDE EFFECTS

Defining Characteristics: Nausea, vomiting, diarrhea, anorexia may occur; rarely, pseudomembranous colitis caused by *C. difficile* resistant to the antibiotic occurs. Rarely, transient increases in LFTs—AST, ALT, alk phos, bili—may occur.

Nursing Implications: Assess baseline nutritional status. Instruct patient to report GI disturbances. Administer and teach patient to self-administer antiemetics, antidiarrheals as needed and as ordered. Teach patient importance of nutritious diet, and suggest small, frequent, high-calorie, high-protein meals as appropriate. Assess baseline LFTs and monitor periodically during treatment. Discuss abnormalities and drug interruption with physician.

III. FUNGAL SUPERINFECTION related to REDISTRIBUTION OF ENDOGENOUS MICROORGANISMS

Defining Characteristics: Vaginal candidiasis, vaginitis may occur as endogenous bacteria are eliminated and normal fungal population expands.

Nursing Implications: Instruct female patient to report vaginal itching or discharge. Discuss appropriate antifungal treatment with physician. Teach perineal hygiene and symptomatic management.

IV. ALTERATIONS IN PROTECTIVE MECHANISMS (RARE) related to TRANSIENT LEUKOPENIA

Defining Characteristics: Rarely, transient leukopenia, lymphocytosis, anemia, eosinophilia may occur. Prolonged PT, prolonged APTT, and hypoprothrombinemia have occurred rarely, especially in elderly or debilitated patients, or in individuals with vitamin K deficiency.

Nursing Implications: Assess baseline laboratory parameters, and monitor periodically during treatment. Assess patient for response to antibiotics. Discuss abnormalities with physician. Assess for signs/symptoms of bleeding. If they occur, especially in elderly or debilitated patients, discuss vitamin K administration with physician. Instruct patient to avoid aspirin. If taking oral anticoagulants, assess for increased PT, signs/symptoms of bleeding.

V. ALTERATIONS IN SENSORY/PERCEPTUAL PATTERNS related to DIZZINESS, SOMNOLENCE

Defining Characteristics: Dizziness, headache, somnolence occur rarely.

Nursing Implications: Assess baseline neurologic function and comfort, and monitor during treatment. Instruct patient to report any changes. Discuss any abnormalities with physician.

VI. ALTERATIONS IN COMFORT related to LOCAL INJECTION IRRITATION

Defining Characteristics: Pain, induration, and sterile abscesses may form in IM injection sites; phlebitis may develop in IV sites.

Nursing Implications: Rotate IM injection sites, and administer drug deep IM in large muscle mass (e.g., gluteus maximus). Use IM injection when IV administration is not possible. Change IV sites q 48 h, and assess for signs/symptoms of phlebitis prior to each administration. Administer drug slowly. Apply warm packs to increase comfort.

Drug: cefuroxime (Ceftin; Kefurox; Zinacef)

Class: Second-generation cephalosporin antibiotic.

Mechanism of Action: Semisynthetic derivative of cephalosporin C; contains β-lactam ring, and is related to penicillins and cephamycins. Bactericidal through inhibition of cell wall synthesis by binding to one or more of the penicillin-binding proteins (PSPs) that in turn inhibit the final transpeptidation step of peptidoglycan synthesis in bacterial cell walls, thus inhibiting cell wall biosynthesis. Bacteria eventually lyse due to ongoing activity of cell wall autolytic enzymes (autolysins and murein hydrolases) while cell wall assembly is arrested.

Metabolism: Widely distributed in body tissues, fluids; crosses blood–brain barrier; therapeutic concentrations achieved in cerebrospinal fluid even when meninges are not inflamed; readily crosses placenta and is excreted in breast milk. Unchanged drug rapidly excreted by the kidneys.

Dosage/Range:
- Oral (adult): 250–500 mg twice daily for 10 days.
- IM and IV (adult): 750 mg to 1.5 g/dose every 8 hours or 100–150 mg/kg/day in divided doses every 6–8 hours; maximum dose—6 g/24 hours.

Drug Preparation:
- Refrigerate suspension; solution stable for 48 hours.
- IV infusion in NS or D5W solution stable for 7 days when refrigerated.

Drug Interactions:
- Probenecid: increased serum concentrations of cefotetan, but does not usually require dose reduction of antibiotic.
- Aminoglycosides: can increase nephrotoxicity.

Lab Effects/Interference:
- Serum ALT (SGPT), serum alk phos, serum AST (SGOT), and serum bilirubin—values may be increased.
- BUN and serum creatinine—concentrations may be increased.

Special Considerations:

- Use cautiously if renal impairment is present.
- Contraindicated if hypersensitive to other cephalosporins, or if has had angioedema response to penicillin.

Potential Toxicities/Side Effects and the Nursing Process

I. POTENTIAL FOR INJURY related to HYPERSENSITIVITY REACTION

Defining Characteristics: Urticaria, pruritus, rash (maculopapular or erythematous), fever and chills, eosinophilia, myalgia, edema, erythema, angioedema. Increased risk in individuals allergic to penicillin.

Nursing Implications: Assess allergy to cephalosporin antibiotics and penicillin: if patient states "yes," determine actual response, e.g., "swollen lips = angioedema." If angioedema, patient SHOULD NOT receive drug. Discuss other patient responses with physician to determine whether drug should be given. Assess baseline skin condition, including integrity and allergy history to drugs. Teach patient to report rash, itching, and other skin changes. Teach patient skin care and symptomatic measures as appropriate. If skin rash develops, discuss drug discontinuance with physician.

II. ALTERATION IN NUTRITION, LESS THAN BODY REQUIREMENTS, related to GI SIDE EFFECTS

Defining Characteristics: Nausea, vomiting, diarrhea, and anorexia may occur. May cause transient increases in LFTs.

Nursing Implications: Assess baseline nutritional status. Teach patient to report GI disturbances. Administer and teach patient to self-administer antiemetics as needed and as ordered. Teach patient importance of nutritious diet, and suggest small, frequent, high-calorie, high-protein meals as appropriate. Assess baseline LFTs and monitor periodically during treatment. Discuss abnormalities and drug interruption with physician.

III. FUNGAL SUPERINFECTION related to REDISTRIBUTION OF ENDOGENOUS MICROORGANISMS

Defining Characteristics: Vaginal moniliasis, vaginitis may occur as endogenous bacteria are eliminated and normal fungal population expands.

Nursing Implications: Teach female patient to report vaginal itching or discharge. Discuss appropriate antifungal treatment with physician. Teach perineal hygiene and symptomatic management.

IV. KNOWLEDGE DEFICIT related to SELF-ADMINISTRATION OF MEDICATION

Defining Characteristics: Increased compliance when patient is instructed in self-care activities.

Nursing Implications: Assess knowledge regarding infection and planned treatment. Teach about drug action, potential side effects, and when and how to take drug. Teach patient to report any possible side effects that occur.

Drug: cephalexin (Biocef; Keflex; Keftab)

Class: First-generation cephalosporin antibacterial.

Mechanism of Action: Semisynthetic derivative of cephalosporin C, contains β-lactam ring, and is related to penicillins and cephamycins. Bactericidal through inhibition of cell wall synthesis by binding to one or more of the penicillin-binding proteins (PBPs) that in turn inhibits the final transpeptidation step of peptidoglycan synthesis in bacterial cell walls, thus inhibiting cell wall biosynthesis. Bacteria eventually lyse due to ongoing activity of cell wall autolytic enzymes (autolysins and murein hydrolases) while cell wall assembly is arrested.

Metabolism: Well absorbed from GI tract; delayed GI absorption if taken with food, but total amount of drug absorption is the same. Widely distributed in body tissues, fluids except cerebrospinal fluid; readily crosses placenta and is excreted in breast milk. Unchanged drug rapidly excreted by the kidneys.

Dosage/Range:
- Adults: 250–1000 mg every 6 hours, maximum—4 g/day.
- Dose reduce if creatinine clearance is reduced per manufacturer's recommendations.

Drug Preparation:
- Store suspension in refrigerator, discard after 14 days.
- Oral administration.

Drug Interactions:
- Aminoglycosides increase nephrotic potential and increase toxicity.
- Probenecid may decrease cephalosporin elimination and increase effect.

Lab Effects/Interference:
- Serum SGPT, serum alk phos, serum SGOT, serum bilirubin, or serum LDH—values may be increased.
- BUN and serum creatinine—concentrations may be increased.

Special Considerations:

- Use with caution in patients with renal dysfunction—dose reduction required if severe impairment exists.
- Contraindicated in patients hypersensitive to other cephalosporin antibiotics.
- Use cautiously if sensitive to penicillin; contraindicated if angioedema reaction to penicillin.
- Obtain ordered specimen and send for culture and sensitivity prior to first drug dose.

Potential Toxicities/Side Effects and the Nursing Process

I. POTENTIAL FOR INJURY related to HYPERSENSITIVITY REACTION

Defining Characteristics: Urticaria, pruritus, rash (maculopapular or erythematous), fever and chills, eosinophilia, myalgia, edema, erythema, angioedema. Increased risk in individuals allergic to penicillin.

Nursing Implications: Assess allergy to cephalosporin antibiotics and penicillin: if patient states "yes," determine actual response, e.g., "swollen lips = angioedema." If angioedema, patient SHOULD NOT receive drug. Discuss other patient responses with physician to determine whether drug should be given. Assess baseline skin condition, including integrity and allergy history to drugs. Teach patient to report rash, itching, other skin changes. Teach patient skin care and symptomatic measures as appropriate. If skin rash develops, discuss drug discontinuance with physician.

II. ALTERATION IN NUTRITION, LESS THAN BODY REQUIREMENTS, related to GI SIDE EFFECTS

Defining Characteristics: Nausea and vomiting and diarrhea and anorexia may occur. Rarely, transient increases in LFTs—AST (SGOT), ALT (SGPT), alk phos, bili—may occur.

Nursing Implications: Assess baseline nutritional status. Teach patient to report GI disturbances. Administer and teach patient to self-administer medication as needed and as ordered. Teach patient importance of nutritious diet, and suggest small, frequent, high-calorie, high-protein meals as appropriate. Assess baseline LFTs and monitor periodically during treatment. Discuss abnormalities and drug interruption with physician.

III. FUNGAL SUPERINFECTION related to REDISTRIBUTION OF ENDOGENOUS MICROORGANISMS

Defining Characteristics: Vaginal moniliasis, vaginitis may occur as endogenous bacteria are eliminated and normal fungal population expands.

Nursing Implications: Teach female patient to report vaginal itching or discharge. Discuss appropriate antifungal treatment with physician. Teach perineal hygiene and symptomatic management.

Drug: cephapirin (Cefadyl; Cephapirin Sodium)

Class: First-generation cephalosporin antibacterial.

Mechanism of Action: Semisynthetic derivative of cephalosporin C, contains β-lactam ring, and is related to penicillins and cephamycins. Bactericidal through inhibition of cell wall synthesis by binding to one or more of the penicillin-binding proteins (PBPs) that in turn inhibit the final transpeptidation step of peptidoglycan synthesis in bacterial cell walls, thus inhibiting cell wall biosynthesis. Bacteria eventually lyse due to ongoing activity of cell wall autolytic enzymes (autolysins and murein hydrolases) while cell wall assembly is arrested.

Metabolism: Well absorbed from GI tract; delayed GI absorption if taken with food, but total amount of drug absorption is the same. Widely distributed in body tissues, fluids except cerebrospinal fluid; readily crosses placenta and is excreted in breast milk. Unchanged drug rapidly excreted by the kidneys.

Dosage/Range:

- Adults: 500–1000 mg every 6 hours, maximum—4 g/day
- Dose reduce if creatinine clearance is reduced per manufacturer's recommendations.

Drug Preparation:

- Reconstituted solution is stable for 10 days when refrigerated.
- IV infusion in NS or D5W solution stable for 10 days when refrigerated.

Drug Interactions:

- Aminoglycosides increase nephrotic potential and increase toxicity.
- Probenecid may decrease cephalosporin elimination and increase effect.

Lab Effects/Interference:

- Serum SGPT, serum alk phos, serum SGOT, serum bilirubin, or serum LDH—values may be increased.
- BUN and serum creatinine—concentrations may be increased.

Special Considerations:

- Use with caution in patients with renal dysfunction—dose reduction required if severe impairment exists.
- Contraindicated in patients hypersensitive to other cephalosporin antibiotics.
- Use cautiously if sensitive to penicillin; contraindicated if angioedema reaction to penicillin.
- Obtain ordered specimen and send for culture and sensitivity prior to first drug dose.

Potential Toxicities/Side Effects and the Nursing Process

I. POTENTIAL FOR INJURY related to HYPERSENSITIVITY REACTION

Defining Characteristics: Urticaria, pruritus, rash (maculopapular or erythematous), fever and chills, eosinophilia, myalgia, edema, erythema, angioedema. Increased risk in individuals allergic to penicillin.

Nursing Implications: Assess allergy to cephalosporin antibiotics and penicillin: if patient states "yes," determine actual response, e.g., "swollen lips = angioedema." If angioedema, patient SHOULD NOT receive drug. Discuss other patient responses with physician to determine whether drug should be given. Assess baseline skin condition, including integrity and allergy history to drugs. Teach patient to report rash, itching, other skin changes. Teach patient skin care and symptomatic measures as appropriate. If skin rash develops, discuss drug discontinuance with physician.

II. ALTERATION IN NUTRITION, LESS THAN BODY REQUIREMENTS, related to GI SIDE EFFECTS

Defining Characteristics: Nausea and vomiting and diarrhea and anorexia may occur. Rarely, transient increases in LFTs—AST (SGOT), ALT (SGPT), alk phos, bili—may occur.

Nursing Implications: Assess baseline nutritional status. Teach patient to report GI disturbances. Administer and teach patient to self-administer medication as needed and as ordered. Teach patient importance of nutritious diet, and suggest small, frequent, high-calorie, high-protein meals as appropriate. Assess baseline LFTs and monitor periodically during treatment. Discuss abnormalities and drug interruption with physician.

III. FUNGAL SUPERINFECTION related to REDISTRIBUTION OF ENDOGENOUS MICROORGANISMS

Defining Characteristics: Vaginal moniliasis, vaginitis may occur as endogenous bacteria are eliminated and normal fungal population expands.

Nursing Implications: Teach female patient to report vaginal itching or discharge. Discuss appropriate antifungal treatment with physician. Teach perineal hygiene and symptomatic management.

Drug: cephradine (Anspor, Velosef)

Class: First-generation cephalosporin antibacterial.

Mechanism of Action: Semisynthetic derivative of cephalosporin C (produced by fungus); contains β-lactam ring and is related to penicillins and cephamycins (e.g., cefoxitin). Bactericidal through inhibition of cell wall synthesis, with resulting cell wall instability and cell lysis. Active against many gram-positive aerobic cocci (streptococci, staphylococci) and has limited gram-negative activity (*Klebsiella, H. influenzae, E. coli, Proteus*). Used in treatment of infections of respiratory tract, GU tract, skin, bone and joint, and in meningitis, sepsis.

Metabolism: Poorly absorbed from GI tract so must be given parenterally. Widely distributed throughout body tissues and fluids, including CSF; 65–79% protein-bound. Crosses placenta and is excreted in breast milk. Metabolized in liver and kidneys and is excreted in the urine.

Dosage/Range:

Adult:
- 500 mg–1 g IM or IV q 4–6 h; and in life-threatening infections, 2 g q 4 h.
- Dose reduction in renal insufficiency according to manufacturer's package insert.

Drug Preparation:
- Store vial of powder for injection at < 40°C (< 104°F), and frozen injection containers at ≤ −20° (−4°F).
- IV: Reconstitute with at least 10 mL sterile water for injection according to manufacturer's package insert. Further dilute in 100 mL 0.9% sodium chloride or 5% dextrose injection and administer over 30–60 minutes.
- IM: Reconstitute each gram of drug with 4 mL sterile water for injection. Administer deep IM in large muscle mass (e.g., gluteus maximus).

Drug Interactions:
- Probenecid: increased serum concentrations of antibiotic; monitor and decrease dose if needed.
- Aminoglycosides, penicillins: may have synergistic antibacterial effect against some organisms.
- Nephrotoxic drugs (aminoglycosides, colistin, vancomycin): may increase risk of renal dysfunction; avoid if possible.

Lab Effects/Interference:

Major clinical significance:
- Coombs' (antiglobulin) tests: a positive reaction frequently appears in patients who receive large doses of cephalosporins; hemolysis rarely occurs, but it has been reported; test may be positive in neonates whose mothers received cephalosporins before delivery.

- Urine glucose: some cephalosporins (cephradine) may produce a false-positive or falsely elevated test results with copper sulfate tests (Benedict's, Fehling's, or Clinitest); glucose enzymatic tests (Clinistix and Testape) are not affected.
- PT: may be prolonged; cephalosporins may inhibit vitamin K synthesis by suppressing gut flora.

Clinical significance:

- Serum ALT, serum alk phos, serum AST, serum bili, or serum LDH values may be increased.
- BUN and serum creatinine concentrations may be increased.
- CBC or platelet count: transient leukopenia, neutropenia, agranulocytosis, thrombocytopenia, eosinophilia, lymphocytosis, and thrombocytosis have been seen on rare occasions.

Special Considerations:

- Use with caution in patients with renal dysfunction; dose reduction required if severe impairment exists.
- Use cautiously if history of colitis exists.
- Contraindicated in patients hypersensitive to other cephalosporin antibiotics.
- Use cautiously if sensitive to penicillin; contraindicated if angioedema reaction to penicillin.
- Obtain specimen and send for culture and sensitivity prior to first drug dose.
- May cause false-positive direct Coombs' test.
- May cause false-positive Clinitest glucose result.

Potential Toxicities/Side Effects and the Nursing Process

I. POTENTIAL FOR INJURY related to HYPERSENSITIVITY REACTION

Defining Characteristics: Urticaria, pruritus, rash (maculopapular or erythematous), fever and chills, eosinophilia, myalgia, edema, erythema, angioedema, Stevens-Johnson syndrome, and exfoliative skin reactions occur in 5% of patients. Increased risk in individuals allergic to penicillin.

Nursing Implications: Assess allergy to cephalosporin antibiotics and penicillin: if patient states "yes," determine actual response, e.g., "swollen lips = angioedema." If angioedema, patient SHOULD NOT receive drug. Discuss other patient responses with physician to determine whether drug should be given. Assess baseline skin condition, including integrity and allergy history to drugs. Instruct patient to report rash, itching, other skin changes. Teach patient skin care and symptomatic measures as appropriate. If skin rash develops, discuss drug discontinuance with physician. If rash progresses, drug should be discontinued, as fatal Stevens-Johnson syndrome may develop. Be prepared to treat severe acute hypersensitivity reactions with airway management, oxygen, epinephrine, corticosteroids, antihistamines as ordered.

II. ALTERATION IN NUTRITION, LESS THAN BODY REQUIREMENTS, related to GI SIDE EFFECTS

Defining Characteristics: Nausea, vomiting, diarrhea, anorexia may occur; rarely, pseudomembranous colitis caused by *C. difficile* resistant to the antibiotic occurs. Rarely, transient increases in LFTs—AST, ALT, alk phos, bili—may occur.

Nursing Implications: Assess baseline nutritional status. Instruct patient to report GI disturbances. Administer and teach patient to self-administer antiemetics as needed and as ordered. Teach patient importance of nutritious diet, and suggest small, frequent, high-calorie, high-protein meals as appropriate. Assess baseline LFTs and monitor periodically during treatment. Discuss abnormalities and drug interruption with physician.

III. FUNGAL SUPERINFECTION related to REDISTRIBUTION OF ENDOGENOUS MICROORGANISMS

Defining Characteristics: Vaginal candidiasis, vaginitis may occur as endogenous bacteria are eliminated and normal fungal population expands.

Nursing Implications: Instruct female patient to report vaginal itching or discharge. Discuss appropriate antifungal treatment with physician. Teach perineal hygiene and symptomatic management.

IV. ALTERATIONS IN PROTECTIVE MECHANISMS (RARE) related to TRANSIENT LEUKOPENIA

Defining Characteristics: Rarely, transient leukopenia, lymphocytosis, anemia, eosinophilia may occur. Prolonged PT, prolonged APTT, and hypoprothrombinemia have occurred rarely, especially in elderly or debilitated patients, or in individuals with vitamin K deficiency.

Nursing Implications: Assess baseline laboratory parameters, and monitor periodically during treatment. Assess patient for response to antibiotics. Discuss abnormalities with physician.

V. ALTERATIONS IN SENSORY/PERCEPTUAL PATTERNS related to DIZZINESS, SOMNOLENCE

Defining Characteristics: Dizziness, headache, somnolence occur rarely.

Nursing Implications: Assess baseline neurologic function and comfort, and monitor during treatment. Instruct patient to report any changes. Discuss any abnormalities with physician.

VI. ALTERATIONS IN COMFORT related to LOCAL INJECTION IRRITATION

Defining Characteristics: Pain, induration, sterile abscesses may form in IM injection sites; phlebitis may develop in IV sites.

Nursing Implications: Rotate IM injection sites, and administer drug deep IM in large muscle mass (e.g., gluteus maximus). Use IM injection when IV administration is not possible. Change IV sites q 48 h, and assess for signs/symptoms of phlebitis prior to each administration. Administer drug slowly. Apply warm packs to increase comfort.

VII. KNOWLEDGE DEFICIT related to SELF-ADMINISTRATION OF MEDICATION

Defining Characteristics: Increased compliance when patient is instructed in self-care activities.

Nursing Implications: Assess knowledge about infection and planned treatment. Teach about drug action, potential side effects, and when and how to take drug. Teach patient to report any side effects that occur.

Drug: ciprofloxacin (Cipro)

Class: Fluoroquinolone.

Mechanism of Action: Anti-infective; appears to inhibit DNA replication in susceptible bacteria. Has a broad spectrum, and is active against most gram-negative bacteria (e.g., *Enterobacter, Pseudomonas*), some gram-positive organisms (e.g., methicillin-resistant staphylococci), and some mycobacteria.

Metabolism: Well absorbed from GI tract; rate decreased by food but not extent of absorption. Widely distributed in body tissues and fluids with highest concentrations in organs, such as liver, kidneys, and lungs. Partially metabolized in liver; excreted in urine and feces. Crosses placenta and is excreted in breast milk.

Dosage/Range:
- 250–750 mg q 12 h × 1–2 weeks.
- IV: 200–400 mg q 12 h × 1–2 weeks (IV used if patient unable to take oral formulation).
- Dose modification necessary if renal impairment exists.

Drug Preparation:
- Oral: Take drug with 1 large glass of fluid, preferably 2 hours after meal/food. Encourage oral fluids of 2–3 qt/day.
- IV: Further dilute drug in 0.9% sodium chloride or 5% dextrose in water to final concentration of < 2 mg/mL. Administer over 60 minutes.

Drug Interactions:

- Antacids (containing magnesium, aluminum, or calcium): decrease oral ciprofloxacin serum level; do not administer concurrently. If must administer antacids, administer at least 2 hours apart.
- Other anti-infectives: potential synergism with clindamycin, aminoglycosides, β-lactam antibiotics against certain organisms.
- Probenecid: 50% increase in ciprofloxacin serum levels; decrease ciprofloxacin dose if given concurrently.
- Theophylline: increases theophylline serum level; avoid if possible since fatal reactions have occurred. Otherwise, monitor theophylline level very closely and decrease theophylline dose as needed.
- Caffeine: delays caffeine clearance from body. Instruct patient to limit coffee, tea, soft drinks, especially if CNS side effects.

Lab Effects/Interference:

- Serum ALT, serum alk phos, serum AST, and serum LDH values may be increased.

Special Considerations:

- Used in the treatment of infections of urinary and lower respiratory tract, skin, bone and joint, and GI tract, as well as gonorrhea.
- Contraindicated in pregnancy and in women who are breast-feeding.
- Obtain ordered specimen for culture and sensitivity prior to first drug dose.
- Use cautiously in patients with seizure disorders.
- Use cautiously in patients receiving concurrent theophylline, as cardiopulmonary arrest has occurred.

Potential Toxicities/Side Effects and the Nursing Process

I. ALTERATION IN NUTRITION, LESS THAN BODY REQUIREMENTS, related to GI SIDE EFFECTS

Defining Characteristics: 2–10% incidence of nausea, vomiting, abdominal discomfort, diarrhea, anorexia.

Nursing Implications: Assess baseline nutritional and elimination status. Instruct patient to report GI disturbances. Administer and teach patient to self-administer antiemetics, antidiarrheals as needed and as ordered. Teach patient importance of nutritious diet, and suggest small, frequent, high-calorie, high-protein meals as appropriate. Assess baseline LFTs and monitor periodically during treatment. Discuss abnormalities and drug interruption with physician. Assess whether taking other hepatotoxic drugs. (See Special Considerations section.)

II. ALTERATIONS IN SENSORY/PERCEPTUAL PATTERNS related to CNS EFFECTS

Defining Characteristics: 1–2% incidence of headache, restlessness. Dizziness, hallucinations, and seizures may also occur. Exacerbated by caffeine, as ciprofloxacin delays caffeine excretion.

Nursing Implications: Assess baseline neurologic function and comfort, and monitor during treatment. Instruct patient to report any changes. Discuss any abnormalities with physician. Teach patient to limit or restrict all caffeine containing fluids, medications, e.g., tea, coffee, soft drinks containing caffeine.

III. ALTERATION IN SKIN INTEGRITY related to ALLERGY/HYPERSENSITIVITY

Defining Characteristics: 1–4% incidence of rash; other manifestations include eosinophilia, urticaria, flushing, fever, chills, photosensitivity, angioedema. Fatal hypersensitivity reactions have occurred rarely. Direct exposure to sunlight can cause sunburn (moderate to severe phototoxicity).

Nursing Implications: Assess baseline skin condition, including integrity and drug allergy history. Instruct patient to report rash, itching, other skin changes. Teach patient skin care and symptomatic measures as appropriate. If skin rash develops, discuss drug discontinuance with physician. If rash progresses, especially in HIV-infected patients, drug should be discontinued as fatal Stevens-Johnson syndrome may develop. Be prepared to treat severe acute hypersensitivity reactions with airway management, oxygen, epinephrine, corticosteroids, antihistamines as ordered. Instruct patient to avoid excessive sun exposure and to use skin protection factor (SPF) 15 or higher.

IV. ALTERATION IN URINARY ELIMINATION related to RENAL TOXICITY

Defining Characteristics: Increased BUN and creatinine, crystal and stone formation in urine, interstitial nephritis, and renal failure may occur.

Nursing Implications: Assess baseline renal function; expect that drug dose will be decreased in presence of renal dysfunction. Instruct patient to take drug with at least 8 oz (240 mL) of water, and to increase oral fluids to 2–3 qt/day.

V. ALTERATION IN COMFORT related to IV ADMINISTRATION

Defining Characteristics: Drug may cause pain, inflammation, and rare thrombophlebitis at IV site.

Nursing Implications: Change IV site q 48 h. Assess for phlebitis, discomfort, and IV patency prior to each administration. Administer drug slowly over 60–90 minutes in large volume of 5% dextrose (see Drug Preparation). Apply heat to promote comfort.

VI. FUNGAL SUPERINFECTION related to REDISTRIBUTION OF ENDOGENOUS MICROORGANISMS

Defining Characteristics: Vaginal candidiasis, vaginitis may occur as endogenous bacteria are eliminated and normal fungal population expands.

Nursing Implications: Instruct female patient to report vaginal itching or discharge. Discuss appropriate antifungal treatment with physician. Teach perineal hygiene and symptomatic management.

Drug: clarithromycin (Biaxin; Biaxin XL)

Class: Antibacterial (macrolide).

Mechanism of Action: Clarithromycin exerts its antibacterial action by binding to 50S ribosomal subunit resulting in inhibition of protein synthesis. The 14-OH metabolite of clarithromycin is twice as active as the parent compound against certain organisms.

Metabolism: Rapidly and widely distributed throughout the body. Highly stable in presence of gastric acid (unlike erythromycin); food delays but does not affect extent of absorption. Widely distributed in body tissues but does not cross blood–brain barrier into CSF. Metabolized by liver and excreted by kidneys into urine.

Dosage/Range:
- Adults: Usual dosage 250–500 mg every 12 hours or 1000 mg (two 500 mg extended release tablets) once daily for 7–14 days.
- Children ≥ 6 months: 15 mg/kg/day divided every 12 hours for 10 days.

Drug Preparation:
- Store tablets and granules for oral suspension at controlled room temperature.
- Reconstituted oral suspension should not be refrigerated because it might gel.
- Microencapsulated particles of clarithromycin in suspension are stable for 14 days when stored at room temperature.

Drug Interactions:

- Alfentanil (and possible other narcotic analgesics): Serum levels may be increased by clarithromycin—monitor for increased effect.
- Astemizole: Concomitant use is contraindicated—may lead to QT prolongation or torsade de pointes.
- Benzodiazepines (those metabolized CYP3A4, including alprazolam and triazolam): Serum levels may be increased by clarithromycin—somnolence and confusion have been reported.
- Bromocriptine: Serum levels may be increased by clarithromycin—monitor for increased effect.
- Buspirone: Serum levels may be increased by clarithromycin— monitor.
- Calcium-channel blockers (felodipine, verapamil, and potentially others metabolized by CYP3A4): Serum levels may be increased by clarithromycin—monitor.
- Carbamazepine: Serum levels may be increased by clarithromycin—monitor.
- Cisapride: Serum levels may be increased by clarithromycin—monitor.
- Cilostazol: Serum levels may be increased by clarithromycin—monitor.
- Clozapine: Serum levels may be increased by clarithromycin—monitor.
- Cyclosporine: Serum levels may be increased by clarithromycin—monitor serum levels.
- Delavirdine: Serum levels may be increased by clarithromycin.
- Digoxin: Serum levels may be increased by clarithromycin; digoxin toxicity and potentially fatal arrhythmias have been reported; monitor digoxin levels.
- Disopyramide: Serum levels may be increased by clarithromycin—monitor.
- Ergot alkaloids: Concurrent use may lead to acute ergot toxicity (severe peripheral vasospasm and dysesthesia).
- Fluconazole: Increases clarithromycin levels and AUC by ~25%.
- Indinavir: Serum levels may be increased by clarithromycin—monitor.
- Loratadine: Serum levels may be increased by clarithromycin—monitor.
- Neuromuscular-blocking agents: May be potentate by clarithromycin (case reports).
- Oral contraceptives: Serum levels may be increased by clarithromycin—monitor.
- Phenytoin: Serum levels may be increased by clarithromycin; other evidence suggests phenytoin levels may be decreased in some patients—monitor.
- Pimozide: Serum levels may be increased, leading to malignant arrhythmias; concomitant use is contraindicated.
- Quinolone antibiotics (sparfloxacin, gatifloxacin, or moxifloxacin): Concomitant use may increase the risk of malignant arrhythmias—avoid concomitant use.
- Rifabutin: Serum levels may be increased by clarithromycin—monitor.
- Ritonavir: Concurrent use results in a 77% increase in clarithromycin levels (100% increase in metabolite levels); may be given together without dosage adjustment in patients with normal renal function; dosage of clarithromycin must be decreased in renal impairment.
- Sildenafil: Serum levels may be increased by clarithromycin—monitor.

- Tacrolimus: Serum levels may be increased by clarithromycin—monitor serum concentrations.
- Terfenadine: Serum levels may be increased by clarithromycin; may lead to QT prolongation, ventricular tachycardia, ventricular fibrillation or torsade de pointes; concomitant use is contraindicated.
- Theophylline: Serum levels may be increased by clarithromycin (by as much as 20%)—monitor.
- Valproic acid (and derivatives): Serum levels may be increased by clarithromycin—monitor.
- Warfarin: Effects may be potentiated—monitor INR closely and adjust warfarin dose as needed or choose another antibiotic.
- Zidovudine: Peak levels (but not AUC) of zidovudine may be increased—other studies suggest levels may be decreased.
- St. John's wort: May decrease clarithromycin levels.
- CYP3A3/4 enzyme substrate—CYP1A2 and 3A3/4 enzyme inhibitor.

Lab Effects/Interference:
- PT/INR—may be prolonged.
- Serum SGPT, serum alk phos, serum SGOT, serum bilirubin, or serum LDH—values may be increased.
- BUN and serum creatinine—concentrations may be increased.

Special Considerations:
- Use with caution in patients with renal dysfunction—dose reduction required if severe impairment exists.
- Do not use when there is known hypersensitivity to erythromycins or other macrolides.
- Obtain ordered specimen and send for culture and sensitivity prior to first drug dose.

Potential Toxicities/Side Effects and the Nursing Process

I. POTENTIAL FOR INJURY related to HYPERSENSITIVITY REACTION

Defining Characteristics: Urticaria, pruritus, rash (maculopapular or erythematous), fever and chills, eosinophilia, myalgia, edema, erythema, angioedema.

Nursing Implications: Assess allergy to erythromycin: if patient states "yes," determine actual response, e.g., "swollen lips = angioedema." If angioedema, patient SHOULD NOT receive drug. Discuss other patient responses with physician to determine whether drug should be given. Assess baseline skin condition, including integrity and allergy history to drugs. Teach patient to report rash, itching, other skin changes. Teach patient skin care and symptomatic measures as appropriate. If skin rash develops, discuss drug discontinuance with physician.

II. ALTERATION IN NUTRITION, LESS THAN BODY REQUIREMENTS, related to GI SIDE EFFECTS

Defining Characteristics: Abdominal pain, diarrhea, nausea, and vomiting may occur.

Nursing Implications: Assess baseline nutritional status, preexisting nausea/vomiting, anorexia. Assess baseline LFTs and monitor periodically during treatment. Teach patient to report GI disturbances. Administer and teach patient to self-administer symptomatic interventions if side effects occur; discuss with physician use of alternative drug(s).

III. FUNGAL SUPERINFECTION related to REDISTRIBUTION OF ENDOGENOUS MICROORGANISMS

Defining Characteristics: Vaginal moniliasis, vaginitis may occur as endogenous bacteria are eliminated and normal fungal population expands.

Nursing Implications: Teach female patient to report vaginal itching or discharge. Discuss appropriate antifungal treatment with physician. Teach perineal hygiene and symptomatic management.

IV. ALTERATIONS IN PROTECTIVE MECHANISMS (RARE)

Defining Characteristics: Prolonged PT, prolonged INR, and hypoprothrombinemia have occurred rarely, especially in elderly or debilitated patients, or in individuals with vitamin K deficiency.

Nursing Implications: Assess baseline laboratory parameters, and monitor periodically during treatment. Assess patient for response to antibiotics. Discuss abnormalities with physician. Assess for signs/symptoms of bleeding. If they occur, especially in elderly or debilitated patients, discuss vitamin K administration with physician. Teach patient to avoid aspirin. If taking oral anticoagulants, assess for increased PT, signs/symptoms of bleeding.

Drug: clindamycin phosphate (Cleocin)

Class: Antibacterial (systemic); antiprotozoal.

Mechanism of Action: Bacteriostatic or bactericidal depending on drug concentration or when used against highly susceptible organisms; binds to bacterial ribosomes and prevent peptide bond formation, thus inhibiting protein synthesis. Active against gram-positive cocci (e.g., staphylococci, streptococci) and some anaerobic gram-positive and gram-negative bacilli (e.g., clostridia, mycobacteria).

Metabolism: Well absorbed (90% of dose) from GI tract. Food may delay absorption but does not affect amount absorbed. Widely distributed in body tissues and fluids, including bile. Crosses placenta and is excreted in breast milk. Excreted in urine, bile, and feces.

Dosage/Range:

Adult:

- Oral: 150–450 mg PO q 6 h; IM/IV: 300 mg q 6–12 h (maximum 2.7 g/day).

Drug Preparation:

- Oral: Administer with 8 oz (240 mL) of water to prevent esophageal irritation.
- IM: Single dose should not exceed 600 mg.
- Further dilute in 0.9% sodium chloride or 5% dextrose in water to final concentration < 12 mg/mL, and infuse over 20 minutes (600-mg dose) or 30–40 minutes (1.2-g dose). Maximum 1.2 gm in single 1-hour period. May be given as continuous infusion.

Drug Interactions:

- Neuromuscular blocking agents (tubocurarine, ether, pancuronium): may increase neuromuscular blockade; use concurrently with caution.
- Erythromycin: decreases bactericidal activity of clindamycin.
- Kaolin: decreases GI absorption of clindamycin. Avoid concurrent administration, or administer at least 2 hours apart.

Lab Effects/Interference:

- Serum ALT, serum alk phos, and serum AST concentrations may be increased.

Special Considerations:

- Contraindicated in patients with hypersensitivity to clindamycin or lincomycin; contraindicated in patients with history of colitis.
- Can cause severe, sometimes fatal colitis. Stop drug if diarrhea develops, or if necessary, continue only under close monitoring and endoscopy.
- Used in the treatment of serious infections of respiratory tract, skin/soft tissues, female pelvic/genital tract. May be used investigationally with other drugs in treatment of *Mycobacterium avium* complex (MAC); also may be used to treat *P. carinii* pneumonia, cryptosporidiosis, and toxoplasmosis in AIDS patients.
- Also used for prophylaxis of bacterial endocarditis in penicillin-allergic, erythromycin-intolerant patients.
- DO NOT GIVE rapid IVB: cardiopulmonary arrest has occurred.
- Avoid use in pregnant or breast-feeding women.

Potential Toxicities/Side Effects and the Nursing Process

I. ALTERATION IN NUTRITION, LESS THAN BODY REQUIREMENTS, related to GI SIDE EFFECTS

Defining Characteristics: Nausea, vomiting, diarrhea, abdominal pain, and tenesmus may occur. Flatulence, bloating, anorexia, and esophagitis may occur as well. Fatal pseudomembranous colitis has occurred, characterized by severe diarrhea, abdominal cramping, and melena. Usually begins 2–9 days after drug is initiated.

Nursing Implications: Assess elimination and nutrition pattern, baseline and during therapy. Instruct patient to report diarrhea and/or abdominal pain immediately. Discuss drug discontinuance with physician if diarrhea occurs. Guaiac stool for occult blood, and notify physician if positive. If severe diarrhea develops, discuss management plan including endoscopy, fluid and electrolyte replacement. Do not administer antiperistaltic agents such as opiates and diphenoxylate with atropine (Lomotil), since it may worsen condition. Assess for nausea/vomiting, and administer prescribed antiemetic medications. Encourage small, frequent feedings as tolerated. Instruct patient to take oral dose with a full glass of water.

II. ALTERATION IN SKIN INTEGRITY related to HYPERSENSITIVITY

Defining Characteristics: Maculopapular rash, urticaria may occur. Rarely, erythema multiforme may occur. Increased risk of allergic reaction in asthma patients. Anaphylaxis may rarely occur.

Nursing Implications: Assess baseline allergy history. Assess baseline skin integrity. Instruct patient to report rash, pruritus. Teach patient symptomatic management of rash, pruritus. Assess for hypersensitivity reaction: if it occurs, monitor vital signs (VS), discontinue drug, notify physician, and institute supportive measures.

III. ALTERATIONS IN COMFORT related to LOCAL ADMINISTRATION EFFECTS

Defining Characteristics: IM administration may cause pain, induration, sterile abscesses, and transient increase in creatine phosphokinase (CPK) due to muscle injury. IV administration may cause erythema, pain, swelling, and thrombophlebitis.

Nursing Implications: Administer maximum 600-mg dose IM deeply in large muscle mass (e.g., gluteus maximus). Rotate sites. Assess IV site prior to each dose for phlebitis or swelling, and change site at least q 48 h. Administer dose slowly: 300–600 mg in 50 mL over 20–30 minutes, and 900–1200-mg dose in 100 mL IV over 40–60 minutes. Apply heat to painful IV sites as ordered.

IV. ALTERATION IN HEPATIC FUNCTION related to TRANSIENT INCREASE LFTs

Defining Characteristics: Transient increases in serum bili, AST, alk phos have occurred.

Nursing Implications: Assess baseline LFTs, and monitor during therapy.

V. FUNGAL SUPERINFECTION related to REDISTRIBUTION OF ENDOGENOUS MICROORGANISMS

Defining Characteristics: Vaginal candidiasis, vaginitis may occur as endogenous bacteria are eliminated, and normal fungal population expands.

Nursing Implications: Instruct female patient to report vaginal itching or discharge. Discuss appropriate antifungal treatment with physician. Teach perineal hygiene and symptomatic management.

Drug: co-trimoxazole; trimethoprim and sulfamethoxazole (Bactrim, Bactrim DS, Cotrim, Septra)

Class: Sulfonamide antibacterial (systemic); antiprotozoal.

Mechanism of Action: Bactericidal by preventing folic acid synthesis so microorganism cannot undergo cell division (sequential inhibition of folic acid synthesis, first by sulfamethoxazole, then by trimethoprim). Active against gram-positive bacteria (streptococci, *S. aureus, Nocardia*), gram-negative bacteria (*Enterobacter, E. coli, Proteus, Klebsiella, Shigella*), and protozoa (*P. carinii*).

Metabolism: Rapidly absorbed from GI tract. Widely distributed into body tissues and fluids; crosses the placenta and is excreted in breast milk. Highly protein-bound. Metabolized by the liver and excreted in the urine.

Dosage/Range:

Adult:

- Oral: Trimethoprim 160 mg and sulfamethoxazole 800 mg (double-strength tablet DS) q 12 h × 7–14 days (depending on infection).
- Oral: *P. carinii* pneumonia prophylaxis: 1 DS tablet twice daily 2 days per week (typically consecutive) or 1 DS tablet every other day.
- IV: 10–20 mg/kg in two to four divided doses q 6–8 h (usually 21 days for *P. carinii* pneumonia in AIDS patients).
- Dose modification if renal impairment exists.

Drug Preparation:

- Oral tablets should be stored in tight, light-resistant containers; vials of powder for injection and suspension should be stored at 15–30°C (59–86°F).

Drug Administration:

Oral: Administer with full (8 oz or 240 mL) glass of water.

- IV: Add each 5 mL of drug to 125 mL of 5% dextrose in water ONLY. Stable for 6 hours. If patient is fluid restricted, can mix each 5 mL in 75 mL of 5% dextrose immediately prior to administration and give within 2 hours. DO NOT REFRIGERATE. Administer over 60–90 minutes.

Drug Interactions:

- Warfarin: increases PT. Monitor PT closely and decrease dose of warfarin as needed.
- Sulfonylureas: increases hypoglycemic effect. Monitor blood glucose closely and reduce sulfonylurea dose as needed.
- Phenytoin: increases and prolongs serum levels. Monitor serum phenytoin level closely and reduce dose as needed.
- Thiazide diuretics (in elderly): increases toxicity (thrombocytopenia with purpura). AVOID CONCURRENT USE.
- Cyclosporine: decreases cyclosporine effect; increases risk of nephrotoxicity. AVOID CONCURRENT USE when possible.
- Methotrexate: increases methotrexate level and potential toxicity (e.g., bone marrow depression). Monitor levels or decrease methotrexate dose as needed.
- Oral contraceptives: decreases contraceptive effect. Monitor for breakthrough bleeding and counsel patient to use barrier contraceptive in addition during antibiotic therapy.
- Ammonium chloride or ascorbic acid: causes antibiotic drug precipitation in kidneys. AVOID CONCURRENT USE.

Lab Effects/Interference:

- Jaffe alkaline picrate reaction overestimation of creatinine by 10%.

Special Considerations:

- Drug is teratogenic, so should not be used in pregnant women if avoidable.
- Drug is excreted in breast milk and can cause kernicterus in infants. Alternative drug should be used or mother should interrupt breast-feeding during drug use.
- Contraindicated if patient has porphyria.
- Contraindicated in patients with hypersensitivity to sulfites, sulfonamides, or to trimethoprim.
- Contraindicated if severe renal failure (creatinine clearance < 15 mL/minute).
- Use with caution at reduced dosage in patients with glucose-6-phosphate dehydrogenase deficiency (G6PD); hemolysis may occur. Also, use with caution in patients with impaired renal or hepatic function, severe allergy, bronchial asthma, and blood dyscrasias.

- Use cautiously in patients with known hypersensitivity to sulfonamide-derivative drugs such as thiazides, acetazolamide, tolbutamide.
- Increased incidence of adverse side effects in AIDS patients, especially allergic, hematologic reactions. Monitor closely for toxicity.
- Drug is first line treatment for *P. carinii* pneumonia; it is at least as effective as pentamidine, with a cure rate of 70–80%.
- Send specimen for culture and sensitivity prior to initial drug dose, as appropriate.

Potential Toxicities/Side Effects and the Nursing Process

I. ALTERATION IN SKIN INTEGRITY related to HYPERSENSITIVITY REACTION

Defining Characteristics: Skin reactions ranging from mild maculopapular rash with urticaria, pruritus to erythema multiforme, exfoliative dermatitis, and Stevens-Johnson syndrome. Risk for rash is increased in AIDS patients; usually occurs 7–14 days after beginning drug. Other allergic manifestations include fever, chills, photosensitivity, angioedema, and anaphylaxis.

Nursing Implications: Assess for prior hypersensitivity to drug. Assess for signs/symptoms of drug allergy. Instruct patient to report rash, allergic reaction immediately. Discuss any drug continuance with physician if rash appears. Teach patient symptomatic management of discomfort and skin irritation. Be prepared to treat severe acute hypersensitivity reactions with airway management, oxygen, epinephrine, corticosteroids, antihistamines as ordered.

II. POTENTIAL FOR INFECTION, BLEEDING, AND FATIGUE related to HEMATOLOGIC TOXICITY

Defining Characteristics: Leukopenia, neutropenia, and thrombocytopenia are common in AIDS patients. Agranulocytosis, aplastic and megaloblastic anemia, thrombocytopenia, hemolytic anemia, neutropenia, hypoprothrombinemia, and eosinophilia may occur less commonly. Increased risk exists in folate-deficient patients: elderly, alcoholic, malnourished; also, patients receiving folate antimetabolites, e.g., phenytoin, methotrexate, or thiazide diuretics; or in patients with renal dysfunction.

Nursing Implications: Assess baseline risk, CBC, and monitor CBC periodically during treatment. Assess for and teach patient to monitor signs/symptoms of infection, bleeding, fatigue, and to report these. If side effects occur, discuss with physician use of folinic acid (leucovorin).

III. ALTERATION IN NUTRITION, LESS THAN BODY REQUIREMENTS, related to GI TOXICITY

Defining Characteristics: Nausea, vomiting, and anorexia are most common; pseudomembranous colitis, glossitis, stomatitis, abdominal pain, diarrhea may occur.

Nursing Implications: Assess GI function. Teach patient to assess for and instruct to report GI side effects, and to administer prescribed antiemetics or antidiarrheals as needed. Assess oral mucosa, and if stomatitis develops, discuss with physician use of leucovorin (folinic acid). Teach patient oral hygiene. Take drug with 8 oz (240 mL) water to prevent esophageal ulcerations. Discuss food preferences, use of spices, and suggest small, frequent meals if anorexia develops.

IV. SENSORY/PERCEPTUAL DYSFUNCTION related to FATIGUE, WEAKNESS

Defining Characteristics: Headache, vertigo, insomnia, fatigue, weakness, mental depression, seizures, and hallucinations may occur.

Nursing Implications: Assess baseline neurologic function and comfort, and monitor during treatment. Instruct patient to report any changes. Discuss any abnormalities with physician.

V. ALTERATION IN URINARY ELIMINATION related to RENAL TOXICITY

Defining Characteristics: Increased BUN and creatinine, crystal and stone formation in urine, interstitial nephritis, and renal failure may occur.

Nursing Implications: Assess baseline renal function; expect that drug dose will be decreased in presence of renal dysfunction. Instruct patient to take drug with at least 8 oz water and to increase oral fluids to 2–3 qt/day.

VI. ALTERATION IN COMFORT related to IV ADMINISTRATION

Defining Characteristics: Drug may cause pain, inflammation, and rare thrombophlebitis at IV site.

Nursing Implications: Change IV site q 48 h. Assess for phlebitis, discomfort, and IV patency prior to each administration. Administer drug slowly over 60–90 minutes in large volume of 5% dextrose (see Drug Administration). Apply heat to promote comfort.

VII. FUNGAL SUPERINFECTION related to REDISTRIBUTION OF ENDOGENOUS MICROORGANISMS

Defining Characteristics: Vaginal candidiasis, vaginitis may occur as endogenous bacteria are eliminated and normal fungal population expands.

Nursing Implications: Instruct female patient to report vaginal itching or discharge. Discuss appropriate antifungal treatment with physician. Teach perineal hygiene and symptomatic management.

Drug: daptomycin (Cubicin)

Class: Cyclic lipopeptide antibiotic.

Mechanism of Action: This antibiotic is the first in a new structural class. It is derived from the fermentation of *Streptomyces roseosporus*. The mechanism of action is not fully understood. Daptomycin binds to bacterial membranes and causes a rapid depolarization of membrane potential. This loss of membrane potential leads to inhibition of protein, DNA, and RNA synthesis resulting in bacterial cell death. It acts against gram-positive bacteria, and retains in vitro potency against isolates resistant to methicillin, vancomycin, and linezolid.

Metabolism: Excreted by the kidney. Renal excretion is primary route of elimination.

Dosage/Range:

Adult:

- 4 mg/kg by IV infusion q d for 7–14 days.
- Drug dose should be reduced or adjusted in patients with severe renal insufficiency.

Drug Preparation:

- 0.9% sodium chloride injection.
- Administer over 30 minutes.

Drug Interactions:

- Tobramycin: interaction between daptomycin and tobramycin is unknown. Caution is warranted when daptomycin is coadministered with tobramycin.
- Warfarin: anticoagulant activity in patients receiving daptomycin and warfarin should be monitored for the first several days.

Lab Effects/Interference:

- There are no reported drug-laboratory test interactions.

Special Considerations:

- Contraindicated in patients with known hypersensitivity to daptomycin.
- Obtain ordered specimen and send for culture and sensitivity prior to first antibiotic dose.
- Consider alternative antibiotic therapy if anemia, drug rash or fever, arthralgia, or unexplained rise in BUN and serum creatinine occur.

Potential Toxicities/Side Effects and the Nursing Process

I. ALTERATION IN NUTRITION, LESS THAN BODY REQUIREMENTS, related to GI SIDE EFFECTS

Defining Characteristics: Constipation, nausea, diarrhea, vomiting, dyspepsia.

Nursing Implications: Assess baseline nutritional status, preexisting nausea/vomiting, anorexia. Assess baseline bowel pattern. Administer symptomatic interventions if side effects occur; discuss with physician use of alternative drug(s).

II. POTENTIAL FOR INJURY related to HYPERSENSITIVITY REACTION

Defining Characteristics: Rash, urticaria, pruritus, and fever can occur in individuals with hypersensitivity to daptomycin.

Nursing Implications: Assess for drug allergies prior to drug administration. Instruct patient to report any allergic reactions. Assess for signs/symptoms of allergic reaction after drug dose.

III. SENSORY/PERCEPTUAL ALTERATIONS related to CNS EFFECTS OF DIZZINESS AND HEADACHE

Defining Characteristics: Dizziness, headache and insomnia may occur.

Nursing Implications: Assess baseline neurological status. Teach patient about side effects and to report dizziness or headache. If signs/symptoms arise, discuss drug discontinuance with physician.

Drug: demeclocycline hydrochloride (Declomycin)

Class: Antibacterial (systemic); tetracycline; antiprotozoal.

Mechanism of Action: Bacteriostatic but may be bactericidal at high concentrations. Binds to bacterial ribosomes and prevents protein synthesis. Active against broad range of gram-negative and gram-positive organisms. Demeclocycline hydrochloride may also be used in special cases of fluid retention (SIADH). A syndrome of polyuria, polydipsia, and weakness has been shown to be nephrogenic, dose-dependent, and reversible on discontinuation of therapy.

Metabolism: Absorbed from the GI tract. Widely distributed into body tissues and fluids. Crosses placenta and is excreted in breast milk. Concentrated in the liver, excreted into the bile. The rate of demeclocycline hydrochloride clearance is less than half that of tetracycline.

Dosage/Range:

Adult:

- Oral: 150 mg q 6 hours or 300 mg q 12 hours.
- Duration of therapy depends on indication.
- As treatment for hyponatremia: 600–1200 mg daily.
- Drug dose should be reduced or adjusted in patients with hepatic or renal insufficiency.

Drug Preparation:

- Oral: Take 1 hour before meals or 2 hours after meals. Dose reduce in patients with renal and liver impairment.

Drug Interactions:

- Oral anticoagulants: increase PT. Monitor patient closely and decrease anticoagulant dose as needed.
- Concurrent use of tetracyclines with oral contraceptives may render oral contraceptives less effective. Advise patient to use barrier contraceptive as well during a course of tetracycline therapy.
- Methoxyflurane: fatal renal toxicity has been reported with concurrent use.
- Iron preparations: decreases oral absorption. Administer iron preparations 3 hours after or 2 hours before any tetracycline.
- Antacids and antidiarrheals: may decrease absorption of tetracyclines. Avoid concurrent use.

Lab Effects/Interference:

- There are no reported drug-laboratory test interactions.
- SGPT, alk phos, Amylase, SGOT, and bilirubin: serum concentrations may be increased.

Special Considerations:

- Avoid use in pregnant or lactating women.
- Contraindicated in patients with known hypersensitivity to tetracyclines.
- Obtain ordered specimen and send for culture and sensitivity prior to first antibiotic dose.

Potential Toxicities/Side Effects and the Nursing Process

I. ALTERATION IN NUTRITION, related to GI SIDE EFFECTS

Defining Characteristics: Anorexia, nausea, vomiting, diarrhea, glossitis, dysphagia, enterocolitis, pancreatitis.

Nursing Implications: Assess baseline nutritional status. Assess for and teach patient to report any symptoms. Administer and teach patient self-administration of prescribed antiemetic or antidiarrheal medication as appropriate. Administer and teach to self-administer oral dose with at least 8 oz of water at least 1 hour before or 2 hours after a meal or sleep.

II. ALTERATION IN SKIN INTEGRITY related to RASH, PHOTOSENSITIVITY

Defining Characteristics: Maculopapular and erythematous rash may occur. Photosensitivity risk (exaggerated sunburn) persists 1–2 days after completion of drug therapy.

Nursing Implications: Teach patient about potential side effects, to avoid sunlight during drug therapy, and to report rash, and other abnormalities. Teach symptomatic skin care as appropriate.

III. INJURY related to HYPERSENSITIVITY

Defining Characteristics: Urticaria, angioneurotic edema, anaphylaxis may occur; also fever, arthralgias, eosinophilia, and pericarditis.

Nursing Implications: Assess drug allergy history. Assess baseline allergy history. Assess baseline skin integrity. Teach patient to report rash, pruritus. Teach patient symptomatic management of rash, pruritus. Assess for hypersensitivity reaction: if it occurs, monitor VS, discontinues drug, notify physician, and institute supportive measures.

IV. FUNGAL SUPERINFECTION related to REDISTRIBUTION OF ENDOGENOUS MICROORGANISMS

Defining Characteristics: Vaginal moniliasis, vaginitis may occur as endogenous bacteria are eliminated and normal fungal population expands.

Nursing Implications: Teach female patient to report vaginal itching or discharge. Discuss appropriate antifungal treatment with physician. Teach perineal hygiene and symptom management.

Drug: dicloxacillin sodium (Dycill, Dynapen, Pathocil)

Class: Penicillin antibacterial.

Mechanism of Action: Semisynthetic antibiotic prepared from fungus *Penicillium*. Contains β-lactam ring and is bactericidal by inhibiting cell wall synthesis. Penicillinase-resistant and active against penicillin-resistant staphylococci, which produce the enzyme penicillinase. Used to treat upper and lower respiratory tract and skin infections.

Metabolism: Well absorbed from GI tract, but food decreases rate and extent of absorption. Widely distributed through body tissues and fluids; crosses placenta and is excreted in breast milk; 95–99% bound to serum proteins. Excreted in urine and bile.

Dosage/Range:
- Adult: 125 mg–500 mg PO q 6 h × 14 days (depends on severity of infection).

Drug Preparation:
- Store in tight containers at < 40°C (104°F).

Drug Administration:
- Oral: administer at least 1 hour before or 2 hours after meals.

Drug Interactions:
- Aminoglycosides: synergism.
- Rifampin: possible antagonism, only at high doses of penicillin.
- Probenecid: increased serum level of penicillin; may be coadministered to exert this effect.

Lab Effects/Interference:

Major clinical significance:
- Urine glucose: high urinary concentrations of a penicillin may produce false-positive or falsely elevated test results with copper sulfate tests (Benedict's, Clinitest, or Fehling's); glucose enzymatic tests (Clinistix or Testape) are not affected.

Clinical significance:
- Coombs' (direct antiglobulin) test: false-positive result may occur during therapy with any penicillin.
- ALT, alk phos, AST, serum LDH values may be increased.
- WBC: leukopenia or neutropenia is associated with the use of all penicillins; the effect is more likely to occur with prolonged therapy and severe hepatic function impairment.

Special Considerations:
- Contraindicated in patients with prior hypersensitivity to penicillins. Use with caution in patients sensitive to other β-lactams (e.g., cephalosporins) since partial cross-allergenicity exists.
- Obtain ordered specimen and send for culture and sensitivity prior to first antibiotic dose.
- Consider alternative antibiotic therapy if eosinophilia, drug fever or rash, arthralgia, hematuria, or unexplained rise in BUN and serum creatinine occur.
- Monitor electrolytes and renal, hepatic, and hematologic laboratory parameters during extended treatment periods.
- Use with caution in pregnancy or with nursing women.

Potential Toxicities/Side Effects and the Nursing Process

I. POTENTIAL FOR INJURY related to HYPERSENSITIVITY REACTION

Defining Characteristics: Urticaria, pruritus, rash (maculopapular or erythematous), fever and chills, eosinophilia, myalgia, edema, erythema, angioedema, Stevens-Johnson syndrome, and exfoliative skin reactions occur in 5% of patients. Increased risk exists in individuals allergic to cephalosporin antibiotics.

Nursing Implications: Assess allergy to cephalosporin antibiotics and penicillin: if patient states "yes," determine actual response, e.g., "swollen lips = angioedema." If angioedema, patient SHOULD NOT receive drug. Discuss other patient responses with physician to determine whether drug should be given. Assess baseline skin condition, including integrity and allergy history to drugs. Instruct patient to report rash, itching, and other skin changes. Teach patient skin care and symptomatic measures as appropriate. If skin rash develops, discuss drug discontinuance with physician. If rash progresses, drug should be discontinued as fatal Stevens-Johnson syndrome may develop. Be prepared to treat severe acute hypersensitivity reactions with airway management, oxygen, epinephrine, corticosteroids, antihistamines as ordered.

II. ALTERATION IN NUTRITION, LESS THAN BODY REQUIREMENTS, related to GI SIDE EFFECTS

Defining Characteristics: Nausea, vomiting, diarrhea may occur; rarely, pseudomembranous colitis caused by *C. difficile* resistant to the antibiotic occurs. Rarely, transient increases in LFTs—AST, ALT, alk phos, bili—may occur.

Nursing Implications: Assess baseline nutritional status. Instruct patient to report GI disturbances. Administer and teach patient to self-administer antiemetics as needed and as ordered. Teach patient importance of nutritious diet, and suggest small, frequent, high-calorie, high-protein meals as appropriate. Assess baseline LFTs, and monitor periodically during treatment. Discuss abnormalities and drug interruption with physician.

III. FUNGAL SUPERINFECTION related to REDISTRIBUTION OF ENDOGENOUS MICROORGANISMS

Defining Characteristics: Vaginal candidiasis, vaginitis may occur as endogenous bacteria are eliminated and normal fungal population expands.

Nursing Implications: Instruct female patient to report vaginal itching or discharge. Discuss appropriate antifungal treatment with physician. Teach perineal hygiene and symptomatic management.

IV. ALTERATIONS IN PROTECTIVE MECHANISMS (RARE) related to TRANSIENT LEUKOPENIA

Defining Characteristics: Rarely, transient leukopenia, lymphocytosis, anemia, eosinophilia may occur. Prolonged PT, prolonged APTT, and hypoprothrombinemia have occurred rarely, especially in elderly or debilitated patients, or in individuals with vitamin K deficiency.

Nursing Implications: Assess baseline laboratory parameters, and monitor periodically during treatment. Assess patient for response to antibiotics. Discuss abnormalities with physician.

V. KNOWLEDGE DEFICIT related to SELF-ADMINISTRATION OF MEDICATION

Defining Characteristics: Increased compliance when patient is instructed in self-care activities.

Nursing Implications: Assess knowledge about infection and planned treatment. Teach about drug action, potential side effects, and when and how to take drug (take medication as directed, 1 hour before or 2 hours after food). Instruct patient to report any possible drug side effects that occur.

Drug: doxycycline hyclate (Vibramycin, Doryx, MonoDox)

Class: Antibacterial (systemic); antiprotozoal.

Mechanism of Action: Bacteriostatic but may be bactericidal at high concentrations. Binds to bacterial ribosomes and prevents protein synthesis. Active against broad range of gram-positive and gram-negative bacteria, *Chlamydia*, and *Mycoplasma*.

Metabolism: Absorbed (60%–80%) from GI tract. Widely distributed into body tissues and fluids. Crosses placenta and is excreted in breast milk. Excreted unchanged in urine.

Dosage/Range:

Adult:

- Oral: 100 mg q 12 hours for the first day, then 100–200 mg once daily, or 50–100 mg q 12 hours. Duration of therapy depends on indication.
- IV: 200 mg daily or 100 mg q 12 hours for the first day, then 100–200 mg daily or 50–100 mg q 12 hours. Duration of therapy depends on indication.

Drug Preparation:

- Oral: may be taken with food, water, milk, or carbonated beverages.
- IV: add 10 mL sterile water for injection to 100-mg vial or 20 mL to each 200-mg vial. Further dilute in 100 to 1000 mL or in 200 to 2000 ml, respectively, of lactated Ringer's injection or 5% dextrose and lactated Ringer's injection. Infuse over 1 to 4 hours.
- CONCENTRATIONS LESS THAN 100 MICROGRAMS/ML OR GREATER THAN 1 MG/ML ARE NOT RECOMMENDED.
- AVOID RAPID ADMINISTRATION.
- Solution stable for 6 hours, so use after mixing. Avoid exposure to heat or sunlight. Convert to oral preparation as soon as possible as there is risk of thrombophlebitis.
- DO NOT ADMINISTER INTRAMUSCULARLY OR SUBCUTANEOUSLY.

Drug Interactions:

- Hepatotoxic drugs: may increase hepatotoxicity if given concurrently. Assess baseline and periodically during treatment.
- Iron preparations: decrease oral and possibly IV absorption. Administer iron preparations 3 hours after or 2 hours before any tetracycline.

- Oral anticoagulants: increase PT. Monitor patient closely and decrease anticoagulant dose as needed.
- Antidiarrheals (containing kaolin, pectate, or bismuth): may decrease absorption of tetracyclines. Avoid concurrent use.
- Oral contraceptives: decreased effectiveness of contraceptive and increased incidence of breakthrough bleeding. Advise patient to use barrier contraceptive as well during a course of tetracycline therapy.
- Lithium: may decrease lithium levels. Monitor serum levels and increase dose as needed.

Lab Effects/Interference:
- Urine catecholamine determinations: may produce false elevations of urinary catecholamines because of interfering fluorescence in the Hingerty method.
- SGPT, alk phos, Amylase, SGOT, and bilirubin: serum concentrations may be increased.

Special Considerations:
- Use cautiously in patients with myasthenia gravis: may increase muscle weakness.
- Avoid use in pregnant or lactating women.
- Obtain ordered specimen for culture and sensitivity prior to first dose.
- IV preparation contains ascorbic acid and may cause false-positive result using Clinitest, or false-negative result when using Clinistix and Testape.
- Drug has affinity for ischemic, necrotic tissue, and may localize in tumors.

Potential Toxicities/Side Effects and the Nursing Process

I. ALTERATION IN NUTRITION related to GI SIDE EFFECTS

Defining Characteristics: Nausea, vomiting, diarrhea, anorexia, abdominal discomfort, epigastric burning and distress, glossitis, black hairy tongue may occur.

Nursing Implications: Assess baseline nutritional status. Assess for and teach patient to report any symptoms. Administer and teach patient self-administration of prescribed antiemetic or antidiarrheal medication as appropriate. Administer and teach patient to self-administer oral dose with at least 8 oz of water taken at least 1 hour before lying down for sleep.

II. ALTERATION IN SKIN INTEGRITY related to RASH, PHOTOSENSITIVITY

Defining Characteristics: Maculopapular and erythematous rashes may occur. Rarely, exfoliative dermatitis, onycholysis, and nail discoloration. Photosensitivity risk (exaggerated sunburn) persists 1–2 days after completion of drug therapy.

Nursing Implications: Teach patient about potential side effects, to avoid sunlight during drug therapy, and to report rash, other abnormalities. Teach symptomatic skin care as appropriate.

III. INJURY related to HYPERSENSITIVITY

Defining Characteristics: Urticaria, angioneurotic edema, anaphylaxis may occur; also, fever, rash, arthralgias, eosinophilia, and pericarditis.

Nursing Implications: Assess drug allergy history. Assess baseline allergy history. Assess baseline skin integrity. Teach patient to report rash, pruritus. Teach patient symptomatic management of rash, pruritus. Assess for hypersensitivity reaction: if it occurs, monitor VS, discontinue drug, notify physician, and institute supportive measures.

IV. FUNGAL SUPERINFECTION related to REDISTRIBUTION OF ENDOGENOUS MICROORGANISMS

Defining Characteristics: Vaginal moniliasis, vaginitis may occur as endogenous bacteria are eliminated, and normal fungal population expands.

Nursing Implications: Teach female patient to report vaginal itching or discharge. Discuss appropriate antifungal treatment with physician. Teach perineal hygiene and symptomatic management.

V. ALTERATION IN HEPATIC FUNCTION

Defining Characteristics: Associated with high IV doses (> 2 gm/day): hepatotoxicity and cholestasis may occur.

Nursing Implications: Assess baseline LFTs and monitor during therapy.

VI. INFECTION AND BLEEDING related to NEUTROPENIA, THROMBOCYTOPENIA

Defining Characteristics: Neutropenia, leukocytosis, leukopenia, atypical lymphocytes, thrombocytopenia, thrombocytopenic purpura, hemolytic anemia occur rarely with long-term therapy.

Nursing Implications: Assess baseline WBC, hematocrit, and platelets, and monitor periodically during long-term therapy.

VII. ALTERATIONS IN COMFORT related to LOCAL ADMINISTRATION EFFECTS

Defining Characteristics: IM administration may cause pain, induration due to muscle injury. IV administration may cause erythema, pain, swelling, and thrombophlebitis.

Nursing Implications: Rotate sites. Apply ice as ordered to painful buttock. Assess IV site prior to each dose for phlebitis or swelling and change site at least q 48 hours. Apply heat to painful IV sites as ordered.

VIII. SENSORY/PERCEPTUAL ALTERATION

Defining Characteristics: Light-headedness, dizziness, headache may occur.

Nursing Implications: Assess baseline neurological status. Teach patient to report any changes and discuss them with physician.

Drug: ertapenem sodium (Invanz)

Class: antibiotic, carbapenem.

Mechanism of Action: The bactericidal activity results from the inhibition of cell wall synthesis. Penetrates the cell wall of most gram-positive and gram-negative bacteria to reach penicillin-binding protein (PBP) targets.

Metabolism: Widely distributed in body tissues and fluids, excreted in urine.

Dosage/Range:

Adult:

- Acute pelvic infection: 1 gram IV/IM once a day for 3–10 days.
- Community acquired pneumonia: 1 gram IV/IM once a day for 10–14 days.
- Intra-abdominal infection: 1 gram IV/IM once a day for 5–14 days.
- Skin/skin structure infections: 1 gram IV/IM once a day for 7–14 days.
- Urinary tract infections: 1 gram IV/IM once a day for 10–14 days.
- Adjust dose in patients with renal impairment and on hemodialysis.

Drug Administration:

- IV infusion for up to 14 days.
- IV infusion for up to 14 days.
- IM injection for up to 7 days.
- DO NOT DILUTE WITH diluents containing dextrose.

Drug Interactions:

- Probenecid competes with ertapenem for active tubular secretion; increasing AUC by 25% and reducing the plasma and renal clearances by 20% and 35% respectively.

Lab Effects/Interference:

- Ertapenem posses the characteristic low toxicity of the β-lactam group of antibiotics.
- Periodically assess organ system function: renal, hepatic, and hematopoietic.

Potential Toxicities/Side Effects and the Nursing Process

I. POTENTIAL FOR INJURY related to HYPERSENSITIVITY REACTION and LOCAL REACTIONS (pain at injection site)

Defining Characteristics: Urticaria, pruritus, rash (maculopapular or erythematous), fever and chills, eosinophilia, myalgia, edema, erythema, angioedema.

Nursing Implications: Assess allergy to cephalosporin antibiotics and penicillin; if patient states "yes," determine actual response, e.g., "swollen lips = angioedema." If angioedema, patient SHOULD NOT receive drug. Discuss other patient responses with physician to determine whether drug should be given. Assess baseline skin condition, including integrity and allergy history to drugs. Instruct patient to report rash, itching, and other skin changes. Teach patient skin care and symptomatic measures as appropriate. If skin rash develops, discuss drug discontinuance with physician. Be prepared to treat severe acute hypersensitivity reactions with airway management, oxygen, epinephrine, corticosteroids, antihistamines as ordered.

II. ALTERATION IN NUTRITION, LESS THAN BODY REQUIREMENTS, related to GI SIDE EFFECTS

Defining Characteristics: Nausea, vomiting, diarrhea may occur; rarely, pseudomembranous colitis caused by antibiotic resistance occurs.

Nursing Implications: Assess baseline nutritional status. Instruct patient to report GI disturbances. Administer and teach patient to self-administer antiemetics as needed and as ordered. Teach patient importance of nutritious diet, and suggest small, frequent, high-calorie, high-protein meals as appropriate. Assess baseline LFTs, and monitor periodically during treatment. Discuss abnormalities and drug interruption with physician.

III. FUNGAL SUPERINFECTION related to REDISTRIBUTION OF ENDOGENOUS MICROORGANISMS

Defining Characteristics: Vaginal candidiasis, vaginitis may occur as endogenous bacteria are eliminated, and normal fungal population expands.

Nursing Implications: Instruct female patient to report vaginal itching or discharge. Discuss appropriate antifungal treatment with physician. Teach perineal hygiene and symptomatic management.

Drug: erythromycin (ERYC, E-Mycin, Ilotycin, Erythrocin)

Class: Antibacterial (macrolide).

Mechanism of Action: Erythromycin is a broad spectrum antibiotic with activity against gram-positive and gram-negative bacteria, and other infectious agents, including *Chlamydia trachomatis*, mycoplasmas (*Mycoplasma pneumoniae* and *Ureaplasma urealyticum*), and spirochetes (*Treponema pallidum* and *Borrelia* species). Erythromycin has good activity against *S. pyogenes, Streptococcus pneumoniae (group A beta-hemolytic streptococci)*, and *Staphylococcus aureus*.

Erythromycin is a bacteriostatic macrolide antibiotic. It may be bactericidal in high concentrations or when used against highly susceptible organisms. It is thought to penetrate the bacterial cell membrane and to reversibly bind to the 50 S ribosomal subunit. It does not directly inhibit peptide formation rather, it inhibits the translocation of peptides from the acceptor site on the ribosome to the donor site, inhibiting subsequent protein synthesis. Effective against actively dividing organisms.

Metabolism: 90% of the drug is metabolized by the liver; may accumulate in patients with severe hepatic disease. Primarily excreted into the bile. Between 2 to 5% is excreted unchanged by the kidneys following oral administration; 12 to 15% excreted unchanged following IV administration. Erythromycins cross the placental barrier in pregnancy; can be found in breast milk.

Dosage/Range:
- Oral: 250 mg once q 6 h for 10 days; or 500 mg q 6 h for 10 days; or 333 mg q 8 h.
- IV: 500 mg q 6 h; up to 1000 mg q 6 h (Legionnaires' disease).

Drug Preparation:
- Further dilute in 0.9% sodium chloride to a concentration of 1–5 mg/mL (500 mg/100 mL, 1000 mg/250 mL).
- Reconstitute 500 mg or 1 g vials with 10 or 20 mL, respectively, of sterile water for injection only (no preservatives).

Drug Administration:
- Must not be given IV push.
- Intermittent IV infusion over 1 hour is appropriate.

Drug Interactions:
- Use of alcohol concurrently with IV erythromycin increases peak blood alcohol concentrations by 40%; this is thought to be related to rapid gastric emptying, less exposure to alcohol dehydrogenase in the gastric mucosa, and slower small intestine transit time.
- Concurrent use of astemizole or terfenadine with erythromycins is contraindicated and may increase risk of cardiotoxicity, such as torsades de points, ventricular tachycardia, and death.

- Erythromycins may inhibit carbamazepine and valproic acid metabolism, resulting in increased anticonvulsant plasma concentration and toxicity.
- Concurrent use of chloramphenicol, lincomycins, and erythromycins is not recommended due to their antagonizing effects. It is best to avoid concurrent use of bactericidal and bacteriostatic drugs until culture and sensitivity results are determined.
- Erythromycin can increase cyclosporin plasma concentrations and may increase the risk of nephrotoxicity.
- Erythromycins inhibit the metabolism of ergotamine and increase the vasospasm associated with ergotamines.
- Simultaneous administration of erythromycin and lovastatin should be used with caution since concurrent use may increase the risk of rhabdomyolysis.
- Concurrent use of midazolam and triazolam with erythromycins can increase the pharmacological effect of these drugs.
- Erythromycins may cause prolonged prothrombin time and increased risk of hemorrhage, especially in the elderly.
- Use of erythromycins and xanthines (i.e., Aminophylline, caffeine, Oxtriphylline, and Theophylline) may lead to increased serum levels of xanthines and toxicity.

Lab Effects/Interference:
- Serum SGPT, serum SGOT serum bilirubin, and alkaline phosphatase—values may be increased by all erythromycins.
- Urinary catecholamines may produce false positive results when patient is on erythromycin.

Special Considerations:
- Do not use when there is a known hypersensitivity to erythromycins.
- Use with caution in patients with impaired hepatic function.
- Patients with a history of hearing loss, may be at risk of further hearing loss especially if hepatic or renal function is present or if on high dose erythromycins, or if patient is elderly.

Potential Toxicities/Side Effects and the Nursing Process

I. ALTERATION IN NUTRITION related to GI SIDE EFFECTS

Defining Characteristics: Nausea, vomiting, anorexia have occurred frequently. Also, transient increase LFTs—AST (SGOT), ALT (SGPT), LDH, alk phos, bili—has occurred. Hepatotoxicity (fever, nausea, skin rash, stomach pain, severe and unusual tiredness or weakness, yellow eyes or skin, and vomiting) has occurred less frequently. Pancreatitis (severe abdominal pain, nausea and vomiting) has occurred but is rare.

Nursing Implications: Assess baseline nutritional status, preexisting nausea/vomiting, anorexia. Assess baseline LFTs and monitor periodically during treatment. Teach patient to report side effects. Provide symptomatic interventions if side effects occur; discuss with physician use of alternative drug(s).

II. POTENTIAL FOR INJURY related to HYPERSENSITIVITY REACTION

Defining Characteristics: Urticaria, pruritus, rash (maculopapular or erythematous), fever and chills, eosinophilia, myalgia, edema, erythema, angioedema.

Nursing Implications: Assess for drug allergies to erythromycin or macrolide antibiotic prior to drug administration. Teach patient to report any allergic reactions. Assess for signs/symptoms of allergic reaction after drug dose. Assess baseline skin integrity and presence of drug allergies; monitor patient closely during drug infusions. Teach patient to report immediately signs/symptoms of rash, pruritus, shortness of breath, any adverse sensation. Teach patient skin care and symptomatic measures as appropriate. If skin rash develops, discuss drug discontinuance with physician. If rash progresses, especially in human immunodeficiency virus (HIV)-infected patients, drug should be discontinued as fatal Stevens-Johnson syndrome may develop. Be prepared to treat severe acute hypersensitivity reactions with airway management, oxygen, epinephrine, corticosteroids, antihistamines as ordered.

III. ALTERATIONS IN COMFORT related to LOCAL INJECTION IRRITATION

Defining Characteristics: Incidence of phlebitis, thrombophlebitis, and pain when administering IV.

Nursing Implications: Change IV sites q 48 hours, and assess for signs/symptoms of phlebitis prior to each administration. Administer drug slowly. Apply warm packs to increase comfort.

IV. ALTERATIONS IN CARDIAC OUTPUT related to CARDIOVASCULAR CHANGES

Defining Characteristics: Rare incidence of cardiac arrhythmias, electrocardiogram (EKG) changes (e.g., QT prolongation), torsades de points (irregular or slow heart rate, recurrent fainting, sudden death).

Nursing Implications: Assess baseline heart rate and blood pressure (BP); monitor during therapy, at least with initial dose.

V. SENSORY/PERCEPTUAL ALTERATIONS related to OTOTOXICITY

Defining Characteristics: Damage to eighth cranial nerve (auditory) may result in dizziness, nystagmus, vertigo, ataxia (vestibular damage), and more commonly tinnitus, roaring sound in ears, and impaired hearing (auditory damage). Hearing loss usually begins with high-frequency loss, followed by clinical hearing loss, then permanent hearing loss if damage continues. Increased risk in elderly, renally, hepatically impaired patients.

Nursing Implications: Assess baseline hearing (ability to hear spoken voice) and continue to assess during therapy. Teach patient potential side effects, and instruct patient to report any hearing/perceptual problems (e.g., tinnitus, vertigo, decreased hearing). Discuss drug discontinuance and audiogram with physician to confirm hearing dysfunction if symptoms arise. Assess for increased risk if given concurrently with other ototoxic medications (e.g., cisplatin, furosemide).

VI. FUNGAL SUPERINFECTION related to REDISTRIBUTION OF ENDOGENOUS MICROORGANISMS

Defining Characteristics: Vaginal candidiasis (sore mouth or tongue; white patches in mouth and/or tongue); vaginitis (vaginal candidiasis); vaginal itching and discharge may occur as endogenous bacteria are eliminated and normal fungal population expands.

Nursing Implications: Teach female patient to report vaginal itching or discharge. Discuss appropriate antifungal treatment with physician. Teach perineal hygiene and symptomatic management.

Drug: gatifloxacin (Tequin)

Class: Quinolone.

Mechanism of Action: Gatifloxacin is a broad-spectrum anti-infective, active against a wide range of aerobic gram-positive and gram-negative organisms. Acts intracellularly by inhibiting DNA gyrase (bacterial topoisomerase IV).

Metabolism: Widely distributed to most body fluids and tissues with highest concentrations in organs such as kidneys, gallbladder, lungs, liver, gynecological tissue, prostatic tissue, phagocytic cells, urine, sputum, and bile. Well absorbed from GI tract. Metabolized in liver; excreted in urine and feces. Crosses placenta and is excreted in breast milk.

Dosage/Range:
- 400 mg PO or IV daily.

Drug Preparation:
- Oral: Take drug with large glass of water; preferably 2 hours after meal/food. Encourage oral fluids of 2–3 qt/day.
- IV: Further dilute drug in 0.9% sodium chloride or 5% dextrose in water to final concentration of 2 mg/mL.

Drug Interactions:

- Antacids (containing magnesium, aluminum, or calcium) and iron decrease absorption of serum level of gatifloxacin; do not administer concurrently. If must administer antacids or iron, administer at least 4 hours apart. The administration of antacids containing aluminum, magnesium, calcium, sucralfate, zinc, or iron may substantially reduce the absorption of gatifloxacin; do not administer concurrently.
- Serum digoxin concentrations should be monitored; gatifloxacin may raise serum levels in some patients.
- Probenecid: decreases the renal tubular secretion of gatifloxacin resulting in a prolonged elimination half-life and increased risk of toxicity.
- Gatifloxacin may have the potential to prolong the Q-T interval of the EKG in some patients. Gatifloxacin should not be used in patients with prolonged Q-T interval; patients with uncorrected hypokalemia; and patients taking quinidine, procainamide, amiodarone, and sotalol (antiarrhythmic agents).
- Increased intracranial pressure and psychosis have been reported along with CNS stimulation.
- Hypersensitivity reactions have been reported.

Lab Effects/Interference:

- Serum SGPT, serum alk phos, serum SGOT, and serum LDH: values may be increased.

Special Considerations:

- Used in treatment of infections of urinary and lower respiratory tracts, skin, bone and joint, and GI tract, as well as gonorrhea.
- Contraindicated in pregnancy or in women who are breast-feeding.
- Obtain ordered specimen for culture and sensitivity prior to first drug dose.
- Use cautiously in patients with seizure disorders.
- Used in the treatment of infections or most bacterial infections.

Potential Toxicities/Side Effects and the Nursing Process

I. ALTERATION IN NUTRITION related to GI SIDE EFFECTS

Defining Characteristics: Incidence of nausea, vomiting, abdominal discomfort, diarrhea, anorexia.

Nursing Implications: Assess baseline nutritional and elimination status. Teach patient to report GI disturbances. Administer and teach patient to self-administer antiemetics and antidiarrheals as needed and as ordered. Teach patient importance of nutritious diet, and suggest small, frequent, high-calorie, high-protein meals as appropriate. Assess baseline LFTs and monitor periodically during treatment. Discuss abnormalities and drug interruption with physician. Assess taking other hepatotoxic drugs (see Special Considerations).

II. SENSORY/PERCEPTUAL ALTERATIONS related to CNS EFFECTS

Defining Characteristics: Incidence of headache, restlessness. Dizziness, hallucinations, and seizures may also occur. Exacerbated by caffeine as quinolones delay caffeine excretion.

Nursing Implications: Assess baseline neurological function and comfort, and monitor during treatment. Teach patient to report any changes. Discuss any abnormalities with physician. Teach patient to limit or restrict all medications and caffeine-containing fluids (e.g., tea, coffee, caffeinated soft drinks).

III. ALTERATION IN SKIN INTEGRITY related to ALLERGY/HYPERSENSITIVITY

Defining Characteristics: Incidence of rash; other manifestations include eosinophilia, urticaria, flushing, fever, chills, photosensitivity, angioedema. Fatal hypersensitivity reactions have occurred rarely. Direct exposure to sunlight can cause sunburn (moderate to severe phototoxicity).

Nursing Implications: Assess baseline skin condition, including integrity and drug allergy history. Teach patient to report rash, itching, other skin changes. Teach patient skin care and symptomatic measures as appropriate. If skin rash develops, discuss drug discontinuance with physician. Be prepared to treat severe acute hypersensitivity reactions with airway management, oxygen, epinephrine, corticosteroids, antihistamines as ordered. Teach patient to avoid excessive sun exposure and to use skin protection factor (SPF) 15 or higher. If rash progresses, especially in HIV-infected patients, drug should be discontinued as fatal Stevens-Johnson syndrome may develop.

IV. FUNGAL SUPERINFECTION related to REDISTRIBUTION OF ENDOGENOUS MICROORGANISMS

Defining Characteristics: Vaginal moniliasis, vaginitis may occur as endogenous bacteria are eliminated and normal fungal population expands.

Nursing Implications: Teach female patient to report vaginal itching or discharge. Discuss appropriate antifungal treatment with physician. Teach perineal hygiene and symptomatic management.

V. ALTERATION IN URINARY ELIMINATION related to RENAL TOXICITY

Defining Characteristics: Increased BUN and creatinine, crystal and stone formation in urine, interstitial nephritis, and renal failure may occur.

Nursing Implications: Assess baseline renal function; expect that drug dose will be decreased in presence of renal dysfunction. Teach patient to take drug with at least 8 oz of water, and to increase oral fluids to 2–3 qt/day.

VI. ALTERATIONS IN COMFORT related to IV ADMINISTRATION

Defining Characteristics: Drug may cause pain, inflammation, and rare thrombophlebitis at IV site.

Nursing Implications: Change IV site q 48 hours. Assess for phlebitis, discomfort, and IV patency prior to each administration. Administer drug slowly over 60–90 minutes in large volume of 5% dextrose (see Drug Preparation). Apply heat to promote comfort.

Drug: gemifloxacin mesylate (Factive)

Class: Quinolone.

Mechanism of Action: Gemifloxacin is a broad-spectrum anti-infective, active against a wide range of aerobic gram-positive and gram-negative organisms. Acts inhibiting DNA synthesis through the inhibition of DNA gyrase and topoisomerase IV, which are essential for bacterial growth.

Metabolism: Widely distributed to most body fluids and tissues after oral administration. Gemifloxacin penetrates well into lung tissues and fluids. Well absorbed from GI tract. Metabolized to a limited extent in the liver; excreted in urine and feces. The safety in pregnant women has not been established. The drug is excreted in breast milk in animal studies.

Dosage/Range:
- 320 mg orally once a day for 5–7 days.

Drug Preparation:
- Oral: Take drug with or without food. Take with large glass of water; encourage oral fluids of 2–3 qt/day.

Drug Interactions:
- Antacids (containing magnesium, aluminum, or calcium) and iron decrease absorption of serum level of gemifloxacin; do not administer concurrently. If must administer antacids or iron, administer at least 3 hours before or 2 hours after. The administration of antacids containing aluminum, magnesium, calcium, sucralfate, zinc, or iron may substantially reduce the absorption of gemifloxacin; do not administer concurrently.
- Probenecid: decreases the renal tubular secretion of gemifloxacin resulting in a prolonged elimination half-life and increased risk of toxicity.

- Gemifloxacin may have the potential to prolong the Q-T interval of the EKG in some patients. Gemifloxacin should not be used in patients with prolonged Q-T interval; patients with uncorrected hypokalemia or hypomagnesemia; and patients taking quinidine, procainamide, amiodarone, and sotalol (Class 1A antiarrhythmic agents).
- Increased intracranial pressure and psychosis have been reported along with CNS stimulation.
- Hypersensitivity reactions have been reported.
- Fluoroquinolones have been shown to cause arthropathy and osteochondrosis in animal studies. Discontinue if patient experiences pain, inflammation, or rupture of a tendon. Elderly patients, athletes, and patients taking corticosteroids are more prone to tendonitis.
- Pseudomembranous colitis has been reported and may range from mild to life-threatening.

Lab Effects/Interference:

- Serum SGPT, serum alk phos, serum SGOT, and serum LDH: values may be increased.

Special Considerations:

- Used in treatment of infections of lower respiratory tracts.
- Contraindicated in pregnancy or in women who are breast-feeding.
- Obtain ordered specimen for culture and sensitivity prior to first drug dose.
- Use cautiously in patients with seizure disorders.
- Used in the treatment of infections or most bacterial infections.

Potential Toxicities/Side Effects and the Nursing Process

I. ALTERATION IN NUTRITION related to GI SIDE EFFECTS

Defining Characteristics: Incidence of nausea, vomiting, abdominal discomfort, diarrhea, anorexia.

Nursing Implications: Assess baseline nutritional and elimination status. Teach patient to report GI disturbances. Administer and teach patient to self-administer antiemetics and antidiarrheals as needed and as ordered. Teach patient importance of nutritious diet, and suggest small, frequent, high-calorie, high-protein meals as appropriate. Assess baseline LFTs and monitor periodically during treatment. Discuss abnormalities and drug interruption with physician. Assess taking other hepatotoxic drugs.

II. SENSORY/PERCEPTUAL ALTERATIONS related to CNS EFFECTS

Defining Characteristics: Incidence of headache, restlessness. Dizziness, hallucinations, and seizures may also occur. Exacerbated by caffeine, as quinolones delay caffeine excretion.

Nursing Implications: Assess baseline neurological function and comfort, and monitor during treatment. Teach patient to report any changes. Discuss any abnormalities with physician. Teach patient to limit or restrict all medications and caffeine-containing fluids (e.g., tea, coffee, caffeinated soft drinks).

III. ALTERATION IN SKIN INTEGRITY related to ALLERGY/HYPERSENSITIVITY

Defining Characteristics: Incidence of rash; other manifestations include eosinophilia, urticaria, flushing, fever, chills, photosensitivity, angioedema. Fatal hypersensitivity reactions have occurred rarely. Direct exposure to sunlight can cause sunburn (moderate to severe phototoxicity).

Nursing Implications: Assess baseline skin condition, including integrity and drug allergy history. Teach patient to report rash, itching, and other skin changes. Teach patient skin care and symptomatic measures as appropriate. If skin rash develops, discuss drug discontinuance with physician. Be prepared to treat severe acute hypersensitivity reactions with airway management, oxygen, epinephrine, corticosteroids, antihistamines as ordered. Teach patient to avoid excessive sun exposure and to use skin protection factor (SPF) 15 or higher. If rash progresses, especially in HIV-infected patients, drug should be discontinued as fatal Stevens-Johnson syndrome may develop.

IV. FUNGAL SUPERINFECTION related to REDISTRIBUTION OF ENDOGENOUS MICROORGANISMS

Defining Characteristics: Vaginal moniliasis, vaginitis may occur as endogenous bacteria are eliminated and normal fungal population expands.

Nursing Implications: Teach female patient to report vaginal itching or discharge. Discuss appropriate antifungal treatment with physician. Teach perineal hygiene and symptomatic management.

V. ALTERATION IN URINARY ELIMINATION related to RENAL TOXICITY

Defining Characteristics: Increased BUN and creatinine, crystal and stone formation in urine, interstitial nephritis, and renal failure may occur.

Nursing Implications: Assess baseline renal function; expect that drug dose will be decreased in presence of renal dysfunction. Teach patient to take drug with at least 8 oz of water, and to increase oral fluids to 2–3 qt/day.

Drug: gentamicin sulfate (Garamycin, Gentamicin)

Class: Aminoglycoside antibacterial.

Mechanism of Action: Derived from *Micromonospora*; bactericidal, most probably by inhibition of protein synthesis. Active against aerobic microorganisms: many sensitive gram-negative organisms (including *Acinetobacter, Brucella, Citrobacter, Enterobacter, E. coli, Klebsiella, Proteus, Pseudomonas, Salmonella, Serratia,* and *Shigella*) and some sensitive gram-positive organisms (*S. aureus* and *S. epidermidis*). Over time, bacterial resistance may develop, either naturally or acquired.

Metabolism: Well absorbed following IV administration, but variability in absorption after IM injection (peak serum level 0.5–2 hours, duration 8–12 hours). Widely distributed into body fluids. Minimally protein-bound. Readily crosses placenta and into breast milk. Drug excreted unchanged in the urine.

Dosage/Range:
- IM, IV: Loading dose, 2 mg/Kg, then 3–6 mg/Kg/day in one daily dose, 2 equal doses in split 8-hour dosing.
- IT: 4–8 mg (preservative-free).
- Desired peak serum concentration 4–10 μg/mL, and trough serum concentration is 1–2 μg/mL.
- DOSE REDUCTION IF RENAL DYSFUNCTION.

Drug Preparation:
- Store injectable at < 40°C (104°F). Stable for 24 hours at room temperature in 0.9% sodium chloride or 5% dextrose.

Drug Administration:
- Do not mix with other drugs.
- IV: Mix in 50–200 mL 0.9% sodium chloride or 5% dextrose injection and infuse over 30 minutes to 2 hours. Can also be given IM.

Drug Administration:
- Increased risk of toxicity with other ototoxic drugs: acyclovir, other aminoglycosides, amphotericin B, bacitracin, cephalosporins, colistin, cisplatin, ethacrynic acid, furosemide, vancomycin.
- Potentiation of neuromuscular blockade when given concurrently with general anesthetics (succinylcholine, tubocurarine); use cautiously, observe for signs/symptoms of respiratory depression.
- Synergism with extended-spectrum penicillins, but must be administered separately.

Lab Effects/Interference:
- Serum ALT, serum alk phos, serum AST, serum bili, and serum LDH values may be increased.
- BUN and serum creatinine concentrations may be increased.

- Serum Ca++, serum Mg++, serum K+, and serum Na+ concentrations may be decreased.

Special Considerations:

- Used as first-line treatment in short-term treatment of serious gram-negative infections (e.g., septicemia, respiratory tract infections).
- Use against gram-positive organisms only as second-line treatment.
- Use in pregnancy only if infection is life-threatening and no safer drug exists; drug crosses placenta and may cause fetal toxicity.

Potential Toxicities/Side Effects and the Nursing Process

I. ALTERATIONS IN SENSORY/PERCEPTUAL PATTERNS related to OTOTOXICITY

Defining Characteristics: Damage to eighth cranial nerve (auditory) may result in dizziness, nystagmus, vertigo, ataxia (vestibular damage), and more commonly tinnitus, roaring sound in ears, and impaired hearing (auditory damage). Hearing loss usually begins with high-frequency loss, followed by clinical hearing loss, then permanent hearing loss if damage continues. Increased risk in elderly or renally impaired patients.

Nursing Implications: Assess baseline hearing (ability to hear spoken voice) and continue to access during therapy. Teach patient potential side effects and instruct patient to report any hearing/perceptual problems (e.g., tinnitus, vertigo, decreased hearing). Discuss drug discontinuance and audiogram with physician to confirm hearing dysfunction if symptoms arise. Assess for increased risk if given concurrently with other ototoxic medications (e.g., cisplatin, furosemide).

II. ALTERATION IN URINARY ELIMINATION related to NEPHROTOXICITY

Defining Characteristics: Renal damage characterized by tubular necrosis with increased serum BUN, creatinine; decreased urine creatinine clearance and specific gravity; proteinuria and casts in urine. Azotemia usually not associated with oliguria. Rarely, electrolyte wasting with hypomagnesemia, hypocalcemia, and hypokalemia may occur. Renal dysfunction is usually reversible after drug discontinuance. Increased risk exists in elderly and if preexisting renal dysfunction. Risk low in well-hydrated patients with normal renal function when normal doses given.

Nursing Implications: Assess baseline renal function and electrolytes, and monitor periodically during therapy. Discuss any abnormalities with physician, as drug should be dose-reduced or discontinued if renal dysfunction develops. Assess baseline total body fluid balance, weight, and monitor periodically during antibiotic therapy.

Monitor hydration status to keep patient well hydrated. Assess drug peak and trough levels as ordered so that drug dosage is correctly titrated. Increased risk of toxicity if peak serum concentration > 10–12 μg/mL. Draw blood for peak drug concentration 30 minutes after end of 30-minute infusion or at the end of a 60-minute infusion; draw trough immediately before next dose.

III. ALTERATIONS IN SENSORY/PERCEPTUAL PATTERNS related to CNS EFFECTS, NEUROMUSCULAR BLOCKADE

Defining Characteristics: Headache, tremor, lethargy may occur. Peripheral neuropathy or encephalopathy (numbness, skin tingling, muscle twitching) may occur rarely. Neuromuscular blockade is dose-related, self-limiting, and uncommon; risk is greater with topical application or when drug is administered to patient with neuromuscular disease (myasthenia gravis) or hypocalcemia.

Nursing Implications: Assess baseline neurologic status. Assess coexisting risk factors, neuromuscular blockade medications. Teach patient about side effects and to report headache, tremor, lethargy. Observe for respiratory depression. If signs/symptoms arise, discuss drug discontinuance with physician.

IV. POTENTIAL FOR INJURY related to HYPERSENSITIVITY

Defining Characteristics: Rash, urticaria, pruritus, fever, eosinophilia have occurred rarely. CROSS-SENSITIVITY between AMINOGLYCOSIDES exists!

Nursing Implications: Assess for drug allergies to any aminoglycoside—amikacin, gentamicin, kanamycin, neomycin, netilmicin, streptomycin, tobramycin—prior to drug administration. Instruct patient to report any allergic reactions. Assess for signs/symptoms of allergic reaction after drug dose.

V. ALTERATION IN NUTRITION, LESS THAN BODY REQUIREMENTS, related to GI SIDE EFFECTS

Defining Characteristics: Nausea, vomiting, anorexia have occurred rarely. Also, transient hepatomegaly with increased LFTs—AST, ALT, LDH, alk phos, bili—has occurred.

Nursing Implications: Assess baseline nutritional status, preexisting nausea/vomiting, anorexia. Assess baseline LFTs and monitor periodically during treatment. Instruct patient to report side effects. Provide symptomatic interventions if side effects occur; discuss with physician use of alternative drug(s).

VI. POTENTIAL FOR FATIGUE, INFECTION, AND BLEEDING related to BONE MARROW INJURY

Defining Characteristics: Anemia, leukopenia, granulocytopenia, and thrombocytopenia may occur. Also, patients receiving antibiotics are at risk for overgrowth of nonsusceptible microorganisms, such as fungi (superinfection). Rare.

Nursing Implications: Assess baseline CBC, differential, and monitor periodically during treatment. Instruct patient to report signs/symptoms of fatigue, infection, or bleeding immediately. Assess for signs/symptoms of superinfection. Discuss any adverse effects with physician.

Drug: imipenem/cilastatin sodium (Primaxin)

Class: Antibacterial. Imipenem is a β-lactam antibiotic, carbapenem type; cilastatin inhibits an enzyme in the kidneys that breaks down imipenem, increasing drug potency and protecting kidneys.

Mechanism of Action: Semisynthetic derivative of cephalosporin C (produced by fungus); contains β-lactam ring and is related to penicillins and cephamycins (e.g., cefoxitin). Bactericidal through inhibition of cell wall synthesis, with resulting cell wall instability and cell lysis. Active against most anaerobic and aerobic gram-positive and gram-negative organisms. These include *Staphylococcus, Streptococcus, E. coli, P. aeruginosa, Proteus, Klebsiella, Enterobacter*. Some activity against *Mycobacterium*. Resists hydrolysis by β-lactamase enzymes produced by microorganisms, so resistance to these organisms is much less than other β-lactam antibiotics (e.g., cephalosporins, penicillins). Used in treatment of serious infections of lower respiratory tract, urinary tract, abdomen, female pelvis, skin, bone, and joint, as well as polymicrobial infections and infections resistant to other antibiotics.

Metabolism: Not well absorbed from GI tract, so must be given IV. Incompletely absorbed after IM injection. Widely distributed in body tissues and fluids, including bile; does not result in significant CSF drug levels. Crosses placenta and is excreted in breast milk. Cilastatin decreases renal metabolism of imipenem; both drugs are excreted in urine, and to a lesser degree in feces.

Dosage/Range:

Adult:

- IV: 250 mg–1 g q 6–8 h (maximum 50 mg/kg or 4 g/day, whichever is less).
- IM (if unable to give IV): 500–750 mg q 12 h (maximum 1.5 g/day). Reduce dose if renal insufficiency, according to manufacturer's package insert.

Drug Preparation:

- Store vial of sterile powder at < 30°C (86°F).
- IV: Reconstitute according to manufacturer's package insert and further dilute in 100 mL 0.9% sodium chloride or 5% dextrose injection. Infuse over 60 minutes for each gram of drug administered. Slow infusion if nausea/vomiting develop.
- IM: Reconstitute drug with lidocaine HCl 1% injection (without epinephrine) as directed by package insert. Administer deep IM in large muscle mass (e.g., gluteus maximus). Assess allergy to lidocaine. IM preparation SHOULD NOT BE USED FOR IV ADMINISTRATION.

Drug Interactions:

- Probenecid: increases serum concentrations of imipenem. DO NOT USE CONCURRENTLY.
- Aminoglycosides: may have synergistic antimicrobial effect.
- β-lactam antibiotics (cephalosporins, extended-spectrum penicillins): Antagonism. Imipenem stimulates production of β-lactamase enzymes by the bacteria that inactivate the cephalosporins and penicillins. DO NOT USE CONCURRENTLY.
- Ganciclovir: may decrease seizure threshold. Do not use concurrently unless critical for life-saving treatment.
- Co-trimoxazole: possible synergy against *Nocardia asteroides*.
- Chloramphenicol: possible antagonism. Consider chloramphenicol administration 2+ hours after imipenem (requires clinical study).

Lab Effects/Interference:

- Serum ALT, serum alk phos, and serum AST values may be transiently increased.

Clinical significance:

- Coombs' (direct antiglobulin) tests: may occur during therapy.
- Serum LDH values may be transiently increased.
- Serum bili, BUN concentrations, and serum creatinine concentrations may be transiently increased.
- HCT and Hgb concentrations may be decreased.

Special Considerations:

- Contraindicated in patients hypersensitive to imipenem or cilastatin. Use cautiously in patients sensitive to penicillin or other β-lactams, as partial cross-allergenicity exists.
- Do not give IM preparation reconstituted with 1% lidocaine if hypersensitive to lidocaine.
- Drug may cause false-positive glucose determination when using Clinitest.
- Ensure specimen sent for culture and sensitivity prior to first antibiotic dose.
- Drug has significantly broad antibacterial properties.
- Drug dosage needs to be reduced if severe renal insufficiency.
- Slow IV infusion if nausea/vomiting develops.

Potential Toxicities/Side Effects and the Nursing Process

I. POTENTIAL FOR INJURY related to HYPERSENSITIVITY REACTION

Defining Characteristics: Urticaria, pruritus, rash (maculopapular or erythematous), fever and chills, eosinophilia, myalgia, edema, erythema, angioedema, Stevens-Johnson syndrome, and exfoliative skin reactions occur in 5% of patients. Increased risk in individuals allergic to penicillin.

Nursing Implications: Assess allergy to cephalosporin antibiotics and penicillin: if patient states "yes," determine actual response, e.g., "swollen lips = angioedema." If angioedema, discuss with physician RISK versus benefit prior to drug administration, as there is partial cross-allergenicity. Discuss other patient responses with physician to determine whether drug should be given. Assess baseline skin condition, including integrity and allergy history to drugs. Instruct patient to report rash, itching, other skin changes. Teach patient skin care and symptomatic measures as appropriate. If skin rash develops, discuss drug discontinuance with physician. If rash progresses, drug should be discontinued, as fatal Stevens-Johnson syndrome may develop. Be prepared to treat severe acute hypersensitivity reactions with airway management, oxygen, epinephrine, corticosteroids, antihistamines as ordered.

II. ALTERATION IN NUTRITION, LESS THAN BODY REQUIREMENTS, related to GI SIDE EFFECTS

Defining Characteristics: Nausea, vomiting occurs more frequently than diarrhea, anorexia; rarely, pseudomembranous colitis caused by *C. difficile* resistant to the antibiotic occurs. Rarely, transient increases in LFTs—AST, ALT, alk phos, bili—may occur.

Nursing Implications: Assess baseline nutritional status. Instruct patient to report GI disturbances. Administer and teach patient to self-administer antiemetics as needed and as ordered. Teach patient importance of nutritious diet and suggest small, frequent, high-calorie, high-protein meals as appropriate. Assess baseline LFTs and monitor periodically during treatment. Discuss abnormalities and drug interruption with physician.

III. FUNGAL SUPERINFECTION related to REDISTRIBUTION OF ENDOGENOUS MICROORGANISMS

Defining Characteristics: Vaginal candidiasis, vaginitis may occur as endogenous bacteria are eliminated and normal fungal population expands.

Nursing Implications: Instruct female patient to report vaginal itching or discharge. Discuss appropriate antifungal treatment with physician. Teach perineal hygiene and symptomatic management.

IV. ALTERATIONS IN PROTECTIVE MECHANISMS (RARE) related to TRANSIENT LEUKOPENIA

Defining Characteristics: Rarely, transient leukopenia, lymphocytosis, anemia, eosinophilia may occur. Prolonged PT, prolonged APTT, and hypoprothrombinemia have occurred rarely, especially in elderly or debilitated patients, or in individuals with vitamin K deficiency.

Nursing Implications: Assess baseline laboratory parameters, and monitor periodically during treatment. Assess patient for response to antibiotics. Discuss abnormalities with physician.

V. ALTERATIONS IN SENSORY/PERCEPTUAL PATTERNS related to DIZZINESS, SOMNOLENCE

Defining Characteristics: Dizziness, headache, somnolence, seizures occur rarely. Most seizures have occurred in patients with preexisting CNS problems, those who had received higher-than-recommended IV doses, the elderly, and patients with impaired renal function.

Nursing Implications: Assess baseline neurologic function and comfort, and monitor during treatment. Instruct patient to report any changes. Discuss any abnormalities with physician. Institute seizure precautions. If seizures occur, discuss with physician anticonvulsant therapy or discontinuance of antibiotic.

VI. ALTERATIONS IN COMFORT related to LOCAL INJECTION IRRITATION

Defining Characteristics: Pain, induration, sterile abscesses may form in IM injection sites; phlebitis may develop in IV sites.

Nursing Implications: Rotate IM injection sites, and administer drug deep IM in large muscle mass (e.g., gluteus maximus). Use IM injection when IV administration is not possible. Change IV sites q 48 h, and assess for signs/symptoms of phlebitis prior to each administration. Administer drug slowly. Apply warm packs to increase comfort.

Drug: kanamycin sulfate (Kantrex)

Class: Aminoglycoside antibacterial.

Mechanism of Action: Synthetic antibiotic derived from *Streptomyces*; bactericidal, most probably by inhibition of protein synthesis. Active against aerobic microorganisms: many sensitive gram-negative organisms (including *Acinetobacter, Citrobacter, Enterobacter, E. coli, Klebsiella, Proteus, Salmonella, Serratia, and Shigella*) and some sensitive gram-positive organisms (*S. aureus* and *S. epidermidis*). Over time, bacterial resistance may develop, either naturally or acquired.

Metabolism: Well absorbed following parenteral administration, but variable absorption after IM injection (peak serum level 0.5–2 hours, duration 8–12 hours). Widely distributed into body fluids. Minimally protein-bound. Readily crosses placenta and into breast milk. Drug excreted unchanged in the urine.

Dosage/Range:
- IM, IV: 15 mg/kg/day in equally divided doses at 8- or 12-hour intervals.
- Desired peak serum concentration 15–30 μg/mL, and trough serum concentration is 5–10 μg/mL.
- DOSE REDUCTION IF RENAL IMPAIRMENT.

Drug Preparation:
- Store capsules in tight containers at temperature < 40°C (104°F).
- Injection should be stored at < 40°C (104°F), preferably 15–30°C (59–86°F).
- Mix 500 mg in 100–200 mL of IV infusion solution. Stable for 24 hours at room temperature in 0.9% sodium chloride or 5% dextrose. DO NOT MIX WITH OTHER MEDICATIONS.

Drug Administration:
- Deep IM: upper outer quadrant of buttock.
- IV: Infuse over 30–60 minutes.
- Orally (preoperative bowel sterilization): 1 g PO qh × four doses, then q 4 h × four doses.
- Wound irrigation: 2–2.5 mg/mL in 0.9% sodium chloride irrigant.

Drug Interactions:
- Increased risk of toxicity with other ototoxic drugs: acyclovir, other aminoglycosides, amphotericin B, bacitracin, cephalosporins, colistin, cisplatin, ethacrynic acid, furosemide, vancomycin.
- Potentiation of neuromuscular blockade when given concurrently with general anesthetics (succinylcholine, tubocurarine); use cautiously, observe for signs/symptoms of respiratory depression.
- Synergism with extended-spectrum penicillins, but must be administered separately.

Lab Effects/Interference:

- Serum ALT, serum alk phos, serum AST, serum bili, and serum LDH values may be increased.
- BUN and serum creatinine concentrations may be increased.
- Serum Ca++, serum Mg++, serum K+, and serum Na+ concentrations may be decreased.

Special Considerations:

- Used as first-line treatment in short-term treatment of serious gram-negative infections (e.g., septicemia, respiratory tract infections).
- Use against gram-positive organisms only as second-line treatment.
- Use in pregnancy only if infection is life-threatening and no safer drug exists; drug crosses placenta and may cause fetal toxicity.

Potential Toxicities/Side Effects and the Nursing Process

I. ALTERATION IN SENSORY/PERCEPTUAL PATTERNS related to OTOTOXICITY

Defining Characteristics: Damage to eighth cranial nerve (auditory) may result in dizziness, nystagmus, vertigo, ataxia (vestibular damage), and less commonly tinnitus, roaring sound in ears, and impaired hearing (auditory damage). Hearing loss usually begins with high-frequency loss, followed by clinical hearing loss, then permanent hearing loss if damage continues. Increased risk in elderly or renally impaired patients.

Nursing Implications: Assess baseline hearing (ability to hear spoken voice) and continue during therapy. Teach patient potential side effects, and instruct patient to report any hearing/perceptual problems (e.g., tinnitus, vertigo, decreased hearing). Discuss drug discontinuance and audiogram with physician to confirm hearing dysfunction if symptoms arise. Assess for increased risk if given concurrently with other ototoxic medications (e.g., cisplatin, furosemide).

II. ALTERATION IN URINARY ELIMINATION related to NEPHROTOXICITY

Defining Characteristics: Renal damage characterized by tubular necrosis with increased serum BUN, creatinine; decreased urine creatinine clearance and specific gravity; proteinuria and casts in urine. Azotemia usually not associated with oliguria. Rarely, electrolyte wasting with hypomagnesemia, hypocalcemia, and hypokalemia may occur. Renal dysfunction usually reversible after drug discontinuance. Increased risk exists in elderly and if there is preexisting renal dysfunction. Risk is low in well-hydrated patients with normal renal function when normal doses given.

Nursing Implications: Assess baseline renal function and electrolytes, and monitor periodically during therapy. Discuss any abnormalities with physician, as drug should be dose-reduced or discontinued if renal dysfunction develops. Assess baseline total body fluid balance, weight, and monitor periodically during antibiotic therapy. Monitor hydration status to keep patient well hydrated. Assess drug peak and trough levels as ordered so that drug dosage is correctly titrated. Increased risk of toxicity if peak serum concentration > 30–35 μg/mL. Draw blood for peak drug concentration 30 minutes after end of 30-minute infusion or at the end of a 60-minute infusion; draw trough immediately before next dose.

III. ALTERATIONS IN SENSORY/PERCEPTUAL PATTERNS related to CNS EFFECTS, NEUROMUSCULAR BLOCKADE

Defining Characteristics: Headache, tremor, lethargy may occur. Peripheral neuropathy or encephalopathy (numbness, skin tingling, muscle twitching) may occur rarely. Neuromuscular blockade is dose-related, self-limiting, and uncommon; risk is greater with topical application or when drug is administered to patient with neuromuscular disease (myasthenia gravis) or hypocalcemia.

Nursing Implications: Assess baseline neurologic status. Assess coexisting risk factors, neuromuscular blockade medications. Teach patient about side effects, and instruct to report headache, tremor, lethargy. Observe for respiratory depression. If signs/symptoms arise, discuss drug discontinuance with physician.

IV. POTENTIAL FOR INJURY related to HYPERSENSITIVITY

Defining Characteristics: Rash, urticaria, pruritus, fever, eosinophilia have occurred rarely. CROSS-SENSITIVITY between AMINOGLYCOSIDES exists!

Nursing Implications: Assess for drug allergies to any aminoglycoside—amikacin, gentamicin, kanamycin, neomycin, netilmicin, streptomycin, tobramycin—prior to drug administration. Instruct patient to report any allergic reactions. Assess for signs/symptoms of allergic reaction after drug dose.

V. ALTERATION IN NUTRITION, LESS THAN BODY REQUIREMENTS, related to GI SIDE EFFECTS

Defining Characteristics: Nausea, vomiting, anorexia have occurred rarely. Also, transient hepatomegaly with increased LFTs—AST, ALT, alk phos—has occurred.

Nursing Implications: Assess baseline nutritional status, preexisting nausea/vomiting, anorexia. Assess baseline LFTs and monitor periodically during treatment. Instruct patient to report side effects. Provide symptomatic interventions if side effects occur; discuss with physician use of alternative drug(s).

VI. POTENTIAL FOR FATIGUE, INFECTION, AND BLEEDING related to BONE MARROW INJURY

Defining Characteristics: Anemia, leukopenia, granulocytopenia, and thrombocytopenia may occur. Also, patients receiving antibiotics are at risk for overgrowth of nonsusceptible microorganisms, such as fungi (superinfection). Rare.

Nursing Implications: Assess baseline CBC, differential, and monitor periodically during treatment. Instruct patient to report signs/symptoms of fatigue, infection, or bleeding immediately. Assess for signs/symptoms of superinfection. Discuss any adverse effects with physician.

Drug: levofloxacin (Levaquin)

Class: Fluoroquinolone antibiotic.

Mechanism of Action: Drug is a synthetic, broad-spectrum antibacterial agent. Inhibits DNA gyrase (bacterial topoisomerase II), which is necessary for DNA replication, transcription, and repair. Has activity against a wide range of gram-negative and gram-positive bacteria, as well as against some bacteria resistant to β-lactam antibiotics.

Metabolism: Drug is well absorbed from the GI tract without regard to food, with 99% bioavailability; peak serum levels occur in 1–2 hours. Steady-state is reached in 48 hours. Drug is not extensively metabolized, with 87% of drug excreted largely unchanged in the urine at 48 hours. Terminal half-life is 6–8 hours.

Dosage/Range:
- 500 mg daily × 7 days (acute bacterial exacerbation of chronic bronchitis), × 7–14 days (community-acquired pneumonia), × 7–10 days (uncomplicated skin and skin structure infection), × 10–14 days (acute maxillary sinusitis), × 10 days (uncomplicated UTI, acute pyelonephritis).

Drug Preparation:
- Oral, available in 250-mg and 500-mg tablets.
- IV: Administer over 60 min to prevent hypotension; IV available in premixed 250-mg or 500-mg bags, or 20-mL vial containing 500 mg that is further diluted in 5% dextrose, 0.9% sodium chloride.

Drug Administration:
- Administer without regard to food.
- Dose-reduce if renal compromise (see Special Considerations section).
- Administer oral doses at least 2 hours before or 2 hours after antacids containing magnesium or aluminum, as well as sucralfate, metal cations such as iron, and multivitamins containing zinc.

Drug Interactions:

- Antacids containing magnesium or aluminum, sucralfate, iron, multivitamins containing zinc: may decrease serum levels of levofloxacin; take any of these agents at least 2 hours before or 2 hours after levofloxacin.
- Theophylline: possible increase in theophylline serum levels; monitor levels and change dose accordingly.
- Warfarin: theoretically could enhance effects of oral anticoagulants; monitor INR closely and modify dose accordingly.
- NSAIDs: possible increase in the risk of CNS stimulation and seizures; assess patient risk for seizures, and use cautiously if at all in patients at risk.
- Antidiabetic agents: changes in glucose (hyper- or hypoglycemia); monitor blood sugar closely, and modify dose accordingly.

Lab Effects/Interference:

- Decreased glucose, decreased lymphocytes.

Special Considerations:

- Indicated for the treatment of acute maxillary sinusitis due to *Streptococcus pneumoniae*, *Haemophilus influenzae*, *Moraxella catarrhalis*; acute bacterial exacerbation of chronic bronchitis due to *Staphylococcus aureus*, *Streptococcus pneumoniae*, *Haemophilus influenzae*, *Haemophilus parainfluenzae*, or *Moraxella catarrhalis*; community-acquired pneumonia due to *Staphylococcus aureus*, *Streptococcus pneumoniae*, *Haemophilus influenzae*, *Haemophilus parainfluenzae*, *Klebsiella pneumoniae*, *Moraxella catarrhalis*, *Chlamydia pneumoniae*, *Legionella pneumophila*, or *Mycoplasma pneumoniae*.
- Active against the above as well as aerobic gram-positive *Enterococcus faecalis* and *Streptococcus pyogenes* and aerobic gram-negative microorganisms *Enterobacter cloacae*, *Escherichia coli*, *Proteus mirabilis*, and *Pseudomonas aeruginosa*.
- Dose modifications for renal dysfunction:

Acute Bacterial Exacerbation of:	Chronic Bronchitis, Community-Acquired	Pneumonia, Acute Maxillary Sinusitis, Uncomplicated Skin Infections
Renal status	Initial dose	Subsequent dose
Cr cl 20–49 mL/min	500 mg	250 mg q 24 h
Cr cl 10–19 mL/min	500 mg	250 mg q 48 h
Hemodialysis	500 mg	250 mg q 48 h
CAPD	500 mg q 48 h	250 mg q 48 h
Uncomplicated UTI/Acute Pyelonephritis		
Cr cl 10–19 mL/min	250 mg	250 mg q 48 h

- Use drug cautiously, if at all, in the following patients: (1) known or suspected CNS or seizure disorder (e.g., severe cerebral arteriosclerosis or epilepsy); (2) possess factors lowering seizure threshold (e.g., renal dysfunction, other drug therapy); (3) pregnant or nursing mothers; (4) children < 18 years old.
- Obtain ordered specimen for culture and sensitivity prior to first drug dose.

Potential Toxicities/Side Effects and the Nursing Process

I. ALTERATION IN NUTRITION related to GI SIDE EFFECTS

Defining Characteristics: 0.1–3.0% incidence of nausea, vomiting, abdominal discomfort, diarrhea, anorexia. As with all antibiotics, pseudomembranous colitis may occur, ranging in severity from mild to life-threatening. Treatment with antibiotics changes the intestinal microflora, so *C. difficile* bacteria may overgrow. Once diagnosis is made, mild diarrhea may stop with cessation of drug; if moderate to severe, it will require hydration, electrolyte replacement, nutritional support, and antibacterial coverage against *C. difficile*.

Nursing Implications: Assess baseline nutritional and elimination status. Teach patient to report GI disturbances. Teach patient to report diarrhea immediately, and consider whether this is pseudomembranous colitis and send stool specimen for *C. difficile*; if positive, discuss drug discontinuance with physician. Administer and teach patient to self-administer antiemetics, antidiarrheals as needed and as ordered. Teach patient importance of nutritious diet, and suggest small, frequent, high-calorie, high-protein meals as appropriate. Assess baseline LFTs and monitor periodically during treatment. Discuss abnormalities and drug interruption with physician.

II. SENSORY/PERCEPTUAL ALTERATIONS related to CNS EFFECTS

Defining Characteristics: 1–2% incidence of insomnia, dizziness, taste perversion, headache, nervousness, anxiety, tremors, and seizures may also occur.

Nursing Implications: Assess baseline neurological function and comfort, and monitor during treatment. Teach patient to report any changes. Discuss any abnormalities with physician. Teach patient to avoid caffeine-containing fluids, medications, e.g., tea, coffee, soft drinks.

III. ALTERATION IN SKIN INTEGRITY related to ALLERGY/HYPERSENSITIVITY

Defining Characteristics: 1–4% incidence of rash; other manifestations include eosinophilia, urticaria, flushing, fever, chills, photosensitivity, angioedema. Fatal hypersensitivity reactions have occurred rarely. Direct exposure to sunlight can cause sunburn (moderate-to-severe phototoxicity).

Nursing Implications: Assess baseline skin condition, including integrity and drug allergy history. Teach patient to report rash, itching, other skin changes. Teach patient skin care and symptomatic measures as appropriate. If skin rash develops, discuss drug discontinuance with physician. If rash progresses, especially in HIV-infected patients, drug should be discontinued, as fatal Stevens-Johnson syndrome may develop. Be prepared to treat severe acute hypersensitivity reactions with airway management, oxygen, epinephrine, corticosteroids, antihistamines as ordered. Teach patient to avoid excessive sun exposure and to use skin protection factor (SPF) 15 or higher.

IV. FUNGAL SUPERINFECTION related to REDISTRIBUTION OF ENDOGENOUS MICROORGANISMS

Defining Characteristics: Vaginal moniliasis, vaginitis may occur as endogenous bacteria are eliminated and normal fungal population expands.

Nursing Implications: Teach female patient to report vaginal itching or discharge. Discuss appropriate antifungal treatment with physician. Teach perineal hygiene and symptomatic management.

Drug: linezolid (Zyvox)

Class: Oxazolidinone class of antibiotic.

Mechanism of Action: Linezolid inhibits initiation of protein synthesis by preventing the formation of the fmet-tRNA:mRNA:30S subunit ternary complex. Oxazolidinones bind to the 50S subunit in a region shared with the peptidyl transferase inhibitor chloramphenicol. Oxazolidinones are not peptidyl transferase inhibitors, and it is not known which specific ribosome reaction is inhibited by 50S subunit binding. Linezolid has a specific mechanism of action against bacteria resistant to other antibiotics, including methicillin-resistant *Staphylococcus aureus* (MRSA), multiresistant strains of *Streptococcus pneumoniae*, and vancomycin-resistant *enterococcus faecium* (VRE).

Metabolism: Primarily metabolized by oxidation of the morpholine ring, resulting in two inactive carboxylic acid metabolites. Only about 30% of a dose is excreted unchanged in the urine.

Dosage/Range:
- Oral: 400–600 mg q 12 h for 10 to 14 days; up to 28 days for VRE.
- IV: 600 mg q 12 h for 10–14 days; up to 28 days for VRE.

Drug Preparation:

- Available in single-use, ready-to-use infusion bags.

Drug Administration:

- IV infusion over 30–120 minutes.
- Linezolid has the potential to interact with adrenergic (phenylpropanolamine, pseudoephedrine) and serotonergic agents since it is a reversible, nonselective monoamine oxidase inhibitor.
- Large quantities of foods or beverages with high tyramine content should be avoided.

Lab Effects/Interference:

- Thrombocytopenia has been seen when this drug is administered long-term (up to 28 days).

Special Considerations:

- IV and PO doses are the same.

Potential Toxicities/Side Effects and the Nursing Process

I. ALTERATION IN NUTRITION related to GI SIDE EFFECTS

Defining Characteristics: Nausea, vomiting, anorexia have occurred frequently.

Nursing Implications: Assess baseline nutritional status, preexisting nausea/vomiting, anorexia. Teach patient to report side effects. Provide symptomatic interventions if side effects occur; discuss with physician use of alternative drug(s).

II. POTENTIAL FOR INJURY related to HYPERSENSITIVITY REACTION

Defining Characteristics: Urticaria, pruritus, rash (maculopapular or erythematous), fever and chills, eosinophilia, myalgia, edema, erythema, angioedema.

Nursing Implications: Assess for drug allergies to erythromycin or macrolide antibiotic prior to drug administration. Teach patient to report any allergic reactions. Assess for signs/symptoms of allergic reaction after drug dose. Assess baseline skin integrity and presence of drug allergies; monitor patient closely during drug infusions. Teach patient to report immediately signs/symptoms of rash, pruritus, shortness of breath, any adverse sensation. Teach patient skin care and symptomatic measures as appropriate. If skin rash develops, discuss drug discontinuance with physician. If rash progresses, especially in human immunodeficiency virus (HIV)-infected patients, drug should be discontinued, as fatal Stevens-Johnson syndrome may develop. Be prepared to treat severe acute hypersensitivity reactions with airway management, oxygen, epinephrine, corticosteroids, antihistamines as ordered.

III. ALTERATIONS IN COMFORT related to HEADACHE

Defining Characteristics: Headache has occurred in some patients.

Nursing Implications: Assess baseline hearing (ability to hear spoken voice) and continue to assess during therapy. Teach patient potential side effects, and instruct patient to report any hearing/perceptual problems (e.g., tinnitus, vertigo, decreased hearing). Discuss drug discontinuance and audiogram with physician to confirm hearing dysfunction if symptoms arise. Assess for increased risk if given concurrently with other ototoxic medications (e.g., cisplatin, furosemide).

IV. FUNGAL SUPERINFECTION related to REDISTRIBUTION OF ENDOGENOUS MICROORGANISMS

Defining Characteristics: Vaginal or oral candidiasis (sore mouth or tongue; white patches in mouth and/or tongue); vaginitis (vaginal candidiasis); vaginal itching and discharge may occur as endogenous bacteria are eliminated and normal fungal population expands.

Nursing Implications: Teach female patient to report vaginal itching or discharge. Discuss appropriate antifungal treatment with physician. Teach perineal hygiene and symptomatic management.

Drug: meropenem (Merrem)

Class: antibiotic, carbapenem.

Mechanism of Action: The bactericidal activity results from the inhibition of cell wall synthesis. Penetrates the cell wall of most gram-positive and gram-negative bacteria to reach penicillin-binding protein (PBP) targets.

Metabolism: Widely distributed in body tissues and fluids, excreted in urine.

Dosage/Range:

Adult:

- Intra-abdominal infection: 1 gram IV every 8 hours.
- Meningitis: bacterial 2 grams IV every 8 hours.

Drug Preparation:

- IV bolus, dilute with 5–20 ml. Sterile water for injection and give over 3–5 minutes.
- IV infusion dilute with D5W or normal saline, infuse over 15–30 minutes, maximum concentration 50 mg/ml.

Drug Interactions:

- Probenecid competes with meropenem for active tubular secretion and thus inhibits the renal excretion of meropenem.
- Meropenem may reduce serum levels of valproic acid to subtherapeutic levels.

Lab Effects/Interference:

- Meropenem possesses the characteristic low toxicity of the β-lactam group of antibiotics.
- Periodically assess organ system function; renal, hepatic and hematopoietic.

Potential Toxicities/Side Effects and the Nursing Process

I. POTENTIAL FOR INJURY related to HYPERSENSITIVITY REACTION and LOCAL REACTIONS (pain at injection site)

Defining Characteristics: Urticaria, pruritus, rash (maculopapular or erythematous), fever and chills, eosinophilia, myalgia, edema, erythema, angioedema.

Nursing Implications: Assess allergy to cephalosporin antibiotics and penicillin: if patient states "yes," determine actual response, e.g., "swollen lips = angioedema." If angioedema, patient SHOULD NOT receive drug. Discuss other patient responses with physician to determine whether drug should be given. Assess baseline skin condition, including integrity and allergy history to drugs. Instruct patient to report rash, itching, and other skin changes. Teach patient skin care and symptomatic measures as appropriate. If skin rash develops, discuss drug discontinuance with physician. Be prepared to treat severe acute hypersensitivity reactions with airway management, oxygen, epinephrine, corticosteroids, antihistamines as ordered.

II. ALTERATION IN NUTRITION, LESS THAN BODY REQUIREMENTS, related to GI SIDE EFFECTS

Defining Characteristics: Nausea, vomiting, diarrhea may occur; rarely, pseudomembranous colitis caused by antibiotic resistance occurs.

Nursing Implications: Assess baseline nutritional status. Instruct patient to report GI disturbances. Administer and teach patient to self-administer antiemetics as needed and as ordered. Teach patient importance of nutritious diet, and suggest small, frequent, high-calorie, high-protein meals as appropriate. Assess baseline LFTs, and monitor periodically during treatment. Discuss abnormalities and drug interruption with physician.

III. FUNGAL SUPERINFECTION related to REDISTRIBUTION OF ENDOGENOUS MICROORGANISMS

Defining Characteristics: Vaginal candidiasis, vaginitis may occur as endogenous bacteria are eliminated, and normal fungal population expands.

Nursing Implications: Instruct female patient to report vaginal itching or discharge. Discuss appropriate antifungal treatment with physician. Teach perineal hygiene and symptomatic management.

Drug: metronidazole hydrochloride (Flagyl)

Class: Antibacterial (systemic); antiprotozoal.

Mechanism of Action: Disrupts DNA, inhibits nucleic acid synthesis in susceptible organisms. Active against anaerobic gram-negative (*Bacteroides*) and gram-positive bacilli (*Clostridium*), and protozoa (*Trichomonas, Giardia*).

Metabolism: Well absorbed after oral administration; rate affected by food, but not amount absorbed. Oral and IV serum levels are similar. Widely distributed in body tissues and fluids, including CSF, placenta, breast milk. Excreted in urine (60–80%) and feces.

Dosage/Range:

Adult:

- Oral: 250–750 mg PO tid × 7–10 days or single dose of 2 g PO (trichomoniasis).
- Pseudomembranous colitis: 250 mg PO qid × 7–14 days or 500 mg PO tid × 7–14 days.
- IV: Loading dose of 15 mg/kg IV over 1 hour (1 g); then maintenance dose of 7.5 mg/kg IV (500 mg) q 8 h (maximum 4 g/day).

Drug Preparation:

- Oral: Store in light-resistant container at < 30°C (86°F).
- IV: Protect from light and freezing. Reconstitute according to manufacturer's package insert. Further dilute with 0.9% sodium chloride or 5% dextrose to concentration of ≤ 8 mg/mL. Do not use aluminum needles. Administer over 30–60 minutes. May be given as continuous or intermittent infusion.

Drug Interactions:

- Coumarin anticoagulants: increase anticoagulant effect. Avoid concurrent use if possible; otherwise, monitor PT closely and decrease anticoagulant drug dose as needed.

- Alcohol: inhibits alcohol metabolism, causing a disulfiram-like reaction (flushing, headache, nausea, vomiting, abdominal cramps, diaphoresis). Avoid alcohol and alcohol-containing medications for 48 hours after last metronidazole dose.
- Disulfiram: causes acute psychoses and confusion. Avoid concurrent use and separate use by 2 weeks.
- Phenobarbital/phenytoin: decrease metronidazole activity. Monitor effectiveness and increase metronidazole dose as needed.
- Cimetidine: increases metronidazole levels with potential for increased toxicity. Avoid concurrent administration.

Lab Effects/Interference:

- Serum ALT, serum AST, and LDH: metronidazole has a high absorbance at the wavelength at which NADH is determined; therefore, elevated liver enzyme concentrations may appear to be suppressed by metronidazole when measured by continuous-flow methods based on endpoint decrease.

Special Considerations:

- Carcinogenic in rodents, so drug is used only when necessary.
- Contraindicated in first trimester of pregnancy and administered only as salvage therapy in second and third trimesters when other agents have failed; lactating mothers should interrupt breast-feeding during treatment with drug.
- Use with caution in patients with a history of blood dyscrasias, CNS disorders/dysfunction, hepatic dysfunction, or alcoholism.
- May interfere with laboratory determinations of LFTs (AST, ALT, LDH).

Potential Toxicities/Side Effects and the Nursing Process

I. ALTERATION IN NUTRITION, LESS THAN BODY REQUIREMENTS, related to GI SIDE EFFECTS

Defining Characteristics: Nausea (with/without headache), anorexia, dry mouth, metallic taste in mouth have occurred; less frequently, vomiting, diarrhea, epigastric distress, or constipation. Rare pseudomembranous colitis.

Nursing Implications: Assess baseline nutritional and elimination status. Instruct patient to report GI disturbances. Administer and teach patient to self-administer antiemetics, antidiarrheals as needed and as ordered. Teach patient importance of nutritious diet, and suggest small, frequent, high-calorie, high-protein meals as appropriate. Assess baseline LFTs and monitor periodically during treatment. Discuss abnormalities and drug interruption with physician. Assess whether taking other hepatotoxic drugs (see Special Considerations section). Instruct patient to avoid alcohol and alcohol-containing medications for 48 hours after last drug dose.

II. ALTERATIONS IN SENSORY/PERCEPTUAL PATTERNS related to PERIPHERAL NEUROPATHY

Defining Characteristics: Peripheral neuropathy (numbness, tingling, paresthesia) is reversible with drug discontinuance. Headache, dizziness, ataxia, confusion, mood changes have also occurred.

Nursing Implications: Assess baseline neurologic function and comfort, and monitor during treatment. Instruct patient to report any changes. Discuss abnormalities and drug discontinuance with physician.

III. ALTERATIONS IN SKIN INTEGRITY related to SENSITIVITY REACTIONS

Defining Characteristics: Urticaria, erythematous rash, pruritus, flushing, transient joint pain may occur.

Nursing Implications: Assess drug allergy history. Assess baseline skin integrity. Instruct patient to report rash, pruritus. Teach patient symptomatic management of rash, pruritus.

IV. ALTERATIONS IN URINARY ELIMINATION related to DYSURIA

Defining Characteristics: Urethral burning, dysuria, cystitis, polyuria, incontinence, sensation of pelvic pressure may occur with oral dose. Urine may be dark or reddish-brown.

Nursing Implications: Assess baseline elimination status. Instruct patient to report side effects, and to increase oral fluids to 2–3 qt/day. Reassure patient urine color change is related to drug and will disappear when drug therapy is completed.

V. ALTERATIONS IN SEXUALITY related to DECREASED LIBIDO, DYSPAREUNIA

Defining Characteristics: Decreased libido, dyspareunia, dryness of vagina and vulva may occur.

Nursing Implications: Assess pattern of sexuality. Inform patient and partner that these effects, if they occur, are temporary. Suggest frequent perineal hygiene as needed to relieve dryness and use of lubricants during intercourse.

VI. FUNGAL SUPERINFECTION related to REDISTRIBUTION OF ENDOGENOUS MICROORGANISMS

Defining Characteristics: Vaginal candidiasis, vaginitis may occur as endogenous bacteria are eliminated and normal fungal population expands.

Nursing Implications: Instruct female patient to report vaginal itching or discharge. Discuss appropriate antifungal treatment with physician. Teach perineal hygiene and symptomatic management.

VII. ALTERATIONS IN COMFORT related to PHLEBITIS

Defining Characteristics: Phlebitis and thrombophlebitis may occur with IV administration.

Nursing Implications: Assess IV site prior to each dose for phlebitis, erythema, swelling, and change site at least q 48 h. Apply heat to painful IV site as ordered.

Drug: mezlocillin sodium (Mezlin)

Class: Antibacterial (extended spectrum penicillin).

Mechanism of Action: Semisynthetic antibiotic prepared from fungus *Penicillium*. Contains β-lactam ring and is bactericidal by inhibiting cell wall synthesis. Active against most gram-positive (except penicillinase-producing strains) and most gram-negative bacilli. Used in the treatment of serious gram-negative infections, especially *P. aeruginosa*–related infections of lower respiratory tract, urinary tract, and skin.

Metabolism: Poorly absorbed from GI tract, so must be given parenterally. Widely distributed in body tissues and fluids. Crosses placenta and is excreted in breast milk. Excreted via urine and bile.

Dosage/Range:

Adult:

- IV: 200–300 mg/kg/day in four to six divided doses (usual dose 3 g q 4–6 h).
- Dose modification if severe renal insufficiency; refer to manufacturer's package insert.

Drug Preparation:

- IV: Reconstitute each gram with at least 10 mL sterile water for injection. Further dilute in 50–100 mL 0.9% sodium chloride or 5% dextrose injection. Administer over 30 minutes.

- IM: Reconstitute each gram with 3–4 mL sterile water for injection or 0.5–1% lidocaine HCl (without epinephrine). Maximum dose is 2 g. Divide dose into two injections, as needed, and administer deep IM in large muscle mass. Administer slowly. Make certain patient is NOT ALLERGIC to lidocaine.

Drug Interactions:
- Aminoglycosides: synergism.
- Aminoglycosides (e.g., gentamicin): incompatible when mixed together; administer at separate sites at different times. Also, penicillinase-resistant penicillins can inactivate aminoglycoside serum samples from patients receiving both drugs.
- Clavulanic acid (inhibits β-lactamase): increases antibacterial action.
- Probenecid: increased serum level of mezlocillin; may be coadministered to exert this effect.

Lab Effects/Interference:
Major clinical significance:
- Urine glucose: high urinary concentrations of a penicillin may produce false-positive or falsely elevated test results with copper sulfate tests (Benedict's, Clinitest, or Fehling's); glucose enzymatic tests (Clinistix or Testape) are not affected.

Clinical significance:
- Coombs' (direct antiglobulin) test: false-positive result may occur during therapy with any penicillin.
- Urine protein: high urinary concentrations of mezlocillin may produce false-positive protein reactions (pseudoproteinuria) with the sulfosalicylic acid and boiling test, the acetic acid test, the biuret reaction, and the nitric acid test; bromophenol blue reagent test strips (Multistix) are reportedly unaffected.
- ALT, alk phos, AST, serum LDH values may be increased.
- Serum bili: an increase has been associated with mezlocillin.
- BUN and serum creatinine: an increase has been associated with mezlocillin.
- Serum K+: hypokalemia may occur following the administration of parenteral mezlocillin, which may act as a non-reabsorbable anion in the distal renal tubules; this may cause an increase in pH and result in increased urinary K+ loss. The risk of hypokalemia increases with the use of larger doses.
- Serum Na+: hypernatremia may occur following administration of large doses of parenteral mezlocillin because of the high Na+ content of these medications.
- WBC: leukopenia or neutropenia is associated with the use of all penicillins; the effect is more likely to occur with prolonged therapy and severe hepatic function impairment.

Special Considerations:
- Contraindicated in patients with prior hypersensitivity to penicillins. Use with caution in patients sensitive to other β-lactams (e.g., cephalosporins) since partial cross-allergenicity exists.

- Obtain ordered specimen, and send for culture and sensitivity test prior to first antibiotic dose.
- Consider alternative antibiotic therapy if eosinophilia, drug fever or rash, arthralgia, hematuria, or unexplained rise in BUN and serum creatinine occur.
- Monitor electrolytes and renal, hepatic, and hematologic laboratory parameters during extended treatment periods.
- Use with caution in pregnancy or with nursing women.
- Na content is 1.85 mEq/g of drug.

Potential Toxicities/Side Effects and the Nursing Process

I. POTENTIAL FOR INJURY related to HYPERSENSITIVITY REACTION

Defining Characteristics: Urticaria, pruritus, rash (maculopapular or erythematous), fever and chills, eosinophilia, myalgia, edema, erythema, angioedema, Stevens-Johnson syndrome, and exfoliative skin reactions occur in 5% of patients. Increased risk in individuals allergic to cephalosporin antibiotics.

Nursing Implications: Assess allergy to cephalosporin antibiotics and penicillin: if patient states "yes," determine actual response, e.g., "swollen lips = angioedema." If angioedema, patient SHOULD NOT receive drug. Discuss other patient responses with physician to determine whether drug should be given. Assess baseline skin condition, including integrity and allergy history to drugs. Instruct patient to report rash, itching, and other skin changes. Teach patient skin care and symptomatic measures as appropriate. If skin rash develops, discuss drug discontinuance with physician. If rash progresses, drug should be discontinued, as fatal Stevens-Johnson syndrome may develop. Be prepared to treat severe acute hypersensitivity reactions with airway management, oxygen, epinephrine, corticosteroids, antihistamines as ordered.

II. ALTERATION IN NUTRITION, LESS THAN BODY REQUIREMENTS, related to GI SIDE EFFECTS

Defining Characteristics: Nausea, vomiting, diarrhea may occur; rarely, pseudomembranous colitis caused by *C. difficile* resistant to the antibiotic occurs. Rarely, transient increases in LFTs—AST, ALT, alk phos, bili—may occur.

Nursing Implications: Assess baseline nutritional status. Instruct patient to report GI disturbances. Administer and teach patient to self-administer antiemetics as needed and as ordered. Teach patient importance of nutritious diet, and suggest small, frequent, high-calorie, high-protein meals as appropriate. Assess baseline LFTs, and monitor periodically during treatment. Discuss abnormalities and drug interruption with physician.

III. FUNGAL SUPERINFECTION related to REDISTRIBUTION OF ENDOGENOUS MICROORGANISMS

Defining Characteristics: Vaginal candidiasis, vaginitis may occur as endogenous bacteria are eliminated and normal fungal population expands.

Nursing Implications: Instruct female patient to report vaginal itching or discharge. Discuss appropriate antifungal treatment with physician. Teach perineal hygiene and symptomatic management.

IV. ALTERATIONS IN PROTECTIVE MECHANISMS (RARE) related to TRANSIENT LEUKOPENIA

Defining Characteristics: Rarely, transient leukopenia, lymphocytosis, anemia, eosinophilia may occur. Prolonged PT, prolonged APTT, and hypoprothrombinemia have occurred rarely, especially in elderly or debilitated patients, or in individuals with vitamin K deficiency.

Nursing Implications: Assess baseline laboratory parameters, and monitor periodically during treatment. Assess patient for response to antibiotics. Discuss abnormalities with physician. Assess for signs/symptoms of bleeding.

V. ALTERATIONS IN SENSORY/PERCEPTUAL PATTERNS related to DIZZINESS, SOMNOLENCE

Defining Characteristics: Dizziness, headache, somnolence occur rarely. Neuromuscular irritability and seizures may occur with high drug serum levels.

Nursing Implications: Assess baseline neurologic function and comfort, and monitor during treatment. Instruct patient to report any changes. Discuss any abnormalities with physician. Institute seizure precautions.

VI. ALTERATIONS IN COMFORT related to LOCAL INJECTION IRRITATION

Defining Characteristics: Vein irritation (pain, erythema), phlebitis, and thrombophlebitis may occur at IV administration site.

Nursing Implications: Change IV sites q 48 h, and assess for signs/symptoms of phlebitis prior to each administration. Administer drug slowly. Apply warm packs to increase comfort. Discuss central line with patient and physician to facilitate administration.

VII. ALTERATION IN FLUID AND ELECTROLYTE BALANCE related to HYPOKALEMIA AND INCREASED SODIUM INTAKE

Defining Characteristics: Prolonged therapy may cause hypokalemia; also, drug is prepared as sodium salt. Frequent IV infusions increase fluid intake.

Nursing Implications: Assess baseline electrolytes, fluid balance, weight, and monitor throughout therapy. Monitor renal function studies, especially if patient has preexisting renal dysfunction.

Drug: minocycline hydrochloride (Minocin, Vectrin, Dynacin)

Class: Antibacterial (systemic); antiprotozoal.

Mechanism of Action: Bacteriostatic, but may be bactericidal at high concentrations. Binds to bacterial ribosomes and prevents protein synthesis. Active against broad range of gram-positive and gram-negative bacteria, Chlamydia, and Mycoplasma.

Metabolism: Absorbed (60%–80%) from GI tract. Widely distributed into body tissues and fluids. Crosses placenta and is excreted in breast milk. Excreted unchanged in urine.

Dosage/Range:

Adult:

- Oral: 200 mg initially, then 100 mg q 12 h for 5–15 days; or 100–200 mg initially, then 50 mg q 6 h for 5–15 days.
- IV: 200 mg initially, then 100 mg q 12 h for 5–15 days (depends on indication).
- Dose modification necessary if renal dysfunction exists.

Drug Preparation:

- Oral: may be taken with food, water, or milk.
- IV: add 5–10 mL sterile water for injection to 100-mg vial. Further dilute in 500 to 1000 mL of 0.9% sodium chloride injection, dextrose injection, dextrose and sodium chloride injections, Ringer's injection, or lactated Ringer's injection. Do not use other calcium-containing solutions, since precipitate may form.
- AVOID RAPID ADMINISTRATION.
- Solution stable for 24 hours at room temperature. Avoid exposure to heat or sunlight. Convert to oral preparation as soon as possible, as there is risk of thrombophlebitis.
- DO NOT ADMINISTER INTRAMUSCULARLY or SUBCUTANEOUSLY.

Drug Interactions:

- Hepatotoxic drugs: may increase hepatotoxicity if given concurrently. Assess baseline and periodically during treatment.
- Iron preparations: decrease oral and possibly IV absorption. Administer iron preparations 3 hours after or 2 hours before any tetracycline.

- Oral anticoagulants: increase PT. Monitor patient closely and decrease anticoagulant dose as needed.
- Antidiarrheals (containing kaolin, pectate, or bismuth): may decrease absorption of tetracyclines. Avoid concurrent use.
- Oral contraceptives: decreased effectiveness of contraceptive and increased incidence of breakthrough bleeding. Advise patient to use barrier contraceptive as well during a course of tetracycline therapy.
- Lithium: may decrease lithium levels. Monitor serum levels and increase dose as needed.

Lab Effects/Interference:
- Urine catecholamine determinations: may produce false elevations of urinary catecholamines because of interfering fluorescence in the Hingerty method.
- SGPT, alk phos, amylase, SGOT, and bilirubin: serum concentrations may be increased.

Special Considerations:
- May cause dizziness, lightheadedness, or unsteadiness (CNS toxicity).
- Pigmentation of skin and mucous membranes may occur.
- Use cautiously in patients with myasthenia gravis: may increase muscle weakness.
- Avoid use in pregnant or lactating women.
- Obtain ordered specimen for culture and sensitivity prior to first dose.
- IV preparation contains ascorbic acid and may cause false-positive result using Clinitest, or false-negative when using Clinistix and Testape.
- Drug has affinity for ischemic, necrotic tissue, and may localize in tumors.

Potential Toxicities/Side Effects and the Nursing Process

I. ALTERATION IN NUTRITION related to GI SIDE EFFECTS

Defining Characteristics: Nausea, vomiting, diarrhea, anorexia, abdominal discomfort, epigastric burning and distress, glossitis, black hairy tongue may occur.

Nursing Implications: Assess baseline nutritional status. Assess for and teach patient to report any symptoms. Administer and teach patient self-administration of prescribed antiemetic or antidiarrheal medication as appropriate. Administer and teach patient to self-administer oral dose with at least 8 oz of water taken at least 1 hour before lying down for sleep.

II. ALTERATION IN SKIN INTEGRITY related to RASH, PHOTOSENSITIVITY

Defining Characteristics: Maculopapular and erythematous rashes may occur. Rarely, exfoliative dermatitis, onycholysis, and nail discoloration. Photosensitivity risk (exaggerated sunburn) persists 1–2 days after completion of drug therapy.

Nursing Implications: Teach patient about potential side effects, to avoid sunlight during drug therapy, and to report rash, other abnormalities. Teach symptomatic skin care as appropriate.

III. INJURY related to HYPERSENSITIVITY

Defining Characteristics: Urticaria, angioneurotic edema, anaphylaxis may occur; also, fever, rash, arthralgias, eosinophilia, and pericarditis.

Nursing Implications: Assess drug allergy history. Assess baseline allergy history. Assess baseline skin integrity. Teach patient to report rash, pruritus. Teach patent symptomatic management of rash, pruritus. Assess for hypersensitivity reaction; if it occurs, monitor VS, discontinue drug, notify physician, and institute supportive measures.

IV. FUNGAL SUPERINFECTION related to REDISTRIBUTION OF ENDOGENOUS MICROORGANISMS

Defining Characteristics: Vaginal moniliasis, vaginitis may occur as endogenous bacteria are eliminated and normal fungal population expands.

Nursing Implications: Teach female patient to report vaginal itching or discharge. Discuss appropriate antifungal treatment with physician. Teach perineal hygiene and symptomatic management.

V. ALTERATION IN HEPATIC FUNCTION

Defining Characteristics: Associated with high IV doses (> 2 g/day): hepatotoxicity and cholestasis may occur.

Nursing Implications: Assess baseline LFTs and monitor during therapy.

VI. INFECTION AND BLEEDING related to NEUTROPENIA, THROMBOCYTOPENIA

Defining Characteristics: Neutropenia, leukocytosis, leukopenia, atypical lymphocytes, thrombocytopenia, thrombocytopenic purpura, hemolytic anemia occur rarely with long-term therapy.

Nursing Implications: Assess baseline WBC, HCT, and platelets, and monitor periodically during long-term therapy.

VII. ALTERATION IN COMFORT related to LOCAL ADMINISTRATION EFFECTS

Defining Characteristics: IM administration may cause pain, induration due to muscle injury. IV administration may cause erythema, pain, swelling, and thrombophlebitis.

Nursing Implications: Rotate sites. Apply ice as ordered to painful buttock. Assess IV site prior to each dose for phlebitis or swelling, and change site at least q 48 h. Apply heat to painful IV sites as ordered.

VIII. SENSORY/PERCEPTUAL ALTERATION

Defining Characteristics: Light-headedness, dizziness, headache may occur.

Nursing Implications: Assess baseline neurological status. Teach patient to report any changes and discuss them with physician.

Drug: moxifloxacin (ABC Pack; Avelox)

Class: Antibiotic; Quinolone.

Mechanism of Action: Moxifloxacin is a broad-spectrum anti-infective, active against a wide range of aerobic gram-positive and gram-negative organisms. Acts intracellularly by inhibiting DNA gyrase and bacterial topoisomerase IV. DNA gyrase is required for DNA replication and transcription, DNA repair, recombination, and transposition; inhibition is bactericidal.

Metabolism: Widely distributed to most body fluids and tissues with highest concentrations in organs, such as kidneys, gallbladder, lungs, liver, gynecological tissue, prostatic tissue, phagocytic cells, urine, sputum, and bile. Well absorbed from GI tract. Metabolized in liver; excreted in urine and feces. Crosses placenta and is excreted in breast milk.

Dosage/Range:
- 400 mg PO or IV daily.

Drug Preparation:
- Oral: Take drug with large glass of water, preferably 2 hours after meal/food. Encourage oral fluids of 2–3 qt/day.
- IV: Further dilute drug in 0.9% sodium chloride or 5% dextrose in water to final concentration of 2 mg/mL. Administer over 60 minutes, do not infuse by rapid or bolus intravenous infusion.
- Do not refrigerate.

Drug Interactions:

- Antacids (containing magnesium, aluminum, or calcium) and iron decrease absorption of serum level of moxifloxacin; do not administer concurrently. If must administer antacids or iron, administer at least 4 hours apart. The administration of antacids containing aluminum, magnesium, calcium, sucralfate, zinc, or iron may substantially reduce the absorption of moxifloxacin; do not administer concurrently.
- Serum digoxin concentrations should be monitored; moxifloxacin may raise serum levels in some patients.
- Probenecid: decreases the renal tubular secretion of moxifloxacin, resulting in a prolonged elimination half-life and increased risk of toxicity.
- Moxifloxacin may have the potential to prolong the Q-T interval of the EKG in some patients. Moxifloxacin should not be used in patients with prolonged Q-T interval; patients with uncorrected hypokalemia; and patients on quinidine, procainamide, amiodarone, and sotalol (antiarrhythmic agents).
- Increased intracranial pressure and psychosis has been reported along with CNS stimulation.
- Hypersensitivity reactions have been reported.

Lab Effects/Interference:

- Serum SGPT, serum alk phos, serum SGOT, and serum LDH—values may be increased.

Special Considerations:

- Used in the treatment of respiratory tract infections (acute bacterial exacerbation of chronic bronchitis, acute bacterial sinusitis, and commonly acquired pneumonia).
- Used in the treatment of uncomplicated infections of the skin and skin structures.
- Contraindicated in pregnancy or women who are breast-feeding.
- Obtain ordered specimen for culture and sensitivity prior to first drug dose.
- Use cautiously in patients with seizure disorders.

Potential Toxicities/Side Effects and the Nursing Process

I. ALTERATION IN NUTRITION related to GI SIDE EFFECTS

Defining Characteristics: Incidence of nausea, vomiting, abdominal discomfort, diarrhea, anorexia.

Nursing Implications: Assess baseline nutritional and elimination status. Teach patient to report GI disturbances. Administer and teach patient to self-administer antiemetics, antidiarrheals as needed and as ordered. Teach patient importance of nutritious diet, and suggest small, frequent, high-calorie, high-protein meals as appropriate. Assess baseline LFTs and monitor periodically during treatment. Discuss abnormalities and drug interruption with physician.

II. SENSORY/PERCEPTUAL ALTERATIONS related to CNS EFFECTS

Defining Characteristics: Incidence of headache, restlessness. Dizziness, hallucinations, and seizures may also occur. Exacerbated by caffeine as quinolones delay caffeine excretion.

Nursing Implications: Assess baseline neurological function and comfort, and monitor during treatment. Teach patient to report any changes. Discuss any abnormalities with physician. Teach patient to limit or restrict all caffeine-containing fluids, medications, e.g., tea, coffee, soft drinks.

III. ALTERATION IN SKIN INTEGRITY related to ALLERGY/HYPERSENSITIVITY

Defining Characteristics: Incidence of rash; other manifestations include eosinophilia, urticaria, flushing, fever, chills, photosensitivity, angioedema. Fatal hypersensitivity reactions have occurred rarely. Direct exposure to sunlight can cause sunburn (moderate to severe phototoxicity).

Nursing Implications: Assess baseline skin condition, including integrity and drug allergy history. Teach patient to report rash, itching, and other skin changes. Teach patient skin care and symptomatic measures as appropriate. If skin rash develops, discuss drug discontinuance with physician. Be prepared to treat severe acute hypersensitivity reactions with airway management, oxygen, epinephrine, corticosteroids, antihistamines as ordered. Teach patient to avoid excessive sun exposure and to use skin protection factor (SPF) 15 or higher. If rash progresses, especially in HIV-infected patients, drug should be discontinued as fatal Stevens-Johnson syndrome may develop.

IV. FUNGAL SUPERINFECTION related to REDISTRIBUTION OF ENDOGENOUS MICROORGANISMS

Defining Characteristics: Vaginal moniliasis, vaginitis may occur as endogenous bacteria are eliminated and normal fungal population expands.

Nursing Implications: Teach female patient to report vaginal itching or discharge. Discuss appropriate antifungal treatment with physician. Teach perineal hygiene and symptomatic management.

V. ALTERATION IN URINARY ELIMINATION related to RENAL TOXICITY

Defining Characteristics: Increased BUN and creatinine, crystal and stone formation in urine, interstitial nephritis, and renal failure may occur.

Nursing Implications: Assess baseline renal function; expect that drug dose will be decreased in presence of renal dysfunction. Teach patient to take drug with at least 8 oz of water, and to increase oral fluids to 2–3 qt/day.

VI. ALTERATION IN COMFORT related to LOCAL ADMINISTRATION

Defining Characteristics: Drug may cause pain, inflammation, and rare thrombophlebitis at IV site.

Nursing Implications: Change IV site q 48 hours. Assess for phlebitis, discomfort, and IV patency prior to each administration. Administer drug slowly over 60–90 minutes in large volume of 5% dextrose (see Drug Preparation). Apply heat to promote comfort.

Drug: nafcillin sodium (Unipen)

Class: Antibacterial (systemic).

Mechanism of Action: Semisynthetic antibiotic. Contains β-lactam ring and is bactericidal by inhibiting cell wall synthesis. Penicillinase-resistant penicillin; active against penicillin-resistant staphylococci that produce the enzyme penicillinase.

Metabolism: Incompletely absorbed from GI tract; rapidly absorbed when given IM or IV. Widely distributed in body tissues and fluid, including bile. Crosses placenta and is excreted in breast milk; 70–90% bound to serum proteins. Metabolized in liver, excreted in bile, and to a lesser degree in the urine.

Dosage/Range:
Adult:
- Oral: 500 mg–1 g PO q 6 h.
- IM/IV: 500 mg–2 g q 4 h.

Drug Preparation:
- Oral: Reconstitute per manufacturer's recommendation or by capsules or tablets. Administer 1 hour before meals or 2 hours after meals.
- IM: Reconstitute with sterile or bacteriostatic water for injection, and give deep IM in large muscle (e.g., gluteus maximus).
- IV: Reconstitute with sterile water for injection or 0.9% sodium chloride for injection according to manufacturer's package insert. Further dilute in 100 mL IV solution and infuse over 40–60 minutes.

Drug Interactions:

- Aminoglycosides: synergism.
- Aminoglycosides (e.g., gentamicin): incompatible when mixed together; administer at separate sites at different times. Also, penicillinase-resistant penicillins can inactivate aminoglycoside serum samples from patients receiving both drugs.
- Rifampin: possible antagonism, only at high doses of penicillin.
- Probenecid: increased serum level of nafcillin; may be coadministered to exert this effect.

Lab Effects/Interference:

Major clinical significance:

- Urine glucose: high urinary concentrations of a penicillin may produce false-positive or falsely elevated test results with copper sulfate tests (Benedict's, Clinitest, or Fehling's); glucose enzymatic tests (Clinistix or Testape) are not affected.

Clinical significance:

- Coombs' (direct antiglobulin) test: false-positive result may occur during therapy with any penicillin.
- ALT, alk phos, AST, serum LDH: values may be increased.
- WBC: leukopenia or neutropenia is associated with the use of all penicillins; the effect is more likely to occur with prolonged therapy and severe hepatic function impairment.

Special Considerations:

- Contraindicated in patients with prior hypersensitivity to penicillins. Use with caution in patients sensitive to other β-lactams (e.g., cephalosporins) since partial cross-allergenicity exists.
- Obtain ordered specimen and send for culture and sensitivity prior to first antibiotic dose.
- Consider alternative antibiotic therapy if eosinophilia, drug fever or rash, arthralgia, hematuria, or unexplained rise in BUN and serum creatinine occur.
- Monitor electrolytes and renal, hepatic, and hematologic laboratory parameters during extended treatment periods.
- Use with caution in pregnancy or with nursing women.

Potential Toxicities/Side Effects and the Nursing Process

I. POTENTIAL FOR INJURY related to HYPERSENSITIVITY REACTION

Defining Characteristics: Urticaria, pruritus, rash (maculopapular or erythematous), fever and chills, eosinophilia, myalgia, edema, erythema, angioedema, Stevens-Johnson syndrome, and exfoliative skin reactions occur in 5% of patients. Increased risk in individuals allergic to cephalosporin antibiotics.

Nursing Implications: Assess allergy to cephalosporin antibiotics and penicillin: if patient states "yes," determine actual response, e.g., "swollen lips = angioedema."

If angioedema, patient SHOULD NOT receive drug. Discuss other patient responses with physician to determine whether drug should be given. Assess baseline skin condition, including integrity and allergy history to drugs. Instruct patient to report rash, itching, other skin changes. Teach patient skin care and symptomatic measures as appropriate. If skin rash develops, discuss drug discontinuance with physician. If rash progresses, drug should be discontinued, as fatal Stevens-Johnson syndrome may develop. Be prepared to treat severe acute hypersensitivity reactions with airway management, oxygen, epinephrine, corticosteroids, antihistamines as ordered.

II. ALTERATION IN NUTRITION, LESS THAN BODY REQUIREMENTS, related to GI SIDE EFFECTS

Defining Characteristics: Nausea, vomiting, diarrhea may occur; rarely, pseudomembranous colitis caused by *C. difficile* resistant to the antibiotic occurs. Rarely, transient increases in LFTs—AST, ALT, alk phos, bili—may occur.

Nursing Implications: Assess baseline nutritional status. Instruct patient to report GI disturbances. Administer and teach patient to self-administer antiemetics, antidiarrheals as needed and as ordered. Teach patient importance of nutritious diet, and suggest small, frequent, high-calorie, high-protein meals as appropriate. Assess baseline LFTs and monitor periodically during treatment. Discuss abnormalities and drug interruption with physician.

III. FUNGAL SUPERINFECTION related to REDISTRIBUTION OF ENDOGENOUS MICROORGANISMS

Defining Characteristics: Vaginal candidiasis, vaginitis may occur as endogenous bacteria are eliminated and normal fungal population expands.

Nursing Implications: Instruct female patient to report vaginal itching or discharge. Discuss appropriate antifungal treatment with physician. Teach perineal hygiene and symptomatic management.

IV. ALTERATIONS IN PROTECTIVE MECHANISMS (RARE) related to TRANSIENT LEUKOPENIA

Defining Characteristics: Rarely, transient leukopenia, lymphocytosis, anemia, eosinophilia may occur. Prolonged PT, prolonged APTT, and hypoprothrombinemia have occurred rarely, especially in elderly or debilitated patients, or in individuals with vitamin K deficiency.

Nursing Implications: Assess baseline laboratory parameters, and monitor periodically during treatment. Assess patient for response to antibiotics. Discuss abnormalities with physician.

V. ALTERATIONS IN COMFORT related to PHLEBITIS

Defining Characteristics: Phlebitis and thrombophlebitis may occur with IV administration. Increased risk in elderly.

Nursing Implications: Assess IV site prior to each dose for phlebitis, erythema, swelling, and change site at least q 48 h. Apply heat to painful IV site as ordered.

Drug: oxacillin sodium (Bactocill, Prostaphlin)

Class: Antibacterial (systemic).

Mechanism of Action: Semisynthetic antibiotic. Contains β-lactam ring and is bactericidal by inhibiting cell wall synthesis. Penicillinase-resistant penicillin and active against penicillin-resistant staphylococci, which produce the enzyme penicillinase.

Metabolism: Incompletely absorbed from GI tract; rapidly absorbed when given IM or IV. Widely distributed in body tissues and fluid, including bile. Crosses placenta and is excreted in breast milk; 89–94% bound to serum proteins. Metabolized in liver, excreted in urine.

Dosage/Range:

Adult:

- Oral: 500 mg–1 g PO q 6 h.
- IM/IV: 500 mg–2 g q 4 h.

Drug Preparation:

- Oral: Reconstitute per manufacturer's package insert or by capsules or tablets. Administer 1 hour before meals or 2 hours after meals.
- IM: Reconstitute with sterile or bacteriostatic water for injection, and give deep IM in large muscle (e.g., gluteus maximus).
- IV: Reconstitute with sterile water for injection or 0.9% sodium chloride for injection according to manufacturer's package insert. Further dilute in 100 mL IV solution and infuse over 40–60 minutes.

Drug Interactions:

- Aminoglycosides: synergism.
- Aminoglycosides (e.g., gentamicin): incompatible when mixed together; administer at separate sites at different times. Also, penicillinase-resistant penicillins can inactivate aminoglycoside serum samples from patients receiving both drugs.
- Rifampin: possible antagonism, only at high doses of oxacillin.
- Probenecid: increased serum level of oxacillin; may be coadministered to exert this effect.

Lab Effects/Interference:

Major clinical significance:

- Urine glucose: high urinary concentrations of a penicillin may produce false-positive or falsely elevated test results with copper sulfate tests (Benedict's, Clinitest, or Fehling's); glucose enzymatic tests (Clinistix or Testape) are not affected.

Clinical significance:

- Coombs' (direct antiglobulin) test: false-positive result may occur during therapy with any penicillin.
- ALT, alk phos, AST, serum LDH values may be increased.
- WBC: leukopenia or neutropenia is associated with the use of all penicillins; the effect is more likely to occur with prolonged therapy and severe hepatic function impairment.

Special Considerations:

- Contraindicated in patients with prior hypersensitivity to penicillins. Use with caution in patients sensitive to other β-lactams (e.g., cephalosporins) since partial cross-allergenicity.
- Obtain ordered specimen and send for culture and sensitivity prior to first antibiotic dose.
- Consider alternative antibiotic therapy if eosinophilia, drug fever or rash, arthralgia, hematuria, or unexplained rise in BUN and serum creatinine occur.
- Monitor electrolytes and renal, hepatic, and hematologic laboratory parameters during extended treatment periods.
- Use with caution in pregnant or nursing women.

Potential Toxicities/Side Effects and the Nursing Process

I. POTENTIAL FOR INJURY related to HYPERSENSITIVITY REACTION

Defining Characteristics: Urticaria, pruritus, rash (maculopapular or erythematous), fever and chills, eosinophilia, myalgia, edema, erythema, angioedema, Stevens-Johnson syndrome, and exfoliative skin reactions occur in 5% of patients. Increased risk in individuals allergic to cephalosporin antibiotics.

Nursing Implications: Assess allergy to cephalosporin antibiotics and penicillin: if patient states "yes," determine actual response, e.g., "swollen lips = angioedema." If angioedema, patient SHOULD NOT receive drug. Discuss other patient responses with physician to determine whether drug should be given. Assess baseline skin condition, including integrity and allergy history to drugs. Instruct patient to report rash, itching, and other skin changes. Teach patient skin care and symptomatic measures as appropriate. If skin rash develops, discuss drug discontinuance with physician. If rash progresses, drug should be discontinued, as fatal Stevens-Johnson syndrome may develop. Be prepared to treat severe acute hypersensitivity reactions with airway management, oxygen, epinephrine, corticosteroids, antihistamines as ordered.

II. ALTERATION IN NUTRITION, LESS THAN BODY REQUIREMENTS, related to INCREASED LFTs

Defining Characteristics: Oral lesions may occur, as may hepatitis (rare) and increased LFTs.

Nursing Implications: Assess baseline oral mucosa, and LFTs—AST, ALT, alk phos, bili. Teach patient to practice oral hygiene after meals and at bedtime, and instruct to report any oral lesions. Monitor LFTs periodically during treatment, and discuss abnormalities with physician.

III. FUNGAL SUPERINFECTION related to REDISTRIBUTION OF ENDOGENOUS MICROORGANISMS

Defining Characteristics: Vaginal candidiasis, vaginitis may occur as endogenous bacteria are eliminated and normal fungal population expands.

Nursing Implications: Instruct female patient to report vaginal itching or discharge. Discuss appropriate antifungal treatment with physician. Teach perineal hygiene and symptomatic management.

IV. ALTERATIONS IN PROTECTIVE MECHANISMS (RARE) related to TRANSIENT LEUKOPENIA

Defining Characteristics: Rarely, transient leukopenia, lymphocytosis, anemia, eosinophilia may occur. Prolonged PT, prolonged APTT, and hypoprothrombinemia have occurred rarely, especially in elderly or debilitated patients, or in individuals with vitamin K deficiency.

Nursing Implications: Assess baseline laboratory parameters, and monitor periodically during treatment. Assess patient for response to antibiotics. Discuss abnormalities with physician.

V. ALTERATIONS IN COMFORT related to PHLEBITIS

Defining Characteristics: Phlebitis and thrombophlebitis may occur with IV administration. Increased risk in elderly.

Nursing Implications: Assess IV site prior to each dose for phlebitis, erythema, swelling, and change site at least q 48 h. Apply heat to painful IV site as ordered.

VI. ALTERATIONS IN URINARY ELIMINATION related to RENAL DAMAGE

Defining Characteristics: Interstitial nephritis, transient proteinuria, hematuria may occur.

Nursing Implications: Assess baseline liver, renal function tests (e.g., serum BUN, creatinine, and urinalysis), and monitor during therapy.

VII. ALTERATIONS IN SENSORY/PERCEPTUAL PATTERNS related to NEUROPATHY

Defining Characteristics: Neuropathy, seizures, neuromuscular irritability may occur rarely.

Nursing Implications: Assess baseline neurologic function and comfort, and monitor during treatment. Instruct patient to report any changes. Discuss any abnormalities with physician.

Drug: penicillin G (PenG Potassium, PenG Sodium, Intravenous; PenVK, Oral Preparation)

Class: Natural penicillin.

Mechanism of Action: Produced by fermentation of *Penicillium chrysogenum*. Active against many gram-positive bacteria (streptococci, staphylococci) but resistant to *S. aureus* and *S. epidermidis* strains that produce penicillinases. Also active against some gram-negative bacteria (*Neisseria, H. influenzae*), and spirochetes.

Metabolism: Decreased oral absorption, but IM or IV absorption is quite rapid and complete. Widely distributed in body tissues and fluids; 45–68% bound to proteins. Eliminated in urine and bile.

Dosage/Range:
- Oral: 250–500 mg qid.
- IV: 200,000–4 million U q 4 h.
- Dose modification may be necessary in patients with renal impairment.

Drug Preparation:
- Oral: Administer at least 1 hour before or 2 hours after meals.
- IM: Reconstitute drug as directed. Administration of greater than 100,000 U is likely to result in some discomfort. Give IM deep in large muscle mass.
- IV: Reconstitute drug as directed. Further dilute in 0.9% sodium chloride or 5% dextrose in water, and administer over 1–2 hours.

Drug Interactions:
- Aminoglycosides: synergism.
- Aminoglycosides (e.g., gentamicin): incompatible when mixed together; administer at separate sites at different times. Also, penicillinase-resistant penicillins can inactivate aminoglycoside serum samples from patients receiving both drugs.
- Rifampin: possible antagonism, only at high doses of penicillin.

- Probenecid: increased serum level of penicillin; may be coadministered to exert this effect.

Lab Effects/Interference:
Major clinical significance:
- Urine glucose: high urinary concentrations of a penicillin may produce false-positive or falsely elevated test results with copper sulfate tests (Benedict's, Clinitest, or Fehling's); glucose enzymatic tests (Clinistix or Testape) are not affected.

Clinical significance:
- Coombs' (direct antiglobulin) test: false-positive result may occur during therapy with any penicillin.
- ALT, alk phos, AST, serum LDH values may be increased.
- Serum K+: hyperkalemia may occur following administration of parenteral penicillin G potassium because of the high potassium content.
- Serum Na+: hypernatremia may occur following administration of large doses of parenteral penicillin G sodium because of the high sodium content.
- WBC: leukopenia or neutropenia is associated with the use of all penicillins; the effect is more likely to occur with prolonged therapy and severe hepatic function impairment.

Special Considerations:
- Contraindicated in patients with prior hypersensitivity to penicillins. Use with caution in patients sensitive to other β-lactams (e.g., cephalosporins) since partial cross-allergenicity exists.
- Obtain ordered specimen and send for culture and sensitivity test prior to first antibiotic dose.
- Consider alternative antibiotic therapy if eosinophilia, drug fever or rash, arthralgia, hematuria, or unexplained rise in BUN and serum creatinine occur.
- Monitor electrolytes and renal, hepatic, and hematologic laboratory parameters during extended treatment periods.
- Hyperkalemia may occur with high dose therapy: monitor serum K+.
- Use with caution in pregnant or nursing women.
- Penicillin G benzathine should never be given IV (suspension); give IM only.

Potential Toxicities/Side Effects and the Nursing Process

I. POTENTIAL FOR INJURY related to HYPERSENSITIVITY REACTION

Defining Characteristics: Urticaria, pruritus, rash (maculopapular or erythematous), fever and chills, eosinophilia, myalgia, edema, erythema, angioedema, Stevens-Johnson syndrome, and exfoliative skin reactions occur in 5% of patients. Increased risk exists in individuals allergic to cephalosporin antibiotics.

Nursing Implications: Assess allergy to cephalosporin antibiotics and penicillin: if patient states "yes," determine actual response, e.g., "swollen lips = angioedema." If angioedema, patient SHOULD NOT receive drug. Discuss other patient responses with physician to determine whether drug should be given. Assess baseline skin condition, including integrity and allergy history to drugs. Instruct patient to report rash, itching, and other skin changes. Teach patient skin care and symptomatic measures as appropriate. If skin rash develops, discuss drug discontinuance with physician. If rash progresses, drug should be discontinued, as fatal Stevens-Johnson syndrome may develop. Be prepared to treat severe acute hypersensitivity reactions with airway management, oxygen, epinephrine, corticosteroids, antihistamines as ordered.

II. ALTERATION IN NUTRITION, LESS THAN BODY REQUIREMENTS, related to GI SIDE EFFECTS

Defining Characteristics: Rarely, nausea, vomiting, diarrhea, and pseudomembranous colitis caused by *C. difficile* resistant to the antibiotic may occur. Rarely, transient increases in LFTs—AST, ALT, alk phos, bili—may occur.

Nursing Implications: Assess baseline nutritional status. Instruct patient to report GI disturbances. Administer and teach patient to self-administer antiemetics as needed and as ordered. Teach patient importance of nutritious diet, and suggest small, frequent, high-calorie, high-protein meals as appropriate. Assess baseline LFTs and monitor periodically during treatment. Discuss abnormalities and drug interruption with physician.

III. FUNGAL SUPERINFECTION related to REDISTRIBUTION OF ENDOGENOUS MICROORGANISMS

Defining Characteristics: Vaginal candidiasis, vaginitis may occur as endogenous bacteria are eliminated and normal fungal population expands.

Nursing Implications: Instruct female patient to report vaginal itching or discharge. Discuss appropriate antifungal treatment with physician. Teach perineal hygiene and symptomatic management.

IV. ALTERATIONS IN PROTECTIVE MECHANISMS (RARE) related to RARE LEUKOPENIA

Defining Characteristics: Rarely, hemolytic anemia, leukopenia, thrombocytopenia may occur.

Nursing Implications: Assess baseline laboratory parameters, and monitor periodically during treatment. Assess patient for response to antibiotics. Discuss abnormalities with physician.

V. ALTERATIONS IN SENSORY/PERCEPTUAL PATTERNS related to NEUROPATHY

Defining Characteristics: Neuropathy, seizures may occur with high doses.

Nursing Implications: Assess baseline neurologic function and comfort, and monitor during treatment. Instruct patient to report any changes. Discuss any abnormalities with physician.

VI. ALTERATIONS IN COMFORT related to LOCAL INJECTION IRRITATION

Defining Characteristics: Pain, induration may form in IM injection sites; phlebitis may develop in IV sites.

Nursing Implications: Rotate IM injection sites, and administer drug deep IM in large muscle mass (e.g., gluteus maximus). Use IM injection when IV administration is not possible. Change IV sites q 48 h, and assess for signs/symptoms of phlebitis prior to each administration. Administer drug slowly. Apply warm packs to increase comfort.

Drug: piperacillin sodium (Pipracil); combined with tazobactam sodium (Zosyn)

Class: Antibacterial (systemic) (extended-spectrum penicillin).

Mechanism of Action: Semisynthetic antibiotic prepared from fungus *Penicillium*. Contains β-lactam ring and is bactericidal by inhibiting cell wall synthesis. Active against most gram-positive (except penicillinase-producing strains) and most gram-negative bacilli. Used in the treatment of serious gram-negative infections, especially *P. aeruginosa*–related infections of lower respiratory tract, urinary tract, and skin. When combined with tazobactam sodium, which inhibits β-lactamases, piperacillin sodium is effective against resistant bacteria.

Metabolism: Poorly absorbed from GI tract, so must be given parenterally. Widely distributed in body tissues and fluids. Crosses placenta and is excreted in breast milk. Excreted via urine and bile.

Dosage/Range:
- IV route preferred.

Adult:

Piperacillin sodium:
- IV: 3–4 g q 4–6 h (maximum 24 g, but higher doses may be used in severe infection); IM: maximum 2 g/per dose.

Zosyn:
- 3 g piperacillin and 0.375 g tazobactam (3.375 g)–4 g piperacillin and 0.50 g tazobactam (4.50 g) q 6 h IV × 7–10 days.

- Moderate-to-severe pneumonia caused by piperacillin-resistant s. aureus that produces β-lactamase: 3.375 g IV q 6 h plus aminoglycoside × 7–10 days.
- Dose modification necessary if severe renal insufficiency exists.

Drug Preparation:
- IV: Reconstitute each gram of drug with at least 5 mL of sterile or bacteriostatic water. Further dilute in 50–100 mL 0.9% sodium chloride or 5% dextrose injection and infuse over 30 minutes.
- IM: Reconstitute with 2 mL of sterile or bacteriostatic water, or 0.5–1.0% lidocaine HCl (without epinephrine), with final concentration 1 g/2.5 mL. Administer as deep IM injection in large muscle mass (e.g., gluteus maximus). Make certain patient is NOT ALLERGIC to lidocaine.

Drug Interactions:
- Aminoglycosides: synergism.
- Aminoglycosides (e.g., gentamicin): incompatible when mixed together; administer at separate sites at different times. Also, penicillinase-resistant penicillins can inactivate aminoglycoside serum samples from patients receiving both drugs.
- Clavulanic acid (inhibits β-lactamase): increases antibacterial action.
- Probenecid: increased serum level of piperacillin; may be coadministered to exert this effect.
- Tazobactam: inhibits β-lactamase, thus broadening drug's antimicrobial effectiveness.

Lab Effects/Interference:
Major clinical significance:
- Urine glucose: high urinary concentrations of a penicillin may produce false-positive or falsely elevated test results with copper sulfate tests (Benedict's, Clinitest, or Fehling's); glucose enzymatic tests (Clinistix or Testape) are not affected.
- PTT and PT: an increase has been associated with intravenous piperacillin.

Clinical significance:
- Coombs' (direct antiglobulin) test: false-positive result may occur during therapy with any penicillin.
- Urine protein: high urinary concentrations of piperacillin may produce false-positive protein reactions (pseudoproteinuria) with the sulfosalicylic acid and boiling test; bromophenol blue reagent test strips (Multistix) are reportedly unaffected.
- ALT, alk phos, AST, serum LDH values may be increased.
- Serum bili: an increase has been associated with piperacillin.
- BUN and serum creatinine: increased concentrations have been associated with piperacillin.
- Serum K+: hypokalemia may occur following administration of parenteral piperacillin, which may act as a non-reabsorbable anion in the distal tubals; this may cause an increase in pH and result in increased urinary potassium loss: the risk of hypokalemia increases with use of larger doses.

- WBC: leukopenia or neutropenia is associated with the use of all penicillins; the effect is more likely to occur with prolonged therapy and severe hepatic function impairment.

Special Considerations:

- Contraindicated in patients with prior hypersensitivity to penicillins. Use with caution in patients sensitive to other β-lactams (e.g., cephalosporins), since partial cross-allergenicity exists.
- Obtain ordered specimen, and send for culture and sensitivity test prior to first antibiotic dose.
- Consider alternative antibiotic therapy if eosinophilia, drug fever or rash, arthralgia, hematuria, or unexplained rise in BUN and serum creatinine occur.
- Monitor electrolytes and renal, hepatic, and hematologic laboratory parameters during extended treatment periods.
- Use with caution in pregnant or nursing women.
- Low Na content: 1.98 mEq/g of drug.
- Increased activity against *P. aeruginosa*.

Potential Toxicities/Side Effects and the Nursing Process

I. POTENTIAL FOR INJURY related to HYPERSENSITIVITY REACTION

Defining Characteristics: Urticaria, pruritus, rash (maculopapular or erythematous), fever and chills, eosinophilia, myalgia, edema, erythema, angioedema, Stevens-Johnson syndrome, and exfoliative skin reactions occur in 5% of patients. Increased risk exists in individuals allergic to cephalosporin antibiotics.

Nursing Implications: Assess allergy to cephalosporin antibiotics and penicillin: if patient states "yes," determine actual response, e.g., "swollen lips = angioedema." If angioedema, patient SHOULD NOT receive drug. Discuss other patient responses with physician to determine whether drug should be given. Assess baseline skin condition, including integrity and allergy history to drugs. Instruct patient to report rash, itching, other skin changes. Teach patient skin care and symptomatic measures as appropriate. If skin rash develops, discuss drug discontinuance with physician. If rash progresses, drug should be discontinued, as fatal Stevens-Johnson syndrome may develop. Be prepared to treat severe acute hypersensitivity reactions with airway management, oxygen, epinephrine, corticosteroids, antihistamines as ordered.

II. ALTERATION IN NUTRITION, LESS THAN BODY REQUIREMENTS, related to GI SIDE EFFECTS

Defining Characteristics: Nausea, vomiting, diarrhea may occur; rarely, pseudomembranous colitis caused by *C. difficile* resistant to the antibiotic occurs. Rarely, transient increases in LFTs—AST, ALT, alk phos, bili—may occur.

Nursing Implications: Assess baseline nutritional status. Instruct patient to report GI disturbances. Administer and teach patient to self-administer antiemetics as needed and as ordered. Teach patient importance of nutritious diet, and suggest small, frequent, high-calorie, high-protein meals as appropriate. Assess baseline LFTs and monitor periodically during treatment. Discuss abnormalities and drug interruption with physician.

III. FUNGAL SUPERINFECTION related to REDISTRIBUTION OF ENDOGENOUS MICROORGANISMS

Defining Characteristics: Vaginal candidiasis, vaginitis may occur as endogenous bacteria are eliminated and normal fungal population expands.

Nursing Implications: Instruct female patient to report vaginal itching or discharge. Discuss appropriate antifungal treatment with physician. Teach perineal hygiene and symptomatic management.

IV. ALTERATIONS IN PROTECTIVE MECHANISMS (RARE) related to HEMATOLOGIC ABNORMALITIES

Defining Characteristics: Rarely, transient leukopenia, lymphocytosis, anemia, eosinophilia may occur. Prolonged PT, prolonged APTT, and hypoprothrombinemia have occurred rarely, especially in elderly or debilitated patients, or in individuals with vitamin K deficiency.

Nursing Implications: Assess baseline laboratory parameters, and monitor periodically during treatment. Assess patient for response to antibiotics. Discuss abnormalities with physician. Assess for signs/symptoms of bleeding.

V. ALTERATIONS IN SENSORY/PERCEPTUAL PATTERNS related to DIZZINESS, SOMNOLENCE

Defining Characteristics: Dizziness, headache, somnolence occur rarely. Neuromuscular irritability and seizures may occur with high drug serum levels.

Nursing Implications: Assess baseline neurologic function and comfort, and monitor during treatment. Instruct patient to report any changes. Discuss any abnormalities with physician. Institute seizure precautions.

VI. ALTERATIONS IN COMFORT related to LOCAL INJECTION IRRITATION

Defining Characteristics: Vein irritation (pain, erythema), phlebitis, and thrombophlebitis may occur at IV administration site.

Nursing Implications: Change IV sites q 48 h, and assess for signs/symptoms of phlebitis prior to each administration. Administer drug slowly. Apply warm packs to increase comfort. Discuss central line with patient and physician to facilitate administration.

VII. ALTERATION IN FLUID AND ELECTROLYTE BALANCE related to HYPOKALEMIA AND INCREASED SODIUM INTAKE

Defining Characteristics: Prolonged therapy may cause hypokalemia; also, drug is prepared as sodium salt. Frequent IV infusions increase fluid intake.

Nursing Implications: Assess baseline electrolytes, fluid balance, weight, and monitor throughout therapy. Monitor renal function studies, especially if patient has preexisting renal dysfunction.

Drug: quinupristin and dalfopristin (Synercid)

Class: Macrolide-lincoasmide-streptogram (MLS) class of antibiotic.

Mechanism of Action: Synercid inhibits bacterial protein synthesis by each component irreversibly binding to different sites on the 50S bacterial ribosome subunit to form stable quinupristin-ribosome-dalfopristin tertiary complex. Quinupristin inhibits peptide chain formation and results in early termination, while dalfopristin directly interferes with peptidyl transferase and inhibits peptide chain elongation. Active against gram-positive aerobic microorganisms, e.g., *Enterococcus faecium*, including vancomycin- and teicoplanin-resistant organisms and vancomycin-resistant, but teicoplanin-susceptible organisms; staphylococci; streptococci; some anaerobes and respiratory pathogens.

Metabolism: Quinupristin and dalfopristin are rapidly converted in the liver to several active metabolites. Quinupristin is broken down into two active metabolites: one glutathione-conjugated metabolite and one cysteine-conjugated metabolite. Dalfopristin has one active metabolite formed by drug hydrolysis. Elimination half-life is approximately 0.9 and 0.75 hours for quinupristin and dalfopristin, respectively. Protein binding for quinupristin ranges from 55–78%, and from 11–26% for dalfopristin. Excreted in feces (75–77%) and urine (15% of quinupristin and 19% dalfopristin).

Dosage/Range:

- Recommended dose is 7.5 mg/kg of actual body weight in D5W over 60 minutes q 8–12 h, depending upon the type and severity of infection.

Drug Preparation:
- Reconstitute single-dose vial by slowly adding 5 mL of solution or preservative-free sterile water for injection. CAUTION: FURTHER DILUTION IS REQUIRED PRIOR TO ADMINSTRATION.
- According to patient weight, Synercid solution should be added to 250 mL of D5W solution within 30 minutes of initial reconstitution.
- Stability of the prepared infusate is 5 h at room temperature or 54 h under refrigeration at 2–8°C (36–46°F).
- Drug is NOT compatible with 0.9% sodium chloride or heparin-containing solutions.
- Desired dose should be administered IV over 60 minutes. If drug is administered through a common IV line, flush with 5% dextrose prior to and following administration.

Drug Interactions:
- Synercid should not be physically mixed with or added to other drugs since compatibility has not been established.
- Drugs metabolized by CYP450 3A4 isoenzyme system: drug is metabolized by CYP450 3A4 isoenzymes and is an inhibitor of CYP450 3A4, and thus may increase the serum concentrations of drugs metabolized by this isoenzyme, e.g., nifedipine, cyclosporin. Use together with caution and assess for toxicity.

Lab Effects/Interference:
- Eosinophils, BUN, GGT (gamma glutamyl transferase), LDH, CPK, AST, ALT, blood glucose, alk phos, and creatinine: concentrations may be increased.
- Hemoglobin and hematocrit: may be decreased.
- Serum K+ and platelet count: may be increased or decreased.

Special Considerations:
- Infusion via central line preferred to decrease incidence of local infusion reactions.

Potential Toxicities/Side Effects and the Nursing Process

I. ALTERATION IN NUTRITION related to GI SIDE EFFECTS

Defining Characteristics: Nausea, vomiting, diarrhea, constipation, abdominal pain, dyspepsia, stomatitis, and pseudomembranous enterocolitis may occur.

Nursing Implications: Assess elimination and nutrition pattern, baseline and during therapy. Teach patient to report diarrhea and/or abdominal pain immediately. Discuss drug discontinuance with physician if diarrhea occurs. Guaiac stool for occult blood, and notify physician if positive. If severe diarrhea develops, discuss management plan, including endoscopy, fluid and electrolyte replacement. Assess for nausea/vomiting, and administer prescribed antiemetic medications. Encourage small, frequent feedings as tolerated.

II. ALTERATION IN SKIN INTEGRITY related to HYPERSENSITIVITY

Defining Characteristics: Maculopapular rash and urticaria may occur. Allergic reactions (anaphylactic-like) may rarely occur.

Nursing Implications: Assess baseline allergy history. Assess baseline skin integrity. Teach patient to report rash, pruritus. Teach patient symptomatic management of rash, pruritus. Assess for hypersensitivity reaction: if it occurs, monitor VS, discontinue drug, notify physician, and institute supportive measures.

III. ALTERATION IN COMFORT related to LOCAL ADMINISTRATION EFFECTS

Defining Characteristics: IV administration may cause erythema, pain, swelling, and thrombophlebitis.

Nursing Implications: Assess IV site prior to each dose for phlebitis or swelling, and change site at least q 48 hours. Administer dose slowly over 60 minutes. Apply heat to painful IV sites as ordered. Infuse via central line if possible.

IV. ALTERATION IN COMFORT

Defining Characteristics: Myalgias and arthralgias may occur.

Nursing Implications: Assess baseline T, VS, neurologic status, and comfort level and monitor q 4–6 hours if patient in hospital. Teach patient self-care measures, including use of prescribed medications as well as use of heat or cold for myalgias and arthralgias.

V. ALTERATION IN HEPATIC FUNCTION

Defining Characteristics: Transient increases in serum BR, AST (SGOT), alk phos have occurred.

Nursing Implications: Assess baseline LFTs and monitor during therapy.

VI. FUNGAL SUPERINFECTION related to REDISTRIBUTION OF ENDOGENOUS MICROORGANISMS

Defining Characteristics: Vaginal moniliasis, vaginitis, and oral moniliasis may occur as endogenous bacteria are eliminated and normal fungal population expands.

Nursing Implications: Teach female patient to report vaginal itching or discharge. Discuss appropriate antifungal treatment with physician. Teach perineal hygiene and symptomatic management.

Drug: rifaximin (Xifaxan)

Class: Anti-infective, antidiarrheals, gastrointestinal, rifamycin.

Mechanism of Action: Acts by binding to the beta-subunit of bacterial DNA-dependent RNA polymerase resulting in inhibition of bacterial RNA synthesis. Structural analog of rifampin. Active against *Escherichia coli* (enterotoxigenic and enteroaggregative strains).

Metabolism: Well absorbed following PO administration. Poorly absorbed from the gastrointestinal tract. Drug excreted unchanged in the feces.

Dosage/Range:
- Traveler's diarrhea: 200 mg orally three times daily for 3 days.

Drug Preparation:
- Oral preparation.

Drug Administration:
- May be taken with or without food.

Drug Interactions:
- Rifaximin has not been shown to significantly affect intestinal or hepatic CYP3A4 activity.
- Rifaximin has not been shown to effect contraceptives containing ethinyl estradiol and norgestimate.

Lab Effects/Interference:
- None reported.

Special Considerations:
- Rifaximin was teratogenic in animal studies. There are no adequate and well-controlled studies in pregnant women.

Potential Toxicities/Side Effects and the Nursing Process

I. ALTERATION IN NUTRITION related to GI SIDE EFFECTS

Defining Characteristics: Gas, abdominal pain, nausea, vomiting, constipation, and pseudomembranous enterocolitis may occur.

Nursing Implications: Assess elimination and nutrition pattern, baseline and during therapy. Teach patient to report changes in diarrhea and/or abdominal pain immediately. Guaiac stool for occult blood, and notify physician if positive. Discuss management plan, including fluid and electrolyte replacement. Assess for nausea/vomiting, and administer prescribed antiemetic medications. Encourage small, frequent feedings as tolerated.

Drug: streptomycin sulfate

Class: Antibacterial; antimycobacterial (systemic).

Mechanism of Action: Synthetic antibiotic derived from *Streptomyces*; bactericidal, most probably by inhibition of protein synthesis; active against *Mycobacterium tuberculosis*. Active as second-line agent against sensitive microorganisms (including *Brucella, Nocardia, M. avium-intracellulare*).

Metabolism: Well absorbed following IM administration. Widely distributed into body fluids; 35% bound to plasma proteins. Readily crosses placenta and into breast milk. Drug excreted unchanged in the urine.

Dosage/Range:

- Antituberculosis regimen: Adults: 15 mg/kg/day or 1 g/day IM × 2–3 months, then 1 g 2 3 × per week. Elderly: dose may be limited to 10 mg/kg (or 750 mg). Desired serum peak is 5–25 μg/mL, and trough < 5 μg/mL.

Drug Preparation:

- Prepare a solution with concentration of ≤ 500 mg/mL, using sterile water for injection or 0.9% sodium chloride. Use within 2 days if kept at room temperature, or within 2 weeks if refrigerated at 2–8°C (36–46°F).

Drug Administration:

- Deep IM: into large muscle mass; rotate sites as sterile abscesses may form. DO NOT GIVE IV.

Drug Interactions:

- Increased risk of toxicity with other ototoxic drugs: acyclovir, other aminoglycosides, amphotericin B, bacitracin, cephalosporins, colistin, cisplatin, ethacrynic acid, furosemide, vancomycin.
- Potentiation of neuromuscular blockade when given concurrently with general anesthetics (succinylcholine, tubocurarine)—use cautiously, observe for signs/symptoms of respiratory depression.
- Synergism with extended-spectrum penicillins, but must be administered separately.

Lab Effects/Interference:

- Serum ALT, serum alk phos, serum AST, serum bili, and serum LDH values may be increased.
- BUN and serum creatinine concentrations may be increased.
- Serum Ca++, serum Mg++, serum K+, and serum Na+ concentrations may be decreased.

Special Considerations:

- Used parenterally with at least one other agent in treatment of tuberculosis.
- Use in pregnancy only if infection is life-threatening and no safer drug exists; drug crosses placenta and may cause fetal toxicity.

Potential Toxicities/Side Effects and the Nursing Process

I. ALTERATIONS IN SENSORY/PERCEPTUAL PATTERNS related to OTOTOXICITY

Defining Characteristics: Damage to eighth cranial nerve (auditory) may result in dizziness, nystagmus, vertigo, ataxia (vestibular damage), and more commonly, tinnitus, roaring sound in ears, and impaired hearing (auditory damage). Hearing loss usually begins with high-frequency loss, followed by clinical hearing loss, then permanent hearing loss if damage continues. Increased risk in elderly or renally impaired patients.

Nursing Implications: Assess baseline hearing (ability to hear spoken voice) and continue during therapy. Teach patient potential side effects, and instruct patient to report any hearing/perceptual problems (e.g., tinnitus, vertigo, decreased hearing). Discuss drug discontinuance and audiogram with physician to confirm hearing dysfunction if symptoms arise. Assess for increased risk if given concurrently with other ototoxic medications (e.g., cisplatin, furosemide).

II. ALTERATION IN URINARY ELIMINATION related to NEPHROTOXICITY

Defining Characteristics: Risk of nephrotoxicity is less than with other aminoglycosides. Renal damage characterized by tubular necrosis with increased serum BUN, creatinine; decreased urine creatinine clearance and specific gravity; proteinuria and casts in urine. Azotemia usually not associated with oliguria. Rarely, electrolyte wasting with hypomagnesemia, hypocalcemia, and hypokalemia may occur. Renal dysfunction is usually reversible after drug discontinuance. Increased risk exists in elderly and if there is preexisting renal dysfunction. Risk is low in well-hydrated patients with normal renal function when normal doses are given.

Nursing Implications: Assess baseline renal function and electrolytes, and monitor periodically during therapy. Discuss any abnormalities with physician, as drug should be dose-reduced or discontinued if renal dysfunction develops. Assess baseline total body fluid balance, weight, and monitor periodically during antibiotic therapy. Monitor hydration status to keep patient well hydrated. Assess drug peak and trough levels as ordered so that drug dosage is correctly titrated. Increased risk of toxicity if peak serum concentration > 40 μg/mL. Draw blood for peak drug concentration 30 minutes after end of 30-minute infusion or at the end of a 60-minute infusion; draw trough immediately before next dose.

III. ALTERATIONS IN SENSORY/PERCEPTUAL PATTERNS related to CNS EFFECTS, NEUROMUSCULAR BLOCKADE

Defining Characteristics: Headache, tremor, lethargy may occur. Peripheral neuropathy or encephalopathy (numbness, skin tingling, muscle twitching) may occur rarely. Neuromuscular blockade is dose-related, self-limiting, and uncommon. Risk is greater with topical application or when drug is administered to patient with neuromuscular disease (myasthenia gravis) or hypocalcemia.

Nursing Implications: Assess baseline neurologic status. Assess coexisting risk factors, neuromuscular blockade medications. Teach patient about side effects and instruct to report headache, tremor, lethargy. Observe for respiratory depression. If signs/symptoms arise, discuss drug discontinuance with physician.

IV. POTENTIAL FOR INJURY related to HYPERSENSITIVITY

Defining Characteristics: Rash, urticaria, pruritus, fever, eosinophilia have occurred rarely. CROSS-SENSITIVITY between AMINOGLYCOSIDES exists! Handling of drug can cause sensitization to the drug.

Nursing Implications: Assess for drug allergies to any aminoglycoside—amikacin, gentamicin, kanamycin, neomycin, netilmicin, streptomycin, tobramycin—prior to drug administration. Instruct patient to report any allergic reactions. Assess for signs/symptoms of allergic reaction after drug dose. Take special care in preparing drug or wear gloves.

V. ALTERATION IN NUTRITION, LESS THAN BODY REQUIREMENTS, related to GI SIDE EFFECTS

Defining Characteristics: Nausea, vomiting, anorexia have occurred rarely. Also, transient hepatomegaly with increased LFTs—AST, ALT, LDH, alk phos—has occurred.

Nursing Implications: Assess baseline nutritional status, preexisting nausea/vomiting, anorexia. Assess baseline LFTs and monitor periodically during treatment. Instruct patient to report side effects. Provide symptomatic interventions if side effects occur; discuss with physician use of alternative drug(s).

VI. POTENTIAL FOR FATIGUE, INFECTION, AND BLEEDING related to BONE MARROW INJURY

Defining Characteristics: Anemia, leukopenia, granulocytopenia, and thrombocytopenia may occur. Also, patients receiving antibiotics are at risk for overgrowth of nonsusceptible microorganisms, such as fungi (superinfection). Rare.

Nursing Implications: Assess baseline CBC, differential, and monitor periodically during treatment. Instruct patient to report signs/symptoms of fatigue, infection, or bleeding immediately. Assess for signs/symptoms of superinfection. Discuss any adverse effects with physician.

VII. ALTERATION IN SKIN INTEGRITY related to IRRITATION AT INJECTION SITE, EXFOLIATIVE DERMATITIS

Defining Characteristics: Exfoliative dermatitis rarely occurs; may develop pain, irritation, and sterile abscesses at injection site.

Nursing Implications: Assess skin integrity and presence of lesions. Monitor for changes during treatment, and instruct patient to report them. Rotate injection sites and give injection deeply into large muscle mass, e.g., upper outer quadrant of buttock. Administer solutions of ≤ 500 mg/mL.

Drug: telithromycin (Ketek)

Class: Antimicrobial agent. This antibiotic is a new structural class called ketolides.

Mechanism of Action: Similar to that of macrolides and is related to the 50S-ribosomal subunit binding with inhibition of bacterial protein synthesis. Telithromycin appears to have greater affinity for the ribosomal binding site than macrolides. Demonstrated efficacy against *Staphylococcus aureus, Streptococcus aureus, Streptococcus pneumoniae, Haemophilus influenzae, Moraxella catarrhalis, Chlamydia pneumoniae*, and *Mycoplasma pneumoniae*.

Metabolism: Absorbed from the GI tract. Eliminated by multiple pathways: 7% of the dose is excreted unchanged by biliary and/or intestinal secretion; 13% of the dose is excreted unchanged in urine; and 37% of the dose is metabolized by the liver. May accumulate in patients with severe hepatic disease.

Dosage/Range:

- Adult: Oral: 800 mg daily for 5–10 days. Duration of therapy depends on indication. Drug dose should be reduced or adjusted in patients with hepatic or renal insufficiency.

Drug Preparation:

- Oral: Administration of telithromycin with food had no significant effect on extent or rate of oral absorption in healthy subjects.

Drug Interactions:

- Class I, IA, & III Anti-arrhythmic Agents: Concomitant use is contraindicated as it may lead to QT prolongation. Serum levels may be increased.

- CYP 3A4 inhibitors: Itraconazole and Ketoconazole: Increases telithromycin levels and AUC by ~54% and 95%, respectively.
- CYP3A4 substrates: Cisapride, Simvastin, and Midazolam: Increases serum concentration of cisapride by 95%; significantly increases serum concentration of simvastin and midazolam. These drugs SHOULD NOT be used when a patient is taking telithromycin.
- CYP 2D6 substrates: Metoprolol: Increases serum concentrations. Administer with caution. Rifampin: Decreases serum concentrations. Digoxin: Increases serum concentration. Theophylline: Increases serum concentrations. Take 1 hour apart to decrease the gastrointestinal side effects. Sotalol: Decreases serum concentrations.

Lab Effects/Interference:

- There are no reported drug-laboratory test interactions. SGPT, alk phos, Amylase, SGOT, and bilirubin: serum concentrations may be increased in patients with preexisting hepatic disease.

Special Considerations:

- Avoid use in pregnant or lactating women.
- Contraindicated in patients with known hypersensitivity, patients with previous history of hepatitis and/or jaundice associated with the use of this drug or any macrolide antibiotic, such as azithromycin (Zithromax), erythromycin, clarithromycin (Biaxin), or dirithromycin (Dynabac).
- Acute hepatic failure and severe liver injury (in some cases fatal) have been reported in patients immediately during or immediately after receiving this drug. Monitor closely (for jaundice, hyperbilirubinuria, acholic stools, liver tenderness or hepatomegaly) and teach patient to report signs/symptoms (fatigue, malaise, anorexia, nausea, jaundice, dark amber urine). If patient has any signs or symptoms, drug must be stopped and the patient evaluated for this (LFTs, physical exam). The drug should be discontinued if hepatitis or transaminase elevations plus symptoms occur.
- Use with caution, if at all, in patients with myasthenia gravis, as they may have worsening symptoms of the disease (such as death and life-threatening breathing difficulties within a few hours of the first dose).
- Obtain ordered specimen and send for culture and sensitivity prior to first antibiotic dose.

Potential Toxicities/Side Effects and the Nursing Process

I. ALTERATION IN NUTRITION related to GI SIDE EFFECTS

Defining Characteristics: Anorexia, nausea, vomiting, diarrhea, glossitis, dysphagia, gastroenteritis, gastritis, constipation.

Nursing Implications: Assess baseline nutritional status. Assess for and teach patient to report any symptoms. Administer and teach patient self-administration of prescribed antiemetic or antidiarrheal medication as appropriate.

II. ALTERATION IN PROTECTIVE MECHANISMS

Defining Characteristics: Prolonged PT, prolonged INR, cardiac arrhythmias including atrial arrhythmias, bradycardia, and hypotension.

Nursing Implications: Monitor and teach patient about potential side effects and to report abnormalities such as fainting and dizziness.

III. POTENTIAL FOR INJURY related to VISUAL DISTURBANCES

Defining Characteristics: Blurred vision and difficulty focusing.

Nursing Implications: Assess baseline visual and neurologic status. Teach patient to report any changes in vision. If signs/symptoms arise, discuss discontinuance with physician, and institute supportive measures.

IV. FUNGAL SUPERINFECTION related to REDISTRIBUTION OF ENDOGENOUS MICROORGANISMS

Defining Characteristics: Vaginal moniliasis, vaginitis may occur as endogenous bacteria are eliminated and normal fungal population expands.

Nursing Implications: Teach female patient to report vaginal itching or discharge. Discuss appropriate antifungal treatment with physician. Teach perineal hygiene and symptom management.

Drug: ticarcillin disodium (Ticar); combined with clavulanate potassium (Timentin)

Class: Antibacterial (systemic) (extended spectrum penicillin).

Mechanism of Action: Semisynthetic antibiotic prepared from fungus *Penicillium*. Contains β-lactam ring and is bactericidal by inhibiting cell wall synthesis. Active against most gram-positive (except penicillinase-producing strains) and most gram-negative bacilli. Used in the treatment of serious gram-negative infections, especially *P. aeruginosa*–related infections of lower respiratory tract, urinary tract, and skin. When combined with clavulanate potassium, the drug is protected from breakdown by bacterial β-lactamase enzymes, thus keeping therapeutic antibiotic serum levels.

Metabolism: Poorly absorbed from GI tract, so must be given parenterally. Widely distributed in body tissues and fluids. Crosses placenta and is excreted in breast milk. Excreted via urine and bile.

Dosage/Range:
- IV dosing preferred but drug can be given IM or IV.

Adult:

Ticarcillin disodium:
- 3 g q 4–6 h (200–300 mg/kg/day in divided doses).
- Dosage modification required if renal insufficiency exists; refer to manufacturer's package insert.

Timentin:
- 3 g ticarcillin plus 0.1 g clavulanic acid (3.1 g) IV q 4–6 h × 10–14 days if weight < 60 kg: 200–300 mg ticarcillin/kg/d in divided doses q 4–6 h IV.

Drug Preparation:
- IV: reconstitute each gram with 4 mL 0.9% sodium chloride or 5% dextrose injection. Further dilute in 50–100 mL IV solution and infuse over 30 minutes to 2 hours.
- IM: reconstitute each gram with 2 mL sterile water for injection or 1% lidocaine HCl (without epinephrine). Ensure patient is NOT ALLERGIC to lidocaine. Inject drug deep IM in large muscle mass (e.g., gluteus maximus). Maximum 2 g at one site.

Drug Interactions:
- Aminoglycosides: synergism.
- Aminoglycosides (e.g., gentamicin): incompatible when mixed together; administer at separate sites at different times. Also, penicillinase-resistant penicillins can inactivate aminoglycoside serum samples from patients receiving both drugs.
- Probenecid: increased serum level of penicillin; may be coadministered to exert this effect.
- Clavulanic acid (β-lactamase inhibitor): Synergistic bacterial effect.

Lab Effects/Interference:

Major clinical significance:
- Urine glucose: high urinary concentrations of a penicillin may produce false-positive or falsely elevated test results with copper sulfate tests (Benedict's, Clinitest, or Fehling's); glucose enzymatic tests (Clinistix or Testape) are not affected.
- PTT and PT: an increase has been associated with ticarcillin.

Clinical significance:
- Coombs' (direct antiglobulin) test: false-positive result may occur during therapy with any penicillin.
- Urine protein: high urinary concentrations of ticarcillin may produce false-positive protein reactions (pseudoproteinuria) with the sulfosalicylic acid and boiling test; bromophenol blue reagent test strips (Multistix) are reportedly unaffected.
- ALT, alk phos, AST, serum LDH values may be increased.
- Serum bili: an increase has been associated with ticarcillin.
- BUN and serum creatinine: increased concentrations have been associated with ticarcillin.

- Serum K+: hypokalemia may occur following administration of parenteral ticarcillin, which may act as a non-reabsorbable anion in the distal tubules; this may cause an increase in pH and result in increased urinary potassium loss. The risk of hypokalemia increases with use of larger doses.
- WBC: leukopenia or neutropenia is associated with the use of all penicillins; the effect is more likely to occur with prolonged therapy and severe hepatic function impairment.

Special Considerations:

- Contraindicated in patients with prior hypersensitivity to penicillins. Use with caution in patients sensitive to other β-lactams (e.g., cephalosporins) since partial cross-allergenicity exists.
- Obtain ordered specimen, and send for culture and sensitivity test prior to first antibiotic dose.
- Consider alternative antibiotic therapy if eosinophilia, drug fever or rash, arthralgia, hematuria, or unexplained rise in BUN and serum creatinine occur.
- Monitor electrolytes and renal, hepatic, and hematologic laboratory parameters during extended treatment periods.
- Use with caution in pregnant or nursing women.
- Decreased incidence of hypokalemia, and less salt load, than other extended spectrum penicillins.

Potential Toxicities/Side Effects and the Nursing Process

I. POTENTIAL FOR INJURY related to HYPERSENSITIVITY REACTION

Defining Characteristics: Urticaria, pruritus, rash (maculopapular or erythematous), fever and chills, eosinophilia, myalgia, edema, erythema, angioedema, Stevens-Johnson syndrome, and exfoliative skin reactions occur in 5% of patients. Increased risk in individuals allergic to cephalosporin antibiotics.

Nursing Implications: Assess allergy to cephalosporin antibiotics and penicillin: if patient states "yes," determine actual response, e.g., "swollen lips = angioedema." If angioedema, patient SHOULD NOT receive drug. Discuss other patient responses with physician to determine whether drug should be given. Assess baseline skin condition, including integrity and allergy history to drugs. Instruct patient to report rash, itching, other skin changes. Teach patient skin care and symptomatic measures as appropriate. If skin rash develops, discuss drug discontinuance with physician. If rash progresses, drug should be discontinued, as fatal Stevens-Johnson syndrome may develop. Be prepared to treat severe acute hypersensitivity reactions with airway management, oxygen, epinephrine, corticosteroids, antihistamines as ordered.

II. ALTERATION IN NUTRITION, LESS THAN BODY REQUIREMENTS, related to GI SIDE EFFECTS

Defining Characteristics: Nausea, vomiting, diarrhea may occur; rarely, pseudomembranous colitis caused by *C. difficile* resistant to the antibiotic occurs. Rarely, transient increases in LFTs—AST, ALT, alk phos, bili—may occur.

Nursing Implications: Assess baseline nutritional status. Instruct patient to report GI disturbances. Administer and teach patient to self-administer antiemetics, antidiarrheals as needed and as ordered. Teach patient importance of nutritious diet, and suggest small, frequent, high-calorie, high-protein meals as appropriate. Assess baseline LFTs, and monitor periodically during treatment. Discuss abnormalities and drug interruption with physician.

III. FUNGAL SUPERINFECTION related to REDISTRIBUTION OF ENDOGENOUS MICROORGANISMS

Defining Characteristics: Vaginal candidiasis, vaginitis may occur as endogenous bacteria are eliminated, and normal fungal population expands.

Nursing Implications: Instruct female patient to report vaginal itching or discharge. Discuss appropriate antifungal treatment with physician. Teach perineal hygiene and symptomatic management.

IV. ALTERATIONS IN PROTECTIVE MECHANISMS (RARE) related to TRANSIENT LEUKOPENIA

Defining Characteristics: Rarely, transient leukopenia, lymphocytosis, anemia, eosinophilia may occur. Prolonged PT, prolonged APTT, and hypoprothrombinemia have occurred rarely, especially in elderly or debilitated patients, or in individuals with vitamin K deficiency.

Nursing Implications: Assess baseline laboratory parameters, and monitor periodically during treatment. Assess patient for response to antibiotics. Discuss abnormalities with physician. Assess for signs/symptoms of bleeding.

V. ALTERATIONS IN SENSORY/PERCEPTUAL PATTERNS related to DIZZINESS, SOMNOLENCE

Defining Characteristics: Dizziness, headache, somnolence occur rarely. Neuromuscular irritability and seizures may occur with high drug serum levels.

Nursing Implications: Assess baseline neurologic function and comfort, and monitor during treatment. Instruct patient to report any changes. Discuss any abnormalities with physician. Institute seizure precautions.

VI. ALTERATIONS IN COMFORT related to LOCAL INJECTION IRRITATION

Defining Characteristics: Vein irritation (pain, erythema), phlebitis, and thrombophlebitis may occur at IV administration site.

Nursing Implications: Change IV sites q 48 h, and assess for signs/symptoms of phlebitis prior to each administration. Administer drug slowly. Apply warm packs to increase comfort. Discuss central line with patient and physician to facilitate administration.

VII. ALTERATION IN FLUID AND ELECTROLYTE BALANCE related to HYPOKALEMIA AND INCREASED SODIUM INTAKE

Defining Characteristics: Prolonged therapy may cause hypokalemia; also, drug is prepared as sodium salt. Frequent IV infusions increase fluid intake.

Nursing Implications: Assess baseline electrolytes, fluid balance, weight, and monitor throughout therapy. Monitor renal function studies, especially if patient has preexisting renal dysfunction.

Drug: tigecycline (Tygacil)

Class: Antimicrobial agent. This antibiotic is the first in a new class called glycylcyclines. This novel IV antibiotic has a broad spectrum of antimicrobial activity, including activity against the drug-resistant bacteria methicillin-resistant Staphylococcus aureus (MRSA).

Mechanism of Action: Inhibits protein transplantation in bacteria by binding to the 30S ribosomal subunit and blocking entry of amino-acyl tRNA molecules into the A site of the ribosome. Demonstrated efficacy against methicillin-susceptible and -resistant *Staphylococcus aureus* (MRSA), *Escherichia coli*, *Enterococcus faecalis* (vancomycin-resistant isolates), *Streptococcus anginosus*, *Streptococcus intermedius*, *Streptococcus constellatus*, *Bacteroides fragilis*, *Bacteroides thetaiotaomicron*, *Bacteroides uniformis*, *Bacteroides vulgatus*, *Clostridium perfringens*, and *Peptostreptococcus micros*.

Metabolism: Is not extensively metabolized. Eliminated by multiple pathways: 7% of the dose is excreted unchanged by biliary and/or intestinal secretion; 59% of the dose is excreted unchanged in bile/feces and 33% of the dose is excreted in the urine. May accumulate in patients with severe hepatic disease.

Dosage/Range:

Adult:

- Initial dose 100 mg IV, followed by 50 mg every 12 hours.
- Duration of therapy depends on indication.
- Drug dose should be reduced or adjusted in patients with severe hepatic insufficiency.

Drug Preparation:

- Intravenous injection should be administered over 30–60 minutes every 12 hours.

Drug Interactions:

- Monitor prothrombin time if administered with warfarin.
- Concurrent use of antibacterial drugs with oral contraceptives may render the oral contraceptives less effective.

Lab Effects/Interference:

- There are no reported drug-laboratory test interactions. SGPT, alk phos, Amylase, SGOT, and bilirubin: serum concentrations may be increased in patients with preexisting hepatic disease.

Special Considerations:

- Avoid use in pregnant or lactating women.
- Contraindicated in patients with known hypersensitivity.
- Obtain ordered specimen and send for culture and sensitivity prior to first antibiotic dose.

Potential Toxicities/Side Effects and the Nursing Process

I. ALTERATION IN NUTRITION related to GI SIDE EFFECTS

Defining Characteristics: Anorexia, nausea, vomiting, diarrhea, glossitis, dysphagia, gastroenteritis, gastritis, constipation.

Nursing Implications: Assess baseline nutritional status. Assess for and teach patient to report any symptoms. Administer and teach patient self-administration of prescribed antiemetic or antidiarrheal medication as appropriate.

II. POTENTIAL FOR INJURY related to HYPERSENSITIVITY REACTION

Defining Characteristics: Urticaria, pruritus, rash (maculopapular or erythematous), fever and chills, eosinophilia, myalgia, edema, erythema, angioedema, Stevens-Johnson syndrome, and exfoliative skin reactions occur.

Nursing Implications: Assess allergy to antibiotics: if patient states "yes," determine actual response, e.g., "swollen lips = angioedema." If angioedema, patient SHOULD

NOT receive drug. Discuss other patient responses with physician to determine whether drug should be given. Assess baseline skin condition, including integrity and allergy history to drugs. Instruct patient to report rash, itching, and other skin changes. Teach patient skin care and symptomatic measures as appropriate. If skin rash develops, discuss drug discontinuance with physician. If rash progresses, drug should be discontinued, as fatal Stevens-Johnson syndrome may develop. Be prepared to treat severe acute hypersensitivity reactions with airway management, oxygen, epinephrine, corticosteroids, and antihistamines as ordered.

III. ALTERATIONS IN COMFORT related to LOCAL INJECTION IRRITATION

Defining Characteristics: Vein irritation (pain, erythema), phlebitis, and thrombophlebitis may occur at IV administration site.

Nursing Implications: Change IV sites q 48 h, and assess for signs/symptoms of phlebitis prior to each administration. Administer drug slowly. Apply warm packs to increase comfort. Discuss central line with patient and physician to facilitate administration.

IV. FUNGAL SUPERINFECTION related to REDISTRIBUTION OF ENDOGENOUS MICROORGANISMS

Defining Characteristics: Vaginal moniliasis, vaginitis may occur as endogenous bacteria are eliminated and normal fungal population expands.

Nursing Implications: Teach female patient to report vaginal itching or discharge. Discuss appropriate antifungal treatment with physician. Teach perineal hygiene and symptom management.

Drug: tobramycin sulfate (Nebcin)

Class: Aminoglycoside antibacterial (systemic).

Mechanism of Action: Synthetic antibiotic derived from *Streptomyces*; bactericidal, most probably by inhibition of protein synthesis. Active against aerobic microorganisms: many sensitive gram-negative (including *Acinetobacter, Citrobacter, Enterobacter, E. coli, Klebsiella, Proteus, Pseudomonas, Salmonella, Serratia,* and *Shigella*) and some sensitive gram-positive organisms (*S. aureus* and *S. epidermidis*). Over time, bacterial resistance may develop, either naturally or acquired.

Metabolism: Well absorbed following parenteral administration, but variability in absorption after IM injection (peak serum level 0.5–2 hours, duration 8–12 hours).

Widely distributed into body fluids. Minimally protein-bound. Readily crosses placenta and into breast milk. Drug excreted unchanged in the urine.

Dosage/Range:

- 3 mg/kg/day given in equally divided doses q 8 h.
- Desired peak serum concentration is 4–10 μg/mL, and trough serum concentration is 1–2 μg/mL.
- May use 5–6 mg/kg/day in three equally divided doses to treat life-threatening infections.
- If loading dose required, 2 mg/kg; usual dosing q 8 h, but q 12 or q 24 dosing may also be used.
- DOSE-REDUCE IF RENAL IMPAIRMENT.

Drug Preparation:

- Store unreconstituted vials at 15–30°C (59–86°F).
- Store injections at 25°C (77°F).
- Store reconstituted solution (using sterile water for injection, with final concentration 40 mg/mL) at room temperature (stable 24 hours) or in refrigerator at 2–8°C (36–46°F) (stable 96 hours).

Drug Administration:

- IV: further dilute by adding dose to 50–100 mL in 0.9% sodium chloride and administer over 30–60 minutes.

Drug Interactions:

- Increased risk of toxicity with other ototoxic drugs: acyclovir, other aminoglycosides, amphotericin B, bacitracin, cephalosporins, colistin, cisplatin, ethacrynic acid, furosemide, vancomycin.
- Potentiation of neuromuscular blockade when given concurrently with general anesthetics (succinylcholine, tubocurarine); use cautiously; observe for signs/symptoms of respiratory depression.
- Synergism with extended-spectrum penicillins, but must be administered separately.

Lab Effects/Interference:

- Serum ALT, serum alk phos, serum AST, serum bili, and serum LDH values may be increased.
- BUN and serum creatinine concentrations may be increased.
- Serum Ca++, serum Mg++, serum K+, and serum Na+ concentrations may be decreased.

Special Considerations:

- Used as first-line treatment in short-term treatment of serious gram-negative infections (e.g., septicemia, respiratory tract infections).
- Use against gram-positive organisms only as second-line treatment.
- Use in pregnancy only if infection is life-threatening and no safer drug exists; drug crosses placenta and may cause fetal toxicity.

Potential Toxicities/Side Effects and the Nursing Process

I. ALTERATIONS IN SENSORY/PERCEPTUAL PATTERNS related to OTOTOXICITY

Defining Characteristics: Damage to eighth cranial nerve (auditory) may result in dizziness, nystagmus, vertigo, ataxia (vestibular damage), and more commonly, tinnitus, roaring sound in ears, and impaired hearing (auditory damage). Hearing loss usually begins with high-frequency loss, followed by clinical hearing loss, then permanent hearing loss if damage continues. Increased risk in elderly or renally-impaired patients.

Nursing Implications: Assess baseline hearing (ability to hear spoken voice) and continue during therapy. Teach patient potential side effects, and instruct patient to report any hearing/perceptual problems (e.g., tinnitus, vertigo, decreased hearing). Discuss drug discontinuance and audiogram with physician to confirm hearing dysfunction if symptoms arise. Assess for increased risk if given concurrently with other ototoxic medications (e.g., cisplatin, furosemide).

II. ALTERATION IN URINARY ELIMINATION related to NEPHROTOXICITY

Defining Characteristics: Risk of nephrotoxicity is less than with other aminoglycosides. Renal damage characterized by tubular necrosis with increased serum BUN, creatinine; decreased urine creatinine clearance and specific gravity; proteinuria and casts in urine. Azotemia usually not associated with oliguria. Rarely, electrolyte wasting with hypomagnesemia, hypocalcemia, and hypokalemia may occur. Renal dysfunction is usually reversible after drug discontinuance. Increased risk exists in elderly and if there is preexisting renal dysfunction. Risk is low in well-hydrated patients with normal renal function when normal doses given.

Nursing Implications: Assess baseline renal function and electrolytes, and monitor periodically during therapy. Discuss any abnormalities with physician, as drug should be dose-reduced or discontinued if renal dysfunction develops. Assess baseline total body fluid balance, weight, and monitor periodically during antibiotic therapy. Monitor hydration status to keep patient well hydrated. Assess drug peak and trough levels as ordered so that drug dosage is correctly titrated. Increased risk of toxicity if peak serum concentration > 10–12 μg/mL. Draw blood for peak drug concentration 30 minutes after end of 30-minute infusion or at the end of a 60-minute infusion; draw trough immediately before next dose.

III. ALTERATIONS IN SENSORY/PERCEPTUAL PATTERNS related to CNS EFFECTS, NEUROMUSCULAR BLOCKADE

Defining Characteristics: Headache, tremor, lethargy may occur. Peripheral neuropathy or encephalopathy (numbness, skin tingling, muscle twitching) may occur rarely. Neuromuscular blockade is dose-related, self-limiting, and uncommon. Risk is greater with topical application or when drug is administered to patient with neuromuscular disease (myasthenia gravis) or hypocalcemia.

Nursing Implications: Assess baseline neurologic status. Assess coexisting risk factors, neuromuscular blockade medications. Teach patient about side effects, and instruct to report headache, tremor, lethargy. Observe for respiratory depression. If signs/symptoms arise, discuss drug discontinuance with physician.

IV. POTENTIAL FOR INJURY related to HYPERSENSITIVITY

Defining Characteristics: Rash, urticaria, pruritus, fever, eosinophilia have occurred rarely. CROSS-SENSITIVITY between AMINOGLYCOSIDES exists!

Nursing Implications: Assess for drug allergies to any aminoglycoside—amikacin, gentamicin, kanamycin, neomycin, netilmicin, streptomycin, tobramycin—prior to drug administration. Instruct patient to report any allergic reactions. Assess for signs/symptoms of allergic reaction after drug dose.

V. ALTERATION IN NUTRITION, LESS THAN BODY REQUIREMENTS, related to GI SIDE EFFECTS

Defining Characteristics: Nausea, vomiting, anorexia have occurred rarely. Also, transient hepatomegaly with increased LFTs—AST, ALT, LDH, alk phos—has occurred.

Nursing Implications: Assess baseline nutritional status, preexisting nausea/vomiting, anorexia. Assess baseline LFTs and monitor periodically during treatment. Instruct patient to report side effects. Provide symptomatic interventions if side effects occur; discuss with physician use of alternative drug(s).

VI. POTENTIAL FOR FATIGUE, INFECTION, AND BLEEDING related to BONE MARROW INJURY

Defining Characteristics: Anemia, leukopenia, granulocytopenia, and thrombocytopenia may occur. Also, patients receiving antibiotics are at risk for overgrowth of nonsusceptible microorganisms, such as fungi (superinfection). Rare.

Nursing Implications: Assess baseline CBC, differential, and monitor periodically during treatment. Instruct patient to report signs/symptoms of fatigue, infection, or bleeding immediately. Assess for signs/symptoms of superinfection. Discuss any adverse effects with physician.

Drug: vancomycin hydrochloride (Vancocin)

Class: Antibacterial (systemic).

Mechanism of Action: Derived from cultures of *Streptomyces orientalis*; drug is bactericidal by binding to bacterial cell wall, thus blocking protein polymerization and cell wall synthesis. Also damages cell membrane and acts at a different site than the penicillins. Bacteriostatic for enterococci. Active against many gram-positive organisms (staphylococci, group A β-hemolytic streptococci, *S. pneumoniae, C. difficile,* enterococci, *Corynebacterium, Clostridium*).

Metabolism: Not well absorbed from the GI tract—except in those patients with colitis—especially if patient has renal compromise. Effective when administered IV and is widely distributed in body tissues and fluid, including bile. Crosses placenta; unknown whether drug is excreted in breast milk; 52–60% bound to plasma proteins. IV dose excreted primarily by kidneys and, to a small degree, in bile; oral dose excreted in feces.

Dosage/Range:

Adult:

- Oral (for use in pseudomembranous colitis): capsules or powder: 0.5–1 g/day in four divided doses × 7–10 days.
- IV: 500 mg or 1 g q 12 h.
- Desired peak serum concentration is 20 to 40 mg/mL; and trough serum concentration is 5–15 μg/ml.
- Dose reduction necessary if renal dysfunction; see manufacturer's package insert.

Drug Preparation:

- Oral dose for treatment of *C. difficile* pseudomembranous colitis. Oral dose not recommended for treating systemic infections.
- Reconstituted by adding 10 mL of sterile water to 500-mg vial (20 mL to 1-g vial). Further dilute in at least 100 mL 0.9% sodium chloride or 5% dextrose in water, and infuse over 1 hour (central line).
- For peripheral lines, further dilution in 250 mL is recommended.
- Causes tissue necrosis if given IM; DO NOT ADMINISTER IM.

Drug Interactions:

- Nephrotoxic drugs (aminoglycoside antibiotics, amphotericin B, cisplatin, colistin): increased risk of nephrotoxicity; avoid concurrent use if possible.

Lab Effects/Interference:

- BUN concentrations may be increased.

Special Considerations:

- Use cautiously in patients with renal dysfunction.
- DO NOT USE in patients with hearing loss—or use at reduced doses if necessary in life-threatening infections.
- Contraindicated in patients with known hypersensitivity.
- Obtain ordered specimen for culture and sensitivity prior to first antibiotic dose.
- Use with caution in pregnancy, as fetal effects are unknown, and in lactating mothers, as drug may be excreted in breast milk.

Potential Toxicities/Side Effects and the Nursing Process

I. ALTERATIONS IN SENSORY PERCEPTUAL PATTERNS related to OTOTOXICITY

Defining Characteristics: IV drug appears to damage eighth cranial nerve (auditory). First symptom of ototoxicity is tinnitus and may progress to deafness; may also be associated with vertigo and dizziness (vestibular branch). High risk exists in patients with renal impairment who are receiving concurrent ototoxic drugs (e.g., cisplatin) or prolonged therapy, or those whose age > 60 years old.

Nursing Implications: Assess baseline hearing (ability to hear spoken voice) or audiogram if patient is at high risk—both at baseline and throughout therapy. Monitor serum drug concentrations during therapy if at high risk. Teach patient potential side effects, and instruct patient to report any hearing/perceptual problems (e.g., tinnitus, decreased hearing, vertigo). Discuss drug discontinuance with physician if symptoms arise.

II. ALTERATION IN URINARY ELIMINATION related to NEPHROTOXICITY

Defining Characteristics: Renal damage may occur, characterized by transient increases in serum BUN or creatinine, hyaline casts, and albuminuria. May cause acute interstitial nephritis. High risk in patients with renal impairment who are receiving concurrent nephrotoxic drugs (e.g., cisplatin) or prolonged therapy, or those whose age > 60 years.

Nursing Implications: Assess baseline renal function and electrolytes, and monitor periodically during therapy. Discuss any abnormalities with physician, as drug should be dose-reduced or discontinued if renal dysfunction develops. Assess baseline hydration status, including urinary output, total body balance, daily weights; keep patient well hydrated.

III. ALTERATION IN COMFORT related to LOCAL TISSUE EFFECTS

Defining Characteristics: Vesicant if given IM (causing tissue necrosis). Irritating to veins when given IV, causing pain and thrombophlebitis.

Nursing Implications: Administer drug IV *NOT* IM. Assess IV site prior to each dose and at completion of dose; instruct patient to report pain or burning; change IV site if irritation, phlebitis develop. Change site at least q 48 h and consider central line for prolonged therapy. AVOID EXTRAVASATION.

IV. ALTERATION IN CARDIAC OUTPUT related to RAPID IV INFUSION

Defining Characteristics: Rapid IV administration may cause histamine release and "red-neck" syndrome, characterized by rapid onset of hypotension, flushing, and erythematous or maculopapular rash of neck, face, chest. May be associated with wheezing, dyspnea, angioedema, urticaria, pruritus. Rarely, seizures and cardiac arrest may occur. Syndrome occurs minutes after beginning infusion, but may occur at end; usually resolves spontaneously over 2+ hours, but may require antihistamines, corticosteroids, or IV fluids. Rare when drug is administered over 1 hour.

Nursing Implications: Monitor temperature, VS at baseline, 5 minutes into IV administration, and at end of infusion, at least with the initial dose; infuse over at least 1 hour, using infusion controller if necessary. Observe patient during first 5 minutes, and instruct patient to report rash, wheezing, itching immediately. If reaction occurs, stop infusion, assess VS, and notify physician. Patient may be treated with antihistamine or IV fluids, or both. Completion of dose and subsequent doses may be ordered at very slow rate. Document episode in medical record and update care plan/medication sheet to reflect change in drug administration.

V. INJURY related to BONE MARROW SUPPRESSION

Defining Characteristics: Rarely, leukopenia, thrombocytopenia, agranulocytosis may occur, especially with cumulative doses > 25 g.

Nursing Implications: Monitor baseline and periodic WBC, differential, platelet count, especially if receiving other bone marrow-suppressive drugs. Discuss abnormalities with physician.

VI. INFECTION related to OVERGROWTH OF NONSUSCEPTIBLE MICROORGANISMS

Defining Characteristics: Normal microflora populations altered by drug, with possible overgrowth by nonsusceptible microorganisms, i.e., fungi, gram-negative bacteria.

Nursing Implications: Assess for signs/symptoms of other infections of skin, mucous membranes. Instruct patient to report signs/symptoms. Discuss further antimicrobial therapy with physician.

ANTIFUNGALS

Drug: amphotericin B (deoxycholate) (Fungizone); amphotericin B lipid complex (Abelcet); amphotericin B cholesteryl sulfate complex (Amphotec); liposomal amphotericin B (AmBisome)

Class: Antifungal (systemic); antiprotozoal.

Mechanism of Action: Produced by *Streptomyces*; binds to sterol molecule in fungal membrane, causing disruption and leakage of intracellular ions. Is fungistatic (prevents replication at normal doses) and fungicidal (kills fungi at high doses). Active against systemic fungal infections (*Aspergillus, Candida, Cryptococcus, Histoplasma capsulatum*); used to treat fungal meningitis and *Leishmania* (protozoan) infections.

Metabolism: Poorly absorbed from GI tract so must be given IV. Crosses BBB and the placenta; 90–95% bound to serum proteins. Single-dose elimination half-life is 24 hours, while following long-term administration is 15 days.

Dosage/Range:
Adult:
Amphotericin B (deoxycholate):
- Initial: 0.25 mg/kg IV (or first dose of 1 mg IV) over 6-hour period (may use 2–4 hours).
- Gradual increase in daily dosage, (e.g., over 1 week) to dose of 0.5 mg/kg/day to 1 mg/kg/day or 1.5 mg/kg on alternate days (maximum 1.5 mg/kg/day).
- If dose is interrupted for > 1 week, reinstitute at 0.25 mg/kg/day and titrate up.
- Intrathecal: 25 µg (0.1 mL diluted with 10–20 mL CSF) 2–3×/week.
- Oral: oral candida: amphotericin B oral suspension: 1 mL (100 mg) qid.

Lipid-based amphotericin B (infection refractory or pt has renal impairment):
- Amphotec: test dose 1.6–8.3 mg/10 mL IV over 15–30 min, 3–4 mg/kg/d prepared as a 0.6 mg/mL infusion IV at 1 mg/kg/hr.
- Abelcet: 5 mg/kg/day (1–2 mg/mL) IV at 2.5 mg/kg/hr; if infusion time > 2 hr, shake to remix q 2 h.
- AmBisome: 3–5 mg/kg/day IV (1–2 mg/mL) over 1–2 hours.
- Bladder irrigation: 50 micrograms/mL solution given into bladder intermittently or as a continuous irrigation × 5–20 days.

Drug Preparation (amphotericin B deoxycholate):
- Use sterile water for injection (NO PRESERVATIVES) to reconstitute drug; for peripheral line only further dilute to a concentration of 0.1 mg/mL using 500 mL

of 5% dextrose injection. Manufacturer recommends protecting from light, but appears to be stable for 24 hours in room light.

Drug Administration:

- Administer slowly over 2–6 hours.
- If an inline filter is used, it must have a mean pore diameter of ≥ 1 μm or drug will be filtered out; no filter for Amphotec, Abelcet.
- Protect from light during infusion.

Drug Interactions:

- Norfloxacin: possible enhanced antifungal action.
- Additive nephrotoxic effects when combined with other nephrotoxic drugs: aminoglycosides, cisplatin, cyclosporine, pentamidine, vancomycin, so concurrent administration should be avoided.
- Enhanced hypokalemic effects when combined with other drugs that lower serum potassium: corticosteroids.
- Enhanced digitoxin: toxicity related to amphotericin-induced hypokalemia.
- Synergism with flucytosine with increased drug effect.
- Antagonism with miconazole: do not use together.
- Nitrogen mustard: increases toxicity (renal, bronchospasm, hypotension)—avoid concurrent administration.
- Granulocyte transfusions: acute pulmonary dysfunction may occur if given concurrently or close together. Time administration far apart and monitor pulmonary function.

Lab Effects/Interference:

- Increased AST, ALT, alk phos, creatinine, BUN.
- Hypomagnesemia, hypokalemia, hypocalcemia.
- Hypoglycemia, hyperglycemia.

Special Considerations:

- Use with caution in patients with renal dysfunction.
- Contraindicated if hypersensitive to amphotericin.
- Safety in pregnancy has not been established—use with caution and only if benefits outweigh risks.
- Drug encapsulation in liposome decreases toxicity, including renal toxicity. Amphotericin B lipid complex injection is approved for the treatment of aspergillosis in patients refractory or intolerant to conventional amphotericin B.

Potential Toxicities/Side Effects and the Nursing Process

I. POTENTIAL FOR INJURY related to DRUG ADMINISTRATION

Defining Characteristics: Headache, hypotension, malaise, myalgias, tachypnea, cramping, nausea, and vomiting may occur. Fever and chills usually begin 1–3 hours after infusion is started, and tolerance develops with subsequent doses. Rapid IV administration may cause hypertension and shock, hypokalemia, and arrhythmias.

Nursing Implications: Assess baseline comfort level, temperature, VS. Teach patient potential side effects, and instruct to report any changes. Discuss premedication with physician, such as ibuprofen (inhibits prostaglandin PGE_2) and/or hydrocortisone. Discuss with physician use of IV meperidine HCl (Demerol) for management of rigor if it develops. Administer test dose (e.g., 1 mg/250 mL 5% dextrose IV over 1–4 hours) and monitor temperature, heart rate, BP, respiratory rate during infusion. Administer drug slowly (over 2–6 hours) and escalate dose slowly. Administer antiemetic agents as needed, then prophylactically.

II. ALTERATION IN URINARY ELIMINATION related to NEPHROTOXICITY

Defining Characteristics: 80% incidence; multiple toxic effects (vasoconstriction, lytic action on renal tubular cell membranes, calcium deposits in distal nephron); hypokalemia may precede azotemia with increased BUN and creatinine, decreased creatinine clearance, and increased excretion of K+, uric acid, and protein. Renal tubular acidosis may occur. Renal impairment usually diminishes after drug discontinuance, but some degree of impairment may be permanent.

Nursing Implications: Assess baseline renal function and electrolytes; monitor every other day during dosage escalation, then at least weekly. Discuss any abnormalities with physician. Drug should be dose-reduced if renal dysfunction develops. Slowly administer initial test dose, then gradually increase doses over first week. Assess fluid status and total body balance closely to keep patient well hydrated. Assess for signs/symptoms of hypokalemia: arthralgia, myalgia, muscle weakness. Administer potassium and magnesium replacements as ordered.

III. FATIGUE related to ANEMIA

Defining Characteristics: High incidence of reversible normocytic, normochromic anemia that rarely requires transfusion.

Nursing Implications: Assess baseline CBC, HCT; monitor Hgb and HCT during treatment. Instruct patient to report fatigue, shortness of breath, headache. Transfuse red blood cells as needed and ordered by physician.

IV. ALTERATION IN COMFORT, PAIN related to PAIN AT INJECTION SITE

Defining Characteristics: Drug may cause pain at injection site, phlebitis, thrombophlebitis; extravasation causes local irritation.

Nursing Implications: Select veins for IV administration distally and then more proximally, avoiding phlebitic veins or small veins. Apply heat to increase comfort. Administer drug slowly.

V. ALTERATION IN CARDIAC OUTPUT related to CARDIOPULMONARY DYSFUNCTION

Defining Characteristics: Rarely, hypertension, ventricular fibrillation, cardiac arrest, failure, pulmonary edema may occur. Pulmonary hypersensitivity may occur with bronchospasm, wheezing, or pulmonary pneumonitis.

Nursing Implications: Monitor VS closely, noting heart rate and rhythm, BP, breath sounds at baseline and during infusion. Instruct patient to report dyspnea, other changes in breathing pattern, or general feeling state ASAP. Discuss any changes, abnormalities with physician. Administer granulocyte transfusions as far apart from amphotericin administration as possible, and monitor pulmonary status closely. Be prepared to provide basic life support/resuscitation if needed.

VI. ALTERATIONS IN SENSORY/PERCEPTUAL PATTERNS related to PERIPHERAL AND CNS DYSFUNCTION

Defining Characteristics: Rarely, hearing loss, tinnitus, transient vertigo, blurred vision or diplopia, peripheral neuropathy, and seizures may occur. Following intrathecal drug administration, headache, lumbar nerves, arachnoiditis, and visual changes may occur.

Nursing Implications: Assess baseline neurologic function and monitor during drug administration and over time, especially when drug is given intrathecally. Notify physician if abnormalities occur. Discuss with physician coadministration of small doses of intrathecal corticosteroids to decrease CNS irritation.

VII. ALTERATION IN NUTRITION, LESS THAN BODY REQUIREMENTS, related to GI TOXICITY

Defining Characteristics: Anorexia, nausea, vomiting, dyspepsia, cramping, epigastric pain, and diarrhea may occur. Rarely, melena and hemorrhagic gastroenteritis may occur. Elevated LFTs may occur.

Nursing Implications: Assess baseline nutritional status, including weight and usual weight. Administer antiemetics as ordered and needed, then prophylactically prior to infusion if nausea and/or vomiting develop. Administer antidiarrheal medicine as ordered and needed. Instruct patient to report any symptoms; teach/reinforce importance of high-calorie, high-protein diet; suggest family/significant other bring in favorite foods from home as appropriate. Assess LFT results at base line and periodically during treatment as elevated serum aminotransferase, bili, and alk phos may occur. Discuss abnormalities with physician. Encourage patient to eat favorite foods, especially those high in calories, protein, potassium, and magnesium. Monitor daily weight during treatment, and discuss weight loss with dietitian, patient, and physician to revise nutritional plan.

VIII. ALTERATION IN PROTECTIVE MECHANISMS related to BONE MARROW INJURY

Defining Characteristics: Rarely, thrombocytopenia, leukopenia, agranulocytosis, and coagulation defects may occur.

Nursing Implications: Assess baseline CBC, differential. Assess for any signs/symptoms of bleeding or infection, and discuss with physician if they occur. Teach patient general self-assessment guidelines, such as taking temperature and reporting any changes from baseline condition.

Drug: anidulafungin (Eraxis)

Class: Antifungal.

Mechanism of Action: Semisynthetic lipopeptide synthesized from fermentation products of *Aspergillus nidulans*. Fungistatic by damaging fungal cell membrane increasing permeability, altering cell metabolism, and inhibiting cell growth. Fungicidal at high concentrations. Inhibits the synthesis of β(1, 3)-D-glucan synthase, resulting in selective inhibition of the synthesis of glucan, an integral component of the fungal cell wall.

Metabolism: Unique among echinocandins because it slowly degrades in human plasma, undergoing a process of biotransformation rather than metabolism. Degradation products pass into the feces via the biliary tree.

Dosage/Range:

- Esophageal Candidiasis: 100 mg/day (loading dose), followed by 50 mg/day × 14 days or × 7 days after resolution of symptoms.
- Candidemia and other deep tissue Candida infections: 200 mg on day 1, followed by 100 mg/day × 14 days after the last positive blood culture.

Drug Preparation:

- Do not mix or co-infuse with other medications.
- No dose adjustment is required in patients based on age, sex, weight, disease state, concomitant drug therapy, or renal or hepatic insufficiency.

- IV: Use manufacturer's suggested dilution guideline.
- Infuse slowly; histamine-mediated reactions have been observed related to infusion rate.

Drug Interactions:
- Contraindications: hypersensitivity to anidulafungin, other echinocandins, or any component of the formulation.
- Anidulafungin was found to be safe and was not affected by concomitant treatment with substrates, inhibitors, or inducers of the cytochrome P450 metabolic pathway, including rifampin and cyclosporine in clinical trials.

Lab Effects/Interference:
Major clinical significance:
- Elevated liver function tests, hepatitis, and worsening hepatic failure have been reported.

Special Considerations:
- Used in treatment of fungal infections.
- On the basis of a lack of interactions with amphotericin B and voriconazole, anidulafungin is well suited to be used in combination with other antifungal agents.
- Histamine-mediated reactions (urticaria, flushing, hypotension) have been observed related to infusion rate.

Potential Toxicities/Side Effects and the Nursing Process

I. POTENTIAL FOR INJURY related to INFUSION-RELATED ADVERSE EVENTS

Defining Characteristics: Infusion-related adverse events occurred in 1.3% (N=6) of the patients in clinical trials. Hypotension with tachycardia, dyspnea, rash, urticaria, flushing, pruritus, dyspnea, hypotension, and dizziness may occur.

Nursing Implications: Assess baseline VS and monitor throughout infusion. Instruct patient to report signs/symptoms immediately. Assess for signs/symptoms: nausea, generalized itching, crampy abdominal pain, chest tightness, anxiety, agitation, sense of impending doom, wheezing, and dizziness.

II. ALTERATION IN NUTRITION, LESS THAN BODY REQUIREMENTS, related to GI SIDE EFFECTS

Defining Characteristics: Nausea, vomiting, diarrhea, and anorexia may occur.

Nursing Implications: Assess baseline nutritional and elimination status. Instruct patient to report GI disturbances. Administer and teach patient to self-administer antiemetics, antidiarrheals as needed and as ordered. Teach patient importance of nutritious diet, and suggest small, frequent, high-calorie, high-protein meals as appropriate.

III. ALTERATIONS IN SENSORY/PERCEPTUAL PATTERNS related to CNS, ENDOCRINE EFFECTS

Defining Characteristics: Dizziness, headache, and somnolence may occur. Hypokalemia occurs in 3% of patients.

Nursing Implications: Assess baseline neurologic function and comfort, and monitor during treatment. Instruct patient to report any changes. Discuss any abnormalities with physician.

Drug: caspofungin (Cancidas)

Class: Echinocandin; glucan synthesis inhibitor.

Mechanism of Action: Caspofungin inhibits the synthesis of β-(1, 3)-D-glucan, an integral component of the fungal cell wall of susceptible filamentous fungi. It has demonstrated activity in regions of active cell growth of *Aspergillus fumigatus*.

Metabolism: Caspofungin is slowly metabolized by hydrolysis and N-acetylation. Elimination route is via feces and urine.

Dosage/Range:

- The recommended dose of caspofungin is a 70-mg loading dose on the first day, followed by 50 mg/daily.
- No dosage adjustment is necessary for the elderly.
- No dosage adjustment is necessary for patients with renal insufficiency. Caspofungin is not dialyzable.
- No dosage adjustment is recommended for patients with mild hepatic insufficiency (Child-Pugh score 5 to 6). In those with moderate hepatic insufficiency (Child-Pugh score 7 to 9), a daily dose of 35 mg after the 70-mg loading dose is recommended.

Drug Administration:

- Caspofungin should be given as a slow IV infusion in 250 ml 0.9% sodium chloride over 1 hour.
- Caspofungin is not compatible with dextrose-containing solutions.

Drug Interactions:

- Transient increase in AST and ALT have been observed when caspofungin and cyclosporine are coadministered. Therefore, concomitant use of these two agents is not recommended unless the potential benefit outweighs the potential risk.

Potential Toxicities/Side Effects and the Nursing Process

I. ALTERATIONS IN COMFORT related to LOCAL VEIN IRRITATION (IV ADMINISTRATION)

Defining Characteristics: Erythema, irritation, pain, swelling, phlebitis may occur at injection site. Consider use of central line.

Nursing Implications: Assess IV site for patency, irritation prior to each dose. Change IV site at least q 48 hours. Apply warmth/heat to painful area as needed.

II. POTENTIAL FOR INJURY related to HYPERSENSITIVITY REACTION

Defining Characteristics: Fever and erythema. Increased risk in allergic individuals.

Nursing Implications: Assess allergy/allergic potential to drug. Discuss other patient responses with physician to determine whether drug should be given. Assess baseline skin condition, including integrity and allergy history to drugs. Teach patient to report rash, itching, and other skin changes. Teach patient skin care and symptomatic measures as appropriate. If reaction occurs, discuss drug discontinuance with physician.

III. ALTERATION IN NUTRITION, LESS THAN BODY REQUIREMENTS, related to GI SIDE EFFECTS

Defining Characteristics: Nausea and vomiting may occur. Rarely, transient increases in LFTs—AST (SGOT), ALT (SGPT), alk phos, bili—may occur with coadministration of cyclosporine.

Nursing Implications: Assess baseline nutritional status. Teach patient to report GI disturbances. Administer and teach patient to self-administer antiemetics as needed and as ordered. Teach patient importance of nutritious diet, and suggest small, frequent, high-calorie, high-protein meals as appropriate. Assess baseline LFTs and monitor periodically during treatment. Discuss abnormalities and drug interruption with physician.

IV. SENSORY/PERCEPTUAL ALTERATIONS

Defining Characteristics: Headache.

Nursing Implications: Assess baseline neurological function and comfort, and monitor during treatment. Teach patient to report any changes. Discuss any abnormalities with physician.

Drug: fluconazole (Diflucan)

Class: Azole, antifungal (systemic).

Mechanism of Action: Fungistatic; causes increased permeability of fungal cell membrane, so intracellular nutrients leak out (potassium, amino acids) and cell is unable to take in nutrients to make DNA (precursors for purine, pyrimidines). Active against most fungi, including yeast.

Metabolism: Drug is rapidly and highly absorbed from GI tract, with > 90% of drug bioavailable. GI absorption is unaffected by food or gastric pH. Steady-state plasma levels achieved in 5–10 days, or by second day if loading dose given. Widely distributed in body tissues and fluids, including CSF. There is minimal protein binding. It is unknown whether drug crosses the placenta or is excreted in human milk; 60–80% of drug is excreted unchanged in the urine. Renal dysfunction results in higher circulating serum levels with prolonged drug effect and potential toxicity. Drug elimination in elderly clients may be decreased.

Dosage/Range:

- Oral and parenteral dosages are the same; IV dosage recommended for patients unable to take oral form. Dose is a single daily dose.
- Dosage depends on fungal infection. Candidiasis (oropharyngeal or esophageal): 200 mg day 1, followed by 100 mg/day (may titrate based on patient's response up to 400 mg/day) × 2 weeks (oropharyngeal); × 3 weeks or at least × 2 weeks after symptoms resolve (esophageal). Candidiasis (systemic): 400 mg day 1, followed by 200 mg/day × 4 weeks at least, then × 2 weeks after symptoms resolve (esophageal). Cryptococcal infections: Initial: 400 mg day 1, followed by 200–400 mg/day × 10–12 weeks after CSF cultures for *Cryptococcus* are negative. Maintenance (AIDS patients): 200 mg/day indefinitely.
- DOSE-REDUCE AFTER LOADING DOSE IF RENAL COMPROMISE based on creatinine clearance (e.g., 21–50 mL/min, dose-reduce 50%; if 11–20 mL/min, dose-reduce 75%).

Drug Preparation:

- Oral: store in tight containers at < 30°C (86°F).
- Parenteral: glass vials for injection should be stored at 5–30°C, (41–86°F); protect from freezing. Plastic containers should be stored at 5–25°C (41–77°F). Inspect for any discoloration, particulate matter, or leaks in plastic bags. If found, do not use.

Drug Administration:

- Oral: once daily without regard to food intake.
- IV: once daily at a rate ≤ 200 mg/hour. DO NOT ADD ADDITIVES. DO NOT ADMINISTER IV IN SERIES THAT COULD INTRODUCE AIR EMBOLISM.

Drug Interactions:
- Coumarin anticoagulants: increased PT; monitor PT closely.
- Cyclosporine: increased cyclosporine serum levels; monitor closely and adjust dose.
- Phenytoin: increased phenytoin serum level; monitor closely and reduce phenytoin dose as needed.
- Rifampin: decreased fluconazole serum level; increase fluconazole dose when given concurrently.
- Sulfonylurea antidiabetic agents (tolbutamide, glyburide, glipizide): increased drug serum levels; monitor blood glucose levels closely and decrease dose as needed.
- Thiazide diuretics: increased fluconazole serum level; do not appear to increase fluconazole toxicity so dose adjustment not necessary.
- Rifampin, isoniazid, phenytoin, valproic acid, oral sulfonylurea: increased risk of elevated hepatic transaminases exists.

Lab Effects/Interference:
Major clinical significance:
- ALT, alk phos, AST, and serum bili values may be elevated.

Special Considerations:
- Drug is being studied as a prophylactic antifungal agent in patients at risk for neutropenia and fungal infections (cancer patients receiving myelosuppressive chemotherapy, bone marrow transplant patients).
- Use cautiously in patients with renal dysfunction; dose reduction based on creatinine clearance (see Dosage/Range section).
- Absorption NOT affected by gastric pH or food intake.
- Risk of drug toxicity may be higher in patients with HIV infection.

Potential Toxicities/Side Effects and the Nursing Process

I. ALTERATION IN NUTRITION, LESS THAN BODY REQUIREMENTS, related to GI SIDE EFFECTS

Defining Characteristics: 2–8% incidence of mild-to-moderate nausea, vomiting, abdominal pain, diarrhea is seen; anorexia, dyspepsia, dry mouth, flatus, bloating occur rarely; 5–7% incidence of mild, transient increases in LFTs, which are reversible with drug discontinuance.

Nursing Implications: Assess baseline nutritional and elimination status. Instruct patient to report GI disturbances. Administer and teach patient to self-administer antiemetics, antidiarrheals as needed and as ordered. Teach patient importance of nutritious diet, and suggest small, frequent, high-calorie, high-protein meals as appropriate. Assess baseline LFTs and monitor periodically during treatment. Discuss abnormalities and drug interruption with physician. Assess whether patient is taking other hepatotoxic drugs (see Special Considerations section).

II. ALTERATION IN SKIN INTEGRITY related to ALLERGY/ HYPERSENSITIVITY

Defining Characteristics: 5% incidence is seen of rash, often diffuse, associated with eosinophilia and pruritus; rarely, exfoliative dermatitis and Stevens-Johnson syndrome may occur in patients receiving multiple drugs.

Nursing Implications: Assess baseline skin condition, including integrity and drug allergy history. Instruct patient to report rash, itching, and other skin changes. Teach patient skin care and symptomatic measures as appropriate. If skin rash develops, discuss drug discontinuance with physician. If rash progresses, especially in HIV-infected patients, drug should be discontinued, as fatal Stevens-Johnson syndrome may develop. Be prepared to treat severe acute hypersensitivity reactions with airway management, oxygen, epinephrine, corticosteroids, antihistamines as ordered.

III. ALTERATIONS IN SENSORY/PERCEPTUAL PATTERNS related to CNS EFFECTS

Defining Characteristics: Dizziness and headache occur in 2% of patients. Rarely, somnolence, delirium/coma, dysesthesia, malaise, fatigue, seizure, and psychiatric disturbance may occur.

Nursing Implications: Assess baseline neurologic function and comfort, and monitor during treatment. Instruct patient to report any changes. Discuss any abnormalities with physician.

Drug: flucytosine (Ancobon)

Class: Antifungal (systemic).

Mechanism of Action: Nonantibiotic antifungal; enters fungal cell and undergoes deamination to fluorouracil, which acts as an antimetabolite, preventing RNA and protein synthesis; may also interfere with DNA synthesis. Active against *Candida* and *Cryptococcus*.

Metabolism: Oral preparation well absorbed from GI tract; decreased rate of absorption when taken with food. Widely distributed into body tissues and fluids, including CSF; 75–90% of dose excreted unchanged by kidneys, with increased serum levels and toxicity in patients with renal dysfunction.

Dosage/Range:

- Oral: 50–150 mg/kg/day in four equally divided doses given q 6 h × weeks or months until fungal studies are negative. Dose may be 150–250 mg/kg/day in *Cryptococcus* meningitis.

- Dose must be reduced in patients with renal dysfunction:
- Dose must be determined by flucytosine levels (therapeutic range is 25–120 μg/mL).
- Dose may be determined by creatinine clearance. Individual dose of 12.5–37.5 mg/kg given:
  - q 12 h if creatinine clearance is 20–40 mL/min.
  - q 24 h if creatinine clearance is 10–20 mL/min.
  - q 24–48 h if creatinine clearance is < 10 mL/min.

Drug Preparation:
- Store in tight, light-resistant container at < 40°C (104°F).
- Oral.

Drug Interactions:
- Amphotericin B: theoretical synergism.
- Norfloxacin: theoretical synergism.

Lab Effects/Interference:
- Rare anemia, leukopenia, agranulocytosis, thrombocytopenia, pancytopenia, eosinophilia.

Special Considerations:
- Use only in severe infections, as drug is toxic.
- Theoretically synergistic with amphotericin, but some studies do not show significant benefit of combination.
- Therapeutic response (negative fungal cultures) may take weeks to months.
- Drug has no antineoplastic activity.
- Drug is teratogenic, capable of causing fetal malformations when given to pregnant women. Risks and benefits should be carefully considered before drug is used in a pregnant patient.

Potential Toxicities/Side Effects and the Nursing Process

I. POTENTIAL FOR INFECTION, BLEEDING, AND FATIGUE related to BONE MARROW DEPRESSION

Defining Characteristics: Anemia, leukopenia, thrombocytopenia may occur; agranulocytosis and aplastic anemia occur rarely. Increased risk exists with increased serum flucytosine levels (100 μg/mL), especially in patients with renal compromise or those receiving concurrent amphotericin B.

Nursing Implications: Assess baseline CBC, differential, BUN, and creatinine, and monitor closely during therapy, especially if receiving concurrent amphotericin B. Assess for signs/symptoms of bleeding, fatigue, infection during therapy. Teach patient to self-assess for signs/symptoms of infection, bleeding, and instruct to report them immediately. Discuss dose with physician; dose modification is needed if renal dysfunction occurs. Monitor flucytosine therapeutic levels (to maintain level of 25–100 μg/mL).

II. ALTERATION IN NUTRITION, LESS THAN BODY REQUIREMENTS, related to MUCOSITIS, NAUSEA, VOMITING

Defining Characteristics: Frequently dividing epithelial cells of GI mucosa are damaged, leading to diarrhea and possible bowel perforation (rare). Nausea, vomiting, anorexia, abdominal bloating may also occur. Elevated LFTs may occur, but are dose-related and reversible; liver enlargement may occur.

Nursing Implications: Assess elimination and nutritional status, baseline and throughout treatment. Assess baseline LFTs. Instruct patient to report diarrhea, nausea, vomiting immediately, and teach self-administration of prescribed antiemetics and antidiarrheal medication. Monitor weight, and teach patient importance of high-protein, high-calorie diet. Instruct patient to administer dose over 15 minutes to decrease nausea and vomiting. If weight loss occurs/persists, refer to dietitian/nutritionist. Monitor LFTs during treatment: AST, ALT, bili, and alk phos.

III. INJURY related to ANAPHYLAXIS

Defining Characteristics: Rare anaphylaxis has occurred in patients with AIDS, characterized by diffuse erythema, pruritus, injection of conjunctiva, fever, tachycardia, hypotension, edema, and abdominal pain.

Nursing Implications: Instruct AIDS patients to report any signs/symptoms of rash, pruritus, conjunctivitis, abdominal pain immediately. Use drug cautiously in AIDS patients. Monitor any adverse sensations over time. Assess for signs/symptoms.

IV. ALTERATION IN SENSORY/PERCEPTUAL PATTERNS related to CNS CHANGES

Defining Characteristics: Confusion, sedation, hallucinations, and headaches occur infrequently.

Nursing Implications: Assess baseline mental status. Instruct patient to report headaches, abnormal thoughts, mental status changes. Discuss alternative drug if mental status changes occur.

Drug: itraconazole (Sporanox)

Class: Azole; antifungal.

Mechanism of Action: Fungistatic; may be fungicidal, depending on concentration; azole antifungals interfere with cytochrome P-450 activity, which is necessary for the demethylation of 14-α-methylsterols to ergosterol. Ergosterol, the principal sterol in the fungal cell membrane, becomes depleted. This damages the cell membrane, producing alterations in membrane function and permeability. In *Candida albicans*, azole antifungals inhibit transformation of blastospores into invasive mycelial form.

Metabolism: Rapidly absorbed from GI tract in acid environment. Decreased absorption in patients with gastric hypochlorhydria or achlorhydria, or in patients taking medications that raise pH (antacids, H_2 antagonists).

Dosage/Range:

- Oral: 100–200 mg/day × 7–14 days (candidiasis); longer for other infections (400 mg/day in severe infections).
- Although studies did not provide a loading dose, in life-threatening situations a loading dose of 200 mg three times a day (600 mg/day) for the first 3 days is recommended, based on pharmacokinetic data.
- Doses above 200 mg/day should be given in two divided doses.
- IV: 200 mg bid × 4 doses followed by 200 mg daily; gave each dose over 1 hour—do not use for more than 14 days.

Drug Preparation:

- Store in tightly closed container at < 40°C (104°F).
- Itraconazole injection must be diluted prior to IV infusion. The entire 250 mg ampule should be diluted in the 50 mL bag of 0.9% sodium chloride provided by the manufacturer. The final concentration of the solution is 3.33 mg/mL (250 mg/75 mL).

Drug Administration:

- Orally in single or split dose, depending on total daily dose.
- Should take with meals to increase absorption of medication.
- Oral solution should be taken on an empty stomach to increase absorption of the medication.
- To administer a 200 mg dose of itraconazole, 60 mL should be given by IV infusion over 60 minutes. The infusion should be given using a controlled infusion device, the manufacturer-provided infusion set, and a dedicated IV line. When the infusion is complete, the manufacturer recommends that the infusion set be flushed via the 2-way stopcock using 15–20 mL of 0.9% sodium chloride over 30 seconds to 15 minutes. The entire IV line should then be discarded.

Drug Interactions:

- Drugs that increase gastric pH: antacids, anticholinergics/antispasmodics, histamine H_2-receptor antagonists, or omeprazole will decrease the absorption of itraconazole.

- Didanosine contains a buffer to increase its absorption; this will decrease the absorption of itraconazole since itraconazole needs an acidic environment.
- Use with oral antidiabetic agents has increased the plasma concentration of these sulfonylurea agents, leading to hypoglycemia.
- Use with carbamazepine may decrease itraconazole plasma concentrations, leading to clinical failure or relapse.
- Itraconazole may increase digoxin concentrations, leading to digoxin toxicity.
- Use with lovastatin or simvastatin may increase the plasma concentrations of these cholesterol-lowering agents and may increase the risk of rhabdomyolysis.
- Use with midazolam or triazolam may potentiate the hypnotic and sedative effects of these benzodiazepines.

Lab Effects/Interference:

Major clinical significance:

- ALT, alk phos, AST, serum bili values may be elevated.
- Serum K+: hypokalemia has occurred in approximately 2–6% of patients treated with itraconazole and has resulted in ventricular fibrillation, especially in higher doses.

Special Considerations:

- High failure rate in HIV-infected patients due to achlorhydria.

Potential Toxicities/Side Effects and the Nursing Process

I. ALTERATION IN NUTRITION, LESS THAN BODY REQUIREMENTS, related to GI SIDE EFFECTS

Defining Characteristics: Increased LFTs may occur: AST, ALT, alk phos. Hepatotoxicity is less common, is usually reversible, and is rarely fatal.

Nursing Implications: Assess baseline nutritional and elimination status. Instruct patient to report GI disturbances. Administer and teach patient to self-administer antiemetics, antidiarrheals as needed and as ordered. Teach patient importance of nutritious diet, and suggest small, frequent, high-calorie, high-protein meals as appropriate. Assess baseline LFTs and monitor periodically during treatment. Discuss abnormalities and drug interruption with physician. Assess whether taking other hepatotoxic drugs (see Special Considerations section). Assess for increased fatigue, jaundice, dark urine, pale stools (signs of hepatotoxicity), and discuss drug discontinuance immediately with physician.

II. ALTERATION IN SKIN INTEGRITY related to ALLERGIC REACTION

Defining Characteristics: Rash, dermatitis, purpura, urticaria occur; rarely, anaphylaxis may occur.

Nursing Implications: Assess baseline skin condition and integrity. Instruct patient to report itch, rash, other skin changes. Teach patient skin care and symptomatic measures. If rash or dermatitis progresses, discuss drug discontinuance with physician. Assess for signs/symptoms of anaphylaxis.

Drug: ketoconazole (Nizoral)

Class: Azole; antifungal (systemic).

Mechanism of Action: Fungistatic by damaging fungal cell membrane and increasing permeability, altering cell metabolism, and inhibiting cell growth. Fungicidal at high concentrations. Active against mucocutaneous candidiasis, histoplasmosis, coccidioidomycosis, and blastomycosis.

Metabolism: Rapidly absorbed from GI tract in acid environment. Decreased absorption in patients with gastric hypochlorhydria (25% of all AIDS patients) or in patients taking medications that raise pH (antacids, H_2 antagonists). Distributed widely but cerebrospinal penetration is unpredictable. Drug is ~90% protein-bound. Partially metabolized in liver, and mostly excreted in the feces via bile.

Dosage/Range:
- Oral: 200 mg/day × 7–14 days (candidiasis); longer for other infections (400 mg/day in severe infections).

Drug Preparation:
- Store in tightly closed container at < 40°C (104°F).

Drug Administration:
- Orally in single dose.
- May take with meals to decrease GI side effects (unclear if food increases absorption).
- In patients with gastric achlorhydria, patient may be instructed to dissolve ketoconazole in 4 mL aqueous solution of 0.2 N hydrochloric acid and drink through a straw; follow with 4 oz (120 mL) water.

Drug Interactions:
- Drugs that increase gastric pH: antacids, cimetidine, ranitidine, famotidine, sucralfate decrease ketoconazole absorption; give these drugs at least 2 hours after ketoconazole.
- Other hepatotoxic drugs: use cautiously, and monitor liver function studies closely.
- Rifampin or rifampin plus isoniazid: decreased ketoconazole levels, especially if isoniazid is taken as well. Increase ketoconazole dose.
- Acyclovir: synergism and increased antiviral action against herpes simplex virus.
- Norfloxacin: theoretically increases antifungal action of ketoconazole, but studies are inconsistent.

- Coumarin anticoagulants: increased PT; monitor patient closely and decrease anticoagulant dose accordingly.
- Cyclosporine: increased cyclosporine serum level; monitor serum level and decrease cyclosporine dose accordingly.
- Phenytoin: may have altered serum levels of phenytoin or ketoconazole; monitor serum levels of each and adjust dosages accordingly.
- Theophylline: may decrease theophylline serum concentrations; monitor serum levels and increase dosage accordingly.
- Corticosteroids: may increase corticosteroid serum level; may need to decrease dosage.

Lab Effects/Interference:

Major clinical significance:

- ALT, alk phos, AST, serum bili values may be elevated.
- ACTH-induced serum corticosteroid concentrations and serum testosterone concen trations may be decreased by doses of 800 mg/day of ketoconazole; serum testosterone concentrations are abolished by values of 1.6 g/day of ketoconazole, but return to baseline values when ketoconazole is discontinued.

Special Considerations:

- Monitor liver function studies.
- High failure rate in HIV-infected patients due to achlorhydria.

Potential Toxicities/Side Effects and the Nursing Process

I. ALTERATION IN NUTRITION, LESS THAN BODY REQUIREMENTS, related to GI SIDE EFFECTS

Defining Characteristics: Nausea, vomiting is seen in 3–10% of patients. Diarrhea, abdominal pain, flatulence, constipation may occur less frequently. Increased LFTs may occur: AST, ALT, alk phos. Hepatotoxicity is less common, is usually reversible, and is rarely fatal.

Nursing Implications: Assess baseline nutritional and elimination status. Instruct patient to report GI disturbances. Administer and teach patient to self-administer antiemetics, antidiarrheals as needed and as ordered. Teach patient importance of nutritious diet, and suggest small, frequent, high-calorie, high-protein meals as appropriate. Assess baseline LFTs and monitor periodically during treatment. Discuss abnormalities and drug interruption with physician. Assess whether taking other hepatotoxic drugs (see Special Considerations section). Assess for increased fatigue, jaundice, dark urine, pale stools (signs of hepatotoxicity), and discuss drug discontinuance immediately with physician.

II. ALTERATION IN COMFORT related to GYNECOMASTIA AND BREAST TENDERNESS

Defining Characteristics: Breast enlargement and tenderness may occur in some men, lasting weeks to duration of therapy.

Nursing Implications: Assess for occurrence in male patients. Assess comfort level, degree of tenderness, and self-care measures used to increase comfort. Assess impact on body image.

III. ALTERATION IN SKIN INTEGRITY related to ALLERGIC REACTION

Defining Characteristics: Rash, dermatitis, purpura, urticaria occur in 1% of patients; rarely, anaphylaxis may occur.

Nursing Implications: Assess baseline skin condition and integrity. Teach patient to report itch, rash, and other skin changes. Teach patient skin care and symptomatic measures. If rash or dermatitis progresses, discuss drug discontinuance with physician. Assess for signs/symptoms of anaphylaxis.

IV. ALTERATIONS IN SENSORY/PERCEPTUAL PATTERNS related to CNS EFFECTS

Defining Characteristics: Dizziness, headache, nervousness, insomnia, lethargy, somnolence, and paresthesia have occurred in ~1% of patients.

Nursing Implications: Assess baseline neurologic function and comfort, and monitor during treatment. Instruct patient to report any changes. Discuss any abnormalities with physician.

Drug: micafungin sodium (Mycamine)

Class: Antifungal.

Mechanism of Action: Fungistatic by damaging fungal cell membrane increasing permeability, altering cell metabolism, and inhibiting cell growth. Fungicidal at high concentrations. Inhibits the synthesis of 1,3-β-D-glucan, an integral component of the fungal cell wall.

Metabolism: Metabolized by liver and excreted in urine.

Dosage/Range:
- Esophageal candidiasis: 150 mg/day × 15 days.
- Prophylaxis of candida infections in HSCT recipients 50 mg/day × 19 days.

Drug Preparation:

- Do not mix or co-infuse with other medications. Mycafungin has been shown to precipitate when mixed directly with a number of other commonly used medications.
- No dose adjustment is required with concomitant use of mycophenolate mofetil, cyclosporine, tacrolimus, prednisolone, Sirolimus, nifedipine, fluconazole, ritonavir, or rifampin.
- A loading dose is not required; typically, 85% of the steady-state is achieved after three daily doses.
- IV: Dilute in 0.9% sodium chloride, USP (without a bacteriostatic agent) or 5% dextrose injection, USP.
- Infuse over 1 hour. Stable × 24 hours at room temperature.

Drug Interactions:

- Coumarin anticoagulants: increased PT. Monitor patient closely and decrease anticoagulant dose accordingly.
- Norfloxacin: may increase antifungal action.
- Cyclosporine: increased cyclosporine serum level. Monitor serum level and decrease cyclosporine dose accordingly.

Lab Effects/Interference:

Major clinical significance:

- ALT, alk phos, AST, serum bili values may be elevated.

Special Considerations:

- Used in treatment of fungal infections.
- Monitor HCT, Hgb, serum electrolytes, and lipids, as changes may occur during treatment.

Potential Toxicities/Side Effects and the Nursing Process

I. POTENTIAL FOR INJURY related to ANAPHYLAXIS

Defining Characteristics: Anaphylaxis with tachycardia, arrhythmias, and cardiac arrest may occur.

Nursing Implications: Assess baseline VS and monitor throughout infusion. Instruct patient to report signs/symptoms immediately. Assess for signs/symptoms: nausea, generalized itching, crampy abdominal pain, chest tightness, anxiety, agitation, sense of impending doom, wheezing, and dizziness.

II. ALTERATION IN COMFORT related to PRURITUS, PHLEBITIS, SKIN ERUPTIONS, FEVER

Defining Characteristics: Phlebitis, pruritus with or without rash may occur.

Nursing Implications: Assess temperature, skin integrity, and comfort prior to drug administration, and monitor throughout treatment. Discuss with physician use of diphenhydramine to decrease itching. Change IV sites q 48 h to decrease phlebitis, or discuss with patient and physician use of central line. If rash and pruritus worsen, discuss with physician drug discontinuance.

III. ALTERATION IN NUTRITION, LESS THAN BODY REQUIREMENTS, related to GI SIDE EFFECTS

Defining Characteristics: Nausea, vomiting, diarrhea, and anorexia may occur.

Nursing Implications: Assess baseline nutritional and elimination status. Instruct patient to report GI disturbances. Administer and teach patient to self-administer antiemetics, antidiarrheals as needed and as ordered. Teach patient importance of nutritious diet, and suggest small, frequent, high-calorie, high-protein meals as appropriate.

IV. ALTERATIONS IN SENSORY/PERCEPTUAL PATTERNS related to CNS, ENDOCRINE EFFECTS

Defining Characteristics: Dizziness, headache, and somnolence may occur.

Nursing Implications: Assess baseline neurologic function and comfort, and monitor during treatment. Instruct patient to report any changes. Discuss any abnormalities with physician.

Drug: miconazole nitrate (Monistat)

Class: Azole; antifungal (systemic).

Mechanism of Action: Fungistatic by damaging fungal cell membrane and increasing permeability, altering cell metabolism, and inhibiting cell growth. Fungicidal at high concentrations. Active against most fungi, especially candidiasis, coccidioidomycosis, cryptococcosis.

Metabolism: Limited (50%) oral absorption so usually given parenterally; 91–93% protein-bound to plasma proteins. Unpredictable penetration into CSF, so must be given intrathecally to achieve therapeutic levels. Metabolized by liver and excreted in urine.

Dosage/Range:

IV:

- Coccidioidomycosis: 1.8–3.6 g/day × 3–20+ weeks.
- Cryptococcosis: 1.2–2.4 g/day × 3–12+ weeks.

- Candidiasis: 600 mg–1.8 g/day × 1–20+ weeks.
- Intrathecal: refer to protocol; usually 20 mg q 1–2 days, or q 3–7 days if given by lumbar puncture.
- Intravesical: 200 mg in dilute solution 2–4 × day or by continuous bladder irrigation.

Drug Preparation:

- IV: Dilute in 200 mL of 0.9% sodium chloride (preferred) or 5% dextrose injection and infuse over 30–60 min; daily dosage usually given in three divided doses q 8 h. Stable × 24 hours at room temperature.
- Intrathecal: is administered undiluted.
- Intravesical: as above (dosage) in conjunction with IV drug as well.

Drug Interactions:

- Coumarin anticoagulants: increased PT. Monitor patient closely and decrease anticoagulant dose accordingly.
- Norfloxacin: may increase antifungal action.
- Oral sulfonylureas: increased hypoglycemia effect. Monitor blood glucose and decrease dose of oral sulfonylurea.
- Rifampin or rifampin plus isoniazid: decreased miconazole levels, especially if isoniazid taken as well. Increase miconazole dose.
- Phenytoin: may have altered serum levels of phenytoin or miconazole.
- Monitor serum levels of each and adjust dosages accordingly.
- Cyclosporine: increased cyclosporine serum level. Monitor serum level and decrease cyclosporine dose accordingly.

Lab Effects/Interference:

Major clinical significance:

- ALT, alk phos, AST, serum bili values may be elevated.

Clinical significance:

- Serum lipid profile: hyperlipidemia has occurred in patients receiving intravenous miconazole; this is reportedly due to the vehicle in the miconazole solution, PEG 40 castor oil (Cremophor EL).

Special Considerations:

- Used in treatment of severe fungal infections.
- Initial dose should be in hospital with resuscitation equipment available to determine hypersensitivity (cardiac arrest has occurred with initial dose). Drug is suspended in castor oil base, which stimulates allergic reaction. Subsequent dosing can be safely given to selected patients in ambulatory settings.
- IV push injection of drug may cause arrhythmias, so drug must be diluted (200+ mL) and administered over 30–60 minutes.
- Monitor HCT, Hgb, serum electrolytes, and lipids, as changes may occur during treatment.

Potential Toxicities/Side Effects and the Nursing Process

I. POTENTIAL FOR INJURY related to ANAPHYLAXIS

Defining Characteristics: Anaphylaxis with tachycardia, arrhythmias, and cardiac arrest may occur on first IV dose, probably related to suspension medium of drug (castor oil).

Nursing Implications: Ensure first dose is given in inpatient setting with resuscitation equipment and physician available. Assess baseline VS and monitor throughout infusion. Instruct patient to report signs/symptoms immediately. Assess for signs/symptoms: nausea, generalized itching, crampy abdominal pain, chest tightness, anxiety, agitation, sense of impending doom, wheezing, and dizziness.

II. ALTERATION IN COMFORT related to PRURITUS, PHLEBITIS, SKIN ERUPTIONS, FEVER

Defining Characteristics: Phlebitis, pruritus with or without rash may occur.

Nursing Implications: Assess temperature, skin integrity, and comfort prior to drug administration, and monitor throughout treatment. Discuss with physician use of diphenhydramine to decrease itching. Change IV sites q 48 h to decrease phlebitis, or discuss with patient and physician use of central line. If rash and pruritus worsen, discuss with physician drug discontinuance.

III. ALTERATION IN NUTRITION, LESS THAN BODY REQUIREMENTS, related to GI SIDE EFFECTS

Defining Characteristics: Nausea, vomiting, diarrhea, anorexia, and bitter taste may occur.

Nursing Implications: Assess baseline nutritional and elimination status. Instruct patient to report GI disturbances. Administer and teach patient to self-administer antiemetics, antidiarrheals as needed and as ordered. Teach patient importance of nutritious diet, and suggest small, frequent, high-calorie, high-protein meals as appropriate.

IV. ALTERATIONS IN SENSORY/PERCEPTUAL PATTERNS related to CNS, ENDOCRINE EFFECTS

Defining Characteristics: Dizziness, flushing, anxiety, increased libido, blurred vision, eye dryness, headache may occur.

Nursing Implications: Assess baseline neurologic function and comfort, and monitor during treatment. Instruct patient to report any changes. Discuss any abnormalities with physician.

Drug: nystatin (Mycostatin, Nilstat)

Class: Antifungal.

Mechanism of Action: Binds to sterol molecule in fungi cell membrane, increasing permeability so that potassium and other intracellular ions are lost. Active against yeast and fungi, especially Candida.

Metabolism: Drug is not absorbed from intact skin, mucous membranes, and is poorly absorbed from GI tract. Excreted as unchanged drug in the feces.

Dosage/Range:

- Oral (for treatment of oral or intestinal candidiasis): 500,000–1 million U tid; continue therapy for 48 hours after clinical remission to prevent recurrence.
- Powder: topical for candidal rash infections.
- Vaginal: 100,000 U as vaginal tablet, inserted into vagina daily or bid × 14 days.

Drug Preparation:

- Oral suspension and tablets should be stored in tight, light-resistant containers < 40°C (104°F).

Drug Administration:

- Oral suspension. Instruct patient to:
  - — Rinse mouth with oral hygiene solution to clean food debris.
  - — Hold suspension in mouth and swish for 1–2 minutes, then swallow or spit solution.
  - — Do not rinse mouth or eat for 15–30 minutes.

Drug Interactions:

- None.

Lab Effects/Interference:

- None known.

Special Considerations:

- For patients with oral thrush who have difficulty taking oral suspension:
  - — Oral suspension can be frozen in medicine cups so it is easier to administer if the patient has stomatitis.
  - — Vaginal suppository may be sucked as this increases mucosal contact with drug.
  - — Cannot be used to treat systemic infections.
  - — Adverse effects are infrequent.

Potential Toxicities/Side Effects and the Nursing Process

I. ALTERATION IN NUTRITION, LESS THAN BODY REQUIREMENTS, related to GI SIDE EFFECTS

Defining Characteristics: High oral doses may cause nausea, vomiting, diarrhea.

Nursing Implications: Assess baseline nutritional status. Instruct patient to report GI disturbances. Administer and teach patient to self-administer antiemetics, antidiarrheals as needed and as ordered. Teach patient importance of nutritious diet, and suggest small, frequent, high-calorie, high-protein meals as appropriate.

II. KNOWLEDGE DEFICIT related to SELF-ADMINISTRATION OF MEDICATION

Defining Characteristics: Increased compliance when patient is instructed in self-care activities.

Nursing Implications: Assess knowledge about infection and planned treatment. Teach about drug action, potential side effects, and when and how to take drug. Instruct patient to rinse mouth with saline gargle (or other rinse) to remove food debris prior to taking nystatin suspension; solution should be swished in mouth 1–2 minutes, then swallowed or spit out. Patient should not eat or rinse mouth for 15–30 minutes.

Drug: posaconazole (Noxafil)

Class: Triazole; antifungal (systemic).

Mechanism of Action: Fungistatic; inhibits fungi by blocking ergosterol synthesis through inhibition of the enzyme lanosterol 14 alpha-demethylase (CYP51). Ergosterol depletion coupled with the accumulation of methylated sterol precursors results in inhibition of fungal cell growth, fungal death by damaging fungal cell membrane and increasing permeability, altering cell metabolism, and inhibiting cell growth. Fungicidal at high concentrations. Active against invasive Candida species, Aspergillus species, non-Aspergillus hyalohyphomycetes, phaeohyphomycetes, zygomycetes, and endemic fungi.

Metabolism: Absorbed from GI tract when administered as an oral suspension. Partially metabolized in liver, and mostly excreted in the feces via bile.

Dosage/Range:

- Oral: 200 mg q 6 hours for 7 days (loading dose) and then 400 mg q 12 hours daily (maintenance therapy) dose may be increased if there is an inadequate response to infections.

Drug Preparation:
- Drug is given orally.

Drug Administration:
- Orally. May take 1 hour before meals or 1 hour after meals.
- Absorption enhanced by co-administration with food and nutritional supplements.

Drug Interactions:
- Drugs that increase gastric pH: antacids, cimetidine, ranitidine, and sucralfate have minor or no significant effect on posaconazole.
- Hepatotoxic drugs: use cautiously, and monitor liver function studies closely.
- Coumarin anticoagulants: increases PT; monitor patient closely and decrease anticoagulant dose accordingly.
- Potential interactions could occur with concomitant use of posaconazole and cisapride, astemizole, terfenadine, quinidine, pimozide, bepridil, sertindole, dofetilide, and halofantrine.
- Well tolerated in pediatric and elderly patients.

Lab Effects/Interference:

Major clinical significance:
- ALT, alk phos, AST, serum bili values may be elevated.

Special Considerations:
- Monitor liver function studies.

Potential Toxicities/Side Effects and the Nursing Process

I. ALTERATION IN NUTRITION, LESS THAN BODY REQUIREMENTS, related to GI SIDE EFFECTS

Defining Characteristics: Nausea, vomiting is seen in 18% of patients. Diarrhea, abdominal pain, flatulence, constipation may occur less frequently. Increased LFTs may occur: AST, ALT, alk phos. Hepatotoxicity is less common, is usually reversible, and is rarely fatal.

Nursing Implications: Assess baseline nutritional and elimination status. Instruct patient to report GI disturbances. Administer and teach patient to self-administer antiemetics, antidiarrheals as needed and as ordered. Teach patient importance of nutritious diet, and suggest small, frequent, high-calorie, high-protein meals as appropriate. Assess baseline LFTs and monitor periodically during treatment. Discuss abnormalities and drug interruption with physician. Assess whether taking other hepatotoxic drugs (see Special Considerations section). Assess for increased fatigue, jaundice, dark urine, pale stools (signs of hepatotoxicity), and discuss drug discontinuance immediately with physician.

II. ALTERATION IN SENSORY/PERCEPTUAL PATTERNS related to HEADACHE

Defining Characteristics: Treatment-related disturbances are common (17%). Generally mild and rarely result in discontinuing treatment.

Nursing Implications: Assess for occurrence. Assess comfort level. Educate patient about this side effect. Assess impact on body image.

III. ALTERATION IN COMFORT related to PRURITUS, DRY SKIN, and FLUSHING

Defining Characteristics: Rash, dry skin, and flushing.

Nursing Implications: Assess temperature, skin integrity, and comfort before drug administration, and monitor throughout course of treatment. Discuss with physician use of diphenhydramine to decrease itching and cream or lotions to smooth skin and maintain skin integrity. If rash and skin condition worsens, discuss with physician drug discontinuance.

Drug: voriconazole (VFEND)

Class: Triazole; antifungal (systemic).

Mechanism of Action: Fungistatic by damaging fungal cell membrane and increasing permeability, altering cell metabolism, and inhibiting cell growth. Fungicidal at high concentrations. Active against invasive *Aspergillus fumigatus*, *Fusarium* spp. infection, and *Scedosporium apiospermum* infection.

Metabolism: Rapidly absorbed from GI tract in acid environment. Partially metabolized in liver, and mostly excreted in the feces via bile.

Dosage/Range:
- Oral: 200 mg q 12 hours for 7–14 days; dose may be increased if there is an inadequate response to infections (300 mg q 12 hours).
- IV preparation is available. The final voriconazole preparation must be infused over 1–2 hours at a maximum rate of 3 mg/kg per hour.

Drug Preparation:
- Once reconstituted, drug should be used immediately, or it can be stored for no longer than 24 hours at 2–8°C (37–46°F).

Drug Administration:
- Orally. May take 1 hour before meals or 1 hour after meals.

- The final voriconazole preparation must be infused over 1–2 hours at a maximum rate of 3 mg/kg per hour.

Drug Interactions:
- Drugs that increase gastric pH: antacids, cimetidine, ranitidine have minor or no significant effect on voriconazole.
- Hepatotoxic drugs: use cautiously, and monitor liver function studies closely.
- Rifampin decreases the steady state of voriconazole.
- Coumarin anticoagulants: increases PT; monitor patient closely and decrease anticoagulant dose accordingly.
- Cyclosporine: increases cyclosporine serum level; monitor serum level and decrease cyclosporine dose accordingly.
- Phenytoin: may have altered serum levels of phenytoin or ketoconazole; monitor serum levels of each and adjust dosages accordingly.
- Carbamazepine and long-acting barbiturates and macrolide antibiotics reduce the efficacy of voriconazole.

Lab Effects/Interference:
Major clinical significance:
- ALT, alk phos, AST, serum bili values may be elevated.

Special Considerations:
- Monitor liver function studies.

Potential Toxicities/Side Effects and the Nursing Process

I. ALTERATION IN NUTRITION, LESS THAN BODY REQUIREMENTS, related to GI SIDE EFFECTS

Defining Characteristics: Nausea, vomiting is seen in 3–10% of patients. Diarrhea, abdominal pain, flatulence, constipation may occur less frequently. Increased LFTs may occur: AST, ALT, alk phos. Hepatotoxicity is less common, is usually reversible, and is rarely fatal.

Nursing Implications: Assess baseline nutritional and elimination status. Instruct patient to report GI disturbances. Administer and teach patient to self-administer antiemetics, antidiarrheals as needed and as ordered. Teach patient importance of nutritious diet, and suggest small, frequent, high-calorie, high-protein meals as appropriate. Assess baseline LFTs and monitor periodically during treatment. Discuss abnormalities and drug interruption with physician. Assess whether taking other hepatotoxic drugs (see Special Considerations section). Assess for increased fatigue, jaundice, dark urine, pale stools (signs of hepatotoxicity), and discuss drug discontinuance immediately with physician.

II. ALTERATION IN SENSORY/PERCEPTUAL PATTERNS related to VISUAL DISTURBANCES

Defining Characteristics: Treatment-related visual disturbances are common (30%). Generally mild and rarely result in discontinuing treatment.

Nursing Implications: Assess for occurrence. Assess comfort level. Educate patient about this side effect. Assess impact on body image.

III. ALTERATION IN SKIN INTEGRITY related to ALLERGIC REACTION

Defining Characteristics: Rash, dermatitis, purpura, urticaria occur in 6% of patients.

Nursing Implications: Assess baseline skin condition and integrity. Teach patient to report itch, rash, and other skin changes. Teach patient skin care and symptomatic measures. If rash or dermatitis progresses, discuss drug discontinuance with physician. Assess for signs/symptoms of anaphylaxis.

ANTIVIRALS

Drug: acyclovir (Zovirax)

Class: Antiviral (systemic).

Mechanism of Action: Interferes with DNA synthesis so that viral replication cannot occur. Active against herpes simplex virus (HSV-1, HSV-2), varicella-zoster virus (VZV) (shingles), Epstein-Barr virus (EBV), and cytomegalovirus (CMV).

Metabolism: Variable GI absorption; unaffected by food. Widely distributed in body tissue and fluids, including CSF. Variable protein-binding (9–33%).Crosses placenta and is excreted in breast milk.

Dosage/Range:

Adult:

- Oral: 200 mg PO q 4 h (genital herpes) to 800 mg PO 5 ×/day (acute herpes zoster).
- IV (initial/recurrent infections in immunocompromised patients): 5–10 mg/kg q 8 h × 7 days; 5 mg/kg q 8 h × 7–14 days (herpes simplex); 10 mg/kg q 8 h × 7–14 days (herpes zoster, herpes encephalitis).
- Use ideal body weight for dose calculation.
- Avoid doses greater than 1000 mg/dose.
- Dose modification is required if renal dysfunction is present.

Drug Preparation:

- Oral: store in tight, light-resistant containers at 15–25°C (59–77°F).

- IV: reconstitute with sterile water for injection per manufacturer's directions and further dilute in 50–100 mL IV fluid; a final concentration of 7 mg/mL or less is recommended to minimize the incidence of phlebitis; infuse over 1 hour.

Drug Interactions:

- Zidovudine: potentiates antiretroviral activity of zidovudine, but may cause increased neurotoxicity (drowsiness, lethargy) in AIDS patients. Monitor for increased neurotoxicity.
- Probenecid: may increase plasma half-life. Monitor for increased acyclovir toxicity.
- Antifungals: potential antiviral synergy.
- Interferon: potential synergistic antiviral effect, potential increased neurotoxicity. Use together with caution.
- Methotrexate (intrathecal): possible increased neurotoxicity. Use together with caution.

Lab Effects/Interference:

Major clinical significance:

- BUN and serum creatinine concentrations required prior to and during therapy, since intravenous acyclovir may be nephrotoxic; if acyclovir is given by rapid intravenous injection or its urine solubility is exceeded, precipitation of acyclovir crystals may occur in renal tubules; renal tubular damage may occur and may progress to acute renal failure.

Clinical significance:

- Pap test: although clear association has not been shown to date, patients with genital herpes may be at increased risk of developing cervical cancer. Pap test should be done at least once a year to detect early cervical changes.

Special Considerations:

- Use cautiously in patients with preexisting renal dysfunction or dehydration; underlying neurologic dysfunction or neurologic reactions to cytotoxic drugs, intrathecal methotrexate, or interferon and in patients with hepatic dysfunction.
- It is imperative that patients be well hydrated, with adequate urine output prior to and for up to 2 hours after IV dosing.
- Administer with caution if patient is receiving other nephrotoxic drugs.
- Contraindicated in patients hypersensitive to drug.
- Minimal injury to normal cells, so few adverse effects exist.

Potential Toxicities/Side Effects and the Nursing Process

I. ALTERATION IN URINARY ELIMINATION related to RENAL TOXICITY

Defining Characteristics: Transient increase is seen in renal function tests (serum BUN, creatinine) and decreased urine creatinine clearance, as drug may precipitate in renal tubules during dehydration or rapid IV drug administration. Increased risk exists if preexisting renal disease or concurrent administration of nephrotoxic drugs.

Nursing Implications: Assess baseline renal function, and monitor periodically during therapy. Notify physician of any abnormalities before administering next dose. Ensure adequate hydration and urine output prior to and for 2 hours after IV drug administration. Administer IV drug slowly over 1 hour.

II. ALTERATIONS IN SENSORY/PERCEPTUAL PATTERNS related to ENCEPHALOPATHY

Defining Characteristics: IV administration: encephalopathy (lethargy, tremors, confusion, agitation, seizures, dizziness) may occur rarely. Oral: headache occurs in 13% of patients receiving chronic suppressive treatment.

Nursing Implications: Assess baseline neurologic function and comfort, and monitor during treatment. Instruct patient to report any changes. Discuss any abnormalities with physician.

III. ALTERATIONS IN COMFORT related to LOCAL VEIN IRRITATION (IV ADMINISTRATION)

Defining Characteristics: Erythema, irritation, pain, swelling, phlebitis may occur at injection site.

Nursing Implications: Assess IV site for patency, irritation prior to each dose. Change IV site at least q 48 h. Apply warmth/heat to painful area as needed.

IV. ALTERATION IN NUTRITION, LESS THAN BODY REQUIREMENTS, related to GI SIDE EFFECTS (ORAL DOSAGE)

Defining Characteristics: Nausea, vomiting, and diarrhea occur in 2–5% of patients receiving chronic therapy.

Nursing Implications: Assess history of nausea/vomiting, diarrhea, and instruct patient to report any occurrence. Teach patient self-medication of prescribed antinausea or antidiarrheal medicines. Discuss drug discontinuance with physician if symptoms are severe.

V. ALTERATION IN SKIN INTEGRITY related to RASH

Defining Characteristics: Rash, urticaria, pruritus may occur.

Nursing Implications: Assess baseline history of drug allergy and skin integrity. Instruct patient to report any occurrence of rash, pruritus. Teach symptomatic management measures unless severe; if severe, discuss drug discontinuance with physician.

VI. KNOWLEDGE DEFICIT related to (ORAL) DRUG ADMINISTRATION

Defining Characteristics: Patient may not realize drug does not cure viral infection, nor does it prevent spread of virus to others. Prodrome of tingling, itching, or pain can herald mucocutaneous herpes.

Nursing Implications: Teach patient about herpetic infection and goal of therapy to suppress infection. When used to treat recurrent episodes of chronic infection, teach patient to recognize prodromal symptoms and to take prescribed drug then or within two days of onset of lesions. Teach patient about routes of viral spread, and instruct to avoid contacts with others that may lead to viral spread.

Drug: cidofovir (Vistide)

Class: Antiviral (systemic).

Mechanism of Action: Suppresses CMV replication by selective inhibition of viral DNA synthesis.

Metabolism: Less than 6% bound to plasma proteins. Renal clearance is reduced with the concomitant administration of probenecid.

Dosage/Range:
- Weekly induction regimen: 5 mg/kg infused every week × 2 weeks.
- Twice monthly maintenance regimen: 5 mg/kg infused every other week.

Drug Preparation:
- Requires chemotherapy safety handling (drug is mutagenic, tumorigenic, embryotoxic).
- Reconstitute drug (single use, nonpreserved); vial contains 75 mg/mL.
- Further dilute in 100 mL 0.9% sodium chloride.

Drug Administration:
- Administer 2 g probenecid (four 500-mg tabs) 3 hours prior to drug infusion.
- Infuse 1 L of 0.9% sodium chloride over 1–2 hours immediately prior to drug infusion.
- Infuse IV drug over 1 hour.
- As ordered by physician, may administer second liter of 0.9% sodium chloride at the start of the drug infusion, and continue for 1–3 hours.

- Two hours after end of drug infusion, administer 1 g probenecid (two 500-mg tabs).
- Eight hours after end of the drug infusion, administer 1 g probenecid (two 500-mg tabs).

Drug Interactions:

- Probenecid: interacts with the metabolism or renal tubular excretion of acetaminophen, acyclovir, angiotensin-converting enzyme (ACE) inhibitors, barbiturates, NSAIDs, theophylline, zidovudine.
- Increased nephrotoxicity when combined with other nephrotoxic drugs.

Lab Effects/Interference:

- Serum creatinine levels may be elevated.

Special Considerations:

- Indicated for the treatment of AIDS patients who have newly diagnosed or relapsed CMV retinitis.
- Dose-limiting toxicity is nephrotoxicity evidenced by proteinuria and increased serum creatinine.
- Treatment requires prehydration and posthydration use of concomitant probenecid.
- Drug contraindicated in patients with baseline serum creatinine > 1.5 mg/dL, creatinine clearance ≤ 55 mL/min, proteinuria ≥ 3+, past severe hypersensitivity to probenecid or other sulfa-containing medications, hypersensitivity to cidofovir, and patients who are pregnant or breast-feeding.

DOSE REDUCTIONS:

- (a) Patients with baseline normal renal function:

Renal Abnormality	Cidofovir Dosage
Serum creatinine 0.3–0.4 mg/dL > baseline	3 mg/kg
Serum creatinine = 0.5 mg/dL above baseline	discontinue cidofovir
Proteinuria ≥ 3+	discontinue cidofovir

- (b) Patients with baseline renal impairment:

Creatinine Clearance (mL/min)	Induction (once a week × 2 weeks)	Maintenance (once every 2 weeks)
41–55	2.0 mg/kg	2.0 mg/kg
30–40	1.5 mg/kg	1.1 mg/kg
20–29	1.0 mg/kg	1.0 mg/kg
≤ 19	0.5 mg/kg	0.1 mg/kg

- Patient teaching:
  - — Encourage increased oral intake of fluids to 1–3 L as tolerated.
  - — Return to clinic for appointments (induction: weekly × 2 weeks, maintenance every other week).
  - — Report side effects immediately.
  - — Ophthalmologic appointments as scheduled for intraocular pressure (IOP), visual acuity monitoring.

Potential Toxicities/Side Effects and the Nursing Process

I. POTENTIAL FOR INJURY related to NEUTROPENIA

Defining Characteristics: Neutropenia (< 750/mm^2) may occur in 28% of patients, and < 500/mm^3 occurred in 20% of patients. Infections occurred in 25% of patients.

Nursing Implications: Monitor WBC and ANC prior to each drug dose, and hold treatment if neutropenic. Discuss with physician use of G-CSF. If the patient is receiving zidovudine, the zidovudine should be temporarily discontinued or dose decreased by 50% on days of probenecid therapy. Instruct patient to monitor temperature and to report fever > 101°F immediately. Discuss use of G-CSF with physician as needed (up to 34% required G-CSF in clinical trials).

II. ALTERATION IN NUTRITION, LESS THAN BODY REQUIREMENTS, related to NAUSEA/VOMITING

Defining Characteristics: Nausea/vomiting occurs in about 65% of patients.

Nursing Implications: Encourage patients to eat food prior to each dose of probenecid. Discuss antiemetic prior to the first dose of probenecid, and then during period of probenecid therapy.

III. ALTERATION IN COMFORT related to FEVER, CHILLS, RASH, HEADACHE FROM PROBENECID

Defining Characteristics: Fever occurs in up to 57% of patients, rash in 30%, headache in 27%, chills in 24%. Asthenia (46% incidence), diarrhea (27%), alopecia (25%), anorexia (22%), dyspnea (22%), abdominal pain (17%), and anemia (20%). In clinical trials, 25% of patients withdrew from treatment due to adverse events.

Nursing Implications: Assess baseline comfort, and instruct patient to report symptoms. Discuss symptom management with physician, such as antihistamine and/or antipyretic (acetaminophen) for fever, and then use prophylactically in subsequent doses.

IV. ALTERATION IN ELIMINATION related to RENAL TOXICITY

Defining Characteristics: Creatinine elevations to > 1.5 mg/dL occur in approximately 17% of patients, proteinuria in 80% of patients, and decreased serum bicarbonate in > 5% of patients.

Nursing Implications: Encourage patients to increase their daily oral fluid intake to 2–3 L. Closely monitor renal function; patients who have received foscarnet are at increased risk for nephrotoxicity. Ensure that patient receives prehydration and posthydration, and is able to take oral fluids. Discuss dose reductions based on alterations in renal function with physician. Check urine for protein. If positive, discuss additional hydration and rechecking of urine for blood with physician.

V. ALTERATIONS IN SENSORY/PERCEPTUAL PATTERNS related to OCULAR HYPOTONY

Defining Characteristics: OCULAR HYPOTONY occurs rarely, may be increased risk for patients with concomitant diabetes mellitus.

Nursing Implications: Patients should see ophthalmologist for IOP assessments and visual acuity periodically.

VI. METABOLIC ACIDOSIS related to DECREASED SERUM BICARBONATE

Defining Characteristics: Occurs rarely (2%).

Nursing Implications: Assess for decreases in serum bicarbonate < 16 mEq/L associated with evidence of renal tubular damage (incidence 9%). Serious metabolic acidosis in association with liver failure, mucormycosis, aspergillus, and disseminated MAC has occurred, with subsequent death in one patient. Monitor baseline chemistries, and review results prior to each treatment.

Drug: famciclovir (Famvir)

Class: Antiviral (systemic).

Mechanism of Action: Rapidly transformed into antiviral penciclovir, which inhibits herpes simplex types HSV-1, HSV-2, or VZV by inhibiting HSV-2 polymerase. Herpes viral DNA synthesis and viral replication are selectively inhibited.

Metabolism: Oral bioavailability is 77%, with peak plasma levels 30–90 minutes after dosing. Plasma half-life is 2.3 hours. In the virus, the active form of the drug has a long intracellular half-life. Low protein binding and rapid and complete elimination in the urine (73%) and feces (27%).

Dosage/Range:
- Herpes zoster: 500 mg q 8 h × 7 days.
- Genital herpes: 125 mg bid × 5 days.

Drug Preparation:
- Available in 125-, 250-, 500-mg tablets.

Drug Administration:
- Oral, without regard to meals.

Drug Interactions:
- None.

Lab Effects/Interference:
- None known.

Special Considerations:
- Treatment of herpes zoster: viral shedding stopped 50% faster than with placebo, with full crusting in < 1 week, and shorter time to relief from acute pain. In addition, drug significantly reduces the duration of postherpetic neuralgia by two months compared to placebo.
- Dose should be reduced in patients with renal impairment according to schedule below:

Condition	Creatinine Clearance cc/min	Dose
Herpes zoster	40–59	500 mg q 12 h
	20–39	500 mg q 24 h
	< 20	250 mg q 48 h
Recurrent genital herpes	20–39	125 mg q 24 h
	< 20	125 mg q 48 h

Potential Toxicities/Side Effects and the Nursing Process

I. ALTERATION IN COMFORT related to HEADACHE, NAUSEA

Defining Characteristics: Headache occurred in approximately 22% of patients. Nausea occurred in 12% of patients.

Nursing Implications: Teach patient that side effects may occur and are usually mild. Instruct patient to report headache that does not resolve with acetaminophen, or nausea that does not resolve with diet modification.

Drug: foscarnet sodium (Foscavir)

Class: Antiviral (systemic).

Mechanism of Action: Inhibits binding sites on virus-specific DNA polymerases and reverse transcriptases without affecting cellular DNA polymerases. Thus, prevents viral replication of all known herpes viruses: CMV, HSV-1, HSV-2, EBV, and VZV. Active against resistant herpes simplex viruses that are resistant via thymidine kinase deficiency. Indicated for treatment of CMV retinitis in AIDS patients.

Metabolism: 14–17% bound to plasma proteins, and excreted into urine 80–90% unchanged by kidneys. Variable penetration into CSF.

Dosage/Range:

Adult (normal renal function):

- IV induction: 60 mg/kg IV over 1 hour q 8 h × 2–3 weeks.
- Maintenance: 90–120 mg/kg/day IV over 2 hours.
- Dose modification is necessary if renal insufficiency. See manufacturer's package insert.

Drug Preparation:

- Add drug solution (24 mg/mL) to 0.9% sodium chloride or 5% dextrose to achieve a final concentration = 12 mg/mL.
- Administer via rate controller or infusion pump over 1 hour (induction) or 2 hours (maintenance) via peripheral or central vein.
- Do not administer or give concurrently with other drugs or solutions.

Drug Interactions:

- Incompatible with $D_{30}W$, amphotericin B, Ringer's lactate, total parenteral nutrition (TPN), acyclovir, ganciclovir, trimetrexate, pentamidine, vancomycin, trimethoprim/sulfamethoxazole, diazepam, digoxin, phenytoin, leucovorin, pro-chlorperazine.
- Pentamidine: potentially fatal HYPOCALCEMIA; seizures have occurred; AVOID CONCURRENT USE.
- Nephrotoxic drugs (amphotericin B, aminoglycosides): additive nephrotoxicity; AVOID CONCURRENT USE.
- Hypocalcemic agents: additive hypocalcemia; AVOID CONCURRENT USE.
- Zidovudine: increased anemia; monitor patient closely and transfuse with red blood cells as ordered.

Lab Effects/Alterations:

Major clinical significance:

- Serum calcium (ionized), serum calcium (total), and serum phosphate: concentrations of phosphate may be increased or decreased; concentrations of total calcium may be decreased; although the total calcium concentration may also appear normal, the level of ionized calcium may be decreased and result in symptomatic hypocalcemia.

- Serum creatinine concentrations may be increased.
- Serum Mg++ concentrations may be decreased.

Clinical significance:

- ALT, alk phos, AST, and serum bili values may be increased.
- Serum K+ concentrations may be decreased.

Special Considerations:

- Contraindicated in patients hypersensitive to foscarnet.
- DO NOT administer concomitantly with IV pentamidine.
- Avoid use during pregnancy; lactating women should interrupt breast-feeding while receiving the drug.
- Regular monitoring of renal function IMPERATIVE; dose modifications must be made if renal insufficiency exists.
- Use measures for safe handling of cytotoxic drugs (see Appendix 1).

Potential Toxicities/Side Effects and the Nursing Process

I. ALTERATION IN URINARY ELIMINATION related to RENAL TOXICITY

Defining Characteristics: Abnormal renal function occurs commonly; increased serum creatinine, decreased creatinine clearance, acute renal failure may occur.

Nursing Implications: Assess baseline elimination pattern and renal function studies, and monitor closely throughout treatment. Manufacturer suggests creatinine clearance be calculated 2–3 × per week (induction) and q 1–2 weeks (maintenance). Creatinine clearance can be calculated from modified Cockcroft and Gault equation:

$$\text{For male: } \frac{140 - \text{age}}{\text{serum creatinine} \times 72}$$

$$\text{For female: } \frac{140 - \text{age}}{\text{serum creatinine} \times 72} \times 0.085$$

Discuss dose modifications with physician if renal dysfunction occurs. Ensure adequate hydration and urinary output prior to and following dose; administer drug slowly over 1–2 hours, at no more than 1 mg/kg/min. Teach patient to increase oral fluids as tolerated to clear drug from kidneys.

II. ALTERATION IN ELECTROLYTE BALANCE related to METABOLIC ABNORMALITIES

Defining Characteristics: Hypocalcemia, hypophosphatemia, hyperphosphatemia, hypomagnesemia, and hypokalemia occur. Transient decreased ionized calcium may not appear in serum total calcium value. Tetany and seizures may occur, especially in patients receiving foscarnet and IV pentamidine. Increased risk exists if renal impairment or neurologic impairment.

Nursing Implications: Assess baseline calcium, phosphorus, magnesium, potassium, and concurrent drugs that might affect these values. Assess patient for signs/symptoms of hypocalcemia, such as perioral tingling, numbness, or paresthesias during or after infusion. Instruct patient to report these signs/symptoms immediately. If signs/symptoms occur, stop infusion, notify physician, and evaluate serum electrolyte, renal studies. Administer ordered electrolyte repletion.

III. ALTERATIONS IN SENSORY/PERCEPTUAL PATTERNS related to NEUROLOGIC CHANGES

Defining Characteristics: Headache, paresthesia, dizziness, involuntary muscle contractions, hypoesthesia, neuropathy, and seizures (including grand mal) have occurred. Increased risk exists of hypocalcemia (ionized Ca++) and renal insufficiency.

Nursing Implications: Assess baseline risk factors and neurologic status, and monitor during treatment. Assess for and instruct patient to report signs/symptoms. Discuss abnormalities with physician, and possible drug discontinuance.

IV. FATIGUE related to ANEMIA

Defining Characteristics: Anemia occurs in 33% of patients, and in 60% of patients receiving concomitant zidovudine.

Nursing Implications: Assess baseline HCT/Hgb, activity tolerance, cardiopulmonary status, and monitor during therapy. Instruct patient to report increasing fatigue, headache, irritability, shortness of breath, chest pain. Transfuse RBCs as ordered by physician. Discuss with clinic patient self-care ability; refer for home health assistance as needed.

V. ALTERATION IN NUTRITION, LESS THAN BODY REQUIREMENTS, related to GI SIDE EFFECTS

Defining Characteristics: Nausea, vomiting, diarrhea are common; anorexia, abdominal pain may also occur.

Nursing Implications: Assess baseline nutrition, liver function and monitor during therapy. Instruct patient to report GI side effects. Administer or teach patient to self-administer prescribed antiemetic or antidiarrheal medications. Encourage adequate oral or IV hydration. Notify physician of abnormal LFTs. If anorexia occurs, encourage favorite foods and small, frequent meals as tolerated.

VI. INFECTION related to NEUTROPENIA

Defining Characteristics: May occur in 17% of patients; increased risk when receiving concurrent zidovudine.

Nursing Implications: Assess baseline WBC, ANC, and temperature; monitor during therapy. Assess for signs/symptoms of infection and discuss these with physician. Instruct patient to report signs/symptoms of infection.

VII. ALTERATIONS IN COMFORT related to LOCAL VEIN IRRITATION (IV ADMINISTRATION)

Defining Characteristics: Erythema, irritation, pain, swelling, phlebitis may occur at injection site. Consider use of central line.

Nursing Implications: Assess IV site for patency, irritation prior to each dose. Change IV site at least q 48 h. Apply warmth/heat to painful area as needed.

VIII. ALTERATION IN SKIN INTEGRITY related to RASH

Defining Characteristics: Rash, sweating may occur. Also, rarely, local irritation and ulcerations of penile epithelium in males, and vulvovaginal mucosa in females has occurred—perhaps related to drug in urine.

Nursing Implications: Assess skin integrity baseline and during treatment. Instruct patient to report any irritation or lesions. Teach patient to perform frequent perineal hygiene.

Drug: ganciclovir (Cytovene)

Class: Antiviral (systemic).

Mechanism of Action: Interferes with DNA synthesis so that viral replication cannot occur. Active against HSV-1, HSV-2, VZV (shingles), EBV, and CMV.

Metabolism: Poorly absorbed from GI tract. Appears to be widely distributed, concentrates in kidneys, and is well distributed to the eyes. Crosses BBB. Drug crosses placenta and is excreted in breast milk in animals. Excreted unchanged in urine. Active against CMV infections, especially in the retina.

Dosage/Range:

Adult:

- IV induction: 5 mg/kg IV q 12 h × 14–21 days.
- Maintenance: 5 mg/kg IV 7 days/week or 6 mg/kg/day × 5 days/week.

- Intravitreous by ophthalmologist (investigational).
- DOSE MUST BE REDUCED IN RENAL IMPAIRMENT.

Drug Preparation:
- Drug is CARCINOGENIC and TERATOGENIC: use chemotherapy handling precautions (see Appendix 1) when preparing and administering ganciclovir.
- Administer only if ANC is > 500 cells/mm^3 and platelet count > 25,000/mm^3.
- Add 10 mL of sterile water for injection to 500-mg vial. Further dilute dose in 50–250 mL of IV fluid and infuse over at least 1 hour.

Drug Interactions:
- Zidovudine: increased hematologic toxicity (neutropenia, anemia); do not use together if possible. Consider didanosine (ddI) instead of zidovudine (AZT) or concomitant use of neutrophil growth factor (e.g., G-CSF or GM-CSF).
- Foscarnet: additive or synergistic antiviral activity.
- Probenecid: may increase ganciclovir serum levels. Monitor closely and decrease ganciclovir dose as needed.
- Immunosuppressant (corticosteroids, cyclosporine, azathioprine): increased bone marrow suppression; dose reduce or hold immunosuppressants during ganciclovir treatment.
- Interferon: potent synergism against herpes virus, VZV.
- Imipenem/cilastatin: increase neurotoxicity with seizures. AVOID CONCURRENT USE.
- Cytotoxic antineoplastic agents: additive toxicity in bone marrow, gonads, GI epithelium/mucosa.
- Other cytotoxic drugs (dapsone, pentamidine, flucytosine, amphotericin B, trimethoprim-sulfamethoxazole): increase toxicity. Use cautiously if unable to avoid concurrent use.

Lab Effects/Interference:
- Serum ALT, serum alk phos, serum AST, and serum bili values may be increased.
- BUN and serum creatinine values may be increased.

Special Considerations:
- Do not use in pregnancy.
- Patient should be well hydrated; use with caution at reduced doses if renal insufficiency exists.
- Drug is mutagenic; patient should use barrier contraceptive.
- For CMV retinitis patient, should see ophthalmologist at least every 6 weeks during ganciclovir therapy.
- Administer over at least 1 hour.
- Monitor blood counts frequently (3 × per week).

Potential Toxicities/Side Effects and the Nursing Process

I. INFECTION, BLEEDING related to BONE MARROW DEPRESSION

Defining Characteristics: Neutropenia (< 1000/mm^3) occurs in 25–50% of patients, especially in patients with AIDS or those undergoing bone marrow transplant. Thrombocytopenia (< 50,000/mm^3) occurs in 20% of patients. Anemia occurs in 1% of patients.

Nursing Implications: Assess baseline WBC, ANC, and platelet count; monitor throughout therapy (every other day initially, then 3 × per week). Hold ganciclovir if ANC < 500/mm^3, platelet count < 25,000/mm^3. Assess for signs/symptoms of infection or bleeding; instruct patient in signs/symptoms of infection and bleeding, and instruct to report these immediately. Teach patient self-care measures to minimize risk of infection, bleeding, including avoidance of OTC aspirin-containing medicines. Administer or teach patient to self-administer prescribed G-CSF or GM-CSF. Assess Hgb/HCT and signs/symptoms of fatigue. Instruct patient to alternate rest and activity periods.

II. ALTERATIONS IN SENSORY/PERCEPTUAL PATTERNS related to SENSORY CHANGES

Defining Characteristics: Retinal detachment may occur in 30% of patients treated for CMV retinitis. Local reactions (foreign body sensation, conjunctival or vitreal hemorrhage) may occur with intravitreal injection. CNS effects include headache, confusion, altered dreams, ataxia, dizziness, and affect 5–17% of patients.

Nursing Implications: Assess baseline neurologic status, including vision, and monitor during treatment. Patient should see ophthalmologist at least every six weeks. Instruct patient to report any abnormalities and discuss them with physician.

III. ALTERATION IN NUTRITION, LESS THAN BODY REQUIREMENTS, related to GI SIDE EFFECTS

Defining Characteristics: Nausea, vomiting, diarrhea, anorexia may occur in 2% of patients. Elevated LFTs may occur due to drug, but may be difficult to distinguish from CMV infection of liver or biliary tree.

Nursing Implications: Assess baseline nutrition, liver function, and monitor during therapy. Instruct patient to report GI side effects. Administer or teach patient to self-administer prescribed antiemetic or antidiarrheal medications. Encourage adequate oral or IV hydration. Notify physician of abnormal LFTs. If anorexia occurs, encourage favorite foods and small, frequent meals as tolerated.

IV. ALTERATION IN URINARY ELIMINATION related to RENAL TOXICITY

Defining Characteristics: 2% of patients have increased serum BUN, creatinine, hematuria. Increased risk exists in elderly or patients with renal insufficiency.

Nursing Implications: Ensure adequate hydration with urinary output prior to drug administration and infuse drug over at least 1 hour. Dose should be reduced in patients with decreased renal function.

V. ALTERATIONS IN COMFORT related to LOCAL VEIN IRRITATION (IV ADMINISTRATION)

Defining Characteristics: Inflammation, phlebitis, pain occur often at IV infusion site due to high pH of drug.

Nursing Implications: Assess IV site for patency, irritation, prior to each dose. Change IV site at least q 48 h. Apply warmth/heat to painful area as needed. Assess need for tunneled central line. Avoid drug extravasation.

VI. ALTERATION IN CARDIAC OUTPUT related to CHANGES IN BP

Defining Characteristics: Rarely, hypotension, or hypertension, arrhythmia, myocardial infarction, arrest occur.

Nursing Implications: Assess baseline VS and monitor throughout treatment. Notify physician of any changes from baseline.

VII. ALTERATION IN SEXUALITY/REPRODUCTIVE PATTERNS related to REPRODUCTIVE HAZARD

Defining Characteristics: Drug is carcinogenic, mutagenic, and teratogenic; may produce infertility in males. It is unknown whether drug crosses placenta and is excreted in breast milk.

Nursing Implications: Assess sexuality/reproductive patterns. Teach patient and partner about reproductive hazards; offer contraceptive counseling or refer for counseling, as barrier contraceptive should be used by patient.

Drug: valacyclovir hydrochloride (Valtrex)

Class: Antiviral (systemic).

Mechanism of Action: Drug is well absorbed and rapidly converted to acyclovir. Drug interferes with DNA synthesis so that viral replication cannot occur. Active against HSV-1, HSV-2, VZV (shingles), EBV, and CMV.

Metabolism: Widely distributed in body tissues and fluids including the CNS.

Dosage/Range:
- Herpes zoster: 1 g tid × 7 days.

Drug Preparation:
- Available in 500-mg caplets.
- Oral, without regard to meals.

Drug Interactions:
- Cimetidine and probenecid decrease renal clearance of valacyclovir.

Lab Effects/Interference:
- None known.

Special Considerations:
- Dose-reduce for renal impairment:

Creatinine Clearance (cc/min)	Dose
≥ 50	1 g q 8 h
30–49	1 g q 12 h
10–29	1 g q 24 h
< 10	500 mg q 24 h

- Treatment should be started within 48 hours of rash onset.
- AVOID DRUG IN IMMUNOCOMPROMISED PATIENTS, as patients with advanced HIV infection, and those undergoing bone marrow and renal transplants, have developed thrombotic thrombocytopenic purpura/hemolytic uremic syndrome (TTP/HUS).

Potential Toxicities/Side Effects and the Nursing Process

I. ALTERATION IN COMFORT related to HEADACHE, NAUSEA

Defining Characteristics: Headache occurred in approximately 22% of patients. Nausea occurred in 12% of patients.

Nursing Implications: Teach patient that side effects may occur and are usually mild. Patient should report headache that does not resolve with acetaminophen or nausea that does not resolve by diet modification.

Chapter 12
Constipation

Constipation is a decreased frequency of defecation that is difficult or uncomfortable (Walsh 1989). Levy (1992) reports five causes of constipation in cancer patients:

- Disease itself: i.e., primary bowel cancers, paraneoplastic autonomic neuropathy.
- Disease sequelae: i.e., dehydration, paralysis, immobility, alterations in bowel elimination patterns.
- Prior history of laxative abuse, hemorrhoids/anal fissures, other diseases.
- Cancer therapy: chemotherapy (vinca alkaloids, e.g., vincristine, vinblastine); bowel surgery.
- Medications used to manage symptoms: opioids, antihistamines, tricyclic antidepressants, aluminum antacids.

Complications of constipation can be severe (i.e., bowel perforation), extremely painful, and compromise quality of life. Nurses play an enormous role in preventing morbidity from constipation in patients with cancer. Assessment of the patient's previous and current nutrition and elimination patterns, along with assessment of probable etiology of constipation, are critical, as is patient/family teaching about constipation management and prevention. Teaching should include dietary modifications to include high-fiber intake (fruits, vegetables, or nutritional supplements high in fiber); fluid intake of 3 L/day; and moderate exercise as tolerated. Patients receiving drugs (i.e., opioids) that are likely to be constipating should also receive a bowel regimen to prevent constipation. Available laxatives include the following types:

- *Bulk-forming laxatives* cause the stool to retain water, and thus increase peristalsis (fiber, bran, psyllium, methylcellulose).
- *Lubricants* coat and soften the stool so it can move more smoothly through the intestines (mineral oil).
- *Saline laxatives* pull water into the gut and into the stool, increasing peristalsis (magnesium citrate, sodium biphosphate, magnesium hydroxide).
- *Osmotic laxatives* work through colonic bacteria that metabolize osmotic laxatives causing increased osmotic pressure gradient, pulling water into the gut and then into the stool, thus increasing peristalsis (glycerin, lactulose, sorbitol).
- *Detergent laxatives* reduce surface tension of the colonic cells, so water and fats enter the stool; in addition, electrolyte and water absorption is decreased (docusate salts).
- *Stimulant laxatives* irritate the gut, increasing gut motility (senna, bisacodyl).

New approaches to opioid-induced constipation prevention and management include the use of opioid antagonists, such as methylnaltrexone, which is now FDA approved under the trade name Relistor.

References

Levy MH. Constipation and Diarrhea in Cancer Patients, Part I. *Prim Care Cancer* 1992; 12(4) 11–18

Massey RL, Haylock PJ, Curtiss C. *Constipation*, Chapter 27. Yarbro CH, Frogge MH, Goodman M. *Cancer Symptom Management*, 3rd ed. Sudbury, MA: Jones and Bartlett, 2003

Twycross RG, Harcourt JMV. The Use of Laxatives at a Palliative Care Centre. *Pallia Med* 1991; 5 27–33

Walsh TD. Constipation. Walsh TD. *Symptom Control*. Cambridge: Blackwell Scientific Publications Inc., 1989; 331–381

Drug: bisacodyl (Dulcolax)

Class: Stimulant laxative.

Mechanism of Action: Stimulates/irritates smooth muscle of intestines, increasing peristalsis; increases fluid accumulation in colon and small intestines. Indicated for relief of constipation and bowel preparation prior to bowel surgery.

Metabolism: Minimal oral absorption. Evacuation occurs in 6–10 hours when taken orally, or within 15 minutes to 1 hour when administered rectally.

Dosage/Range:

Adult:

- Oral: 5–15 mg at bedtime or early morning. Bowel preparation may use up to 30 mg.
- Suppository: 10 mg PR.

Drug Preparation:

- Administer oral tablet > 1 hour after antacids or milk.
- Insert suppository as high as possible against wall of rectum.

Drug Interactions:

- None.

Lab Effects/Interference:

- None known.

Special Considerations:

- Contraindicated in patients with signs/symptoms of acute abdomen (nausea, vomiting, abdominal pain), intestinal obstruction, fecal impaction, or ulcerative bowel lesions.

Potential Toxicities/Side Effects and the Nursing Process

I. ALTERATIONS IN BOWEL ELIMINATION related to CHRONIC USE

Defining Characteristics: Removes defecation reflexes when used chronically (laxative dependence). Narcotic analgesics and vinca alkaloid chemotherapy may predispose to constipation.

Nursing Implications: Assess baseline elimination pattern. Teach patient how to self-administer laxative. Encourage patient to normalize bowel habits through adequate fluid intake (2–3 L/day), diet high in fiber and bulk (bran, cereals, fruits, and vegetables), and exercise as tolerated. Teach patient bowel regimen when on narcotics or vinca alkaloids to promote regular evacuation.

II. ALTERATION IN NUTRITION, LESS THAN BODY REQUIREMENTS, related to GI SIDE EFFECTS

Defining Characteristics: Constipation or drug may cause nausea, vomiting, abdominal pain; rectal suppository may cause burning in rectum as it is absorbed.

Nursing Implications: Assess comfort level and GI distress related to constipation. Encourage patient to drink cold fluids or ginger ale as tolerated. Encourage patient to try resting in different positions; warm packs may decrease abdominal pain. Teach patient to expect burning sensation with suppository use; reassure that it will resolve in 5–10 minutes.

III. ALTERATION IN FLUID AND ELECTROLYTE BALANCE related to LAXATIVE ABUSE

Defining Characteristics: Diarrhea resulting from laxative abuse can deplete fluid volume, nutrients, and electrolytes.

Nursing Implications: Teach patient regular bowel regimen when receiving constipating drugs (narcotics, vinca alkaloids). Teach patient to replace lost fluids and electrolytes (encourage chicken soup, sports drink).

Drug: docusate calcium, docusate potassium, docusate sodium (Dioctyl Calcium Sulfosuccinate, Dioctyl Potassium Sulfosuccinate, Dioctyl Sodium Sulfosuccinate, Colace, Diocto-K, Diosuccin, DOK-250, Doxinate, Duosol, Laxinate 100, Regulax SS, Stulex)

Class: Stool softener.

Mechanism of Action: The calcium, sodium, and potassium salts of docusate soften stool by decreasing surface tension, emulsification, and wetting action, thus increasing stool absorption of water in the bowel.

Metabolism: Appears to be absorbed somewhat in the duodenum and jejunum, and excreted in bile. Stool softening occurs in 1–3 days.

Dosage/Range:

Adult:

- Oral: 50–360 mg/day, in single or divided doses, depending on stool-softening response.

Drug Preparation:

- Oral: store gelatin capsule in tight container; store syrup in light-resistant containers.
- Rectal: according to manufacturer's package insert.

Drug Interactions:

- Mineral oil: increased mineral oil absorption; AVOID CONCURRENT USE.

Lab Effects/Interference:

- None known.

Special Considerations:

- Useful in prevention of straining-at-stool in patients receiving narcotics; when combined with other agents/laxatives, prevents constipation in these patients.
- Does not increase intestinal peristalsis; stop drug if severe abdominal cramping occurs.
- Is effective only in prevention of constipation, not in treating constipation.

Potential Toxicities/Side Effects and the Nursing Process

I. KNOWLEDGE DEFICIT related to BOWEL ELIMINATION

Defining Characteristics: Oncology patients who are receiving narcotic analgesics, vinca alkaloid chemotherapy (vincristine, vinblastine, vindesine), or who are dehydrated or hypercalcemic are at increased risk of constipation.

Nursing Implications: Assess baseline elimination pattern. Teach patient need for bowel movement at least every other day, depending on usual pattern. Teach patient importance of adequate fluid intake (2–3 L/day), diet high in fiber and bulk (bran, cereals, fruits, vegetables, and supplements with fiber), and exercise as tolerated. Teach self-administration of stool softeners and prescribed laxatives.

Drug: glycerin suppository (Fleet Babylax, Sani-Supp)

Class: Hyperosmotic laxative.

Mechanism of Action: Local irritant, with hyperosmotic action, drawing water from tissues into feces and stimulating fecal evacuation within 15–30 minutes.

Metabolism: Poorly absorbed from rectum.

Dosage/Range:

Adult:

- Rectal suppository: 2–3 g PR.
- Enema: 5–15 mL PR.

Drug Preparation:

- Rectal administration must be retained for 15 minutes.

Drug Interactions:

- None.

Lab Effects/Interference:

- None known.

Special Considerations:

- Contraindicated in patients with undiagnosed abdominal pain, intestinal obstruction.

Potential Toxicities/Side Effects and the Nursing Process

I. ALTERATIONS IN BOWEL ELIMINATION related to CHRONIC USE

Defining Characteristics: Removes defecation reflexes when used chronically (laxative dependence). Narcotic analgesics and vinca alkaloid chemotherapy may predispose to constipation.

Nursing Implications: Assess baseline elimination pattern. Teach patient how to self-administer laxative. Encourage patient to normalize bowel habits through adequate fluid intake (2–3 L/day), diet high in fiber and bulk (bran, cereals, fruits, and vegetables), and exercise as tolerated. Teach patient bowel regimen when on narcotics or vinca alkaloids to promote regular evacuation.

II. ALTERATION IN FLUID AND ELECTROLYTE BALANCE related to LAXATIVE ABUSE

Defining Characteristics: Diarrhea resulting from laxative abuse can deplete fluid volume, nutrients, and electrolytes.

Nursing Implications: Teach patient regular bowel regimen when receiving constipating drugs (narcotics, vinca alkaloids). Teach patient to replace lost fluids and electrolytes (encourage chicken soup, sports drink).

III. ALTERATION IN COMFORT related to CRAMPING PAIN, RECTAL IRRITATION, OR DISCOMFORT

Defining Characteristics: Cramping pain, rectal irritation, and inflammation or discomfort may occur.

Nursing Implications: Teach patient this may occur. If discomfort is not self-limited, suggest sitz bath, warm or cold packs, and position changes.

Drug: lactulose (Cholac, Constilac, Constulose, Duphalac)

Class: Hyperosmolar sugar.

Mechanism of Action: Delivers osmotically active molecules to intestine, drawing fluid into colon and causing distension; this stimulates peristalsis and evacuation in 24–48 hours. Also used to lower blood ammonia in hepatic encephalopathy.

Metabolism: Less than 3% absorbed; metabolized by bacteria in colon into lactic acid.

Dosage/Range:

Adult:

- Oral: 10–20 g (15–30 mL)/day to 40 g (60 mL)/day.

Drug Preparation:

- Store solution at 15–30°C (59–86°F).
- Give with juice.

Drug Interactions:

- Antacids: may decrease lactulose effect; avoid administering together.

Special Considerations:

- Diarrhea indicates overdosage; dose should be reduced.

Potential Toxicities/Side Effects and the Nursing Process

I. ALTERATION IN COMFORT related to GI SIDE EFFECTS

Defining Characteristics: Gaseous distension, flatulence, abdominal pain may occur.

Nursing Implications: Encourage patient to find comfortable position; apply warmth to decrease abdominal pain; reassure that symptoms will resolve.

II. ALTERATION IN FLUID AND ELECTROLYTE BALANCE related to DIARRHEA

Defining Characteristics: Diarrhea resulting from laxative abuse can deplete fluid volume, nutrients, and electrolytes.

Nursing Implications: Teach patient regular bowel regimen when receiving constipating drugs (narcotics, vinca alkaloids). Teach patient to replace lost fluids and electrolytes (encourage chicken soup, sports drink).

Drug: magnesium citrate

Class: Saline laxative.

Mechanism of Action: Draws water into small intestinal lumen, stimulating peristalsis and evacuation in 3–6 hours.

Metabolism: 15–30% absorbed, excreted in urine.

Dosage/Range:

Adult:

- Oral: 11–25 g (5–10 oz or 150–300 mL)/day as single or divided dose at bedtime.

Drug Preparation:

- Refrigerate and serve with ice. Taste can be masked by adding small amount of juice.

Drug Interactions:

- None.

Lab Effects/Interference:

- None known.

Special Considerations:

- Contraindicated in patients with signs/symptoms of acute abdomen (nausea, vomiting, abdominal pain), intestinal obstruction, fecal impaction, or ulcerative bowel lesions.
- Contraindicated in patients with rectal fissures, myocardial infarction, renal disease.

Potential Toxicities/Side Effects and the Nursing Process

I. ALTERATIONS IN BOWEL ELIMINATION related to CHRONIC USE

Defining Characteristics: Removes defecation reflexes when used chronically (laxative dependence). Narcotic analgesics and vinca alkaloid chemotherapy may predispose to constipation.

Nursing Implications: Assess baseline elimination pattern. Teach patient how to self-administer laxative. Encourage patient to normalize bowel habits through adequate fluid intake (2–3 L/day), diet high in fiber and bulk (bran, cereals, fruits, and vegetables), and exercise as tolerated. Teach patient bowel regimen when on narcotics or vinca alkaloids to promote regular evacuation.

II. ALTERATION IN NUTRITION, LESS THAN BODY REQUIREMENTS, related to GI SIDE EFFECTS

Defining Characteristics: Constipation or drug may cause nausea and abdominal pain.

Nursing Implications: Assess comfort level and GI distress related to constipation. Encourage patient to drink cold fluids or ginger ale as tolerated. Encourage patient to try resting in different positions; warm packs may decrease abdominal pain.

III. ALTERATION IN FLUID AND ELECTROLYTE BALANCE related to LAXATIVE ABUSE

Defining Characteristics: Diarrhea resulting from laxative abuse can deplete fluid volume, nutrients, and electrolytes.

Nursing Implications: Teach patient regular bowel regimen when receiving constipating drugs (narcotics, vinca alkaloids). Teach patient to replace lost fluids and electrolytes (encourage chicken soup, sports drink).

Drug: methylcellulose (Citrucel)

Class: Bulk-producing laxative.

Mechanism of Action: Absorbs water; bulk expansion stimulates peristalsis and evacuation in 12–24 hours. May also be used to slow diarrhea.

Metabolism: Not absorbed by GI tract.

Dosage/Range:

Adult:

- Oral: up to 6 g/day PO in 2–3 divided doses.

Drug Preparation:

- Administer each dose with at least 250 mL of water or juice.

Drug Interactions:

- None.

Lab Effects/Interference:

- None known.

Special Considerations:

- Safest and most physiologically normal laxative.

Potential Toxicities/Side Effects and the Nursing Process

I. ALTERATIONS IN BOWEL ELIMINATION related to CHRONIC USE

Defining Characteristics: Removes defecation reflexes when used chronically (laxative dependence). Narcotic analgesics and vinca alkaloid chemotherapy may predispose to constipation.

Nursing Implications: Assess baseline elimination pattern. Teach patient how to self-administer laxative. Encourage patient to normalize bowel habits through adequate fluid intake (2–3 L/day), diet high in fiber and bulk (bran, cereals, fruits, and vegetables), and exercise as tolerated. Teach patient bowel regimen when on narcotics or vinca alkaloids to promote regular evacuation.

II. ALTERATION IN NUTRITION, LESS THAN BODY REQUIREMENTS, related to GI SIDE EFFECTS

Defining Characteristics: Constipation or drug may cause nausea, vomiting, cramps.

Nursing Implications: Assess comfort level and GI distress related to constipation. Encourage patient to drink cold fluids or ginger ale as tolerated. Encourage patient to try resting in different positions; warm packs may decrease abdominal pain. Teach patient laxative effect may take 12–24 hours, and assess need for other cathartic(s).

Drug: methylnaltrexone bromide (Relistor)

Class: Selective, peripherally acting opioid antagonist.

Mechanism of Action: Mu opioid antagonist that competes with opioid analgesics for opioid receptors in the periphery, such as in the gut, but not in the CNS, as it is unable to cross the blood–brain barrier. Thus, it does not interfere with opioid pain relief, which is centrally mediated. Drug inhibits opioid induced delayed intestinal transit time.

Metabolism: Absorbed rapidly with peak serum level in 30 minutes. Drug is metabolized in the liver and is excreted by the kidneys (about 50%) and in the feces; 85% of the drug is excreted intact. The terminal half-life is 8 hours.

Dosage Range:

- 8 mg SQ every other day (weight 32–62 kg [84–136 lbs]) or 12 mg for patients weighing 62–114 kg (136–251 lbs), as needed. For patients weighing more or less, determine dose at 0.15 mg/kg SQ every other day as needed.
- If needed more frequently than every other day, maximum frequency is once every 24 hours.
- Dose reduce 50% if patient has renal impairment (creatinine clearance < 30 mL/min).

Drug Preparation:

- Drug is available as 12 mg in 0.6 mL in a single dose vial. Aseptically draw up ordered amount.
- Once drawn up, if not used right away, may be stored at ambient room temperature for 24 hours.
- Store vial at controlled room temperature and protect from light.

Drug Administration:

- Subcutaneous injection (8 mg dose is 0.4 mL and 12 mg dose is 0.6 mL) in upper arm, abdomen, or thigh.

Drug Interactions:

- Is a weak inhibitor of cytochrome P450 (CYP) isozyme CYP2D6 activity but did not interact with dextromethorphan.

Special Considerations:

- Indicated for the treatment of opioid-induced constipation in patients with advanced illness receiving palliative care when the response to laxative therapy has not been sufficient (not studied beyond 4 months of treatment).
- Contraindicated in patients with known or suspected mechanical GI obstruction. Approved only for adult use. Drug has not been studied in patients with peritoneal catheters.
- Oral and IV formulations are being developed and studied.

- Most common side effects are abdominal pain, flatulence, nausea, dizziness, and diarrhea.
- No difference in efficacy or safety profile in older patients.
- Thirty percent of patients have laxation within 30 minutes of drug administration, and 48–62% have laxation within 4 hours of first dose.

Potential Toxicities/Side Effects and the Nursing Process

I. ALTERATION IN NUTRITION, POTENTIAL, related to GI SIDE EFFECTS

Defining Characteristics: Drug may cause nausea (11.5%), abdominal pain (28.5%), flatulence (13.3%), and diarrhea (5.5%).

Nursing Implications: Assess comfort level and GI distress related to constipation. Encourage patient to drink cold fluids or ginger ale as tolerated. Encourage patient to try resting in different positions; warm packs may decrease abdominal pain. Teach patient to call nurse or physician if abdominal pain, nausea, or vomiting become more severe or if new symptoms develop. If patient develops persistent or severe diarrhea, stop drug and discuss with physician.

Drug: mineral oil (Fleet Mineral Oil)

Class: Lubricant laxative.

Mechanism of Action: Lubricates intestine, preventing fecal fluid from being absorbed in colon; water retention distends colon, stimulating peristalsis and evacuation in 6–8 hours.

Metabolism: Minimal GI absorption occurs following oral or rectal administration.

Dosage/Range:
Adult:
- Oral: 15–45 mL PO in single or divided doses.
- Rectal enemas: 120 mL PR as a single dose.

Drug Preparation:
- Administer plain mineral oil at bedtime on an empty stomach.
- Administer mineral oil emulsion with food if desired at bedtime.
- May mix with juice to mask taste.

Drug Interactions:
- Docusate salts: increase mineral oil absorption; DO NOT ADMINISTER CONCURRENTLY.
- Fat-soluble vitamins: decrease absorption with chronic mineral oil administration.

Lab Effects/Interference:
- Decreased fat-soluble vitamins, e.g., vitamins A, D, E, K with chronic drug administration.

Special Considerations:
- Contraindicated in patients with signs/symptoms of acute abdomen (nausea, vomiting, abdominal pain), intestinal obstruction, fecal impaction, or ulcerative bowel lesions.
- Do not use for more than 1 week.

Potential Toxicities/Side Effects and the Nursing Process

I. ALTERATIONS IN BOWEL ELIMINATION related to CHRONIC USE

Defining Characteristics: Removes defecation reflexes when used chronically (laxative dependence). Narcotic analgesics and vinca alkaloid chemotherapy may predispose to constipation.

Nursing Implications: Assess baseline elimination pattern. Teach patient how to self-administer laxative. Encourage patient to normalize bowel habits through adequate fluid intake (2–3 L/day), diet high in fiber and bulk (bran, cereals, fruits, and vegetables), and exercise as tolerated. Teach patient bowel regimen when on narcotics or vinca alkaloids to promote regular evacuation.

II. ALTERATION IN NUTRITION, LESS THAN BODY REQUIREMENTS, related to GI SIDE EFFECTS

Defining Characteristics: Constipation or drug may cause nausea, vomiting, cramps.

Nursing Implications: Assess comfort level and GI distress related to constipation. Encourage patient to drink cold fluids or ginger ale as tolerated. Encourage patient to try resting in different positions; warm packs may decrease abdominal pain. Teach patient to expect burning sensation with suppository use; reassure that it will resolve in 5–10 minutes.

Drug: polyethylene glycol 3350, NF powder (Miralax®)

Class: Osmotic cathartic.

Mechanism of Action: Drug is an osmotic agent that pulls water into the intestines with the stool, softening the stool and causing peristalsis and evacuation in 2–4 days.

Metabolism: Is not fermented by colonic microflora and does not affect intestinal absorption or secretion of glucose or electrolytes.

Dosage/Range:
- 17 g (1 heaping T) (product comes with a measuring cup).

Drug Preparation:
- Mix in 8 oz of water and take orally once a day.

Drug Administration:
- Oral. Available in 14-oz and 26-oz containers.
- Store at room temperature.

Drug Interactions:
- None.

Lab Effects/Interference:
- None.

Special Considerations:
- Contraindicated in patients with bowel obstruction.
- Indicated for the treatment of occasional constipation for up to 2 weeks.
- Use during pregnancy only if clearly needed.
- Excessive or frequent use or use > 2 weeks may result in electrolyte imbalance and dependence on laxatives.

Potential Toxicities/Side Effects and the Nursing Process

I. ALTERATIONS IN BOWEL ELIMINATION related to CHRONIC USE

Defining Characteristics: Removes defecation reflexes when used chronically (laxative dependence). Narcotic analgesics and vinca alkaloid chemotherapy may predispose to constipation.

Nursing Implications: Assess baseline elimination pattern. Teach patient how to self-administer laxative. Encourage patient to normalize bowel habits through adequate fluid intake (2–3 L/day), diet high in fiber and bulk (bran, cereals, fruits, and vegetables), and exercise as tolerated. Teach patient bowel regimen when on narcotics or vinca alkaloids to promote regular evacuation.

II. ALTERATION IN NUTRITION related to GI SIDE EFFECTS

Defining Characteristics: Constipation or drug may cause nausea, cramps, abdominal bloating, flatulence. High doses may cause diarrhea, especially in the elderly. Continued use beyond 2 weeks may cause electrolyte imbalance.

Nursing Implications: Assess comfort level and GI distress related to constipation. Encourage patient to drink cold fluids or ginger ale as tolerated. Encourage patient to try resting in different positions; warm packs may decrease abdominal pain. Teach patient laxative effect may take 2–4 days and assess need for other cathartic(s).

Drug: senna (Senexon, Senokot)

Class: Irritant/stimulant laxative.

Mechanism of Action: Stimulates/irritates smooth muscle of intestines, increasing peristalsis; increases fluid accumulation in colon and small intestines. Indicated for relief of constipation or bowel preparation prior to bowel surgery.

Metabolism: Minimal oral absorption occurs. Evacuation occurs in 6–10 hours when taken orally.

Dosage/Range:
- Senexon: 2 tablets at bedtime (187 mg senna).
- Senokot: 2–4 tablets bid (187 mg senna); 1–2 tsp granules bid (326 mg senna); 1 suppository at bedtime, repeat PRN in 2 hours (652 mg senna).
- Black-Draught: 2 tablets (600 mg senna) or 1/4–1/2 level tsp granules (1.65 gm senna).

Drug Preparation:
- Store in a tightly closed bottle.

Drug Interactions:
- None.

Lab Effects/Interference:
- None known.

Special Considerations:
- Contraindicated in patients with signs/symptoms of acute abdomen (nausea, vomiting, abdominal pain), intestinal obstruction, fecal impaction, or ulcerative bowel lesions.
- Senna is very effective as part of bowel regimen for patients receiving narcotic analgesic medication.

Potential Toxicities/Side Effects and the Nursing Process

I. ALTERATIONS IN BOWEL ELIMINATION related to CHRONIC USE

Defining Characteristics: Removes defecation reflexes when used chronically (laxative dependence). Narcotic analgesics and vinca alkaloid chemotherapy may predispose to constipation.

Nursing Implications: Assess baseline elimination pattern. Teach patient how to self-administer laxative. Encourage patient to normalize bowel habits through adequate fluid intake (2–3 L/day), diet high in fiber and bulk (bran, cereals, fruits, and vegetables), and exercise as tolerated. Teach patient bowel regimen when on narcotics or vinca alkaloids to promote regular evacuation.

II. ALTERATION IN NUTRITION, LESS THAN BODY REQUIREMENTS, related to GI SIDE EFFECTS

Defining Characteristics: Constipation or drug may cause nausea, vomiting, abdominal pain; rectal suppository may cause burning in rectum as it is absorbed.

Nursing Implications: Assess comfort level and GI distress related to constipation. Encourage patient to drink cold fluids or ginger ale as tolerated. Encourage patient to try resting in different positions; warm packs may decrease abdominal pain. Teach patient to expect burning sensation with suppository use; reassure that it will resolve in 5–10 minutes.

III. ALTERATION IN FLUID AND ELECTROLYTE BALANCE related to LAXATIVE ABUSE

Defining Characteristics: Diarrhea resulting from laxative abuse can deplete fluid volume, nutrients, and electrolytes.

Nursing Implications: Teach patient regular bowel regimen when receiving constipating drugs (narcotics, vinca alkaloids). Teach patient to replace lost fluids and electrolytes (encourage chicken soup, sports drink).

Drug: sorbitol

Class: Hyperosmotic laxative.

Mechanism of Action: Local irritant, with hyperosmotic action, drawing water from tissues into feces and stimulating fecal evacuation within 15–30 minutes.

Metabolism: Poorly absorbed from GI tract.

Dosage/Range:

Adult:

- Oral: 15 mL of 70% solution repeated until diarrhea starts.
- Rectal: 120 mL if a 25–30% solution is used.

Drug Preparation:

- Keep stored in tightly closed bottle.

Drug Interactions:
- None.

Lab Effects/Interference:
- None known.

Special Considerations:
- Contraindicated in patients with undiagnosed abdominal pain, intestinal obstruction.
- Oral 70% sorbitol may be as effective as lactulose in relieving constipation.

Potential Toxicities/Side Effects and the Nursing Process

I. ALTERATIONS IN BOWEL ELIMINATION related to CHRONIC USE

Defining Characteristics: Removes defecation reflexes when used chronically (laxative dependence). Narcotic analgesics and vinca alkaloid chemotherapy may predispose to constipation.

Nursing Implications: Assess baseline elimination pattern. Teach patient how to self-administer laxative. Encourage patient to normalize bowel habits through adequate fluid intake (2–3 L/day), diet high in fiber and bulk (bran, cereals, fruits, and vegetables), and exercise as tolerated. Teach patient bowel regimen when on narcotics or vinca alkaloids to promote regular evacuation.

II. ALTERATION IN FLUID AND ELECTROLYTE BALANCE related to LAXATIVE ABUSE

Defining Characteristics: Diarrhea resulting from laxative abuse can deplete fluid volume, nutrients, and electrolytes.

Nursing Implications: Teach patient regular bowel regimen when receiving constipating drugs (narcotics, vinca alkaloids). Teach patient to replace lost fluids and electrolytes (encourage chicken soup, sports drink).

III. ALTERATION IN COMFORT related to CRAMPING PAIN, RECTAL IRRITATION OR DISCOMFORT

Defining Characteristics: Cramping pain, rectal irritation, and inflammation or discomfort may occur.

Nursing Implications: Teach patient this may occur. If discomfort is not self-limited, suggest sitz bath, warm or cold packs, and position changes.

Chapter 13
Diarrhea

Rutledge and Engleking (1998) define diarrhea as an abnormal increase in liquidity and frequency, and occurring as acute (within 24–48 hours of a stimulus, resolving in 7–14 days) or chronic (late onset, lasting > 2–3 weeks). Diarrhea occurring in patients with cancer is most often related to osmotic, malabsorptive, secretory, exudative, dysmotility-associated, or chemotherapy-induced (Levy, 1992; Engleking, 2003). Engleking (2003) gives examples of each.

- *Osmotic diarrhea* occurs as a result of hyperosmolar or non-absorbable substances, which draw large volumes of fluid into the intestines, producing watery stools that usually resolve with removal of the cause. Causative factors include high osmolality tube feedings, lactulose or sorbital, and gastrointestinal hemorrhage.
- *Malabsorptive diarrhea* results from changes in mucosal integrity causing changes in membrane permeability, or loss of absorptive surfaces, resulting in diarrhea that is large volume, frothy, and foul-smelling (steatorrhea). Causes include deficiency of an enzyme responsible for digestion of fats (lactose intolerance, pancreatic insufficiency) or surgical resection or removal of the intestines.
- *Secretory diarrhea* results from intestinal hypersecretion of large volumes (> 1 L/day) of watery stool with an osmolality equal to that in the plasma. Causes are endocrine tumors (VIPoma and carcinoid), enterotoxin-producing pathogens such as *C. difficile*, acute graft-versus-host disease, and short gut syndrome.
- *Exudative diarrhea* is caused by inflammation or ulceration of the bowel mucosa, resulting in stools containing mucous, blood, and serum protein; the patient experiences frequent stooling, although the total volume is usually < 1 L/day. Unfortunately, this type of diarrhea is associated with hypoalbuminemia and anemia. Causes are radiation to the bowel (radiation enteritis) or opportunistic infection in the denuded bowel, such as with neutropenic typhlitis.
- *Dysmotility-associated diarrhea* is related to factors which increase or decrease normal peristalsis, such as with irritable bowel syndrome, the ingestion of food or medication that affects peristalsis, or psychological factors such as anxiety or fear that cause parasympathetic stimulation. Diarrhea of this type is usually semi-solid to liquid, small, and frequent.
- *Chemotherapy-induced diarrhea* occurs as a result of chemotherapy-induced cell death of the intestinal mucosa causing over-stimulation of intestinal water and electrolyte secretion. The patient experiences frequent watery to semi-solid stools within 24–96 hours of chemotherapy administration. With irinotecan chemotherapy, acute diarrhea occurs initially during or soon after administration related to cholinergic stimulation, and then

delayed diarrhea occurs about 9–12 days later. In combination with 5-fluorouracil, the delayed diarrhea can lead to dehydration, and together with neutropenia, sepsis. Nurses play a very important role in teaching patients about the potential life-threatening diarrhea that may occur from this chemotherapy, self-administration of anti-diarrheal medicines, increased fluid and diet modifications, and triage if these efforts are not effective.

Nurses are key in the management of diarrhea. Nurses play a significant role in patient assessment and patient/family teaching. Assessment of the patient's previous and current nutrition and elimination patterns, as well as assessment of probable etiology of diarrhea, are critical, as is patient/family teaching about the management and prevention of diarrhea.

Patient teaching includes (Wadler et al, 1998):

- Diet modification: recommend low-residue foods high in protein and calories; high fluid intake of 3 L/day; avoidance of milk and milk products, foods high in potassium.
- Care of irritated skin, mucosa in perirectal area; critical in neutropenic or immunocompromised patients.
- Self-administration of prescribed antidiarrheal medication(s).
- Need for blood tests to assess electrolyte imbalance and hydration if diarrhea is severe. Diarrhea can lead to severe fluid and electrolyte imbalance, as well as significant patient discomfort. Common electrolyte imbalances related to diarrhea include metabolic acidosis, hypokalemia, hyperchloremia, hypocalcemia, and hypomagnesemia.

Ippoliti (1998) describes antidiarrheal agents as:

- *Intraluminal agents*: Decrease water in gut by absorption, increasing bulk of the stool, and protecting intestinal mucosa; includes absorbents such as activated charcoal and mucilloid preparations, and adsorbents such as psyllium, kaolin and pectate; less commonly used as more effective agents available without possible drug interactions or difficulty ingesting them.
- *Intestinal transit inhibitors*: Primarily anti-cholinergic (atropine sulfate and scopolamine) and opiate agonists (DTO and the synthetic opioids diphenoxylate and loperamide), which slow intestinal peristalsis and increasing fluid absorption.
- *Proabsorptive agents*: Intraluminal absorbent agents as above.
- *Antisecretory agents*: Octreotide (Sandostatin) is a synthetic somatostatin analogue that inhibits the secretion of gut hormones like serotonin and motilin, and thus slows transit time and improves regulation of water and electrolyte movement in the gut. Bismuth subsalicylate (Pepto-Bismol) also works to decrease gut mucosal inflammation and hypermotility by binding to toxins and inhibition of prostaglandin synthesis.

References

Engleking C. Diarrhea, Chapter 28. In Yarbro CH, Frogge MH, Goodman M. *Cancer Symptom Management* 3rd ed. Sudbury, MA: Jones and Bartlett Publishers 2003

Harris AG. Consensus Statement Recommendations: Octreotide Dose Titration in Secretory Diarrhea. *Dig Dis Sci* 1995; 40(7) 1464–1473

Ippoliti C. Antidiarrheal Agents for the Management of Treatment-related Diarrhea in Cancer Patients. *Am J Health Syst Pharm* 1998; 55(15) 1573–80
Levy MH. Constipation and Diarrhea, Part II. *Prim Care Cancer* 1992; 12(5) 53–58
Rutledge D, Engleking C. Cancer-related Diarrhea: Selected Findings of a National Survey of Oncology Nurse Experiences. *Oncol Nurs Forum* 1998; 25 861–878
Wadler S, Benson AB, Engelking C. Recommended Guidelines for the Treatment of Chemotherapy-Induced Diarrhea. *J Clin Oncol* 1998; 16(9) 3169–3178

Drug: deodorized tincture of opium (DTO, Laudanum)

Class: Opium antidiarrheal agent.

Mechanism of Action: Increases GI smooth muscle tone and inhibits GI motility, delaying movement of intestinal contents; water is absorbed from fecal contents, decreasing diarrhea.

Metabolism: Variable absorption from GI tract; metabolized by liver and excreted in urine.

Dosage/Range:
Adult:
- Oral: 0.3–1 mL qid (maximum 6 mL/day).

Drug Preparation:
- Store in tight, light-resistant bottle. Administer with water or juice.

Drug Interactions:
- None.

Lab Effects/Interference:
- None known.

Special Considerations:
- DTO contains 25 times more morphine than paregoric.
- Physical dependence may develop if drug is used chronically (e.g., colitis).
- Controlled substance.
- May be used in combination with kaolin and pectin mixtures.
- Do not use in diarrhea that results from poisoning until poison is removed (e.g., by lavage or cathartics).

Potential Toxicities/Side Effects and the Nursing Process

I. ALTERATION IN NUTRITION, LESS THAN BODY REQUIREMENTS, related to GI SIDE EFFECTS

Defining Characteristics: Nausea, vomiting may occur.

Nursing Implications: Assess baseline nutrition, GI status. If nausea/vomiting appears to follow dose administration, administer DTO with juice to disguise taste.

Drug: diphenoxylate hydrochloride and atropine (Lomotil)

Class: Antidiarrheal agent.

Mechanism of Action: Diphenoxylate is a synthetic opiate agonist that inhibits intestinal smooth muscle activity, thereby slowing peristalsis so that excess water is absorbed from feces. Atropine discourages deliberate overdosage.

Metabolism: Well absorbed from GI tract. Metabolized in liver. Excreted principally via feces in bile. Onset of action 45 minutes to 1 hour; duration 3–4 hours.

Dosage/Range:

Adult:

- Oral: 5 mg PO qid then titrate to response × 2 days (if no response in 48 hours, drug ineffective).

Drug Preparation:

- Oral: one tablet contains 2.5 mg diphenoxylate HCl and 0.025 mg atropine sulfate.

Drug Interactions:

- CNS depressants (alcohol, barbiturates): potentiate CNS depressant action; use together cautiously.
- MAOIs: may cause hypertensive crisis (similar structure to meperidine); use together cautiously.

Lab Effects/Interference:

- None known.

Special Considerations:

- May be habit-forming when used in high doses (40–60 mg); physical dependence.
- Use with extreme caution in patients with hepatic cirrhosis, as drug may precipitate hepatic coma, and in patients with acute ulcerative colitis.
- Contraindicated in patients with jaundice, diarrhea resulting from poisoning or pseudomembranous colitis caused by antibiotics.

Potential Toxicities/Side Effects and the Nursing Process

I. ALTERATION IN NUTRITION, LESS THAN BODY REQUIREMENTS, related to GI SIDE EFFECTS

Defining Characteristics: Nausea, vomiting, abdominal distension or discomfort, anorexia, mouth dryness, and (rarely) paralytic ileus may occur.

Nursing Implications: Assess baseline nutrition and elimination status. Instruct patient to report signs and symptoms. Discuss drug discontinuance with physician. Instruct patient that drug should be used for two days and physician notified if diarrhea persists.

II. ALTERATIONS IN SENSORY/PERCEPTUAL PATTERNS related to SEDATION

Defining Characteristics: Sedation, dizziness, lethargy, restlessness or insomnia, headache, paresthesia occur rarely with higher doses and prolonged therapy. Blurred vision may occur due to mydriasis.

Nursing Implications: Teach patient that drug is for short-term relief of diarrhea. Assess for and instruct patient to report signs/symptoms. Discuss drug discontinuance with physician if symptoms are severe.

III. ALTERATION IN SKIN INTEGRITY related to RASH, SENSITIVITY

Defining Characteristics: Pruritus, angioedema (swelling of lips, face, gums), giant urticaria may occur.

Nursing Implications: Assess for and instruct patient to report signs/symptoms immediately. Drug should be discontinued if angioedema or giant urticaria occurs.

Drug: kaolin/pectin (Kaodene, K-P, Kaopectate, K-Pek)

Class: Antidiarrheal agent.

Mechanism of Action: Drug acts as absorbent and protectant; decreases stool fluidity but not total amount of fluid excreted.

Metabolism: Not absorbed from GI tract and excreted in stool.

Dosage/Range:

Adult:

- Oral: 60–120 mL regular or 45–90 mL concentrated suspension after each loose bowel movement < 48 hours.

Drug Preparation:

- Shake well prior to administration.

Drug Interactions:

- Oral lincomycin: decreases lincomycin absorption; administer kaolin/pectin at least 2 hours before or 3–4 hours after lincomycin dose.
- Oral digoxin: decreases digoxin absorption; administer kaolin/pectin 2 hours after digoxin dose.

Lab Effects/Interference:

- None known.

Special Considerations:
- Few adverse effects.
- Used for temporary relief of diarrhea.

Potential Toxicities/Side Effects and the Nursing Process

I. KNOWLEDGE DEFICIT related to SELF-ADMINISTRATION

Defining Characteristics: Transient constipation may occur.

Nursing Implications: Assess understanding of medication and self-administration schedule. Instruct patient in self-administration and to notify nurse/physician if diarrhea persists beyond 48 hours or fever develops. Reinforce need to drink fluids, especially in elderly or debilitated patients, to prevent constipation.

Drug: loperamide hydrochloride (Imodium)

Class: Antidiarrheal agent.

Mechanism of Action: Slows intestinal motility by inhibiting peristalsis (direct effect on circular and longitudinal intestinal muscles); increases stool bulk and viscosity.

Metabolism: Well absorbed from GI tract. Metabolized and small amounts are excreted in urine and feces as intact drug.

Dosage/Range:
Adult:
- Oral: 4 mg followed by 2 mg after each unformed stool (maximum 16 mg or higher if under direction of a physician; 8 mg per 24-hour period if self-medicating).

Drug Preparation:
- Oral.

Drug Interactions:
- None.

Lab Effects/Interference:
- None known.

Special Considerations:
- Reduces electrolyte and fluid loss from intestines; may be used to reduce volume of ileostomy drainage. 2–3 times more potent than diphenoxylate.
- Use cautiously in patients with acute ulcerative colitis; drug should be discontinued if abdominal distension occurs (risk of megacolon).
- Intended for self-medication × 48 hours; patients should be taught to notify nurse/physician if symptoms persist or fever occurs.

- Contraindicated in diarrhea due to pseudomembranous colitis (antibiotic related), in acute diarrhea caused by mucosal-penetrating organisms (*Shigella, E. coli, Salmonella*), or if hypersensitivity to drug exists.
- Use cautiously in pregnant or nursing women.

Potential Toxicities/Side Effects and the Nursing Process

I. ALTERATION IN NUTRITION, LESS THAN BODY REQUIREMENTS, related to GI SIDE EFFECTS

Defining Characteristics: Less frequent adverse reactions occur than with diphenoxylate/atropine. Nausea, vomiting, abdominal pain, and distension may occur.

Nursing Implications: Assess baseline nutrition and elimination status. Instruct patient to report signs and symptoms. Discuss drug discontinuance with physician. Instruct patient that drug should be used for two days and physician notified if diarrhea persists.

II. ALTERATIONS IN SENSORY/PERCEPTUAL PATTERNS related to DROWSINESS

Defining Characteristics: Drowsiness, dizziness, fatigue may occur.

Nursing Implications: Teach patient that drug is for short-term relief of diarrhea. Assess for and instruct patient to report signs/symptoms. Discuss drug discontinuance with physician if symptoms are severe.

III. ALTERATION IN SKIN INTEGRITY related to RASH, SENSITIVITY

Defining Characteristics: Rarely, rash may develop.

Nursing Implications: Assess baseline skin integrity. Instruct patient to report rash. Discuss drug discontinuance with physician.

Drug: octreotide acetate (Sandostatin)

Class: Cyclic octapeptide that mimics the pharmacologic actions of the natural hormone somatostatin and is long-acting.

Mechanism of Action: Drug is a more potent inhibitor than somatostatin of growth hormone, glucagon, insulin; also suppresses LH (luteinizing hormone) response to GnRH (gonadotropin-releasing hormone); decreases splanchnic blood flow; and inhibits release of serotonin, gastrin, vasoactive intestinal peptide (VIP), secretin, motilin, and pancreatic-polypeptide–like somatostatin. Stimulates fluid and electrolyte absorption from GI tract, and lengthens transit time of intestinal contents. Controls symptoms associated with carcinoid syndrome (e.g., flushing, levels of serotonin metabolite 5-HIAA), and VIP-secreting adenomas (e.g., watery diarrhea).

Metabolism: Absorbed rapidly and completely after injection, with peak concentrations after 24 minutes. Protein binding 65%, and eliminated from plasma with a half-life of 1.7 hours (natural hormone is 1–3 minutes). Duration of action approximately 12 hours depending upon tumor type. Excreted in urine, with decreased clearance by 26% in the elderly. LAR Depot consists of biodegradable microspheres that slowly release octreotide from the injection site over 4 weeks. After IM injection, serum octreotide concentration reaches a transient initial peak within 1 hour, then declines over the next 3–5 days, then slowly increases to plateau 2–3 weeks post-injection. Steady state is reached by the 3rd monthly injection.

Dosage/Range:

Adult (immediate release injection):

- Carcinoid: Starting dose of 100–600 micrograms/day (median 450 micrograms/day) in 2–4 divided doses SQ.
- VIPoma: 200–300 mcg/day SQ in 2–4 divided doses during initial 2 weeks, then titrated to response with range of 150–750 mcg/day to control symptoms.
- Acromegaly: 50 micrograms SQ tid, titrated to need every 2 weeks based on IGF (somatomedin C) levels.
- AIDS-related diarrhea: 500 mcg SQ q 8 h.
- Chemotherapy-induced diarrhea (high dose): 300 micrograms/day continuous infusion.
- Radiation-induced diarrhea: 50 micrograms SQ q 8 h.
- Graft-versus-host disease (GVHD): 100 micrograms IV q 8 h.
- Short bowel syndrome: 50 micrograms SQ q 8 h.
- Chronic idiopathic secretory diarrhea: 100 micrograms SQ q 8 h.

Sandostatin LAR Depot:

- Renal failure: drug half-life may be increased requiring dosage adjustment.

Carcinoid Tumors and VIPomas:

- If patient is not currently on octreotide acetate, begin therapy with immediate release dosing for 2 weeks: Carcinoid: 100–600 micrograms/da SQ in 2–4 divided doses (mean daily dose 300 micrograms) although some patients may require up to 1500 micrograms/da; VIPoma: 200–300 micrograms/da SQ in 2–4 divided doses (range 150–750 micrograms) and dosage may be individualized to control symptoms, but usually does not exceed 450 micrograms/da.
- For patients who respond to the initial 2 week therapy, switch to Sandostatin LAR Depot 20 mg IM q 4 weeks × 2 months. In addition, since it will take at least 2 weeks to achieve steady state, the patient should ALSO continue to receive Sandostatin immediate release dosing SQ for at least 2 weeks at the same dose as in the first

2 weeks. After 2 months of Sandostatin LAR Depot 20 mg, the dose may be increased to 30 mg q 4 weeks if symptoms are not controlled. Some patients who have their symptoms controlled on 20 mg q 4 weeks, may be decreased to 10 mg q 4 weeks.
- Some patients may have exacerbation of symptoms and require temporary additional immediate release in addition to the LAR Depot to control the increase in symptoms.

Acromegaly:
- If patient is not currently on octreotide acetate, begin therapy with immediate release dosing q 8 h at an initial dose of 50 micrograms tid, and gradually increase as needed (based on growth hormone [GH] levels) as the goal is to normalize GH and IGF-1 (somatomedin C) levels. After 2 weeks, tolerability and response should be evident, so that patient can be changed to LAR Depot at a dose of 20 mg q 4 weeks if tolerance and effectiveness positive.
- For patients currently on octreotide, they can be changed directly to LAR Depot q 4 weeks, and at the end of 3 months, the LAR Depot dose should be titrated based on growth hormone level:
  - — GH ≤ 2.5 ng/mL, IGF-1 (somatomedin C) normal and controlled symptoms, 20 mg IM (intragluteally) q 4 weeks.
  - — GH > 2.5 ng/mL, IGF-1 elevated and/or uncontrolled symptoms, increase dose to 30 mg IM q 4 weeks.
  - — GH ≤ 1 ng/mL, IGF-1 normal and controlled symptoms, reduce dose to 10 mg IM q 4 weeks.

Drug Preparation:
- Available in 1-mL (50 micrograms, 100 micrograms, 500 micrograms) ampules, and 5-mL (1000 micrograms and 5000 micrograms) multidose vials. Immediate release injection: administer SQ, IV over 15–30 minutes, or IVP over 3 minutes.
- Stable in solution in 0.9% sodium chloride or 5% dextrose in water for 24 hours; dilute drug in 50–200 mL of 0.9% sodium chloride or 5% dextrose for IV infusions over 15–30 minutes.
- Patient may develop pain, stinging, tingling, or burning sensation at injection site, with redness and swelling.
- Patient may develop pain, stinging, tingling, or burning sensation at injection site, with redness and swelling.

LAR Depot:
- Available in (5-mL) vials containing 10, 20, or 30 mg octreotide free peptide; injection kit includes a syringe containing 2.5 mL of diluent, 2 sterile 1.5 inch 19 gauge needles, and 2 alcohol wipes as well as instruction booklet.
- Allow drug vial and diluent-filled syringe to reach room temperature (30–60 minutes) prior to preparation of drug suspension.
- Drug must be administered immediately after mixing.
- Tap vial to ensure drug has settled to bottom of vial; aseptically inject diluent slowly down the inside wall of the vial while rotating the vial to evenly distribute the diluent using one of the needles. Allow to sit for 5 minutes or longer to assure full saturation

of the drug powder; once saturated, swirl the vial gently for 30–60 seconds until a milky uniform suspension appears (DO NOT shake vigorously or invert the vial). Aseptically withdraw the ordered dose, holding the vial at 45 degrees. There will be some remaining suspension as the vial has over-fill. Add a small amount of air into the syringe, and gently rock back and forth until the patient is given the injection (DO NOT invert syringe). Eliminate air from the syringe.
- Replace needle with second needle, and aseptically administer drug immediately.
- Administer IM in gluteal muscle as other sites too painful (never give IV or SC) q 28 days.
- Record injection site and rotate sites.

Drug Interactions:
- May affect absorption of orally administered drugs.
- Cyclosporine: decreased serum levels of cyclosporine, resulting in transplant rejection.
- Insulin, oral hypoglycemic agents, beta-blockers, calcium-channel blockers: assess patient response and need for dosage adjustment of these drugs.

Lab Effects/Interference:
- Hypoglycemia or hyperglycemia: suppression of TSH may result in hypothyroidism and decreased total/free T_4 (generally patients with acromegaly receiving long-term therapy).
- Decreased vitamin B_{12} levels (Shilling's test).

Special Considerations:
- Sandostatin LAR Depot is indicated for patients in whom initial treatment with Sandostatin Injection has been shown to be effective and tolerated: (1) carcinoid tumors: the long-term treatment of severe diarrhea and flushing episodes, (2) VIPomas: long-term treatment of profuse watery diarrhea, (3) acromegaly: long-term maintenance therapy who require medical treatment.
- Octreotide acetate is appropriate when other conventional antidiarrheal medications have failed, and other treatable causes of diarrhea have been excluded (e.g., obstruction, infection).
- Patient should be taught sterile SQ injection technique for immediate release preparations.
- Laboratory test monitoring (efficacy) based on treatment intent:
  - —Carcinoid: 5-HIAA (urinary 5-hydroxyindoleacetic acid), plasma substance P and serotonin.
  - —VIPoma: VIP (plasma vasoactive intestinal peptide).
  - —Acromegaly: growth hormone, IGF-1 (somatomedin C).
- Adverse reactions of diabetes mellitus, hypothyroidism, and cardiovascular disease occur in patients treated for acromegaly.
- May change to long-acting depot if already controlled on immediate-release preparation, or in a new patient, after response is assessed after 2 weeks of immediate-release dosing.

- Drug inhibits gallbladder contraction and decreases bile secretion in 63% of patients with acromegaly or psoriasis when treated for long periods of time.
- Drug may rarely cause alterations in hormonal levels, so patients receiving long-term therapy should be monitored baseline and periodically during treatment: glucose, glucose tolerance in patients receiving antidiabetic drugs, thyroid function (TSH, total and/or free T_4), B_{12} level, and zinc level in patients receiving TPN.
- In patients with acromegaly or carcinoid, drug may rarely cause cardiac abnormalities such as bradycardia, QT prolongation, non-specific ST segment changes, and worsening of CHF; drug may cause visual field defects in patients with growth hormone secreting tumors.

Potential Toxicities/Side Effects (dose and schedule dependent) and the Nursing Process

I. ALTERATION IN NUTRITION, LESS THAN BODY REQUIREMENTS, related to CARBOHYDRATE METABOLISM

Defining Characteristics: Rarely, transient hypoglycemia or hyperglycemia due to altered balance between hormones regulating serum glucose (insulin, glucagon, growth hormone). Rarely, diarrhea, nausea and vomiting, abdominal pain or discomfort. Incidence 3–10%.

Nursing Implications: Assess baseline nutritional balance. Instruct patient to report any changes, and assess for hyperglycemia (drowsiness, dry mouth, flushing, dry skin, fruity breath, polyuria, polydipsia, polyphagia, weight loss, stomach ache, nausea/vomiting, fatigue), hypoglycemia (anxiety, chills, cool/pale skin, difficulty concentrating, headache, hunger, shakiness, diaphoresis, fatigue, weakness, nausea). If patient is hypoglycemic, teach patient to carry candy. Monitor serum glucose, and discuss alterations with physician. Treat nausea and vomiting symptomatically, and discuss need for antiemetic if significant.

II. ALTERATION IN COMFORT related to HEADACHE, FLUSHING

Defining Characteristics: Rarely (1–3%) patient may experience lightheadedness, dizziness, fatigue, pedal edema, headache, flushing of the face, weakness.

Nursing Implications: Assess baseline comfort, and instruct patient to report any changes. Assess safety, and manage symptoms symptomatically. If unrelieved or significant, discuss with physician.

Appendix 1
Controlling Occupational Exposure to Hazardous Drugs

A. Introduction

In response to numerous inquiries,[1] OSHA published guidelines for the management of cytotoxic (antineoplastic) drugs in the workplace in 1986.[106] At that time, surveys indicated little standardization in the use of engineering controls and personal protective equipment (PPE).[56,73] Although practices have improved in subsequent years, problems still exist.[111] In addition, the occupational management of these chemicals has been further clarified. These trends, in conjunction with many information requests, have prompted OSHA to revise its recommendations for hazardous drug handling. In addition, some of these agents are covered under the Hazard Communication Standard (HCS) [29 CFR 1910.1200].[107] In order to provide recommendations consistent with current scientific knowledge, this informational guidance document has been expanded to cover hazardous drugs (HD), in addition to the cytotoxic drugs (CD) that were covered in the 1986 guidelines. The recommendations apply to all settings where employees are occupationally exposed to HDs, such as hospitals, physicians' offices, and home health care agencies. This review will:

- provide criteria for classifying drugs as hazardous,
- summarize the evidence supporting the management of HDs as an occupational hazard,
- discuss the equipment and worker education recommended as well as the legal requirements of standards for the protection of workers exposed and potentially exposed to HDs,
- update the important aspects of medical surveillance, and
- list some common HDs currently in use.

Anesthetic agents have not been considered in this review. However, exposure to some of these agents is a recognized health hazard,[104] and they have been considered in a separate Technical Manual Chapter.

B. Categorization of Drugs as Hazardous

The purpose of this section is to describe the biological effects of those pharmaceuticals that are considered hazardous. A number of pharmaceuticals in the healthcare setting may pose occupational risk to employees through acute and chronic workplace exposure. Past attention focused on drugs used to treat cancer. However, it is clear that many other agents also have toxicity profiles of concern. This recognition prompted the American Society of Hospital Pharmacists (ASHP) to define a class of agents as "hazardous drugs."[3] That report specified concerns about antineoplastic and nonantineoplastic hazardous drugs in use in most institutions throughout the country. OSHA shares this concern. The ASHP Technical Assistance Bulletin (TAB) described four drug characteristics, each of which could be considered hazardous:

- genotoxicity,
- carcinogenicity,
- teratogenicity or fertility impairment, and
- serious organ or other toxic manifestation at low doses in experimental animals or treated patients.

Table A.1 of this review lists some common drugs that are considered hazardous by the above criteria. There is no standardized reference for this information, nor is there complete consensus on all agents listed. Professional judgment by personnel trained in pharmacology/toxicology is essential in designating drugs as hazardous, and reference 65 provides information regarding the development of such a list at one institution. Some drugs, which have a long history of safe use in humans despite *in vitro* or animal evidence to toxicity, may be excluded by the institution's experts by considerations such as those used to formulate GRAS (*Generally Regarded as Safe*) lists by the FDA under the Food, Drug, and Cosmetics Act.

Table A.1 Some Common Drugs Considered Hazardous

Chemical/Generic Name	Source*
ALTRETAMINE	C
AMINOGLUTETHIMIDE	A
AZATHIOPRINE	ACE
L-ASPARAGINASE	ABC
BLEOMYCIN	ABC
BUSULFAN	ABC
CARBOPLATIN	ABC
CARMUSTINE	ABC
CHLORAMBUCIL	ABCE
CHLORAMPHENICOL	E
CHLOROTRIANISENE	B
CHLOROZOTOCIN	E
CYCLOSPORIN	E
CISPLATIN	ABCE

(continued)

Table A.1 *(Continued)*

Chemical/Generic Name	Source*
CYCLOPHOSPHAMIDE	ABCE
CYTARABINE	ABC
DACARBAZINE	ABC
DACTINOMYCIN	ABC
DAUNORUBICIN	ABC
DIETHYLSTILBESTROL	BE
DOXORUBICIN	ABCE
ESTRADIOL	B
ESTRAMUSTINE	AB
ETHINYL ESTRADIOL	B
ETOPOSIDE	ABC
FLOXURIDINE	AC
FLUOROURACIL	ABC
FLUTAMIDE	BC
GANCICLOVIR	AD
HYDROXYUREA	ABC
IDARUBICIN	AC
IFOSFAMIDE	ABC
INTERFERON-α	BC
ISOTRETINOIN	D
LEUPROLIDE	BC
LEVAMISOLE	C
LOMUSTINE	ABCE
MECHLORETHAMINE	BC
MEDROXYPROGESTERONE	B
MEGESTROL	BC
MELPHALAN	ABCE
MERCAPTOPURINE	ABC
METHOTREXATE	ABC
MITOMYCIN	ABC
MITOTANE	ABC

(continued)

Table A.1 *(Continued)*

Chemical/Generic Name	Source*
MITOXANTRONE	ABC
NAFARELIN	C
PIPOBROMAN	C
PLICAMYCIN	BC
PROCARBAZINE	ABCE
RIBAVIRIN	D
STREPTOZOCIN	AC
TAMOXIFEN	BC
TESTOLACTONE	BC
THIOGUANINE	ABC
THIOTEPA	ABC
URACIL MUSTARD	ACE
VIDARABINE	D
VINBLASTINE	ABC
VINCRISTINE	ABC
ZIDOVUDINE	D

**Sources*:
A The National Institutes of Health, Clinical Center Nursing Department
B Antineoplastic drugs in the *Physicians' Desk Reference*
C American Hospital Formulary, Antineoplastics
D Johns Hopkins Hospital E International Agency for Research on Cancer

Table A.1 is not all inclusive, should not be construed as complete, and represents an assessment of some, but not all, marketed drugs at a fixed point in time. Table A.1 was developed through consultation with institutions that have assembled teams of pharmacists and other healthcare personnel to determine which drugs should be used with caution. These teams reviewed product literature and drug information when considering each product.

Sources for this appendix are the *Physicians' Desk Reference,* Section 10:00 in the American Hospital Formulary Service Drug Information,[68] IARC publications (particularly Volume 50),[43] the Johns Hopkins Hospital, and the National Institutes of Health, Clinical Center Nursing Department. No attempt to include investigational drugs was made, but they should be prudently handled as hazardous drugs until adequate information becomes available to exclude them. Any determination of the hazard status of drug should be periodically reviewed and updated as new information becomes available. Importantly, new drugs should routinely undergo a hazard assessment.

List of Abbreviations

ANSI	American National Standards Institute
ASHP	American Society of Hospital Pharmacists
BSC	Biological Safety Cabinet
CD	Cytotoxic Drug
EPA	Environmental Protection Agency
HD	Hazardous Drug
HCS	Hazard Communication Standard
HEPA	High Efficiency Particulate Air
IARC	International Agency for Research on Cancer
MSDS	Material Safety Data Sheet
NIOSH	National Institute for Occupational Safety and Health
NTP	National Toxicology Program
OSHA	Occupational Safety and Health Administration
PPE	Personal Protective Equipment

In contrast, investigational drugs are new chemicals for which there is often little information on potential toxicity. Structure or activity relationships with similar chemicals and in vitro data can be considered in determining potential toxic effects. Investigational drugs should be prudently handled as HDs unless adequate information becomes available to exclude them.

Some major considerations by professionals trained in pharmacology/toxicology[65] in designating a drug as hazardous are:

- Is the drug designated as Therapeutic Category 10:00 (Antineoplastic Agent) in the American Hospital Formulary Service Drug Information?[68]
- Does the manufacturer suggest the use of special isolation techniques in its handing, administration, or disposal?
- Is the drug known to be a human mutagen, carcinogen, teratogen, or reproductive toxicant?
- Is the drug known to be carcinogenic or teratogenic in animals (drugs known to be mutagenic in multiple bacterial systems or animals should also be considered hazardous)?
- And, is the drug known to be acutely toxic to an organ system?

C. Background: Hazardous Drugs as Occupational Risk

Preparation, administration, and disposal of HDs may expose pharmacists, nurses, physicians, and other healthcare workers to potentially significant workplace levels of these chemicals. The literature establishing these agents as occupational hazards deals primarily with CDs; however, documentation of adverse exposure effects from other HDs is rapidly accumulating.[15,40,41,42,43,59] The degree of absorption that takes place during work and the significance of secondary early biological effects on each individual encounter are difficult to assess and may vary depending on the HD. As a result, it is difficult to set safe levels of exposure on the basis of current scientific information.

However, there are several lines of evidence supporting the toxic potential of these drugs if handled improperly. Therefore, it is essential to minimize exposure to all HDs. Summary tables of much of the data presented below can be found in Sorsa[95] and Rogers.[84]

1. Mechanism of Action

Most HDs either bind directly to genetic material in the cell nucleus or affect cellular protein synthesis. Cytotoxic drugs may not distinguish between normal and cancerous cells. The growth and reproduction of the normal cells are often affected during treatment of cancerous cells.

2. Animal Data

Numerous studies document the carcinogenic, mutagenic, and teratogenic effects of HD exposure in animals. They are well summarized in the pertinent IARC publications.[37–43] Alkylating agents present the strongest evidence of carcinogenicity (e.g., *cyclophosphamide, mechlorethamine hydrochloride [nitrogen mustard]*). However, other classes, such as some antibiotics, have been implicated as well. Extensive evidence for mutagenic and reproductive effects can be found in all antineoplastic classes. The antiviral agent *ribavirin* has additionally been shown to be teratogenic in all rodent species tested.[31,49] The ASHP recommends that all pharmaceutical agents that are animal carcinogens be handled as if human carcinogens.

3. Human Data at Therapeutic Levels

Many HDs are known human carcinogens, for which there is no safe level of exposure. The development of secondary malignancies is a well-documented side effect of chemotherapy treatment.[52,86,90,115] Leukemia has been most frequently observed. However, other secondary malignancies, such as bladder cancer and lymphoma, have been documented in patients treated for other, usually solid, primary malignancies.[52,114] Chromosomal aberrations can result from chemotherapy treatment as well. One study, on *chlorambucil,* reveals chromosomal damage in recipients to be cumulative and related to both dose and duration of therapy.[77]

Numerous case reports have linked chemotherapeutic treatment to adverse reproductive outcomes.[7,88,91,98] Testicular and ovarian dysfunction, including permanent sterility, have occurred in male and female patients who have received CDs either singly or in combination.[14] In addition, some antineoplastic agents are known or suspected to be transmitted to infants through breast milk.[79]

The literature also documents the effects of these drugs on other organ systems. Extravasation of some agents can cause severe soft-tissue injury, consisting of necrosis and sloughing of exposed areas.[23,78,87] Other HDs, such as *pentamidine* and *zidovudine* (formerly AZT), are known to have significant side effects (i.e., hematologic abnormalities), in treated patients.[4,33] Serum transaminase elevation has also been reported in treated patients.[4,33]

4. Occupational Exposure—Airborne Levels

Monitoring efforts for cytotoxic drugs have detected measurable air levels when exhaust biological safety cabinets (BSC) were not used for preparation or when monitoring was performed inside the BSC.[50,73]

Concentrations of *fluorouracil* ranging from 0.12 to 82.26 ng/m^3 have been found during monitoring of drug preparation without a BSC implying an opportunity for respiratory exposure.[73] Elevated concentrations of *cyclophosphamide* were found by these authors as well. *Cyclophosphamide* has also been detected on the HEPA filters of flow hoods used in HD preparation, demonstrating aerosolization of the drug and an exposure opportunity mitigated by effective engineering controls.[81]

A recent study has reported wipe samples of *cyclophosphamide,* one of the Class I IARC carcinogens, on surfaces of work stations in an oncology pharmacy and outpatient treatment areas (sinks and countertops). Concentrations ranged from 0.005 to 0.03 μg/cm^2, documenting opportunity for dermal exposure.[60]

Administration of drugs via aerosolization can lead to measurable air concentrations in the breathing zone of workers providing treatment. Concentrations up to 18 μg/m^3 have been found by personal air sampling of workers administering *pentamidine.*[67] Similar monitoring for *ribavirin* has found concentrations as high as 316 μg/m.[3,31]

5. Occupational Exposure—Biological Evidence of Absorption

Urinary Mutagenicity

Falk et al. were the first to note evidence of mutagenicity in the urine of nurses who handled cytotoxic drugs.[26] The extent of this effect increased over the course of the work week. With improved handling practices, a decrease in mutagenic activity was seen.[27] Researchers have also studied pharmacy personnel who reconstitute antineoplastic drugs. These employees showed increasingly mutagenic urine over the period of exposure; when they stopped handling the drugs, activity fell within 2 days to the level of unexposed controls.[5,76] They also found mutagenicity in workers using horizontal laminar flow BSCs that decreased to control levels with the use of vertical flow containment BSCs.[76] Other studies have failed to find a relationship between exposure and urine mutagenicity.[25] Sorsa[95] summarizes this information and discusses the factors, such as differences in urine collection timing and variations in the use of PPE, which could lead to disparate results. Differences may also be related to smoking status; smokers exposed to CDs exhibit greater urine mutagenicity than exposed non-smokers or control smokers, suggesting contamination of the work area by CDs and some contribution of smoking to their mutagenic profile.[9]

Urinary Thioethers

Urinary thioethers are glutathione conjugated metabolites of alkylating agents that have been evaluated as an indirect means of measuring exposure. Workers who handle cytotoxic drugs have been reported to have increased levels compared to controls and also have increasing thioether levels over a five-day work week.[44,48] Other studies of nurses who handle CDs and of treated patients have yielded variable results that could be due to confounding by smoking, PPE, and glutathione-S-transferase activity.[11]

Urinary Metabolites

Venitt[112] assayed the urine of pharmacy and nursing personnel handling cisplatin and found platinum concentrations at or below the limit of detection for both workers and controls. Hirst[35] found *cyclophosphamide* in the urine of two nurses who handled the drug, documenting worker absorption. (Hirst also documented skin absorption in human volunteers by using gas chromatography after topical application of the drug.) Urinary *pentamidine* recovery has also been reported in exposed healthcare workers.[94]

6. Occupational Exposure—Human Effects

Cytogenetic Effects

A number of studies have examined the relationship of exposure to CDs in the workplace to chromosomal aberrations. These studies have looked at a variety of markers for damage, including sister chromatid exchanges (SCE), structural aberrations (e.g., gaps, breaks, translocations), and micronuclei in peripheral blood lymphocytes. The results have been somewhat conflicting. Several authors found increases in one or more markers.[74,75,88,113] Increased mutilation frequency has been reported as well.[17] Other studies have failed to find a significant difference between workers and controls.[99,101] Some researchers have found higher individual elevations[28] or a relationship between number of drugs handled and SCEs.[8] These disparate results are not unexpected. The difficulties in quantitating exposure have resulted in different exposure magnitudes between studies; workers in several negative studies appear to have a lower overall exposure.[10] In addition, differences in the use of PPE and work technique will alter absorption of CDs and resultant biologic effects.

Finally, techniques for SCE measurement may not be optimal. A recent study that looked at correlation of phosphoramide-induced SCE levels with duration of anticancer drug handling found a statistically significant correlation coefficient of 0.[63,66]

Taken together, the evidence indicates an excess of markers of mutagenic exposure in unprotected workers.

Reproductive Effects

Reproductive effects associated with occupational exposure to CDs have been well documented. Hemminki et al.[32] found no difference in exposure between nurses who had spontaneous abortions and those who had normal pregnancies. However, the study group consisted of nurses who were employed in surgical or medical floors of a general hospital. When the relationship between CD exposure and congenital malformations was explored, the study group was expanded to include oncology nurses, among others, and an odds ratio of 4:7 was found for exposures of more than once per week. This observed odds ratio is statistically significant. Selevan et al.[39] found a relationship between CD exposure and spontaneous abortion in a case-control study of Finnish nurses. This well-designed study reviewed the reproductive histories of 568 women (167 cases) and found a statistically significant odds ratio of 2:3. Similar results were obtained in another large case-control study of French nurses,[102] and a study of Baltimore area nurses found a significantly higher proportion of adverse pregnancy outcomes when exposure to antineoplastic agents occurred during the pregnancy.[85] The nurses involved in these studies usually prepared and administered the drugs. Therefore, workplace exposure of these groups of professionals to such products has been associated with adverse reproductive outcomes in several investigations.

Other Effects

Hepatocellular damage has been reported in nurses working in an oncology ward; the injury appeared to be related to intensity and duration of work exposure to CDs.[96] Symptoms such as light-headedness, dizziness, nausea, headache, and allergic reactions have also been described in employees after the preparation and administration of antineoplastic drugs in unventilated areas.[22,96] In occupational settings, these agents are known to be toxic to the skin and mucous membranes, including the cornea.[69,82]

Pentamidine has been associated with respiratory damage in one worker who administered the aerosol. The injury consisted of a decrease in diffusing capacity that improved after exposure ceased.[29] The onset of bronchospasm in a pentamidine-exposed worker has also been reported.[22] Employees involved in the aerosol administration of *ribavirin* have noted symptoms of respiratory tract irritation.[55] A number of medications including *psyllium* and various antibiotics are known respiratory and dermal sensitizers. Exposure in susceptible individuals can lead to asthma or allergic contact dermatitis.

D. Work Areas

Risks to personnel working with HDs are a function of the drugs' inherent toxicity and the extent of exposure. The main routes of exposure are: inhalation of dusts or aerosols, dermal absorption, and ingestion. Contact with contaminated food or cigarettes represents the primary means of ingestion. Opportunity for exposure to HDs may occur at many points in the handling of these drugs.

1. Pharmacy or Other Preparation Areas

In large oncology centers, HDs are usually prepared in the pharmacy. However, in small hospitals, outpatient treatments areas, and physicians' offices they have been prepared by physicians or nurses without appropriate engineering controls and protective apparel.[16,20] Many HDs must be reconstituted, transferred from one container to another, or manipulated before administration to patients. Even if care is taken, opportunity for absorption through inhalation or direct skin contact can occur.[35,36,73,116] Examples of manipulations that can cause splattering, spraying, and aerosolization include:

- withdrawal of needles from drug vials,
- drug transfer using syringes and needles or filter straws,
- breaking open of ampules,
- expulsion of air from a drug-filled syringe.

Evaluation of these preparation techniques, using fluorescent dye solutions, has shown contamination of gloves and the sleeves and chest of gowns.[97]

Horizontal airflow work benches provide an aseptic environment for the preparation of injectable drugs. However, these units provide a flow of filtered air originating at the back of the workspace and exiting toward the employee using the unit. Thus, they increase the likelihood of drug exposure for both the preparer and other personnel in the room. As a result, the use of horizontal BSCs is contraindicated in the preparation of HDs. Smoking, drinking, applying cosmetics, and eating where these drugs are prepared, stored, or used also increase the chance of exposure.

2. Administration of Drugs to Patients

Administration of drugs to patients is generally performed by nurses or physicians. Drug injection into the IV line, clearing of air from the syringe or infusion line, and leakage at the tubing, syringe, or stopcock connection present opportunities for skin contact and aerosol generation. Clipping used needles and crushing used syringes can produce considerable aerosolization as well.

Such techniques where needles and syringes are contaminated with blood or other potentially infectious material are prohibited by the Bloodborne Pathogens Standard.[109] Prohibition of clipping or crushing of any needle or syringe is sound practice.

Excreta from patients who have received certain antineoplastic drugs may contain high concentrations of the drug or its hazardous metabolites. For example, patients receiving *cyclophosphamide* excrete large amounts of the drug and its mutagenic metabolites.[46,92] Patients treated with *cisplatin* have been shown to excrete potentially hazardous amounts of the drug.[112] Unprotected handling of urine or urine-soaked sheets by nursing or housekeeping personnel poses a source of exposure.

3. Disposal of Drugs and Contaminated Materials

Contaminated materials used in the preparation and administration of HDs, such as gloves, gowns, syringes, and vials, present a hazard to support and housekeeping staff. The use of properly labeled, sealed, and covered disposal containers, handled by trained and protected personnel, should be routine, and is required under the Bloodborne Pathogens Standard[109] if such items are contaminated with blood or other potentially infectious materials. HDs and contaminated materials should be disposed of in accordance with federal, state, and local laws. Disposal of some of these drugs is regulated by the EPA. Those drugs that are unused commercial chemical products and are considered by the EPA to be toxic wastes must be disposed of in accordance with 40 CFR part 261.33.[24] Spills can also represent a hazard; the employer should ensure that all employees are familiar with appropriate spill procedures.

4. Survey of Current Work Practices

Surveys of U.S. cancer centers and oncology clinics reveal wide variation in work practices, equipment, or training for personnel preparing CDs.[56,73] This lack of standardization results in a high prevalence of potential occupational exposure to CDs. One survey found that 40% of hospital pharmacists reported a skin exposure to CDs at least once a month, and only 28% had medical surveillance programs in their workplace.[16] Nurses, particularly those in outpatient settings, were found to be even less well protected than pharmacists.[111] Such findings emphasize current lack of protection for all personnel who risk potential exposure to HDs.

E. Prevention of Employee Exposure

1. Hazardous Drug Safety and Health Plan

Where hazardous drugs, as defined in this review, are used in the workplace, sound practice would dictate that a written *Hazardous Drug Safety and Health Plan* be developed. Such a plan assists in:

- protecting employees from health hazards associated with HDs,
- keeping exposures as low as reasonably achievable.

When a *Hazardous Drug Safety and Health Plan* is developed, it should be readily available and accessible to all employees, including temporary employees, contractors, and trainees.

The ASHP recommends that the plan include each of the following elements and indicate specific measures that the employer is taking to ensure employee protection:[3]

- standard operating procedures relevant to safety and health considerations to be followed when healthcare workers are exposed to hazardous drugs,
- criteria that the employer uses to determine and implement control measures to reduce employee exposure to hazardous drugs including engineering controls, the use of personal protective, equipment, and hygiene practices,

- a requirement that ventilation systems and other protective equipment function properly, and specific measures to ensure proper and adequate performance of such equipment,
- provision for information and training,
- the circumstances under which the use of specific HDs (that is, FDA investigational drugs) require prior approval from the employer before implementation,
- provision for medical examinations of potentially exposed personnel,
- designation of personnel responsible for implementation of the *Hazardous Drug Safety and Health Plan,* including the assignment of a Hazardous Drug Officer (who is an industrial hygienist, nurse, or pharmacist health and safety representative); and, if appropriate, establishment of a Hazardous Drug Committee or a joint Hazardous Drug Committee/Chemical Committee.

The ASHP further recommends that specific consideration of the following provisions be included where appropriate:

- establishment of a designated HD handling area,
- use of containment devices such as biological safety cabinets,
- procedures for safe removal of contaminated waste,
- decontamination procedures.

The ASHP recommends that the *Hazardous Drug Safety and Health Plan* be reviewed and its effectiveness reevaluated at least annually and updated as necessary.

A comparison of OSHA 200 log entries to employee medical clinic appointment or visit rosters can be made[3] to establish if there is evidence of disorders that could be hazardous drug-related.

Previous health and safety inspections by local health departments, fire departments, regulatory or accrediting agencies may be helpful for the facility's planning purposes as well as any OSHA review of hazards and programs in the facility. Joint Commission on Accreditation of Healthcare Organizations (JCAHO), or College of American Pathologists (CAP) review of facilities may contain information on hazardous drugs used in the facility.

2. Drug Preparation Precautions

Work Area

The ASHP recommends that HD preparation be performed in a restricted, preferably centralized, area. Signs restricting the access of unauthorized personnel are to be prominently displayed. Eating, drinking, smoking, chewing gum, applying cosmetics, and storing food in the preparation area should be prohibited.[71] The ASHP recommends that procedures for spills and emergencies, such as skin or eye contact, be available to workers, preferably posted in the area.[3]

Biological Safety Cabinets

Class II or III Biological Safety Cabinets (BSC) that meet the current National Sanitation Foundation Standard[49,70,72] should minimize exposure to HDs during preparation. Although these cabinets are designed for biohazards, several studies have documented reduced urine mutagenicity in CD-exposed workers or reduce environmental levels after the institution of BSCs.[5,51,61] If a BSC is unavailable, for example in private practice office, accepted medical practice is the sharing of a cabinet (e.g., several medical offices share a cabinet) or sending the patient to a center where HDs can be prepared in a BSC. Alternatively, preparation can be performed in a facility with a BSC and the drugs transported to the area of administration. Use of a dedicated BSC, where only HDs are prepared, is prudent medical practice.

Types of BSCs

Four main types of Class II BSCs are available. They all have downward airflow and HEPA filters. They are differentiated by the amount of air recirculated within the cabinet, whether this air is vented to the room or the outside, and whether contaminated ducts are under positive or negative pressure. These four types are:

- Type A cabinets recirculate approximately 70% of cabinet air through HEPA filters back into the cabinet; the rest is discharged through a HEPA filter into the preparation room. Contaminated ducts are under positive pressure.
- Type B1 cabinets have higher velocity air inflow, recirculate 30% of the cabinet air, and exhaust the rest to the outside through HEPA filters. They have negative pressure contaminated ducts and plenums.
- Type B2 systems are similar to Type B1 except that no air is recirculated.
- Type B3 cabinets are similar to Type A in that they recirculate approximately 70% of cabinet air. However, the other 30% is vented to the outside and the ducts are under negative pressure.

Class III cabinets are totally enclosed with gas-tight construction. The entire cabinet is under negative pressure, and operations are performed through attached gloves. All air is HEPA-filtered.

Class II, type B, or Class III BSCs are recommended since they vent to the outside.[3] Those without air recirculation are the most protective. If the BSC has an outside exhaust, it should be vented away from air intake units.

The blower on the vertical airflow hood should be on at all times. If the BSC is turned off, it should be decontaminated and covered in plastic until airflow is resumed.[3,72] Each BSC should be equipped with a continuous monitoring device to allow confirmation of adequate air flow and cabinet performance. The cabinet should be in an area with minimal air turbulence; this will reduce leakage to the environment.[6,70] Additional information on design and performance testing of BSCs can be found in papers by Avis and Levchuck,[6] Bryan and Marback,[10] and the National Sanitation Foundation.[70] Practical information regarding space needs and conversion possibilities is contained in the ASHP's 1990 technical assistance bulletins.[3]

Ventilation and biosafety cabinets installed should be maintained and evaluated for proper performance in accordance with the manufacturer's instructions.

Decontamination

The cabinet should be cleaned according to the manufacturer's instructions. Some manufacturers have recommended weekly decontamination as well as whenever spills occur or when the cabinet requires moving, service, or certification.

Decontamination should consist of surface cleaning with water and detergent, followed by thorough rinsing. The use of detergent is recommended because there is no single accepted method of chemical deactivation for all agents involved.[13,45] Quaternary ammonium cleaners should be avoided due to the possibility of vapor build-up in recirculated air.[3] Ethyl alcohol or 70% isopropyl alcohol may be used with the cleaner if the contamination is soluble only in alcohol.[3] Alcohol vapor build-up has also been a concern, so the use of alcohol should be avoided in BSCs where air is recirculated.[3] Spray cleaners should also be avoided due to the risk of spraying the HEPA filter. Ordinary decontamination procedures, which include fumigation with a germicidal agent, are inappropriate in a BSC used for HDs because such procedures do not remove or deactivate the drugs.

Removable work trays, if present, should be lifted in the BSC, so the back and the sump below can be cleaned. During cleaning, the worker should wear PPE similar to that used for spills. *Ideally, the sash should remain down during cleaning; however, a NIOSH-approved respirator appropriate for the hazard must be worn by the worker if the sash will be lifted during the process.* The exhaust fan/blower should be left on. Cleaning should proceed from least to most contaminated areas. The drain spillage trough area should be cleaned twice since it can be heavily contaminated. All materials from the decontamination process should be handled as HDs and disposed of in accordance with federal, state, and local laws.

Service and Certification

The ASHP recommends that BSCs be serviced and certified by a qualified technician every 6 months or any time the cabinet is moved or repaired.[3,71] Technicians servicing these cabinets or changing the HEPA filters should be aware of HD risk through hazard communication training from their employers and should use the same personal protective equipment as recommended for large spills. Certification of the BSC includes performance testing as outlined in the procedures of the National Sanitation Foundation's Standard Number 49.[70] Helpful information on such testing can be found in the ASHP 1990 technical assistance bulletins,[3] the BSC manufacturer's equipment manuals, and Bryan and Marback's paper.[10] HEPA filters should be changed when they restrict air flow or if they are contaminated by an accidental spill. They should be bagged in plastic and disposed of as HDs. Any time the cabinet is turned off or transported, it should be sealed with plastic.

Personal Protective Equipment

1. Gloves

Research indicates that the thickness of gloves used in handling HDs is more important than the type of material, since all materials tested have been found to be permeable to some HDs.[3,19,53] The best results are seen with latex gloves. Therefore, latex gloves should be used for the preparation of HDs unless the drug-product manufacturer specifically stipulates that some other glove provides better protection.[19,53,72,93,100] Thicker, longer latex gloves that cover the gown cuff are recommended for the use with HDs. *Individuals with latex allergy should consider the use of vinyl or nitrile gloves or glove liners.* Gloves with minimal or no powder are preferred since the powder may absorb contamination.[3,104]

The above referenced sources have noted great variability in permeability within and between glove lots. Therefore, double gloving is recommended if it does not interfere with an individual's technique.[3] Because all gloves are permeable to some extent and their permeability increases with time, they should be changed regularly (hourly) or immediately if they are torn, punctured, or contaminated with a spill. Hands should always be washed before gloves are put on and after they are removed. Employees need thorough training in proper methods for contaminated glove removal.

2. Gowns

A protective disposable gown made of lint-free, low-permeability fabric with a closed front, long sleeves, and elastic or knit closed cuff should be worn. The cuffs should be tucked under the gloves. If double gloves are worn, the outer glove should be over the gown cuff and the inner glove should be under the gown cuff. When the gown is removed, the inner glove should be removed last. Gowns and gloves in use in the HD preparation area should not be used outside the HD preparation area.[3]

As with gloves, there is no ideal material. Research has found non-porous Tyvek and Kaycel to be more permeable than Saranex-laminated Tyvek and polyethylene-coated Tyvek after 4 hours of exposure to the CDs tested.[54] However, little airflow is allowed with the latter materials. As a result, manufacturers have produced gowns with Saranex or polyethylene reinforced sleeves and front in an effort to decrease permeability in the most exposure-prone areas, but little data exists on decreasing exposure.

3. Respiratory Protection

A BSC is essential for the preparation of HDs. Where a BSC is not currently available, a *NIOSH-approved respirator*[*] *appropriate for the hazard must be worn to afford protection until the BSC is installed.* The use of respirators must comply with OSHA's Respiratory Protection Standard,[105] which outlines the aspects of a respirator program, including selection, fit testing, and worker training. Surgical masks are *not appropriate* since they *do not prevent* aerosol inhalation. Permanent respirator use, in lieu of BSCs, is imprudent practice and should not be a substitute for engineering controls.

---

[*]NIOSH recommendation at the time of this publication is for a respirator with a high-efficiency filter, preferably a powered air-purifying respirator.

4. Eye and Face Protection

Whenever splashes, sprays, or aerosols of HDs may be generated, which can result in eye, nose, or mouth contamination, chemical barrier face and eye protection must be provided and used in accordance with 29 CFR 1910.133. Eye glasses with temporary side shields are inadequate protection.

When a respirator is used to provide temporary protection as described above, and splashes, sprays, or aerosols are possible, employee protection should be:

- a respirator with a full face piece, or
- a plastic face shield or splash goggles complying with ANSI standards[2] when using a respirator of less than full face piece design.

Eyewash facilities should also be made available.

5. PPE Disposal and Decontamination

All gowns, gloves, and disposable materials used in preparation should be disposed of according to the hospital's hazardous drug waste procedures and as described under this review's section on Waste Disposal. Goggles, face shields, and respirators may be cleaned with mild detergent and water for reuse.

Work Equipment

NIH has recommended the work with HDs be carried out in a BSC on a disposable, plastic-backed paper liner. The liner should be changed after preparation is completed for the day, or after a shift, whichever comes first. Liners should also be changed after a spill.[103]

Syringes and IV sets with Luer-Lok fittings should be used for HDs. Syringe size should be large enough so that they are not full when the entire drug dose is present.

A covered disposable container should be used to contain excess solution. A covered sharps container should be in the BSC.

The ASHP recommends that HD-labeled plastic bags be available for all contaminated materials (including gloves, gowns, and paper liners), so that contaminated material can be immediately placed in them and disposed of in accordance with ASHP recommendations.[3]

Work Practices

Correct work practices are essential to worker protection. *Aseptic technique* is assumed as a standard practice in drug preparation. The general principles of aseptic technique, therefore, will not be detailed here. It should be noted, however, that BSC benches differ from horizontal flow units in several ways that require special precautions. Manipulations should not be performed close to the work surface of a BSC. Unsterilized items, including liners and hands, should be kept downstream from the working area. Entry and exit of the cabinet should be perpendicular to the front. Rapid lateral hand movements should be avoided. Additional information can be found in the National Sanitation Foundation Standard 49 for Class II (Laminar Flow) Biohazard Cabinetry[70] and Avis and Levchuck's paper.[6] All operators should be trained in these containment-area protocols.

All PPE should be donned before work is started in the BSC. All items necessary for drug preparation should be placed within the BSC before work is begun. Extraneous items should be kept out of the work area.

1. Labeling

In addition to standard pharmacy labeling practices, all syringes and IV bags containing HDs should be labeled with a distinctive warning label such as

SPECIAL HANDLING/Disposal Precautions

In addition, those HDs covered under HCS must have labels in accordance with section (f) of the standard to warn employees handling the drug(s) of the hazards.

2. Needles

The ASHP recommends that all syringes and needles used in the course of preparation be placed in *"sharps"* containers for disposal without being crushed, clipped, or capped.[3,103]

3. Priming

Prudent practice dictates that drug administration sets be attached and primed within the BSC, prior to addition of the drug. This eliminates the need to prime the set in a less well-controlled environment and ensures that any fluid that escapes during priming contains no drug. If priming must occur at the site of administration, the intravenous line should be primed with non-drug containing fluid, or backflow closed system should be used.[3]

4. Handling Vials

Extremes of positive and negative pressure in medication vials should be avoided, e.g., attempting to withdraw 10 mL of fluid from a 10-mL vial or placing 10 mL of a fluid into an air filled 10-mL vial. The use of large-bore needles, #18 or #20, avoids *high-pressure syringing* of solutions. However, some experienced personnel believe that large-bore needles are more likely to drip. Multi-use dispensing pins are recommended to avoid these problems.

Venting devices such as filter needles or dispensing pins permit outside air to replace the withdrawn liquid. Proper worker education is essential before using these devices.[3] Although venting devices are recommended, another technique is to add diluent slowly to the vial by alternately injecting small amounts and allowing displaced air to escape into the syringe. When all diluent has been added, a small amount of additional air may be withdrawn to create a slight negative pressure in the vial. This should not be expelled into room air because it may contain drug residue. It should either be injected into a vacuum vial or remain in the syringe to be discarded.

If any negative pressure must be applied to withdraw a dosage from a stoppered vial and handling safety is compromised, an air-filled syringe should be used to equalize pressure in the stoppered vial. The volume of drug to be withdrawn can be replaced by injecting small amounts of air into the vial and withdrawing equal amounts of liquid until the required volume is withdrawn. The drug should be cleared from the needle and hub (neck) of the syringe before separating to reduce spraying on separation.

5. Handling Ampules

Prudent practice requires that ampules with dry material should be "*gently tapped down*" before opening to move any material in the top of the ampule to the bottom quantity. A sterile gauze pad should be wrapped around the ampule neck before breaking the top.[3] This can protect against cuts and catch airborne powder or aerosol. If diluent is to be added, it should be injected slowly down the inside wall of the ampule. The ampule should be tilted gently to ensure that all the powder is wet before agitating it to dissolve the contents.

After the solution is withdrawn from the ampule with a syringe, the needle should be cleared of solution by holding it vertically with the point upwards; the syringe should be tapped to remove air bubbles. Any bubbles should be expelled into a closed container.

6. Packaging HDs for Transport

The outside of bags or bottles containing the prepared drug should be wiped with moist gauze.

Entry ports should be wiped with moist alcohol pads and capped. Transport should occur in sealed plastic bags and in containers designed to avoid breakage.

HDs that are shipped and that are subject to EPA regulation as hazardous waste are also subject to Department of Transportation (DOT) regulations as specified in 49 CFR Part 172.101.

7. Non-liquid HDs

The handling of non-liquid forms of HDs requires special precautions as well. Tablets that may produce dust or potential exposure to the handler should be counted in a BSC. Capsules, i.e., gel caps or coated tablets, are unlikely to produce dust unless broken in handling.

These are counted in a BSC on equipment designated for HDs only, because even manual counting devices may be covered with dust from the drugs handled. Automated counting machines should not be used unless an enclosed process isolates the hazard from the employee(s).

Compounding should also occur in a BSC. A gown and gloves should be worn. *(If a BSC is unavailable, an appropriate NIOSH-approved respirator must be worn.)*

Drug Administration

1. Personal Protective Equipment

The National Study Commission on Cytotoxic Exposure has recommended that personnel administering HDs wear gowns, latex gloves, and chemical splash goggles or equivalent safety glasses as described under the PPE Section, Preparation.[71] *NIOSH-approved respirators should be worn when administering aerosolized drugs.*

2. Administration Kit

Protective and administration equipment may be packaged together and labeled as an HD administration kit. Such a kit should include:

- personal protective equipment,
- gauze (4 × 4) for cleanup,
- alcohol wipes,
- disposable plastic-backed absorbent liner,
- puncture-resistant container for needles and syringes,
- a thick sealable plastic bag (with warning label),
- accessory warning labels.

3. Work Practices

Safe work practices when handling HDs should include:

- Hands should be washed before donning and after removing gloves. Gowns or gloves that become contaminated should be changed immediately. Employees should be trained in proper methods to remove contaminated gloves and gowns. After use, gloves and gowns should be disposed of in accordance with ASHP recommendations.
- Infusion sets and pumps, which should have Luer-Lok fittings, should be observed for leakage during use. A plastic-backed absorbent pad should be placed under the tubing during administration to catch any leakage. Sterile gauze should be placed around any push sites; IV tubing connection sites should be taped.
- Priming IV sets or expelling air from syringes should be carried out in a BSC. If done at the administration site, ASHP recommends that the line be primed with non-drug-containing solution or that a backflow closed system be used. IV containers with venting tubes should not be used.[3]
- Syringes, IV bottles and bags, and pumps should be wiped clean of any drug contamination with sterile gauze. Needles and syringes should not be crushed or clipped. They should be placed in a puncture-resistant container then into the HD disposal bag with all other HD contaminated materials. Administration sets should be disposed of intact. Disposal of the waste bag should follow HD disposal requirements. Unused drugs should be returned to the pharmacy.
- Protective goggles should be cleaned with detergent and properly rinsed. All protective equipment should be disposed of upon leaving the patient care area.

- Nursing stations where these drugs will be administered should have spill and emergency skin and eye decontamination kits available and relevant MSDSs for guidance. The HCS requires MSDSs to be readily available in the workplace to all employees working with hazardous chemicals.
- PPE should be used during the administration of oral HDs if splashing is possible.

A large number of investigational HDs are under clinical study in healthcare facilities. Personnel not directly involved in the investigation should not administer these drugs unless they have received adequate instructions regarding safe handling procedures. Literature regarding potential toxic effects of investigational drugs should be evaluated prior to the drug's introduction into the workplace.[65]

The increased use of HDs in the home environment necessitates special precautions. Employees involved in home care delivery should follow the above work practices, and employers should make administration and spill kits available. Home healthcare workers should have emergency protocols with them as well as phone numbers and addresses in the event emergency care becomes necessary.[3] Waste disposal for drugs delivered for home use and other home-contaminated material should also be considered by the employer and should follow applicable regulations.

4. Aerosolized Drugs

The administration of aerosolized HDs requires special engineering controls to prevent exposure to healthcare workers and others in the vicinity. In the case of *pentamidine,* these controls include treatment booths with local exhaust ventilation designed specifically for its administration. A variety of ventilation methods have also been used for the administration of *ribavirin.* These include isolation rooms with separate HEPA-filtered ventilation systems and administration via endotracheal tube.[30,47] Engineering controls used to manage employee exposure to anesthetic gases is a traditional example of occupational chemical management. Both isolation and ventilation are used for these volatile HDs.

Caring for Patients Receiving HDs

In accordance with the Bloodborne Pathogens Standard, universal precautions must be observed to prevent contact with blood or other potentially infectious materials. Under circumstances in which differentiation between body fluid types is difficult or impossible, all body fluids should be considered potentially infectious materials and must be managed as dictated in the Bloodborne Pathogens Standard.[109]

1. Personal Protective Equipment

Personnel dealing with excreta, primarily urine, from patients who have received HDs in the last 48 hours should be provided with and wear latex or other appropriate gloves and disposable gowns, to be discarded after each use or whenever contaminated, as detailed under Waste Disposal. Eye protection should be worn if splashing is possible.

Such excreta contaminated with blood, or other potentially infectious materials as well, should be managed according to the Bloodborne Pathogen Standard. Hands should be washed after removal of gloves or after contact with the above substances.

2. Linen

Linen contaminated with HDs or excreta from patients who have received HDs in the past 48 hours is a potential source of exposure to employees. Linen soiled with blood or other potentially infectious materials as well as contaminated with excreta must also be managed according to the Bloodborne Pathogens Standard.[109] Linen contaminated with HDs should be placed in specially marked laundry bags and then placed in a labeled, impervious bag. The laundry bag and its contents should be prewashed, and then the linens added to other laundry for a second wash. Laundry personnel should wear latex gloves and gowns while handling prewashed material.

3. Reusable Items

Glassware or other contaminated reusable items should be washed twice with detergent by a trained employee wearing double latex gloves and a gown.

Waste Disposal

1. Equipment

Thick, leakproof plastic bags, colored differently from other hospital trash bags, should be used for routine accumulation and collection of used containers, discarded gloves, gowns, and any other disposable material. Bags containing hazardous chemicals (as defined by Section C of HCS), shall be labeled in accordance with Section F of the Hazard Communication Standard where appropriate. Where the Hazard Communication Standard does not apply, labels should indicate that bags contain HD-related wastes.

Needles, syringes, and breakable items not contaminated with blood or other potentially infectious materials should be placed in a "*sharps*" container before they are stored in the waste bag. Such items that are contaminated with blood or other potentially infectious material *must* be placed in a "*sharps*" container. Similarly, needles should not be clipped or capped nor syringes crushed. If contaminated by blood or other potentially infectious material, such needles/syringes *must not* be clipped, capped, or crushed (except as on a rare instance where a *medical* procedure requires recapping). The waste bag should be kept inside a covered waste container clearly labeled "HD Waste Only." At least one such receptacle should be located in every area where the drugs are prepared or administered. Waste should not be moved from one area to another. The bag should be sealed when filled and the covered waste container taped.

2. Handling

Prudent practice dictates that every precaution be taken to prevent contamination of the exterior of the container. Personnel disposing of HD waste should wear gowns and protective gloves when handling waste containers with contaminated exteriors. Prudent practice further dictates that such a container with a contaminated exterior be placed in a second container in a manner that eliminates contamination of the second container. HD waste handlers should also receive hazard communication training as discussed in Section H.

3. Disposal

Hazardous drug-related wastes should be handled separately from other hospital trash and disposed of in accordance with applicable EPA, state, and local regulations for hazardous waste.[24,110] This disposal can occur at either an incinerator or a licensed sanitary landfill for toxic wastes, as appropriate. Commercial waste disposal is performed by a licensed company. While awaiting removal, the waste should be held in a secure area in covered, labeled drums with plastic liners.

Chemical inactivation traditionally has been a complicated process that requires specialized knowledge and training. The MSDS should be consulted regarding specific advice on cleanup (IARC13 and Lunn et al.)[56] have validated inactivation procedures for specific agents that are effective. However, these procedures vary from drug to drug and may be impractical for small amounts. Care must be taken because of unique problems presented by the cleanup of some agents, such as byproduct formation.[57] Serious consideration should be given to alternative disposal methods.

Spills

Emergency procedures to cover spills or inadvertent release of hazardous drugs should be included in the facility's overall health and safety program.

Incidental spills and breakages should be cleaned up immediately by a properly protected person trained in the appropriate procedures. The area should be identified with a warning sign to limit access to the area. Incident Reports should be filed to document the spill and those exposed.

1. Personnel Contamination

Contamination of protective equipment or clothing, or direct skin or eye contact should be treated by:

- Immediately removing the gloves or gown,
- Immediate cleansing of the affected skin with soap and water,
- Flooding an affected eye at an eyewash fountain or with water or isotonic eyewash designated for that purpose for at least 15 minutes, for eye exposure,
- Obtaining medical attention [Protocols for emergency procedures should be maintained at the designated sites for such medical care. Medical attention should also be sought for inhalation of HDs in powder form.],
- Documenting the exposure in the employee's medical record.

2. Cleanup of Small Spills

The ASHP considers small spills to be those less than 5 mL. The 5 mL volume of material should be used to categorize spills as large or small. Spills of less than 5 mL or 5 gm outside a BSC should be cleaned up immediately by personnel wearing gowns, double latex gloves, and splash goggles. *An appropriate NIOSH-approved respirator should be used for either powder or liquid spills where airborne powder or aerosol is or has been generated.*

- Liquids should be wiped with absorbent gauze pads; solids should be wiped with wet absorbent gauze. The spill areas should then be cleaned three times using a detergent solution followed by clean water.
- Any broken glass fragments should be picked up using a small scoop (never the hands) and placed in a "*sharps*" container. The container should then go into a HD disposal bag, along with used absorbent pads and any other contaminated waste.
- Contaminated reusable items, for example glassware and scoops, should be treated as outlined above under Reusable Items.

3. Cleanup of Large Spills

When a large spill occurs, the area should be isolated and aerosol generation avoided. For spills larger than 5 mL, liquid spread is limited by gently covering with absorbent sheets or spill-control pads or pillows. If a powder is involved, damp cloths or towels should be used. Specific individuals should be trained to clean up large spills.

- Protective apparel, including respirators, should be used as with small spills when there is any suspicion of airborne powder or that an aerosol has been or will be generated. Most CDs are not volatile; however, this may not be true for all HDs. The volatility of the drug should be assessed in selecting the type of respiratory protection.
- As discussed under Waste Disposal, chemical inactivation should be avoided in this setting.
- All contaminated surfaces should be thoroughly cleaned three times with detergent and water.
- All contaminated absorbent sheets and other materials should be placed in the HD disposal bag.

4. Spills in BSCs

Extensive spills within a BSC necessitate decontamination of all interior BSC surfaces after completion of the spill cleanup. The ASHP3 recommends this action for spills larger than 150 mL or the contents of one vial. If the HEPA filter of a BSC is contaminated, the unit should be labeled and sealed in plastic until the filter can be changed and disposed of properly by trained personnel wearing appropriate protective equipment.

5. Spill Kits

Spill kits, clearly labeled, should be kept in or near preparation and administrative areas. The MSDSs include sections on emergency procedures, including appropriate personal protective equipment. The ASHP recommends that kits include: chemical splash goggles, two pairs of gloves, utility gloves, a low-permeability gown, two sheets (12″ × 12″) of absorbent material, 250-mL and liter spill control pillows, a "*sharps*" container, a small scoop to collect glass fragments, and two large HD waste-disposal bags.[3]

Prior to cleanup, appropriate protective equipment should be donned. Absorbent sheets should be incinerable. Protective goggles and respirators should be cleaned with mild detergent and water after use.

Storage and Transport

1. Storage Areas

Access to areas where HDs are stored should be limited to authorized personnel with signs restricting entry.[72] A list of drugs covered by HD policies and information on spill and emergency contact procedures should be posted or easily available to employees. Facilities used for storing HDs should not be used for other drugs, and should be designed to prevent containers from falling to the floor, e.g., bins with barrier fronts. Warning labels should be applied to all HD containers, as well as the shelves and bins where these containers are permanently stored.

2. Receiving Damaged HD Packages

Damaged shipping cartons should be opened in an isolated area or a BSC by a designated employee wearing double gloves, a gown, goggles, and appropriate respiratory protection. Individuals must be trained to process damaged packages as well.

The ASHP recommends that broken containers and contaminated packaging mats be placed in a "*sharps*" container and then into HD disposal bags.[3] The bags should then be closed and placed in receptacles as described under Waste Disposal.

The appropriate protective equipment and waste disposal materials should be kept in the area where shipments are received, and employees should be trained in their use and the risks of exposure to HDs.

3. Transport

HDs should be securely capped or sealed, placed in sealed clear plastic bags, and transported in containers designed to avoid breakage.

Personnel involved in transporting HDs should be trained in spill procedures, including sealing off the contaminated area and calling for appropriate assistance.

All HD containers should be labeled as noted in Drug Preparation Work Practices. If transport methods that produce stress on contents, such as pneumatic tubes are used, guidance from the OSHA clarification of 1910.1030 with respect to transport (M.4.b.(8)(c)) should be followed. This clarification provides for use of packaging material inside the tube to prevent breakage. These recommendations that pertain to the Bloodborne Pathogens Standard are prudent practice for HDs, e.g., padded inserts for carriers.

F. Medical Surveillance

Workers who are potentially exposed to chemical hazards should be monitored in a systematic program or medical surveillance intended to prevent occupational injury and disease.[3,7] The purpose of surveillance is to identify the earliest reversible biologic effects so that exposure can be reduced or eliminated before the employee sustains irreversible damage. The occurrence of exposure-related disease or other adverse health effects should prompt immediate re-evaluation of primary preventive measures (e.g., engineering controls, personal protective equipment). In this manner, medical surveillance acts as a check on the appropriateness of controls already in use.[62]

For detection and control of work-related health effects, *job-specific* medical evaluations should be performed:

- before job placement,
- periodically during employment,
- following acute exposures,
- at the time of job termination or transfer (exit examination).

This information should be collected and analyzed in a systematic fashion to allow early detection of disease patterns in individual workers and groups of workers.

1. Preplacement Medical Examinations

Sound medical practice dictates that employees who will be working with HDs in the workplace have an initial evaluation consisting of a history, physical exam, and laboratory studies.

Information made available, by the employer, to the examining physician should be:

- a description of the employee's duties as they relate to the employee's exposure,
- the employee's exposure levels or anticipated exposure levels,
- a description of any personal protective equipment used or to be used,
- information from previous medical examinations of the employee, which is not readily available to the examining physician.

The history details the individual's medical and reproductive experience with emphasis on potential risk factors, such as past hematopoietic, malignant, or hepatic disorders. It also includes a complete occupational history with information on extent of past exposures (including environmental sampling data, if possible) and use of protective equipment. Surrogates for worker exposure, in the absence of environmental sampling data, include:

- records of drugs and quantities handled,
- hours spent handling these drugs per week,
- number of preparations/administrations per week.

The physical examination should be complete, but the skin, mucous membranes, cardiopulmonary, lymphatic system, and liver should be emphasized. An evaluation for respirator use must be performed in accordance with 29 CFR 1910.134, if the employee will wear a respirator. The laboratory assessment may include a complete blood count with differential, liver function tests, blood urea nitrogen, creatinine, and a urine dipstick. Other aspects of the physical and laboratory evaluation should be guided by known toxicities of the HD of exposure. Due to poor reproducibility, interindividual variability, and lack of prognostic value regarding disease development, no biological monitoring tests (e.g., genotoxic markers) are currently recommended for routine use in employee surveillance. Biological marker testing should be performed only within the context of a research protocol.

2. Periodic Medical Examinations

Recognized occupational medicine experts in the HD area recommend these exams to update the employee's medical, reproductive, and exposure histories. They are recommended on a yearly basis or every 2–3 years. The interval between exams is a function of the opportunity for exposure, duration of exposure, and possibly the age of the worker at the discretion of the occupational medicine physician, guided by the worker's history. Careful documentation of an individual's routine exposure and any acute accidental exposures are made. The physical examination and laboratory studies follow the format outlined in the pre-placement examination.[54]

3. Post-exposure Examinations

Post-exposure evaluation is tailored to the type of exposure (e.g., spills or needle sticks from syringes containing HDs). An assessment of the extent of exposure is made and included in the confidential database (discussed in the "Exposure/Health Outcome Linkage" section) and in an incident report. The physical examination focuses on the involved area as well as other organ systems commonly affected (i.e., for CDs the skin and mucous membranes; for aerosolized HDs the pulmonary system). Treatment and laboratory studies follow as indicated and should be guided by emergency protocols.

4. Exit Examinations

The exit examination completes the information on the employee's medical, reproductive, and exposure histories. Examination and laboratory evaluation should be guided by the individual's history of exposures and follow the outline of the periodic evaluation.

5. Exposure/Health Outcome Linkage

Exposure assessment of all employees who have worked with HDs is important, and the maintenance of records is required by 29 CFR 1910.20. The use of previously outlined exposure surrogates is acceptable, although actual environmental or employee monitoring data is preferable. An MSDS can serve as an exposure record. Details of the use of personal protective equipment and engineering controls present should be included. A confidential database should be maintained with information regarding the individual's medical and reproductive history, with linkage to exposure information to facilitate epidemiologic review.

6. Reproductive Issues

The examining physician should consider the reproductive status of employees and inform them regarding relevant reproductive issues. The reproductive toxicity of hazardous drugs should be carefully explained to all workers who will be exposed to these chemicals, and is required for those chemicals covered by the HCS. Unfortunately, no information is available regarding the reproductive risks of HD handling with the current use of BSCs and PPE. However, as discussed earlier, both spontaneous abortion and congenital malformation excesses have been documented among workers handling some of these drugs without currently recommended engineering controls and precautions. The facility should have a policy regarding reproductive toxicity of HDs and worker exposure in male and female employees and should follow that policy.

G. Hazard Communication

This section is for informational purposes only and is not a substitute for the requirements of the Hazard Communication Standard.

The Hazard Communication Standard (HCS),[107] is applicable to some drugs. It defines a hazardous chemical as *any chemical that is a physical hazard or a health hazard.*

Physical hazard refers to characteristics such as combustibility or reactivity. A health hazard is defined as *a chemical for which there is statistically significant evidence based on at least one study conducted in accordance with established scientific principles that acute or chronic health effects may occur in exposed employees.* Appendixes A and B of the HCS outline the criteria used to determine whether an agent is hazardous.

According to HCS Appendix A, agents with any of the following characteristics would be considered hazardous:

- carcinogens,
- corrosives,

- toxic or highly toxic (defined on the basis of median lethal doses),
- irritants,
- sensitizers, or
- target organ effectors, including reproductive toxins, hepatotoxins, nephrotoxins, neurotoxins, agents that act on the hematopoietic system, and agents that damage the lungs, skin, eyes, or mucous membranes.

Both human and animal data are to be used in this determination. HCS Appendix C lists sources of toxicity information.

As a result of the February 21, 1990 Supreme Court decision,[21] all provisions of the Hazard Communication Standard [29 CFR 1910.1200][107] are now in effect for all industrial segments. This includes the coverage of drugs and pharmaceuticals in the non-manufacturing sector. On February 9, 1994, OSHA issued a revised Hazard Communication Final Rule with technical clarification regarding drugs and pharmaceutical agents.

The Hazard Communication Standard (HCS) requires that drugs posing a health hazard (with the exception of those in solid, final form for direct administration to the patient, i.e., tablets or pills) be included on lists of hazardous chemicals to which employees are exposed.[107] Their storage and use locations can be confirmed by reviewing purchasing office records of currently used and past used agents such as those in Table A.1. Employee exposure records, including workplace monitoring, biological monitoring, and MSDSs, as well as employee medical records related to drugs posing a health hazard must be maintained and access to them provided to employees in accordance with 29 CFR 1910.20. Training required under the HCS should include all employees potentially exposed to these agents, not only healthcare professional staff, but also physical plant, maintenance, or support staff.

MSDSs are required to be prepared and transmitted with the initial shipment of all hazardous chemicals including covered drugs and pharmaceutical products. This excludes drugs defined by the Federal Food, Drug and Cosmetic Act, which are in solid, final form for direct administration to the patient (e.g., tablets, pills, or capsules) or which are packaged for sale to consumers in a retail establishment. Package inserts and the *Physicians' Desk Reference* are not acceptable in lieu of requirements of MSDSs under the Standard. Items mandated by the Standard will use the term *shall* instead of *should.*

1. Written Hazard Communication Program

Employers shall develop, implement, and maintain at the workplace, a written hazard communication program for employees handling or otherwise exposed to chemicals, including drugs that represent a health hazard to employees. The written program will describe how the criteria specified in the Standard concerning labels and other forms of warning, MSDSs, and employee information and training will be met. This also includes the following:

- a list of the covered hazardous drugs known to be present using an identity that is referenced on the appropriate MSDS,

- the methods the employer will use to inform employees of the hazards of non-routine tasks in their work areas,
- the methods the employer will use to inform employees of other employers of hazards at the worksite.

The employer shall make the written hazard communication program available, upon request, to employees, their designated representatives, and the Assistant Secretary of OSHA in accordance with requirements of the HCS.

2. MSDSs

In accordance with requirements in the Hazard Communication Standard, the employer must maintain MSDSs accessible to employees for all covered HDs used in the hospital. Specifics regarding MSDS content are contained in the Standard. Essential information includes: health hazards, primary exposure routes, carcinogenic evaluations, acute exposure treatment, chemical inactivators, solubility, stability, volatility, PPE-required and spill procedures for each covered HD. MSDSs shall also be made readily available upon request to employees, their designated representatives, or the Assistant Secretary of OSHA.

H. Training and Information Dissemination

In compliance with the Hazard Communication Standard, all personnel involved in any aspect of the handling of covered HDs (physicians, nurses, pharmacists, housekeepers, employees involved in receiving, transport, or storage) must receive information and training to apprise them of the hazards of HDs present in the work area.[71] Such information should be provided at the time of an employee's initial assignment to a work area where HDs are present and prior to assignments involving new hazards. The employer should provide annual refresher information and training.

The National Study Commission on Cytotoxic Exposure has recommended that knowledge and competence of personnel be evaluated after the first orientation or training session, and then yearly, or more often if a need is perceived.[71] Evaluation may involve direct observation of an individual's performance on the job. In addition, non-HD solutions should be used for evaluation of preparation technique; quinine, which will fluoresce under ultraviolet light, provides an easy mechanism for evaluation of technique.

1. Employee Information

Employees must be informed of the requirements of the Hazard Communication Standard, 29 CFR 1910.1200:

- any operation/procedure in their work area where drugs that present a hazard are present,
- the location and availability of the written hazard communication program.

In addition, they should be informed regarding:

- any operations or procedure in their work area where other HDs are present,
- the location and availability of any other plan regarding HDs.

2. Employee Training

Employee training must include at least:

- methods of observations that may be used to detect the presence or release of a HCS-covered hazardous drug in the work area (such as monitoring conducted by the employer, continuous monitoring devices, visual appearance, or odor of covered HDs being released, etc.),
- the physical and health hazards of the covered HDs in the area.
- the measures employees can take to protect themselves from these hazards. This includes specific procedures that the employer has implemented to protect the employees from exposure to such drugs, such as identification of covered drugs and those to be handled as hazardous, appropriate work practices, emergency procedures (for spills or employee exposure), and personal protective equipment, and
- the details of the hazard communication program developed by the employer, including an explanation of the labeling system and the MSDS, and how employees can obtain and use the appropriate hazard information.

It is essential that workers understand the carcinogenic potential and reproductive hazards of these drugs. Both females and males should understand the importance of avoiding exposure, especially early in pregnancy, so they can make informed decisions about the hazards involved. In addition, the facility's policy regarding reproductive toxicity of HDs should be explained to workers. Updated information should be provided to employees on a regular basis and whenever their jobs involve new hazards. Medical staff and other personnel who are not hospital employees should be informed of hospital policies and of the expectation that they will comply with these policies.

I. Record Keeping

Any workplace-exposure record created in connection with HD handling shall be kept, transferred, and made available for at least thirty years, and medical records shall be kept for the duration of employment plus thirty years in accordance with the Access to Employee Exposure and Medical Records Standard (29 CFR 1910.20).[108] In addition, sound practice dictates that training records should include the following information:

- the dates of the training sessions,
- the contents or a summary of the training sessions,
- the names and qualifications of the persons conducting the training,
- the names and job titles of all persons attending the training sessions.

Training records should be maintained for three years from the date on which the training occurred.

Position Statement

For the handling of cytotoxic agents by women who are pregnant, attempting to conceive, or breast-feeding. There are substantial data regarding the mutagenic, teratogenic, and abortifacient properties of certain cytotoxic agents both in animals and humans who have received therapeutic doses of these agents. Additionally, the scientific literature suggests a possible association of occupational exposure to certain cytotoxic agents during the first trimester of pregnancy with fetal loss or malformation. These data suggest the need for caution when women who are pregnant, or attempting to conceive, handle cytotoxic agents. Incidentally, there is no evidence relating male exposure to cytotoxic agents with adverse fetal outcome. There are no studies that address the possible risk associated with the occupational exposure to cytotoxic agents and the passage of these agents into breast milk. Nevertheless, it is prudent that women who are breast-feeding should exercise caution in handling cytotoxic agents.

If all procedures for safe handling, such as those recommended by the Commission, are complied with, the potential for exposure will be minimized. Personnel should be provided with information to make an individual decision. This information should be provided in written form, and it is advisable that a statement of understanding be signed. It is essential to refer to individual state right-to-know laws to ensure compliance.

Approved by the National Study Commission on Cytotoxic Exposure, September 1987.

References

1. American Medical Association Council on Scientific Affairs. Guidelines for handling parenteral antineoplastics. *JAMA* 1985; 253 1590–2
2. American National Standards Institute. Occupational and Educational Eye and Face Protection. *ANSI* 1968; Z87 1
3. American Society of Hospital Pharmacists. ASHP Technical Assistance Bulletin on Handling Cytotoxic and Hazardous Drugs. *Am. J. Hosp. Pharm.* 1990; 47 1033–49
4. Andersen R, Boedicker M, Ma M, Goldstein EJC. Adverse Reactions Associated with Pentamidine Isethionate in AIDS Patients: Recommendations for Monitoring Therapy. *Drug Intell. Clin. Pharm.* 1986; 20 862–8
5. Anderson RW, Puckett WH, Dana WJ, et al. Risk of handling injectable antineoplastic agents. *Am. J. Hosp. Pharm.* 1982; 39 1881–87
6. Avis KE, Levchuck JW. Special considerations in the use of vertical laminar flow workbenches. *Am. J. Hosp. Pharm.* 1984; 41 81–7
7. Barber RK. Fetal and neonatal effects of cytotoxic agents. *Obstet. Gynecol.* 1981; 51 41S–47S
8. Benhamou S, Pot-Deprun J, Sancho-Garnier H, Chouroulinkov I. Sister chromatid exchanges and chromosomal aberrations in lymphocytes of nurses handling cytostatic drugs. *Int. J. Cancer* 1988; 41 350–3

9. Bos RP, Leenars AO, Theuws JL, Henderson PT. Mutagenicity of urine from nurses handling cytostatic drugs, influence of smoking. *Int. Arch. Occ. Envir. Health* 1982; 50 359–69
10. Bryan D, Marback RC. Laminar-airflow equipment certification: What the pharmacist needs to know. *Am. J. Hosp. Pharm.* 1984; 41 1343–9
11. Burgaz S, Ozdamar YN, Karakaya AE. A signal assay for the detection of toxic compounds: Application on the urines of cancer patients on chemotherapy and of nurses handling cytotoxic drugs. *Human Toxicol.* 1988; 7 557–60
12. California Department of Health Services Occupational Health Surveillance and Evaluation Program. *Health care worker exposure to ribavirin aerosol: field investigation FI-86-009.* Berkeley: California Department of Health Services. 1986
13. Castegnaro M, Adams J, Armour MA, eds, et al. Laboratory decontamination and destruction of carcinogens in laboratory wastes: Some antineoplastic agents. International Agency for Research on Cancer. Scientific Publications No. 73. Lyons, France: IARC 1985
14. Chapman RM. Effect of cytotoxic therapy on sexuality and gonadal function. Perry MC, Yarbro JW, (eds), *Toxicity of Chemotherapy* Orlando: Grune & Stratton. 1984 343–363
15. Chen CH, Vazquez-Padua M, Cheng YC. Effect of antihuman immunodeficiency virus nucleoside analogs on mDNA and its implications for delayed toxicity. *Mol. Pharm.* 1990; 39 625–628
16. Christensen CJ, Lemasters GK, Wakeman MA. Work practices and policies of hospital pharmacists preparing antineoplastic agents. *J. Occup. Med.* 1990; 32 508–12
17. Chrysostomou A, Morley AA, Seshadri R. Mutation frequency in nurses and pharmacists working with cytotoxic drugs. *Aust. N. Z. J. Med.* 1984; 14 831–4
18. Connor JD, Hintz M, Van Dyke R. Ribavirin pharmacokinetics in children and adults during therapeutic trials. Smith RA, Knight V, Smith JAD (eds), In *Clinical Applications of Ribavirin.* Orlando: Academic Press, 1984
19. Connor TH, Laidlaw JL, Theiss JC, et al. Permeability of latex and polyvinyl chloride gloves to carmustine. *Am. J. Hosp. Pharm.* 1984; 41 676–9
20. Crudi CB. A compounding dilemma: I've kept the drug sterile but have I contaminated myself? *Nat. Intra. Therapy J.* 1980; 3 77–80
21. Dole v. United Steelworkers. 1990; 494 U.S.26.
22. Doll C. Aerosolised pentamidine. *Lancet* 1989; ii 1284–5
23. Duvall E, Baumann B. An unusual accident during the administration of chemotherapy. *Cancer Nurs.* 1980; 3 305–6
24. Environmental Protection Agency. *Discarded commercial chemical products, off specification species, container residues, and spill residues thereof.* 40 CFR 1991; 261.33(f)
25. Everson RB, Ratcliffe JM, Flack PM et al. Detection of low levels of urinary mutagen excretion by chemotherapy workers which was not related to occupational drug exposures. *Cancer Research* 1985; 45 6487–97
26. Falck K, Grohn P, Sorsa M, et al. Mutagenicity in urine of nurses handling cytostatic drugs. *Lancet* 1979; i 1250–1
27. Falck K, Sorsa M, Vainio H. Use of the bacterial fluctuation test to detect mutagenicity in urine of nurses handling cytostatic drugs (abstract). *Mutation Res.* 1981; 85 236–7
28. Ferguson LR, Everts R, Robbie MA, et al. The use within New Zealand of cytogenetic approaches to monitoring of hospital pharmacists for exposure to cytotoxic drugs: Report of a pilot study in Auckland. *Aust J Hosp Pharm.* 1988; 18 228–33
29. Gude JK. Selective delivery of pentamidine to the lung by aerosol. *Am. Rev. Resp. Dis.* 1989; 139 1060
30. Guglielmo BJ, Jacobs RA, Locksley RM. The exposure of health care workers to ribavirin aerosol. *JAMA* 1989; 261 1880–1

31. Harrison R, Bellows J, Rempel D, et al. Assessing exposures of health-care personnel to aerosols of ribavirin—California. *Morbidity and Mortality Weekly Report* 1988; 37 560–3
32. Hemminki K, Kyyronen P, Lindbohm ML. Spontaneous abortions and malformations in the offspring of nurses exposed to anaesthetic gases, cytostatic drugs, and other potential hazards in hospitals, based on registered information of outcome. *J. Epidem. Comm. Health* 1985; 39 141–7
33. Henderson DK, Gerberding JL. Prophylactic zidovudine after occupational exposure to the human immunodeficiency virus: An interim analysis. *J. Infectious Diseases* 1989; 160 321–7
34. Hillyard IW. The preclinical toxicology and safety of ribavirin. Smith RA, Kirkpatrick W, (eds), *In Ribavirin: a broad spectrum antiviral agent*. New York: Academic Press 1980
35. Hirst M, Tse S, Mills DG, et al. Occupational exposure to cyclophosphamide. *Lancet* 1984; i 186–8
36. Hoy RH, Stump LM. Effect of an air-venting filter device on aerosol production from vials. *Am. J. Hosp. Pharm.* 1984; 41 324–6
37. International Agency for Research on Cancer. *IARC Monographs on the Evaluation of the Carcinogenic Risk of Chemicals to Man: Some Aziridines, N-, S-, and O-mustards and selenium.* Lyons, France. 1975; Vol. 9
38. International Agency for Research on Cancer. *IARC Monographs on the Evaluation of the Carcinogenic Risk of Chemicals to Man: Some naturally occurring substances.* Lyons, France: IARC. 1976; Vol. 10
39. International Agency for Research on Cancer. *IARC Monographs on the Evaluation of the Carcinogenic Risk of Chemicals to Humans: Some Antineoplastic and Immunosuppressive Agents.* Lyons, France: IARC. 1981; Vol. 26
40. International Agency for Research on Cancer. *IARC Monographs on the Evaluation of the Carcinogenic Risk of Chemicals to Humans: Chemicals, Industrial Processes and Industries Associated with Cancer in Humans.* Lyons, France: IARC. 1982; Vol. 1–29 (Suppl. 4)
41. International Agency for Research on Cancer. *IARC Monographs on the Evaluation of the Carcinogenic Risk of Chemicals to Humans: Genetic and related effects: An updating of selected IARC Monographs from Volumes 1–42.* Lyons, France: IARC. 1987; Vol. 1–42 (Suppl. 6)
42. International Agency for Research on Cancer. *IARC Monographs on the Evaluation of the Carcinogenic Risk of Chemicals to Humans; Overall evaluations of carcinogenicity: An updating of IARC Monographs Volumes 1 to 42.* Lyons, France: IARC. 1987; Vol. 1–42 (Suppl. 7)
43. International Agency for Research on Cancer. *IARC Monographs on the Evaluation of the Carcinogenic Risk of Chemicals to Humans: Pharmaceutical Drugs.* Lyons, France: IARC
44. Jagun O, Ryan M, Waldron HA. Urinary thioether excretion in nurses handling cytotoxic drugs. *Lancet* 1982; i 443–4
45. Johnson EG, Janosik JE. Manufacturer's recommendations for handling spilled antineoplastic agents. *Am. J. Hosp. Pharm.* 1989; 46 318–9
46. Juma FD, Rogers HJ, Trounce JR, Bradbrook ID. Pharmacokinetics of intravenous cyclophosphamide in man, estimated by gas-liquid chromatography. *Cancer Chemother. Pharmacol.* 1978; 1 229–31
47. Kacmarek RM. Ribavirin and pentamidine aerosols: Caregiver beware! *Respiratory Care* 1990; 35 1034–6
48. Karakaya AE, Burgaz S, Bayhan A. The significance of urinary thioethers as indicators of exposure to alkylating agents. *Arch. Toxicol.* 1989; 13(suppl) 117–9
49. Kilham L, Ferm VH. Congenital anomalies induced in hamster embryos with ribavirin. *Science* 1977; 195 413–4
50. Kleinberg ML, Quinn MJ. Airborne drug levels in a laminar-flow hood. *Am. J. Hosp. Pharm.* 1981; 38 1301–3

51. Kolmodin-Hedman B, Hartvig P, Sorsa M, Falck K. Occupational handling of cytostatic drugs. *Arch. Toxicol.* 1983; 54 25–33
52. Kyle RA. Second malignancies associated with chemotherapy. Perry MC, Yarbro JW, (eds), *Toxicity of Chemotherapy*. Orlando: Grune & Stratton. 1984; 479–506
53. Laidlaw JL, Connor TH, Theiss JC, et al. Permeability of latex and polyvinyl chloride gloves to 20 antineoplastic drugs. *Am. J. Hosp. Pharm.* 1984; 41 2618–23
54. Laidlaw JL, Connor TH, Theiss JC, et al. Permeability of four disposable protective clothing materials to seven antineoplastic drugs. *Am. J. Hosp. Pharm.* 1985; 42 2449–54
55. Lee SB. Ribavirin—Exposure to health care workers. *Am. Ind. Hyg. Assoc.* 1988; 49 A13–A14
56. LeRoy ML, Roberts MJ, Theisen JA. Procedures for handling antineoplastic injections in comprehensive cancer centers. *Am. J. Hosp. Pharm.* 1983; 40 601–3
57. Lunn G, Sansone EB. Validated methods for handling spilled antineoplastic agents. *Am. J. Hosp. Pharm.* 1989; 46 1131
58. Lunn G, Sansone EB, Andrews AW, Hellwig LC. Degradation and disposal of some antineoplastic drugs. *J. Pharm. Sciences.* 1989; 78 652–9
59. Matthews T, Boehme R. Antiviral activity and mechanism of action of ganciclovir. *Rev. Infect. Diseases* 1988; 10 (suppl 3) S490–94
60. McDevitt JJ, Lees PSJ, McDiarmid MA. Exposure of hospital pharmacists and nurses to antineoplastic agents. *J. Occup. Med.* 1993; 35 57–60
61. McDiarmid MA, Egan T, Furio M, et al. Sampling for airborne fluorouracil in a hospital drug preparation area. *Am. J. Hosp. Pharm.* 1988; 43 1942–5
62. McDiarmid MA, Emmett EA. Biological monitoring and medical surveillance of workers exposed to antineoplastic agents. *Seminars in Occup. Med.* 1987; 2 109–17
63. McDiarmid MA, Jacobson-Kram D. Aerosolized pentamidine and public health. *Lancet* 1989; ii 863
64. McDiarmid MA. Medical surveillance for antineoplastic-drug handlers. *Am. J. Hosp. Pharm.* 1990; 47 1061–6
65. McDiarmid MA, Gurley HT, Arrington D. Pharmaceuticals as hospital hazards: Managing the risks. *J. Occup. Med.* 1991; 33 155–8
66. McDiarmid MA, Kolodner K, Humphrey F, et al. Baseline and phosphoramide mustard-induced sister chromatid exchanges in pharmacists handling anti-cancer drugs. *Mutation Research* 1992; 279 199–204
67. McDiarmid MA, Schaefer J, Richard CL, Chaisson RE, Tepper BS. Efficacy of engineering controls in reducing occupational exposure to aerosolized pentamidine. *Chest* 1992; 102 1764–6
68. McEvoy GK, ed. *American Hospital Formulary Service Drug Information.* Bethesda: American Society of Hospital Pharmacists, 1993
69. McLendon BF, Bron AF. Corneal toxicity from vinblastine solution. *Br. J. Ophthalmol.* 1978; 62 97–9
70. National Sanitation Foundation. *Standard No. 49 for Class II (Laminar Flow) Biohazard Cabinetry.* Ann Arbor: National Sanitation Foundation, 1990
71. National Study Commission on Cytotoxic Exposure. Louis P Jeffrey Sc. D Chairman, (eds), *Recommendations for Handling Cytotoxic Agents*. Providence, Rhode Island: Rhode Island Hospital, 1983
72. National Study Commission on Cytotoxic Exposure. Consensus Responses to Unresolved Questions Concerning Cytotoxic Agents. Louis P Jeffrey -Sc. D, (eds), Providence, Rhode Island. Chairman, Rhode Island Hospital, 1984
73. Neal AD, Wadden RA, Chiou WL. Exposure of hospital workers to airborne antineoplastic agents. *Am. J. Hosp. Pharm.* 1983; 40 597–601

74. Nikula E, Kiviniitty K, Leisti J, Taskinen P. Chromosome aberrations in lymphocytes of nurses handling cytostatic agents. *Scand. J. Work Environ. Health.* 1984; 10 71–4
75. Norppa H, Sorsa M, Vainio H, et al. Increased sister chromatid exchange frequencies in lymphocytes of nurses handling cytostatic drugs. *Scand. J. Work Environ. Health* 1980; 6 299–301
76. Nguyen TV, Theiss JC, Matney TS. Exposure of pharmacy personnel to mutagenic antineoplastic drugs. *Cancer Research* 42 4792–6
77. Palmer RG, Dore CJ, Denman AM. Chlorambucil-induced chromosome damage to human lymphocytes is dose-dependent and cumulative. *Lancet* 1984; i 246–9
78. Perry MC, Yarbro JW, eds. *Toxicity of Chemotherapy*. Orlando: Grune & Stratton. 1984
79. Physicians' Desk Reference. Barnhart ER, (eds), *Physicians' Desk Reference*, 45th ed. Oradell, New Jersey: Medical Economics Data. 1991; 730
80. Pohlova H, Cerna M, Rossner P. Chromosomal aberrations, SCE and urine mutagenicity in workers occupationally exposed to cytostatic drugs. *Mutation Res.* 1986; 174 213–7
81. Pyy L, Sorsa M, Hakala E. Ambient monitoring of cyclophosphamide in manufacture and hospitals. *Am. Ind. Hyg. Assoc. J.* 1988; 49 314–7
82. Reich SD, Bachur NR. Contact dermatitis associated with adriamycin (NSC-123127) and daunorubicin (NSC-82151). *Cancer Chemotherap. Reports* 1975; 59 677–8
83. Reynolds RD, Ignoffo R, Lawrence J, et al. Adverse reactions to AMSA in medical personnel. *Cancer Treat. Rep.* 1982; 66 1885
84. Rogers B. Health hazards to personnel handling antineoplastic agents. *Occupational Medicine: State of the Art Reviews* 1987; 2 513–24
85. Rogers B, Emmett EA. Handling antineoplastic agents: Urine mutagenicity in nurses. *IMAGE Journal of Nursing Scholarship.* 1987; 19 108–113
86. Rosner F. Acute leukemia as a delayed consequence of cancer chemotherapy. *Cancer* 1976; 37 1033–6
87. Rudolph R, Suzuki M, Luce JK. Experimental skin necrosis produced by adriamycin. *Cancer Treat. Reports* 1979; 63 529–37
88. Schafer AI. Teratogenic effects of antileukemic therapy. *Arch. Int. Med.* 1981; 141 514–5
89. Selevan SG, Lindbolm ML, Homung RW, Hemminki K. A study of occupational exposure to antineoplastic drugs and fetal loss in nurses. *New Engl. J. Med.* 1985; 313 1173–8
90. Sieber SM. Cancer chemotherapeutic agents and carcinogenesis. *Cancer Chemotherap. Reports* 1975; 59 915–8
91. Sieber SM, Adamson RH. Toxicity of antineoplastic agents in man: Chromosomal aberrations, antifertility effects, congenital malformations, and carcinogenic potential. *Adv. Cancer Res.* 1975; 22 57–155
92. Siebert D, Simon U. Cyclophosphamide: Pilot study of genetically active metabolites in the urine of a treated human patient. *Mutat. Res.* 1973; 19 65–72
93. Slevin ML, Ang LM, Johnston A, Turner P. The efficiency of protective gloves used in the handling of cytotoxic drugs. *Cancer Chemo. Pharmacol.* 1984; 12 151–3
94. Smaldone GC, Vincicuerra C, Marchese J. Detection of inhaled pentamidine in health care workers. *New Engl. J. Med.* 1991; 325 891–2
95. Sorsa M, Hemminki K, Vanio H. Occupational exposure to anticancer drugs—Potential and real hazards. *Mut. Res.* 1985; 154 135–49
96. Sotaniemi EA, Sutinen S, Arranto AJ, et al. Liver damage in nurses handling cytostatic agents. *Acta Med. Scand.* 1983; 214 181–9
97. Stellman JM. The spread of chemotherapeutic agents at work: Assessment through stimulation. *Cancer Investigation* 1987; 5 75–81
98. Stephens JD, Golbus MS, Miller TR, et al. Multiple congenital abnormalities in a fetus exposed to 5-fluorouracil during the first trimester. *Am. J. Obstet. Gynecol.* 1980; 137 747–9

99. Stiller A, Obe G, Bool I, Pribilla W. No elevation of the frequencies of chromosomal aberrations as a consequence of handling cytostatic drugs. *Mut. Res.* 1983; 121 253–9
100. Stoikes ME, Carlson JD, Farris FF, Walker PR. Permeability of latex and polyvinyl chloride gloves to fluorouracil and methotrexate. *Am. J. Hosp. Pharm.* 1987; 44 1341–6
101. Stucker I, Hirsch A, Doloy T, et al. Urine mutagenicity, chromosomal abnormalities and sister chromatid exchanges in lymphocytes of nurses handling cytostatic drugs. *Int. Arch. Occup. Environ. Health* 1986; 57 195–205
102. Stucker I, Caillard JF, Collin R, et al. Risk of spontaneous abortion among nurses handling antineoplastic drugs. *Scand. J. Work Environ. Health* 1990; 16 102–7
103. U.S. Department of Health and Human Services. Public Health Service. National Institutes of Health. *Recommendations for the Safe Handling of Cytotoxic Drugs*. NIH Publication No. 92-2621. 1992
104. U.S. Department of Health and Human Services. Public Health Service. Centers for Disease Control. National Institute for Occupational Safety and Health. *Guidelines for Protecting the Safety and Health of Health Care Workers*. DHHS (NIOSH) Publication No. 88–119. 1988
105. U.S. Department of Labor, Occupational Safety and Health Administration. Respiratory Protection Standard. 1984; 29 CFR 1910.134
106. U.S. Department of Labor, Occupational Safety and Health Administration. Work practice guidelines for personnel dealing with cytotoxic (antineoplastic) drugs. OSHA Publication #8-1.1. 1986
107. U.S. Department of Labor, Occupational Safety and Health Administration. *Hazard Communication Standard*. 1989; 29 CFR 1910.1200, as amended February 9, 1994.
108. U.S. Department of Labor, Occupational Safety and Health Administration. *Access to Employee and Medical Records Standard*. 1990; 29 CFR 1910.20
109. U.S. Department of Labor, Occupational Safety and Health Administration. *Occupational Exposure to Bloodborne Pathogens Standard*. 1991; 29 CFR 1910.1030
110. Vaccari FL, Tonat K, DeChristoforo R, et al. Disposal of antineoplastic waste at the NIH. *Am. J. Hosp. Pharm.* 1984; 41 87–92
111. Valanis B, Vollmer WM, Labuhn K, Glass A, Corelle C. Antineoplastic drug handling protection after OSHA guidelines: Comparison by profession, handling activity, and work site. *J. Occup. Med.* 1992; 34 149–55
112. Venitt S, Crofton-Sleigh C, Hunt J, et al. Monitoring exposure of nursing and pharmacy personnel to cytotoxic drugs. Urinary mutation assays and urinary platinum as markers of absorption. *Lancet* 1984; i:74 6
113. Waksvik H, Klepp O, Brogger A. Chromosome analyses of nurses handling cytostatic agents. *Cancer Treat. Reports* 1981; 65 607–10
114. Wall RL, Clausen KP. Carcinoma of the urinary bladder in patients receiving cyclophosphamide. *New Engl. J. Med.* 1975; 293 271–3
115. Weisburger JH, Griswold DP, Prejean JD, et al. Tumor induction by cytostatics. The carcinogenic properties of some of the principal drugs used in clinical cancer chemotherapy. *Recent Results Cancer Res.* 1975; 52 1–17
116. Zimmerman PF, Larsen RK, Barkley EW, Gallelli JF. Recommendations for the safe handling of injectable antineoplastic drug products. *Am. J. Hosp. Pharm.* 1981; 38 1693–5

Appendix 2
Common Toxicity Criteria for Adverse Events v. 3.0 (CTCAE)

Source: From *Cancer Therapy Evaluation Program (CTEP)* [Online], Common Technology Criteria for Adverse Events v. 3.0, 2003. Available: http://ctep.cancer.gov/forms/CTCAEv3.pdf, accessed October 29, 2007

ALLERGY/IMMUNOLOGY						
		Grade				
Adverse Event	**Short Name**	**1**	**2**	**3**	**4**	**5**
Allergic reaction/hypersensitivity (including drug fever)	Allergic reaction	Transient flushing or rash; drug fever <38°C (<100.4°F)	Rash; flushing; urticaria; dyspnea; drug fever ≥38°C (≥100.4°F)	Symptomatic bronchospasm, with or without urticaria; parenteral medication(s) indicated; allergy-related edema/angioedema; hypotension	Anaphylaxis	Death
Remark: Urticaria with manifestations of allergic or hypersensitivity reaction is graded as Allergic reaction/hypersensitivity (including drug fever). Also Consider: Cytokine release syndrome/acute infusion reaction.						
Allergic rhinitis (including sneezing, nasal stuffiness, postnasal drip)	Rhinitis	Mild, intervention not indicated	Moderate, intervention indicated	—	—	—
Remark: Rhinitis associated with obstruction or stenosis is graded as Obstruction/stenosis of airway – *Select* in the PULMONARY/UPPER RESPIRATORY CATEGORY.						

(continued)

Appendix 2 *(Continued)*

ALLERGY/IMMUNOLOGY						
		Grade				
Adverse Event	**Short Name**	**1**	**2**	**3**	**4**	**5**
Autoimmune reaction	Autoimmune reaction	Asymptomatic and serologic or other evidence of autoimmune reaction, with normal organ function and intervention not indicated	Evidence of autoimmune reaction involving a nonessential organ or function (e.g., hypothyroidism)	Reversible autoimmune reaction involving function of a major organ or other adverse event (e.g., transient colitis or anemia)	Autoimmune reaction with life-threatening consequences	Death
ALSO CONSIDER: Colitis; Hemoglobin; Hemolysis (e.g., immune hemolytic anemia, drug-related hemolysis); Thyroid function, low (hypothyroidism).						
Serum sickness	Serum sickness	—	—	Present	—	Death
NAVIGATION NOTE: Splenic function is graded in the BLOOD/BONE MARROW CATEGORY.						
NAVIGATION NOTE: Urticaria as an isolated symptom is graded as Urticaria (hives, welts, wheals) in the DERMATOLOGY/SKIN CATEGORY.						
Vasculitis	Vasculitis	Mild, intervention not indicated	Symptomatic, nonsteroidal medical intervention indicated	Steroids indicated	Ischemic changes; amputation indicated	Death
Allergy/Immunology – Other (Specify, _______)	Allergy – Other (Specify)	Mild	Moderate	Severe	Life-threatening; disabling	Death

(continued)

AUDITORY/EAR						
		Grade				
Adverse Event	**Short Name**	**1**	**2**	**3**	**4**	**5**
NAVIGATION NOTE: Earache (otalgia) is graded as Pain – *Select* in the PAIN CATEGORY.						
Hearing: patients with/without baseline audiogram and enrolled in a monitoring program[1]	Hearing (monitoring program)	Threshold shift or loss of 15–25 dB relative to baseline, averaged at 2 or more contiguous test frequencies in at least one ear; or subjective change in the absence of a Grade 1 threshold shift	Threshold shift or loss of >25–90 dB, averaged at 2 contiguous test frequencies in at least one ear	Adult only: Threshold shift of >25–90 dB, averaged at 3 contiguous test frequencies in at least one ear Pediatric: Hearing loss sufficient to indicate therapeutic intervention, including hearing aids (e.g., ≥20 dB bilateral HL in the speech frequencies; ≥30 dB unilateral HL; and requiring additional speech-language related services)	Adult only: Profound bilateral hearing loss (>90 dB) Pediatric: Audiologic indication for cochlear implant and requiring additional speech-language related services	—
REMARK: Pediatric recommendations are identical to those for adults, unless specified. For children and adolescents (≤18 years of age) without a baseline test, pre-exposure/pretreatment hearing should be considered to be <5 dB loss.						

(continued)

Appendix 2 *(Continued)*

AUDITORY/EAR						
		Grade				
Adverse Event	**Short Name**	**1**	**2**	**3**	**4**	**5**
Hearing: patients without baseline audiogram and not enrolled in a monitoring program[1]	Hearing (without monitoring program)	—	Hearing loss not requiring hearing aid or intervention (i.e., not interfering with ADL)	Hearing loss requiring hearing aid or intervention (i.e., interfering with ADL)	Profound bilateral hearing loss (>90 dB)	—
REMARK: Pediatric recommendations are identical to those for adults, unless specified. For children and adolescents (≤18 years of age) without a baseline test, pre-exposure/pretreatment hearing should be considered to be <5 dB loss.						
Otitis, external ear (non-infectious)	Otitis, external	External otitis with erythema or dry desquamation	External otitis with moist desquamation, edema, enhanced cerumen or discharge; tympanic membrane perforation; tympanostomy	External otitis with mastoiditis; stenosis or osteomyelitis	Necrosis of soft tissue or bone	Death
ALSO CONSIDER: Hearing: patients with/without baseline audiogram and enrolled in a monitoring program.[1] Hearing: patients without baseline audiogram and not enrolled in a monitoring program.[1]						
Otitis, middle ear (non-infectious)	Otitis, middle	Serous otitis	Serous otitis, medical intervention indicated	Otitis with discharge; mastoiditis	Necrosis of the canal soft tissue or bone	Death

(continued)

AUDITORY/EAR						
		Grade				
Adverse Event	**Short Name**	**1**	**2**	**3**	**4**	**5**
Tinnitus	Tinnitus	—	Tinnitus not interfering with ADL	Tinnitus interfering with ADL	Disabling	—
ALSO CONSIDER: Hearing: patients with/without baseline audiogram and enrolled in a monitoring program.[1] Hearing: patients without baseline audiogram and not enrolled in a monitoring program.[1]						
Auditory/Ear – Other (Specify, ________)	Auditory/Ear – Other (Specify)	Mild	Moderate	Severe	Life-threatening; disabling	Death

BLOOD/BONE MARROW						
		Grade				
Adverse Event	**Short Name**	**1**	**2**	**3**	**4**	**5**
Bone marrow cellularity	Bone marrow cellularity	Mildly hypocellular or ≤25% reduction from normal cellularity for age	Moderately hypocellular or >25–≤50% reduction from normal cellularity for age	Severely hypocellular or >50–≤75% reduction cellularity from normal for age	—	Death
CD4 count	CD4 count	<LLN–500/mm^3 <LLN–0.5 × 10^9/L	<500–200/mm^3 <0.5–0.2 × 10^9/L	<200–50/mm^3 <0.2–0.05 × 10^9/L	<50/mm^3 <0.05 × 10^9/L	Death
Haptoglobin	Haptoglobin	<LLN	—	Absent	—	Death
Hemoglobin	Hemoglobin	<LLN–10.0 g/dL <LLN–6.2 mmol/L <LLN–100 g/L	<10.0–8.0 g/dL <6.2–4.9 mmol/L <100–80g/L	<8.0–6.5 g/dL <4.9–4.0 mmol/L <80–65 g/L	<6.5 g/dL <4.0 mmol/L <65 g/L	Death

(continued)

Appendix 2 *(Continued)*

BLOOD/BONE MARROW						
		Grade				
Adverse Event	**Short Name**	**1**	**2**	**3**	**4**	**5**
Hemolysis (e.g., immune hemolytic anemia, drug-related hemolysis)	Hemolysis	Laboratory evidence of hemolysis only (e.g., direct antiglobulin test [DAT, Coombs'] schistocytes)	Evidence of red cell destruction and ≥2 gm decrease in hemoglobin, no transfusion	Transfusion or medical intervention (e.g., steroids) indicated	Catastrophic consequences of hemolysis (e.g., renal failure, hypotension, bronchospasm, emergency splenectomy)	Death
ALSO CONSIDER: Haptoglobin; Hemoglobin.						
Iron overload	Iron overload	—	Asymptomatic iron overload, intervention not indicated	Iron overload, intervention indicated	Organ impairment (e.g., endocrinopathy, cardiopathy)	Death
Leukocytes (total WBC)	Leukocytes	<LLN–3000/mm^3 <LLN–3.0 × 10^9/L	<3000–2000/mm^3 <3.0–2.0 × 10^9/L	<2000–1000/mm^3 <2.0–1.0 × 10^9/L	<1000/mm^3 <1.0 × 10^9/L	Death
Lymphopenia	Lymphopenia	<LLN–800/mm^3 <LLN × 0.8–10^9/L	<800–500/mm^3 <0.8–0.5 × 10^9/L	<500–200 mm^3 <0.5–0.2 × 10^9/L	<200/mm^3 <0.2 × 10^9/L	Death

(continued)

BLOOD/BONE MARROW						
		Grade				
Adverse Event	**Short Name**	**1**	**2**	**3**	**4**	**5**
Myelodysplasia	Myelodysplasia	—	—	Abnormal marrow cytogenetics (marrow blasts $\leq$5%)	RAEB or RAEB-T (marrow blasts $>$5%)	Death
Neutrophils/granulocytes (ANC/AGC)	Neutrophils	$<$LLN–1500/mm^3 $<$LLN–1.5 × 10^9/L	$<$1500–1000/mm^3 $<$1.5–1.0 × 10^9/L	$<$1000–500/mm^3 $<$1.0–0.5 × 10^9/L	$<$500/mm^3 $<$0.5 × 10^9/L	Death
Platelets	Platelets	$<$LLN–75,000/mm^3 $<$LLN–75.0 × 10^9/L	$<$75,000–50,000/mm^3 $<$75.0–50.0 × 10^9/L	$<$50,000–25,000/mm^3 $<$50.0–25.0 × 10^9/L	$<$25,000/mm^3 $<$25.0 × 10^9/L	Death
Splenic function	Splenic function	Incidental findings (e.g., Howell-Jolly bodies)	Prophylactic antibiotics indicated	—	Life-threatening consequences	Death
Blood/Bone Marrow – Other (Specify, _______)	Blood – Other (Specify)	Mild	Moderate	Severe	Life-threatening; disabling	Death

(continued)

Appendix 2 *(Continued)*

CARDIAC ARRYTHMIA						
		Grade				
Adverse Event	**Short Name**	**1**	**2**	**3**	**4**	**5**
Conduction abnormality/ atrioventricular heart block – *Select*: – Asystole – AV Block-First degree – AV Block-Second degree Mobitz Type I (Wenckebach) – AV Block-Second degree Mobitz Type II – AV Block-Third degree (Complete AV block) – Conduction abnormality NOS – Sick Sinus Syndrome – Stokes-Adams Syndrome – Wolff-Parkinson-White Syndrome	Conduction abnormality – *Select*	Asymptomatic intervention not indicated	Non-urgent medical intervention indicated	Incompletely controlled medically or controlled with device (e.g., pacemaker)	Life-threatening (e.g., arrhythmia associated with CHF, hypotension, sycope, shock)	Death
Palpitations	Palpitations	Present	Present with associated symptoms (e.g., lightheadedness, shortness of breath)	—	—	—
REMARK: Grade palpitations only in the absence of a documented arrhythmia.						

(continued)

CARDIAC ARRYTHMIA						
		Grade				
Adverse Event	**Short Name**	**1**	**2**	**3**	**4**	**5**
Prolonged QTc interval	Prolonged QTc	QTc > 0.45–0.47 second	QTc > 0.47–0.50 second; ≥0.06 second above baseline	QTc >0.50 second	QTc >0.50 second; life-threatening signs or symptoms (e.g., arrhythmia, CHF, hypotension, shock syncope); Torsade de pointes	Death
Supraventricular and nodal arrhythmia – *Select*: – Atrial fibrillation – Atrial flutter – Atrial tachycardia/Paroxysmal Atrial Tachycardia – Nodal/Junctional – Sinus arrhythmia – Sinus bradycardia – Sinus tachycardia – Supraventricular arrhythmia NOS – Supraventricular extrasystoles (Premature Atrial Contractions; Premature Nodal/Junctional Contractions) – Supraventricular tachycardia	Supraventricular arrhythmia – *Select*	Asymptomatic, intervention not indicated	Non-urgent medical intervention indicated	Symptomatic and incompletely controlled medically, or controlled with device (e.g., pacemaker)	Life-threatening (e.g., arrhythmia associated with CHF, hypotension, syncope, shock)	Death

(continued)

Appendix 2 *(Continued)*

CARDIAC ARRYTHMIA						
		Grade				
Adverse Event	**Short Name**	**1**	**2**	**3**	**4**	**5**
NAVIGATION NOTE: Syncope is graded as Syncope (fainting) in the NEUROLOGY CATEGORY.						
Vasovagal episode	Vasovagal episode	—	Present without loss of consciousness	Present with loss of consciousness	Life-threatening consequences	Death
Ventricular arrhythmia – *Select*: – Bigeminy – Idioventricular rhythm – PVCs – Torsade de pointes – Trigeminy – Ventricular arrhythmia NOS – Ventricular fibrillation – Ventricular flutter – Ventricular tachycardia	Ventricular arrhythmia – *Select*	Asymptomatic, no intervention indicated	Non-urgent medical intervention indicated	Symptomatic and incompletely controlled medically or controlled with device (e.g., defibrillator)	Life-threatening (e.g., arrhythmia associated with CHF, hypotension, syncope, shock)	Death
Cardiac Arrhythmia – Other (Specify, _______)	Cardiac Arrhythmia – Other (Specify)	Mild	Moderate	Severe	Life-threatening; disabling	Death

(continued)

CARDIAC GENERAL						
		Grade				
Adverse Event	**Short Name**	**1**	**2**	**3**	**4**	**5**
NAVIGATION NOTE: Angina is graded as Cardiac ischemia/infarction in the CARDIAC GENERAL CATEGORY.						
Cardiac ischemia/infarction	Cardiac ischemia/infarction	Asymptomatic arterial narrowing without ischemia	Asymptomatic and testing suggesting ischemia; stable angina	Symptomatic and testing consistent with ischemia; unstable angina; intervention indicated	Acute myocardial infarction	Death
Cardiac troponin I (cTnI)	cTnI	—	—	Levels consistent with unstable angina as defined by the manufacturer	Levels consistent with myocardial infarction as defined by the manufacturer	Death
Cardiac troponin T (cTnT)	cTnT	0.03 to <0.05 ng/mL	0.05 to <0.1 ng/mL	0.1 to <0.2 ng/mL	0.2 ng/mL	Death
Cardiopulmonary arrest, cause unknown (non-fatal)	Cardiopulmonary arrest	—	—	—	Life-threatening	—

REMARK: Grade 4 (non-fatal) is the only appropriate grade. CTCAE provides three alternatives for reporting Death:

1. A CTCAE term associated with Grade 5.
2. A CTCAE 'Other (Specify, _______)' within any CATEGORY.
3. Death not associated with CTCAE term – *Select* in the DEATH CATEGORY.

(continued)

Appendix 2 *(Continued)*

CARDIAC GENERAL						
		Grade				
Adverse Event	**Short Name**	**1**	**2**	**3**	**4**	**5**
NAVIGATION NOTE: Chest pain (non-cardiac and non-pleuritic) is graded as Pain – *Select* in the PAIN CATEGORY.						
NAVIGATION NOTE: CNS ischemia is graded as CNS cerebrovascular ischemia in the NEUROLOGY CATEGORY.						
Hypertension	Hypertension	Asymptomatic, transient (<24 hrs) increase by >20 mmHg (diastolic) or to >150/100 if previously WNL; intervention not indicated Pediatric: Asymptomatic, transient (<24 hrs) BP increase >ULN; intervention not indicated	Recurrent or persistent (≥24 hrs) or symptomatic increase by >20 mmHg (diastolic) or to >150/100 if previously WNL; monotherapy may be indicated Pediatric: Recurrent or persistent (≥24 hrs) BP >ULN; monotherapy may be indicated	Requiring more than one drug or more intensive therapy than previously Pediatric: Same as adult	Life-threatening consequences (e.g., hypertensive crisis) Pediatric: Same as adult	Death
REMARK: Use age and gender-appropriate normal values >95th percentile ULN for pediatric patients.						

(continued)

CARDIAC GENERAL						
		Grade				
Adverse Event	Short Name	1	2	3	4	5
Hypotension	Hypotension	Changes, intervention not indicated	Brief (<24 hrs) fluid replacement or other therapy; no physiologic consequences	Sustained (≥24 hrs) therapy, resolves without persisting physiologic consequences	Shock (e.g., acidemia; impairment of vital organ function)	Death
ALSO CONSIDER: Syncope (fainting).						
Left ventricular diastolic dysfunction	Left ventricular diastolic dysfunction	Asymptomatic diagnostic finding; intervention not indicated	Asymptomatic, intervention indicated	Symptomatic CHF responsive to intervention	Refractory CHF, poorly controlled; intervention such as ventricular assist device or heart transplant indicated	Death
Left ventricular systolic dysfunction	Left ventricular systolic dysfunction	Asymptomatic, resting ejection fraction (EF) <60–50%; shortening fraction (SF) <30–24%	Asymptomatic, resting EF <50–40%; SF <24–15%	Symptomatic CHF responsive to intervention; EF <40–20% SF <15%	Refractory CHF or poorly controlled; EF <20%; intervention such as ventricular assist device, ventricular reduction surgery, or heart transplant indicated	Death
NAVIGATION NOTE: Myocardial infarction is graded as Cardiac ischemia/infarction in the CARDIAC GENERAL CATEGORY.						

(continued)

Appendix 2 *(Continued)*

CARDIAC GENERAL						
		Grade				
Adverse Event	**Short Name**	**1**	**2**	**3**	**4**	**5**
Myocarditis	Myocarditis	—	—	CHF responsive to intervention	Severe or refractory CHF	Death
Pericardial effusion (non-malignant)	Pericardial effusion	Asymptomatic effusion	—	Effusion with physiologic consequences	Life-threatening consequences (e.g., tamponade); emergency intervention indicated	Death
Pericarditis	Pericarditis	Asymptomatic, ECG or physical exam (rub) changes consistent with pericarditis	Symptomatic pericarditis (e.g., chest pain)	Pericarditis with physiologic consequences (e.g., pericardial constriction)	Life-threatening consequences; emergency intervention indicated	Death
NAVIGATION NOTE: Pleuritic pain is graded as Pain – *Select* in the PAIN CATEGORY.						
Pulmonary hypertension	Pulmonary hypertension	Asymptomatic without therapy	Asymptomatic, therapy indicated	Symptomatic hypertension, responsive to therapy	Symptomatic hypertension, poorly controlled	Death

(continued)

CARDIAC GENERAL						
		Grade				
Adverse Event	**Short Name**	**1**	**2**	**3**	**4**	**5**
Restrictive cardiomyopathy	Restrictive cardiomyopathy	Asymptomatic, therapy not indicated	Asymptomatic, therapy indicated	Symptomatic CHF responsive to intervention	Refractory CHF, poorly controlled; intervention such as ventricular assist device, or heart transplant indicated	Death
Right ventricular dysfunction (cor pulmonale)	Right ventricular dysfunction	Asymptomatic without therapy	Asymptomatic, therapy indicated	Symptomatic cor pulmonale, responsive to intervention	Symptomatic cor pulmonale poorly controlled; intervention such as ventricular assist device, or heart transplant indicated	Death
Valvular heart disease	Valvular heart disease	Asymptomatic valvular thickening with or without mild valvular regurgitation or stenosis; treatment other than endocarditis prophylaxis not indicated	Asymptomatic; moderate regurgitation or stenosis by imaging	Symptomatic; severe regurgitation or stenosis; symptoms controlled with medical therapy	Life-threatening; disabling; intervention (e.g., valve replacement, valvuloplasty) indicated	Death

(continued)

Appendix 2 *(Continued)*

CARDIAC GENERAL						
		Grade				
Adverse Event	**Short Name**	**1**	**2**	**3**	**4**	**5**
Cardiac General – Other (Specify, ________)	Cardiac General – Other (Specify)	Mild	Moderate	Severe	Life-threatening; disabling	Death

COAGULATION						
		Grade				
Adverse Event	**Short Name**	**1**	**2**	**3**	**4**	**5**
DIC (disseminated intravascular coagulation)	DIC	—	Laboratory findings with *no* bleeding	Laboratory findings *and* bleeding	Laboratory findings, life threatening or disabling consequences (e.g., CNS hemorrhage, organ damage, or hemodynamically significant blood loss)	Death
REMARK: DIC (disseminated intravascular coagulation) must have increased fibrin split products or D-dimer.						
ALSO CONSIDER: Platelets.						
Fibrinogen	Fibrinogen	<1.0–0.75 × LLN or <25% decrease from baseline	<0.75–0.5 × LLN or 25–<50% decrease from baseline	<0.5–0.25 × LLN or 50–<75% decrease from baseline	<0.25 × LLN or 75% decrease from baseline or absolute value <50 mg/dL	Death
REMARK: Use % decrease only when baseline is ≤LLN (local laboratory value).						

(continued)

CARDIAC GENERAL						
		Grade				
Adverse Event	**Short Name**	**1**	**2**	**3**	**4**	**5**
INR (International Normalized Ratio of prothrombin time)	INR	>1–1.5 × ULN	>1.5–2 × ULN	>2 × ULN	—	—
ALSO CONSIDER: Hemorrhage, CNS; Hemorrhage, GI – *Select*; Hemorrhage, GU – *Select*; Hemorrhage, pulmonary/upper respiratory – *Select*.						
PTT (Partial Thromboplastin Time)	PTT	>1–1.5 × ULN	>1.5–2 × ULN	>2 × ULN	—	—
ALSO CONSIDER: Hemorrhage, CNS; Hemorrhage, GI – *Select*; Hemorrhage, GU – *Select*; Hemorrhage, pulmonary/upper respiratory – Select.						
Thrombotic microangiopathy (e.g., thrombotic thrombocytopenic purpura [TTP] or hemolytic uremic syndrome [HUS])	Thrombotic microangiopathy	Evidence of RBC destruction (schistocytosis) without clinical consequences	—	Laboratory findings present with clinical consequences (e.g., renal insufficiency, petechiae)	Laboratory findings and life-threatening or disabling consequences, (e.g., CNS hemorrhage/bleeding or thrombosis/embolism or renal failure)	Death
REMARK: Must have microangiopathic changes on blood smear (e.g., schistocytes, helmet cells, red cell fragments).						
ALSO CONSIDER: Creatinine; Hemoglobin; Platelets.						
Coagulation – Other (Specify, ______)	Coagulation – Other (Specify)	Mild	Moderate	Severe	Life-threatening; disabling	Death

(continued)

Appendix 2 *(Continued)*

CONSTITUTIONAL SYMPTOMS						
		Grade				
Adverse Event	**Short Name**	**1**	**2**	**3**	**4**	**5**
Fatigue (asthenia, lethargy, malaise)	Fatigue	Mild fatigue over baseline	Moderate or causing difficulty performing some ADL	Severe fatigue interfering with ADL	Disabling	—
Fever (in the absence of neutropenia, where neutropenia is defined as ANC <1.0 × 10^9/L)	Fever	38.0–39.0°C (100.4–102.2°F)	>39.0–40.0°C (102.3–104.0°F)	>40.0°C (>104.0°F) for ≤24 hrs	>40.0°C (>104.0°F) for >24 hrs	Death
REMARK: The temperature measurements listed are oral or tympanic.						
ALSO CONSIDER: Allergic reaction/hypersensitivity (including drug fever).						
NAVIGATION NOTE: Hot flashes are graded as Hot flashes/flushes in the ENDOCRINE CATEGORY.						
Hypothermia	Hypothermia	—	35 to >32°C 95 to >89.6° F	32 to >28°C 89.6 to >82.4° F	≤28 °C 82.4°F or life-threatening consequences (e.g., coma, hypotension, pulmonary edema, acidemia, ventricular fibrillation)	Death

(continued)

CONSTITUTIONAL SYMPTOMS						
		Grade				
Adverse Event	**Short Name**	**1**	**2**	**3**	**4**	**5**
Insomnia	Insomnia	Occasional difficulty sleeping, not interfering with function	Difficulty sleeping, interfering with function but not interfering with ADL	Frequent difficulty sleeping, interfering with ADL	Disabling	—
REMARK: If pain or other symptoms interfere with sleep, do NOT grade as insomnia. Grade primary event(s) causing insomnia.						
Obesity[2]	Obesity	—	BMI 25–29.9 kg/m^2	BMI 30–39.99 kg/m^2	BMI ≥40 kg/m^2	—
REMARK: BMI = (weight [kg])/(height [m])^2						
Odor (patient odor)	Patient odor	Mild odor	Pronounced odor	—	—	—
Rigors/chills	Rigors/chills	Mild	Moderate, narcotics indicated	Severe or prolonged, not responsive to narcotics	—	—
Sweating (diaphoresis)	Sweating	Mild and occasional	Frequent or drenching	—	—	—
ALSO CONSIDER: Hot flashes/flushes.						
Weight gain	Weight gain	5 to <10% of baseline	10 to <20% of baseline	≥20% of baseline	—	—
REMARK: Edema, depending on etiology, is graded in the CARDIAC GENERAL or LYMPHATICS CATEGORIES.						
ALSO CONSIDER: Ascites (non-malignant); Pleural effusion (non-malignant).						

(continued)

Appendix 2 *(Continued)*

CONSTITUTIONAL SYMPTOMS						
		Grade				
Adverse Event	**Short Name**	**1**	**2**	**3**	**4**	**5**
Weight loss	Weight loss	5 to <10% from baseline; intervention not indicated	10 to <20% from baseline; nutritional support indicated	≥20% from baseline; tube feeding or TPN indicated	—	—
Constitutional Symptoms – Other (Specify, _______)	Constitutional Symptoms – Other (Specify)	Mild	Moderate	Severe	Life-threatening; disabling	Death

DEATH						
		Grade				
Adverse Event	**Short Name**	**1**	**2**	**3**	**4**	**5**
Death not associated with CTCAE term –*Select*: – Death NOS – Disease progression NOS – Multi-organ failure – Sudden death	Death not associated with CTCAE term – *Select*	—	—	—	—	Death

REMARK: Grade 5 is the only appropriate grade. 'Death not associated with CTCAE term – *Select*' is to be used where a death:
1. Cannot be attributed to a CTCAE term associated with Grade 5.
2. Cannot be reported within any CATEGORY using a CTCAE 'Other (Specify, _______)'.

(continued)

DERMATOLOGY/SKIN						
		Grade				
Adverse Event	**Short Name**	**1**	**2**	**3**	**4**	**5**
Atrophy, skin	Atrophy, skin	Detectable	Marked	—	—	—
Atrophy, subcutaneous fat	Atrophy, subcutaneous fat	Detectable	Marked	—	—	—
ALSO CONSIDER: Induration/fibrosis (skin and subcutaneous tissue).						
Bruising (in absence of Grade 3 or 4 thrombocytopenia)	Bruising	Localized or in a dependent area	Generalized	—	—	—
Burn	Burn	Minimal symptoms; intervention not indicated	Medical intervention; minimal debridement indicated	Moderate to major debridement or reconstruction indicated	Life-threatening consequences	Death
REMARK: Burn refers to all burns including radiation, chemical, etc.						
Cheilitis	Cheilitis	Asymptomatic	Symptomatic, not interfering with ADL	Symptomatic, interfering with ADL	—	—
Dry skin	Dry skin	Asymptomatic	Symptomatic, not interfering with ADL	Interfering with ADL	—	—
Flushing	Flushing	Asymptomatic	Symptomatic	—	—	—
Hair loss/alopecia (scalp or body)	Alopecia	Thinning or patchy	Complete	—	—	—

(continued)

Appendix 2 *(Continued)*

DERMATOLOGY/SKIN						
		Grade				
Adverse Event	**Short Name**	**1**	**2**	**3**	**4**	**5**
Hyperpigmentation	Hyperpigmentation	Slight or localized	Marked or generalized	—	—	—
Hypopigmentation	Hypopigmentation	Slight or localized	Marked or generalized	—	—	—
Induration/fibrosis (skin and subcutaneous tissue)	Induration	Increased density on palpation	Moderate impairment of function not interfering with ADL; marked increase in density and firmness on palpation with or without minimal retraction	Dysfunction interfering with ADL; very marked density, retraction or fixation	—	—
ALSO CONSIDER: Fibrosis-cosmesis; Fibrosis-deep connective tissue.						
Injection site reaction/ extravasation changes	Injection site reaction	Pain; itching; erythema	Pain or swelling, with inflammation or phlebitis	Ulceration or necrosis that is severe; operative intervention indicated	—	—
ALSO CONSIDER: Allergic reaction/hypersensitivity (including drug fever); Ulceration.						

(continued)

DERMATOLOGY/SKIN						
		Grade				
Adverse Event	**Short Name**	**1**	**2**	**3**	**4**	**5**
Nail changes	Nail changes	Discoloration; ridging (koilonychias); pitting	Partial or complete loss of nail(s); pain in nailbed(s)	Interfering with ADL	—	—
NAVIGATION NOTE: Petechiae is graded as Petechiae/purpura (hemorrhage/bleeding into skin or mucosa) in the HEMORRHAGE/BLEEDING CATEGORY.						
Photosensitivity	Photosensitivity	Painless erythema	Painful erythema	Erythema with desquamation	Life-threatening; disabling	Death
Pruritus/itching	Pruritus	Mild or localized	Intense or widespread	Intense or widespread and interfering with ADL	—	—
ALSO CONSIDER: Rash/desquamation.						
Rash/desquamation	Rash	Macular or papular eruption or erythema without associated symptoms	Macular or papular eruption or erythema with pruritus or other associated symptoms; localized desquamation or other lesions covering <50% of body surface area (BSA)	Severe, generalized erythroderma or macular, papular or vesicular eruption; desquamation covering ≥50% BSA	Generalized exfoliative, ulcerative, or bullous dermatitis	Death
REMARK: Rash/desquamation may be used for GVHD.						

(continued)

Appendix 2 *(Continued)*

DERMATOLOGY/SKIN						
		Grade				
Adverse Event	**Short Name**	**1**	**2**	**3**	**4**	**5**
Rash: acne/acneiform	Acne	Intervention not indicated	Intervention indicated	Associated with pain, disfigurement, ulceration, or desquamation	—	Death
Rash: dermatitis associated with radiation – *Select*: – Chemoradiation – Radiation	Dermatitis – *Select*	Faint erythema or dry desquamation	Moderate to brisk erythema; patchy moist desquamation, mostly confined to skin folds and creases; moderate edema	Moist desquamation other than skin folds and creases; bleeding induced by minor trauma or abrasion	Skin necrosis or ulceration of full thickness dermis; spontaneous bleeding from involved site	Death
Rash: erythema multiforme (e.g., Stevens-Johnson syndrome, toxic epidermal necrolysis)	Erythema multiforme	—	Scattered, but not generalized eruption	Severe (e.g., generalized rash or painful stomatitis); IV fluids, tube feedings, or TPN indicated	Life-threatening; disabling	Death
Rash: hand-foot skin reaction	Hand-foot	Minimal skin changes or dermatitis (e.g., erythema) without pain	Skin changes (e.g., peeling, blisters, bleeding, edema) or pain, not interfering with function	Ulcerative dermatitis or skin changes with pain interfering with function	—	—

(continued)

DERMATOLOGY/SKIN						
		Grade				
Adverse Event	**Short Name**	**1**	**2**	**3**	**4**	**5**
Skin breakdown/ decubitus ulcer	Decubitus	—	Local wound care; medical intervention indicated	Operative debridement or other invasive intervention indicated (e.g., hyperbaric oxygen)	Life-threatening consequences; major invasive intervention indicated (e.g., tissue reconstruction, flap, or grafting)	Death
REMARK: Skin breakdown/decubitus ulcer is to be used for loss of skin integrity or decubitus ulcer from pressure or as the result of operative or medical intervention.						
Striae	Striae	Mild	Cosmetically significant	—	—	—
Telangiectasia	Telangiectasia	Few	Moderate number	Many and confluent	—	—
Ulceration	Ulceration	—	Superficial ulceration <2 cm size; local wound care; medical intervention indicated	Ulceration ≥2 cm size; operative debridement, primary closure or other invasive intervention indicated (e.g., hyperbaric oxygen)	Life-threatening consequences; major invasive intervention indicated (e.g., complete resection, tissue reconstruction, flap, or grafting)	Death

(continued)

Appendix 2 *(Continued)*

DERMATOLOGY/SKIN						
		Grade				
Adverse Event	**Short Name**	**1**	**2**	**3**	**4**	**5**
Urticaria (hives, welts, wheals)	Urticaria	Intervention not indicated	Intervention indicated for <24 hrs	Intervention indicated for ≥24 hrs	—	—
ALSO CONSIDER: Allergic reaction/hypersensitivity (including drug fever).						
Wound complication, non-infectious	Wound complication, non-infectious	Incisional separation of ≤25% of wound, no deeper than superficial fascia	Incisional separation >25% of wound with local care; asymptomatic hernia	Symptomatic hernia without evidence of strangulation; fascial disruption/dehiscence without evisceration; primary wound closure or revision by operative intervention indicated; hospitalization or hyperbaric oxygen indicated	Symptomatic hernia with evidence of strangulation; fascial disruption with evisceration; major reconstruction flap, grafting, resection, or amputation indicated	Death
REMARK: Wound complication, non-infectious is to be used for separation of incision, hernia, dehiscence, evisceration, or second surgery for wound revision.						
Dermatology/Skin – Other (Specify, _______)	Dermatology – Other (Specify)	Mild	Moderate	Severe	Life-threatening; disabling	Death

(continued)

ENDOCRINE						
		Grade				
Adverse Event	**Short Name**	**1**	**2**	**3**	**4**	**5**
Adrenal insufficiency	Adrenal insufficiency	Asymptomatic, intervention not indicated	Symptomatic, intervention indicated	Hospitalization	Life-threatening; disabling	Death
REMARK: Adrenal insufficiency includes any of the following signs and symptoms: abdominal pain, anorexia, constipation, diarrhea, hypotension, pigmentation of mucous membranes, pigmentation of skin, salt craving, syncope (fainting), vitiligo, vomiting, weakness, and weight loss. Adrenal insufficiency must be confirmed by laboratory studies (low cortisol frequently accompanied by low aldosterone).						
ALSO CONSIDER: Potassium, serum-high (hyperkalemia); Thyroid function, low (hypothyroidism).						
Cushingoid appearance (e.g., moon face, buffalo hump, centripetal obesity, cutaneous striae)	Cushingoid	—	Present	—	—	—
ALSO CONSIDER: Glucose, serum-high (hyperglycemia); Potassium, serum-low (hypokalemia).						
Feminization of male	Feminization of male	—	—	Present	—	—
NAVIGATION NOTE: Gynecomastia is graded in the SEXUAL/REPRODUCTIVE FUNCTION CATEGORY.						
Hot flashes/flushes[3]	Hot flashes	Mild	Moderate	Interfering with ADL	—	—
Masculinization of female	Masculinization of female	—	—	Present	—	—

(continued)

Appendix 2 *(Continued)*

ENDOCRINE						
		Grade				
Adverse Event	**Short Name**	**1**	**2**	**3**	**4**	**5**
Neuroendocrine: ACTH deficiency	ACTH	Asymptomatic	Symptomatic, not interfering with ADL; intervention indicated	Symptoms interfering with ADL; hospitalization indicated	Life-threatening consequences (e.g., severe hypotension)	Death
Neuroendocrine: ADH secretion abnormality (e.g., SIADH or low ADH)	ADH	Asymptomatic	Symptomatic, not interfering with ADL; intervention indicated	Symptoms interfering with ADL	Life-threatening consequences	Death
Neuroendocrine: gonadotropin secretion abnormality	Gonadotropin	Asymptomatic	Symptomatic, not interfering with ADL; intervention indicated	Symptoms interfering with ADL; osteopenia; fracture; infertility	—	—
Neuroendocrine: growth hormone secretion abnormality	Growth hormone	Asymptomatic	Symptomatic, not interfering with ADL; intervention indicated	—	—	—
Neuroendocrine: prolactin hormone secretion abnormality	Prolactin	Asymptomatic	Symptomatic, not interfering with ADL; intervention indicated	Symptoms interfering with ADL; amenorrhea; galactorrhea	—	Death

(continued)

ENDOCRINE						
		Grade				
Adverse Event	**Short Name**	**1**	**2**	**3**	**4**	**5**
Pancreatic endocrine: glucose intolerance	Diabetes	Asymptomatic, intervention not indicated	Symptomatic; dietary modification or oral agent indicated	Symptoms interfering with ADL; insulin indicated	Life-threatening consequences (e.g., ketoacidosis, hyperosmolar non-ketotic coma)	Death
Parathyroid function, low (hypoparathyroidism)	Hypoparathyroidism	Asymptomatic, intervention not indicated	Symptomatic; intervention indicated	—	—	—
Thyroid function, high (hyperthyroidism, thyrotoxicosis)	Hyperthyroidism	Asymptomatic, intervention not indicated	Symptomatic, not interfering with ADL; thyroid suppression therapy indicated	Symptoms interfering with ADL; hospitalization indicated	Life-threatening consequences (e.g., thyroid storm)	Death
Thyroid function, low (hypothyroidism)	Hypothyroidism	Asymptomatic, intervention not indicated	Symptomatic, not interfering with ADL; thyroid replacement indicated	Symptoms interfering with ADL; hospitalization indicated	Life-threatening myxedema coma	Death
Endocrine – Other (Specify, _______)	Endocrine – Other (Specify)	Mild	Moderate	Severe	Life-threatening; disabling	Death

(continued)

Appendix 2 *(Continued)*

GASTROINTESTINAL						
		Grade				
Adverse Event	**Short Name**	**1**	**2**	**3**	**4**	**5**
NAVIGATION NOTE: Abdominal pain or cramping is graded as Pain – *Select* in the PAIN CATEGORY.						
Anorexia	Anorexia	Loss of appetite without alteration in eating habits	Oral intake altered without significant weight loss or malnutrition; oral nutritional supplements indicated	Associated with significant weight loss or malnutrition (e.g., inadequate oral caloric and/or fluid intake); IV fluids, tube feedings or TPN indicated	Life-threatening consequences	Death
ALSO CONSIDER: Weight loss.						
Ascites (non-malignant)	Ascites	Asymptomatic	Symptomatic, medical intervention indicated	Symptomatic, invasive procedure indicated	Life-threatening consequences	Death
REMARK: Ascites (non-malignant) refers to documented non-malignant ascites or unknown etiology, but unlikely malignant, and includes chylous ascites.						
Colitis	Colitis	Asymptomatic, pathologic or radiographic findings only	Abdominal pain; mucus or blood in stool	Abdominal pain, fever, change in bowel habits with ileus; peritoneal signs	Life-threatening consequences (e.g., perforation, bleeding, ischemia, necrosis, toxic megacolon)	Death
ALSO CONSIDER: Hemorrhage, GI – *Select*.						

(continued)

GASTROINTESTINAL						
		Grade				
Adverse Event	**Short Name**	**1**	**2**	**3**	**4**	**5**
Constipation	Constipation	Occasional or intermittent symptoms; occasional use of stool softeners, laxatives, dietary modification, or enema	Persistent symptoms with regular use of laxatives or enemas indicated	Symptoms interfering with ADL; obstipation with manual evacuation indicated	Life-threatening consequences (e.g., obstruction, toxic megacolon)	Death
ALSO CONSIDER: Ileus, GI (functional obstruction of bowel, i.e., neuroconstipation); Obstruction, GI – *Select*.						
Dehydration	Dehydration	Increased oral fluids indicated; dry mucous membranes; diminished skin turgor	IV fluids indicated <24 hrs	IV fluids indicated ≥24 hrs	Life-threatening consequences (e.g., hemodynamic collapse)	Death
ALSO CONSIDER: Diarrhea; Hypotension; Vomiting.						
Dental: dentures or prosthesis	Dentures	Minimal discomfort, no restriction in activities	Discomfort preventing use in some activities (e.g., eating), but not others (e.g., speaking)	Unable to use dentures or prosthesis at any time	—	—

(continued)

Appendix 2 *(Continued)*

GASTROINTESTINAL						
		Grade				
Adverse Event	**Short Name**	**1**	**2**	**3**	**4**	**5**
Dental: periodontal disease	Periodontal	Gingival recession or gingivitis; limited bleeding on probing; mild local bone loss	Moderate gingival recession or gingivitis; multiple sites of bleeding on probing; moderate bone loss	Spontaneous bleeding; severe bone loss with or without tooth loss; osteonecrosis of maxilla or mandible	—	—
REMARK: Severe periodontal disease leading to osteonecrosis is graded as Osteonecrosis (avascular necrosis) in the MUSCULOSKELETAL CATEGORY.						
Dental: teeth	Teeth	Surface stains; dental caries; restorable, without extractions	Less than full mouth extractions; tooth fracture or crown amputation or repair indicated	Full mouth extractions indicated	—	—
Dental: teeth development	Teeth development	Hypoplasia of tooth or enamel not interfering with function	Functional impairment correctable with oral surgery	Maldevelopment with functional impairment not surgically correctable	—	—

(continued)

GASTROINTESTINAL						
		Grade				
Adverse Event	**Short Name**	**1**	**2**	**3**	**4**	**5**
Diarrhea	Diarrhea	Increase of <4 stools per day over baseline; mild increase in ostomy output compared to baseline	Increase of 4–6 stools per day over baseline; IV fluids indicated <24hrs; moderate increase in ostomy output compared to baseline; not interfering with ADL	Increase of ≥ 7 stools per day over baseline; incontinence; IV fluids ≥ 24 hrs; hospitalization; severe increase in ostomy output compared to baseline; interfering with ADL	Life-threatening consequences (e.g., hemodynamic collapse)	Death
REMARK: Diarrhea includes diarrhea of small bowel or colonic origin, and/or ostomy diarrhea.						
ALSO CONSIDER: Dehydration; Hypotension.						
Distension/bloating, abdominal	Distension	Asymptomatic	Symptomatic, but not interfering with GI function	Symptomatic, interfering with GI function	—	—
ALSO CONSIDER: Ascites (non-malignant); Ileus, GI (functional obstruction of bowel, i.e., neuroconstipation); Obstruction, GI – *Select*.						

(continued)

Appendix 2 *(Continued)*

GASTROINTESTINAL						
		Grade				
Adverse Event	**Short Name**	**1**	**2**	**3**	**4**	**5**
Dry mouth/salivary gland (xerostomia)	Dry mouth	Symptomatic (dry or thick saliva) without significant dietary alteration; unstimulated saliva flow >0.2 ml/min	Symptomatic and significant oral intake alteration (e.g., copious water, other lubricants, diet limited to purees and/or soft, moist foods); unstimulated saliva 0.1 to 0.2 ml/min	Symptoms leading to inability to adequately aliment orally; IV fluids, tube feedings, or TPN indicated; unstimulated saliva <0.1 ml/min	—	—
Remark: Dry mouth/salivary gland (xerostomia) includes descriptions of grade using both subjective and objective assessment parameters. Record this event consistently throughout a patient's participation on study. If salivary flow measurements are used for initial assessment, subsequent assessments must use salivary flow.						
Also Consider: Salivary gland changes/saliva.						
Dysphagia (difficulty swallowing)	Dysphagia	Symptomatic, able to eat regular diet	Symptomatic and altered eating/swallowing (e.g., altered dietary habits, oral supplements); IV fluids indicated <24 hrs	Symptomatic and severely altered eating/swallowing (e.g., inadequate oral caloric or fluid intake); IV fluids, tube feedings, or TPN indicated ≥24 hrs	Life-threatening consequences (e.g., obstruction, perforation)	Death

(continued)

GASTROINTESTINAL						
			Grade			
Adverse Event	**Short Name**	**1**	**2**	**3**	**4**	**5**
REMARK: Dysphagia (difficulty swallowing) is to be used for swallowing difficulty from oral, pharyngeal, esophageal, or neurologic origin. Dysphagia requiring dilation is graded as Stricture/stenosis (including anastomotic), GI – *Select*.						
ALSO CONSIDER: Dehydration; Esophagitis.						
Enteritis (inflammation of the small bowel)	Enteritis	Asymptomatic, pathologic or radiographic findings only	Abdominal pain; mucus or blood in stool	Abdominal pain, fever, change in bowel habits with ileus; peritoneal signs	Life-threatening consequences (e.g., perforation, bleeding, ischemia, necrosis)	Death
ALSO CONSIDER: Hemorrhage, GI – *Select*; Typhlitis (cecal inflammation).						
Esophagitis	Esophagitis	Asymptomatic pathologic, radiographic, or endoscopic findings only	Symptomatic; altered eating/swallowing (e.g., altered dietary habits, oral supplements); IV fluids indicated <24 hrs	Symptomatic and severely altered eating/swallowing (e.g., inadequate oral caloric or fluid intake); IV fluids, tube feedings, or TPN indicated ≥24 hrs	Life-threatening consequences	Death
REMARK: Esophagitis includes reflux esophagitis.						
ALSO CONSIDER: Dysphagia (difficulty swallowing).						

(continued)

Appendix 2 *(Continued)*

GASTROINTESTINAL						
		Grade				
Adverse Event	**Short Name**	**1**	**2**	**3**	**4**	**5**
Fistula, GI – *Select*: – Abdomen NOS – Anus – Biliary tree – Colon/cecum/appendix – Duodenum – Esophagus – Gallbladder – Ileum – Jejunum – Oral cavity – Pancreas – Pharynx – Rectum – Salivary gland – Small bowel NOS – Stomach	Fistula, GI – *Select*	Asymptomatic, radiographic findings only	Symptomatic; altered GI function (e.g., altered dietary habits, diarrhea, or GI fluid loss); IV fluids indicated <24 hrs	Symptomatic and severely altered GI function (e.g., altered dietary habits, diarrhea, or GI fluid loss); IV fluids, tube feedings, or TPN indicated ≥24 hrs	Life-threatening consequences	Death

REMARK: A fistula is defined as an abnormal communication between two body cavities, potential spaces, and/or the skin. The site indicated for a fistula should be the site from which the abnormal process is believed to have originated. For example, a tracheoesophageal fistula arising in the context of a resected or irradiated esophageal cancer is graded as Fistula, GI – esophagus.

(continued)

GASTROINTESTINAL						
		Grade				
Adverse Event	**Short Name**	**1**	**2**	**3**	**4**	**5**
Flatulence	Flatulence	Mild	Moderate	—	—	—
Gastritis (including bile reflux gastritis)	Gastritis	Asymptomatic radiographic or endoscopic findings only	Symptomatic; altered gastric function (e.g., inadequate oral caloric or fluid intake); IV fluids indicated <24 hrs	Symptomatic and severely altered gastric function (e.g., inadequate oral caloric or fluid intake); IV fluids, tube feedings, or TPN indicated ≥24 hrs	Life-threatening consequences; operative intervention requiring complete organ resection (e.g., gastrectomy)	Death
ALSO CONSIDER: Hemorrhage, GI – *Select*; Ulcer, GI – *Select*.						
NAVIGATION NOTE: Head and neck soft tissue necrosis is graded as Soft tissue necrosis – *Select* in the MUSCULOSKELETAL/SOFT TISSUE CATEGORY.						
Heartburn/dyspepsia	Heartburn	Mild	Moderate	Severe	—	—
Hemorrhoids	Hemorrhoids	Asymptomatic	Symptomatic; banding or medical intervention indicated	Interfering with ADL; interventional radiology, endoscopic, or operative intervention indicated	Life-threatening consequences	Death

(continued)

Appendix 2 *(Continued)*

GASTROINTESTINAL						
		Grade				
Adverse Event	**Short Name**	**1**	**2**	**3**	**4**	**5**
Ileus, GI (functional obstruction of bowel, i.e., neuroconstipation)	Ileus	Asymptomatic, radiographic findings only	Symptomatic; altered GI function (e.g., altered dietary habits); IV fluids indicated <24 hrs	Symptomatic and severely altered GI function; IV fluids, tube feeding, or TPN indicated ≥24 hrs	Life-threatening consequences	Death
REMARK: Ileus, GI is to be used for altered upper or lower GI function (e.g., delayed gastric or colonic emptying).						
ALSO CONSIDER: Constipation; Nausea; Obstruction, GI – *Select*; Vomiting.						
Incontinence, anal	Incontinence, anal	Occasional use of pads required	Daily use of pads required	Interfering with ADL; operative intervention indicated	Permanent bowel diversion indicated	Death
REMARK: Incontinence, anal is to be used for loss of sphincter control as sequelae of operative or therapeutic intervention.						
Leak (including anastomotic), GI – *Select*: – Biliary tree – Esophagus – Large bowel – Leak NOS – Pancreas – Pharynx	Leak, GI – *Select*	Asymptomatic radiographic findings only	Symptomatic; medical intervention indicated	Symptomatic and interfering with GI function; invasive or endoscopic intervention indicated	Life-threatening consequences	Death

(continued)

GASTROINTESTINAL						
		Grade				
Adverse Event	**Short Name**	**1**	**2**	**3**	**4**	**5**
– Rectum – Small bowel – Stoma – Stomach						
REMARK: Leak (including anastomotic), GI – *Select* is to be used for clinical signs/symptoms or radiographic confirmation of anastomotic or conduit leak (e.g., biliary, esophageal, intestinal, pancreatic, pharyngeal, rectal), but without development of fistula.						
Malabsorption	Malabsorption	—	Altered diet; oral therapies indicated (e.g., enzymes, medications, dietary supplements)	Inability to aliment adequately via GI tract (i.e., TPN indicated)	Life-threatening consequences	Death
Mucositis/stomatitis (clinical exam) – *Select*: – Anus – Esophagus – Large bowel – Larynx – Oral cavity – Pharynx – Rectum – Small bowel	Mucositis (clinical exam) – *Select*	Erythema of the mucosa	Patchy ulcerations or pseudomembranes	Confluent ulcerations or pseudomembranes; bleeding with minor trauma	Tissue necrosis; significant spontaneous bleeding; life-threatening consequences	Death

(continued)

Appendix 2 *(Continued)*

GASTROINTESTINAL						
		Grade				
Adverse Event	**Short Name**	**1**	**2**	**3**	**4**	**5**
– Stomach – Trachea						
REMARK: Mucositis/stomatitis (functional/symptomatic) may be used for mucositis of the upper aerodigestive tract caused by radiation, agents, or GVHD.						
Mucositis/stomatitis (functional/symptomatic) – *Select*: – Anus – Esophagus – Large bowel – Larynx – Oral cavity – Pharynx – Rectum – Small bowel – Stomach – Trachea	Mucositis (functional/symptomatic) – *Select*	*Upper aerodigestive tract sites*: Minimal symptoms, normal diet; minimal respiratory symptoms but not interfering with function *Lower GI sites*: Minimal discomfort, intervention not indicated	*Upper aerodigestive tract sites*: Symptomatic but can eat and swallow modified diet; respiratory symptoms interfering with function but not interfering with ADL *Lower GI sites*: Symptomatic, medical intervention indicated but not interfering with ADL	*Upper aerodigestive tract sites*: Symptomatic and unable to adequately aliment or hydrate orally; respiratory symptoms interfering with ADL *Lower GI sites*: Stool incontinence or other symptoms interfering with ADL	Symptoms associated with life-threatening consequences	Death

(continued)

GASTROINTESTINAL						
		Grade				
Adverse Event	**Short Name**	**1**	**2**	**3**	**4**	**5**
Nausea	Nausea	Loss of appetite without alteration in eating habits	Oral intake decreased without significant weight loss, dehydration or malnutrition; IV fluids indicated <24 hrs	Inadequate oral caloric or fluid intake; IV fluids, tube feedings, or TPN indicated ≥24 hrs	Life-threatening consequences	Death
ALSO CONSIDER: Anorexia; Vomiting.						
Necrosis, GI –*Select*: – Anus – Colon/cecum/appendix – Duodenum – Esophagus – Gallbladder – Hepatic – Ileum – Jejunum – Oral – Pancreas – Peritoneal cavity – Pharynx – Rectum	Necrosis, GI – *Select*	—	—	Inability to aliment adequately by GI tract (e.g., requiring enteral or parenteral nutrition); interventional radiology, endoscopic, or operative intervention indicated	Life-threatening consequences; operative intervention requiring complete organ resection (e.g., total colectomy)	Death

(continued)

Appendix 2 *(Continued)*

GASTROINTESTINAL						
		Grade				
Adverse Event	**Short Name**	**1**	**2**	**3**	**4**	**5**
– Small bowel NOS – Stoma – Stomach						
ALSO CONSIDER: Visceral arterial ischemia (non-myocardial).						
Obstruction, GI – *Select*: – Cecum – Colon – Duodenum – Esophagus – Gallbladder – Ileum – Jejunum – Rectum – Small bowel NOS – Stoma – Stomach	Obstruction, GI – *Select*	Asymptomatic radiographic findings only	Symptomatic; altered GI function (e.g., altered dietary habits, vomiting, diarrhea, or GI fluid loss); IV fluids indicated <24 hrs	Symptomatic and severely altered GI function (e.g., altered dietary habits, vomiting, diarrhea, or GI fluid loss); IV fluids, tube feedings, or TPN indicated ≥24 hrs; operative intervention indicated	Life-threatening consequences; operative intervention requiring complete organ resection (e.g., total colectomy)	Death
NAVIGATION NOTE: Operative injury is graded as Intra-operative injury – *Select Organ or Structure* in the SURGERY/INTRA-OPERATIVE INJURY CATEGORY.						
NAVIGATION NOTE: Pelvic pain is graded as Pain – *Select* in the PAIN CATEGORY.						

(continued)

GASTROINTESTINAL						
		Grade				
Adverse Event	**Short Name**	**1**	**2**	**3**	**4**	**5**
Perforation, GI – *Select*: – Appendix – Biliary tree – Cecum – Colon – Duodenum – Esophagus – Gallbladder – Ileum – Jejunum – Rectum – Small bowel NOS – Stomach	Perforation, GI – *Select*	Asymptomatic radiographic findings only	Medical intervention indicated; IV fluids indicated <24 hrs	IV fluids, tube feedings, or TPN indicated ≥24 hrs; operative intervention indicated	Life-threatening consequences	Death
Proctitis	Proctitis	Rectal discomfort, intervention not indicated	Symptoms not interfering with ADL; medical intervention indicated	Stool incontinence or other symptoms interfering with ADL; operative intervention indicated	Life-threatening consequences (e.g., perforation)	Death

(continued)

Appendix 2 *(Continued)*

GASTROINTESTINAL						
		Grade				
Adverse Event	**Short Name**	**1**	**2**	**3**	**4**	**5**
Prolapse of stoma, GI	Prolapse of stoma, GI	Asymptomatic	Extraordinary local care or maintenance; minor revision indicated	Dysfunctional stoma; major revision indicated	Life-threatening consequences	Death
REMARK: Other stoma complications may be graded as Fistula, GI – *Select*; Leak (including anastomotic), GI – *Select*; Obstruction, GI – *Select*; Perforation, GI – *Select*; Stricture/stenosis (including anastomotic), GI – *Select*.						
NAVIGATION NOTE: Rectal or perirectal pain (proctalgia) is graded as Pain – *Select* in the PAIN CATEGORY.						
Salivary gland changes/saliva	Salivary gland changes	Slightly thickened saliva; slightly altered taste (e.g., metallic)	Thick, ropy, sticky saliva; markedly altered taste; alteration in diet indicated; secretion-induced symptoms not interfering with ADL	Acute salivary gland necrosis; severe secretion-induced symptoms interfering with ADL	Disabling	—
ALSO CONSIDER: Dry mouth/salivary gland (xerostomia); Mucositis/stomatitis (clinical exam) – *Select*; Mucositis/stomatitis (functional/symptomatic) – *Select*; Taste alteration (dysgeusia).						
NAVIGATION NOTE: Splenic function is graded in the BLOOD/BONE MARROW CATEGORY.						

(continued)

GASTROINTESTINAL						
		Grade				
Adverse Event	**Short Name**	**1**	**2**	**3**	**4**	**5**
Stricture/stenosis (including anastomotic), GI – *Select*: – Anus – Biliary tree – Cecum – Colon – Duodenum – Esophagus – Ileum – Jejunum – Pancreas/pancreatic duct – Pharynx – Rectum – Small bowel NOS – Stoma – Stomach	Stricture, GI – *Select*	Asymptomatic radiographic findings only	Symptomatic; altered GI function (e.g., altered dietary habits, vomiting, bleeding, diarrhea); IV fluids indicated <24 hrs	Symptomatic and severely altered GI function (e.g., altered dietary habits, diarrhea, or GI fluid loss); IV fluids, tube feedings, or TPN indicated ≥24 hrs; operative intervention indicated	Life-threatening consequences; operative intervention requiring complete organ resection (e.g., total colectomy)	Death
Taste alteration (dysgeusia)	Taste alteration	Altered taste but no change in diet	Altered taste with change in diet (e.g., oral supplements); noxious or unpleasant taste; loss of taste	—	—	—

(continued)

Appendix 2 *(Continued)*

GASTROINTESTINAL						
		Grade				
Adverse Event	**Short Name**	**1**	**2**	**3**	**4**	**5**
Typhlitis (cecal inflammation)	Typhlitis	Asymptomatic, pathologic or radiographic findings only	Abdominal pain; mucus or blood in stool	Abdominal pain, fever, change in bowel habits with ileus; peritoneal signs	Life-threatening consequences (e.g., perforation, bleeding, ischemia, necrosis); operative intervention indicated	Death
ALSO CONSIDER: Colitis; Hemorrhage, GI – *Select*; Ileus, GI (functional obstruction of bowel, i.e., neuroconstipation).						
Ulcer, GI – *Select*: – Anus – Cecum – Colon – Duodenum – Esophagus – Ileum – Jejunum – Rectum – Small bowel NOS – Stoma – Stomach	Ulcer, GI – *Select*	Asymptomatic, radiographic or endoscopic findings only	Symptomatic; altered GI function (e.g., altered dietary habits, oral supplements); IV fluids indicated <24 hrs	Symptomatic and severely altered GI function (e.g., inadequate oral caloric or fluid intake); IV fluids, tube feedings, or TPN indicated ≥24 hrs	Life-threatening consequences	Death
ALSO CONSIDER: Hemorrhage, GI – *Select*.						

(continued)

GASTROINTESTINAL						
		Grade				
Adverse Event	**Short Name**	**1**	**2**	**3**	**4**	**5**
Vomiting	Vomiting	1 episode in 24 hrs	2–5 episodes in 24 hrs; IV fluids indicated <24 hrs	≥6 episodes in 24 hrs; IV fluids, or TPN indicated ≥24 hrs	Life-threatening consequences	Death
ALSO CONSIDER: Dehydration.						
Gastrointestinal – Other (Specify, _______)	GI – Other (Specify)	Mild	Moderate	Severe	Life-threatening; disabling	Death

GROWTH AND DEVELOPMENT						
		Grade				
Adverse Event	**Short Name**	**1**	**2**	**3**	**4**	**5**
Bone age (alteration in bone age)	Bone age	—	±2 SD (standard deviation) from normal	—	—	—
Bone growth: femoral head; slipped capital femoral epiphysis	Femoral head growth	Mild valgus/varus deformity	Moderate valgus/ varus deformity, symptomatic, interfering with function but not interfering with ADL	Mild slipped capital femoral epiphysis; operative intervention (e.g., fixation) indicated; interfering with ADL	Disabling; severe slipped capital femoral epiphysis >60%; avascular necrosis	—

(continued)

Appendix 2 *(Continued)*

GROWTH AND DEVELOPMENT						
		Grade				
Adverse Event	**Short Name**	**1**	**2**	**3**	**4**	**5**
Bone growth: limb length discrepancy	Limb length	Mild length discrepancy <2 cm	Moderate length discrepancy 2–5 cm; shoe lift indicated	Severe length discrepancy >5 cm; operative intervention indicated; interfering with ADL	Disabling; epiphysiodesis	—
Bone growth: spine kyphosis/lordosis	Kyphosis/lordosis	Mild radiographic changes	Moderate accentuation; interfering with function but not interfering with ADL	Severe accentuation; operative intervention indicated; interfering with ADL	Disabling (e.g., cannot lift head)	—
Growth velocity (reduction in growth velocity)	Reduction in growth velocity	10–29% reduction in growth from the baseline growth curve	30–49% reduction in growth from the baseline growth curve	≥50% reduction in growth from the baseline growth curve	—	—
Puberty (delayed)	Delayed puberty	—	No breast development by age 13 yrs for females; no Tanner Stage 2 development by age 14.5 yrs for males	No sexual development by age 14 yrs for girls, age 16 yrs for boys; hormone replacement indicated	—	—

REMARK: Do not use testicular size for Tanner Stage in male cancer survivors.

(continued)

GROWTH AND DEVELOPMENT

		Grade				
Adverse Event	**Short Name**	**1**	**2**	**3**	**4**	**5**
Puberty (precocious)	Precocious puberty	—	Physical signs of puberty <7 years for females, <9 years for males	—	—	—
Short stature	Short stature	Beyond two standard deviations of age and gender mean height	Altered ADL	—	—	—

REMARK: Short stature is secondary to growth hormone deficiency.

ALSO CONSIDER: Neuroendocrine: growth hormone secretion abnormality.

Growth and Development – Other (Specify, ________)	Growth and Development – Other (Specify)	Mild	Moderate	Severe	Life-threatening; disabling	Death

HEMORRHAGE/BLEEDING

		Grade				
Adverse Event	**Short Name**	**1**	**2**	**3**	**4**	**5**
Hematoma	Hematoma	Minimal symptoms, invasive intervention not indicated	Minimally invasive evacuation or aspiration indicated	Transfusion, interventional radiology, or operative intervention indicated	Life-threatening consequences; major urgent intervention indicated	Death

REMARK: Hematoma refers to extravasation at wound or operative site or secondary to other intervention. Transfusion implies pRBC.

ALSO CONSIDER: Fibrinogen; INR (International Normalized Ratio of prothrombin time); Platelets; PTT (Partial Thromboplastin Time).

(continued)

Appendix 2 *(Continued)*

HEMORRHAGE/BLEEDING						
		Grade				
Adverse Event	**Short Name**	**1**	**2**	**3**	**4**	**5**
Hemorrhage/bleeding associated with surgery, intra-operative or postoperative	Hemorrhage with surgery	—	—	Requiring transfusion of 2 units non-autologous (10 cc/kg for pediatrics) pRBCs beyond protocol specification; post-operative interventional radiology, endoscopic, or operative intervention indicated	Life-threatening consequences	Death
Remark: Postoperative period is defined as ≤72 hours after surgery. Verify protocol-specific acceptable guidelines regarding pRBC transfusion.						
Also Consider: Fibrinogen; INR (International Normalized Ratio of prothrombin time); Platelets; PTT (Partial Thromboplastin Time).						
Hemorrhage, CNS	CNS hemorrhage	Asymptomatic, radiographic findings only	Medical intervention indicated	Ventriculostomy, ICP monitoring, intraventricular thrombolysis, or operative intervention indicated	Life-threatening consequences; neurologic deficit or disability	Death
Also Consider: Fibrinogen; INR (International Normalized Ratio of prothrombin time); Platelets; PTT (Partial Thromboplastin Time).						

(continued)

HEMORRHAGE/BLEEDING						
		Grade				
Adverse Event	**Short Name**	**1**	**2**	**3**	**4**	**5**
Hemorrhage, GI – *Select*: – Abdomen NOS – Anus – Biliary tree – Cecum/appendix – Colon – Duodenum – Esophagus – Ileum – Jejunum – Liver – Lower GI NOS – Oral cavity – Pancreas – Peritoneal cavity – Rectum – Stoma – Stomach – Upper GI NOS – Varices (esophageal) – Varices (rectal)	Hemorrhage, GI – *Select*	Mild, intervention (other than iron supplements) not indicated	Symptomatic and medical intervention or minor cauterization indicated	Transfusion, interventional radiology, endoscopic, or operative intervention indicated; radiation therapy (i.e., hemostasis of bleeding site)	Life-threatening consequences; major urgent intervention indicated	Death

REMARK: Transfusion implies pRBC.

ALSO CONSIDER: Fibrinogen; INR (International Normalized Ratio of prothrombin time); Platelets; PTT (Partial Thromboplastin Time).

(continued)

Appendix 2 *(Continued)*

HEMORRHAGE/BLEEDING						
		Grade				
Adverse Event	**Short Name**	**1**	**2**	**3**	**4**	**5**
Hemorrhage, GU – *Select*: – Bladder – Fallopian tube – Kidney – Ovary – Prostate – Retroperitoneum – Spermatic cord – Stoma – Testes – Ureter – Urethra – Urinary NOS – Uterus – Vagina – Vas deferens	Hemorrhage, GU – *Select*	Minimal or microscopic bleeding; intervention not indicated	Gross bleeding, medical intervention, or urinary tract irrigation indicated	Transfusion, interventional radiology, endoscopic, or operative intervention indicated; radiation therapy (i.e., hemostasis of bleeding site)	Life-threatening consequences; major urgent intervention indicated	Death

REMARK: Transfusion implies pRBC.

ALSO CONSIDER: Fibrinogen; INR (International Normalized Ratio of prothrombin time); Platelets; PTT (Partial Thromboplastin Time).

(continued)

HEMORRHAGE/BLEEDING						
		Grade				
Adverse Event	**Short Name**	**1**	**2**	**3**	**4**	**5**
Hemorrhage, pulmonary/upper respiratory – *Select*: – Bronchopulmonary NOS – Bronchus – Larynx – Lung – Mediastinum – Nose – Pharynx – Respiratory tract NOS – Stoma – Trachea	Hemorrhage pulmonary – *Select*	Mild, intervention not indicated	Symptomatic and medical intervention indicated	Transfusion, interventional radiology, endoscopic, or operative intervention indicated; radiation therapy (i.e., hemostasis of bleeding site)	Life-threatening consequences; major urgent intervention indicated	Death
REMARK: Transfusion implies pRBC.						
ALSO CONSIDER: Fibrinogen; INR (International Normalized Ratio of prothrombin time); Platelets; PTT (Partial Thromboplastin Time).						
Petechiae/purpura (hemorrhage/bleeding into skin or mucosa)	Petechiae	Few petechiae	Moderate petechiae; purpura	Generalized petechiae or purpura	—	—
ALSO CONSIDER: Fibrinogen; INR (International Normalized Ratio of prothrombin time); Platelets; PTT (Partial Thromboplastin Time).						
NAVIGATION NOTE: Vitreous hemorrhage is graded in the OCULAR/VISUAL CATEGORY.						
Hemorrhage/Bleeding – Other (Specify, ______)	Hemorrhage – Other (Specify)	Mild without transfusion	—	Transfusion indicated	Catastrophic bleeding, requiring major nonelective intervention	Death

(continued)

Appendix 2 *(Continued)*

HEPATOBILIARY/PANCREAS						
		Grade				
Adverse Event	**Short Name**	**1**	**2**	**3**	**4**	**5**
NAVIGATION NOTE: Biliary tree damage is graded as Fistula, GI – *Select*; Leak (including anastomotic), GI – *Select*; Necrosis, GI – *Select*; Obstruction, GI – *Select*; Perforation, GI – *Select*; Stricture/stenosis (including anastomotic), GI – *Select* in the GASTROINTESTINAL CATEGORY.						
Cholecystitis	Cholecystitis	Asymptomatic, radiographic findings only	Symptomatic, medical intervention indicated	Interventional radiology, endoscopic, or operative intervention indicated	Life-threatening consequences (e.g., sepsis or perforation)	Death
ALSO CONSIDER: Infection (documented clinically or microbiologically) with Grade 3 or 4 neutrophils – *Select*; Infection with normal ANC or Grade 1 or 2 neutrophils – *Select*; Infection with unknown ANC – *Select*.						
Liver dysfunction/failure (clinical)	Liver dysfunction	—	Jaundice	Asterixis	Encephalopathy or coma	Death
REMARK: Jaundice is not an AE, but occurs when the liver is not working properly or when a bile duct is blocked. It is graded as a result of liver dysfunction/failure or elevated bilirubin.						
ALSO CONSIDER: Bilirubin (hyperbilirubinemia).						
Pancreas, exocrine enzyme deficiency	Pancreas, exocrine enzyme deficiency	—	Increase in stool frequency, bulk, or odor; steatorrhea	Sequelae of absorption deficiency (e.g., weight loss)	Life-threatening consequences	Death
ALSO CONSIDER: Diarrhea.						

(continued)

HEPATOBILIARY/PANCREAS						
		Grade				
Adverse Event	**Short Name**	**1**	**2**	**3**	**4**	**5**
Pancreatitis	Pancreatitis	Asymptomatic, enzyme elevation and/or radiographic findings	Symptomatic, medical intervention indicated	Interventional radiology or operative intervention indicated	Life-threatening consequences (e.g., circulatory failure, hemorrhage, sepsis)	Death
ALSO CONSIDER: Amylase.						
NAVIGATION NOTE: Stricture (biliary tree, hepatic or pancreatic) is graded as Stricture/stenosis (including anastomotic), GI – *Select* in the GASTROINTESTINAL CATEGORY.						
Hepatobiliary/Pancreas – Other (Specify, _______)	Hepatobiliary – Other (Specify)	Mild	Moderate	Severe	Life-threatening; disabling	Death

INFECTION						
		Grade				
Adverse Event	**Short Name**	**1**	**2**	**3**	**4**	**5**
Colitis, infectious (e.g., Clostridium difficile)	Colitis, infectious	Asymptomatic, pathologic or radiographic findings only	Abdominal pain with mucus and/or blood in stool	IV antibiotics or TPN indicated	Life-threatening consequences (e.g., perforation, bleeding, ischemia, necrosis or toxic megacolon); operative resection or diversion indicated	Death
ALSO CONSIDER: Hemorrhage, GI – *Select*; Typhlitis (cecal inflammation).						

(continued)

Appendix 2 *(Continued)*

INFECTION						
		Grade				
Adverse Event	**Short Name**	**1**	**2**	**3**	**4**	**5**
Febrile neutropenia (fever of unknown origin without clinically or microbiologically documented infection) (ANC <1.0 × 10^9/L, fever ≥38.5°C)	Febrile neutropenia	—	—	Present	Life-threatening consequences (e.g., septic shock, hypotension, acidosis, necrosis)	Death
Also Consider: Neutrophils/granulocytes (ANC/AGC).						
Infection (documented clinically or microbiologically) with Grade 3 or 4 neutrophils (ANC <1.0 × 10^9/L) – *Select* AEs appear at the end of the CATEGORY.	Infection (documented clinically) – *Select*	—	Localized, local intervention indicated	IV antibiotic, antifungal, or antiviral intervention indicated; interventional radiology or operative intervention indicated	Life-threatening consequences (e.g., septic shock, hypotension, acidosis, necrosis)	Death
Remark: Fever with Grade 3 or 4 neutrophils in the absence of documented infection is graded as Febrile neutropenia (fever of unknown origin without clinically or microbiologically documented infection).						
Also Consider: Neutrophils/granulocytes (ANC/AGC).						

(continued)

INFECTION						
		Grade				
Adverse Event	**Short Name**	**1**	**2**	**3**	**4**	**5**
Infection with normal ANC or Grade 1 or 2 neutrophils – *Select* AEs appear at the end of the CATEGORY.	Infection with normal ANC – *Select*	—	Localized, local intervention indicated	IV antibiotic, antifungal, or antiviral intervention indicated; interventional radiology or operative intervention indicated	Life-threatening consequences (e.g., septic shock, hypotension, acidosis, necrosis)	Death
Infection with unknown ANC – *Select* AEs appear at the end of the CATEGORY.	Infection with unknown ANC – *Select*	—	Localized, local intervention indicated	IV antibiotic, antifungal, or antiviral intervention indicated; interventional radiology or operative intervention indicated	Life-threatening consequences (e.g., septic shock, hypotension, acidosis, necrosis)	Death

REMARK: Infection with unknown ANC – *Select* is to be used in the rare case when ANC is unknown.

(continued)

Appendix 2 *(Continued)*

INFECTION						
		Grade				
Adverse Event	**Short Name**	**1**	**2**	**3**	**4**	**5**
Opportunistic infection associated with ≥Grade 2 Lymphopenia	Opportunistic infection	—	Localized, local intervention indicated	IV antibiotic, antifungal, or antiviral intervention indicated; interventional radiology or operative intervention indicated	Life-threatening consequences (e.g., septic shock, hypotension, acidosis, necrosis)	Death
ALSO CONSIDER: Lymphopenia.						
Viral hepatitis	Viral hepatitis	Present; transaminases and liver function normal	Transaminases abnormal, liver function normal	Symptomatic liver dysfunction; fibrosis by biopsy; compensated cirrhosis	Decompensated liver function (e.g., ascites, coagulopathy, encephalopathy, coma)	Death
REMARK: Non-viral hepatitis is graded as Infection – *Select*.						
ALSO CONSIDER: Albumin, serum-low (hypoalbuminemia); ALT, SGPT (serum glutamic pyruvic transaminase); AST, SGOT (serum glutamic oxaloacetic transaminase); Bilirubin (hyperbilirubinemia); Encephalopathy.						
Infection – Other (Specify, _______)	Infection – Other (Specify)	Mild	Moderate	Severe	Life-threatening; disabling	Death

(continued)

INFECTION – *SELECT*		
AUDITORY/EAR	GENERAL	PULMONARY/UPPER RESPIRATORY
– External ear (otitis externa)	– Blood	– Bronchus
– Middle ear (otitis media)	– Catheter-related	– Larynx
CARDIOVASCULAR	– Foreign body (e.g., graft, implant, prosthesis, stent)	– Lung (pneumonia)
– Artery	– Wound	– Mediastinum NOS
– Heart (endocarditis)	HEPATOBILIARY/PANCREAS	– Mucosa
– Spleen	– Biliary tree	– Neck NOS
– Vein	– Gallbladder (cholecystitis)	– Nose
DERMATOLOGY/SKIN	– Liver	– Paranasal
– Lip/perioral	– Pancreas	– Pharynx
– Peristomal	LYMPHATIC	– Pleura (empyema)
– Skin (cellulitis)	– Lymphatic	– Sinus
– Ungual (nails)	MUSCULOSKELETAL	– Trachea
GASTROINTESTINAL	– Bone (osteomyelitis)	– Upper aerodigestive NOS
– Abdomen NOS	– Joint	– Upper airway NOS
– Anal/perianal	– Muscle (infection myositis)	RENAL/GENITOURINARY
– Appendix	– Soft tissue NOS	– Bladder (urinary)
– Cecum	NEUROLOGY	– Kidney
– Colon	– Brain (encephalitis, infectious)	– Prostate
– Dental-tooth	– Brain + Spinal cord (encephalomyelitis)	– Ureter
– Duodenum	– Meninges (meningitis)	– Urethra
– Esophagus	– Nerve-cranial	– Urinary tract NOS
– Ileum	– Nerve-peripheral	
	– Spinal cord (myelitis)	

(continued)

Appendix 2 *(Continued)*

INFECTION–*SELECT*		
– Jejunum – Oral cavity-gums (gingivitis) – Peritoneal cavity – Rectum – Salivary gland – Small bowel NOS – Stomach	OCULAR – Conjunctiva – Cornea – Eye NOS – Lens	SEXUAL/REPRODUCTIVE FUNCTION – Cervix – Fallopian tube – Pelvis NOS – Penis – Scrotum – Uterus – Vagina – Vulva

LYMPHATICS

		Grade				
Adverse Event	**Short Name**	**1**	**2**	**3**	**4**	**5**
Chyle or lymph leakage	Chyle or lymph leakage	Asymptomatic, clinical or radiographic findings	Symptomatic, medical intervention indicated	Interventional radiology or operative intervention indicated	Life-threatening complications	Death

ALSO CONSIDER: Chylothorax.

(continued)

LYMPHATICS						
		Grade				
Adverse Event	**Short Name**	**1**	**2**	**3**	**4**	**5**
Dermal change lymphedema, phlebolymphedema	Dermal change	Trace thickening or faint discoloration	Marked discoloration; leathery skin texture; papillary formation	—	—	—
REMARK: Dermal change lymphedema, phlebolymphedema refers to changes due to venous stasis.						
ALSO CONSIDER: Ulceration.						
Edema: head and neck	Edema: head and neck	Localized to dependent areas, no disability or functional impairment	Localized facial or neck edema with functional impairment	Generalized facial or neck edema with functional impairment (e.g., difficulty in turning neck or opening mouth compared to baseline)	Severe with ulceration or cerebral edema; tracheotomy or feeding tube indicated	Death

(continued)

Appendix 2 *(Continued)*

LYMPHATICS						
		Grade				
Adverse Event	**Short Name**	**1**	**2**	**3**	**4**	**5**
Edema: limb	Edema: limb	5–10% inter-limb discrepancy in volume or circumference at point of greatest visible difference; swelling or obscuration of anatomic architecture on close inspection; pitting edema	>10–30% inter-limb discrepancy in volume or circumference at point of greatest visible difference; readily apparent obscuration of anatomic architecture; obliteration of skin folds; readily apparent deviation from normal anatomic contour	>30% inter-limb discrepancy in volume; lymphorrhea; gross deviation from normal anatomic contour; interfering with ADL	Progression to malignancy (i.e., lymphangiosarcoma); amputation indicated; disabling	Death
Edema: trunk/genital	Edema: trunk/genital	Swelling or obscuration of anatomic architecture on close inspection; pitting edema	Readily apparent obscuration of anatomic architecture; obliteration of skin folds; readily apparent deviation from normal anatomic contour	Lymphorrhea; interfering with ADL; gross deviation from normal anatomic contour	Progression to malignancy (i.e., lymphangiosarcoma); disabling	Death

(continued)

LYMPHATICS						
		Grade				
Adverse Event	Short Name	1	2	3	4	5
Edema: viscera	Edema: viscera	Asymptomatic; clinical or radiographic findings only	Symptomatic; medical intervention indicated	Symptomatic and unable to aliment adequately orally; interventional radiology or operative intervention indicated	Life-threatening consequences	Death
Lymphedema-related fibrosis	Lymphedema-related fibrosis	Minimal to moderate redundant soft tissue, unresponsive to elevation or compression, with moderately firm texture or spongy feel	Marked increase in density and firmness, with or without tethering	Very marked density and firmness with tethering affecting ≥40% of the edematous area	—	—
Lymphocele	Lymphocele	Asymptomatic, clinical or radiographic findings only	Symptomatic; medical intervention indicated	Symptomatic and interventional radiology or operative intervention indicated	—	—

(continued)

Appendix 2 *(Continued)*

LYMPHATICS						
		Grade				
Adverse Event	**Short Name**	**1**	**2**	**3**	**4**	**5**
Phlebolymphatic cording	Phlebolymphatic cording	Asymptomatic, clinical findings only	Symptomatic; medical intervention indicated	Symptomatic and leading to contracture or reduced range of motion	—	—
Lymphatics – Other (Specify, ________)	Lymphatics – Other (Specify)	Mild	Moderate	Severe	Life-threatening; disabling	Death

METABOLIC/LABORATORY						
		Grade				
Adverse Event	**Short Name**	**1**	**2**	**3**	**4**	**5**
Acidosis (metabolic or respiratory)	Acidosis	pH <normal, but ≥7.3	—	pH <7.3	pH <7.3 with life-threatening consequences	Death
Albumin, serum-low (hypoalbuminemia)	Hypoalbuminemia	<LLN–3 g/dL <LLN–30 g/L	<3–2 g/dL <30–20 g/L	<2 g/dL <20 g/L	—	Death
Alkaline phosphatase	Alkaline phosphatase	>ULN–2.5 × ULN	>2.5–5.0 × ULN	>5.0–20.0 × ULN	>20.0 × ULN	—

(continued)

METABOLIC/LABORATORY						
		Grade				
Adverse Event	**Short Name**	**1**	**2**	**3**	**4**	**5**
Alkalosis (metabolic or respiratory)	Alkalosis	pH >normal, but ≥7.5	—	pH >7.5	pH >7.5 with life-threatening consequences	Death
ALT, SGPT (serum glutamic pyruvic transaminase)	ALT	>ULN–2.5 × ULN	>2.5–5.0 × ULN	>5.0–20.0 × ULN	>20.0 × ULN	—
Amylase	Amylase	>ULN–1.5 × ULN	>1.5–2.0 × ULN	>2.0–5.0 × ULN	>5.0 × ULN	—
AST, SGOT (serum glutamic oxaloacetic transaminase)	AST	>ULN–2.5 × ULN	>2.5–5.0 × ULN	>5.0–20.0 × ULN	>20.0 × ULN	—
Bicarbonate, serum-low	Bicarbonate, serum-low	<LLN–16 mmol/L	<16–11 mmol/L	<11–8 mmol/L	<8 mmol/L	Death
Bilirubin (hyperbilirubinemia)	Bilirubin	>ULN–1.5 × ULN	>1.5–3.0 × ULN	>3.0–10.0 × ULN	>10.0 × ULN	—

REMARK: Jaundice is not an AE, but may be a manifestation of liver dysfunction/failure or elevated bilirubin. If jaundice is associated with elevated bilirubin, grade bilirubin.

(continued)

Appendix 2 *(Continued)*

METABOLIC/LABORATORY						
		Grade				
Adverse Event	**Short Name**	**1**	**2**	**3**	**4**	**5**
Calcium, serum-low (hypocalcemia)	Hypocalcemia	<LLN–8.0 mg/dL <LLN–2.0 mmol/L Ionized calcium: <LLN–1.0 mmol/L	<8.0–7.0 mg/dL <2.0–1.75 mmol/L Ionized calcium: <1.0–0.9 mmol/L	<7.0–6.0 mg/dL <1.75–1.5 mmol/L Ionized calcium: <0.9–0.8 mmol/L	<6.0 mg/dL <1.5 mmol/L Ionized calcium: <0.8 mmol/L	Death

REMARK: Calcium can be falsely low if hypoalbuminemia is present. Serum albumin is ≤4.0 g/dL, hypocalcemia is reported after the following corrective calculation has been performed: Corrected Calcium (mg/dL) = Total Calcium (mg/dL) – 0.8 [Albumin (g/dL) – 4][4]. Alternatively, direct measurement of ionized calcium is the definitive method to diagnose metabolically relevant alterations in serum calcium.

Adverse Event	**Short Name**	**1**	**2**	**3**	**4**	**5**
Calcium, serum-high (hypercalcemia)	Hypercalcemia	>ULN–11.5 mg/dL >ULN–2.9 mmol/L Ionized calcium: >ULN–1.5 mmol/L	>11.5–12.5 mg/dL >2.9–3.1 mmol/L Ionized calcium: >1.5–1.6 mmol/L	>12.5–13.5 mg/dL >3.1–3.4 mmol/L Ionized calcium: >1.6–1.8 mmol/L	>13.5 mg/dL >3.4 mmol/L Ionized calcium: >1.8 mmol/L	Death
Cholesterol, serum-high (hypercholesteremia)	Cholesterol	>ULN–300 mg/dL >ULN–7.75 mmol/L	>300–400 mg/dL >7.75–10.34 mmol/L	>400–500 mg/dL >10.34–12.92 mmol/L	>500 mg/dL >12.92 mmol/L	Death

(continued)

METABOLIC/LABORATORY						
		Grade				
Adverse Event	**Short Name**	**1**	**2**	**3**	**4**	**5**
CPK (creatine phosphokinase)	CPK	>ULN–2.5 × ULN	>2.5 × ULN – 5 × ULN	>5 × ULN–10 × ULN	>10 × ULN	Death
Creatinine	Creatinine	>ULN–1.5 × ULN	>1.5–3.0 × ULN	>3.0–6.0 × ULN	>6.0 × ULN	Death
REMARK: Adjust to age-appropriate levels for pediatric patients.						
ALSO CONSIDER: Glomerular filtration rate.						
GGT (γ-Glutamyltrans-peptidase)	GGT	>ULN–2.5 × ULN	>2.5–5.0 × ULN	>5.0–20.0 × ULN	>20.0 × ULN	—
Glomerular filtration rate	GFR	<75 – 50% LLN	<50–25% LLN	<25% LLN, chronic dialysis not indicated	Chronic dialysis or renal transplant indicated	Death
ALSO CONSIDER: Creatinine.						
Glucose, serum-high (hyperglycemia)	Hyperglycemia	>ULN–160 mg/dL >ULN–8.9 mmol/L	>160–250 mg/dL >8.9–13.9 mmol/L	>250–500 mg/dL >13.9–27.8 mmol/L	>500 mg/dL >27.8 mmol/L or acidosis	Death
REMARK: Hyperglycemia, in general, is defined as fasting unless otherwise specified in protocol.						
Glucose, serum-low (hypoglycemia)	Hypoglycemia	<LLN–55 mg/dL <LLN–3.0 mmol/L	<55–40 mg/dL <3.0–2.2 mmol/L	<40–30 mg/dL <2.2–1.7 mmol/L	<30 mg/dL <1.7 mmol/L	Death

(continued)

Appendix 2 *(Continued)*

METABOLIC/LABORATORY						
		Grade				
Adverse Event	**Short Name**	**1**	**2**	**3**	**4**	**5**
Hemoglobinuria	Hemoglobinuria	Present	—	—	—	Death
Lipase	Lipase	>ULN–1.5 × ULN	>1.5–2.0 × ULN	>2.0–5.0 × ULN	>5.0 × ULN	—
Magnesium, serum-high (hypermagnesemia)	Hypermagne-semia	>ULN–3.0 mg/dL >ULN–1.23 mmol/L	—	>3.0–8.0 mg/dL >1.23–3.30 mmol/L	>8.0 mg/dL >3.30 mmol/L	Death
Magnesium, serum-low (hypomagnesemia)	Hypomagne-semia	<LLN–1.2 mg/dL <LLN–0.5 mmol/L	<1.2–0.9 mg/dL <0.5–0.4 mmol/L	<0.9–0.7 mg/dL <0.4–0.3 mmol/L	<0.7 mg/dL <0.3 mmol/L	Death
Phosphate, serum-low (hypophosphatemia)	Hypophospha-temia	<LLN–2.5 mg/dL <LLN–0.8 mmol/L	<2.5–2.0 mg/dL <0.8–0.6 mmol/L	<2.0–1.0 mg/dL <0.6–0.3 mmol/L	<1.0 mg/dL <0.3 mmol/L	Death
Potassium, serum-high (hyperkalemia)	Hyperkalemia	>ULN–5.5 mmol/L	>5.5–6.0 mmol/L	>6.0–7.0 mmol/L	>7.0 mmol/L	Death
Potassium, serum-low (hypokalemia)	Hypokalemia	<LLN–3.0 mmol/L	—	<3.0–2.5 mmol/L	<2.5 mmol/L	Death
Proteinuria	Proteinuria	1+ or 0.15–1.0 g/24 hrs	2+ to 3+ or >1.0 – 3.5 g/24 hrs	4+ or >3.5 g/24 hrs	Nephrotic syndrome	Death
Sodium, serum-high (hypernatremia)	Hypernatremia	>ULN–150 mmol/L	>150–155 mmol/L	>155–160 mmol/L	>160 mmol/L	Death

(continued)

MUSCULOSKELETAL/SOFT TISSUE						
		Grade				
Adverse Event	**Short Name**	**1**	**2**	**3**	**4**	**5**
Sodium, serum-low (hyponatremia)	Hyponatremia	<LLN–130 mmol/L	—	<130–120 mmol/L	<120 mmol/L	Death
Triglyceride, serum-high (hypertriglyceridemia)	Hypertriglyceridemia	>ULN–2.5 × ULN	>2.5–5.0 × ULN	>5.0–10 × ULN	>10 × ULN	Death
Uric acid, serum-high (hyperuricemia)	Hyperuricemia	>ULN–10 mg/dL ≤0.59 mmol/L without physiologic consequences	—	>ULN–10 mg/dL ≤0.59 mmol/L with physiologic consequences	>10 mg/dL >0.59 mmol/L	Death
ALSO CONSIDER: Creatinine; Potassium, serum-high (hyperkalemia); Renal failure; Tumor lysis syndrome.						
Metabolic/Laboratory – Other (Specify, ______)	Metabolic/Lab – Other (Specify)	Mild	Moderate	Severe	Life-threatening; disabling	Death
Arthritis (non-septic)	Arthritis	Mild pain with inflammation, erythema, or joint swelling, but not interfering with function	Moderate pain with inflammation, erythema, or joint swelling interfering with function, but not interfering with ADL	Severe pain with inflammation, erythema, or joint swelling and interfering with ADL	Disabling	Death
REMARK: Report only when the diagnosis of arthritis (e.g., inflammation of a joint or a state characterized by inflammation of joints) is made. Arthralgia (sign or symptom of pain in a joint, especially non-inflammatory in character) is graded as Pain – *Select* in the PAIN CATEGORY.						

(continued)

Appendix 2 *(Continued)*

MUSCULOSKELETAL/SOFT TISSUE						
		Grade				
Adverse Event	**Short Name**	**1**	**2**	**3**	**4**	**5**
Bone: spine-scoliosis	Scoliosis	≤20 degrees; clinically undetectable	>20–45 degrees; visible by forward flexion; interfering with function but not interfering with ADL	>45 degrees; scapular prominence in forward flexion; operative intervention indicated; interfering with ADL	Disabling (e.g., interfering with cardiopulmonary function)	Death
Cervical spine-range of motion	Cervical spine ROM	Mild restriction of rotation or flexion between 60–70 degrees	Rotation <60 degrees to right or left; <60 degrees of flexion	Ankylosed/fused over multiple segments with no C-spine rotation	—	—
REMARK: 60–65 degrees of rotation is required for reversing a car; 60–65 degrees of flexion is required to tie shoes.						
Exostosis	Exostosis	Asymptomatic	Involving multiple sites; pain or interfering with function	Excision indicated	Progression to malignancy (i.e., chondrosarcoma)	Death

(continued)

MUSCULOSKELETAL/SOFT TISSUE						
		Grade				
Adverse Event	**Short Name**	**1**	**2**	**3**	**4**	**5**
Extremity-lower (gait/walking)	Gait/walking	Limp evident only to trained observer and able to walk ≥1 kilometer; cane indicated for walking	Noticeable limp, or limitation of limb function, but able to walk ≥0.1 kilometer (1 city block); quad cane indicated for walking	Severe limp with stride modified to maintain balance (widened base of support, marked reduction in step length); ambulation limited to walker; crutches indicated	Unable to walk	—
ALSO CONSIDER: Ataxia (incoordination); Muscle weakness, generalized or specific area (not due to neuropathy) – *Select*.						
Extremity-upper (function)	Extremity-upper (function)	Able to perform most household or work activities with affected limb	Able to perform most household or work activities with compensation from unaffected limb	Interfering with ADL	Disabling; no function of affected limb	—
Fibrosis-cosmesis	Fibrosis-cosmesis	Visible only on close examination	Readily apparent but not disfiguring	Significant disfigurement; operative intervention indicated if patient chooses	—	—

(continued)

Appendix 2 *(Continued)*

MUSCULOSKELETAL/SOFT TISSUE						
		Grade				
Adverse Event	**Short Name**	**1**	**2**	**3**	**4**	**5**
Fibrosis-deep connective tissue	Fibrosis-deep connective tissue	Increased density, "spongy" feel	Increased density with firmness or tethering	Increased density with fixation of tissue; operative intervention indicated; interfering with ADL	Life-threatening; disabling; loss of limb; interfering with vital organ function	Death
ALSO CONSIDER: Induration/fibrosis (skin and subcutaneous tissue); Muscle weakness, generalized or specific area (not due to neuropathy) – *Select*; Neuropathy: motor; Neuropathy: sensory.						
Fracture	Fracture	Asymptomatic, radiographic findings only (e.g., asymptomatic rib fracture on plain x-ray, pelvic insufficiency fracture on MRI, etc.)	Symptomatic but nondisplaced; immobilization indicated	Symptomatic and displaced or open wound with bone exposure; operative intervention indicated	Disabling; amputation indicated	Death
Joint-effusion	Joint-effusion	Asymptomatic, clinical or radiographic findings only	Symptomatic; interfering with function but not interfering with ADL	Symptomatic and interfering with ADL	Disabling	Death
ALSO CONSIDER: Arthritis (non-septic).						

(continued)

MUSCULOSKELETAL/SOFT TISSUE						
		Grade				
Adverse Event	**Short Name**	**1**	**2**	**3**	**4**	**5**
Joint-function[5]	Joint-function	Stiffness interfering with athletic activity; ≤25% loss of range of motion (ROM)	Stiffness interfering with function but not interfering with ADL; >25–50% decrease in ROM	Stiffness interfering with ADL; >50–75% decrease in ROM	Fixed or non-functional joint (arthrodesis); >75% decrease in ROM	—
ALSO CONSIDER: Arthritis (non-septic).						
Local complication – device/prosthesis-related	Device/prosthesis	Asymptomatic	Symptomatic, but not interfering with ADL; local wound care; medical intervention indicated	Symptomatic, interfering with ADL; operative intervention indicated (e.g., hardware/device replacement or removal, reconstruction)	Life-threatening; disabling; loss of limb or organ	Death
Lumbar spine-range of motion	Lumbar spine ROM	Stiffness and difficulty bending to the floor to pick up a very light object but able to do activity	Some lumbar spine flexion but requires a reaching aid to pick up a very light object from the floor	Ankylosed/fused over multiple segments with no L-spine flexion (i.e., unable to reach to floor to pick up a very light object)	—	—

(continued)

Appendix 2 *(Continued)*

MUSCULOSKELETAL/SOFT TISSUE						
		Grade				
Adverse Event	**Short Name**	**1**	**2**	**3**	**4**	**5**
Muscle weakness, generalized or specific area (not due to neuropathy) – *Select*: – Extraocular – Extremity-lower – Extremity-upper – Facial – Left-sided – Ocular – Pelvic – Right-sided – Trunk – Whole body/generalized	Muscle weakness – *Select*	Asymptomatic, weakness on physical exam	Symptomatic and interfering with function, but not interfering with ADL	Symptomatic and interfering with ADL	Life-threatening; disabling	Death
ALSO CONSIDER: Fatigue (asthenia, lethargy, malaise).						
Muscular/skeletal hypoplasia	Muscular/skeletal hypoplasia	Cosmetically and functionally insignificant hypoplasia	Deformity, hypoplasia, or asymmetry able to be remediated by prosthesis (e.g., shoe insert) or covered by clothing	Functionally significant deformity, hypoplasia, or asymmetry, unable to be remediated by prosthesis or covered by clothing	Disabling	—

(continued)

MUSCULOSKELETAL/SOFT TISSUE						
		Grade				
Adverse Event	**Short Name**	**1**	**2**	**3**	**4**	**5**
Myositis (inflammation/damage of muscle)	Myositis	Mild pain, not interfering with function	Pain interfering with function, but not interfering with ADL	Pain interfering with ADL	Disabling	Death
REMARK: Myositis implies muscle damage (i.e., elevated CPK).						
ALSO CONSIDER: CPK (creatine phosphokinase); Pain – *Select*.						
Osteonecrosis (avascular necrosis)	Osteonecrosis	Asymptomatic, radiographic findings only	Symptomatic and interfering with function, but not interfering with ADL; minimal bone removal indicated (i.e., minor sequestrectomy)	Symptomatic and interfering with ADL; operative intervention or hyperbaric oxygen indicated	Disabling	Death
Osteoporosis[6]	Osteoporosis	Radiographic evidence of osteoporosis or Bone Mineral Density (BMD) t-score –1 to –2.5 (osteopenia) and no loss of height or therapy indicated	BMD t-score < –2.5; loss of height <2 cm; antiosteoporotic therapy indicated	Fractures; loss of height ≥2 cm	Disabling	Death

(continued)

Appendix 2 *(Continued)*

MUSCULOSKELETAL/SOFT TISSUE						
		Grade				
Adverse Event	**Short Name**	**1**	**2**	**3**	**4**	**5**
Seroma	Seroma	Asymptomatic	Symptomatic; medical intervention or simple aspiration indicated	Symptomatic, interventional radiology or operative intervention indicated	—	—
Soft tissue necrosis – *Select*: – Abdomen – Extremity-lower – Extremity-upper – Head – Neck – Pelvic – Thorax	Soft tissue necrosis–*Select*	—	Local wound care; medical intervention indicated	Operative debridement or other invasive intervention indicated (e.g., hyperbaric oxygen)	Life-threatening consequences; major invasive intervention indicated (e.g., tissue reconstruction, flap, or grafting)	Death
Trismus (difficulty, restriction, or pain when opening mouth)	Trismus	Decreased range of motion without impaired eating	Decreased range of motion requiring small bites, soft foods or purees	Decreased range of motion with inability to adequately aliment or hydrate orally	—	—
NAVIGATION NOTE: Wound-infectious is graded as Infection – *Select* in the INFECTION CATEGORY.						
NAVIGATION NOTE: Wound non-infectious is graded as Wound complication, non-infectious in the DERMATOLOGY/SKIN CATEGORY.						
Musculoskeletal/Soft Tissue – Other (Specify, ______)	Musculoskeletal – Other (Specify)	Mild	Moderate	Severe	Life-threatening; disabling	Death

(continued)

NEUROLOGY						
		Grade				
Adverse Event	**Short Name**	**1**	**2**	**3**	**4**	**5**
NAVIGATION NOTE: ADD (Attention Deficit Disorder) is graded as Cognitive disturbance.						
NAVIGATION NOTE: Aphasia, receptive and/or expressive, is graded as Speech impairment (e.g., dysphasia or aphasia).						
Apnea	Apnea	—	—	Present	Intubation indicated	Death
Arachnoiditis/meningismus/radiculitis	Arachnoiditis	Symptomatic, not interfering with function; medical intervention indicated	Symptomatic (e.g., photophobia, nausea) interfering with function but not interfering with ADL	Symptomatic, interfering with ADL	Life-threatening; disabling (e.g., paraplegia)	Death
ALSO CONSIDER: Fever (in the absence of neutropenia, where neutropenia is defined as ANC $\leq 1.0 \times 10^9/L$); Infection (documented clinically or microbiologically) with Grade 3 or 4 neutrophils (ANC $<1.0 \times 10^9/L$) – *Select*; Infection with normal ANC or Grade 1 or 2 neutrophils – *Select*; Infection with unknown ANC – *Select*; Pain – *Select*; Vomiting.						
Ataxia (incoordination)	Ataxia	Asymptomatic	Symptomatic, not interfering with ADL	Symptomatic, interfering with ADL; mechanical assistance indicated	Disabling	Death
REMARK: Ataxia (incoordination) refers to the consequence of medical or operative intervention.						

(continued)

Appendix 2 *(Continued)*

NEUROLOGY						
		Grade				
Adverse Event	**Short Name**	**1**	**2**	**3**	**4**	**5**
Brachial plexopathy	Brachial plexopathy	Asymptomatic	Symptomatic, not interfering with ADL	Symptomatic, interfering with ADL	Disabling	Death
CNS cerebrovascular ischemia	CNS ischemia	—	Asymptomatic, radiographic findings only	Transient ischemic event or attack (TIA) ≤24 hrs duration	Cerebral vascular accident (CVA, stroke), neurologic deficit >24 hrs	Death
NAVIGATION NOTE: CNS hemorrhage/bleeding is graded as Hemorrhage, CNS in the HEMORRHAGE/BLEEDING CATEGORY.						
CNS necrosis/cystic progression	CNS necrosis	Asymptomatic, radiographic findings only	Symptomatic, not interfering with ADL; medical intervention indicated	Symptomatic and interfering with ADL; hyperbaric oxygen indicated	Life-threatening; disabling; operative intervention indicated to prevent or treat CNS necrosis/cystic progression	Death
Cognitive disturbance	Cognitive disturbance	Mild cognitive disability; not interfering with	Moderate cognitive disability; interfering with work/	Severe cognitive disability; significant impairment	Unable to perform ADL; full-time specialized	Death

(continued)

NEUROLOGY						
		Grade				
Adverse Event	**Short Name**	**1**	**2**	**3**	**4**	**5**
		work/school/life performance; specialized educational services/devices not indicated	school/life performance but capable of independent living; specialized resources on part-time basis indicated	of work/school/life performance	resources or institutionalization indicated	
REMARK: Cognitive disturbance may be used for Attention Deficit Disorder (ADD).						
Confusion	Confusion	Transient confusion, disorientation, or attention deficit	Confusion, disorientation, or attention deficit interfering with function, but not interfering with ADL	Confusion or delirium interfering with ADL	Harmful to others or self; hospitalization indicated	Death
REMARK: Attention Deficit Disorder (ADD) is graded as Cognitive disturbance.						
NAVIGATION NOTE: Cranial neuropathy is graded as Neuropathy-cranial – *Select*.						
Dizziness	Dizziness	With head movements or nystagmus only; not interfering with function	Interfering with function, but not interfering with ADL	Interfering with ADL	Disabling	—
REMARK: Dizziness includes disequilibrium, lightheadedness, and vertigo.						
ALSO CONSIDER: Neuropathy: cranial – *Select*; Syncope (fainting).						

(continued)

Appendix 2 *(Continued)*

NEUROLOGY						
		Grade				
Adverse Event	**Short Name**	**1**	**2**	**3**	**4**	**5**
NAVIGATION NOTE: Dysphasia, receptive and/or expressive, is graded as Speech impairment (e.g., dysphasia or aphasia).						
Encephalopathy	Encephalopathy	—	Mild signs or symptoms; not interfering with ADL	Signs or symptoms interfering with ADL; hospitalization indicated	Life-threatening; disabling	Death
ALSO CONSIDER: Cognitive disturbance; Confusion; Dizziness; Memory impairment; Mental status; Mood alteration – *Select*; Psychosis (hallucinations/delusions); Somnolence/depressed level of consciousness.						
Extrapyramidal/involuntary movement/ restlessness	Involuntary movement	Mild involuntary movements not interfering with function	Moderate involuntary movements interfering with function, but not interfering with ADL	Severe involuntary movements or torticollis interfering with ADL	Disabling	Death
NAVIGATION NOTE: Headache/neuropathic pain (e.g., jaw pain, neurologic pain, phantom limb pain, post-infectious neuralgia, or painful neuropathies) is graded as Pain – *Select* in the PAIN CATEGORY.						
Hydrocephalus	Hydrocephalus	Asymptomatic, radiographic findings only	Mild to moderate symptoms not interfering with ADL	Severe symptoms or neurological deficit interfering with ADL	Disabling	Death

(continued)

NEUROLOGY						
		Grade				
Adverse Event	**Short Name**	**1**	**2**	**3**	**4**	**5**
Irritability (children <3 years of age)	Irritability	Mild; easily consolable	Moderate; requiring increased attention	Severe; inconsolable	—	—
Laryngeal nerve dysfunction	Laryngeal nerve	Asymptomatic, weakness on clinical examination/testing only	Symptomatic, but not interfering with ADL; intervention not indicated	Symptomatic, interfering with ADL; intervention indicated (e.g., thyroplasty, vocal cord injection)	Life-threatening; tracheostomy indicated	Death
Leak, cerebrospinal fluid (CSF)	CSF leak	Transient headache; postural care indicated	Symptomatic, not interfering with ADL; blood patch indicated	Symptomatic, interfering with ADL; operative intervention indicated	Life-threatening; disabling	Death

REMARK: Leak, cerebrospinal fluid (CSF) may be used for CSF leak associated with operation and persisting 72 hours.

(continued)

Appendix 2 *(Continued)*

NEUROLOGY						
		Grade				
Adverse Event	**Short Name**	**1**	**2**	**3**	**4**	**5**
Leukoencephalopathy (radiographic findings)	Leukoencephalopathy	Mild increase in subarachnoid space (SAS); mild ventriculomegaly; small (+/– multiple) focal T2 hyperintensities, involving periventricular white matter or <1/3 of susceptible areas of cerebrum	Moderate increase in SAS; moderate ventriculomegaly; focal T2 hyperintensities extending into centrum ovale or involving 1/3 to 2/3 of susceptible areas of cerebrum	Severe increase in SAS; severe ventriculomegaly; near total white matter T2 hyperintensities or diffuse low attenuation (CT)	—	—
REMARK: Leukoencephalopathy is a diffuse white matter process, specifically NOT associated with necrosis. Leukoencephalopathy (radiographic findings) does not include lacunas, which are areas that become void of neural tissue.						
Memory impairment	Memory impairment	Memory impairment not interfering with function	Memory impairment interfering with function, but not interfering with ADL	Memory impairment interfering with ADL	Amnesia	—

(continued)

NEUROLOGY						
		Grade				
Adverse Event	**Short Name**	**1**	**2**	**3**	**4**	**5**
Mental status[7]	Mental status	—	1–3 point below age and educational norm in Folstein Mini-Mental Status Exam (MMSE)	>3 point below age and educational norm in Folstein MMSE	—	—
Mood alteration – *Select*: – Agitation – Anxiety – Depression – Euphoria	Mood alteration – *Select*	Mild mood alteration not interfering with function	Moderate mood alteration interfering with function, but not interfering with ADL; medication indicated	Severe mood alteration interfering with ADL	Suicidal ideation; danger to self or others	Death
Myelitis	Myelitis	Asymptomatic, mild signs (e.g., Babinski's or Lhermitte's sign)	Weakness or sensory loss not interfering with ADL	Weakness or sensory loss interfering with ADL	Disabling	Death

NAVIGATION NOTE: Neuropathic pain is graded as Pain – *Select* in the PAIN CATEGORY.

(continued)

Appendix 2 *(Continued)*

NEUROLOGY						
		Grade				
Adverse Event	**Short Name**	**1**	**2**	**3**	**4**	**5**
Neuropathy: cranial – *Select*: – CN I Smell – CN II Vision – CN III Pupil, upper eyelid, extra ocular movements – CN IV Downward, inward movement of eye – CN V Motor-jaw muscles; Sensory-facial – CN VI Lateral deviation of eye – CN VII Motor-face; Sensory-taste – CN VIII Hearing and balance – CN IX Motor-pharynx; Sensory-ear, pharynx, tongue – CN X Motor-palate; pharynx, larynx – CN XI Motor-sternomastoid and trapezius – CN XII Motor-tongue	Neuropathy: cranial – *Select*	Asymptomatic, detected on exam/testing only	Symptomatic, not interfering with ADL	Symptomatic, interfering with ADL	Life-threatening; disabling	Death
Neuropathy: motor	Neuropathy-motor	Asymptomatic, weakness on exam/testing only	Symptomatic weakness interfering with function, but not interfering with ADL	Weakness interfering with ADL; bracing or assistance to walk (e.g., cane or walker) indicated	Life-threatening; disabling (e.g., paralysis)	Death

REMARK: Cranial nerve *motor* neuropathy is graded as Neuropathy: cranial – *Select*.
ALSO CONSIDER: Laryngeal nerve dysfunction; Phrenic nerve dysfunction.

(continued)

NEUROLOGY						
		Grade				
Adverse Event	**Short Name**	**1**	**2**	**3**	**4**	**5**
Neuropathy: sensory	Neuropathy-sensory	Asymptomatic; loss of deep tendon reflexes or paresthesia (including tingling) but not interfering with function	Sensory alteration or paresthesia (including tingling), interfering with function, but not interfering with ADL	Sensory alteration or paresthesia interfering with ADL	Disabling	Death
REMARK: Cranial nerve *sensory* neuropathy is graded as Neuropathy: cranial – *Select*.						
Personality/behavioral	Personality	Change, but not adversely affecting patient or family	Change, adversely affecting patient or family	Mental health intervention indicated	Change harmful to others or self; hospitalization indicated	Death
Phrenic nerve dysfunction	Phrenic nerve	Asymptomatic weakness on exam/testing only	Symptomatic but not interfering with ADL; intervention not indicated	Significant dysfunction; intervention indicated (e.g., diaphragmatic plication)	Life-threatening respiratory compromise; mechanical ventilation indicated	Death
Psychosis (hallucinations/delusions)	Psychosis	—	Transient episode	Interfering with ADL; medication, supervision or restraints indicated	Harmful to others or self; life-threatening consequences	Death

(continued)

Appendix 2 *(Continued)*

NEUROLOGY						
		Grade				
Adverse Event	**Short Name**	**1**	**2**	**3**	**4**	**5**
Pyramidal tract dysfunction (e.g., ↑ tone, hyperreflexia, positive Babinski, ↓ fine motor coordination)	Pyramidal tract dysfunction	Asymptomatic, abnormality on exam or testing only	Symptomatic; interfering with function but not interfering with ADL	Interfering with ADL	Disabling; paralysis	Death
Seizure	Seizure	—	One brief generalized seizure; seizure(s) well controlled by anticonvulsants or infrequent focal motor seizures not interfering with ADL	Seizures in which consciousness is altered; poorly controlled seizure disorder, with breakthrough generalized seizures despite medical intervention	Seizures of any kind which are prolonged, repetitive, or difficult to control (e.g., status epilepticus, intractable epilepsy)	Death
Somnolence/depressed level of consciousness	Somnolence	—	Somnolence or sedation interfering with function, but not interfering with ADL	Obtundation or stupor; difficult to arouse; interfering with ADL	Coma	Death

(continued)

NEUROLOGY						
		Grade				
Adverse Event	**Short Name**	**1**	**2**	**3**	**4**	**5**
Speech impairment (e.g., dysphasia or aphasia)	Speech impairment	—	Awareness of receptive or expressive dysphasia, not impairing ability to communicate	Receptive or expressive dysphasia, impairing ability to communicate	Inability to communicate	—
REMARK: Speech impairment refers to a primary CNS process, not neuropathy or end organ dysfunction.						
ALSO CONSIDER: Laryngeal nerve dysfunction; Voice changes/dysarthria (e.g., hoarseness, loss, or alteration in voice, laryngitis).						
Syncope (fainting)	Syncope (fainting)	—	—	Present	Life-threatening consequences	Death
ALSO CONSIDER: CNS cerebrovascular ischemia; Conduction abnormality/atrioventricular heart block – *Select*; Dizziness; Supraventricular and nodal arrhythmia – *Select*; Vasovagal episode; Ventricular arrhythmia – *Select*.						
NAVIGATION NOTE: Taste alteration (CN VII, IX) is graded as Taste alteration (dysgeusia) in the GASTROINTESTINAL CATEGORY.						
Tremor	Tremor	Mild and brief or intermittent but not interfering with function	Moderate tremor interfering with function, but not interfering with ADL	Severe tremor interfering with ADL	Disabling	—
Neurology – Other (Specify, ________)	Neurology – Other (Specify)	Mild	Moderate	Severe	Life-threatening; disabling	Death

(continued)

Appendix 2 *(Continued)*

OCULAR/VISUAL						
		Grade				
Adverse Event	**Short Name**	**1**	**2**	**3**	**4**	**5**
Cataract	Cataract	Asymptomatic, detected on exam only	Symptomatic, with moderate decrease in visual acuity (20/40 or better); decreased visual function correctable with glasses	Symptomatic with marked decrease in visual acuity (worse than 20/40); operative intervention indicated (e.g., cataract surgery)	—	—
Dry eye syndrome	Dry eye	Mild, intervention not indicated	Symptomatic, interfering with function but not interfering with ADL; medical intervention indicated	Symptomatic or decrease in visual acuity interfering with ADL; operative intervention indicated	—	—
Eyelid dysfunction	Eyelid dysfunction	Asymptomatic	Symptomatic, interfering with function but not ADL; requiring topical agents or epilation	Symptomatic; interfering with ADL; surgical intervention indicated	—	—

REMARK: Eyelid dysfunction includes canalicular stenosis, ectropion, entropion, erythema, madarosis, symblepharon, telangiectasis, thickening, and trichiasis.

ALSO CONSIDER: Neuropathy: cranial – *Select.*

(continued)

OCULAR/VISUAL						
		Grade				
Adverse Event	**Short Name**	**1**	**2**	**3**	**4**	**5**
Glaucoma	Glaucoma	Elevated intraocular pressure (EIOP) with single topical agent for intervention; no visual field deficit	EIOP causing early visual field deficit (i.e., nasal step or arcuate deficit); multiple topical or oral agents indicated	EIOP causing marked visual field deficits (i.e., involving both superior and inferior visual fields); operative intervention indicated	EIOP resulting in blindness (20/200 or worse); enucleation indicated	—
Keratitis (corneal inflammation/corneal ulceration)	Keratitis	Abnormal ophthalmologic changes only; intervention not indicated	Symptomatic and interfering with function, but not interfering with ADL	Symptomatic and interfering with ADL; operative intervention indicated	Perforation or blindness (20/200 or worse)	—
NAVIGATION NOTE: Ocular muscle weakness is graded as Muscle weakness, generalized or specific area (not due to neuropathy) – *Select* in the MUSCULOSKELETAL/SOFT TISSUE CATEGORY.						
Night blindness (nyctalopia)	Nyctalopia	Symptomatic, not interfering with function	Symptomatic and interfering with function but not interfering with ADL	Symptomatic and interfering with ADL	Disabling	—

(continued)

Appendix 2 *(Continued)*

OCULAR/VISUAL						
		Grade				
Adverse Event	**Short Name**	**1**	**2**	**3**	**4**	**5**
Nystagmus	Nystagmus	Asymptomatic	Symptomatic and interfering with function but not interfering with ADL	Symptomatic and interfering with ADL	Disabling	—
ALSO CONSIDER: Neuropathy: cranial – *Select*; Ophthalmoplegia/diplopia (double vision).						
Ocular surface disease	Ocular surface disease	Asymptomatic or minimally symptomatic but not interfering with function	Symptomatic, interfering with function but not interfering with ADL; topical antibiotics or other topical intervention indicated	Symptomatic, interfering with ADL; operative intervention indicated	—	—
REMARK: Ocular surface disease includes conjunctivitis, keratoconjunctivitis sicca, chemosis, keratinization, and palpebral conjunctival epithelial metaplasia.						
Ophthalmoplegia/diplopia (double vision)	Diplopia	Intermittently symptomatic, intervention not indicated	Symptomatic and interfering with function but not interfering with ADL	Symptomatic and interfering with ADL; surgical intervention indicated	Disabling	—
ALSO CONSIDER: Neuropathy: cranial – *Select*.						

(continued)

OCULAR/VISUAL						
		Grade				
Adverse Event	**Short Name**	**1**	**2**	**3**	**4**	**5**
Optic disc edema	Optic disc edema	Asymptomatic	Decreased visual acuity (20/40 or better); visual field defect present	Decreased visual acuity (worse than 20/40); marked visual field defect but sparing the central 20 degrees	Blindness (20/200 or worse)	—
ALSO CONSIDER: Neuropathy: cranial – *Select.*						
Proptosis/enophthalmos	Proptosis/enophthalmos	Asymptomatic, intervention not indicated	Symptomatic and interfering with function, but not interfering with ADL	Symptomatic and interfering with ADL	—	—
Retinal detachment	Retinal detachment	Exudative; no central vision loss; intervention not indicated	Exudative and visual acuity 20/40 or better but intervention not indicated	Rhegmatogenous or exudative detachment; operative intervention indicated	Blindness (20/200 or worse)	—
Retinopathy	Retinopathy	Asymptomatic	Symptomatic with moderate decrease in visual acuity (20/40 or better)	Symptomatic with marked decrease in visual acuity (worse than 20/40)	Blindness (20/200 or worse)	—

(continued)

Appendix 2 *(Continued)*

OCULAR/VISUAL						
		Grade				
Adverse Event	**Short Name**	**1**	**2**	**3**	**4**	**5**
Scleral necrosis/melt	Scleral necrosis	Asymptomatic or symptomatic but not interfering with function	Symptomatic, interfering with function but not interfering with ADL; moderate decrease in visual acuity (20/40 or better); medical intervention indicated	Symptomatic, interfering with ADL; marked decrease in visual acuity (worse than 20/40); operative intervention indicated	Blindness (20/200 or worse); painful eye with enucleation indicated	—
Uveitis	Uveitis	Asymptomatic	Anterior uveitis; medical intervention indicated	Posterior or pan-uveitis; operative intervention indicated	Blindness (20/200 or worse)	—
Vision-blurred vision	Blurred vision	Symptomatic not interfering with function	Symptomatic and interfering with function, but not interfering with ADL	Symptomatic and interfering with ADL	Disabling	—

(continued)

OCULAR/VISUAL						
		Grade				
Adverse Event	**Short Name**	**1**	**2**	**3**	**4**	**5**
Vision-flashing lights/floaters	Flashing lights	Symptomatic not interfering with function	Symptomatic and interfering with function, but not interfering with ADL	Symptomatic and interfering with ADL	Disabling	—
Vision-photophobia	Photophobia	Symptomatic not interfering with function	Symptomatic and interfering with function, but not interfering with ADL	Symptomatic and interfering with ADL	Disabling	—
Vitreous hemorrhage	Vitreous hemorrhage	Asymptomatic, clinical findings only	Symptomatic, interfering with function, but not interfering with ADL; intervention not indicated	Symptomatic, interfering with ADL; vitrectomy indicated	—	—
Watery eye (epiphora, tearing)	Watery eye	Symptomatic, intervention not indicated	Symptomatic, interfering with function but not interfering with ADL	Symptomatic, interfering with ADL	—	—

(continued)

Appendix 2 *(Continued)*

OCULAR/VISUAL						
		Grade				
Adverse Event	**Short Name**	**1**	**2**	**3**	**4**	**5**
Ocular/Visual – Other (Specify, _______)	Ocular – Other (Specify)	Symptomatic not interfering with function	Symptomatic and interfering with function, but not interfering with ADL	Symptomatic and interfering with ADL	Blindness (20/200 or worse)	Death

PAIN						
		Grade				
Adverse Event	**Short Name**	**1**	**2**	**3**	**4**	**5**
Pain – *Select*: *Select* AEs appear at the end of the CATEGORY.	Pain – *Select*	Mild pain not interfering with function	Moderate pain; pain or analgesics interfering with function, but not interfering with ADL	Severe pain; pain or analgesics severely interfering with ADL	Disabling	—
Pain – Other (Specify, _______)	Pain – Other (Specify)	Mild pain not interfering with function	Moderate pain; pain or analgesics interfering with function, but not interfering with ADL	Severe pain; pain or analgesics severely interfering with ADL	Disabling	—

(continued)

PAIN–*SELECT*		
AUDITORY/EAR	HEPATOBILIARY/PANCREAS	PULMONARY/UPPER RESPIRATORY
– External ear	– Gallbladder	– Chest wall
– Middle ear	– Liver	– Chest/thorax NOS
CARDIOVASCULAR	LYMPHATIC	– Larynx
– Cardiac/heart	– Lymph node	– Pleura
– Pericardium	MUSCULOSKELETAL	– Sinus
DERMATOLOGY/SKIN	– Back	– Throat/pharynx/larynx
– Face	– Bone	RENAL/GENITOURINARY
– Lip	– Buttock	– Bladder
– Oral-gums	– Extremity-limb	– Kidney
– Scalp	– Intestine	SEXUAL/REPRODUCTIVE FUNCTION
– Skin	– Joint	– Breast
GASTROINTESTINAL	– Muscle	– Ovulatory
– Abdomen NOS	– Neck	– Pelvis
– Anus	– Phantom (pain associated with missing limb)	– Penis
– Dental/teeth/periodontal	NEUROLOGY	– Perineum
– Esophagus	– Head/headache	– Prostate
– Oral cavity	– Neuralgia/peripheral nerve	– Scrotum
– Peritoneum	OCULAR	– Testicle
– Rectum	– Eye	– Urethra
– Stomach		– Uterus
GENERAL		– Vagina
– Pain NOS		
– Tumor pain		

(continued)

Appendix 2 *(Continued)*

PULMONARY/UPPER RESPIRATORY						
		Grade				
Adverse Event	**Short Name**	**1**	**2**	**3**	**4**	**5**
Adult Respiratory Distress Syndrome (ARDS)	ARDS	—	—	Present, intubation not indicated	Present, intubation indicated	Death
ALSO CONSIDER: Dyspnea (shortness of breath); Hypoxia; Pneumonitis/pulmonary infiltrates.						
Aspiration	Aspiration	Asymptomatic ("silent aspiration"); endoscopy or radiographic (e.g., barium swallow) findings	Symptomatic (e.g., altered eating habits, coughing or choking episodes consistent with aspiration); medical intervention indicated (e.g., antibiotics, suction or oxygen)	Clinical or radiographic signs of pneumonia or pneumonitis; unable to aliment orally	Life-threatening (e.g., aspiration pneumonia or pneumonitis)	Death
ALSO CONSIDER: Infection (documented clinically or microbiologically) with Grade 3 or 4 neutrophils (ANC <1.0 × 10^9/L) – *Select*; Infection with normal ANC or Grade 1 or 2 neutrophils – *Select*; Infection with unknown ANC – *Select*; Laryngeal nerve dysfunction; Neuropathy: cranial – *Select*; Pneumonitis/pulmonary infiltrates.						

(continued)

PULMONARY/UPPER RESPIRATORY						
		Grade				
Adverse Event	**Short Name**	**1**	**2**	**3**	**4**	**5**
Atelectasis	Atelectasis	Asymptomatic	Symptomatic (e.g., dyspnea, cough), medical intervention indicated (e.g., bronchoscopic suctioning, chest physiotherapy, suctioning)	Operative (e.g., stent, laser) intervention indicated	Life-threatening respiratory compromise	Death
ALSO CONSIDER: Adult Respiratory Distress Syndrome (ARDS); Cough; Dyspnea (shortness of breath); Hypoxia; Infection (documented clinically or microbiologically) with Grade 3 or 4 neutrophils (ANC <1.0 × 10^9/L) – *Select*; Infection with normal ANC or Grade 1 or 2 neutrophils – *Select*; Infection with unknown ANC – *Select*; Obstruction/stenosis of airway – *Select*; Pneumonitis/pulmonary infiltrates; Pulmonary fibrosis (radiographic changes).						
Bronchospasm, wheezing	Bronchospasm	Asymptomatic	Symptomatic not interfering with function	Symptomatic interfering with function	Life-threatening	Death
ALSO CONSIDER: Allergic reaction/hypersensitivity (including drug fever); Dyspnea (shortness of breath).						
Carbon monoxide diffusion capacity (DL_{CO})	DL_{CO}	90–75% of predicted value	<75–50% of predicted value	<50–25% of predicted value	<25% of predicted value	Death
ALSO CONSIDER: Hypoxia; Pneumonitis/pulmonary infiltrates; Pulmonary fibrosis (radiographic changes).						

(continued)

Appendix 2 *(Continued)*

PULMONARY/UPPER RESPIRATORY						
		Grade				
Adverse Event	**Short Name**	**1**	**2**	**3**	**4**	**5**
Chylothorax	Chylothorax	Asymptomatic	Symptomatic; thoracentesis or tube drainage indicated	Operative intervention indicated	Life-threatening (e.g., hemodynamic instability or ventilatory support indicated)	Death
Cough	Cough	Symptomatic, nonnarcotic medication only indicated	Symptomatic and narcotic medication indicated	Symptomatic and significantly interfering with sleep or ADL	—	—
Dyspnea (shortness of breath)	Dyspnea	Dyspnea on exertion, but can walk 1 flight of stairs without stopping	Dyspnea on exertion but unable to walk 1 flight of stairs or 1 city block (0.1km) without stopping	Dyspnea with ADL	Dyspnea at rest; intubation/ventilator indicated	Death
ALSO CONSIDER: Hypoxia; Neuropathy: motor; Pneumonitis/pulmonary infiltrates; Pulmonary fibrosis (radiographic changes).						
Edema, larynx	Edema, larynx	Asymptomatic edema by exam only	Symptomatic edema, no respiratory distress	Stridor; respiratory distress; interfering with ADL	Life-threatening airway compromise; tracheotomy, intubation, or laryngectomy indicated	Death
ALSO CONSIDER: Allergic reaction/hypersensitivity (including drug fever).						

(continued)

PULMONARY/UPPER RESPIRATORY						
		Grade				
Adverse Event	**Short Name**	**1**	**2**	**3**	**4**	**5**
FEV_1	FEV_1	90–75% of predicted value	<75–50% of predicted value	<50–25% of predicted value	<25% of predicted	Death
Fistula, pulmonary/upper respiratory – *Select* – Bronchus – Larynx – Lung – Oral cavity – Pharynx – Pleura – Trachea	Fistula, pulmonary – *Select*	Asymptomatic, radiographic findings only	Symptomatic, tube thoracostomy or medical management indicated; associated with altered respiratory function but not interfering with ADL	Symptomatic and associated with altered respiratory function interfering with ADL; or endoscopic (e.g., stent) or primary closure by operative intervention indicated	Life-threatening consequences; operative intervention with thoracoplasty, chronic open drainage or multiple thoracotomies indicated	Death
REMARK: A fistula is defined as an abnormal communication between two body cavities, potential spaces, and/or the skin. The site indicated for a fistula should be the site from which the abnormal process is believed to have arisen. For example, a tracheoesophageal fistula arising in the context of a resected or irradiated esophageal cancer should be graded as Fistula, GI – esophagus in the GASTROINTESTINAL CATEGORY.						
NAVIGATION NOTE: Hemoptysis is graded as Hemorrhage, pulmonary/upper respiratory – *Select* in the HEMORRHAGE/BLEEDING CATEGORY.						
Hiccoughs (hiccups, singultus)	Hiccoughs	Symptomatic, intervention not indicated	Symptomatic, intervention indicated	Symptomatic, significantly interfering with sleep or ADL	—	—

(continued)

Appendix 2 *(Continued)*

PULMONARY/UPPER RESPIRATORY						
		Grade				
Adverse Event	**Short Name**	**1**	**2**	**3**	**4**	**5**
Hypoxia	Hypoxia	—	Decreased O_2 saturation with exercise (e.g., pulse oximeter <88%); intermittent supplemental oxygen	Decreased O_2 saturation at rest; continuous oxygen indicated	Life-threatening; intubation or ventilation indicated	Death
Nasal cavity/paranasal sinus reactions	Nasal/paranasal reactions	Asymptomatic mucosal crusting, blood-tinged secretions	Symptomatic stenosis or edema/narrowing interfering with airflow	Stenosis with significant nasal obstruction; interfering with ADL	Necrosis of soft tissue or bone	Death
ALSO CONSIDER: Infection (documented clinically or microbiologically) with Grade 3 or 4 neutrophils (ANC <1.0 × 10^9/L) – *Select*; Infection with normal ANC or Grade 1 or 2 neutrophils – *Select*; Infection with unknown ANC – *Select*.						
Obstruction/stenosis of airway – *Select*: – Bronchus – Larynx – Pharynx – Trachea	Airway obstruction – *Select*	Asymptomatic obstruction or stenosis on exam, endoscopy, or radiograph	Symptomatic (e.g., noisy airway breathing), but causing no respiratory distress; medical management indicated (e.g., steroids)	Interfering with ADL; stridor or endoscopic intervention indicated (e.g., stent, laser)	Life-threatening airway compromise; tracheotomy or intubation indicated	Death

(continued)

PULMONARY/UPPER RESPIRATORY						
		Grade				
Adverse Event	**Short Name**	**1**	**2**	**3**	**4**	**5**
Pleural effusion (non-malignant)	Pleural effusion	Asymptomatic	Symptomatic, intervention such as diuretics or up to 2 therapeutic thoracenteses indicated	Symptomatic and supplemental oxygen, >2 therapeutic thoracenteses, tube drainage, or pleurodesis indicated	Life-threatening (e.g., causing hemodynamic instability or ventilatory support indicated)	Death
Also Consider: Atelectasis; Cough; Dyspnea (shortness of breath); Hypoxia; Pneumonitis/pulmonary infiltrates; Pulmonary fibrosis (radiographic changes).						
Navigation Note: Pleuritic pain is graded as Pain – *Select* in the PAIN CATEGORY.						
Pneumonitis/pulmonary infiltrates	Pneumonitis	Asymptomatic, radiographic findings only	Symptomatic, not interfering with ADL	Symptomatic, interfering with ADL; O_2 indicated	Life-threatening; ventilatory support indicated	Death
Also Consider: Adult Respiratory Distress Syndrome (ARDS); Cough; Dyspnea (shortness of breath); Hypoxia; Infection (documented clinically or microbiologically) with Grade 3 or 4 neutrophils (ANC $<1.0 \times 10^9$/L) – *Select*; Infection with normal ANC or Grade 1 or 2 neutrophils – *Select*; Infection with unknown ANC – *Select*; Pneumonitis/pulmonary infiltrates; Pulmonary fibrosis (radiographic changes).						
Pneumothorax	Pneumothorax	Asymptomatic, radiographic findings only	Symptomatic; intervention indicated (e.g., hospitalization for observation, tube placement without sclerosis)	Sclerosis and/or operative intervention indicated	Life-threatening, causing hemodynamic instability (e.g., tension pneumothorax); ventilatory support indicated	Death

(continued)

Appendix 2 *(Continued)*

PULMONARY/UPPER RESPIRATORY						
		Grade				
Adverse Event	**Short Name**	**1**	**2**	**3**	**4**	**5**
Prolonged chest tube drainage or air leak after pulmonary resection	Chest tube drainage or leak	—	Sclerosis or additional tube thoracostomy indicated	Operative intervention indicated (e.g., thoracotomy with stapling or sealant application)	Life-threatening; debilitating; organ resection indicated	Death
Prolonged intubation after pulmonary resection (>24 hrs after surgery)	Prolonged intubation	—	Extubated within 24–72 hrs postoperatively	Extubated >72 hrs postoperatively, but before tracheostomy indicated	Tracheostomy indicated	Death
NAVIGATION NOTE: Pulmonary embolism is graded as Grade 4 either as Thrombosis/embolism (vascular access-related) or Thrombosis/thrombus/embolism in the VASCULAR CATEGORY.						
Pulmonary fibrosis (radiographic changes)	Pulmonary fibrosis	Minimal radiographic findings (or patchy or bibasilar changes) with estimated radiographic proportion of total lung volume that is fibrotic of <25%	Patchy or bibasilar changes with estimated radiographic proportion of total lung volume that is fibrotic of 25 to <50%	Dense or widespread infiltrates/consolidation with estimated radiographic proportion of total lung volume that is fibrotic of 50 to <75%	Estimated radiographic proportion of total lung volume that is fibrotic is ≥75%; honeycombing	Death
REMARK: Fibrosis is usually a "late effect" seen >3 months after radiation or combined modality therapy (including surgery). It is thought to represent scar/fibrotic lung tissue. It may be difficult to distinguish from pneumonitis that is generally seen within 3 months of radiation or combined modality therapy.						

(continued)

PULMONARY/UPPER RESPIRATORY						
		Grade				
Adverse Event	**Short Name**	**1**	**2**	**3**	**4**	**5**
Also Consider: Adult Respiratory Distress Syndrome (ARDS); Cough; Dyspnea (shortness of breath); Hypoxia; Infection (documented clinically or microbiologically) with Grade 3 or 4 neutrophils (ANC <1.0 × 10^9/L) – *Select*; Infection with normal ANC or Grade 1 or 2 neutrophils – *Select*; Infection with unknown ANC – *Select*.						
Navigation Note: Recurrent laryngeal nerve dysfunction is graded as Laryngeal nerve dysfunction in the NEUROLOGY CATEGORY.						
Vital capacity	Vital capacity	90–75% of predicted value	<75–50% of predicted value	<50–25% of predicted value	<25% of predicted value	Death
Voice changes/dysarthria (e.g., hoarseness, loss or alteration in voice, laryngitis)	Voice changes	Mild or intermittent hoarseness or voice change, but fully understandable	Moderate or persistent voice changes, may require occasional repetition but understandable on telephone	Severe voice changes including predominantly whispered speech; may require frequent repetition or face-to-face contact for understandability; requires voice aid (e.g., electrolarynx) for ≤50% of communication	Disabling; non-understandable voice or aphonic; requires voice aid (e.g., electrolarynx) for >50% of communication or requires >50% written communication	Death
Also Consider: Laryngeal nerve dysfunction; Speech impairment (e.g., dysphasia or aphasia).						
Pulmonary/Upper Respiratory – Other (Specify, _______)	Pulmonary – Other (Specify)	Mild	Moderate	Severe	Life-threatening; disabling	Death

(continued)

Appendix 2 *(Continued)*

RENAL/GENITOURINARY						
		Grade				
Adverse Event	**Short Name**	**1**	**2**	**3**	**4**	**5**
Bladder spasms	Bladder spasms	Symptomatic, intervention not indicated	Symptomatic, antispasmodics indicated	Narcotics indicated	Major surgical intervention indicated (e.g., cystectomy)	—
Cystitis	Cystitis	Asymptomatic	Frequency with dysuria; macroscopic hematuria	Transfusion; IV pain medications; bladder irrigation indicated	Catastrophic bleeding; major non-elective intervention indicated	Death
ALSO CONSIDER: Infection (documented clinically or microbiologically) with Grade 3 or 4 neutrophils (ANC $<1.0 \times 10^9$/L) – *Select*; Infection with normal ANC or Grade 1 or 2 neutrophils – *Select*; Infection with unknown ANC – *Select*; Pain – *Select*.						
Fistula, GU – *Select*: – Bladder – Genital tract-female – Kidney – Ureter – Urethra – Uterus – Vagina	Fistula, GU – *Select*	Asymptomatic, radiographic findings only	Symptomatic; noninvasive intervention indicated	Symptomatic interfering with ADL; invasive intervention indicated	Life-threatening consequences; operative intervention requiring partial or full organ resection; permanent urinary diversion	Death
REMARK: A fistula is defined as an abnormal communication between two body cavities, potential spaces, and/or the skin. The site indicated for a fistula should be the site from which the abnormal process is believed to have originated.						

(continued)

RENAL/GENITOURINARY						
		Grade				
Adverse Event	**Short Name**	**1**	**2**	**3**	**4**	**5**
Incontinence, urinary	Incontinence, urinary	Occasional (e.g., with coughing, sneezing, etc.), pads not indicated	Spontaneous, pads indicated	Interfering with ADL; intervention indicated (e.g., clamp, collagen injections)	Operative intervention indicated (e.g., cystectomy or permanent urinary diversion)	—
Leak (including anastomotic), GU – *Select*: – Bladder – Fallopian tube – Kidney – Spermatic cord – Stoma – Ureter – Urethra – Uterus – Vagina – Vas deferens	Leak, GU – *Select*	Asymptomatic, radiographic findings only	Symptomatic; medical intervention indicated	Symptomatic, interfering with GU function; invasive or endoscopic intervention indicated	Life-threatening	Death

REMARK: Leak (including anastomotic), GU – *Select* refers to clinical signs and symptoms or radiographic confirmation of anastomotic leak but without development of fistula.

(continued)

Appendix 2 *(Continued)*

RENAL/GENITOURINARY						
		Grade				
Adverse Event	**Short Name**	**1**	**2**	**3**	**4**	**5**
Obstruction, GU – *Select*: – Bladder – Fallopian tube – Prostate – Spermatic cord – Stoma – Testes – Ureter – Urethra – Uterus – Vagina – Vas deferens	Obstruction, GU – *Select*	Asymptomatic, radiographic or endoscopic findings only	Symptomatic but no hydronephrosis, sepsis or renal dysfunction; dilation or endoscopic repair or stent placement indicated	Symptomatic and altered organ function (e.g., sepsis or hydronephrosis, or renal dysfunction); operative intervention indicated	Life-threatening consequences; organ failure or operative intervention requiring complete organ resection indicated	Death
NAVIGATION NOTE: Operative injury is graded as Intra-operative injury – *Select Organ or Structure* in the SURGERY/INTRA-OPERATIVE INJURY CATEGORY.						
Perforation, GU – *Select*: – Bladder – Fallopian tube – Kidney – Ovary – Prostate – Spermatic cord	Perforation, GU – *Select*	Asymptomatic radiographic findings only	Symptomatic, associated with altered renal/GU function	Symptomatic, operative intervention indicated	Life-threatening consequences or organ failure; operative intervention requiring organ resection indicated	Death

(continued)

RENAL/GENITOURINARY						
		Grade				
Adverse Event	**Short Name**	**1**	**2**	**3**	**4**	**5**
– Stoma – Testes – Ureter – Urethra – Uterus – Vagina – Vas deferens						
Prolapse of stoma, GU	Prolapse stoma, GU	Asymptomatic; special intervention, extraordinary care not indicated	Extraordinary local care or maintenance; minor revision under local anesthesia indicated	Dysfunctional stoma; operative intervention or major stomal revision indicated	Life-threatening consequences	Death
REMARK: Other stoma complications may be graded as Fistula, GU – *Select*; Leak (including anastomotic), GU – *Select*; Obstruction, GU – *Select*; Perforation, GU – *Select*; Stricture/stenosis (including anastomotic), GU – *Select*.						
Renal failure	Renal failure	—	—	Chronic dialysis not indicated	Chronic dialysis or renal transplant indicated	Death
ALSO CONSIDER: Glomerular filtration rate.						

(continued)

Appendix 2 *(Continued)*

RENAL/GENITOURINARY						
		Grade				
Adverse Event	**Short Name**	**1**	**2**	**3**	**4**	**5**
Stricture/stenosis (including anastomotic), GU –*Select*: – Bladder – Fallopian tube – Prostate – Spermatic cord – Stoma – Testes – Ureter – Urethra – Uterus – Vagina – Vas deferens	Stricture, anastomotic, GU – *Select*	Asymptomatic, radiographic or endoscopic findings only	Symptomatic but no hydronephrosis, sepsis or renal dysfunction; dilation or endoscopic repair or stent placement indicated	Symptomatic and altered organ function (e.g., sepsis or hydronephrosis, or renal dysfunction); operative intervention indicated	Life-threatening consequences; organ failure or operative intervention requiring organ resection indicated	Death
ALSO CONSIDER: Obstruction, GU – *Select*.						
Urinary electrolyte wasting (e.g., Fanconi's syndrome, renal tubular acidosis)	Urinary electrolyte wasting	Asymptomatic, intervention not indicated	Mild, reversible and manageable with replacement	Irreversible, requiring continued replacement	—	—
ALSO CONSIDER: Acidosis (metabolic or respiratory); Bicarbonate, serum-low; Calcium, serum-low (hypocalcemia); Phosphate, serum-low (hypophosphatemia).						

(continued)

RENAL/GENITOURINARY						
		Grade				
Adverse Event	**Short Name**	**1**	**2**	**3**	**4**	**5**
Urinary frequency/urgency	Urinary frequency	Increase in frequency or nocturia up to 2 × normal; enuresis	Increase >2 × normal but <hourly	≥1 /hr; urgency; catheter indicated	—	—
Urinary retention (including neurogenic bladder)	Urinary retention	Hesitancy or dribbling, no significant residual urine; retention occurring during the immediate postoperative period	Hesitancy requiring medication; or operative bladder atony requiring indwelling catheter beyond immediate postoperative period but for <6 weeks	More than daily catheterization indicated; urological intervention indicated (e.g., TURP, suprapubic tube, urethrotomy)	Life-threatening consequences; organ failure (e.g., bladder rupture); operative intervention requiring organ resection indicated	Death
REMARK: The etiology of retention (if known) is graded as Obstruction, GU – *Select*; Stricture/stenosis (including anastomotic), GU – *Select*. ALSO CONSIDER: Obstruction, GU – *Select*; Stricture/stenosis (including anastomotic), GU – *Select*.						
Urine color change	Urine color change	Present	—	—	—	—
REMARK: Urine color refers to change that is not related to other dietary or physiologic cause (e.g., bilirubin, concentrated urine, and hematuria).						
Renal/Genitourinary – Other (Specify, ______)	Renal – Other (Specify)	Mild	Moderate	Severe	Life-threatening; disabling	Death

(continued)

Appendix 2 *(Continued)*

SECONDARY MALIGNANCY						
		Grade				
Adverse Event	**Short Name**	**1**	**2**	**3**	**4**	**5**
Secondary Malignancy – possibly related to cancer treatment (Specify, ________)	Secondary Malignancy (possibly related to cancer treatment)	—	—	Non-life-threatening basal or squamous cell carcinoma of the skin	Solid tumor, leukemia, or lymphoma	Death

REMARK: Secondary malignancy excludes metastasis from initial primary. Any malignancy possibly related to cancer treatment (including AML/MDS) should be reported via the routine reporting mechanisms outlined in each protocol. Important: Secondary Malignancy is an exception to NCI Expedited Adverse Event Reporting Guidelines. Secondary Malignancy is "Grade 4, present" but NCI does not require AdEERS Expedited Reporting for any (related or unrelated to treatment) Secondary Malignancy. A diagnosis of AML/MDS following treatment with an NCI-sponsored investigational agent is to be reported using the form available from the CTEP Web site at http://ctep.cancer.gov. Cancers not suspected of being treatment-related are not to be reported here.

SEXUAL/REPRODUCTIVE FUNCTION						
		Grade				
Adverse Event	**Short Name**	**1**	**2**	**3**	**4**	**5**
Breast function/lactation	Breast function	Mammary abnormality, not functionally significant	Mammary abnormality, functionally significant	—	—	—
Breast nipple/areolar deformity	Nipple/areolar	Limited areolar asymmetry with no change in nipple/areolar projection	Asymmetry of nipple areolar complex with slight deviation in nipple projection	Marked deviation of nipple projection	—	—

(continued)

SEXUAL/REPRODUCTIVE FUNCTION						
		Grade				
Adverse Event	**Short Name**	**1**	**2**	**3**	**4**	**5**
Breast volume/hypoplasia	Breast	Minimal asymmetry; minimal hypoplasia	Asymmetry exists, ≤1/3 of the breast volume; moderate hypoplasia	Asymmetry exists, >1/3 of the breast volume; severe hypoplasia	—	—
REMARK: Breast volume is referenced with both arms straight overhead.						
NAVIGATION NOTE: Dysmenorrhea is graded as Pain – *Select* in the PAIN CATEGORY.						
NAVIGATION NOTE: Dyspareunia is graded as Pain – *Select* in the PAIN CATEGORY.						
NAVIGATION NOTE: Dysuria (painful urination) is graded as Pain – *Select* in the PAIN CATEGORY.						
Erectile dysfunction	Erectile dysfunction	Decrease in erectile function (frequency/rigidity of erections) but erectile aids not indicated	Decrease in erectile function (frequency/rigidity of erections), erectile aids indicated	Decrease in erectile function (frequency/rigidity of erections) but erectile aids not helpful; penile prosthesis indicated	—	—
Ejaculatory dysfunction	Ejaculatory dysfunction	Diminished ejaculation	An ejaculation or retrograde ejaculation	—	—	—
NAVIGATION NOTE: Feminization of male is graded in the ENDOCRINE CATEGORY.						

(continued)

Appendix 2 *(Continued)*

SEXUAL/REPRODUCTIVE FUNCTION						
		Grade				
Adverse Event	**Short Name**	**1**	**2**	**3**	**4**	**5**
Gynecomastia	Gynecomastia	—	Asymptomatic breast enlargement	Symptomatic breast enlargement; intervention indicated	—	—
ALSO CONSIDER: Pain – *Select*.						
Infertility/sterility	Infertility/sterility	—	Male: oligospermia/low sperm count Female: diminished fertility/ovulation	Male: sterile/azoospermia Female: infertile/anovulatory	—	—
Irregular menses (change from baseline)	Irregular menses	1–3 months without menses	>3–6 months without menses but continuing menstrual cycles	Persistent amenorrhea for >6 months	—	—
Libido	Libido	Decrease in interest but not affecting relationship; intervention not indicated	Decrease in interest and adversely affecting relationship; intervention indicated	—	—	—
NAVIGATION NOTE: Masculinization of female is graded in the ENDOCRINE CATEGORY.						

(continued)

SEXUAL/REPRODUCTIVE FUNCTION						
		Grade				
Adverse Event	**Short Name**	**1**	**2**	**3**	**4**	**5**
Orgasmic dysfunction	Orgasmic function	Transient decrease	Decrease in orgasmic response requiring intervention	Complete inability of orgasmic response; not responding to interventicn	—	—
NAVIGATION NOTE: Pelvic pain is graded as Pain – *Select* in the PAIN CATEGORY.						
NAVIGATION NOTE: Ulcers of the labia or perineum are graded as Ulceration in DERMATOLOGY/SKIN CATEGORY.						
Vaginal discharge (non-infectious)	Vaginal discharge	Mild	Moderate to heavy; pad use indicated	—	—	—
Vaginal dryness	Vaginal dryness	Mild	Interfering with sexual function; dyspareunia; intervention indicated	—	—	—
ALSO CONSIDER: Pain – *Select*.						

(continued)

Appendix 2 *(Continued)*

SEXUAL/REPRODUCTIVE FUNCTION						
		Grade				
Adverse Event	**Short Name**	**1**	**2**	**3**	**4**	**5**
Vaginal mucositis	Vaginal mucositis	Erythema of the mucosa; minimal symptoms	Patchy ulcerations; moderate symptoms or dyspareunia	Confluent ulcerations; bleeding with trauma; unable to tolerate vaginal exam, sexual intercourse or tampon placement	Tissue necrosis; significant spontaneous bleeding; life-threatening consequences	—
Vaginal stenosis/length	Vaginal stenosis	Vaginal narrowing and/or shortening not interfering with function	Vaginal narrowing and/or shortening interfering with function	Complete obliteration; not surgically correctable	—	—
Vaginitis (not due to infection)	Vaginitis	Mild, intervention not indicated	Moderate, intervention indicated	Severe, not relieved with treatment; ulceration, but operative intervention not indicated	Ulceration and operative intervention indicated	—
Sexual/Reproductive Function – Other (Specify, ______)	Sexual – Other (Specify)	Mild	Moderate	Severe	Disabling	Death

(continued)

SURGERY/INTRA-OPERATIVE INJURY						
		Grade				
Adverse Event	**Short Name**	**1**	**2**	**3**	**4**	**5**
NAVIGATION NOTE: Intra-operative hemorrhage is graded as Hemorrhage/bleeding associated with surgery, intra-operative or postoperative in the HEMORRHAGE/BLEEDING CATEGORY.						
Intra-operative injury – *Select Organ or Structure* AEs appear at the end of the CATEGORY.	Intraop injury – *Select*	Primary repair of injured organ/structure indicated	Partial resection of injured organ/structure indicated	Complete resection or reconstruction of injured organ/structure indicated	Life threatening consequences; disabling	—
REMARK: The *Select* AEs are defined as significant, unanticipated injuries that are recognized at the time of surgery. These AEs do not refer to additional surgical procedures that must be performed because of a change in the operative plan based on intra-operative findings. Any sequelae resulting from the intra-operative injury that result in an adverse outcome for the patient must also be recorded and graded under the relevant CTCAE Term.						
Intra-operative Injury – Other (Specify, _______)	Intraop Injury – Other (Specify)	Primary repair of injured organ/structure indicated	Partial resection of injured organ/structure indicated	Complete resection or reconstruction of injured organ/structure indicated	Life threatening consequences; disabling	—
REMARK: Intra-operative Injury – Other (Specify, _______) is to be used only to report an organ/structure not included in the *Select* AEs found at the end of the CATEGORY. Any sequelae resulting from the intra-operative injury that result in an adverse outcome for the patient must also be recorded and graded under the relevant CTCAE Term.						

(continued)

Appendix 2 *(Continued)*

SURGERY/INTRA-OPERATIVE INJURY – *SELECT*		
AUDITORY/EAR	GASTROINTESTINAL	NEUROLOGY *(continued)*
– Inner ear	– Abdomen NOS	*NERVES:*
– Middle ear	– Anal sphincter	– CN IX (glossopharyngeal) sensory ear-pharynx-tongue
– Outer ear NOS	– Anus	– CN X (vagus)
– Outer ear-Pinna	– Appendix	– CN XI (spinal accessory)
CARDIOVASCULAR	– Cecum	– CN XII (hypoglossal)
– Artery-aorta	– Colon	– Cranial nerve or branch NOS
– Artery-carotid	– Duodenum	– Lingual
– Artery-cerebral	– Esophagus	– Lung thoracic
– Artery-extremity (lower)	– Ileum	– Peripheral motor NOS
– Artery-extremity (upper)	– Jejunum	– Peripheral sensory NOS
– Artery-hepatic	– Oral	– Recurrent laryngeal
– Artery-major visceral artery	– Peritoneal cavity	– Sacral plexus
– Artery-pulmonary	– Rectum	– Sciatic
– Artery NOS	– Small bowel NOS	– Thoracodorsal
– Heart	– Stoma (GI)	OCULAR
– Spleen	– Stomach	– Conjunctiva
– Vein-extremity (lower)	HEPATOBILIARY/ PANCREAS	– Cornea
– Vein-extremity (upper)	– Biliary tree-common bile duct	– Eye NOS
– Vein-hepatic	– Biliary tree-common hepatic duct	– Lens
– Vein-inferior vena cava	– Biliary tree-left hepatic duct	– Retina
– Vein-jugular	– Biliary tree-right hepatic duct	PULMONARY/UPPER RESPIRATORY
– Vein-major visceral vein	– Biliary tree NOS	– Bronchus
– Vein-portal vein	– Liver	– Lung
– Vein-pulmonary	– Pancreas	– Mediastinum
– Vein-superior vena cava	– Pancreatic duct	– Pleura

(continued)

SURGERY/INTRA-OPERATIVE INJURY – *SELECT*		
– Vein NOS	MUSCULOSKELETAL	– Thoracic duct
DERMATOLOGY/SKIN	– Bone	– Trachea
– Breast	– Cartilage	– Upper airway NOS
– Nails	– Extremity-lower	RENAL/GENITOURINARY
– Skin	– Extremity-upper	– Bladder
ENDOCRINE	– Joint	– Cervix
– Adrenal gland	– Ligament	– Fallopian tube
– Parathyroid	– Muscle	– Kidney
– Pituitary	– Soft tissue NOS	– Ovary
– Thyroid	– Tendon	– Pelvis NOS
HEAD AND NECK	NEUROLOGY	– Penis
– Gingiva	– Brain	– Prostate
– Larynx	– Meninges	– Scrotum
– Lip/perioral area	– Spinal cord	– Testis
– Face NOS	*NERVES:*	– Ureter
– Nasal cavity	– Brachial plexus	– Urethra
– Nasopharynx	– CN I (olfactory)	– Urinary conduit
– Neck NOS	– CN II (optic)	– Urinary tract NOS
– Nose	– CN III (oculomotor)	– Uterus
– Oral cavity NOS	– CN IV (trochlear)	– Vagina
– Parotid gland	– CN V (trigeminal) motor	– Vulva
– Pharynx	– CN V (trigeminal) sensory	
– Salivary duct	– CN VI (abducens)	
– Salivary gland	– CN VII (facial) motor-face	
– Sinus	– CN VII (facial) sensory (taste)	
– Teeth	– CN VIII (vestibulocochlear)	
– Tongue	– CN IX (glossopharyngeal) motor pharynx	
– Upper aerodigestive NOS		

(continued)

Appendix 2 *(Continued)*

SYNDROMES						
		Grade				
Adverse Event	**Short Name**	**1**	**2**	**3**	**4**	**5**
NAVIGATION NOTE: Acute vascular leak syndrome is graded in the VASCULAR CATEGORY.						
NAVIGATION NOTE: Adrenal insufficiency is graded in the ENDOCRINE CATEGORY.						
NAVIGATION NOTE: Adult Respiratory Distress Syndrome (ARDS) is graded in the PULMONARY/UPPER RESPIRATORY CATEGORY.						
Alcohol intolerance syndrome (antabuse-like syndrome)	Alcohol intolerance syndrome	—	—	Present	—	Death
REMARK: An antabuse-like syndrome occurs with some new anti-androgens (e.g., nilutamide) when patient also consumes alcohol.						
NAVIGATION NOTE: Autoimmune reaction is graded as Autoimmune reaction/hypersensitivity (including drug fever) in the ALLERGY/IMMUNOLOGY CATEGORY.						
Cytokine release syndrome/acute infusion reaction	Cytokine release syndrome	Mild reaction; infusion interruption not indicated; intervention not indicated	Requires therapy or infusion interruption but responds promptly to symptomatic treatment (e.g., antihistamines, NSAIDs, narcotics, IV fluids); prophylactic medications indicated for ≤24 hrs	Prolonged (i.e., not rapidly responsive to symptomatic medication and/or brief interruption of infusion); recurrence of symptoms following initial improvement; hospitalization indicated for other clinical sequelae (e.g., renal impairment, pulmonary infiltrates)	Life-threatening; pressor or ventilatory support indicated	Death

(continued)

SYNDROMES

Adverse Event	Short Name	Grade 1	Grade 2	Grade 3	Grade 4	Grade 5
REMARK: Cytokine release syndromes/acute infusion reactions are different from Allergic/hypersensitive reactions, although some of the manifestations are common to both AEs. An acute infusion reaction may occur with an agent that causes cytokine release (e.g., monoclonal antibodies or other biological agents). Signs and symptoms usually develop during or shortly after drug infusion and generally resolve completely within 24 hrs of completion of infusion. Signs/symptoms may include: Allergic reaction/hypersensitivity (including drug fever); Arthralgia (joint pain); Bronchospasm; Cough; Dizziness; Dyspnea (shortness of breath); Fatigue (asthenia, lethargy, malaise); Headache; Hypertension; Hypotension; Myalgia (muscle pain); Nausea; Pruritus/itching; Rash/desquamation; Rigors/chills; Sweating (diaphoresis); Tachycardia; Tumor pain (onset or exacerbation of tumor pain due to treatment); Urticaria (hives, welts, wheals); Vomiting.						
ALSO CONSIDER: Allergic reaction/hypersensitivity (including drug fever); Bronchospasm, wheezing; Dyspnea (shortness of breath); Hypertension; Hypotension; Hypoxia; Prolonged QTc interval; Supraventricular and nodal arrhythmia – *Select*; Ventricular arrhythmia – *Select*.						
NAVIGATION NOTE: Disseminated intravascular coagulation (DIC) is graded in the COAGULATION CATEGORY.						
NAVIGATION NOTE: Fanconi's syndrome is graded as Urinary electrolyte wasting (e.g., Fanconi's syndrome, renal tubular acidosis) in the RENAL/GENITOURINARY CATEGORY.						
Flu-like syndrome	Flu-like syndrome	Symptoms present but not interfering with function	Moderate or causing difficulty performing some ADL	Severe symptoms interfering with ADL	Disabling	Death
REMARK: Flu-like syndrome represents a constellation of symptoms which may include cough with catarrhal symptoms, fever, headache, malaise, myalgia, prostration, and is to be used when the symptoms occur in a cluster consistent with one single pathophysiological process.						
NAVIGATION NOTE: Renal tubular acidosis is graded as Urinary electrolyte wasting (e.g., Fanconi's syndrome, renal tubular acidosis) in the RENAL/GENITOURINARY CATEGORY.						

(continued)

Appendix 2 *(Continued)*

SYNDROMES						
		Grade				
Adverse Event	**Short Name**	**1**	**2**	**3**	**4**	**5**
Retinoic acid syndrome	Retinoic acid syndrome	Fluid retention; less than 3 kg of weight gain; intervention with fluid restriction and/or diuretics indicated	Mild to moderate signs/symptoms; steroids indicated	Severe signs/symptoms; hospitalization indicated	Life-threatening; ventilatory support indicated	Death
REMARK: Patients with acute promyelocytic leukemia may experience a syndrome similar to "retinoic acid syndrome" in association with other agents such as arsenic trioxide. The syndrome is usually manifested by otherwise unexplained fever, weight gain, respiratory distress, pulmonary infiltrates and/or pleural effusion, with or without leukocytosis.						
ALSO CONSIDER: Acute vascular leak syndrome; Pleural effusion (nonmalignant); Pneumonitis/pulmonary infiltrates.						
NAVIGATION NOTE: SIADH is graded as Neuroendocrine: ADH secretion abnormality (e.g., SIADH or low ADH) in the ENDOCRINE CATEGORY.						
NAVIGATION NOTE: Stevens-Johnson syndrome is graded as Rash: erythema multiforme (e.g., Stevens-Johnson syndrome, toxic epidermal necrolysis) in the DERMATOLOGY/SKIN CATEGORY.						
NAVIGATION NOTE: Thrombotic microangiopathy is graded as Thrombotic microangiopathy (e.g., thrombotic thrombocytopenic purpura [TTP] or hemolytic uremic syndrome [HUS]) in the COAGULATION CATEGORY.						
Tumor flare	Tumor flare	Mild pain not interfering with function	Moderate pain; pain or analgesics interfering with function, but not interfering with ADL	Severe pain; pain or analgesics interfering with function and interfering with ADL	Disabling	Death

(continued)

SYNDROMES						
		Grade				
Adverse Event	**Short Name**	**1**	**2**	**3**	**4**	**5**
REMARK: Tumor flare is characterized by a constellation of signs and symptoms in direct relation to initiation of therapy (e.g., anti-estrogens/androgens or additional hormones). The symptoms/signs include tumor pain, inflammation of visible tumor, hypercalcemia, diffuse bone pain, and other electrolyte disturbances.						
ALSO CONSIDER: Calcium, serum-high (hypercalcemia).						
Tumor lysis syndrome	Tumor lysis syndrome	—	—	Present	—	Death
ALSO CONSIDER: Creatinine; Potassium, serum-high (hyperkalemia).						
Syndromes – Other (Specify, _______)	Syndromes – Other (Specify)	Mild	Moderate	Severe	Life-threatening; disabling	Death

VASCULAR						
		Grade				
Adverse Event	**Short Name**	**1**	**2**	**3**	**4**	**5**
Acute vascular leak syndrome	Acute vascular leak syndrome	—	Symptomatic, fluid support not indicated	Respiratory compromise or fluids indicated	Life-threatening; pressor support or ventilatory support indicated	Death
Peripheral arterial ischemia	Peripheral arterial ischemia	—	Brief (<24 hrs) episode of ischemia managed nonsurgically and without permanent deficit	Recurring or prolonged (≥24 hrs) and/or invasive intervention indicated	Life-threatening, disabling and/or associated with end organ damage (e.g., limb loss)	Death

(continued)

Appendix 2 *(Continued)*

VASCULAR						
		Grade				
Adverse Event	**Short Name**	**1**	**2**	**3**	**4**	**5**
Phlebitis (including superficial thrombosis)	Phlebitis	—	Present	—	—	—
ALSO CONSIDER: Injection site reaction/extravasation changes.						
Portal vein flow	Portal flow	—	Decreased portal vein flow	Reversal/retrograde portal vein flow	—	—
Thrombosis/embolism (vascular access-related)	Thrombosis/embolism (vascular access)	—	Deep vein thrombosis or cardiac thrombosis; intervention (e.g., anticoagulation, lysis, filter, invasive procedure) not indicated	Deep vein thrombosis or cardiac thrombosis; intervention (e.g., anticoagulation, lysis, filter, invasive procedure) indicated	Embolic event including pulmonary embolism or life-threatening thrombus	Death
Thrombosis/thrombus/embolism	Thrombosis/thrombus/embolism	—	Deep vein thrombosis or cardiac thrombosis; intervention (e.g., anticoagulation, lysis, filter, invasive procedure) not indicated	Deep vein thrombosis or cardiac thrombosis; intervention (e.g., anticoagulation, lysis, filter, invasive procedure) indicated	Embolic event including pulmonary embolism or life-threatening thrombus	Death

(continued)

VASCULAR

		Grade				
Adverse Event	**Short Name**	**1**	**2**	**3**	**4**	**5**
Vessel injury-artery – *Select*: – Aorta – Carotid – Extremity-lower – Extremity-upper – Other NOS – Visceral	Artery injury – *Select*	Asymptomatic diagnostic finding; intervention not indicated	Symptomatic (e.g., claudication); not interfering with ADL; repair or revision not indicated	Symptomatic interfering with ADL; repair or revision indicated	Life-threatening; disabling; evidence of end organ damage (e.g., stroke, MI, organ or limb loss)	Death
NAVIGATION NOTE: Vessel injury to an artery intra-operatively is graded as Intra-operative injury – *Select Organ or Structure* in the SURGERY/INTRA-OPERATIVE INJURY CATEGORY.						
Vessel injury-vein – *Select*: – Extremity-lower – Extremity-upper – IVC – Jugular – Other NOS – SVC – Viscera	Vein injury – *Select*	Asymptomatic diagnostic finding; intervention not indicated	Symptomatic (e.g., claudication); not interfering with ADL; repair or revision not indicated	Symptomatic interfering with ADL; repair or revision indicated	Life-threatening; disabling; evidence of end organ damage	Death
NAVIGATION NOTE: Vessel injury to a vein intra-operatively is graded as Intra-operative injury – *Select Organ or Structure* in the SURGERY/INTRA-OPERATIVE INJURY CATEGORY.						
Visceral arterial ischemia (non-myocardial)	Visceral arterial ischemia	—	Brief (<24 hrs) episode of ischemia	Prolonged (≥24 hrs) or recurring	Life-threatening; disabling;	Death

(continued)

Appendix 2 *(Continued)*

VASCULAR						
			Grade			
Adverse Event	**Short Name**	**1**	**2**	**3**	**4**	**5**
			managed medically and without permanent deficit	symptoms and/or invasive intervention indicated	evidence of end organ damage	
ALSO CONSIDER: CNS cerebrovascular ischemia.						
Vascular – Other (Specify, _______)	Vascular – Other (Specify)	Mild	Moderate	Severe	Life-threatening; disabling	Death

[1] Drug-induced ototoxicity should be distinguished from age-related threshold decrements or unrelated cochlear insult. When considering whether an adverse event has occurred, it is first necessary to classify the patient into one of two groups: (1) The patient is under standard treatment/enrolled in a clinical trial <2.5 years, and has a 15 dB or greater threshold shift averaged across two contiguous frequencies; or (2) The patient is under standard treatment/enrolled in a clinical trial >2.5 years, and the difference between the expected age-related and the observed threshold shifts is 15 dB or greater averaged across two contiguous frequencies. Consult standard references for appropriate age- and gender-specific hearing norms, e.g., Morrell et al. Age- and Gender-specific Reference Ranges for Hearing Level and Longitudinal Changes in Hearing Level. *Journal of the Acoustical Society of America* 100:1949–1967, 1996; or Shotland, et al. Recommendations for Cancer Prevention Trials Using Potentially Ototoxic Test Agents. *Journal of Clinical Oncology* 19:1658–1663, 2001.
In the absence of a baseline prior to initial treatment, subsequent audiograms should be referenced to an appropriate database of normals. ANSI. (1996) American National Standard: Determination of occupational noise exposure and estimation of noise-induced hearing impairment, ANSI S 3.44-1996. (Standard S 3.44). New York: American National Standards Institute. The recommended ANSI S3.44 database is Annex B.

[2] NHLBI Obesity Task Force. Clinical Guidelines on the Identification, Evaluation, and Treatment of Overweight and Obesity in Adults, *The Evidence Report,* Obes Res 6:51S–209S, 1998.

[3] Sloan JA, Loprinzi CL, Novotny PJ, Barton DL, Lavasseur BI, Windschitl HJ. Methodologic Lessons Learned from Hot Flash Studies, *J Clin Oncol* 2001; 19(23):4280–90.

[4] Crit Rev Clin Lab Sci 1984;21(1):51–97.

[5] Adapted from the International SFTR Method of Measuring and Recording Joint Motion, International Standard Orthopedic Measurements (ISOM), Jon J. Gerhardt and Otto A.

[6] Assessment of Fracture Risk and its Application to Screening for Postmenopausal Osteoporosis, Report of a *WHO Study Group Technical Report Series*, No. 843, 1994, v + 129.

[7] Folstein MF, Folstein SE, and McHugh PR 1975; Mini-Mental State: A Practical Method for Grading the State of Patients for the Clinician, *Journal of Psychiatric Research*, 12:189–198.

Index

Note: Page numbers followed by f indicate figures; those followed by t indicate tables. Generic drug names are in boldface type.

abarelix for injectable suspension (Plenaxis), 40–42
ABC Pack (**moxifloxacin**), 999–1001
Abelcet (**amphotericin B lipid complex**), 1038–1042
ABX-EGF (**panitumumab**), 560–564
Acephen (**acetaminophen**), 628–629
Acetaminophen (Acephen, Actamin, Anacin-3, Apacet, Anesin, Dapa, Datril, Genapap, Genebs, Gentabs, Halenol, Liquiprin, Meda Cap, Panadol, Panex, Suppap, Tempra, Tenol, Ty Caps, Tylenol), 628–629
Actamin (**acetaminophen**), 628–629
Actimmune (**interferon gamma**), 359–362
Actinomycin D (**dactinomycin**), 122–125
Actiq (**fentanyl citrate**), 667–670
Acyclovir (Zovirax), 1078–1081
Adjuvant agents, 620–627
Adjuvant analgesics, 621
Adrenocorticoids, 23
adrenocorticoids, 42–46
Adriamycin (**doxorubicin hydrochloride**), 144–148
Adrucil (**5-fluorouracil**), 176–179
Advil (**ibuprofen**), 642–645
Aldara® (**Imiquimod, 5% topical cream**), 349–351
aldesleukin (Interleukin-2), 334–339
Aldesleukin (Proleukin), 334–339
Alemtuzumab (campath-1H anti-CD52 Monoclonal Antibody, Humanized IgG1 MoAb), 471–475
Alitretinoin gel 0.1% (Panretin®), 475–476
Alkeran (**melphalan hydrochloride**), 223–226
Alkylating Agents, 13, 26, 29
All-Trans-Retinoic Acid Liposomal (**liposomal tretinoin**), 605–610
All-Trans-Retinoic Acid (**tretinoin**), 602–605
allopurinol sodium (Aloprim, Zyloprim, Zurinol), 410–413
Aloprim (**allopurinol sodium**), 410–413
Aloxi (**palonosetron**), 746–748
alpha-2ndashInterferon (**interferon alfa-2b**), 355–359
Alpha interferon (**interferon alfa**), 351–355
Alprazolam (Xanax), 773–775
altretamine (Hexalen, Hexamethylmelamine), 46–48
Ambien (**zolpidem tartrate**), 842–843
Ambisome (**amphotericin B lipid complex**), 1051–1055
Amethopterin (**methotrexate**), 228–231
amifostine for injection (Ethyol, WR-2721), 413–416
Amikacin sulfate (Amikin), 880–883
aminoglutethimide (Cytadren, Elipten), 48–50
Aminopenicillins, 875
Amitriptyline hydrochloride (Elavil), 775–778
Amoxicillin (Amoxil, Polymox, Trimox, Wymox), 884–887

Amoxicillin plus clavulanic acid (Augmentin), 884–887
Amoxil (**amoxicillin**), 884–887
Amphotec (**amphotericin B lipid complex**), 1051–1055
Amphotericin B cholesteryl sulfate complex (**amphotericin B lipid complex**), 1051–1055
Amphotericin B (Fungizone), 1051–1055
Amphotericin B lipid complex (Abelcet, Ambisome, Amphotec, Amphotericin B), 1051–1055
Ampicillin sodium/sulbactam sodium (UNASYN), 887–890
Amrubicin, 51–52
Anacin-3 (**acetaminophen**), 628–629
Anaphylactic reactions, management of, 24–25
anastrozole (Arimidex), 52–54
Ancef (**cefazolin sodium**), 906–910
Ancobon (**flucytosine**), 1061–1063
Androgens, 23
androgens, 55–56
Anergan (**promethazine hydrochloride**), 751–753
Anesin (**acetaminophen**), 628–629
Angiogenesis, 446–451
Anidulafungin (Eraxis), 1055–1057
Anorexia and Cachexia, 756–765
Anspor (**cephradine**), 950–953
antineoplastic drugs, mechanism of action of, 2
Antineoplastic Treatment Agonists, 385–405
Anxiety and Depression, 766–843
Anzemet (**dolasetron mesylate**), 728–731
Apacet (**acetaminophen**), 628–629
Aprepitant (Emend®), 721–723
Ara-C (**cytarabine, cytosine arabinoside**), 113–117
Aranesp (**darbepoetin alfa**), 339–344
Aredia (**pamidronate disodium**), 861–864
Arimidex (**anastrozole**), 52–54
Aromasin (**exemestane**), 169–171
Arranon (**nelarabine**), 239–243
arsenic trioxide (Trisenox), 56–63
ASA (**aspirin, acetylsalicylic acid**), 629–631
asparaginase (Elspar), 63–66
Aspergum (**aspirin, acetylsalicylic acid**), 629–631
Aspirin, acetylsalicylic acid (ASA, Aspergum, Bayer Aspirin, Easprin, Ecotrin, Empirin), 629–631
Assessment guidelines, prechemotherapy, 2, 4–11, 11
Astramorph (**morphine**), 690–695
Ativan (**lorazepam**), 814–817
Atragen® (**liposomal tretinoin**), 605–610
ATRA (**tretinoin**), 602–605
Atropine and diphenoxylate hydrochloride (Lomotil), 1114–1115
Augmentin (**amoxicillin plus clavulanic acid**), 884–887
Avastin (**bevacizumab**), 478–486
Avelox (**moxifloxacin**), 1013–1016
Aventyl (**nortriptyline hydrochloride**), 824–826
Avinza (**morphine**), 690–695
Axitinib, 477–478
Azactam (**aztreonam**), 892–895
5-azacytidine (Vidaza), 66–69
AZD2171 (**cediranib, Recentin**), 497–498
Azithromycin (Zithromax), 890–891
Aztreonam (Azactam), 892–895

Bactocill (**oxacillin sodium**), 1019–1022
Bactrim (**co-trimoxazole**), 962–966
Bactrim DS (**co-trimoxazole**), 962–966
Bayer Aspirin (**aspirin, acetylsalicylic acid**), 629–631
BCNU (**carmustine**), 93–96
BCNU with polifeprosan 20 implant (Gliadel®), 272–275
Benadryl (**diphenhydramine hydrochloride**), 726–728

bendamustine hydrochloride (Treanda,), 69–73
Bevacizumab (Avastin), 478–486
Bexarotene (Targretin), 486–491
Bexxar™ (**tositumomab**), 589–593
Biaxin (**clarithromycin**), 956–959
Biaxin XL (**clarithromycin**), 956–959
bicalutamide (Casodex), 73–74
BiCNU (**carmustine**), 93–96
Biocef (**cephalexin**), 946–948
Biologic Response Modifier Therapy, 329–384
Bisacodyl (Dulcolax), 1096–1097
Blenoxane (**bleomycin sulfate**), 75–78
bleomycin sulfate (Blenoxane), 75–78
Blood cells, development of, 870
Bortezomib (Velcade), 441–445
Bupropion hydrochloride (Wellbutrin), 778–781
Buspirone hydrochloride (BuSpar), 781–782
busulfan for injection (Busulfex), 80–87
busulfan (Myleran), 78–80
Busulfex (**busulfan for injection**), 80–87

Calcimar (**calcitonin-salmon**), 851–853
Calcitonin-salmon (Calcimar, Miacalcin), 851–853
Calcium, ionized serum, 847
Calcium channel blockers, 957
Campath-1H (Anti-CD52 Monoclonal Antibody, Humanized IgG1 MoAb), 471–475
Camptosar (**irinotecan**), 201–205
Camptothecins, 1319
Cancidas (**caspofungin**), 1057–1058
capecitabine (Xeloda, N4-Pentoxycarbonyl-5-deoxy-5-fluorocytidine), 86–89
Carbenicillin indanyl sodium (Geocillin, Geopen), 895–898
carboplatin (Paraplatin), 89–92
Carcinogenicity, 21
Cardiovascular system prechemotherapy nursing assessment guidelines for, 11, 18
carmustine (BCNU, BiCNU), 93–97
Casodex (**bicalutamide**), 73–74
Casopitant, 723–724
Caspofungin (Cancidas), 1057–1058
CCNU (**lomustine**), 217–219
2-CdA (**cladribine**), 103–107
Ceclor (**cefaclor**), 898–901
Cedax (**ceftibuten**), 939–941
Cediranib (Recentin, AZD2171), 497–499
CeeNU (**lomustine**), 217–219
Cefaclor (Ceclor), 898–901
Cefadroxil (Duracef), 900–902
Cefadyl (**cephapirin**), 948–950
Cefamandole nafate (Mandol), 902–906
Cefazolin sodium (Ancef), 906–909
Cefdinir (Omnicef), 910–913
Cefditoren pivoxil (Spectracef), 913–914
Cefepime (Maxipime), 914–917
Cefixime (Suprax), 917–920
Cefobid (**cefoperazone sodium**), 920–922
Cefoperazone sodium (Cefobid), 920–922
Cefotan (**cefotetan**), 926–928
Cefotaxime sodium (Claforan), 928–931
Cefotetan (Cefotan), 926–928
Cefoxitin sodium (Mefoxin), 928–932
Cefpodoxime proxetil (Vantin), 932–934
Cefprozil (Cefzil), 933–935
Ceftazidime (Fortaz, Tazicef, Tazidime), 935–938
Ceftibuten (Cedax), 939–941
Ceftin (**cefuroxime**), 944–946
Ceftriaxone sodium (Rocephin), 941–944
Cefuroxime (Ceftin; Kefurox; Zinacef), 944–946
Cefzil (**cefprozil**), 933–935
Celebrex (**celecoxib**), 631–635
Celecoxib (Celebrex), 631–635
Celexa® (**citalopram hydrobromide**), 783–787
Cell Biology, 426–432

Cell communication, 432–435
Cell cycle nonspecific agents, 13
Cell cycle specific agents, 12
Cephalexin (Biocef; Keflex; Keftab), 946–948
Cephalosporins, 873, 881
Cephapirin (Cefadyl; Cephapirin Sodium), 948–950
Cephapirin Sodium (**cephapirin**), 948–950
Cephradine (Anspor, Velosef), 950–953
Cerubidine (**daunorubicin hydrochloride**), 128–132
Cesamet (**nabilone**), 742–744
Cetuximab (Erbitux), 498–505
Chemotherapeutic agents, mechanism of action of, 23, 40
Chemotherapy agents, 385
chlorambucil (Leukeran), 96–98
Chlorotrianisene (Tace), 162–164
Cholac (**lactulose**), 1100–1101
Choline magnesium trisalicylate (Trilisate), 635–636
Chromic phosphate P32 suspension (Phosphocoltrade P32), 387–389
Cidofovir (Vistide), 1081–1084
Cinacalcet HCl (Sensipar), 853–856
Cipro (**ciprofloxacin**), 953–956
Ciprofloxacin (Cipro), 953–956
cisplatin (Platinol), 98–103
Citalopram hydrobromide (Celexa®), 783–787
Citrovorum factor (**leucovorin calcium**), 397–399
Citrucel (**methylcellulose**), 1102–1103
cladribine (Leustatin, 2-CdA), 103–107
Claforan (**cefotaxime sodium**), 923–926
Clarithromycin (Biaxin; Biaxin XL), 956–961
Cleocin (**clindamycin phosphate**), 959–961
Clindamycin phosphate (Cleocin), 959–961
clofarabine (Clolar), 107–110
Clolar (clofarabine), 107–110
Clonazepam (Klonopin), 786–789
Clonidine hydrochloride (Duraclon), 637–640
Co-trimoxazole (Bactrim, Bactrim DS, Cotrim, Septra), 962–966
Codaphen [Odalan] (**codeine/acetaminophen**), 660–664
Codeine (Capital and Codeine, Codaphen [Odalan], Phenaphen with Codeine, Tylenol with Codeine), 660–664
Codeine phosphate, 660–664
Codeine sulfate, 660–664
Colace (**docusate calcium, docusate potassium, docusate sodium**), 1097–1098
Compazine (**prochlorperazine**), 749–751
Constilac (**lactulose**), 1100–1101
Constipation, 1095–1110
Constulose (**lactulose**), 1100–1101
Corticosteroids, for pain management, 621
Cortisone (**adrenocorticoids**), 42–46
Cosmegen (**dactinomycin**), 122–125
Cotrim (**co-trimoxazole**), 962–966
Cubicin (**daptomycin**), 966–967
cyclophosphamide (Cytoxan), 109–113
Cymbalta (**duloxetine hydrochloride**), 802–805
Cytadren (**aminoglutethimide**), 48–50
cytarabine, cytosine arabinoside (Ara-C, Cytosar-U), 113–117
cytarabine, liposome injection (DepoCyt), 117–119
Cytoprotective Agents, 406–424
Cytosar-U (**cytarabine, cytosine arabinoside**), 113–117
Cytostatic effects, 2
Cytovene (**ganciclovir**), 1089–1093
Cytoxan (**cyclophosphamide**), 109–113

D6474 (**vandetanib**), 610–611
dacarbazine (DTIC-Dome, Dimethyl-triazeno-imidazole-carboximide), 119–122
Dacogen (**decitabine**), 131–134
dactinomycin (Actinomycin D, Cosmegen), 122–125

Dalfopristin and quinupristin (Synercid), 1029–1031
Dapa (**acetaminophen**), 628–629
Daptomycin (Cubicin), 966–967
darbepoetin alfa (Aranesp), 339, 339–344
Dasatinib (Sprycel, BMS354825), 506–510
Datril (**acetaminophen**), 628–629
Daunomycin HCl (**daunorubicin hydrochloride**), 128–131
daunorubicin citrate liposome injection (DaunoXome), 125–128
daunorubicin hydrochloride (Cerubidine, Daunomycin HCl, Rubidomycin), 128–131
DaunoXome (**daunorubicin citrate liposome injection**), 125–128
Decadron (**dexamethasone**), 724–726
decitabine (Dacogen, 5-aza-2prime-deoxycytidine), 131–134
Declomycin (**demeclocycline hydrochloride**), 967–969
Deferasirox tablets for oral suspension (Exjade), 389–394
Demeclocycline hydrochloride (Declomycin), 967–969
Demerol (**meperidine hydrochloride**), 682–686
4-Demethoxydaunorubicin (**idarubicin**), 195–198
Denileukin diftitox (ONTAK®), 511–516
Denosumab, 855–856
Deodorized tincture of opium (DTO, Laudanum), 1099–1100
2-deoxycoformycin (**pentostatin**), 269–272
Depo-Provera (**medroxyprogesterone acetate**), 279–280
DepoCyt (**cytarabine, liposome injection**), 118–119
Desacetylvinblastine (**vindesine**), 321–324
DES (**diethylstilbestrol**), 164–166
Desipramine hydrochloride (Norpramin, Pertofrane), 789–792
Desvenlafaxine, 792–796
Desyrel (**trazodone hydrochloride**), 835–837
Dexamethasone (**adrenocorticoids**), 42–46
Dexamethasone (Decadron), 724–726
dexrazoxane for injection (Zinecard), 419–420
dexrazoxane for injection, extravasation, 416–420
Diarrhea, 1097–1108
Diazepam (Valium), 797–799
Dicloxacillin sodium (Dycill, Dynapen, Pathocil), 969–972
Didronel (**etidronate disodium**), 834–835
diethylstilbestrol (DES), 162–164
Diflucan (**fluconazole**), 1059–1061
Difluorodeoxycitidine (**gemcitabine hydrochlorid**), 183–187
Dihydropyrimidine dehydrogenase inhibitory fluoropyrimidines, 154
Dilaudid (**hydromorphone**), 674–678
Dimethyl-triazeno-imidazole-carboximide (**dacarbazine**), 119–122
Diocto-K (**docusate calcium, docusate potassium, docusate sodium**), 1097–1098
Diosuccin (**docusate calcium, docusate potassium, docusate sodium**), 1097–1098
Diphenhydramine hydrochloride (Benadryl), 726–728
Diphenoxylate hydrochloride and atropine (Lomotil), 1100–1101
Disalcid (**salsalate**), 654–656
docetaxel (Taxotere), 135–144
Docusate calcium, docusate potassium, docusate sodium (Dioctyl Calcium Sulfosuccinate, Dioctyl Potassium Sulfosuccinate, Dioctyl Sodium Sulfosuccinate, Colace, Diocto-K, Diosuccin, DOK-250, Doxinate, Duosol, Laxinate 100, Regulax SS, Stulex), 1097–1098

Dolasetron mesylate (Anzemet), 728–731
Dolophine (**methadone**), 686–690
Doryx (**doxycycline hyclate**), 972–975
Doxepin hydrochloride (Sinequan), 799–802
Doxil (**doxorubicin hydrochloride liposome injection**), 148–153
Doxinate (**docusate calcium, docusate potassium, docusate sodium**), 1097–1098
doxorubicin hydrochloride (Adriamycin), 144–148
doxorubicin hydrochloride liposome injection (Doxil), 148–153
Doxycycline hyclate (Vibramycin, Doryx, MonoDox), 972–975
Dronabinol (Marinol), 731–732, 759–760
Droperidol (Inapsine), 732–733
Droxia (**hydroxyurea**), 192–195
drugs causing, 729
DTIC-Dome (**dacarbazine**), 119–122
DTO (**deodorized tincture of opium**), 1099–1100
Dulcolax (**bisacodyl**), 1096–1097
Duloxetine hydrochloride (Cymbalta), 802–805
Duosol (**docusate calcium, docusate potassium, docusate sodium**), 1097–1098
Duphalac (**lactulose**), 1100–1101
Duracef (**cefadroxil**), 900–902
Duraclon (**clonidine hydrochloride**), 637–639
Duragesic (**fentanyl transdermal system**), 670–674
Duramorph (**morphine**), 691–696
Dycill (**dicloxacillin sodium**), 969–972
Dynacin (**minocycline hydrochloride**), 1010–1013
Dynapen (**dicloxacillin sodium**), 969–972

E-Mycin (**erythromycin**), 962–965
Easprin (**aspirin, acetylsalicylic acid**), 629–631
Ecotrin (**aspirin, acetylsalicylic acid**), 629–631
Efaproxiral (Efaproxyn, RSR13), 405–406
Efaproxyn (**efaproxiral**), 405–406
Effexor (**venlafaxine hydrochloride**), 837–841
Efudex (**5-fluorouracil**), 176–179
Elavil (**amitriptyline hydrochloride**), 775–778
Eldisine (**vindesine**), 321–324
Elesclomol, 516–518
Elipten (**aminoglutethimide**), 48–50
Ellence (**epirubicin hydrochloride**), 155–160
Eloxatin (**oxaliplatin**), 245–249
Elspar (**asparaginase**), 63–66
Emcyt (**estramustine**), 160–162
Emend® (**aprepitant**), 721–723
Empirin (**aspirin, acetylsalicylic acid**), 629–631
Empirin with Codeine (**codeine/aspirin**, 660–663
Endodan (**oxycodone**), 695–699
eniluracil (776C85), 153–155
Eosinophils, 869, 871
epirubicin hydrochloride (Ellence, Farmorubicin(e), Farmorubicina, Pharmorubicin), 155–160
epoetin alfa (Epogen, Erythropoietin, Procrit), 344–347
Epogen (**epoetin alfa**), 344–347
Equianalgesic dose tablets, 623
Eraxis (**anidulafungin**), 1055–1056
Erbitux (**cetuximab**), 498–506
Ergamisol (**levamisole hydrochloride**), 362–364
Erlotinib (OSI-774, Tarcevatrade), 518–521
Ertapenem sodium (Invanz), 975–976
Erythrocin (**erythromycin**), 977–980
Erythromycin (ERYC, E-Mycin, Ilotycin, Erythrocin), 977–980
Erythropoietin (**epoetin alfa**), 344–347
Escitalalopram oxalate (Lexapro), 805–808
Esorubicin, 34
Estinyl (**ethinyl estradiol**), 162–164
Estracyte (**estramustine**), 160–162
estramustine (Emcyt), 160–162
estramustine (Estracyte, Emcyt), 160–162

estrogen, conjugated (Premarin), 162–164
Estrogens, 23
estrogens, 162–164
Etanidazole, 407–408
ethinyl estradiol (Estinyl), 162–164, 165–169
Ethyol (**amifostine for injection**), 413–416
Etidronate disodium (Didronel), 856–857
Etopophos (**etoposide**), 165–169
etoposide (VP-16, VePesid, Etopophos), 165–169
Eulexin (**flutamide**), 179–180
Everolimus, 521–524
exemestane (Aromasin), 169–171
Exjade (**deferasirox tablets for oral suspension**), 389–394
Extended-spectrum penicillins, 875, 881
Extravasation, 23

Factive (**gemifloxacin mesylate**), 983–985
Famciclovir (Famvir), 1084–1085
Famvir (**famciclovir**), 1084–1085
Fareston (**toremifene citrate**), 306–308
Farmorubicina (**epirubicin hydrochloride**), 155–160
Farmorubicin(e) (**epirubicin hydrochloride**), 155–160
Faslodex (**fulvestrant injection**), 180–183
Femara (**letrozole**), 213–214
Fentanyl buccal tablet (Fentora), 663–667
Fentanyl citrate (Oral Transmucosal Fentanyl, Actiq), 667–670
Fentanyl transdermal system (Duragesic), 670–674
Fentora (**fentanyl buccal tablet**), 663–667
filgrastim (Neupogen, G-CSF), 348–349
Fiorinal with Codeine (**codeine/aspirin**), 660–663
Flagyl (**metronidazole hydrochloride**), 1003–1006
Fleet Babylax (**glycerin suppository**), 1099–1100
Fleet Mineral Oil (**mineral oil**), 1105–1106
floxuridine (FUDR, 2prime-Deoxy-5-fluorouridine), 171–174
Fluconazole (Diflucan), 1059–1061
Flucytosine (Ancobon), 1061–1063
fludarabine phosphate (Fludara), 174–176
Fludara (**fludarabine phosphate**), 174–176
5-fluorouracil (Fluorouracil, Adrucil, 5-FU, Efudex), 179–181
Fluosol DA (20%), 396–397
Fluoxetine hydrochloride (Prozac), 808–811
flutamide (Eulexin), 179–180
Folex (**methotrexate**), 228–231
Folinic factor (**leucovorin calcium**), 397–399
Fortaz (**ceftazidime**), 935–939
Fosaprepitant, 734–736
Foscarnet sodium (Foscavir), 1086–1089
Foscavir (**foscarnet sodium**), 1086–1089
Fourth-generation cephalosporins, 876
5-FU (**5-fluorouracil**), 179–181
FUDR (**floxuridine**), 171–174
fulvestrant injection (Faslodex), 180–183
Furosemide (Lasix), 858–860

G-CSF (**filgrastim**), 348–349
Gabapentin (Neurontin), 639–642
Gallium nitrate (Ganite), 860–861
Ganciclovir (Cytovene), 1089–1093
Ganite (**gallium nitrate**), 860–861
Garamycin (**gentamicin sulfate**), 986–989
Gardasil (**quadrivalent human papillomavirus**), 566–567
Gastrointestinal system prechemotherapy nursing assessment guidelines for, 11, 18
Gatifloxacin (Tequin), 980–983
Gefitinib (Iressa), 524–528
gemcitabine hydrochloride (Gemzar, Difluorodeoxycitidine), 183–187
Gemifloxacin mesylate (Factive), 983–985
Gemtuzumab ozogamicin for injection (Mylotarg), 528–532

Gemzar (**gemcitabine hydrochloride**), 183–187
Genapap (**acetaminophen**), 628–629
Genebs (**acetaminophen**), 628–629
Genitourinary system prechemotherapy nursing assessment guidelines for, 11, 18
Genpril (**ibuprofen**), 642–645
Gentabs (**acetaminophen**), 628–629
Gentamicin (**gentamicin sulfate**), 986–989
Gentamicin sulfate (Garamycin, Gentamicin), 986–989
Geocillin (**carbenicillin indanyl sodium**), 895–897
Geopen (**carbenicillin indanyl sodium**), 895–897
Gleevec (**imatinib mesylate**), 536–541
Gliadelreg (**polifeprosan 20 with carmustine (BCNU) implant**), 272–275
glutamine, 420–421
Glycerin suppository (Fleet Babylax, Sani-Supp), 1099–1100
GM-CSF (**sargramostim**), 375–377
goserelin acetate (Zoladex), 187–190
Granisetron hydrochloride (Kytril), 736–738
Granisetron hydrochloride transdermal (Sancuso, investigational), 738–739

Haldol (**haloperidol**), 739–741
Halenol (**acetaminophen**), 628–629
Haloperidol (Haldol), 739–741
Haltran (**ibuprofen**), 642–645
Herceptin (**trastuzumab**), 594–599
Hexalen (**altretamine**), 46–48
Hexamethylmelamine (**altretamine**), 46–48
histrelin implant (Vantas), 190–192
Hormones, 22, 42
Humanized anti-*Her*-2 Antibody (**trastuzumab**), 594–599
Humanized IgG1 MoAb (**alemtuzumab**), 471–475
Hycamtin (**topotecan hydrochloride for injection**), 302–306
Hydrea (**hydroxyurea**), 192–195
Hydrocodone (Lorcet, Lortab, Vicodin), 625
Hydrocortisone (**adrenocorticoids**), 42–46
Hydromorphone (Dilaudid), 674–678
hydroxyurea (Hydrea, Droxia), 192–195
Hypercalcemia, 846–868
Hypersensitivity reactions, 22–23
Hypoxic cell sensitizers, 385

I^{131} tositumomab (Bexxar™), 589–593
Ibuprin (**ibuprofen**), 642–645
Ibuprofen (Advil, Genpril, Haltran, Ibuprin, Midol 200, Nuprin, Rufen), 642–645
Idamycin (**idarubicin**), 195–198
idarubicin (Idamycin, 4-Demethoxydaunorubicin), 195–198
Ifex (**ifosfamide**), 198–201
IFN-alpha-2b Recombinant (**interferon alfa-2b**), 351–355
IFN-gamma (**interferon gamma**), 359–362
IFN (**interferon alfa**), 351–355
ifosfamide (Ifex), 198–201
Ilotycin (**erythromycin**), 977–980
Imatinib mesylate (Gleevec, STI 571), 536–541
Imipenem/cilastatin sodium (Primaxin), 989–992
Imipramine pamoate (Tofranil-PM), 812–814
Imiquimod, 5% topical cream (Aldarareg), 349–351
Imodium (**loperamide hydrochloride**), 1116–1117
Inapsine (**droperidol**), 732–733
Indocin (**indomethacin**), 645–648
Indocin SR (**indomethacin**), 645–648
Indomethacin (Indocin, Indocin SR, Indotech), 645–648
Indotech (**indomethacin**), 645–648
Infection, 869–922
Infumorph (**morphine**), 690–695

interferon alfa-2b (Intron A, IFN-alpha-2b Recombinant, alpha-2ndashInterferon, rIFN-alpha-2), 351–355
interferon alfa (Alpha interferon, IFN, Interferon alpha-2a, rIFN-A, Roferon A), 351–355
interferon alpha-2a (**interferon alfa**), 351–355355–359
interferon gamma (Actimmune, IFN-gamma, rIFN-gamma), 359–362
Interleukin-2 (Aldesleukin), 334–339
Intron A (**interferon alfa-2b**), 355–359
Invanz (**ertapenem sodium**), 975–976
Invasion, 444–446
Ipilimumab, 541–544
Iressa (**gefitinib**), 524–529
irinotecan (Camptosar, Camptothecan-11, CPT-11), 201–206
Irritants, 2629
Itraconazole (Sporanox), 1064–1066
ixabepilone (Ixempra), 206–209

K-Pek (**kaolin/pectin**), 1115–1116
Kadian Morphine Sulfate Sustained Release (**morphine**), 690–695
Kanamycin sulfate (Kantrex), 993–997
Kantrex (**kanamycin sulfate**), 993–997
Kaodene (**kaolin/pectin**), 1115–1116
Kaolin/pectin (Kaodene, K-P, Kaopectate, K-Pek), 1115–1116
Kaopectate (**kaolin/pectin**), 1115–1116
Keflex (**cephalexin**), 946–948
Keftab (**cephalexin**), 946–948
Kefurox (**cefuroxime**), 944–946
Kepivance (**palifermin**), 368–370
Ketek (**telithromycin**), 1036–1038
ketoconazole, 208–212
Ketoconazole (Nizoral), 1066–1068
Ketorolac tromethamine (Toradol), 648–651
Klonopin (**clonazepam**), 786–789
Kytril (**granisetron hydrochloride**), 736–737

L-PAM (**melphalan hydrochloride**), 223–226
L-Phenylalanine Mustard (**melphalan hydrochloride**), 223–226
L-Sarcolysin (**melphalan hydrochloride**), 223–226
Lactulose (Cholac, Constilac, Constulose, Duphalac), 1100–1101
Lapatinib ditosylate (Tykerb), 544–548
Lasix (**furosemide**), 858–860
Laudanum (**deodorized tincture of opium**), 1113
Laxatives, 1095–1096
Laxinate 100 (**docusate calcium, docusate potassium, docusate sodium**), 1097–1098
Lenalidomide (Revlimid), 548–554
letrozole (Femara), 213–214
Leucovorin calcium (Citrovorum Factor, Folinic Acid), 397–399
Leukeran (**chlorambucil**), 96–98
Leukine (**sargramostim**), 375–377
leuprolide acetate (Lupron, Viadur), 214–217
Leustatin (**cladribine**), 103–107
levamisole hydrochloride (Ergamisol), 362–364
Levaquin (**levofloxacin**), 996–999
Levo-Dromoran (**levorphanol tartrate opioid**), 678–682
Levofloxacin (Levaquin), 996–999
Levoleucovorin, 399–401
Levorphanol tartrate opioid (Levo-Dromoran), 678–682
Lexapro (**escitalalopram oxalate**), 805–808
Linezolid (Zyvox), 999–1001
LipoATRA (**liposomal tretinoin**), 605–610
Liposomal amphotericin B (**amphotericin B lipid complex**), 1051–1055
Liposomal tretinoin (Atragen®, All-Trans-Retinoic Acid Liposomal, AR-623, Lipo-ATRA, Tretinoin Liposomal), 605–610
Liquiprin (**acetaminophen**), 628–629

local tissue damage, 29
Lomotil (**diphenoxylate hydrochloride and atropine**), 1114–1115
lomustine (CCNU, CeeNU), 217–219
Loperamide hydrochloride (Imodium), 1116–1117
Lorazepam (Ativan), 814–817
Lorcet (**hydrocodone**), 625
Lortab (**hydrocodone**), 625
Lupron (**leuprolide acetate**), 214–217
Lyrica (**pregabalin**), 652–654
Lysodren (**mitotane**), 234–236

Magnesium citrate, 1101–1102
Malignant transformation, 435–443
management of, 730
Mandol (**cefamandole nafate**), 902–906
Marinol (**dronabinol**), 731–732, 759–760
Matulane (**procarbazine hydrochloride**), 275–278
Maxipime (**cefepime**), 914–917
mechlorethamine hydrochloride (Mustargen, Nitrogen Mustard, HN2), 219–222
Meda Cap (**acetaminophen**), 628–629
medroxyprogesterone acetate (Provera, Depo-Provera), 278–279
Mefoxin (**cefoxitin sodium**), 928–932
Megace (**megestrol acetate**), 760–762
megakaryocyte growth and development factor (MGDF), 364–365
Megestrol acetate (Megace), 760–762
melphalan hydrochloride (Alkeran, L-Phenylalanine Mustard, L-PAM, L-Sarcolysin), 223–226
Mepergan Fortis (**meperidine hydrochloride**), 682–686
Meperidine hydrochloride (Demerol, Mepergan Fortis), 673–677
mercaptopurine (Purinethol, 6-MP), 226–227
Meropenem (Merrem), 1001–1003
Merrem (**meropenem**), 1001–1003
mesna for injection (Mesnex), 421–423
Mesnex (**mesna for injection**), 421–423
Metastases, 444–446
Methadone (Dolophine, Methadose), 686–690
Methadose (**methadone**), 686–690
methotrexate (Amethopterin, Mexate, Folex), 228–231
Methylcellulose (Citrucel), 1102–1103
Methylnaltrexone bromide, 1104–1105
Methylprednisolone (**adrenocorticoids**), 42–46
Metoclopramide hydrochloride (Reglan), 741–742
Metronidazole hydrochloride (Flagyl), 1003–1006
Mexate (**methotrexate**), 228–231
Mezlin (**mezlocillin sodium**), 1006–1010
Mezlocillin sodium (Mezlin), 992–995
Miacalcin (**calcitonin-salmon**), 851–853
Micafungin sodium (Mycamine), 1068–1070
Miconazole nitrate (Monistat), 1070–1073
Midol 200 (**ibuprofen**), 642–645
Mineral oil (Fleet Mineral Oil), 1105–1106
Minocin (**minocycline hydrochloride**), 1010–1013
Minocycline hydrochloride (Minocin, Vectrin, Dynacin), 1010–1013
Miralax® (**polyethylene glycol 3350, NF powder**), 1106–1108
Mirtazapine (Remeron), 817–821
Mitomycin C (**mitomycin**), 231–234
mitomycin (Mitomycin C, Mutamycin, Mitozytrex), 231–234
mitotane (o, pprime-DDD, Lysodren), 234–236
mitoxantrone (Novantrone), 236–239
Modafinil (Provigil), 707–709
Molecularly Targeted Therapies, 425–618
Monistat (**miconazole nitrate**), 1070–1073
MonoDox (**doxycycline hyclate**), 972–975
Morphelan (**morphine**), 690–695
Morphine, 622

Morphine (Astramorph, Avinza, Duramorph, Infumorph, Kadian Morphine Sulfate Sustained Release, MS Contin, MSIR, Morphelan, Oramorph, Roxanol), 690–695
Moxifloxacin (ABC Pack; Avelox), 1013–1016
6-MP (**mercaptopurine**), 226–227
MS Contin (**morphine**), 690–695
MSIR (**morphine**), 690–695
Mustargen (**mechlorethamine hydrochloride**), 219–222
Mutagenic effects, 21
Mutagenicity, 21
Mutamycin (**mitomycin**), 231–234
Mycamine (**micafungin sodium**), 1068–1070
Mycostatin (**nystatin**), 1073–1074
Myleran (**busulfan**), 78–80
Mylotarg (**gemtuzumab ozogamicin for injection**), 528–532

Nabilone (Cesamet), 742–744
Nafcillin sodium (Unipen), 1016–1019
Narcotic analgesics, 732
Nausea and Vomiting, 710–755
Navelbine (**vinorelbine tartrate**), 324–328
Nebcin (**tobramycin sulfate**), 1044–1048
Nefazodone HCl (Serzone), 821–824
nelarabine (Arranon), 239–243
Neulasta (**pegfilgrastim**), 370–374
Neumega (**oprelvekin**), 365–368
Neupogen (**filgrastim**), 348–349
Neurontin (**gabapentin**), 639–642
Neurotoxicity, 406–409
Neutrexin (**trimetrexate**), 308–311
Neutrophils, 869
Nexavar (**sorafenib**), 572–576
Nilandron (**nilutamide**), 243–244
Nilotinib (Tasigna), 555–560
Nilstat (**nystatin**), 1073–1074
nilutamide (Nilandron), 243–244
Nipent (**pentostatin**), 269–272
Nitrogen Mustard (**mechlorethamine hydrochloride**), 219–222
Nizoral (**ketoconazole**), 1066–1068
Nolvadex (**tamoxifen citrate**), 288–291
Non-opiod Analegics, 628–629
Nonhypoxic cell sensitizers, 385
Norpramin (**desipramine hydrochloride**), 789–792
Nortriptyline hydrochloride (Aventyl, Pamelor), 824–826
Novantrone (**mitoxantrone**), 236–239
Noxafil (**posaconazole**), 1074–1076
Nplate, 374–375
Numorphan (**oxymorphone**), 625
Nuprin (**ibuprofen**), 642–645
nursing care plan, 33–35
Nystatin (Mycostatin, Nilstat), 1073–1074

o, pprime-DDD (**mitotane**), 234–236
Oblimersen sodium (Gentasense, G3139), 551–553
Octreotide acetate (Sandostatin), 1117–1121
Odalon (**codeine/acetaminophen**), 660–663
Omnicef (**cefdinir**), 910–912
Omnitarg (**pertuzumab**), 564–566
Oncovin (**vincristine**), 318–321
Ondansetron hydrochloride (Zofran), 744–746
ONTAK® (**denileukin diftitox**), 511–516
Opana ER (**oxymorphone hydrochloride extended release**), 702–707
Opana (**oxymorphone hydrochloride**), 699–702
oprelvekin (Neumega), 365–368
Oral Transmucosal Fentanyl (**fentanyl citrate**), 667–670
Oramorph (**morphine**), 690–695
Orathecin (**rubitecan**), 282–285
Oxacillin sodium (Bactocill, Prostaphlin), 1019–1022
oxaliplatin (Eloxatin), 245–249
Oxazepam (Serax), 827–829

Oxazolidinones, 877, 878
Oxycodone (Percodan, Endodan, Roxiprin), 695–699
Oxymorphone hydrochloride extended release (Opana ER), 702–707
Oxymorphone hydrochloride (Opana), 699–702

paclitaxel protein bound particles for injectable suspension, 257–261
paclitaxel (Taxol), 250–257
Pain, 620–709
palifermin (Kepivance), 368–370
Palonosetron (Aloxi, injection and capsules), 746–748
Pamelor (**nortriptyline hydrochloride**), 824–826
Pamidronate disodium (Aredia), 861–864
Panadol (**acetaminophen**), 628–629
Panex (**acetaminophen**), 616–618
Panitumumab (Vectibix, ABX-EGF), 560–564
Panretin® (**alitretinoin gel 0.1%**), 475–476
Paraplatin (**carboplatin**), 89–92
Paroxetine hydrochloride (Paxil), 829–832
Pathocil (**dicloxacillin sodium**), 969–972
Patupilone, 262
Paxil (**paroxetine hydrochloride**), 829–832
pegasparaginase, 263–265
pegfilgrastim (Neulasta), 370–374
pemetrexed (Alimta), 266–269
PenG Potassium (**penicillin G**), 1022–1025
PenG Sodium (**penicillin G**), 1022–1025
Penicillin G (PenG Potassium, PenG Sodium), 1022–1025
pentostatin (Nipent, 2-deoxycoformycin), 269–272
PenVK (**penicillin G**), 1022–1025
Percodan (**oxycodone**), 695–699
Perphenazine, 748–749
Perphenazine (Trilafon), 748–749
Pertofrane (**desipramine hydrochloride**), 789–792
Pertuzumab (Omnitarg, rhuMab 2C4), 564–566
Pharmorubicin (**epirubicin hydrochloride**), 155–160
Phenameth (**promethazine hydrochloride**), 751–753
Phenaphen with Codeine (**codeine/acetaminophen**), 660–663
Phenergan (**promethazine hydrochloride**), 751–753
Phosphocoltrade P32 (**chromic phosphate P32 suspension**), 387–389
Photofrin (**porfirmer**), 401–402
Piperacillin sodium (Pipracil), 1025–1029
Piperacillin sodium with tazobactam sodium (Zosyn), 1025–1029
Pipracil (**piperacillin sodium**), 1025–1029
Planaxis (**abarelix for injectable suspension**), 40–42
Platinol (**cisplatin**), 98–103
polifeprosan 20 with carmustine (BCNU) implant (Gliadel®), 272–275
Polyethylene glycol 3350, NF powder (Miralax®), 1106–1108
Polymox (**amoxicillin**), 884–887
Porfirmer (Photofrin), 401–402
Posaconazole (Noxafil), 1074–1075
Prechemotherapy nursing assessment guidelines, 24–11
Prednisolone (**adrenocorticoids**), 42–46
Prednisone (**adrenocorticoids**), 42–46
Pregabalin (Lyrica), 641–644
Premarin (**conjugated estrogen**), 162–164
Prialt (**ziconotide intrathecal infusion**), 656–660
Primaxin (**imipenem/cilastatin sodium**), 989–992
procarbazine hydrochloride (Matulane), 275–278

Prochlorperazine (Compazine), 749–751
Procrit (**epoetin alfa**), 344–347
progestational agents, 278–279
Progesterones, 23
Proleukin (Aldesleukin), 334–339
Promethazine hydrochloride (Anergan, Phenameth, Phenergan), 751–753
Prostaphlin (**oxacillin sodium**), 1019–1022
Provera (**medroxyprogesterone acetate**), 278–279
Provigil (**modafinil**), 707–709
Prozac (**fluoxetine hydrochloride**), 808–811
PTK787/ZK222584 (**vatalanib**), 611–613
Purinethol (**mercaptopurine**), 226–227

Quadrivalent human papillomavirus (Gardasil), 566–567
Quinupristin and dalfopristin (Synercid), 1029–1031

raltitrexed (Tomudex, ZD 1694, investigational), 280–282
Recentin (**cediranib**), 497–498
Reglan (**metoclopramide hydrochloride**), 741–742
Regulax SS (**docusate calcium, docusate potassium, docusate sodium**), 1097–1098
Relistor, 1104–1105
Remeron (**mirtazapine**), 817–821
Respiratory System. *See also* Pulmonary system
prechemotherapy nursing assessment guidelines for, 11, 18
Revlimid (**lenalidomide**), 548–554
rhuMab 2C4 (**pertuzumab**), 564–566
Rifaximin (Xifaxan), 1032
rIFN-A (**interferon alfa**), 351–355
rIFN-alpha-2 (**interferon alfa-2b**), 355–359
rIFN-gamma (**interferon gamma**), 359–362
Rituxan (**rituximab**), 567–572
Rituximab (Rituxan), 567–572
Rocephin (**ceftriaxone sodium**), 941–944
Roferon A (**interferon alfa**), 351–355
Rombiplostim, 374–375
Roxanol (**morphine**), 690–695
Roxiprin (**oxycodone**), 695–699
Rubidomycin (**daunorubicin hydrochloride**), 128–131
rubitecan (9-Nitro-20(S)-Camptothecin, Orathecin, investigational), 282–285
Rufen (**ibuprofen**), 642–645

Salflex (**salsalate**), 654–656
Salsalate (Disalcid, Salsalate, Salflex), 654–656
Salsalate (**salsalate**), 654–656
Sandostatin (**octreotide acetate**), 1117–1121
Sani-Supp (**glycerin suppository**), 1099–1100
sargramostim (Leukine, GM-CSF), 375–377
Scopolamine, 753–754
Senexon (**senna**), 1108–1109
Senna (Senexon, Senokot), 1108–1109
Senokot (**senna**), 1108–1109
Sensipar (**cinacalcet HCl**), 853–855
Septra (**co-trimoxazole**), 962–966
Serax (**oxazepam**), 827–829
Sertraline hydrochloride (Zoloft), 832–835
Serzone (**nefazodone HCl**), 821–824
Sinequan (**doxepin hydrochloride**), 799–802
Soltamox oral solution (**tamoxifen citrate**), 288–291
Sorafenib (Nexavar, BAY 43-9006), 572–576
Sorbitol, 1109–1110
Spectracef (**cefditoren pivoxil**), 913–914
Sporanox (**itraconazole**), 1064–1066
Sprycel (**dasatinib**), 506–510
SR57746A (**xaliproden**), 423–424
STI 571 (**imatinib mesylate**), 536–541
Streptogramins, 873–877
Streptomycin sulfate, 1033–1036
streptozocin (Zanosar), 285–287
Stulex (**docusate calcium, docusate potassium, docusate sodium**), 1097–1098

suberoylanilide hydroxamic acid (**vorinostat**), 615–617
Sunitinib malate (Sutent, U-11248), 576–580
Suppap (**acetaminophen**), 628–629
Suprax (**cefixime**), 917–920
Sutent, U-11248 (**sunitinib malate**), 576–580
Synercid (**dalfopristin and quinupristin**), 1029–1031
Synercid (**quinupristin and dalfopristin**), 1029–1031

Tabloid (**thioguanine**), 298–299
Tace (**chlorotrianisene**), 162–164
tamoxifen citrate (Nolvadex, Soltamox oral solution), 288–291
Tarceva (**erlotinib**), 518–521
Targretin (**bexarotene**), 486–491
Tasigna (**nilotinib**), 555–560
Taxol (**paclitaxel**), 250–257
Taxotere (**docetaxel**), 135–144
Tazicef (**ceftazidime**), 935–939
Tazidime (**ceftazidime**), 935–939
Telithromycin (Ketek), 1036–1038
Temodar® (**temozolomide**), 291–294
temozolomide (Temodar®), 291–294
Tempra (**acetaminophen**), 628–629
Temsirolimus (Torisel, CCI-779), 580–584
teniposide (Vumon, VM-26), investigational, 295–298
Tenol (**acetaminophen**), 628–629
Tequin (**gatifloxacin**), 980–983
Teratogenic effects, 22
Teratogenicity, 22
6-TG (**thioguanine**), 298–299
Thalidomide (Thalomid), 584–587
Thalomid (**thalidomide**), 584–587
Thiethylperazine (Torecan), 754–755
thioguanine (Tabloid, 6-Thioguanine, 6-TG), 298–299
6-Thioguanine (**thioguanine**), 298–299
Thioplex (**thiotepa**), 298–300
thiotepa (Thioplex, Triethylenethiophosphoramide), 298–300
Thyrotropin alfa, 377–380
Ticarcillin disodium (Ticar), 1038–1042
Ticarcillin disodium with clavulanate potassium (Timentin), 1038–1042
Ticar (**ticarcillin disodium**), 1038–1042
Tigecycline (Tygacil), 1042–1044
Timentin (**ticarcillin disodium** with clavulanate potassium), 1038–1042
Tirapazamine, 403–405
TNF (**tumor necrosis factor**), 380–382
Tobramycin sulfate (Nebcin), 1044–1048
Tofranil-PM (**imipramine pamoate**), 812–814
Tomudex (**raltitrexed**), 280–282
Topoisomerase II, 11, 12, 14
topoisomerase II, 2
topotecan hydrochloride for injection (Hycamtin), 302–306
Toradol (**ketorolac tromethamine**), 648–651
Torecan (**thiethylperazine**), 754–755
toremifene citrate (Fareston), 306–308
Torisel (**temsirolimus**), 580–584589–593
Tositumomab, I^{131} tositumomab, 589–593
toxicity, 406–409
Trastuzumab (Humanized anti-*Her*-2 Antibody, rhuMAb HER2, Herceptin), 594–599
Trastuzumab-DMI, 600–602
Trazodone hydrochloride (Desyrel, Trialodine), 835–837
Treanda (**bendamustine hydrochloride**), 69–73
Trelstar Depot (triptorelin pamoate), 311–313
Trelstar LA (triptorelin pamoate), 311–313
Tretinoin Liposomal (**liposomal tretinoin**), 605–610
Tretinoin (Vesanoid®, ATRA, All-Trans-Retinoic Acid), 602–605
Trialodine (**trazodone hydrochloride**), 835–837
Triethylenethiophosphoramide (**thiotepa**), 300–302
Trilafon (**perphenazine**), 748–749

Trilisate (**choline magnesium trisalicylate**), 635–637
trimetrexate (Neutrexin), 308–311
Trimox (**amoxicillin**), 884–887
triptorelin pamoate (Trelstar Depot), 311–313
triptorelin pamoate (Trelstar LA), 311–313
Trisenox (**arsenic trioxide**), 56–63
tumor necrosis factor (TNF), 380–382
Ty Caps (**acetaminophen**), 628–629
Tygacil (**tigecycline**), 1042–1044
Tykerb,(**lapatinib ditosylate**), 544–548
Tylenol (**acetaminophen**), 628–629
Tylenol with Codeine (**codeine/acetaminophen**), 660–663
Tylox (**oxycodone**), 695–699

UNASYN (**ampicillin sodium/sulbactam sodium**), 887–890
Unipen (**nafcillin sodium**), 1016–1019

Valacyclovir hydrochloride (Valtrex), 1093–1094
Valium (**diazepam**), 797–799
valrubicin (Valstar), 313–315
Valstar (**valrubicin**), 313–315
Valtrex (**valacyclovir hydrochloride**), 1093–1094
Vancocin (**vancomycin hydrochloride**), 1048–1051
Vancomycin hydrochloride (Vancocin), 1048–1051
Vandetanib (D6474, Zactima), 610–611
Vantas (**histrelin implant**), 190–192
Vantin (**cefpodoxime proxetil**), 932–933
Vatalanib, 611–613
Vectibix (**panitumumab**), 560–564
Vectrin (**minocycline hydrochloride**), 1010–1013
Velban (**vinblastine**), 315–318
Velcade (**bortezomib**), 491–497
Velosef (**cephradine**), 950–953
Venlafaxine hydrochloride (Effexor), 837–841
VePesid (**etoposide**), 165–169
Vesanoid® (**tretinoin**), 602–605
vesicants/irritants, 27–33, 33
VFEND (**voriconazole**), 1076–1078
Viadur (**leuprolide acetate**), 214–217
Vibramycin (**doxycycline hyclate**), 972–975
Vicodin (**hydrocodone**), 613
Vidaza (**5-azacytidine**), 66–69
vinblastine (Velban), 315–318
Vinca Alkaloids, 1118
vincristine (Oncovin), 318–321
vindesine (Eldisine, Desacetylvinblastine, investigational), 321–324
vinorelbine tartrate (Navelbine), 324–328
Vistide (**cidofovir**), 1081–1084
Volociximab, 613–615
Voriconazole (VFEND), 1076–1078
Vorinostat (Zolinza, suberoylanilide hydroxamic acid, SAHA), 615–617
VP-16 (**etoposide**), 165–169
Vumon (**teniposide**), 295–298

Wellbutrin (**bupropion hydrochloride**), 778–781
WR-2721 (**amifostine for injection**), 413–416
Wymox (**amoxicillin**), 884–887

xaliproden (Xenon, SR57746A), 423–424
Xanax (**alprazolam**), 773–775
Xeloda (**capecitabine**), 86–89
Xenon (**xaliproden**), 423–424
Xifaxan (**rifaximin**), 1032

^{90}Y ibritumomab tiuxetan (Zevalin, IDEC-Y2B8), 533–536

Zactima (**vandetanib**), 610–611
Zanosar (**streptozocin**), 285–287
ZD 1694 (**raltitrexed**), 280–282
Zevalin (**^{90}Y ibritumomab tiuxetan**), 533–536

Ziconotide intrathecal infusion (Prialt), 656–660
Zinacef (**cefuroxime**), 944–946
Zinecard (**dexrazoxane for injection**), 419–420
Zithromax (**azithromycin**), 890–891
Zofran (**ondansetron hydrochloride**), 744–746
Zoladex (**goserelin acetate**), 187–190
Zoledronic acid (Zometa), 864–868
Zolinza (**vorinostat**), 615–617
Zoloft (**sertraline hydrochloride**), 832–835
Zolpidem tartrate (Ambien), 842–843
Zometa (**zoledronic acid**), 864–868
Zostavax (**Zoster vaccine live**, 383–384
Zoster vaccine live (Zostavax), 383–384
Zosyn (**piperacillin sodium with tazobactam sodium**), 1025–1029
Zovirax (**acyclovir**), 1078–1081
Zurinol (**allopurinol sodium**), 410–413
Zyloprim (**allopurinol sodium**), 410–413
Zyvox (**linezolid**), 999–1001